Prostate Pathology

Peter A Humphrey, MD, PhD

To my wife Kay, with love, for her tolerance of stolen time
and for allowing transformation of rooms in our house into rooms dedicated to the book,
and to my wonderful children Tom and Jen.

Prostate Pathology

Peter A Humphrey, MD, PhD

Professor of Pathology and Immunology
Division of Surgical Pathology
Department of Pathology and Immunology
Washington University School of Medicine
St Louis, Missouri

ASCP PRESS

American Society for Clinical Pathology
Chicago

Publishing Team
Erik Tanck (production)
Terri Horning (production)
Erica Haratsaris (production)
Joshua Weikersheimer (consulting publisher)

Printed in Hong Kong

05 04 03 02 01 5 4 3 2 1

Preface viii

Acknowledgments ix

Chapter 1
Prostate Gland Development and Anatomic Structure 2

[1.1] Introduction to Prostate Gland Location and Function **3**
[1.2] Historical Perspective of Anatomy and Concepts of Lobes and Zones **3**
[1.3] Embryology and Development **3**
[1.4] Maldevelopment **5**
[1.5] Adult Prostate Anatomy **7**
[1.6] Prostatic Tissue Ectopia **22**

Chapter 2
Prostatic Tissue Handling and Sampling 30

[2.1] Cytologic Specimens **32**
[2.2] Core Needle Biopsy **32**
[2.3] Transurethral Prostatectomy (TURP) **40**
[2.4] Open Suprapubic or Retropubic Simple Prostatectomy (Enucleation) Tissue **44**
[2.5] Radical Perineal and Retropubic Prostatectomy **44**
[2.6] Cystoprostatectomy **51**
[2.7] Postmortem Examination of the Prostate **51**

Chapter 3
Fine Needle Aspiration Biopsy of the Prostate 58

[3.1] The Cells **59**
[3.2] Benign Diseases of the Prostate **62**
[3.3] Malignant Diseases of the Prostate **64**
[3.4] Variants of Prostatic Carcinoma **68**

Chapter 4
Inflammation and Infection 76

[4.1] Clinical Prostatitis **77**
[4.2] Clinical Bacterial Prostatitis **77**
[4.3] Histologic Acute Inflammation **78**
[4.4] Clinical Chronic Bacterial Prostatitis **80**
[4.5] Clinical Chronic Abacterial Prostatitis (Inflammatory) **80**
[4.6] Histologic Chronic Inflammation **80**
[4.7] Clinical Chronic Abacterial Prostatitis (Noninflammatory), or Prostatodynia **86**
[4.8] Granulomatous Prostatitis **86**
[4.9] Vasculitis **94**
[4.10] Infections Prostatitis: Additional Types **94**

Chapter 5
Atrophy 100

[5.1] Classification **101**
[5.2] Pathologic Features **101**
[5.3] Differential Diagnosis **109**
[5.4] Biological Significance **111**

Chapter 6
Metaplasia 114

[6.1] Squamous Cell Metaplasia **115**
[6.2] Transitional Cell Metaplasia **119**
[6.3] Mucinous Metaplasia **121**
[6.4] Paneth Cell–Like Metaplasia **122**
[6.5] Nephrogenic Metaplasia (Adenoma) and Stromal Metaplasia **123**

Chapter 7
Hyperplasia 126

[7.1] Incidence **127**
[7.2] Etiology **127**
[7.3] Pathogenesis **127**
[7.4] Clinical Features **128**
[7.5] Usual Nodular Epithelial and Stromal Hyperplasia **129**
[7.6] Basal Cell Hyperplasia **140**
[7.7] Cribriform Hyperplasia **144**
[7.8] Mesonephric Remnant Hyperplasia **145**
[7.9] Verumontanum Mucosal Gland Hyperplasia **147**

Chapter 8
Atypical Adenomatous Hyperplasia (Adenosis) 154

[8.1] Atypical Adenomatous Hyperplasia (Adenosis) **155**
[8.2] Sclerosing Adenosis **162**

Chapter 9
Unusual Benign Conditions 166

[9.1] Pigment Disorders: Melanosis, Blue Nevus, and Ochronosis **167**
[9.2] Amyloid in the Prostate **169**
[9.3] Collagenous Spherulosis **169**
[9.4] Postoperative Spindle Cell Nodule **170**
[9.5] Endometriosis **171**
[9.6] Extramedullary Hematopoiesis **171**
[9.7] Teratoma **171**
[9.8] Cowper's Glands **172**

Chapter 10
Pseudoneoplastic Lesions 176

[10.1] Pseudoneoplastic Lesions of Prostate **177**
[10.2] Pseudoneoplastic Lesions of Extraprostatic Tissues **177**

Chapter 11
Prostatic Intraepithelial Neoplasia 182

[11.1] History of Diagnostic Terminology **183**
[11.2] Clinical Presentation **183**
[11.3] Incidence of PIN in Core Needle Biopsies **184**
[11.4] Incidence of High-Grade PIN in TURP Chips and Simple (Open) Prostatectomies **184**
[11.5] Incidence of High-Grade PIN in Whole Prostate Glands **185**
[11.6] Histologic Diagnosis of PIN **186**
[11.7] Low-Grade PIN **186**
[11.8] High-Grade PIN **188**
[11.9] Follow-up and Clinical Management of High-Grade PIN **203**
[11.10] PIN Reporting **205**
[11.11] PIN as Precursor **205**
[11.12] Summary **210**

Chapter 12
Focal Glandular Atypia 218

[12.1] FGA in Needle Biopsy **219**
[12.2] FGA in TURP Chips and Simple Prostatectomy Specimens **224**

Chapter 13
Clinical Aspects of Prostatic Carcinoma, With Histopathologic Correlations 226

[13.1] Etiology **231**
[13.2] Clinical Presentation **234**
[13.3] Natural History and Mortality **241**
[13.4] Treatment **245**

Chapter 14
Adenocarcinoma 258

[14.1] General Approach **259**
[14.2] Diagnosis of Adenocarcinoma in Needle Core Biopsy **275**
[14.3] Diagnosis of Adenocarcinoma in Transurethral Resections and Open Prostatectomies **289**
[14.4] Diagnosis of Adenocarcinoma in Radical Prostatectomy Specimens **294**
[14.5] Diagnosis of Prostatic Adenocarcinoma in Locally Advanced and Metastatic Disease **311**

Chapter 15
Grading of Prostatic Carcinoma 338

[15.1] History **339**
[15.2] World Health Organization (Mostofi) System **340**
[15.3] Gleason System **340**
[15.4] Grading in Metastatic Deposits **355**
[15.5] Grading After Radiation and Hormonal Therapy **355**
[15.6] Grade Progression **356**
[15.7] Prognosis and Grade **356**

Chapter 16
Staging of Prostatic Carcinoma 376

[16.1] TNM AJCC/UICC Staging Classification **377**
[16.2] Clinical Staging **378**
[16.3] Pathologic TNM Staging **379**
[16.4] Pretreatment Models of Pathologic Stage **381**
[16.5] Stage Relationships with Pathologic Findings **382**
[16.6] Stage and Patient Outcome **382**
[16.7] Experimental Staging Procedures **384**
[16.8] Reporting of Pathologic Stage **385**

Chapter 17
Variants of Prostatic Carcinoma 390

[17.1] Prostatic Ductal Adenocarcinoma **391**
[17.2] Mucinous (Colloid) Adenocarcinoma **400**
[17.3] Signet-Ring Carcinoma **403**
[17.4] Adenosquamous and Squamous Carcinomas **406**
[17.5] Basaloid and Adenoid Cystic "Carcinomas" **408**
[17.6] Transitional Cell (Urothelial) Carcinoma **410**
[17.7] Small Cell Carcinoma **414**
[17.8] Sarcomatoid Carcinoma (Carcinosarcoma) **419**
[17.9] Others **422**

Chapter 18
Unusual Prostatic Neoplasms 430

[18.1] Adenomas **431**
[18.2] Soft Tissue (Stromal) Tumors **432**
[18.3] Hematolymphoid Neoplasms **441**
[18.4] Miscellaneous Neoplasms **446**
[18.5] Secondary Neoplasms **446**

Chapter 19
Treatment Effects 456

[19.1] Surgery **457**
[19.2] Hormonal Therapy **457**
[19.3] Radiation Therapy **464**
[19.4] Chemotherapy **468**
[19.5] Miscellaneous Therapies **469**
[19.6] Medical Therapy for BPH **469**
[19.7] Minimally Invasive Therapy for BPH **469**
[19.8] Experimental Prostate Cancer Therapy **470**

Chapter 20
Malignant Neoplasms Mistaken for Benign Conditions 478

Chapter 21
Molecular Biology of Human Prostatic Carcinoma: Clinical and Pathologic Implications 480

[21.1] DNA Content (Ploidy) **481**
[21.2] Chromosomal Alterations **482**
[21.3] Tumor Suppressor Genes **487**
[21.4] Oncogenes **489**
[21.5] Androgen Receptor **490**
[21.6] DNA Methylation **491**
[21.7] Cell Proliferation and Cell Death (Apoptosis) **491**
[21.8] Gene Expression Profiling and Proteomics **494**

Chapter 22
Seminal Vesicles 506

[22.1] Embryology and Development **507**
[22.2] Normal Anatomy **507**
[22.3] Cysts **511**
[22.4] Inflammation and Infection **512**
[22.5] Calcification and Calculi **512**
[22.6] Amyloid Deposits **512**
[22.7] Hyperplasia **513**
[22.8] Primary Benign Neoplasms **513**
[22.9] Primary Neoplasms of Indeterminate (or Low) Malignant Potential **515**
[22.10] Primary Malignant Neoplasms **515**
[22.11] Secondary Neoplasms **516**

Chapter 23
Prostatic Urethra 522

[23.1] Congenital Anomalies **523**
[23.2] Urethritis and Infection **524**
[23.3] Infarcts and Fibrosis **525**
[23.4] Urothelial Metaplasias **526**
[23.5] Prostatic Urethral Epithelial Polyps **530**
[23.6] Urothelial Hyperplasia **531**
[23.7] Benign Neoplasms **531**
[23.8] Dysplasia **532**
[23.9] Malignant Neoplasms **533**

Index 540

"Prostatic cancer is a rare affection"

—Sir Henry Thompson in *The Diseases of the Prostate*, 1883

Preface

No longer. Prostate cancer is now the most common noncutaneous malignancy diagnosed in men in the United States. Worldwide it is the third most common male cancer. Prostate diseases are common afflictions of men: clinical prostatitis and benign prostate hyperplasia (BPH) are especially prevalent disorders. In the last 15 years, due in part to demographic shifts and public awareness, and also to widespread clinical use of serum prostate specific antigen in efforts to detect prostate cancer early, there has been an astonishing increase in the number of prostate needle biopsies performed to assess for prostate cancer presence. Indeed, it is estimated that in 2002 some 750,000 prostate needle biopsies were performed in the United States. In this context the concept for a genuinely comprehensive book on pathology of the prostate originated.

This book presents a practical histopathologic approach to diagnosis of prostatic disease. It also should provide a ready repository of information on prostatic diseases. We hope it will prove useful for practicing pathologists, pathology residents and fellows, urologists and genitourinary oncologists, radiologists, and clinicians and researchers interested in diseases of the prostate. The coverage extends from basic anatomy throughout embryology and developmental diseases through tissue sampling considerations, to the diagnosis of benign and malignant diseases (both common and uncommon) in the prostate. We explore diagnosis of prostatic disease in all tissue sample types, including fine needle aspirates (special thanks to Richard M. DeMay, MD), needle core biopsy, transurethrally resected prostatic chips, open (simple) prostatectomy tissues, radical prostatectomy tissue, and metastatic prostatic cancer samples. The emphasis in the book is on surgical pathology diagnosis and differential diagnosis, using gold standard H&E-stained sections as the foundation for diagnosis. As such, the book contains many hundreds of H&E images, in an effort to portray the diversity, heterogeneity, and spectrum of disease within the prostate gland. Particular attention has been paid throughout the book to pseudoneoplastic and pseudobenign conditions, which are frequently misdiagnosed but infrequently discussed adequately in pathology texts. Clinical presentations, gross findings, and the role of special studies, including relevant molecular biologic and genetic testing, are all integrated into the discussion of each disease entity. And while few molecular genetic tests are currently used in the diagnosis or prognostic stratification of prostate diseases, the useful possibilities of molecular medicine will be felt within the book; indeed, a full chapter (Chapter 21) discusses the molecular biology of prostate cancer.

Readers learn in many different ways, so the presentation comprises images, text, figures, quick reference tables and data-rich, larger tables. Quick reference tables allow for capture, at a glance, of essential facts-the book is "prehighlighted" in a very real sense. The larger tables are designed to satisfy those want more about specific studies culled from the world literature on specific diseases. We hope the book will be a resource for "reference mining": a compendium of key references from all of the last century, and also for the years 2000-2003 of the new. Thus, both classical, historical papers, and the most recent, important publications are gathered (alphabetically) at the end of each chapter. Reference updating finally stopped only in February of 2003, one month prior to going to print. The ASCP Press deserves real praise for this often overlooked commitment to currency. We were able to incorporate numerous references from the year 2002, and several from the year of publication itself. We sought to impart the latest diagnostic information, including typing, Gleason grading, and staging of prostate cancer.

We will have succeeded when the book serves as an asset in the daily practice of diagnostic surgical pathology of the prostate, and again when it serves as the necessary consolidated source for otherwise difficult-to-find knowledge on the many diseases that affect the human prostate gland.

Peter A Humphrey, Author

Joshua Weikersheimer, Consulting Publisher, ASCP Press

Acknowledgments

My deep appreciation goes to:

Joshua Weikersheimer, PhD, Consulting Publisher, ASCP Press, for his patience, wit, and wisdom

Mark R Wick, MD, for originating the concept of this book

Robin Vollmer, MD, a valued friend and collaborator, who inspired my interest in urological pathology

Pepper Dehner, MD, Professor and Director of Anatomic Pathology at Washington University Medical Center, who provided support and the freedom in the form of time (in the Lauren Ackerman model) that made the writing of this book possible

Emil Unanue, MD, Professor and Chairman, Department of Pathology and Immunology at Washington University School of Medicine, for creating a Department where academic pathology thrives

My colleagues in urology at Duke University and Washington University Medical Centers, including David Paulson, MD, Philip Walther, MD, PhD, William Catalona, MD, David Keetch, MD, Adam Kibel, MD, and Gerald Andriole, MD

Joel Picus, MD, of Medical Oncology, Washington University, for reviewing Chapter 13 on the clinical aspects of prostate cancer

Madeleine Kraus, MD, for the review and critique of the hematopathology section of Chapter 18

Mahul Amin, MD, David Grignon, MD, and John Srigley, MD, for discussions and work together on the Gleason grading system

Jeffrey Milbrandt, MD, PhD, for discussions on basic science aspects of the molecular pathogenesis of prostate cancer

Henry Royal, MD, Horacio Maluf, MD, John Srigley, MD, Tom Ulbright, MD, Patricia Troncoso, MD, Adriana Reyes, MD, Michael Kyriakos, MD, J Allan Tucker, MD, Robert Young, MD, Robert B Jenkins, MD, Hung Chiang, MD, Xiaopei Zhu, MD, John Pfeifer, MD, PhD, Daniel Niku, MD, Ganesh Devendra, MD, Gerald Dalgleish, MD, and Mark Watson, MD, PhD, for slides, images, and figures

Margaret Chesney, for expert typing and perseverance

Erik Tanck, for care and skill in producing the book, and the ASCP Press Staff for careful work in handling the book

My parents Loren Humphrey, MD, PhD, and Janice Humphrey for continued support and encouragement throughout my medical career

Prostate Gland Development and Anatomic Structure

CHAPTER 1

[1.1] Introduction to Prostate Gland Location and Function **3**

[1.2] Historical Perspective of Anatomy and Concepts of Lobes and Zones **3**

[1.3] Embryology and Development **3**

[1.4] Maldevelopment **5**

[1.5] Adult Prostate Anatomy **7**

[1.6] Prostatic Tissue Ectopia **22**

"In order to study the Pathology of the Prostate, it is necessary to observe accurately its normal structure, conformation, and anatomical relations."

—Sir Henry Thompson
In: *Diseases of the Prostate. Their Pathology and Treatment*, 1883

[1.1] Introduction to Prostate Gland Location and Function

The human prostate gland is one of the male sex accessory tissues, which include the prostate, seminal vesicles, and bulbourethral glands (Partin 2002).

In females, prostate homologues including paraurethral Skene's glands and a rudimentary prostate gland in the posterior wall of the distal urethra have been described (Sesterhenn 1998, Tepper 1984, Wernert 1992, Zaviacic 1985, 2000A, 2000B). These glands often express prostate-specific antigen and prostatic acid phosphatase (Kamoshida 1990, Pollen 1984, Sesterhenn 1998, Spencer 1990, Tepper 1984, Wernert 1992, Zaviacic 1985) and have a hydrolytic enzyme and oxidoreductase enzyme profile similar to that of the male prostate (Zaviacic 1985). The function, if any, of the "female prostate" is unknown (Wernert 1992). Rarely, hyperplasia and carcinoma have been identified in the female prostate (Sesterhenn 1998, Sloboda 1998).

The prostate gland is important for mammals because this structure has been conserved through evolution in all mammals. However, there is tremendous variability in the comparative anatomy of the prostatic complex between humans and animals (Bartsch 1980, Hayward 1996, Hijikata 1986, Holtz 1978, Jacob 1986, Krongard 1989, Lewis 1981). An appreciation of these differences is crucial when attempts are made to understand human prostatic disease by the development and study of animal models of prostatic disease. An interesting but as yet unexplained observation is that only humans and dogs are naturally predisposed to the development of prostatic intraepithelial neoplasia (PIN) and carcinoma in the prostate (Aquilina 1998, Cornell 2000). Dogs and primates can also develop hyperplasia.

The normal human adult male prostate gland is a horse chestnut–shaped structure or, for the more geometrically inclined, an oblate conoid or truncated cone. It has also been likened to a top lying on its side. It measures 5cm × 4cm × 3cm and weighs 20g between ages 20 and 50 years (McNeal 1997, Partin 2002). The prostate surrounds the urethra immediately below the base of the bladder and is located posterior to the inferior symphysis pubis, superior to the urogenital diaphragm, and anterior to the rectum **f1.1** (Partin 2002).

The main function of the prostate is the formation of secretions that constitute one half to two thirds of the 3mL volume of the ejaculate (Partin 2002). The precise biological purpose of many of the biochemical substances secreted into the seminal plasma is uncertain (Partin 2002). A well-defined role has been established for several enzymes that participate in the clotting and lysis of the seminal plasma clot, including prostate-specific antigen (PSA), which is a serine protease and esterase that cleaves semenogelin, a protein involved in clotting (Sokoll 1997). Additional substances that are found at high concentrations in prostatic fluid include potassium, zinc, citric acid, spermine, amino acids, prostaglandins, and enzymes such as acid phosphatase, diamine oxidase, β-glucuronidase, lactic dehydrogenase, α-amylase, and seminal proteinase (Partin 2002). These secretory products enhance fertility by promoting sperm viability and motility. An antimicrobial role has been suggested for a few of these substances such as zinc, spermine, and proteases. Physically, via mass effect, musculature, and location, the prostate may contribute to control of urine outflow from the bladder. The prostate is not vital for life; the entire gland may be removed in radical surgery (prostatectomy) without consequences in most patients. (In a minority of patients, incontinence and impotence may complicate radical prostatectomy through damage to adjacent structures such as distal urethral sphincter and bladder neck [leading to incontinence] and periprostatic neurovascular bundles [leading to impotence] [Walsh 1998]). Failure of the gland to form, as in 5α-reductase deficiency (Wilson 1981) and testicular feminization (Imperato-McGinley 1974), is not lethal.

[1.2] Historical Perspective of Anatomy and Concepts of Lobes and Zones

The first descriptions of the anatomy of the prostate date back to the third century BC, but it was not until the 1500s that the first accurate anatomic representations were recorded (Bush 1977, Lawson 1993, Timms 1997). Until the early twentieth century the prostate gland was thought to possess 2 to 3 lobes (LeDuc 1939). In 1911, several papers were published that forwarded the notion of 3 to 4 lobes: 2 lateral lobes, a middle lobe, and occasionally an anterior lobe. In 1912, Lowsley (Lowsley 1912) described 5 separate lobes, including a posterior lobe, but this work was based on embryonic and fetal prostates, not adult glands. This model dominated until 1954, when Franks (Franks 1954) put forth the concept of an outer gland (where carcinomas occurred) and a periurethral inner gland. Further evolution of this concept occurred when McNeal developed the zonal model that is currently widely used (McNeal 1968, 1980, 1997). As described later in this chapter, this model defines 3 zones: a central zone, a transition zone, and a peripheral zone. Although fibrous encapsulation of these zones is not apparent in histologic sections of whole prostate glands, this zonal anatomy conceptualization is highly attractive.

The designation of lobes has unfortunately been perpetuated by some in diagnostic terminology so that pathologists may receive biopsies from the "right lobe" or " left lobe." Alternatively, one may receive biopsies from the "right side" or "left side," which is more acceptable, but more preferable is the assignment of disease localization in terms of right transition or peripheral zone and left transition or peripheral zone.

[1.3] Embryology and Development

The prostate is derived from the urogenital sinus and is first recognizable at 9 to 10 weeks of development (McNeal 1997, Shapiro 1989). At this time, testosterone from the embryonic testis stimulates ingrowth of endodermal buds into urogenital sinus mesenchyme. It has been hypothesized that there is a reciprocal interaction of epithelium and mesenchyme during development by which, under the influence of androgens, urogenital sinus mesenchyme induces

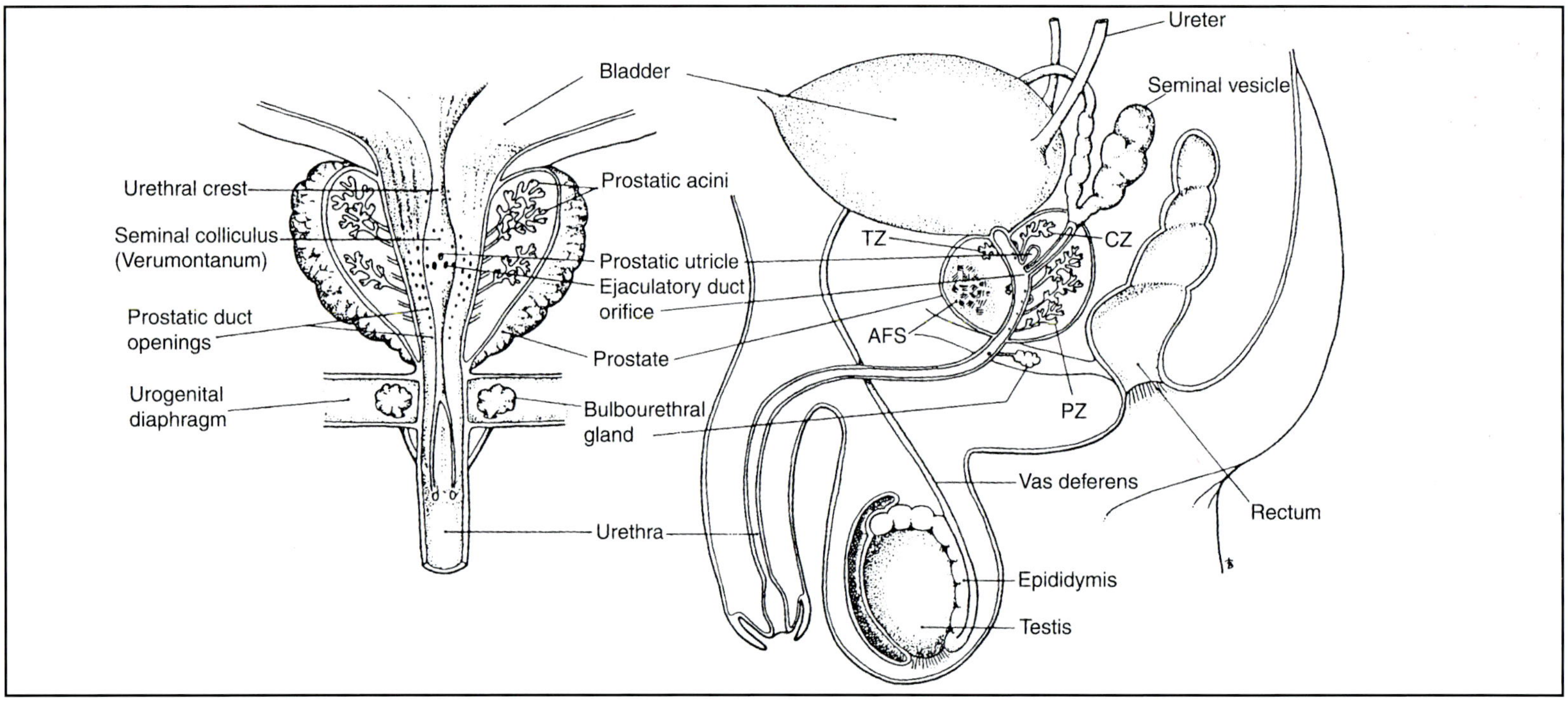

■ **f1.1** *Anatomical relationships of prostate in frontal (left) and sagittal views (right). Abbreviations: TZ: transition zone, CZ: central zone, PZ: peripheral zone, AFS: anterior fibromuscular stroma. (Reprinted with permission from Prostate: Basic and Clinical Aspects. CRC Press).*

urogenital sinus epithelium to undergo prostatic ductal morphogenesis and differentiation (Cunha 1972, Hayward 2000, Timms 1995). The differentiating prostatic epithelium in turn signals the urogenital mesenchyme to differentiate into smooth muscle cells that closely surround the epithelial ducts (Cunha 1996). This dynamic dance of tissue remodeling entails coordinated temporal and spatial processes of ductal budding, branching morphogenesis, cellular proliferation, and secretory function (Timms 1995). By 13 weeks some 70 primary ducts are present. Three stages of development from 20 weeks' gestation to 1 month of age have been delineated (Xia 1990). The bud stage at 20 to 30 weeks' gestation exhibits solid cellular buds at the end of ducts, with spindled cells in the center and columnar cells at the periphery **i1.1.** The bud-tubule stage at 31 to 36 weeks shows small collections of cellular buds and acinar structures **i1.2, i1.3.** The third stage is characterized by more distinct lobular organization of acinotubular clusters. Squamous metaplasia of prostatic ducts and urethra is a common finding in the fetal prostate (Cunha 1972). This metaplasia is gradually lost after birth.

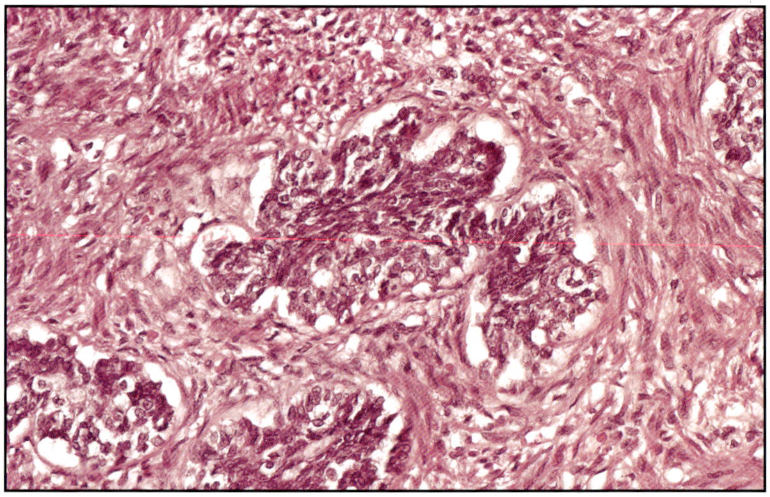

■ **i1.1** *Fetal prostate at 25 weeks, with solid epithelial nests embedded in a dense stroma.*

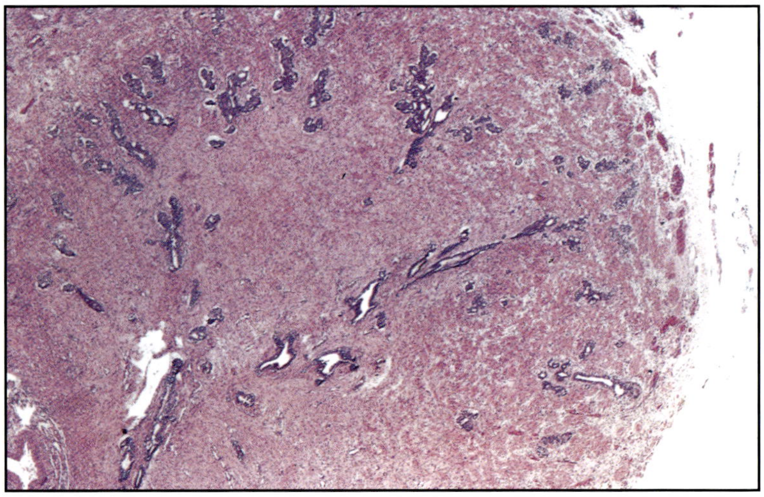

■ **i1.2** *Fetal prostate at 35 weeks demonstrating paucity of epithelial elements.*

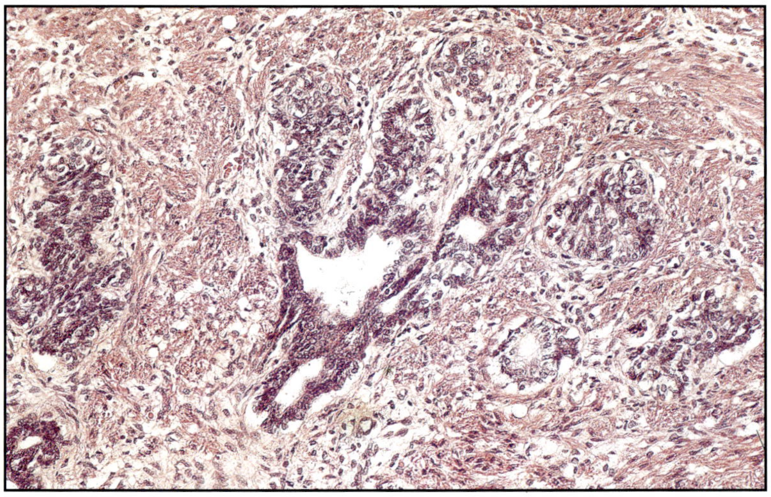

■ **i1.3** *Small glands and solid cellular bands are characteristic of epithelium in the 35-week fetal prostate.*

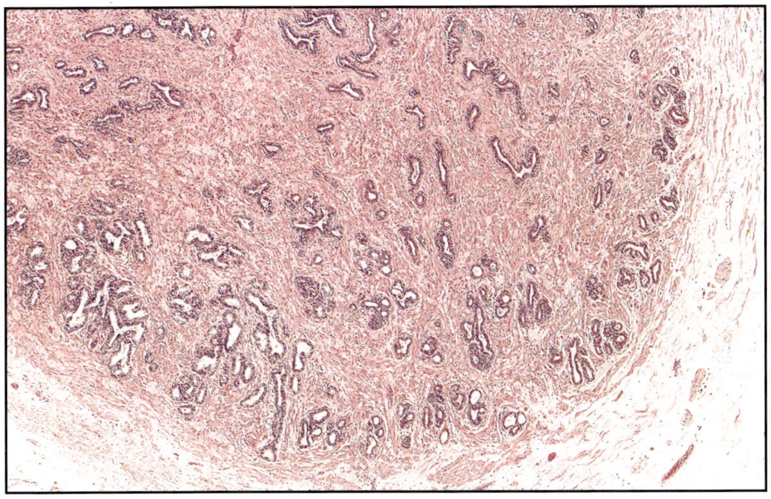

■ **i1.4** *Prostate of a 3-year-old boy, with increased number of glandular units compared to fetal prostate.*

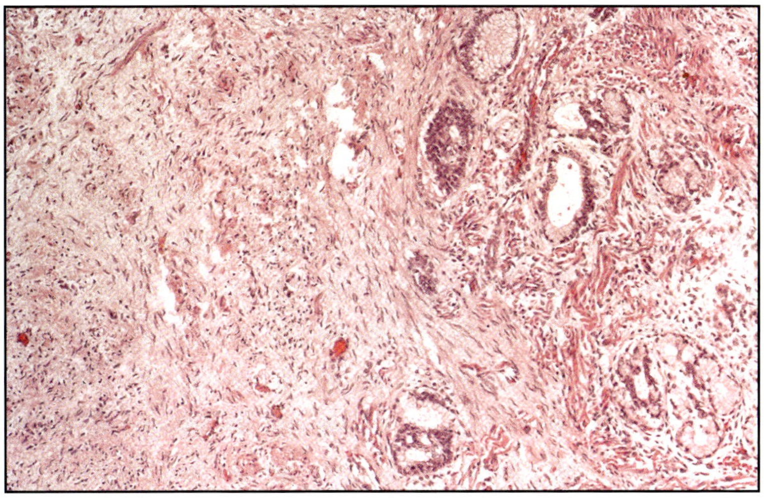

■ **i1.5** *Prostate in prune belly syndrome. Only a few acini are present and there is increased fibrous tissue.*

After birth, there is an infantile resting period until 10 to 12 years of age and then a pubertal maturation period until age 18 years. In the resting period the size of the prostate gland remains stable **t1.1,** but duct formation, solid budding at the periphery, and branching morphogenesis continue **i1.4** (Timms 1995). The pubertal period is marked by substantial androgen-driven increase in gland size **t1.1,** further branching, and differentiation of immature prostatic epithelium into the adult-type basal and secretory cells.

In the adult, prostate size remains stable for roughly 25 to 30 years. Gland size then increases from age 50 on because of transition zone enlargement secondary to benign prostatic hyperplasia (BPH) (Berry 1984, Leissner 1979, McNeal 1992) **t1.1.** Processes related to aging, such as atrophy, inflammation, and hyperplasia, are discussed in later chapters in this book.

The seminal vesicles, epididymis, vas deferens, and ejaculatory ducts are formed from Wolffian (mesonephric) ducts under the influence of testosterone (see Chapter 22, p 507). It has been proposed that the central zone of the prostate is also of mesodermal Wolffian duct origin (Argani 1998, McNeal 1997). In this conceptualization, the prostate gland is of dual embryonic derivation.

■ **t1.1 Prostate Weight by Age**

Age (years)	Mean Weight (grams)
Neonate	0.9
1	1.2
5	1.3
10	1.4
14	3.5
15	5.1
18	11-18
20-50	20
61-67	27
71-80	31
81- >90	39

Aumüller 1998, Haugen 1972, Berry 1984, Leissner 1979

[1.4] Maldevelopment

Clinically manifest developmental abnormalities of the prostate are rare and include aplasia, hypoplasia, cystic change, and abnormal persistence and hyperplasia of mesonephric remnants **t1.2**. Agenesis and hypoplasia of the prostate occur in several conditions including 5α-reductase deficiency (Imperato-McGinley 1974, Walsh 1974), testicular feminization (Griffin 1984, Wilson 1981), and prune belly syndrome (DeKlerk 1978, Hoagland 1988, Manivel 1989, Moerman 1984, Popek 1991, Stephens 1994, Wigger 1977). The first 2 developmental abnormalities are related to deficient androgenic stimulation of prostate growth, but the cause of prune belly syndrome is unclear. In the fetal prostate, testosterone is reduced in the urogenital sinus by the enzyme 5α-reductase to produce the active principal, dihydrotestosterone. Congenital 5α-reductase deficiency results in a rare form of pseudohermaphroditism in which patients have ambiguous external genitalia and small or undetectable prostates. In males with testicular feminization, the androgen receptor is defective, and the prostate is entirely absent. In the prune belly syndrome the prostate is hypoplastic and may not be grossly evident (Popek 1991). There is a pronounced reduction in epithelial elements, a reduction in smooth muscle fibers, and increased fibrous tissue **i1.5.** Concomitantly, the seminal vesicles can be rudimentary or absent and the vas deferens segmentally atretic. The prostatic urethra is markedly dilated in these cases.

Cystic change can develop in the prostatic region secondary to maldevelopment (Angulo 1995, Hendry 1992, Hennessy 1939, Landes 1949, Magri 1960, Moore 1953, Varlet 1992, Workman 1978). These congenital cysts may be classified as utricular (of endodermal origin) and müllerian duct cysts (which are of mesodermal origin), ejaculatory duct cysts, vas deferens cysts, and seminal vesicle cysts (van Poppel 1983). The location of these

■ **t1.2 Maldevelopment of the Prostate**

Agenesis and hypoplasia: In 5-α-reductase deficiency, testicular feminization, prune belly syndrome
Congenital cysts: Utricular, müllerian duct cysts, ejaculatory duct cysts, vas deferens cysts, seminal vesicle cysts
Mesonephric remnants: Often hyperplastic

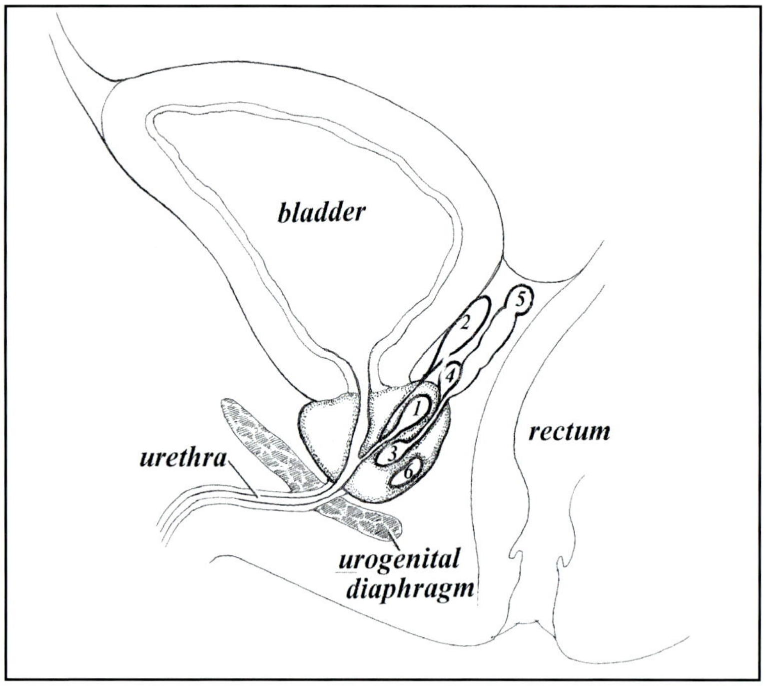

■ **f1.2** *Anatomic location of prostatic and periprostatic cysts:*
1: Utricle cyst
2: Müllerian duct cyst
3: Ejaculatory duct cyst
4: Vas deferens cyst
5: Seminal vesicle cyst
6: Prostatic retention cyst
(Modified with permission from Fig. 3 in van Poppel 1983)

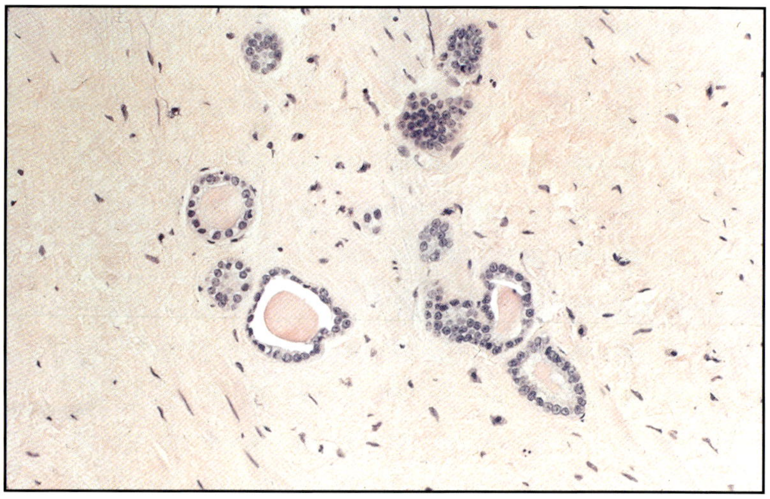

■ **i1.6** *Mesonephric remnants. These tubules contain eosinophilic contents and fail to mark for prostate specific antigen or prostate specific acid phosphatase by immunohistochemistry.*

cysts is given in **f1.2**. Also depicted in this figure is the most common prostatic cyst, which is noncongenital in origin: the retention cyst (Emmett 1936, Riser 1964). Prostatic cysts are not uncommon findings by ultrasonography, with the incidence at 7.9% in one series (Hamper 1990). However, clinical symptoms due to congenital cysts are rare.

Mullerian duct cysts and utricular cysts are uncommon conditions that rarely produce clinical symptoms. Both are midline structures that have been conceptualized as one entity (Schuhrke 1978), although it can be argued that on embryologic and clinical grounds they should be separated (Myers 1969). Embryologically , the prostatic utricle is a remnant of the müllerian duct, but the lining of this small blind epithelial pouch is of endodermal origin. Müllerian ducts are of mesodermal origin. The incidence of utricular cystic dilatation (congenital or postinflammatory) is estimated at 7% (5/70) in newborns and young infants and 1% (7/678) in adults (Moore 1937). Utricular dilatation and cyst formation are associated with intersex abnormalities and hypospadias, whereas true müllerian duct cysts are not (Devine 1980, Howard 1948). Considering the two together, the median age at presentation is 26 to 39 years, and symptomatic patients present most often with hematospermia, recurrent testicular or pelviperineal pain, and irritative lower urinary tract symptoms such as frequency, dysuria, and urgency (Coppens 2002, Schuhrke 1978). These cysts may also be associated with infertility due to ejaculatory duct obstruction (Schuhrke 1978). Aspiration fluid or portions of the cyst obtained by transurethral resection "unroofing" or the complete cyst removed by open surgery may be received in the anatomic pathology laboratory (Shabsigh 1989). Grossly, incidentally detected utricular cysts are 2cm to 3cm in greatest dimension, with a smooth inner wall (Moore 1937). The ejaculatory ducts are displaced laterally, with compression of their lumens. Microscopically, the epithelium lining the cystic cavity has been described as normally columnar or cuboidal (32% of cases), although it may be stratified squamous (19%), transitional (10%), or devoid of epithelium (19%) (Moore 1937, Schuhrke 1978). The cyst walls are composed of smooth muscle or fibrous tissue. In 25% of cases, acini with columnar epithelium have been noted in the cyst wall near the connection with the urethra. Aspiration fluid should not reveal any sperm (unlike the ejaculatory duct cyst). The fluid has been characterized as clear (Moore 1937) or whitish to brown (Schuhrke 1978), with old blood and cellular debris (Angulo 1995). Stones have been found in these cysts (Redman 1978, Warren 1972). Treatment depends on symptoms, and cyst size, and location. Options range from observation for asymptomatic patients to aspiration to surgery (Coppens 2002, Schuhrke 1978). A rare complication in these cysts is the occurrence of malignancy. A few cases of ductal carcinoma (Barringer 1933, Nogueira 1982) and squamous cell carcinoma (Szemes 1968) arising in müllerian duct cysts have been reported.

Congenital seminal vesicle cysts (discussed in Chapter 22, p 511) and ejaculatory duct cysts are also in the differential diagnosis of cystic change in the prostatic region (Borrego 1994, Carter 1989, Elder 1984, Littrup 1987, Loizaga 1994, Malatinsky 1987, Mayersak 1989, Mobilio 1977, Robert 1994, Soh 1995). Congenital ejaculatory duct cysts are rare; in one series where vesiculography was performed in infertile men, the incidence was 0.6% (1/158) (Malatinsky 1987). Ejaculatory duct cysts are not distinguishable from müllerian duct or utricular cysts by radiologic testing, such as ultrasound, because all are midline (Littrup 1987). Aspiration of a midline cyst with spermatozoa identified is consistent with an ejaculatory duct cyst (Elder 1984, Littrup 1987, Robert 1994).

Ejaculatory ducts are absent in many patients with cystic fibrosis (Holsclaw 1971, Olson 1969). Minor congenital anatomic variations of the ejaculatory duct include caudal formation of ejaculatory ducts within the central zone (18% of cases), abnormal posterior penetration of the ejaculatory ducts at the rectal surface (12%), abnormally large muscle bundles in the duct sheath (6%), and ductal dilatation (7%) (Villers 1990).

Finally, as a developmental anomaly, rare examples of mesonephric remnants have been recognized in the prostate, where they may assume pseudoneoplastic status due to florid hyperplasia (Gikas 1993, Jimenez 1998, Val-Bernal 1995) (see Chapter 7 and **t7.16, p 145**). The incidence of nonhyperplastic mesonephric remnants in the prostate is unknown. We have seen a case where the mesonephric tubules were much more focal than the aforementioned mesonephric remnants with hyperplasia **i1.6**; this could represent remnants without superimposed hyperplasia.

■ **t1.3 Prostate Zones are Differentially Affected by Disease**

Prostate zone	Inflammation	Hyperplasia	% of all carcinomas
Central	–	–	5%
Transition	+	+	20%
Peripheral	+	–	75%

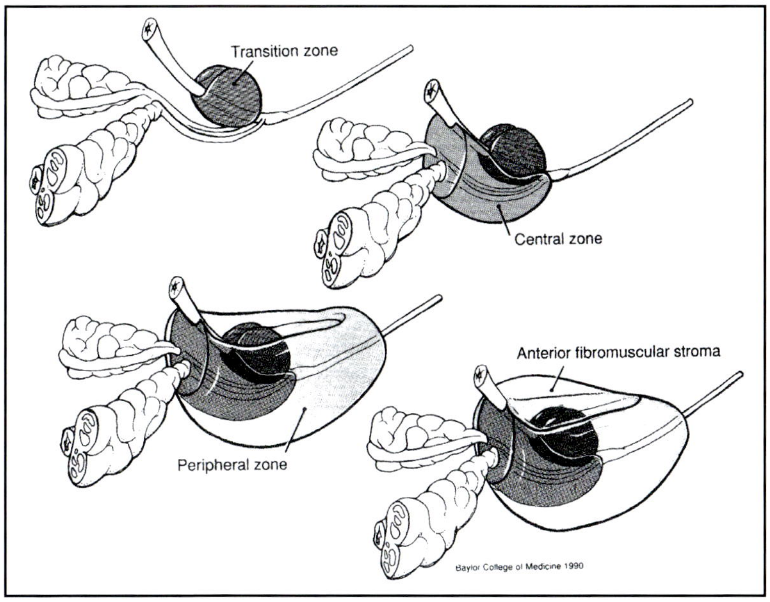

■ **f1.3** *Zonal anatomy of the prostate. (Reprinted with permission from Cancer: Principles and Practice of Oncology, 4th ed. Lippincott Williams and Wilkins.)*

[1.5] Adult Prostate Anatomy

Current concepts hold that the prostate gland is composed of three zones: the central zone, the transition zone, and the peripheral zone **f1.3**. It may be difficult in practice in some cases to grossly and microscopically recognize a sharp demarcation between these zones (Epstein 1997, Kissane 1997, Sesterhenn 1992), but these zones do appear to have structural differences, and diseases differentially affect these zones **t1.3**.

Grossly, the urethra is an important reference point for consideration of the anatomic relationships of these zones (Brooks 2002, McNeal 1968, 1972, 1997). The prostatic urethra is formed at the bladder neck, turns anteriorly 35° at its midpoint (the urethral angle), and exits the prostate at the apex, where it is continuous with the membranous urethra. The urethral angle can vary between 0° and 90° and divides the urethra into proximal (so-called preprostatic) and distal (so-call prostatic) segments. The transition zone, which normally makes up 5% of prostate gland volume, wraps around the proximal urethra **f1.3.** The main ducts of this zone drain into posterolateral recesses of the urethra at a point just proximal to the urethral angle. Some of the more medial ducts penetrate through the thick smooth muscle bundles of preprostatic sphincter. Also found in the smooth muscle of preprostatic sphincter are minute ducts and abortive acinar arrangements of periurethral glands, which constitute only about 1% of the total glandular volume of the prostate. The central zone, depicted next in the layering diagram of **f1.3,** makes up about 25% of the entire prostate gland and is a posteriorly situated conelike structure with the base of cone projecting toward the base of the bladder. The paired ejaculatory ducts run through the central zone from the seminal vesicles to their exit at the posterior urethral protuberance, known as the verumontanum (or colliculus seminalis) **f1.1, i1.7.**The ducts from the central zone drain into the urethra via orifices positioned just next to the ejaculatory duct orifices on the verumontanum. The peripheral zone of the prostate gland is the bulk of the posterior, lateral, and apical portion of the prostate gland and accounts for 70% of the total gland volume. The ducts of this zone empty into the posterior urethral recesses or grooves in a double row from the verumontanum to the prostatic apex **f1.1.** Finally, a patch of nonglandular tissue called the anterior fibromuscular stroma is present anteriorly over the prostate and extends from the bladder neck to the apex of the prostate **f1.3.**

Microscopically, the normal adult prostate in men 20 to 50 years of age comprises a branching duct–acinar glandular system embedded in a dense fibromuscular stroma **i1.8** (McNeal 1968, 1972, 1997). Unlike in

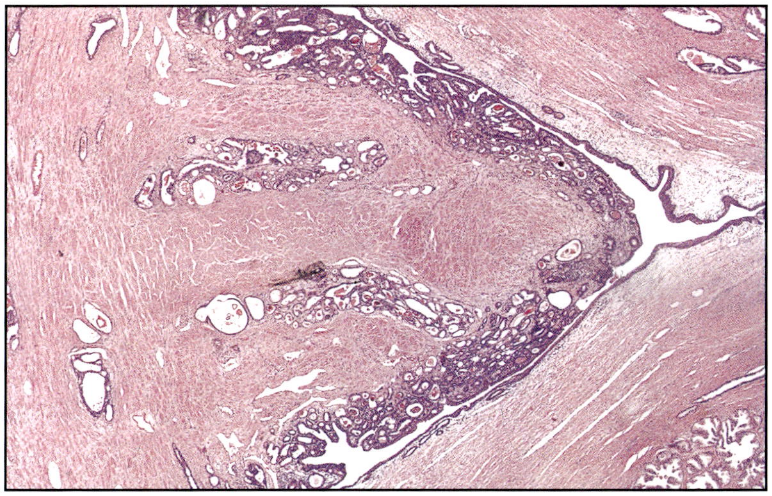

■ **i1.7** *The verumontanum — a mound of tissue projecting into the urethral lumen, which is here compressed into an angulated slit-like space.*

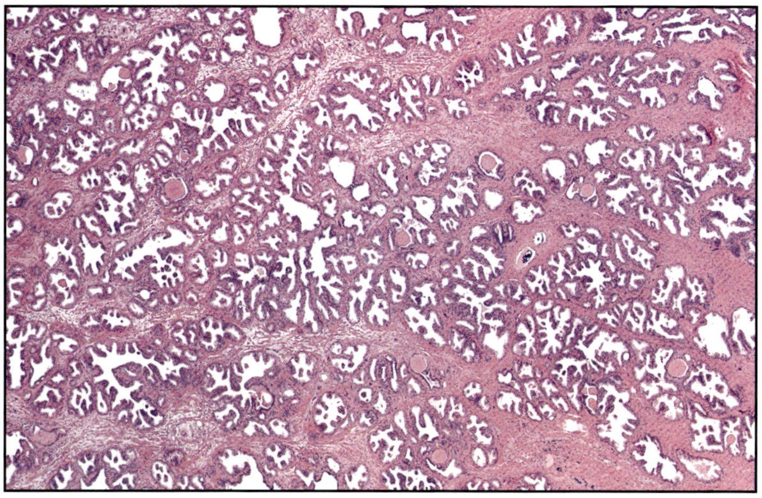

■ **i1.8** *Normal adult prostate — haphazard distribution of complex glands in a fibromuscular stroma.*

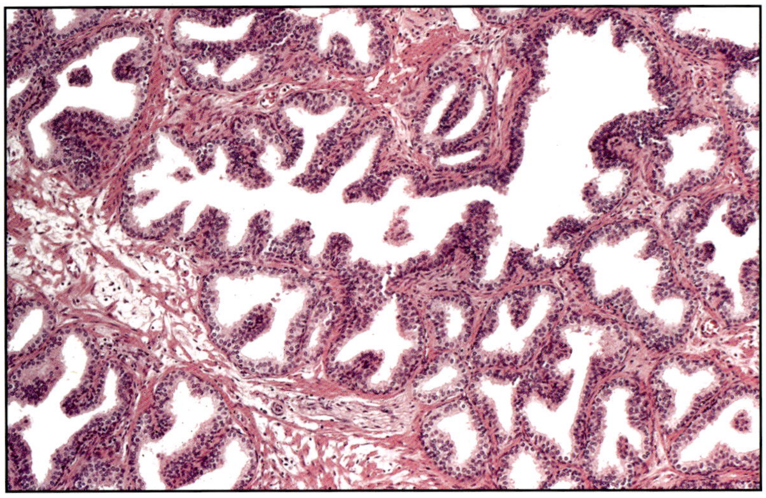

■ **i1.9** *Normal adult prostate: Distinction between ducts and acini may be difficult.*

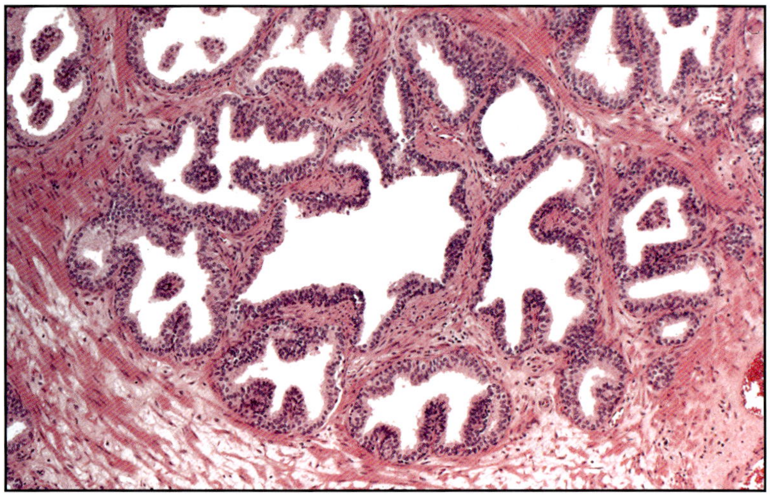

■ **i1.10** *Normal adult prostate: Lobular arrangement of glands, as depicted here, may be difficult to identify.*

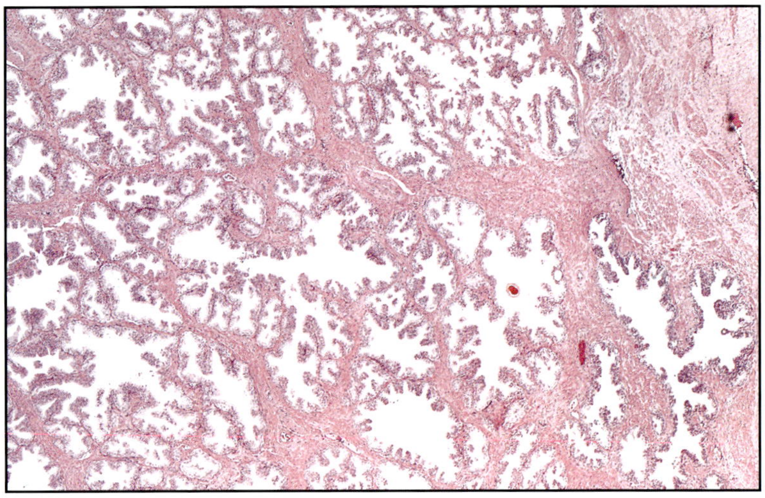

■ **i1.11** *Normal adult peripheral zone: Branching glands.*

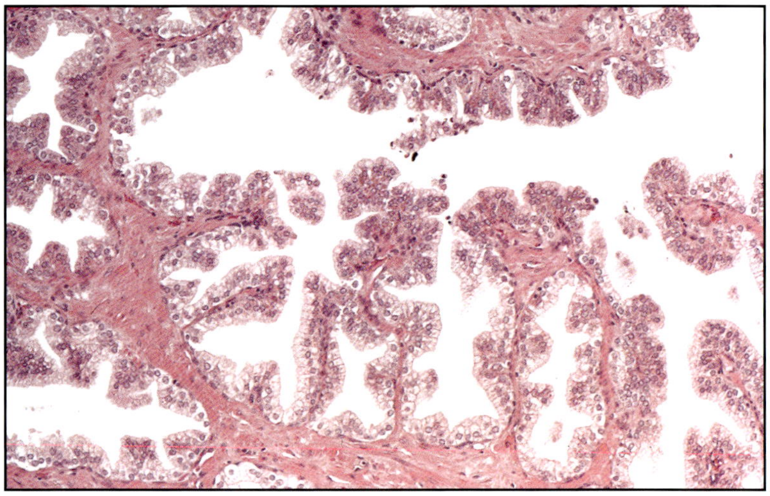

■ **i1.12** *Normal adult peripheral zone: Outpouchings of acini from a duct.*

some other secretory glands in the body, the morphologic separation of ducts from acini usually is not feasible **i1.9**. Also, distinct lobules of glands are not always clearly evident **i1.10**, so defining prostatic diseases as having lobular or nonlobular growth patterns can be challenging.

Zonal architectural differences can be appreciated (McNeal 1968, 1972, 1997). Normally, the peripheral zone ducts and acini are evenly distributed but are irregular in size and shape **i1.11**.The acini appear as rounded outpouchings **i1.12**. The peripheral zone stroma is loosely woven and fibromuscular **i1.13** (McNeal 1997). The normal transition zone glands are similar to the peripheral zone, but the stroma is more compact, with interlacing smooth muscle bundles **i1.14**. The boundary between the transition and peripheral zones can sometimes be appreciated but often is quite indistinct **i1.15, i1.16**. Urologists speak of a "surgical capsule" when they enucleate and remove nodules of hyperplasia (often incorrectly called adenoma) arising in the transition zone (Han 2002), yet although a surgical plane of dissection may exist between the transition and peripheral zones, a true capsule (a discrete fibrous or fibromuscular band of tissue) does not separate these 2 zones. Moreover, the boundary can be completely effaced by disease processes such as hyperplasia, inflammation, and carcinoma. The central zone glands are more densely arranged than the peripheral and transition zone glands. The epithelial-stromal ratio in the central zone is 2:1, compared with 1:1 for the peripheral and transition zone (McNeal 1997). Also, central zone glands are larger and display intraluminal projections with fibrovascular cores **i1.17**. In needle biopsy tissue, central zone epithelium displays tall columnar cells with eosinophilic cytoplasm, a prominent basal cell layer, and on occasion complex intraluminal architecture such as Roman bridge and cribriform formations (Srodon 2002). These findings can be misdiagnosed as atypia or PIN (Srodon 2002).

The normal epithelium of the prostate is classically defined as having two cell layers: a luminal or secretory cell layer and a basal cell layer **i1.18**. A third cell type in normal prostatic epithelium is the neuroendocrine cell (Cohen 1993, di Sant'Agnese 1998).

The basal cell layer separates the secretory cells from the basement membrane and is nearly continuous **i1.19, i1.20** although some secretory cells may rest directly on the basement membrane (deVries 1992, Srigley 1990). Basal cells in the prostatic epithelium often appear as rounded or oblong cells, but can also be flattened, spindled, cuboidal, and triangular (Mao 1966, Srigley 1990). It is critical to recognize this variation in normal morphologic appearance of basal cells because absence of basal cells is an important finding in the diagnosis of invasive carcinoma. Basal cells have a scant amount of dense cytoplasm and small, hyperchromatic nuclei. Small nucleoli may sometimes be seen, especially with the electron microscope (Mao 1966, Srigley 1990).

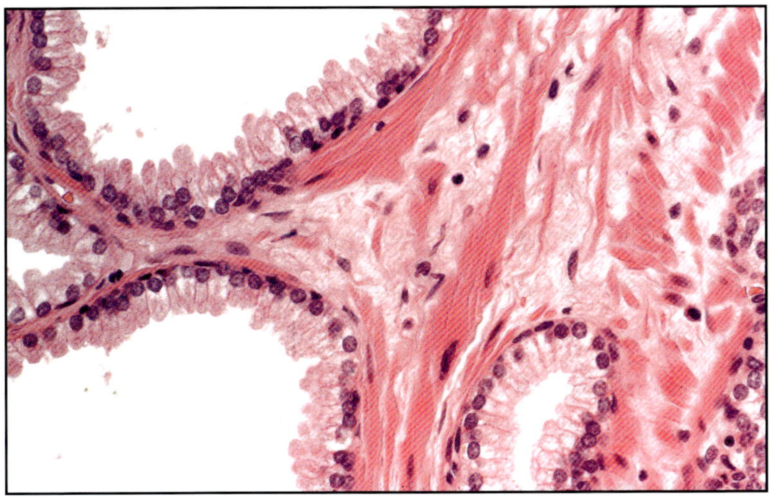

■ **i1.13** *Normal adult peripheral zone: The stroma contains smooth muscle cells and fibroblasts.*

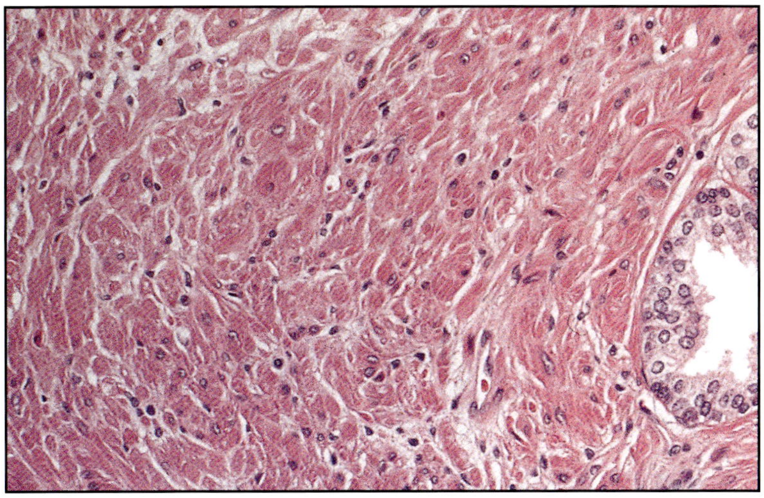

■ **i1.14** *Normal adult transition zone: The stroma is comprised of densely concentrated smooth muscle bundles.*

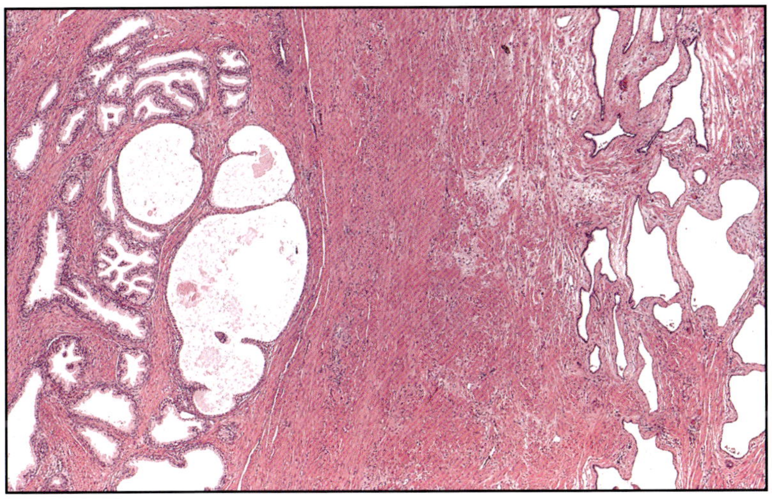

■ **i1.15** *Fibromuscular boundary between transition zone (left) and peripheral zone (right).*

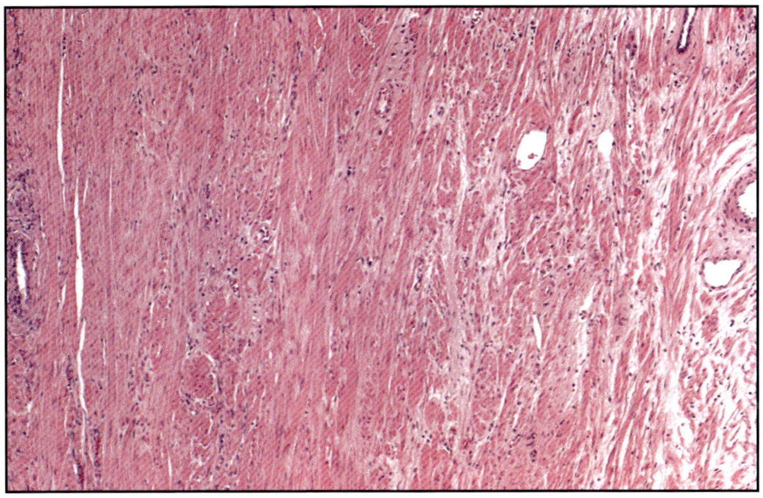

■ **i1.16** *The boundary between the transition and peripheral zones is of variable size and is indistinct, with a gradation from denser transition zone stroma (left) to looser peripheral zone stroma (right) .*

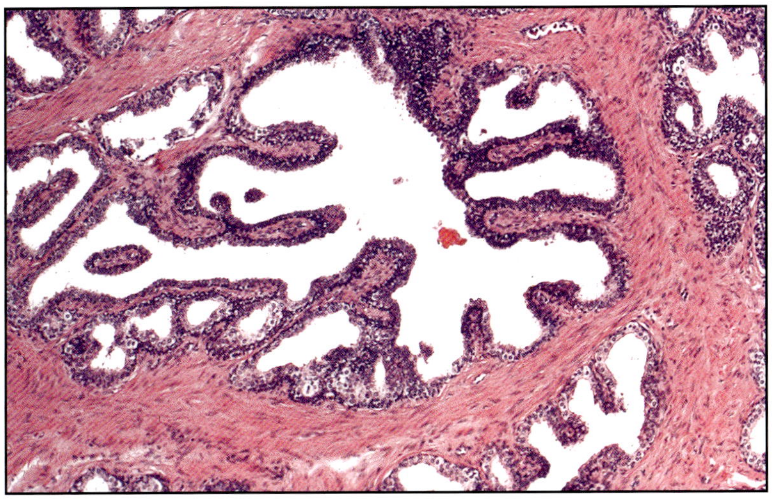

■ **i1.17** *Normal adult central zone: Glands with prominent ridges with stromal cores.*

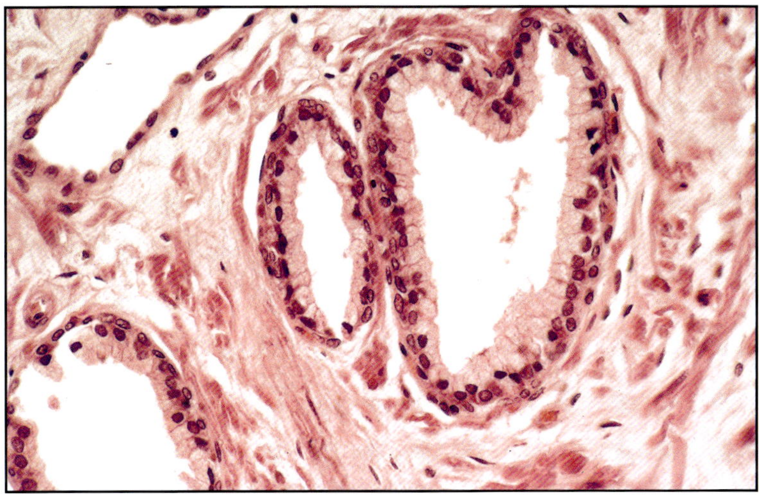

■ **i1.18** *Normal prostatic glands with two cell layers — an inner luminal cell layer and outer basal cell layer.*

The immunophenotype of basal cells **t1.4** is distinctive, is different from luminal secretory cells, and can be of diagnostic utility. Antibodies directed against a large number of cytokeratins, p63, CD40, CD44H, GST-Pi, and bcl-2 react with basal cells, whereas antibodies reactive with neuroendocrine markers, muscle markers, S-100, vimentin, and the secretory products PSA and prostatic acid phosphatase (PAP) are negative (Amin 1994, Bonkhoff 1994A, Devaraj 1993, di Sant'Agnese 1985B, Liu 2002, Magi-Galluzzi 1997, Moghaddami 2001, Nagle 1998, Paradis

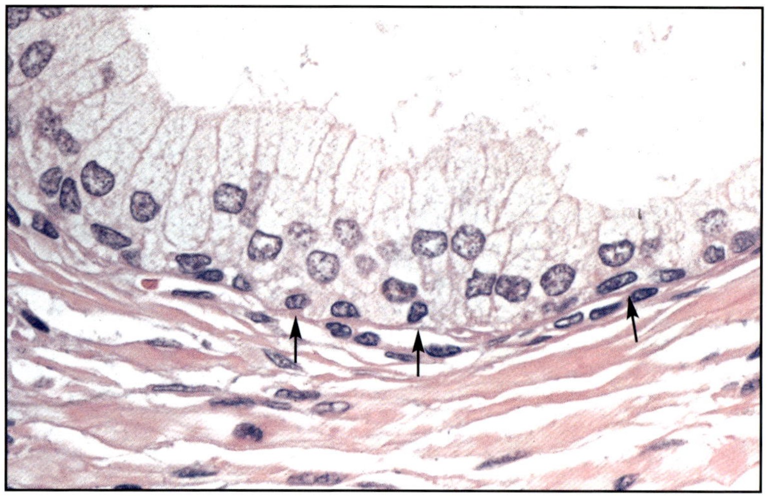

■ **i1.19** *Normal gland with small, rounded to elongated basal cells (arrows) arranged along basement membrane.*

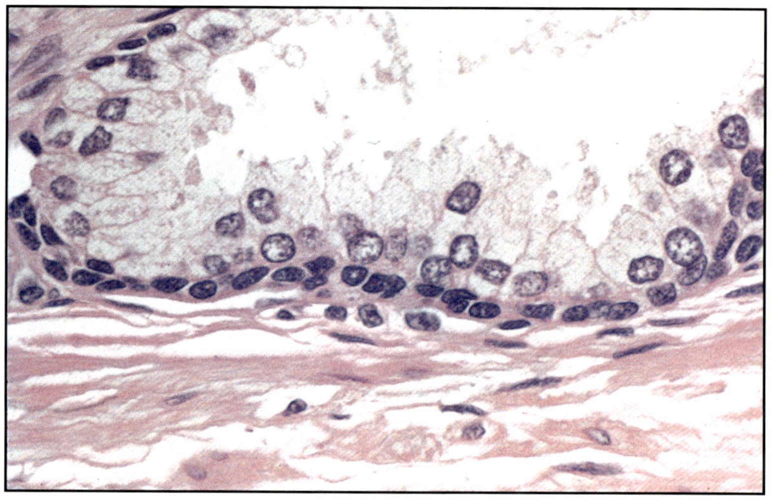

■ **i1.20** *Basal cells in prostatic epithelium can be prominent and, as shown here, can be aligned in a continuous row.*

■ **t1.4 Normal Prostatic Epithelial Cells: Immunophenotype**

	Cell Type		
Marker	**Basal Cell**	**Luminal Cell**	**Neuroendocrine Cell**
Pan-cytokeratin	+	+	+
CK 5,6,10,13,14	+	–	± (focal)
CK 8,18,	– to ± (rare)	+	+
PSA	–	+	+ or –
PAP	–	+	+
Androgen receptor	–	+	+ or –
GST-pi	+	–	NA
bcl-2	+	–	–
chromogranin	–	–	+
MSA, SMA	–	–	–
S-100	–	–	–
Vimentin	–	+	NA
p63	+	–	NA
CD40, CD44H	+	–	NA
CD10, CD57, CDw123	–	+	NA

Pan-cytokeratin: Our pan-cytokeratin cocktail includes antibodies AE1 and AE3. AE1 reacts with cytokeratins 10,14,15,16,19, and AE3 with 1-8.
CK = cytokeratin; PSA = Prostate specific antigen; PAP = Prostatic acid phosphatase; GST-pi = Glutathione-S-transferase-pi; MSA = Muscle-specific actin (HHF35); SMA = Smooth-muscle actin; NA = Not available

1998, Signoretti 2000, Srigley 1990, Wojno 1995). Additional basal cell markers have been identified by in situ hybridization and include pp32 (Kadkol 1998) and prostate stem cell antigen (Reiter 1998).

Basal cells have a more complex keratin expression pattern than luminal cells (Nagle 1998), and basal cell–specific antibodies that bind specific keratin polypeptides have been developed. Of note, this immunophenotype and ultrastructural evidence document that prostatic basal cells are not myoepithelial cells (Srigley 1990). Currently, the most important diagnostic marker of basal cells is monoclonal antibody 34βE12 (Gown 1984) (sometimes incorrectly called antibody 903 or keratin 903), which binds to Moll catalogue (Moll 1982) keratins 1, 5, 10, and 14 (Amin 1994, Brawer 1985, Goldstein 1999, Hedrick 1989, Kahane 1995, Okada 1992, Samaratunga 1997, Shah 1991, Wojno 1995, Yang 1997). This is a basal cell–specific antibody that works well on formalin-fixed, paraffin-embedded tissue sections. The typical pattern of basal cell staining with 34βE12 is continuous **i1.21** (Hedrick 1989, Shah 1991) or continuous with focal disruption (Hedrick 1989), although discontinuity and even lack of staining may be seen in a minority of normal glands (Goldstein 1999) **i1.22**.Because absence of basal cells is an important criterion in the diagnosis of invasive prostatic adenocarcinoma, this lack of staining of basal cells in normal glands constitutes a pitfall for diagnosticians who use this immunohistochemical stain. In normal glandular tissue basal cells must be diagnostically distinguished from periglandular stromal fibroblasts **i1.23**. Periglandular stromal fibroblastic nuclei may be closely apposed to prostatic glands, but these spindled nuclei tend to have pointed ends. Luminal cell nuclei that are basally positioned and poorly preserved, with nuclear shrinkage, may mimic basal cell nuclei. Ultrastructural examination of basal cells reveals a poorly differentiated cell with no secretory vacuoles, numerous mitochondria, and free ribosomes (Mao 1966). The nuclei often assume the overall shape of the cell and have a lobulated nuclear membrane, dispersed chromatin, and occasional small nucleoli (Mao 1966, Srigley 1990). Desmosomal attachments with adjacent secretory cells (Mao 1966, Srigley 1990) and two types of structural attachment of basal cells to underlying basal lamina have been observed (Nagle 1995). Both focal adhesions and hemidesmosome-like structures have been detected; of note, there is a basally polarized distribution of hemidesmosomal-associated proteins, including BP180, BP230, KD1, plectin, laminin-γ2(B2 t), collagen VII,

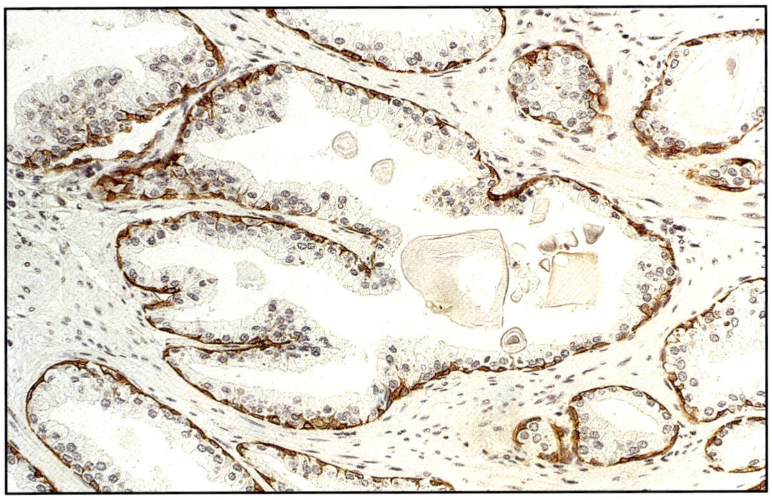

■ **i1.21** *Normal prostatic glands with continuous basal cell layer, as highlighted here by an immunohistochemical reaction using antibody 34βE12.*

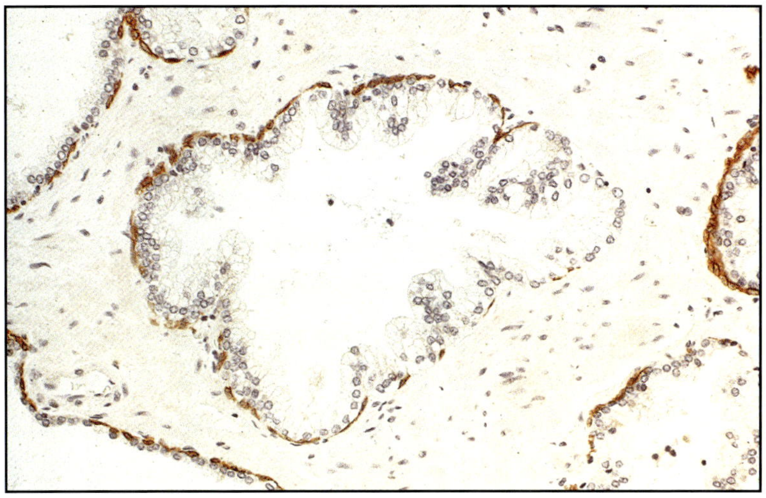

■ **i1.22** *Normal prostate gland with only partial staining of basal cell layer.*

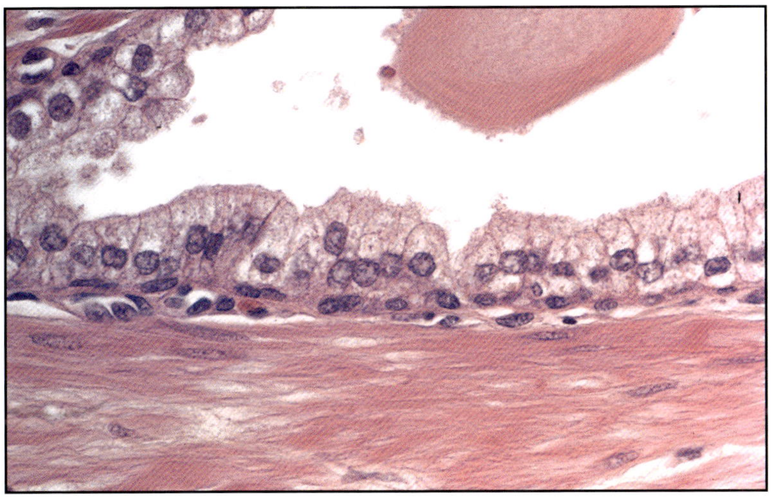

■ **i1.23** *Elongated cells clustered about the basement membrane may be difficult to definitely identify as intraglandular basal cells or periglandular stromal fibroblasts, particularly in thick sections.*

and the corresponding integrin laminin receptors α6β1 and α6β4 (Nagle 1995). Hemidesmosomal structures and some of these proteins are lost in carcinoma (Nagle 1995). The cell adhesion molecule C-CAM is expressed in basal cells and is also lost in prostatic carcinoma (Kleinerman 1995). This suggests a potential diagnostic role for these cellular adhesion alterations, but currently they are experimental. The basal cells are the dominant proliferative cell type in the normal prostate. Even though secretory cells outnumber basal cells 3 to 1 in the normal prostate (Bonkhoff 1994B, McNeal 1995), proliferative basal cells constitute 70% to 80% of proliferating benign epithelium (Bonkhoff 1994B, McNeal 1995). The proliferation index of normal prostatic epithelium is extremely low (Berges 1995, Limas 1994), with 0.2% of cells proliferating per day, which is precisely balanced by a 0.2% cell death rate (Berges 1995). This translates into a continuous replacement or turnover every 500 days (Berges 1995). For basal cells, only 0.2% to 0.7% are in a proliferative state, as assessed by bromodeoxyuridine incorporation or Ki-67 labeling (Bonkhoff 1996A). Mitotic figures are rare in normal prostatic basal cells and epithelium, and their presence in hematoxylin and eosin (H&E)-stained sections should prompt careful scrutiny for epithelial cell atypia.

The precise function of normal prostatic basal cells is unsettled, but it is likely that the basal cell population harbors stem cells (Bonkhoff 1996A, 1996B). Such putative stem cells (Hudson 2000) cannot currently be identified by morphology or markers. Also elusive has been the morphologic identification of intermediate cells with morphologic characteristics of both basal and luminal cells (Srigley 1990). A few cells coexpress basal cell keratins and luminal cell PSA or luminal cell keratins (Bonkhoff 1994A, van Leenders 2000, Verhagan 1992), suggesting that basal cells may differentiate into luminal cells via a transiently proliferating or amplifying cell population. Evidence suggests that such cytodifferentiation requires cell-cell (and specifically stromal cell–basal cell) interaction (Liu 1997). Basal cells could also play a vital role in communicating growth signals (Bonkhoff 1996A) because basal cells express receptors for estrogen, progesterone, epidermal growth factor, and hepatocyte growth factor (Maygarden 1992, Pisters 1996, Wernert 1988). Basal cells could also influence progression of high-grade PIN to invasion via regulation of the balance of expression of proteases (Boag 1993, Sinha 1993) and protease inhibitors (Barsky 1997).

Neuroendocrine (endocrine-paracrine) cells constitute a second population of cells in normal prostatic epithelium (di Sant'Agnese 1995). These cells are a small minority at about 0.4% of the total adult prostatic epithelial cell population (Battaglia 1994, di Sant'Agnese 1995). This is a terminally differentiated, post–mitotic cell population (Bonkhoff 1991B, 1995) that variably expresses androgen receptor (Nakada 1993) and the secretory products PSA and PAP (Aprikian 1993, Bonkhoff 1994A, Cohen 1992) **t1.4.** The keratin expression pattern is more like luminal than basal cells (Xue 1997). These neuroendocrine cells usually are recognizable only by histochemical (Fontana-Masson argentaffin and Churukian-Schenk argyrophil) or immunohistochemical staining (Barsky 1997, Cohen 1992, 1993, di Sant'Agnese 1984B, 1985A, 1986) **i1.24, i1.25.** By immunohistochemical detection of chromogranin and neuron-specific enolase, these cells may be found throughout the prostate but are at highest concentrations in the periurethral region and prostatic ducts **i1.25** (Cohen 1993). A variety of neuroendocrine markers, including chromogranin, neuron-specific enolase, serotonin, thyroid-stimulating hormone–like peptide, calcitonin, bombesin, gastrin-releasing peptide, somatostatin, parathormone-related protein, and neurotensin, have been identified in these cells by immunohistochemistry (di Sant'Agnese 1995). These immunostains highlight the highly interdigitating nature of these cells, which exhibit slender, cytoplasmic dendritic process **i1.24, i1.25** that may be up to 200μm long (di Sant'Agnese 1984B). Most of the neuroendocrine cells are more basally situated without luminal extensions (closed type), but most

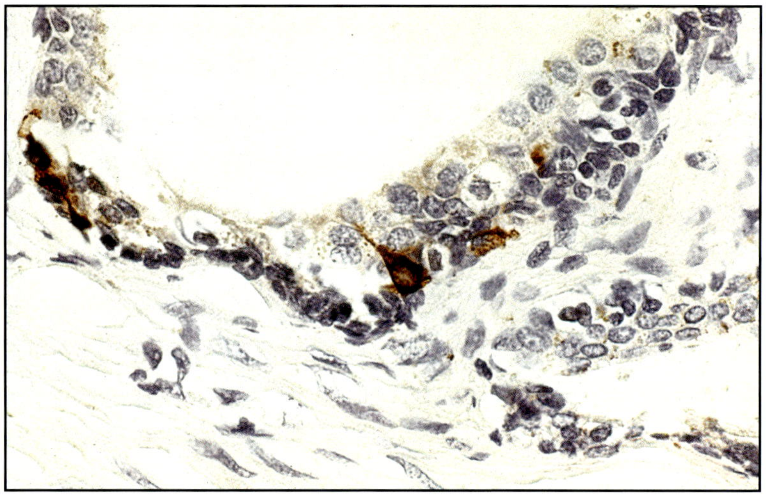

■ **i1.24** *Neuroendocrine cells detected by chromogranin immunolabeling in acinar epithelium.*

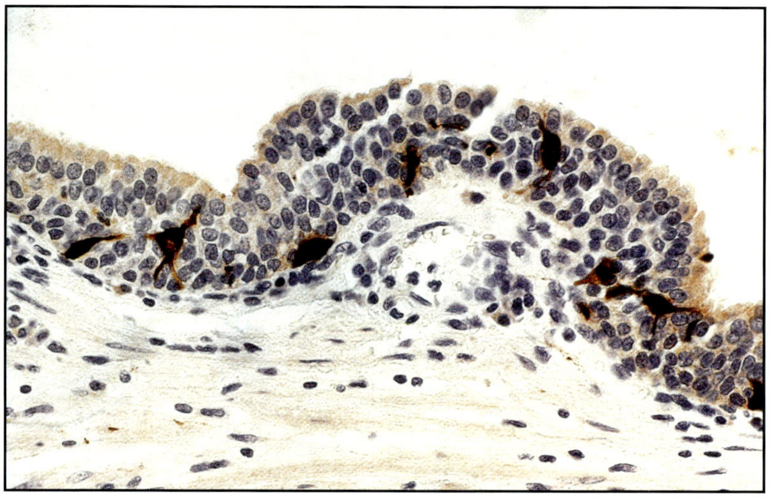

■ **i1.25** *Neuroendocrine cells detected by chromogranin immunostain of a prostatic duct with urothelium (transitional epithelium). Note delicate cytoplasmic processes. These cells are not recognizable as neuroendocrine by H&E-staining.*

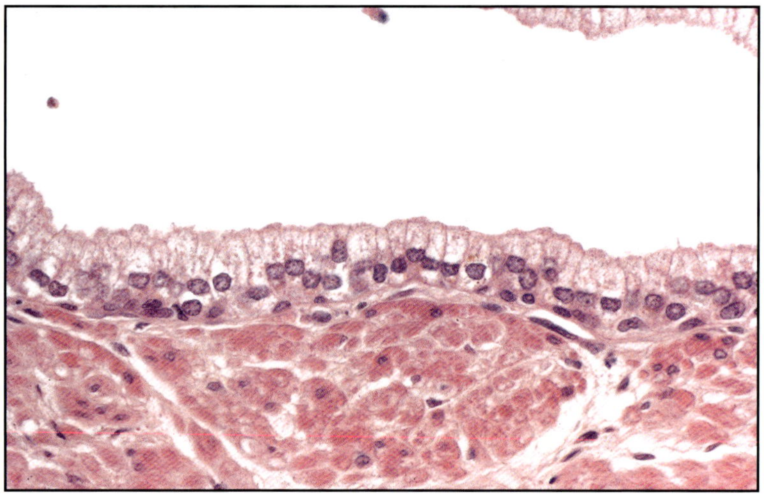

■ **i1.26** *Typical normal luminal cells with abundant pale, cleared to granular cytoplasm and with mainly basally situated, uniform nuclei.*

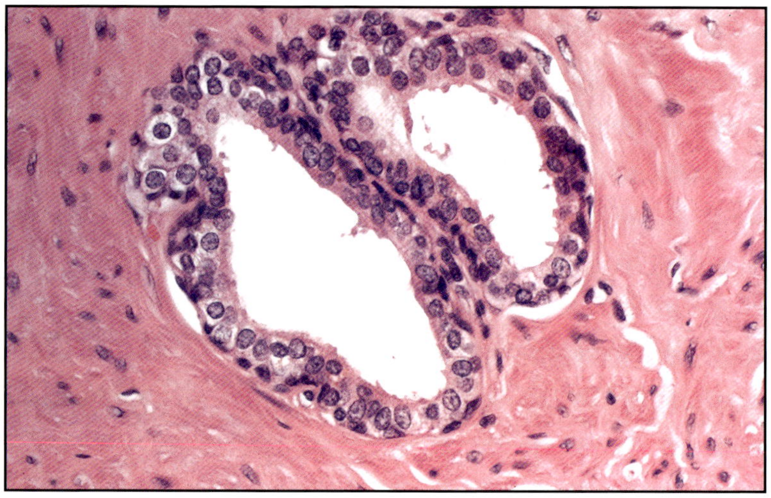

■ **i1.27** *Darker cytoplasm of central zone luminal epithelium.*

are not basal cells because only rarely do basal cells exhibit neuroendocrine differentiation (Bonkhoff 1994A, Devaraj 1993). A few cells are flask-shaped and extend to the luminal surface (so-called open type). Others are more spherical or triangular in shape (Aprikian 1993). Neurosecretory granules of varying sizes are found in these cells by electron microscopy (di Sant'Agnese 1984A). Neuroendocrine differentiation in normal prostatic epithelium may be seen in H&E-stained sections as "Paneth-like" cells, which are cells with bright, eosinophilic intracytoplasmic granules. This is apparently a rare finding in normal prostatic epithelium (Weaver 1992) but may be seen in 10% of carcinomas (Adlakha 1994). The functional significance of neuroendocrine cells in the normal prostate is not clear, but it seems likely that the neuroendocrine products of these cells influence neighboring cells through the elaborate dendritic processes via a paracrine effect (di Sant'Agnese 1995). Autocrine and endocrine influences may also be in operation (di Sant'Agnese 1998).

The secretory or luminal cells of the normal prostate glandular epithelium make up the bulk (73%) of the epithelial volume. The secretory cells are cuboidal to columnar, with nuclei positioned in the basal to midportion of the cell **i1.26** (McNeal 1997). These nuclei are found above basal cell nuclei, but because secretory cell nuclei outnumber basal cell nuclei 3:1, some of the basally positioned secretory cell nuclei may appear to abut the basal lamina, yet here imperceptible (at the H&E level) basal cell cytoplasm usually separates the secretory cell from the basal lamina. Some secretory cells may directly rest on basement membrane (deVries 1992). The luminal border of the secretory cell layer often is irregular.

Cleared cytoplasm is a hallmark of normal prostatic secretory cells **i1.26** because of the presence of a larger number of small clear secretory vacuoles. The central zone secretory cell cytoplasm is somewhat denser because it contains a smaller number of these vacuoles (McNeal 1997) **i1.27**. Cleared cytoplasm in prostatic epithelial cells is somewhat helpful in differential diagnosis (Humphrey 1997) but is not specific for benign or malignant epithelial proliferations. Well-differentiated adenocarcinomas of the prostate of Gleason grade patterns 1 and 2 (and score of 2 to 4) characteristically have cleared cytoplasm (but should not be called clear cell carcinomas). Such cytoplasmic clearing is also not specific for low-grade prostatic carcinoma because higher-grade carcinomas, which usually have amphophilic cytoplasm, may also manifest cleared cytoplasm (Humphrey 1997).

Pigment is common in the cytoplasm of normal prostatic secretory epithelial cells. These granules are 1μm to 3μm in diameter, are apical or subnuclear, and are yellow-brown to gray-brown to blue by H&E staining (Amin 1996, Brennick 1994, Leung 1995) **i1.28, i1.29.** The distribution varies on an individual basis, from focal to diffuse. The histochemical staining characteristics (including positivity for Fontana-Masson,

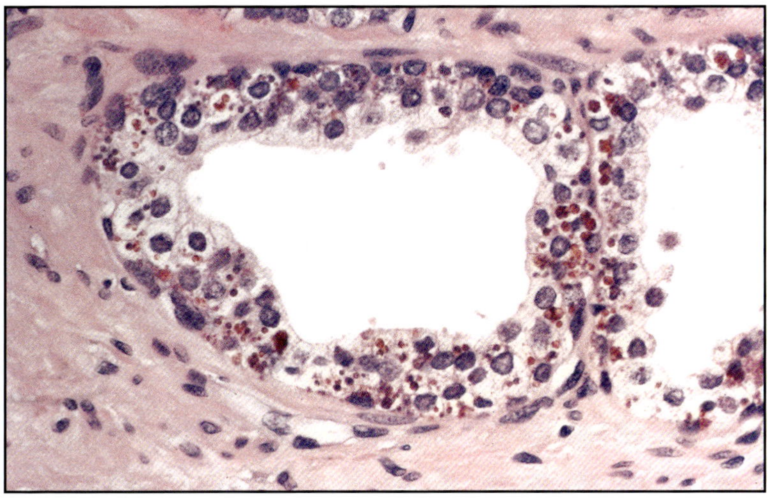

■ **i1.28** *Brownish pigment in benign prostatic epithelium.*

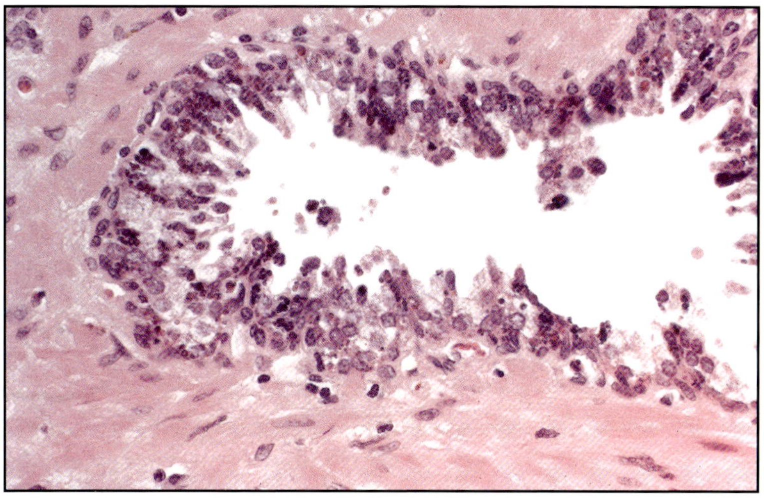

■ **i1.29** *Purple-black intracytoplasmic pigment in benign prostatic luminal epithelial cells.*

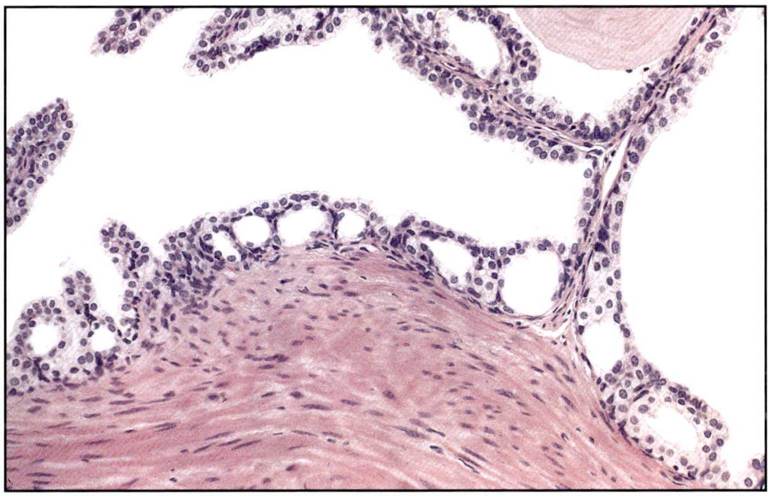

■ **i1.30** *Central zone epithelium with lacunae (tiny spaces or depressions).*

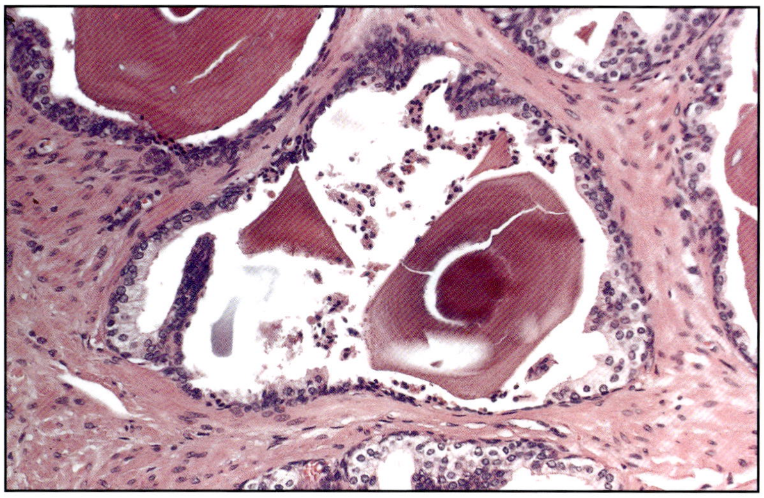

■ **i1.31** *Shed intraluminal epithelial cells and corpora amylacea.*

periodic acid-Schiff with diastase, Congo red, Luxol fast-blue, and Oil-Red-O) and autofluorescence of the pigment are consistent with lipofuscin, which is basically oxidized and polymerized lipid (Brennick 1994), which represents the "wear and tear" or "aging" pigment. This lipofuscin pigment is present in epithelia of all 3 zones of the prostate; one study (Leung 1995) found it to be more common in the central zone. In the past this pigment was though to represent melanin (so-called melanosis of the prostate), but melanin in the prostate is rare (Amin 1996) and is present mainly in blue nevi of the prostate, where melanin is found within dendritic bipolar cells in the stroma. The diagnostic importance of lipofuscin pigment in normal prostatic epithelial cells is twofold. First, although this pigment is more common in benign epithelium, its presence does not exclude neoplasia because it has been detected in high-grade PIN and invasive carcinoma. Second, golden-brown lipofuscin pigment cannot be used to distinguish prostatic epithelium from ejaculatory duct and seminal vesicle epithelium, which also contains golden-brown lipofuscin pigment. Although the seminal vesicle and ejaculatory duct pigment is coarser and more retractile, the best way to distinguish this epithelium from prostatic epithelium is the presence of irregularly distributed atypical hyperchromatic nuclei, which may have intranuclear cytoplasmic protrusions. Distinguishing prostatic from seminal vesicle epithelium is not an uncommon problem: 5% of prostate needle biopsies (Coyne 1987) and 3% of transurethral resection chips (Young 1988) contain seminal vesicle epithelium. If doubt persists regarding epithelial type, a PSA immunostain will be positive in prostatic epithelium but not in ejaculatory duct or seminal vesicle epithelium.

The nuclei of normal prostatic secretory epithelium are small and round with fine, evenly dispersed chromatin. Nucleoli usually are not evident or are pinpoint in size. Nuclei in the central zone usually are larger than those in the peripheral zone and also appear crowded. This results in a pseudostratified nuclear appearance in the central zone and along with the aforementioned denser cytoplasm may yield a false impression of PIN (Srodon 2002).

Central zone epithelium is also distinctive in showing lacunae **i1.30** and in selective expression of pepsinogen II (Reese 1986), lactoferrin (Reese 1992), and lectin-binding sites (McNeal 1988). In contrast, the cytokeratin, BerEP4 and vimentin immunoprofiles of central zone epithelium are not distinctive compared with transition zone and peripheral zone epithelium (Srigley 2000). That the central zone is different morphologically and biochemically from the peripheral and transition zones may result from its proposed different embryologic origin from Wolffian ducts (McNeal 1997).

Intraluminal contents of normal prostatic glands include shed and degenerating epithelial cells **i1.31**, corpora amylacea **i1.31-i1.41**,

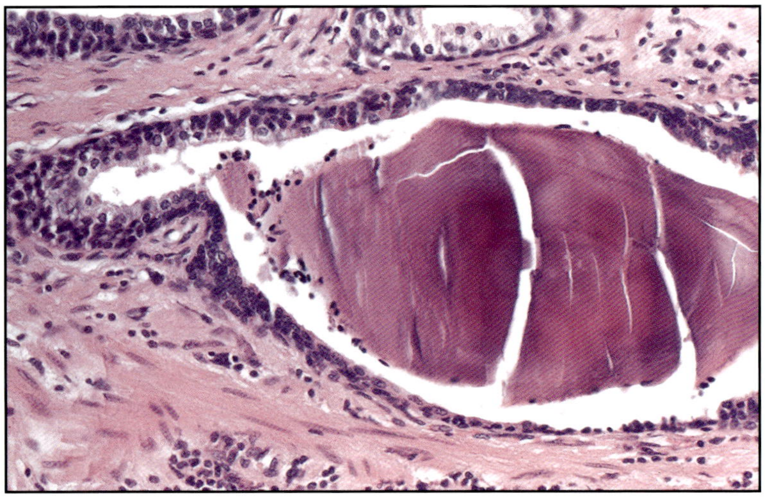

■ **i1.32** *Corpus amylaceum with degenerating, intraluminal epithelial cells at one end.*

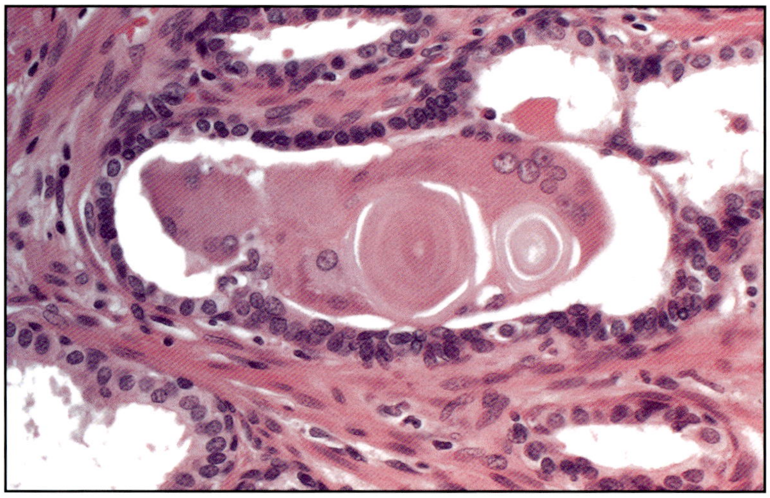

■ **i1.33** *Intraluminal giant cell surrounding corpora amylacea.*

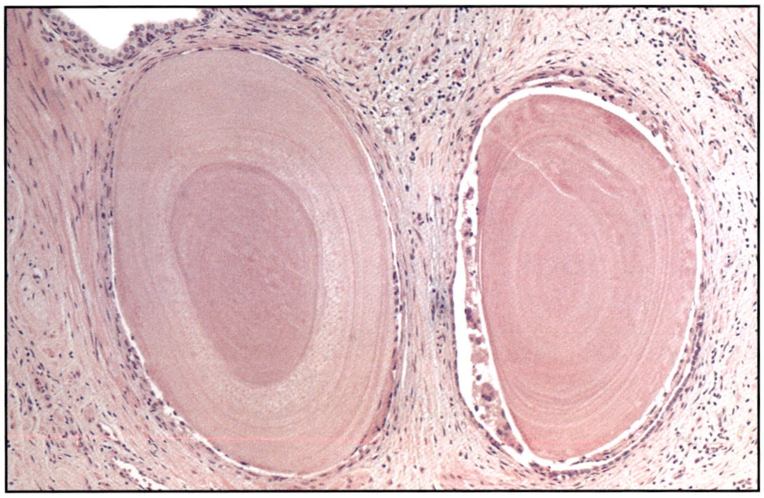

■ **i1.34** *Corpora amylacea can fill and distend glands, with resultant attenuation of the epithelial lining.*

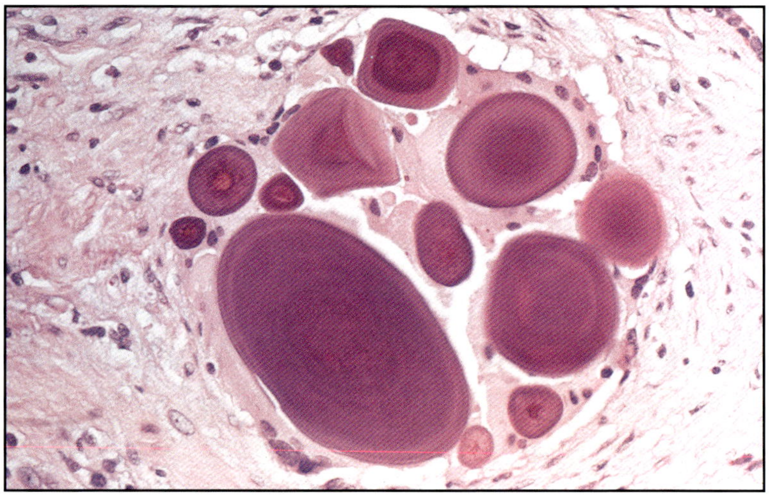

■ **i1.35** *Corpora amylacea in stroma.*

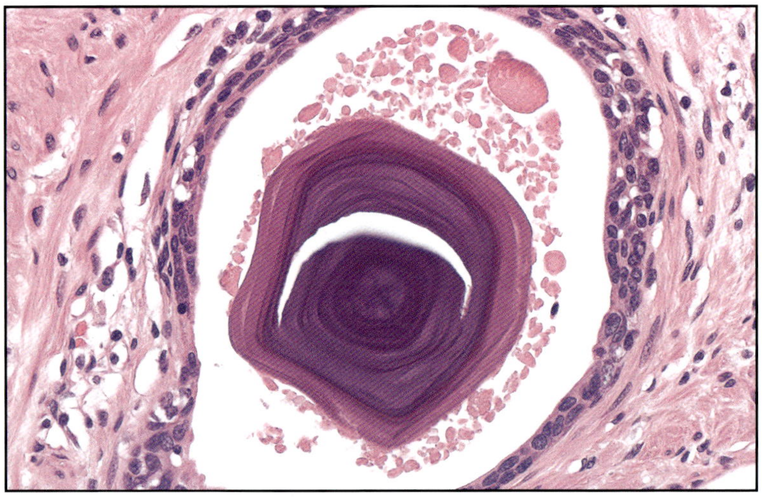

■ **i1.36** *Calcified corpus amylaceum.*

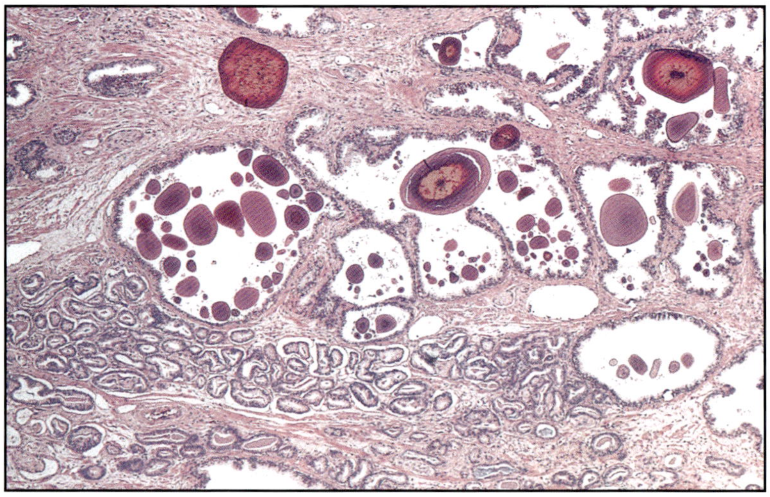

■ **i1.37** *Numerous variably-sized corpora amylacea in benign glands but not in adjacent small acinar adenocarcinoma.*

and calculi **i1.42, i1.43**. Shed and degenerating epithelial cells often are found in association with corpora amylacea and indeed are thought to be related to their formation. These cells may be seen lining the periphery of the corpora **i1.31-i1.33.** Corpora amylacea are inspissated secretions that often assume a concentrically lamellated appearance (Eastman 1897, Humphrey 1990, Marx 1965, Moore 1936A, 1936B, Seaman 1956), like rings in a tree. They are mainly rounded and may vary widely in size **i1.37, i1.38**. Corpora amylacea usually are pink to

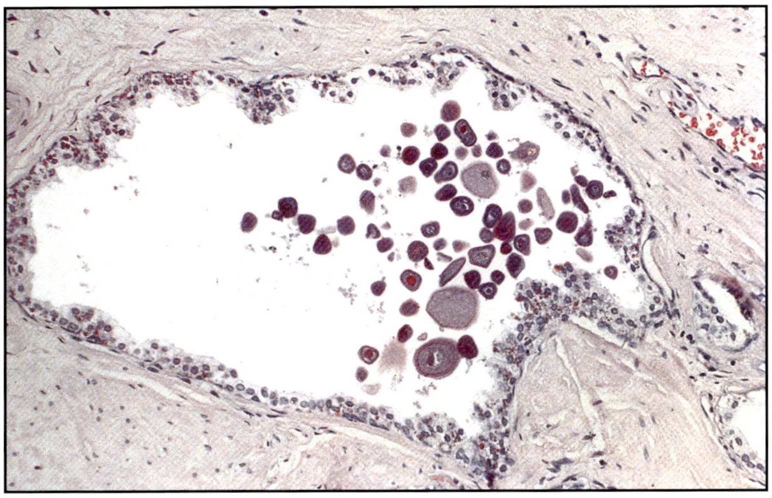

■ **i1.38** *Corpora amylacea may be quite small.*

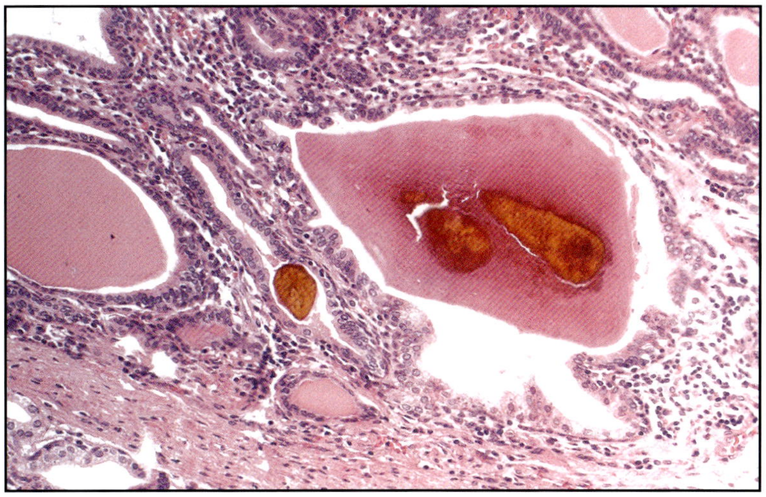

■ **i1.39** *Numerous corpora amylacea can be found within glands of the verumontanum; these sometimes appear yellow-gold to orange.*

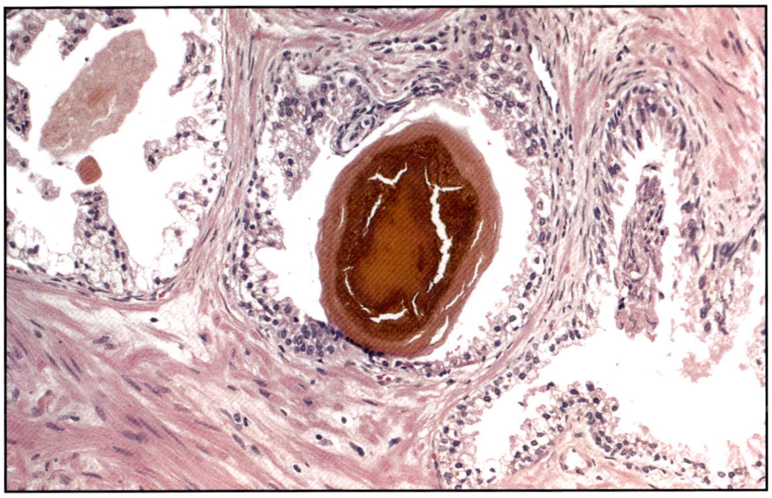

■ **i1.40** *Yellow-gold corpus amylaceum in a peripheral zone gland.*

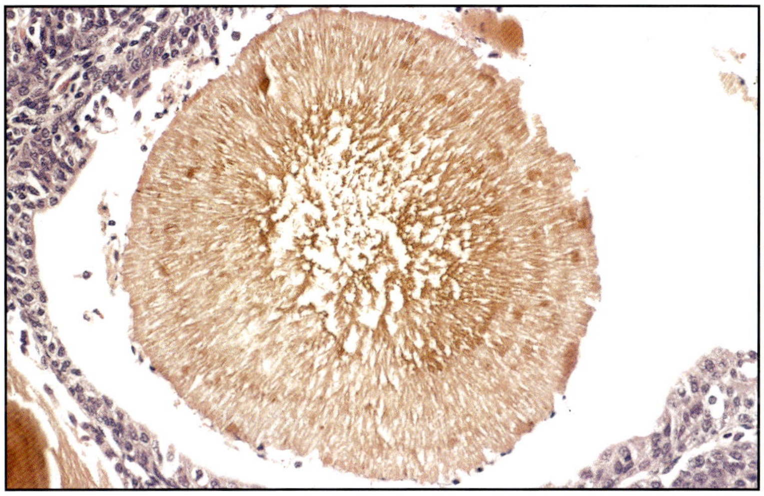

■ **i1.41** *Central "starburst-like" radiations in the center of a corpus amylaceum. Do not confuse these filamentous radiations with fungal hyphae.*

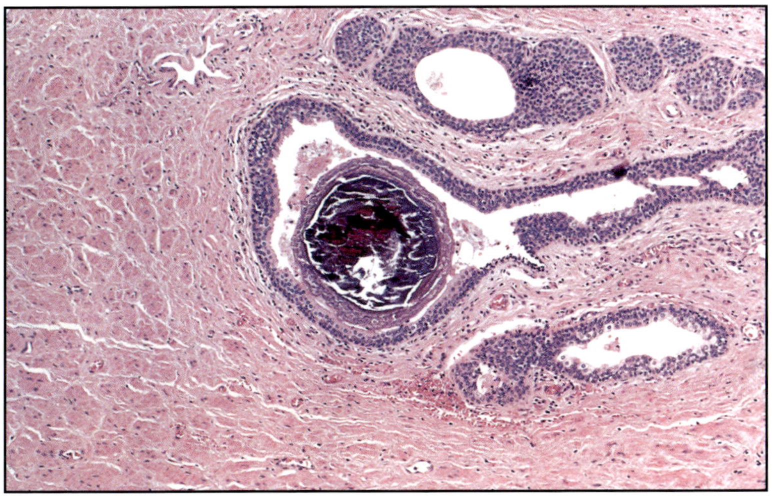

■ **i1.42** *A stone (calcified corpus amylaceum) in a central prostatic duct.*

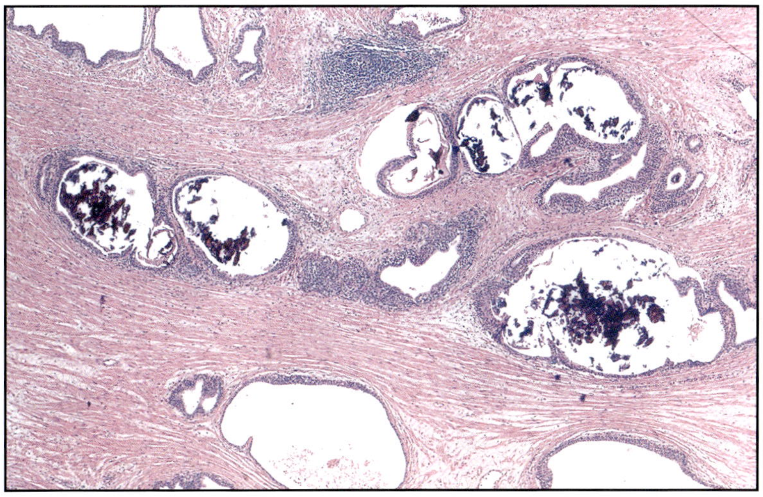

■ **i1.43** *Calcific debris representing stone debris in dilated central prostatic ducts.*

purple but may be yellow-gold to orange, particularly in verumontanum glands **i1.39**. This hue is not specific for corpora in glands of the verumontanum and can be noted in peripheral gland corpora **i1.40**. Although usually corpora have a concentrically lamellated structure, one may uncommonly observe a radiating or starburst pattern within corpora **i1.41**. These radiations should not be confused with fungal organisms. Sometimes corpora can be seen in atrophic glands, with only a thin atrophic epithelial lining

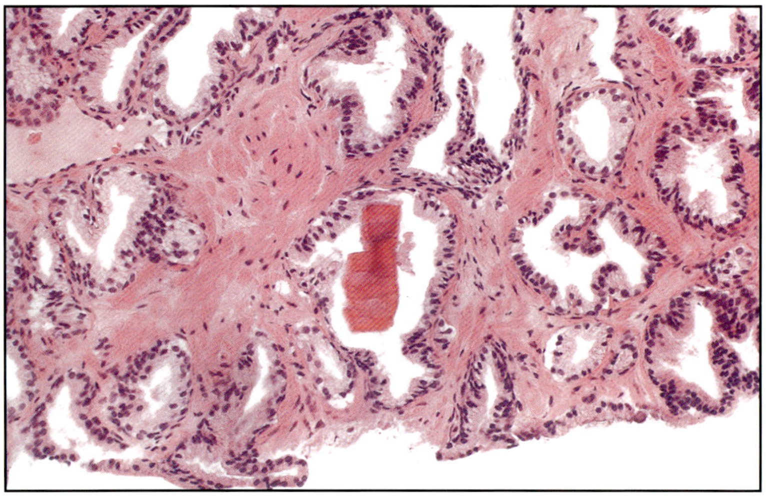

■ **i1.44** *Eosinophilic crystalloid with"sharp" edges in the lumen of a benign gland in needle biopsy tissue.*

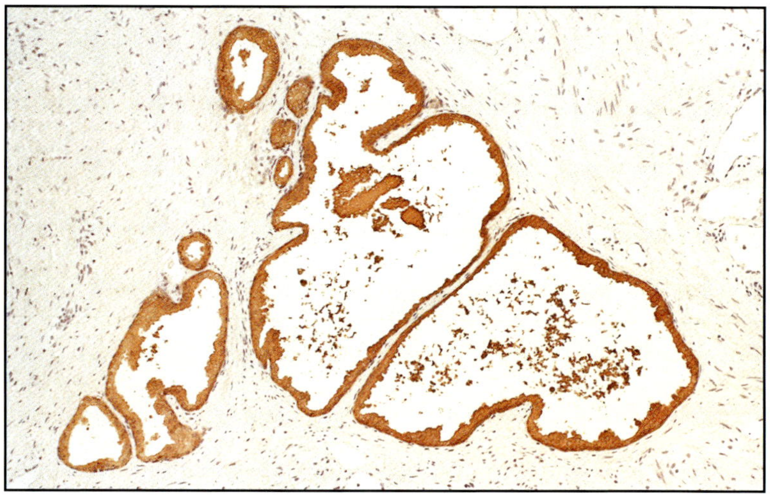

■ **i1.45** *Diffuse, strong immunostaining for prostate specific antigen in benign glands.*

surrounding them **i1.34**, and in spaces without an obvious epithelial lining **i1.35**, or they can be seen in stroma, with or without associated giant cells. Corpora are extremely common in the normal prostate and are found in up to 78% of benign glands (Humphrey 1990). Prostatic corpora appear in the first decade and increase in number with age. They often calcify **i1.36** and probably contribute to the formation of prostatic calculi. Prostatic corpora possess many cellular constituents, including RNA, DNA, lipid, mucopolysaccharide, and protein (Moore 1936A, Seaman 1956); by electron microscopy they show interwoven fibrils arranged in rings (Marx 1965).

Prostatic calculi are extremely common, being detectable in 75% to 100% of men by ultrasonography (Peeling 1984). They are typically found in central, large prostatic ducts. These stones vary in size from microscopic to 4cm in size and grossly are usually multiple, round or ovoid, and brown, with variable white or gray areas (Klimas 1985, Moore 1936B). These prostatic stones mainly contain calcium phosphate, but calcium oxalate, carbonate-apatite, and hydroxyapatite also be present (Klimas 1985, Marx 1965, Moore 1936A). Prostatic calculi are most often seen as incidental findings in the setting of inflammation and BPH. The diagnostic impact of corpora, microcalcifications, and calculi is that they are all more common in benign glands, but their presence does not rule out malignancy. Corpora amylacea have been reported in 11% to 13% of carcinomas (Bostwick 1993, Humphrey 1990), microcalcifications were noted in 2% of carcinomas (Woods 1998), and calculi were found associated with 6% of prostate cancers (Cristol 1944).

Although corpora amylacea are more often seen in benign glands than carcinoma, certain intraluminal materials are, conversely, rare in normal gland lumina but are more common in neoplastic processes. These intraluminal materials include pink amorphous acellular secretions, intraluminal wispy blue mucin (also known as blue-tinged mucinous secretions), and crystalloids. Eosinophilic or pink acellular intraluminal secretions are seen in about one half of prostatic carcinomas and only rarely to occasionally in benign glands (Epstein 1995, Varma 2002). Mucin usually is not visualized in H&E sections of normal glands, but in our experience intraluminal wispy blue mucin is seen in 72% of cases of typical prostatic adenocarcinoma (Kaleem 1998). However, this mucin, which is an acid mucin by histochemical (Alcian blue) staining, is not specific for malignancy and may be seen in mucinous metaplasia, sclerosing adenosis, atypical adenomatous hyperplasia (adenosis), and high-grade PIN. Histochemical staining of normal prostate glands for mucin reveals neutral mucins (periodic acid-Schiff with diastase), whereas neoplastic glands often demonstrate neutral and acidic (Alcian blue, pH 2.5 positive) mucins (Franks 1964, Hukill 1967). However, acid mucin staining is not a "malignant stain" because rare normal glands, adenosis, and PIN stain for acid mucins (Epstein 1992, Franks 1964, Grignon 1993, Hukill 1967, Humphrey 1991, Sentinelli 1993). Luminal acid mucin has also been found in a few cases of postatrophic hyperplasia and basal cell hyperplasia (Grignon 1993); in this same study luminal acid mucin was also found by histochemical staining in one third of areas of transitional cell metaplasia (Grignon 1993). Finally, brightly eosinophilic intraluminal crystalloids often are discovered in malignant prostate glands but only uncommonly in benign glands **i1.44** (Henneberry 1997, Holmes 1977, Jensen 1980, Varma 2002). In two recent series (Anton 1998, Varma 2002), 1% to 5% of benign needle biopsies harbored these crystalloids. These intraluminal materials that are more often found in malignant than normal glands should prompt careful study of the glands containing them as well as surrounding glands. If the glandular epithelium is entirely benign, a diagnosis of benign prostatic tissue should be rendered. The presence of these intraluminal materials alone, without associated epithelial cellular atypia, might prompt one to consider performing additional tissue sampling such as more levels of needle biopsies or submitting more tissue in transurethral resection cases (Sentinelli 1993). The identification of crystalloids alone in normal or benign glands in prostate needle biopsy is not an indication for rebiopsy (Anton 1998, Henneberry 1997).

The immunophenotype of the secretory cell evinces the epithelial, secretory, androgen-responsive, and weakly proliferative nature of this cell type **[t1.4]**. Among the secretory products of the luminal cells, the most important diagnostically is PSA. Normal secretory cells in prostatic epithelium exhibit diffuse, even, and strong immunohistochemical staining for PSA **i1.45** and prostatic acid phosphatase. Antibody reactions against the proliferation markers proliferating cell nuclear antigen and Ki-67 antigen show that only 20% to 30% of proliferating cells in the normal prostatic epithelium are secretory cells and that the proliferation index or growth fraction of those cells is 0.12% (Bonkhoff 1996A, 1996B).

Electron microscopy of normal peripheral zone secretory cells shows tall columnar cells with filling of the cytoplasm by tiny vacuoles of uniform diameter (Srigley 1990). Cytoplasmic organelles and intermediate filaments are compressed in the septae

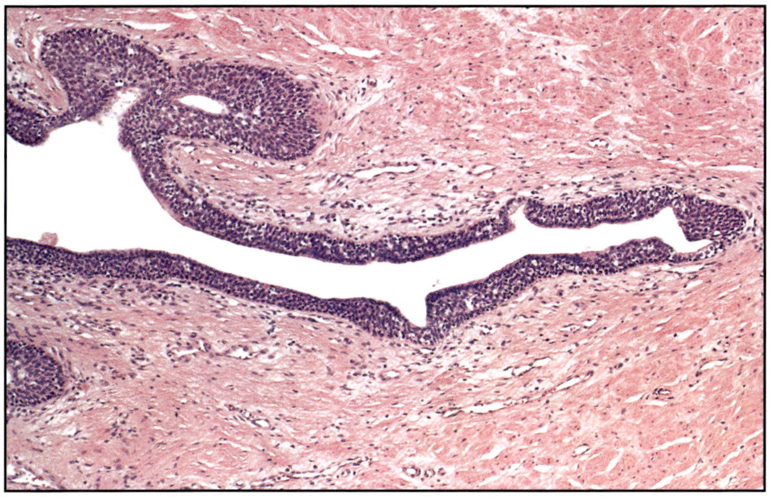

■ **i1.46** *Urothelium (transitional epithelium) in large prostatic duct.*

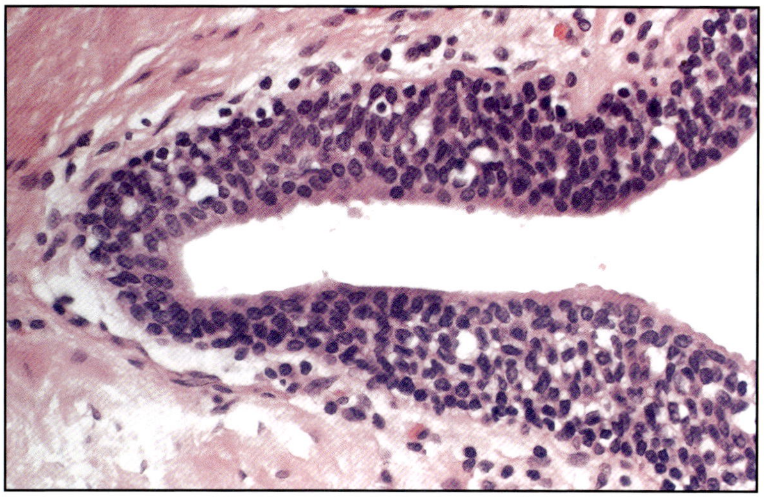

■ **i1.47** *Urothelium in prostatic duct with luminal prostatic secretory epithelial cell layer.*

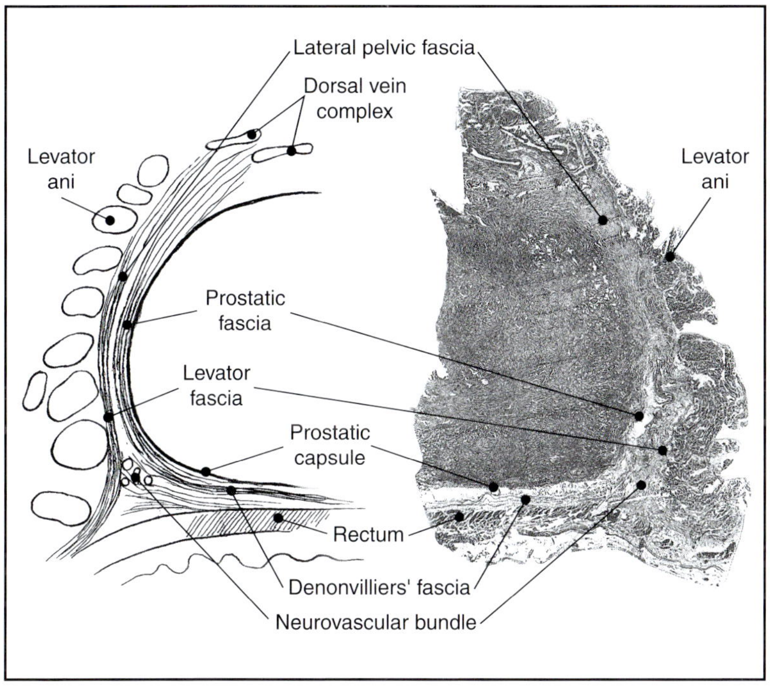

■ **f1.4** *Cross-section of adult prostate demonstrating anatomic relationships of prostate and surrounding fasciae. (Reprinted with permission from* Campbell's Urology, 7th ed. *Copyright Brady Urological Institute.)*

surrounding the vacuoles. Apocrine secretory blebs are prominent at the luminal surface. The nuclei are round, basal, and only rarely have nucleoli.

Transitional cell epithelium (urothelium) is another type of epithelial cell normally found in the prostate. In addition to lining the prostatic urethra, transitional cell epithelium also normally lines major prostatic ducts **i1.46, i1.47**. This ductal lining is variable in extent from one person to the next. The transitional cell epithelium in the prostatic ducts and urethra differs from such lining elsewhere in the urinary tract in that an umbrella layer of cap cells is lacking and is replaced by a single layer of secretory cells **i1.47** that are PSA positive. The transitional cells are PSA negative. Recognition of transitional epithelium usually is straightforward: This is a multilayered epithelium with rounded to elongated nuclei, some of which possess nuclear grooves. A degree of cytoplasmic clearing usually is evident. When transitional epithelium involves acini in the peripheral aspects of the prostate gland, the designation *transitional cell metaplasia* is applied (Yantiss 1997). Here, unlike the normal ductal transitional cell epithelial lining, there is often an associated acute or chronic inflammatory cell infiltrate (Yantiss 1997).

Nonepithelial structures of the prostate include the "capsule", preprostatic sphincter, striated sphincter, anterior fibromuscular stroma, and intraglandular stroma, including smooth muscle cells, fibroblasts, vasculature, and nerves (McNeal 1997).

The outer prostatic "capsule" is actually a band of concentrically placed fibrovascular tissue that is inseparable from prostatic stroma (Ayala 1989, McNeal 1997) and surrounding fasciae. Outside the prostate, this band is also contiguous with pelvic fascia and rectovesical fascia (of Denonvilliers) **f1.4** (Ayala 1989, Krongard 1989). These fascial tissues are important landmarks in radical prostatectomy surgeries. In radical perineal prostatectomy, the lateral and anterior pelvic fasciae are reflected off the prostate, whereas in radical retropubic prostatectomy, the prostate is approached from outside these fascial planes (Walsh 1998). Denonvilliers' fascia is a sheath between the rectum and prostate that covers the posterior aspect of the prostate and seminal vesicles. The complete excision of this fascial tissue at radical prostatectomy is important because prostate cancer can directly extend into it (Villers 1993).

The fibromuscular band ("capsule") of the prostate **i1.48** is 0.5 to 3mm thick and is incomplete, being absent at the apex (Ayala 1989, Di Lollo 1997, Sattar 1995). It is composed mainly of transversely disposed bundles of smooth muscle and collagen. Smooth muscle bundles course between the band and periepithelial stroma inside the prostate gland, without obeying any sort of boundary. Also, the concentration of smooth muscle fibers in the band and prostatic stroma is identical (at 31%) (Sattar 1995). Glands from the prostate approach this band, but the border between the outer limit of epithelium and the band is not often clearly definable under the light microscope **i1.48**. Posteriorly, the band fuses with Denonvilliers' fascia and does not clearly separate prostate from seminal vesicle (Di Lollo 1997) **i1.49**. Posterolaterally, outside the band there is abundant adipose tissue and neurovascular bundles **i1.50, i1.51**. Atherosclerosis **i1.51** and thrombi can be detected as incidental findings in these periprostatic vessels. Peripheral gaping blood vessels **i1.52** have been used as a demarcation landmark between intraprostatic and extraprostatic tissue, but such vessels clearly can extend into the

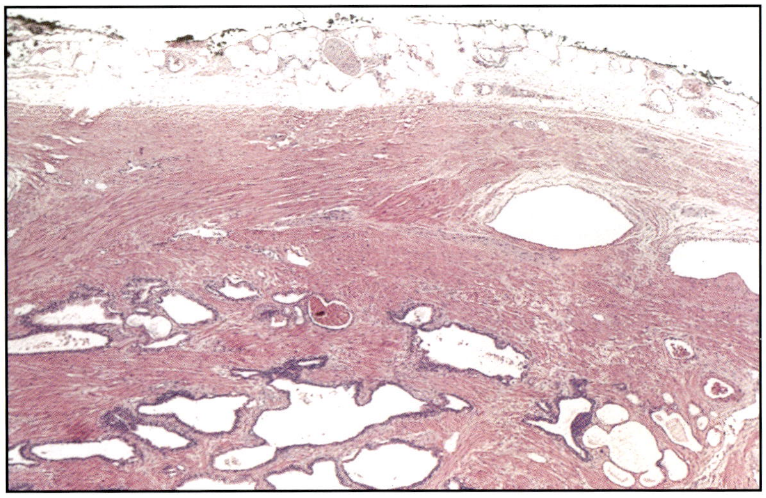

■ **i1.48** *Periphery of prostate with indistinct fibromuscular band between prostatic glands and periprostatic soft tissue.*

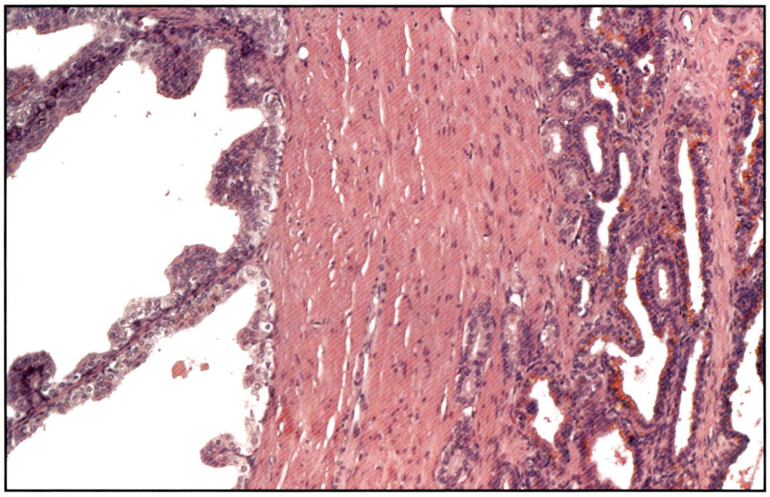

■ **i1.49** *Boundary between prostate (left) and seminal vesicle (right): A smooth muscle band which is not clearly prostatic or seminal vesicle.*

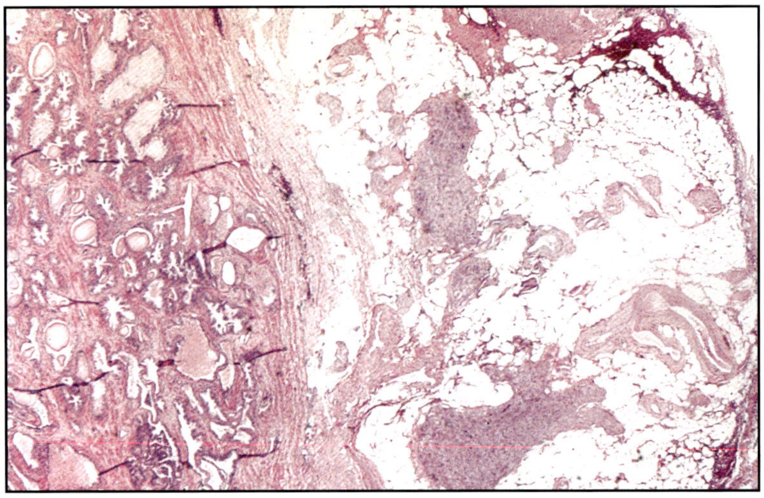

■ **i1.50** *Abundant periprostatic adipose tissue, with large nerves, in posterolateral region.*

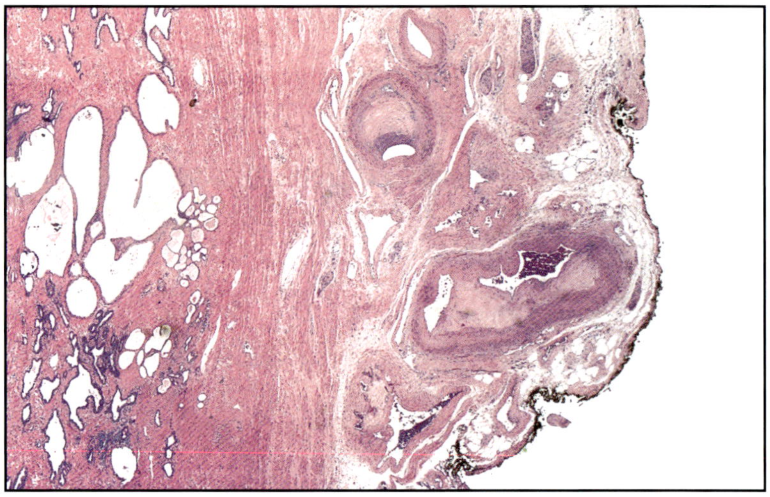

■ **i1.51** *Large blood vessels with atherosclerotic change in periprostatic soft tissue.*

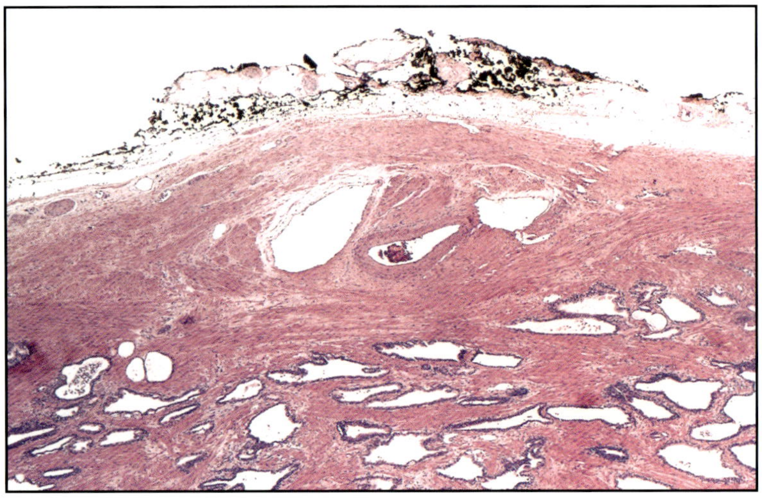

■ **i1.52** *Intracapsular gaping vessels. The "capsule" is ill-defined.*

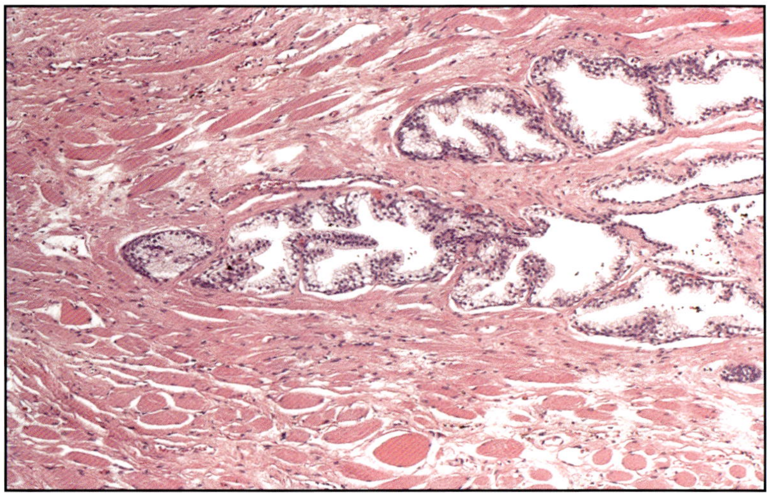

■ **i1.53** *Benign prostatic glands with surrounding smooth and skeletal muscle at apex.*

substance of the prostate and therefore are unreliable as a capsular marker. Anteriorly and anterolaterally, the band blends with the pelvic fascia. Apically, the band is no longer present, and instead there is a jumble of smooth muscle, skeletal muscle, and fibroelastic fibers. Here, it is important to know that the urethral striated sphincter (rhabdosphincter) is in direct continuity with the prostate, and indeed skeletal muscle fibers can normally be found, at an anterior and apical location, within the substance of the gland itself **i1.53, i1.54**

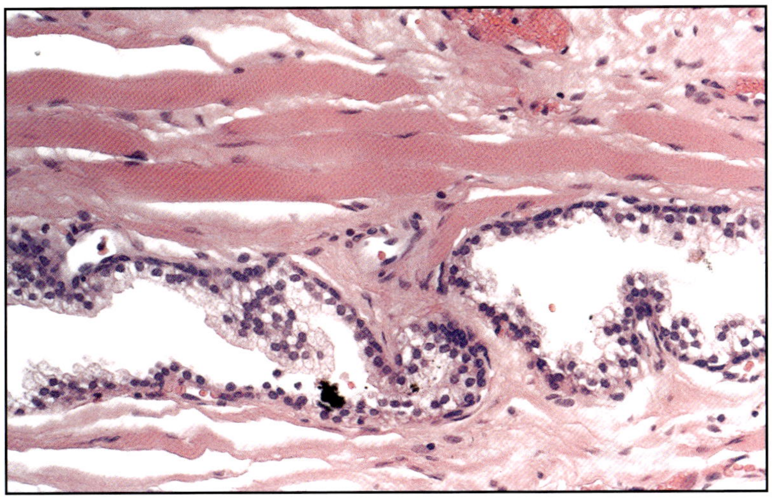

■ **i1.54** *Skeletal muscle fibers can directly abut benign glands in the apex.*

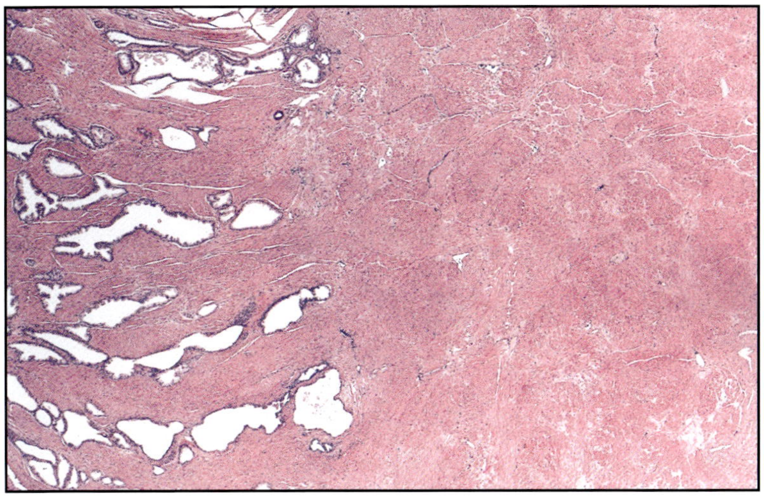

■ **i1.55** *Continuity of fibromuscular stroma of prostate (left) and smooth muscle of bladder neck (right).*

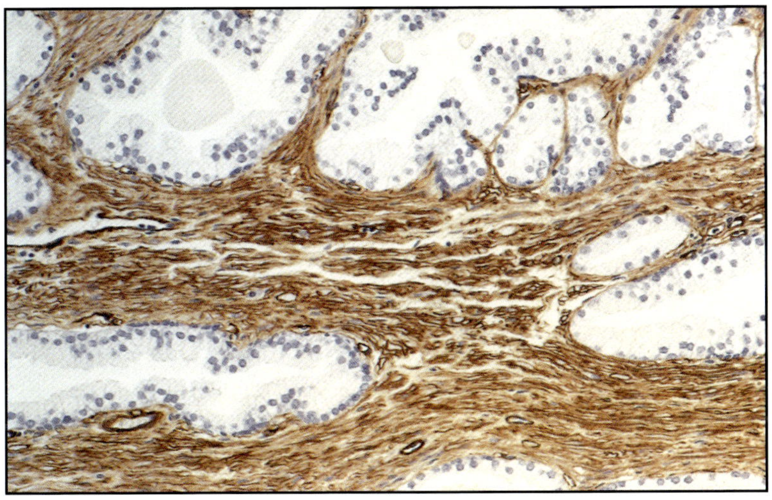

■ **i1.56** *Extensive collagen type IV immunoreactivity in prostatic stroma.*

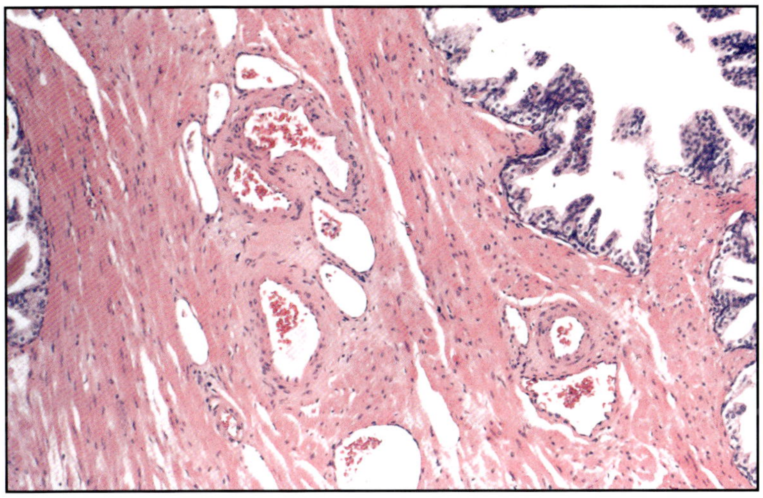

■ **i1.57** *Small arteries and veins in the prostatic stroma.*

(Manley 1966). At the bladder neck, a capsular separation of bladder and prostate also does not exist; rather, there is a fusion of smooth muscle bundles **i1.55**.These anatomic relationships between the prostate proper, the fibromuscular band, and periprostatic tissues are critical in understanding prostate cancer spread and staging.

A thin, delicate basement membrane surrounds ducts and acini of the prostate. This 100-nm-thick membrane is too small to be seen in H&E-stained sections. It contains collagen types IV, V, and VII, laminin, entactin, and heparan sulfate proteoglycan (Bonkhoff 1991A, Bostwick 1995, Dehan 1997, Knox 1994, Nagle 1994, Schultz 1993, Sinha 1989). Antibody binding to heparan sulfate proteoglycan in immunohistochemistry highlights the basement membrane, whereas immunostains for collagen type IV and laminin are less useful because of extensive stromal staining of capillary and smooth muscle external lamina **i1.56** (Bostwick 1995, Schultz 1993). Basement membrane immunostains are currently not of practical utility in diagnosis of prostatic disease because nonneoplastic acini may lose basement membrane secondary to inflammation, and many invasive prostatic carcinomas retain basement membranes (Bonkhoff 1991A, Bostwick 1995, Dehan 1997, Knox 1994, Nagle 1994, Schultz 1993, Sinha 1989). However, this basement membrane does appear abnormal in biochemical composition and cellular attachments (Kadkol 1998).

The stroma in the prostate gland consists chiefly of smooth muscle cells and fibroblasts **i1.13, i1.14**, with ramifications of blood and lymph vessels (Fukuda 2000) as well as nerve bundles and axons (Aumüller 1994, McNeal 1997). In addition to structural support, the normal function of the smooth muscle is to contract upon parasympathetic neural stimulation to promote secretion (McNeal 1968). Additionally, stromal cells modulate normal prostatic epithelial development, growth, and differentiation via dynamic and reciprocal stromal-epithelial interactions (Cunha 1972, 1996, Farnsworth 1999, Liu 1997, Partin 2002, Shapiro 1989, Timms 1995), such as that mediated by diffusible, soluble growth factors. Thus, the stroma is not merely a static scaffold but plays a direct role in normal and disease processes in the prostate.

The extracellular stromal matrix of the prostate is primarily collagen of types I and III, complex polysaccharides, and glycosaminoglycans such as dermatan sulfate, heparin, chondroitin, and hyaluronic acid (Partin 2002). Fibronectin and tenascin polypeptides are also found in prostatic stroma (Ibrahim 1993, Koukoulis 1997). Currently, evaluation of these stromal constituents is not of diagnostic value. Interglandular vessels are easily seen in interglandular stroma **i1.57**, but capillaries adjacent to normal glands are not so readily appreciated on H&E sections **i1.58**, probably because a large number have closed lumina (Montironi 1993). The capillaries are closely associated with the basement membrane and have smooth

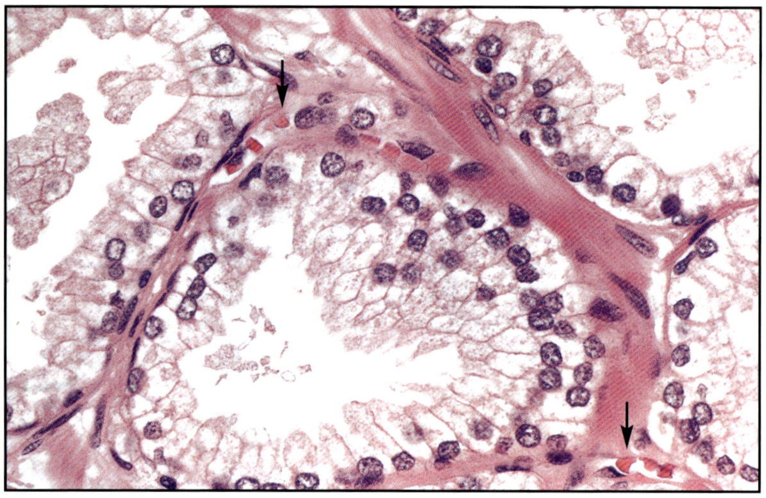

■ **i1.58** *Capillaries adjacent to benign glands (arrows) can be difficult to visualize on H&E-stained sections.*

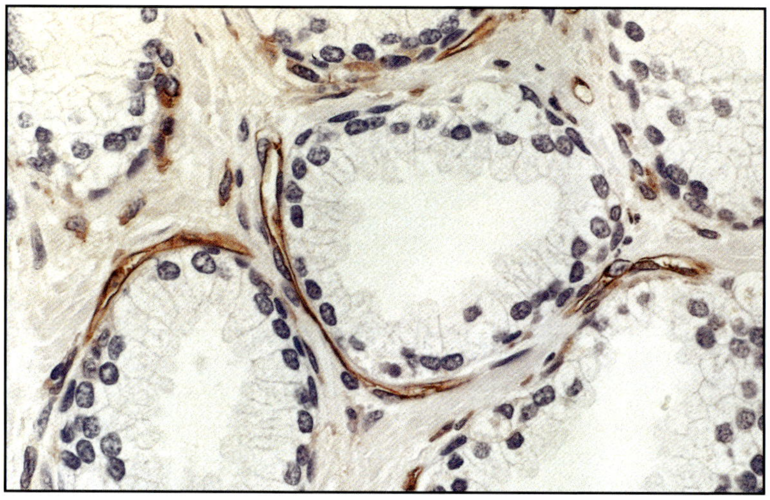

■ **i1.59** *CD31 immunostain for endothelial cells highlights the physical proximity of glandular capillaries and benign glands.*

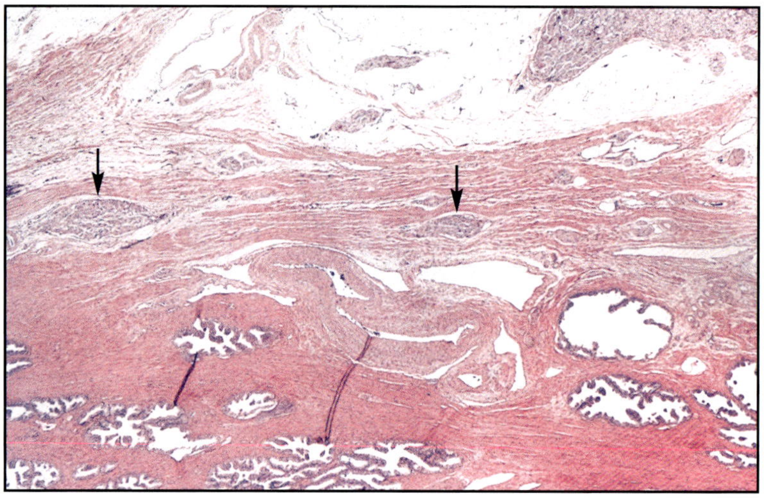

■ **i1.60** *Large periprostatic nerve (upper right) and "intracapsular" nerves (arrows).*

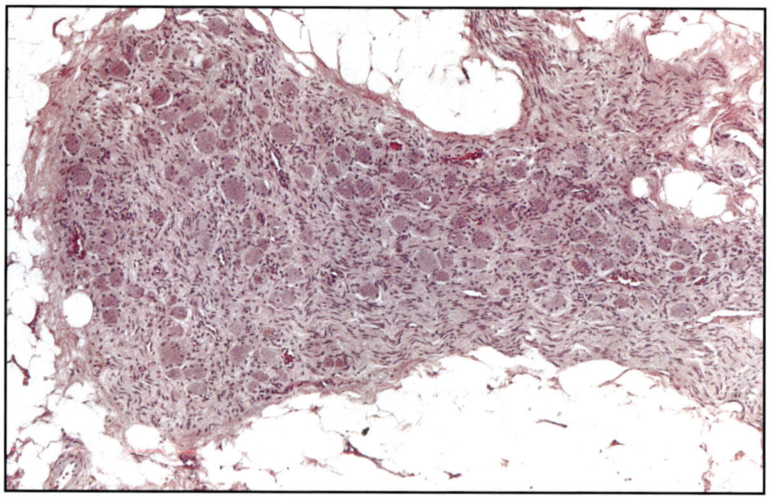

■ **i1.61** *Ganglion in periprostatic adipose tissue.*

outer contours. Immunostains for endothelial cell markers such as factor VIII–related antigen, CD34, and CD31 **i1.59** highlight this vasculature. The formation of new blood vessels (neurovascularity) and abnormal angiogenesis, including structural abnormalities of capillaries and increased microvessel density, occur in prostatic disease states (Montironi 1993, 1996, Siegal 1998). Venous drainage of blood from the prostate is into the plexus of Santorini.

The prostate gland has a rich nerve supply, with sympathetic and parasympathetic innervation arising from the pelvic plexus (McVary 1998). These nerves run with branches of the capsular artery and penetrate the prostate, where parasympathetic fibers course to acini and stimulate secretion and where sympathetic fibers cause contraction of outer band "capsular" and intraprostatic smooth muscle (Brooks 2002). Immediately outside the prostate, bilateral, prominent neurovascular bundles are located posterolateral to the apex, midportion, and base of the prostate **i1.50** (Lepor 1985). Also situated dorsolaterally are nerves that innervate the corpora cavernosa and that are involved in potency (cavernous nerves). These nerves are not excised in nerve-sparing radical prostatectomy operations, where the intent is to preserve potency without compromising cancer extirpation (Catalona 1985, Eggleston 1985, Walsh 1982, 1983). There are specific clinical indications in the decision to spare or excise the neurovascular bundles (Walsh 1998). Histologically, nerves are readily seen in the periprostatic neurovascular bundle **i1.50**, in the outer fibromuscular band **i1.60**, and in the prostate itself. Ganglia **i1.61, i1.62** and paraganglia **i1.63** are usually found outside the gland but may also be found in the outer fibromuscular band and within the prostate itself (Cohen 1995, Denford 1997, Freedman 1975, Ostrowski 1994, Rode 1990, Vaalasti 1980). Paraganglia are most often located in or adjacent to the lateral neurovascular bundles (Ostrowski 1994). They should not be confused with "hypernephroid" prostatic carcinoma. Because ganglia and paraganglia can be found inside the prostate and in the outer fibromuscular band, carcinoma invading around these structures should not necessarily be equated with extraprostatic extension of malignancy. Another diagnostic pitfall is the physical relationship of normal and benign prostatic glands to intraprostatic nerves. Benign prostatic glands can abut nerves (Carstens 1980, McIntire 1986) **i1.64, i1.65** and even be found, in extremely rare cases, within nerves (Cramer 1981). Such glands should not be considered automatically malignant, and a constellation of histomorphologic traits should be used in diagnosis, not solely the physical proximity of prostatic glands and nerves.

Lymphatic drainage from the prostate is principally to the obturator and then internal iliac lymph nodes. A minor amount of drainage occurs through the presacral group and external iliac nodes (Brooks 2002). An uncommon site of flow is through periprostatic or periseminal vesicle lymph nodes, which are found in about 4% of

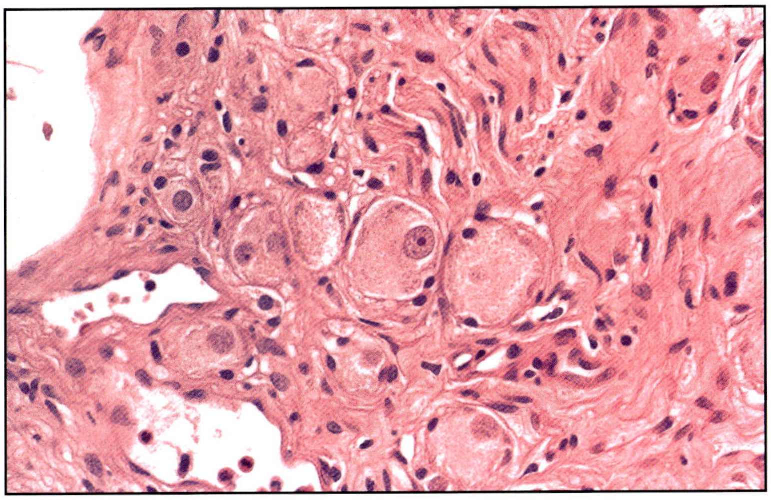

■ **i1.62** *Periprostatic ganglion cells (notice the prominent nucleolus). Such cells should not be mistaken for intraneural spread of prostatic carcinoma cells which classically also have prominent nucleoli.*

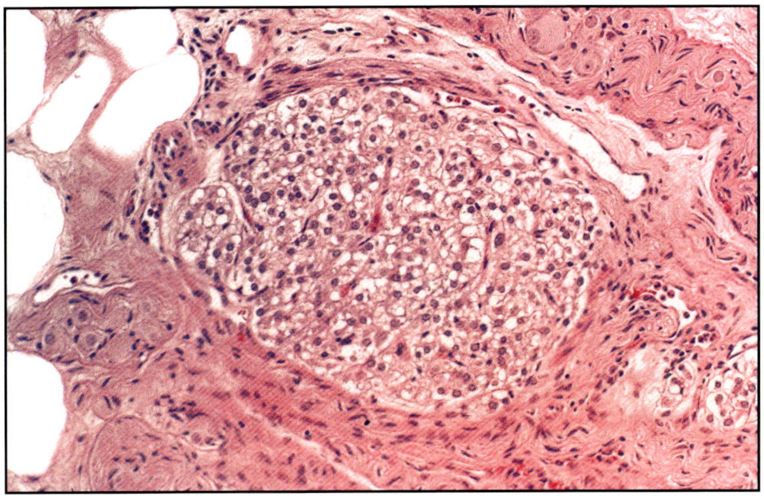

■ **i1.63** *Paraganglion in periprostatic tissue.*

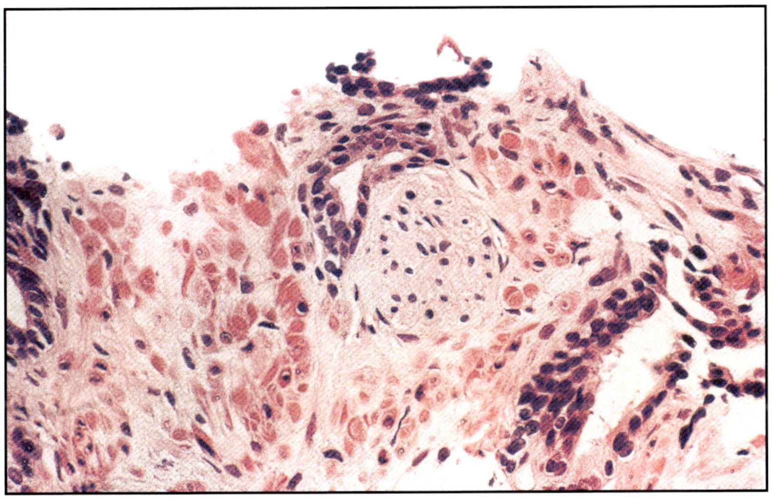

■ **i1.64** *Benign gland appearing to "wrap around" a nerve in a prostate needle biopsy specimen.*

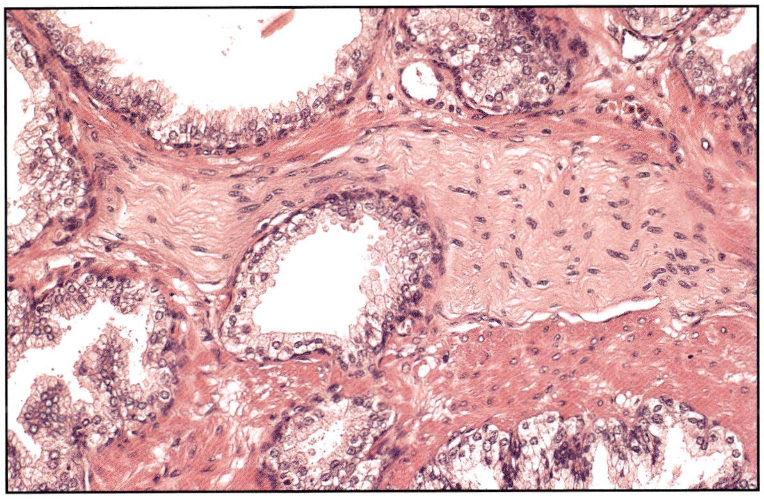

■ **i1.65** *Indentation of intraprostatic nerve by benign gland.*

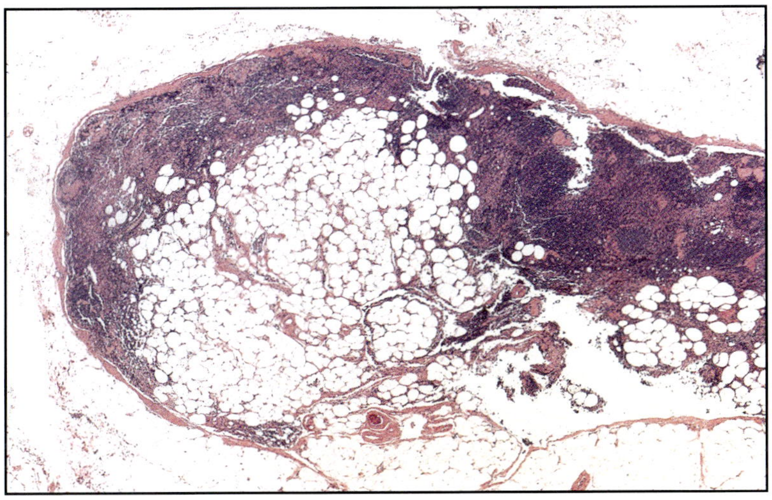

■ **i1.66** *Fatty pelvic (obturator) lymph node excised during a radical prostatectomy operation.*

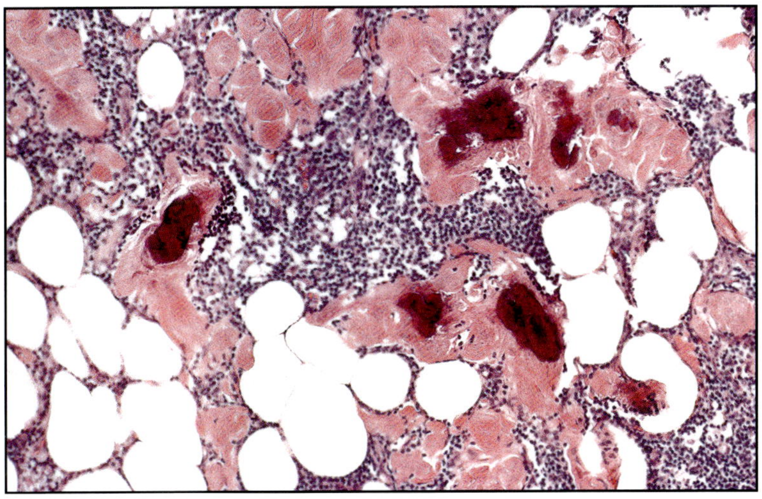

■ **i1.67** *Hyalinized and calcified trabeculae of a pelvic lymph node.*

radical prostatectomy specimens (Kothari 2001). Therefore, for patients with prostate cancer, pelvic lymph node dissection at retropubic radical prostatectomy targets lymph nodes at the angle between the external iliac and hypogastric arteries and obturator lymph nodes (Walsh 1998). Histologically, normal pelvic lymph nodes often contain an appreciable amount of adipose tissue (making frozen sections difficult) **i1.66**. Nodal fibrous trabeculae can be quite hyalinized, with or without calcification **i1.67**.

It is not clear whether the prostate has a normal resident hematolymphoid cell population, but intraepithelial and stromal lymphocytes (mainly T cells) have been found in young patients without substantial associated BPH, florid prostatitis, or cancer (Bostwick 1998). These cells could be related to immune responsiveness in the prostate.

Finally, in extremely rare examples, adipose tissue may be found in prostatic stroma **i1.68** (Cohen 1998). This is important because in the past the presence of malignant glands in adipose tissue has been deemed diagnostic of extraprostatic extension. Clearly, this is almost always but not always true.

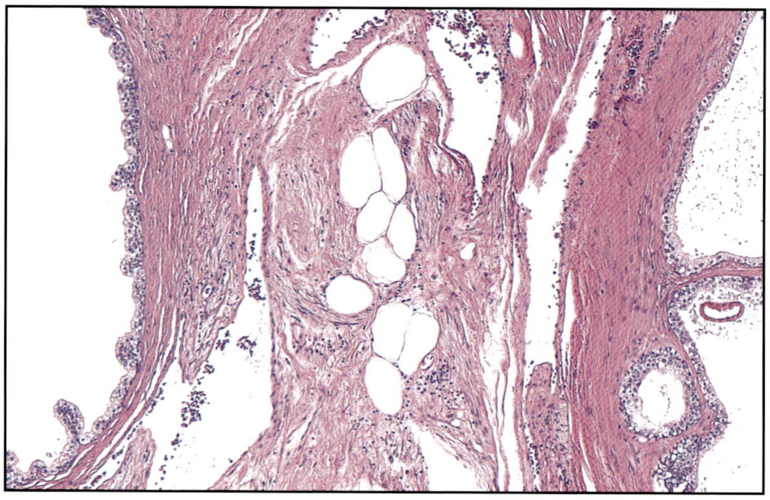

■ **i1.68** *Focal intraprostatic adipose tissue: An extremely rare finding.*

[1.6] Prostatic Tissue Ectopia

Ectopic benign prostatic tissue in males has been found in a number of extraprostatic locations including testis, epididymis, bladder, penile urethra, seminal vesicle, root of the penis, subvesical space, retrovesical space, pericolic fat, anal submucosa, perirectal fat, urachal remnant, and spleen (Bromberg 1991, Congleton 1989, Ewing 1987, Fulton 2001, Kanomata 1997, Klein 1984, Milburn 1994, Morey 1989, Morgan 1992, Salem 1996, Spiro 1994, Vogel 1996,). The most frequently cited type of prostatic ectopia is in the prostatic urethra in the form of prostatic urethral polyps (Chapter 23, p 529) (Butterick 1971, Gledhill 1985, Remick 1984). However, because prostatic epithelium normally can line the urethra in the verumontanum region (Murphy 1997), one could argue that these polyps do not represent ectopia. Furthermore, one should not view Cowper's glands, anal glands, and penile paraurethral glands, which contain immunoreactive PSA (Elgamal 1994, Frazier 1992, Kamoshida 1990), as ectopic prostate tissue. Despite its name, expression of PSA is not specific for prostatic tissue (Chapter 13, p 236).

Prostatic tissue has been reported in females in the posterior wall of the distal urethra, as previously noted, in ovarian hilar mesonephric rests (Smith 1999), in ovarian teratomas **i1.69, i1.70** (Blackwell 1967, Brumback 1985, Buzzi 1994, Halabi 2002, McLachlin 1992, Melniker 1980, Nogales 1995, Uzoaru 1992, Vadmal 1996), and in the cervix (Larraza-Hernandez 1997, Nucci 2000, Rath-Wolfson 1998, Wallace 2001). A single case of ovarian teratoma with prostatic tissue with morphologic features of prostatic carcinoma has been published (Halabi 2002). PSA has been found in normal endometrium (Clements 1994), but this does not reflect prostatic ectopia.

Mature-appearing prostatic tissue has also been rarely reported in neoplasms, including a retroperitoneal lipoma (Tokumitsu 1981) and a testicular teratoma (Unger 1998).

Ectopic prostatic tissue usually presents as an incidental finding but can manifest clinically as a mass **i1.71, i1.72** (Milburn 1994, Yasukawa 1987) or as urinary frequency, voiding difficulty, dysuria, or hematuria (Congleton 1989, Kanomata 1997, Morey 1989, Richter 1991). Although these patients could conceivably present with serum PSA elevation due to ectopic prostate, this event has not been reported. By cystoscopy, ectopic prostatic tissue in the bladder may be confused with cystitis cystica (Ewing 1987). Benign adenomatous (Yasukawa 1987) and malignant (Adams 1993) changes have been described in ectopic prostatic tissue. The precise mechanisms for formation of ectopic prostatic tissue are not definitely established. An embryologic remnant of the ventral portion of the cloaca is a favored possibility (Gledhill 1985), and urothelial metaplasia (Morey 1989) has also been forwarded. The presence of prostatic tissue in ovarian teratomas could be caused by induction by locally produced androgen or tissue-specific genomic imprinting. This remains speculative.

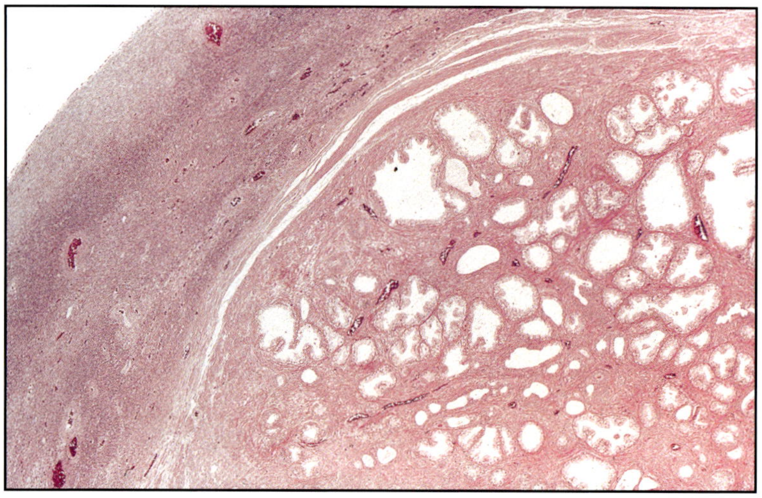

■ **i1.69** *Prostatic tissue in an ovarian teratoma, surrounded by ovarian stroma.*

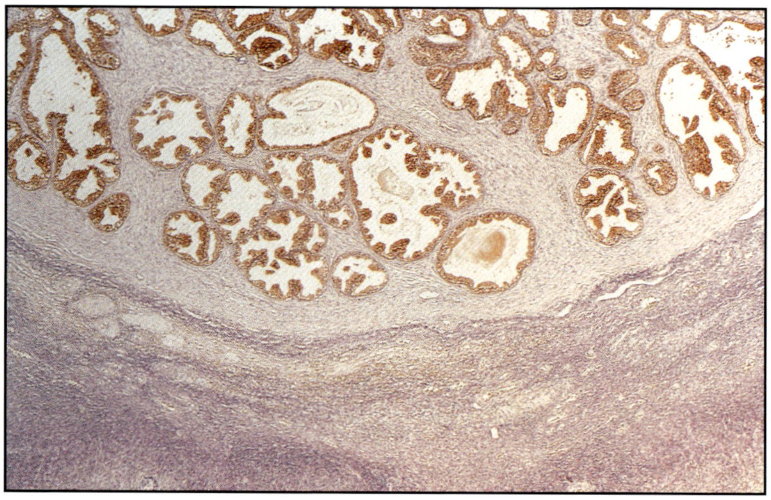

■ **i1.70** *Prostatic tissue in ovarian teratoma exhibiting strong PSA immunoreactivity.*

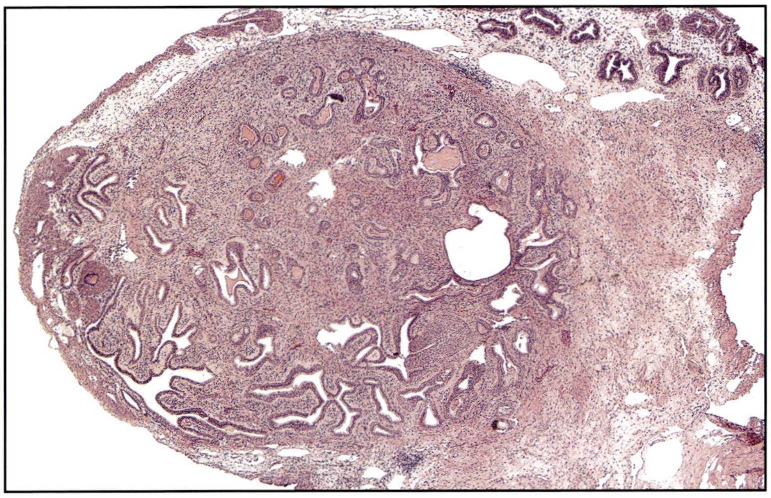

■ **i1.71** *Ectopic prostatic tissue in lamina propria of urinary bladder. Cystoscopically, the nodule appears as a pedunculated lesion at the bladder neck.*

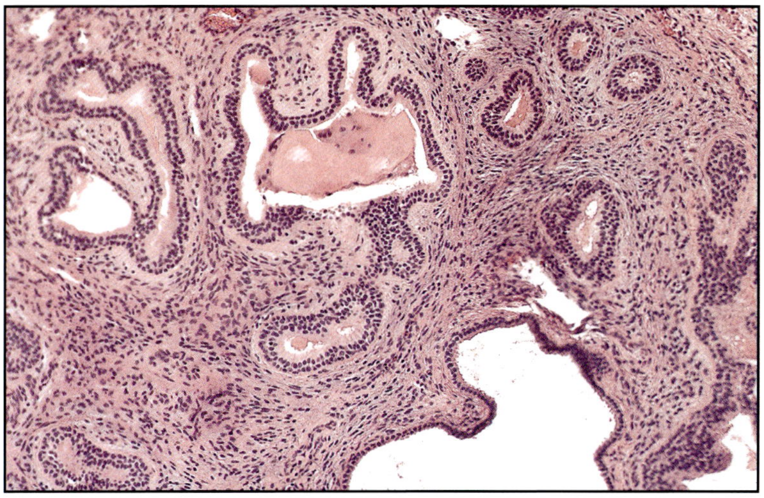

■ **i1.72** *Ectopic prostatic tissue in urinary bladder: Higher power view of* **i1.71**. *A PSA immunostain was positive in some of the glands.*

The diagnostic significance of ectopic prostate tissue is obvious: One should not mistake such ectopia, which is almost always benign, with a metastatic prostatic neoplasm. Prostatic tissue ectopia therefore is a pseudoneoplastic condition. It is included here because most cases probably are caused by an embryologic defect.

References

Adams JR Jr. Adenocarcinoma in ectopic prostatic tissue. *J Urol* 150:1253-1254, 1993.

Adlakha H, Bostwick DG. Paneth cell–like change in prostatic adenocarcinoma represents neuroendocrine differentiation. Report of 30 cases. *Hum Pathol* 25:135-139, 1994.

Amin MB, Schultz DS, Zarbo RJ. Analysis of cribriform morphology in prostatic neoplasia using antibody to high-molecular-weight cytokeratins. *Arch Pathol Lab Med* 118:260-264, 1994.

Amin MB, Bostwick DG. Pigment in prostatic epithelium and adenocarcinoma: a potential source of diagnostic confusion with seminal vesicular epithelium. *Mod Pathol* 9:791-795, 1996.

Angulo JC, Sanchez-Chapado M. Giant müllerian duct cyst mimicking prostatic malignancy. *Scand J Urol Nephrol* 29:229-231, 1995.

Anton RC, Chakraborty S, Wheeler TM. The significance of intraluminal prostatic crystalloids in benign needle biopsies. *Am J Surg Pathol* 22:446-449, 1998.

Aprikian A, Cordon-Cardo C, Fair W, et al. Characterization of neuroendocrine differentiation in human benign prostate and prostatic adenocarcinoma. *Cancer* 71:3952-3965, 1993.

Aquilina JW, McKinney L, Pacelli A, et al. High grade prostatic intraepithelial neoplasia in military working dogs with and without prostate cancer. *Prostate* 36:189-193, 1998.

Argani P, Walsh PC, Epstein JI. Analysis of the prostatic central zone in patients with unilateral absence of wolffian duct structures: further evidence of the mesodermal origin of the prostatic central zone. *J Urol* 160: 2126-2129, 1998.

Aumüller G, Seitz J, Bischof W. Immunohistochemical study on the initiation of acid phosphatase secretion in the human prostate. *J Androl* 4:183-191, 1983.

Aumüller G, Seitz J, Riva A. Functional morphology of prostate gland. In: Riva A, Testa Riva F, Motta PM, eds. *Ultrastructure of Male Urogenital Glands.* Boston: Kluwer Academic; 61-112, 1994.

Aumüller G, Groos S, Renneberg H, et al. Embryology and postnatal development of the prostate. In: Foster CS, Bostwick DG, eds. *Pathology of the Prostate.* Philadelphia: WB Saunders; 10, 1998.

Ayala AG, Ro JY, Babaian R, et al. The prostatic capsule: does it exist? Its importance in the staging and treatment of prostatic carcinoma. *Am J Surg Pathol* 13:21-27, 1989.

Barringer BS. Papillary intracystic adenocarcinoma of prostate and massive benign prostatic cyst. *Am J Surg* 20:51-53, 1933.

Barsky SH, Grossman DA, Huaman JA. Basal cells inhibit prostatic carcinoma invasion: a natural defense against prostatic carcinoma [abstract]. *Mod Pathol* 10:70A, 1997.

Battaglia S, Casali A, Botticelli A. Age-related distribution of endocrine cells in the human prostate: a quantitative study. *Virchows Arch* 424:165-168, 1994.

Berges RR, Vukanovic J, Epstein JI, et al. Implication of cell kinetic changes during the progression of human prostatic cancer. *Clin Cancer Res* 1:473-480, 1995.

Berry SJ, Coffey DS, Walsh PC, et al. The development of human benign prostatic hyperplasia with age. *J Urol* 132:474-479, 1984.

Blackwell WJ, Dockerty MB, Symmonds RE. Benign cystic teratomas. *Obstet Gynecol* 29:719-725, 1967.

Boag AH, Young ID. Immunohistochemical analysis of type IV collagenase expression in prostatic hyperplasia and adenocarcinoma. *Mod Pathol* 6:65-68, 1993.

Bonkhoff H, Wernert N, Dhom G, et al. Basement membranes in fetal, adult normal, hyperplastic and neoplastic human prostate. *Virchows Arch A Pathol Anat* 418:375-381, 1991A.

Bonkhoff H, Wernert N, Dhom G, et al. Relation of endocrine-paracrine cells to cell proliferation in normal, hyperplastic and neoplastic human prostate. *Prostate* 19:91-98, 1991B.

Bonkhoff H, Stein U, Remberger K. Multidirectional differentiation in the normal, hyperplastic and neoplastic human prostate: simultaneous demonstration of cell-specific epithelial markers. *Hum Pathol* 25:42-46, 1994A.

Bonkhoff H, Stein U, Remberger K. The proliferative function of basal cells in the normal and hyperplastic prostate. *Prostate* 24:114-118, 1994B.

Bonkhoff H, Stein U, Remberger K. Endocrine-paracrine cell types in the prostate and prostatic adenocarcinoma are postmitotic cells. *Hum Pathol* 26:167-170, 1995.

Bonkhoff H, Remberger K. Differentiation pathways and histogenetic aspects of normal and abnormal prostatic growth: a stem cell model. *Prostate* 28:98-106, 1996A.

Bonkhoff H. Role of the basal cells in premalignant changes of the human prostate: a stem cell concept for the development of prostate cancer. *Eur Urol* 30:201-205, 1996B.

Borrego J, Fernandez E, Del Hoyo J, et al. Cyst of the ejaculatory duct. *Acta Urol Esp* 18:915-918, 1994.

Bartsch G, Rohr HP. Comparative light and electron microscopic study of the human, dog and rat prostate. *Urol Int* 35:91-104, 1980.

Bostwick DG, Srigley J, Grignon D, et al. Atypical adenomatous hyperplasia of the prostate: morphologic criteria for its distinction from well-differentiated carcinoma. *Hum Pathol* 24:819-832, 1993.

Bostwick DG, Leske DA, Qian J, et al. Prostatic intraepithelial neoplasia and well-differentiated adenocarcinoma maintain an intact basement membrane. *Pathol Res Pract* 191:850-855, 1995.

Bostwick DG, Corica FA, Dundore P, et al. Intraepithelial and stromal lymphocytes in the human prostate [abstract]. *J Urol* 159:126, 1998.

Brawer MK, Peehl DM, Stamey TA, et al. Keratin immunoreactivity in the benign and neoplastic human prostate. *Cancer Res* 45:3663-3667, 1985.

Brennick JB, O'Connell JX, Dickersin GR, et al. Lipofuscin pigmentation (so-called "melanosis") of the prostate. *Am J Surg Pathol* 18:446-454, 1994.

Bromberg WD, Kozlowski JM, Oyasu R. Prostate-type gland in the epididymis. *J Urol* 145:1273-1274, 1991.

Brooks JD: Anatomy of the lower urinary tract and male genitalia. In: Walsh PC, Retik AB, Vaughan ED Jr, et al, eds. *Campbell's Urology.* 8th ed. Philadelphia: Saunders; 41-80, 2002.

Brooks RT Jr. Cyst of the ejaculatory duct: case report. *J Urol* 101:881-883, 1969.

Brumback RA, Brown BS, di Sant'Agnese P. Unique finding of prostatic tissue in a benign cystic ovarian teratoma. *Arch Pathol Lab Med* 109:675-677, 1985.

Bush RB, Bush IM. Early developments in the history of prostatic disorders. In: Tannenbaum M, ed. *Urologic Pathology: The Prostate.* Philadelphia: Lea & Febiger; 7-22, 1977.

Butterick JD, Schnitzer B, Abell MR. Ectopic prostatic tissue in urethra: a clinicopathological entity and a significant cause of hematuria. *J Urol* 105:97-104, 1971.

Buzzi A, Crescini C, Sonzogni A, et al. Prostatic tissue in a cystic teratoma of the ovary [in Italian]. *Minerva Ginecol* 46:49-51, 1994.

Carstens PHB. Perineural glands in normal and hyperplastic prostate. *J Urol* 123:686-688, 1980.

Carter SS, Shinohara K, Lipshultz LI. Transrectal ultrasonography in disorders of the seminal vesicles and ejaculatory ducts. *Urol Clin North Am* 16:773-790, 1989.

Catalona WJ, Dresner SM. Nerve-sparing radical prostatectomy: extra-prostatic tumor extension and preservation of erectile function. *J Urol* 134:1149-1151, 1985.

Clegg EJ. The vascular arrangements within the human prostate gland. *Br J Urol* 28:428-435, 1956.

Clements J, Mukhtar A. Glandular kallikreins and prostate-specific antigen are expressed in the human endometrium. *J Clin Endocrinol Metab* 78:1536-1539, 1994.

Cohen R, Glezerson G, Haffejee Z. Prostatic-specific antigen and prostate-specific acid phosphatase in neuroendocrine cells of prostate cancer. *Arch Pathol Lab Med* 116:65-66, 1992.

Cohen RJ, Glezerson G, Taylor LF, et al. The neuroendocrine cell population of the human prostate gland. *J Urol* 150:365-368, 1993.

Cohen RJ, Nixon JM. Intraprostatic ganglia. *Hum Pathol* 26:807-808, 1995.

Cohen RJ, Stables S. Intraprostatic fat. *Hum Pathol* 29 29:424-425, 1998.

Colombel M, Symmans F, Gil S, et al. Detection of the apoptosis-suppressing oncoprotein bcl-2 in hormone-refractory human prostate cancers. *Am J Pathol* 143:390-400, 1993.

Congleton L, Thomason WB, McMullan DT, et al: Painless hematuria and urethral discharge secondary to ectopic prostate. *J Urol* 142:1554-1555, 1989.

Cookson MS, Reuter VE, Linkov I, et al. Glutathione S-transferase PI (GST-pi) class expression by immunohistochemistry in benign and malignant prostate tissue. *J Urol* 157:673-676, 1997.

Coppens L, Bonnet P, Andrianne R, et al. Adult Mullerian duct or utricle cyst: clinical significance and therapeutic management of 65 cases. *J Urol* 167:1740-1744, 2002.

Cornell KK, Bostwick DG, Cooley DM, et al. Clinical and pathologic aspects of spontaneous canine prostate carcinoma: a retrospective analysis of 76 cases. *Prostate* 45: 173-183, 2000.

Coyne JD, Kealy WF, Annis P. Seminal vesicle epithelium in needle biopsy specimens [letter]. *J Clin Pathol* 40:932, 1987.

Cramer SF. Benign glandular inclusion in prostatic nerve. *Am J Clin Pathol* 75:854-855, 1981.

Cristol DS, Emmett JL. The incidence of coincident prostatic calculi, prostatic hyperplasia and carcinoma of the prostate gland. *JAMA* 124:646, 1944.

Cunha GR. Tissue interactions between epithelium and mesenchyme of urogenital and integumental origin. *Anat Rec* 172:529-542, 1972.

Cunha GR, Hayward SW, Dahiya R, et al. Smooth muscle-epithelial interactions in normal and neoplastic prostatic development. *Acta Anat* 155:63-72, 1996.

DeKlerk DP, Scott WW. Prostatic maldevelopment in the prune belly syndrome: a defect in prostatic stromal-epithelial interaction. *J Urol* 120:341-344, 1978.

Dehan P, Waltregny D, Beschin A, et al. Loss of type IV collagen $\alpha5$ and $\alpha6$ chains in human invasive prostate carcinomas. *Am J Pathol* 15:1097-1104, 1997.

Denford A, Vaughan M, Mayall F. Paraganglia as an unusual mimic of carcinoma in the prostate. *Br J Urol* 80:677-678, 1997.

Devaraj LT, Bostwick DG. Atypical basal cell hyperplasia of the prostate. Immunophenotypic profile and proposed classification of basal cell proliferations. *Am J Surg Pathol* 17:645-659, 1993.

Devine CJ Jr, Gonzalez-Serva L, Stecker JF Jr, et al. Utricular configuration in hypospadias and intersex. *J Urol* 123:407-411, 1980.

deVries CR, McNeal JE, Bensch K. The prostatic epithelial cell in dysplasia: an ultrastructural perspective. *Prostate* 21:209-221, 1992.

Di Lollo S, Menchi I, Brizzi E, et al. The morphology of the prostatic capsule with particular regard to the posterosuperior region: an anatomical and clinical problem. *Surg Radiol Anat* 19:143-147, 1997.

di Sant'Agnese PA, de Mesy Jensen K. Endocrine-paracrine cells of the prostate and prostatic urethra: an ultrastructural study. *Hum Pathol* 15:1034-1041, 1984A.

di Sant'Agnese PA, de Mesy Jensen KL. Somatostatin and/or somatostatinlike immunoreactive endocrine-paracrine cells in the human prostate gland. *Arch Pathol Lab Med* 108:693-696, 1984B.

di Sant'Agnese PA, de Mesy Jensen KL, Churukian CJ, et al. Human prostatic endocrine-paracrine (APUD) cells. *Arch Pathol Lab Med* 109:607-612, 1985A.

di Sant'Agnese PA, de Mesy Jensen, Churukian CJ, et al. Human prostatic endocrine-paracrine (APUD) cells. Distributional analysis with a comparison of serotonin and neuron-specific enolase immunoreactivity and silver stains. *Arch Pathol Lab Med* 109:607-612, 1985B.

di Sant'Agnese PA. Calcitoninlike immunoreactive and bombesinlike immunoreactive endocrine-paracrine cells of the human prostate. *Arch Pathol Lab Med* 110:412-415, 1986.

di Sant'Agnese PA. Neuroendocrine differentiation in prostatic carcinoma. Recent findings and new concepts. *Cancer* 75:1850-1859, 1995.

di Sant'Agnese PA. Identification and pathologic significance of neuroendocrine differentiation in human prostate carcinoma. In: Foster CS, Bostwick DG, eds. *Pathology of the Prostate.* Philadelphia: WB Saunders; 352-363, 1998.

Eastman JR. The origin of corpora amylacea in the prostate gland. *JAMA* 25:158-162, 1897.

Eggleston JC, Walsh PC. Radical prostatectomy with preservation of sexual function: pathological findings in the first 100 cases. *J Urol* 134:1146-1148, 1985.

Elder JS, Mostwin JL. Cyst of the ejaculatory duct/urogenital sinus. *J Urol* 132:768-771, 1984.

Elgamal AA, van de Voorde W, van Poppel H, et al. Immunohistochemical localization of prostate-specific markers within the accessory male sex glands of Cowper, Littre and Morgagni. *Urology* 44:84-91, 1994.

Emmett JL, Bransch WF. Cyst of the prostate gland. *J Urol* 36:236-249, 1936.

Epstein JI, Fynheer J. Acid mucin in the prostate: can it differentiate adenosis from adenocarcinoma? *Hum Pathol* 23:1321-1325, 1992.

Epstein JI. Diagnostic criteria of limited adenocarcinoma of the prostate on needle biopsy. *Hum Pathol* 26:223-229, 1995.

Epstein JI, Murphy WM. Diseases of the prostate gland and seminal vesicles. In: Murphy WM, ed. *Urological Pathology.* 2nd ed. Philadelphia: WB Saunders; 199, 1997.

Ewing R, Harnden-Mayor P, Mason MK, et al. Extra-urethral ectopic prostate. *Br J Urol* 60:433-435, 1987.

Farnsworth WE. Prostate stroma: physiology. *Prostate* 38: 60-72, 1999.

Franks LM. Benign nodular hyperplasia of the prostate: a review. *Ann R Coll Surg* 14:92-106, 1954.

Franks LM , O'Shea JP, Thomson AER. Mucin in the prostate: histochemical study in normal glands, latent, clinical and colloid cancers. *Cancer* 17:983-991, 1964.

Frazier HA, Humphrey PA, Burchette JL, et al. Immunoreactive prostatic specific antigen in male periurethral glands. *J Urol* 147:246-248, 1992.

Freedman SR, Goldman RL. Normal paraganglia in the human prostate. *J Urol* 113:874-875, 1975.

Fukuda H, Yamada T, Kamata S, et al. Anatomic distribution of intraprostatic lymphatics: implications of the lymphatic spread of prostate cancer—a preliminary study. *Prostate* 44: 322-327, 2000.

Fulton RS, Rouse RV, Ranhein EA. Ectopic prostate: case report of a presacral mass presenting with obstructive symptoms. *Arch Pathol Lab Med* 125:286-288, 2001.

Gikas PW, Del Buono EA, Epstein JI. Florid hyperplasia of mesonephric remnants involving prostate and periprostatic tissue. Possible confusion with adenocarcinoma. *Am J Surg Pathol* 17:454-460, 1993.

Gledhill A: Ectopic prostatic tissue. *J Urol* 133:110-111, 1985.

Goldstein NS, Underhill J, Roszka J, et al. Cytokeratin 34βE12 immunoreactivity in benign prostatic acini: quantitation, pattern assessment, and electron microscopic study. *Am J Clin Pathol* 112:69-74, 1999.

Gómez-Ortega J, Val-Bernal JF. Hyperplasia of prostatic mesonephric remnants: a potential pitfall in the evaluation of prostate gland biopsy. *J Urol* 154:1138-1139, 1995.

Gown AM, Vogel AM. Monoclonal antibodies to human intermediate filament proteins: distribution of filament proteins in normal human tissues. *Am J Pathol* 114:309-321, 1984.

Griffin JE, Wilson JD. Disorders of androgen receptor function. *Ann NY Acad Sci* 438:61-71, 1984.

Grignon DJ, O'Malley FP. Mucinous metaplasia in the prostate gland. *Am J Surg Pathol* 17:287-290, 1993

Gutierrez J, Nesbit RM. Ectopic prostatic tissue in bladder. *J Urol* 8:474-478, 1967.

Halabi M, Oliva E, Mazal PR, et al. Prostatic tissue in mature cystic teratomas. A report of 4 cases, including 1 with features of prostatic adenocarcinoma, and cytogenetic studies. *Int J Gynecol Pathol* 21:261-267, 2002.

Hamper UM, Epstein JI, Sheth S, et al. Cystic lesions of the prostate gland. A sonographic-pathologic correlation. *J Ultrasound Med* 9:395-402, 1990.

Han M, Alfert HJ, Partin AW: Retropubic and suprpubic open prostatectomy. In Walsh PC, Retik AB, Vaughan ED Jr, et al, eds. *Campbell's Urology.* 8th ed. Philadelphia: Saunders; 1423-1434, 2002.

Haugen OA, Harbitz TB. Prostatic weight in elderly men. An analysis in an autopsy series. *Acta Pathol Microbiol Scand* 80:769-777, 1972.

Hayward SW, Baskin LS, Haughney PC, et al. Epithelial development in the rat ventral prostate, anterior prostate and seminal vesicle. *Acta Anat* 155:81-93, 1996.

Hayward SW, Cunha GR. The prostate: development and physiology. *Radiol Clin North Am* 38:1-14, 2000.

Hedrick L, Epstein JI. Use of keratin 903 as an adjunct in the diagnosis of prostate carcinoma. *Am J Surg Pathol* 13:389-396, 1989.

Hendry WF, Pryor JP. Müllerian duct (prostatic utricle) cyst: diagnosis and treatment in subfertile males. *Br J Urol* 69:79-82, 1992.

Henneberry JM, Kahane M, Humphrey PA, et al. The significance of intraluminal crystalloids in benign prostatic glands on needle biopsy. *Am J Surg Pathol* 21:725-728, 1997.

Hennessy RA. Müllerian duct cysts. *J Urol* 42:1042-1050, 1939.

Hijikata T, Saito H, Yohro T. Anatomy and histology of the musk shrew *(Suncus murinus)* prostate. *Prostate* 8:277-291, 1986.

Hoagland MH, Frank KA, Hutchins GM. Prune-belly syndrome with prostatic hypoplasia, bladder wall rupture, and massive ascites in a fetus with trisomy 18. *Arch Pathol Lab Med* 112:1126-1128, 1988.

Holmes EJ. Crystalloids of prostatic carcinoma: relationship to Bence-Jones crystals. *Cancer* 39:2073-208, 1977.

Holsclaw DS, Perlmutter AD, Jockin H, et al. Genital abnormalities in male patients with cystic fibrosis. *J Urol* 106:568-574, 1971.

Holtz W, Foote RH. The anatomy of the reproductive system in male dutch rabbits *(Oryctolagus cuniculus)* with special emphasis on the accessory sex glands. *J Morphol* 158:1-20, 1978.

Howard FS. Hypospadias with enlargement of the prostatic utricle. *Surg Gynecol Obstet* 86:307-316, 1948.

Hudson DL, O'Hare M, Watt FM, et al. Proliferation heterogeneity in the human prostate: evidence for epithelial stem cells. *Lab Invest* 80:1243-1250, 2000.

Hukill PB, Vidone RA. Histochemistry of mucus and other polysaccharides in tumors. II. Carcinoma of the prostate. *Lab Invest* 16:395-406, 1967.

Humphrey PA, Vollmer RT. Corpora amylacea in adenocarcinoma of the prostate: prevalence in 100 prostatectomies and clinicopathologic correlations. *Surg Pathol* 3:133-141, 1990.

Humphrey PA. Mucin in severe dysplasia in the prostate. *Surg Pathol* 4:137-143, 1991.

Humphrey PA, Walther PJ. Adenocarcinoma of the prostate. I. Tissue sampling considerations. *Am J Clin Pathol* 97:746-759, 1993.

Humphrey PA. Clear cell neoplasms of the urinary tract and male reproductive system. *Semin Diagn Pathol* 14:240-252, 1997.

Ibrahim SN, Lightner VA, Ventimiglia JB, et al. Tenascin expression in prostatic hyperplasia, intraepithelial neoplasia, and carcinoma. *Hum Pathol* 24:982-989, 1993.

Imperato-McGinley J, Guerrero L, Gautier T, et al. Steroid 5α-reductase deficiency in man: an inherited form of male pseudohermaphroditism. *Science* 186:1213-1215, 1974.

Jacob S, Poddar S. Morphology and histochemistry of the ferret prostate. *Acta Anat* 125:268-273, 1986.

Jensen PE, Gardner WA, Piserchia PV. Prostatic crystalloids: association with adenocarcinoma. *Prostate* 1:25-30, 1980.

Jimenez RE, Raval MFT, Spanta R, et al. Mesonephric remnants hyperplasia: a pitfall in the diagnosis of prostatic adenocarcinoma. *J Urol Pathol* 9:83-92, 1998.

Kadkol SS, Brody JR, Epstein JI, et al. Novel nuclear phosphoprotein pp32 is highly expressed in intermediate- and high-grade prostate cancer. *Prostate* 34:231-237, 1998.

Kahane H, Sharp JW, Shuman GB, et al. Utilization of high molecular weight cytokeratin on prostate needle biopsies in an independent laboratory. *Urology* 45:981-986, 1995.

Kaleem Z, Swanson PE, Vollmer RT, et al. Prostatic adenocarcinoma with atrophic features: a study of 202 consecutive, completely-embedded radical prostatectomy specimens. *Am J Clin Pathol* 109:695-703, 1998.

Kamoshida S, Tsutsumi Y. Extraprostatic localization of prostatic acid phosphatase and prostate-specific antigen: distribution in cloacogenic glandular epithelium and sex-dependent expression in human anal gland. *Hum Pathol* 21:1108-1111, 1990.

Kanomata N, Eble JN, Ohbayashi C, et al. Ectopic prostate in the retrovesical space. *J Urol Pathol* 7:121-126, 1997.

Kissane JM. Development and structure of the urogenital system. In: Murphy WM, ed. *Urological Pathology.* 2nd ed. Philadelphia: WB Saunders; 26, 1997.

Klein HZ, Rosenberg ML. Ectopic prostatic tissue in bladder trigone. A distinctive cause of hematuria. *Urology* 23:81-82, 1984.

Kleinerman DI, Troncoso P, Lin SH, et al. Consistent expression of an epithelial cell adhesion molecule (C-CAM) during human prostate development and loss of expression in prostate cancer: implication as a tumor suppressor. *Cancer Res* 55:1215-1220, 1995.

Klimas R, Bennett B, Gardner WA Jr. Prostatic calculi: a review. *Prostate* 7:91-96, 1985.

Knox JD, Cress A, Clark V, et al. Differential expression of extracellular matrix molecules and the a6-integrins in the normal and neoplastic prostate. *Am J Pathol* 146:167-174, 1994.

Kothari PS, Scardino PT, Ohori M, et al. Incidence, location, and significance of periprostatic and periseminal vesicle lymph nodes in prostate cancer. *Am J Surg Pathol* 25:1429-1432, 2001.

Koukoulis GK, Zardi L, Virtanen I, et al. Immunolocalization of tenascin and fibronectins in the normal, hyperplastic and neoplastic prostate [abstract]. *Mod Pathol* 10:79A, 1997.

Krongard A, Droller MJ. Anatomy of the prostate. In: Fitzpatrick JM, Krane RJ, eds. *The Prostate.* New York: Churchill Livingstone; 17-27, 1989.

Landes RR, Ransom CL. Müllerian duct cysts. *J Urol* 61:1089-1093, 1949.

Larraza-Hernandez O, Molberg KH, Lindberg G, et al. Ectopic prostatic tissue in the uterine cervix. *Int J Gynecol Pathol* 18:291-293, 1997.

Lawson RK. A historical view of prostate disease. In: Lepor H, Lawson RK, eds. *Prostate Disease.* Philadelphia: WB Saunders; 3-7, 1993.

Leav I, McNeal JE, Kwan PW, et al. Androgen receptor expression in prostatic dysplasia (prostatic intraepithelial neoplasia) in the human prostate: an immunohistochemical and in situ hybridization study. *Prostate* 29:137-145, 1996.

LeDuc IE. The anatomy of the prostate and the pathology of early benign hypertrophy. *J Urol* 42:1217-1241, 1939.

Leissner KH, Tisell LE. The weight of the dorsal, lateral and medial prostatic lobes in man. *Scand J Urol Nephrol* 13:223-227, 1979.

Lepor H, Gregerman M, Crosby R, et al. Precise localization of the autonomic nerves from the pelvic plexus to the corpora cavernosa: a detailed anatomical study of the adult male pelvis. *J Urol* 133:207-212, 1985.

Leung CS, Srigley JR. Distribution of lipochrome pigment in the prostate gland: biological and diagnostic implications. *Hum Pathol* 26:1302-1307, 1995.

Lewis RW, Kim JCS, Irani D, et al. The prostate of the nonhuman primate: Normal anatomy and pathology. *Prostate* 2:51-70, 1981.

Limas C, Frizelle SP. Proliferative activity in benign and neoplastic prostatic epithelium. *J Pathol* 174:201-208, 1994.

Littrup PJ, Lee F, McLeary RD, et al. Transrectal ultrasound of the seminal vesicles and ejaculatory ducts: clinical correlation. *Radiology* 168:625-628, 1987.

Liu AY, True LD, LaTray L, et al. Cell-cell interaction in prostate gene regulation and cytodifferentiation. *Proc Natl Acad Sci U S A* 94:10705-10710, 1997.

Liu AY, True LD. Characterization of prostate cell types by CD cell surface molecules. *Am J Pathol* 160:37-43, 2002.

Loizaga Iriarte A, Arceo Santiago R, Garcia Sastre E, et al. Cysts of the ejaculatory ducts. Diagnosis and clinical course after treatment. *Acta Urol Esp* 18:980-982, 1994.

Lowsley OS. The development of the human prostate gland with reference to the development of other structures at the neck of the urinary bladder. *Am J Anat* 13:299-349, 1912.

Lund AJ, Cummings MM. Cyst of the accessory genital tract: a case report with a review of the literature. *J Urol* 51:303-386, 1946.

Magi-Galluzzi C, Xu X, Hlatky L, et al. Heterogeneity of androgen receptor content in advanced prostate cancer. *Mod Pathol* 10:839-845, 1997.

Magri J. Cysts of the prostate gland. *Br J Urol* 32:295-301, 1960.

Malatinsky E, Labady F, Lepies P, et al. Congenital anomalies of the seminal ducts. *Int Urol Nephrol* 19:189-194, 1987.

Manivel JC, Pettinato G, Reinberg Y, et al. Prune belly syndrome: clinicopathologic study of 29 cases. *Pediatr Pathol* 9:691-711, 1989.

Manley CB Jr. The striated muscle of the prostate. *J Urol* 45:234-240, 1966.

Mao P, Angrist A. The fine structure of the basal cell of human prostate. *Lab Invest* 15:1768-1782, 1966.

Marx AJ, Gueft B, Moskal JF. Prostatic corpora amylacea. A study with the electron microscope and electron probe. *Arch Pathol* 80:487-494, 1965.

Mayersak JS. Urogenital sinus-ejaculatory duct cyst: a case report with a proposed clinical classification and review of the literature. *J Urol* 142:1330-1332, 1989.

Maygarden SJ, Strom S, Ware JL. Localization of epidermal growth factor by immunohistochemical methods in human prostatic carcinoma, prostatic intraepithelial neoplasia, and benign hyperplasia. *Arch Pathol Lab Med* 116:269-273, 1992.

McIntire TL, Franzini DA. The presence of benign prostatic glands in perineural spaces. *J Urol* 135:507-509, 1986.

McLachlin CM, Srigley JR. Prostatic tissue in mature cystic teratomas of the ovary. *Am J Surg Pathol* 16:780-786, 1992.

McNeal JE. Regional morphology and pathology of the prostate. *Am J Clin Pathol* 49:347-357, 1968.

McNeal JE. The prostate and prostatic urethra: a morphologic synthesis. *J Urol* 107:1008-1016, 1972.

McNeal JE. Anatomy of the prostate: an historical survey of divergent views. *Prostate* 1:3-13, 1980.

McNeal JE, Leav I, Alroy J, et al. Differential lectin staining of central and peripheral zones of the prostate and alterations in dysplasia. *Am J Clin Pathol* 89:41-48, 1988.

McNeal JE. Pathology of benign prostatic hyperplasia. Insight into etiology. *Urol Clin North Am* 17:477-486, 1992.

McNeal JE, Haillot O, Yemoto C. Cell proliferation in dysplasia of the prostate: analysis by PCNA immunostaining. *Prostate* 27:258-268, 1995.

McNeal JE. Prostate. In: Sternberg SS, ed. *Histology for Pathologists.* 2nd ed. Philadelphia: Lippincott-Raven; 997-1097, 1997.

McVary KT, McKenna KE, Lee C. Prostate innervation. *Prostate* (suppl) 8: 2-13, 1998.

Melniker LA, Slavutin LJ. Prostatic tissue in a benign cystic teratoma of the ovary. *Diagn Gynecol Obstet* 2:139-145, 1980.

Milburn JM, Bluth EI, Mitchell WT Jr. Ectopic prostate in the testicle: an unusual cause of a solid testicular mass on ultrasonography. *J Ultrasound Med* 13:578-580, 1994.

Mobilio G, Cavalli A, Valente M, et al. Cystic duplication of ejaculatory duct: case report. *Br J Urol* 49:319-321, 1977.

Moerman P, Fryns JP, Goddeeris P, et al. Pathogenesis of the prune-belly syndrome: a functional urethral obstruction caused by prostatic hypoplasia. *Pediatrics* 73:470-475, 1984.

Moghaddami M, Cohen P, Stapleton AMF, et al. CD40 is not detected in human prostate cancer cells by immunohistologic techniques. *Urology* 57: 573-578, 2001.

Moll R, Franke WW, Schiller DL, et al. The catalog of human cytokeratins: patterns of expression in normal epithelia, tumors and cultured cells. *Cell* 31:11-24, 1982.

Montironi R, Magi Galluzi C, Diamanti L, et al. Prostatic intra-epithelial neoplasia: qualitative and quantitative analyses of the blood capillary architecture on thin tissue sections. *Pathol Res Pract* 189:542-548, 1993.

Montironi R, Diamanti L, Thompson P, et al. Analysis of the capillary architecture in the precursors of prostate cancer: recent findings and new concepts. *Eur Urol* 30:191-200, 1996.

Moore RA, Hanzel BF. Chemical composition of prostatic corpora amylacea and calculi. *Arch Pathol* 22:41-54, 1936A.

Moore RA. Morphology of prostatic corpora amylacea and calculi. *Arch Pathol* 22:24-40, 1936B.

Moore RA. Pathology of the prostatic utricle. *Arch Pathol* 23:517-524, 1937.

Moore V, Howe GE. Müllerian duct remnants in the male. *J Urol* 70:781-788, 1953.

Morey AF, Kreder KJ, Wikert GA, et al. Ectopic prostate tissue at bladder dome. *J Urol* 141:942-943, 1989.

Morgan MB. Ectopic prostatic tissue of the anal canal. *J Urol* 147:165-166, 1992.

Moskaluk CA, Duray PH, Cowan KH, et al. Immunohistochemical expression of pi-class glutathione s-transferase is down-regulated in adenocarcinoma of the prostate. *Cancer* 79:1595-1599, 1997.

Murphy WM. Diseases of the urinary bladder, urethra, ureters, and renal pelvis. In: Murphy WM, ed. *Urological Pathology.* 2nd ed. Philadelphia: WB Saunders; 114-117, 151, 1997.

Myers GH, Lynn HB, Kelalis PP. Giant cyst of the utricle. *J Urol* 101:369-373, 1969.

Nagle RB, Ahmann FR, McDaniel KM, et al. Cytokeratin characterization of human prostatic carcinoma and its derived cell lines. *Cancer Res* 47:281-286, 1987.

Nagle RB, Knox JD, Wolf C, et al. Adhesion molecules, extracellular matrix, and proteases in prostate carcinoma. *J Cell Biochem* 19(suppl):232-237, 1994.

Nagle RB, Huo J, Knox JD, et al. Expression of hemidesmosomal and extracellular matrix proteins by normal and malignant human prostate tissue. *Am J Pathol* 146:1498-1507, 1995.

Nagle RB. Intermediate filament expression in prostate cancer. *Cancer Metastasis Rev* 15:473-482, 1998.

Nakada SY, di Sant'Agnese PA, Moynes RA, et al. The androgen receptor status of neuroendocrine cells in human benign and malignant prostatic tissue. *Cancer Res* 53:1967-1970, 1993.

Nogales FF, Vergara E, Medina MT. Prostate in ovarian mature cystic teratoma. *Histopathology* 26:373-375, 1995.

Nogueira March JL, Figueiredo L, Mata J, et al. Coexisting cyst of the utricle and carcinoma of the endometrial type in the prostate. *Eur Urol* 8:42-44, 1982.

Nucci MR, Ferry JA, Young RH. Ectopic prostatic tissue in the urine cervix. A report of four cases and review of ectopic prostatic tissue. *Am J Surg Pathol* 24: 1224-1230, 2000.

Okada H, Tsubura A, Okamura A, et al. Keratin profiles in normal/hyperplastic prostates and prostate carcinoma. *Virchows Arch A Pathol Anat* 421:157-161, 1992.

Olson JR, Weaver DK. Congenital mesonephric defects in male infants with cystic fibrosis. *J Clin Pathol* 22:725-730, 1969.

Ostrowski ML, Wheeler TM. Paraganglia of the prostate. Location, frequency and differentiation from prostatic adenocarcinoma. *Am J Surg Pathol* 18:412-4290, 1994.

Paradis V, Eschwege P, Loric S, et al. De novo expression of CD44 in prostate carcinoma is correlated with systemic dissemination of prostate cancer. *J Clin Pathol* 51: 798-802, 1998.

Partin AW, Coffey DS. The molecular biology, endocrinology, and physiology of the prostate and seminal vesicles. In: Walsh PC, Retik AB, Vaughan ED Jr, et al, eds. *Campbell's Urology.* 8th ed. Philadelphia: Saunders; 1237-1296, 2002.

Peeling WB, Griffiths GJ. Imaging of the prostate by ultrasound. *J Urol* 132:217-224, 1984.

Pisters LL, Troncoso P, Zhau HE, et al. c-met Proto-oncogene expression in benign and malignant human prostate tissues. *J Urol* 154:293-298, 1996.

Pollen J, Dreilinger A. Immunohistochemical identification of prostatic acid phosphatase and prostate specific antigen in female periurethral glands. *Urology* 23:303-304, 1984.

Popek EJ, Tyson RW, Miller GJ, et al. Prostate development in prune belly syndrome (PBS) and posterior urethral valves (PUV): etiology of PBS-lower urinary tract obstruction or primary mesenchymal defect? *Pediatr Pathol* 11:1-29, 1991.

Rath-Wolfson L, Koren R, Amiel A, et al. The "female prostate" in cervix uteri. A case report. *Appl Immunohistochem* 6:50-53, 1998.

Redman JF, Bissada NK. Milk-of-calcium calculi in müllerian duct cyst. *Urology* 11:495-497, 1978.

Reese JH, McNeal JE, Redwine EA, et al. Differential distribution of pepsinogen II between zones of the human prostate and seminal vesicle. *J Urol* 136:1148-1152, 1986.

Reese JH, McNeal JE, Goldenberg L, et al. Distribution of lactoferrin in the normal and inflamed human prostate: an immunohistochemical study. *Prostate* 20:73-85, 1992.

Reiter RE, Gu ZN, Watabe T, et al. Prostate stem cell antigen: a cell surface marker overexpressed in prostate cancer. *Proc Natl Acad Sci U S A* 95:1735-1740, 1998.

Remick DG Jr, Kumar NB. Benign polyps with prostatic-type epithelium of the urethra and urinary bladder. A suggestion of histogenesis based on histologic and immunohistochemical studies. *Am J Surg Pathol* 8:833-839, 1984.

Richter S, Saghi N, Nissenkorn I. Supratrigonal ectopic prostate: case report and review of the literature. *Urol Int* 46:96-98, 1991.

Riser C, Griffin TL. Cysts of the prostate. *J Urol* 91:282-286, 1964.

Robert Y, Rigot JM, Rocourt N, et al. MR findings of ejaculatory duct cysts. *Acta Radiol* 35:459-462, 1994.

Rode J, Bentley A, Parkinson C. Paraganglial cells of urinary bladder and prostate: potential diagnostic problem. *J Clin Pathol* 43:13-16, 1990.

Sakatoku J, Komatsu Y, Okabe T. Congenital bilateral absence of ejaculatory duct with ectopic seminal vesicles. *Hinyokika Kiyo* 14:210-214, 1968.

Salem CE, Gibbs DM, Highshaw RA, et al. Benign ectopic prostatic tissue involving the seminal vesicle in a patient with prostate cancer: recognition and implications for staging. *Urology* 48:490-493, 1996.

Samaratunga H, Singh M. Distribution pattern of basal cells detected by cytokeratin 34 Beta E12 in primary prostatic duct adenocarcinoma. *Am J Surg Pathol* 21:435-440, 1997.

Sattar AA, Noël JC, Vanderhaeghen JJ, et al. Prostate capsule: computerized morphometric analysis of its components. *Urology* 46:178-181, 1995.

Schultz DS, Amin MB, Zarbo RJ. Basement membrane type IV collagen immunohistochemical staining in prostatic neoplasia. *Appl Immunohistochem* 1:123-126, 1993.

Schuhrke TD, Kaplan GW. Prostatic utricle cysts (Müllerian duct cysts). *J Urol* 119:765-767, 1978.

Seaman AR. Cytochemical observations on corpora amylacea of human prostate gland. *J Urol* 76:99-106, 1956.

Sentinelli S. Mucins in prostatic intra-epithelial neoplasia and prostatic carcinoma. *Histopathology* 22:271-274, 1993.

Sesterhenn IA, Mostofi FK, Mattrey RR, et al. Preliminary results of three-dimensional reconstruction of previously imaged prostates. *Prostate* 4(suppl):33-41, 1992.

Sesterhenn IA, Davis CJ Jr, Mostofi FK. Benign prostate, prostatic hyperplasia, and prostatic carcinoma in female patients [abstract]. *Mod Pathol* 11:95A, 1998.

Shabsigh R, Lerner S, Fishman IJ, et al. The role of transrectal ultrasonography in the diagnosis and management of prostatic and seminal vesicle cysts. *J Urol* 141:1206-1209, 1989.

Shah IA, Schlageter MO, Stinnett P. Cytokeratin immunohistochemistry as a diagnostic tool for distinguishing malignant from benign epithelial lesions of the prostate. *Mod Pathol* 4:220-224, 1991.

Shapiro E. Prostatic morphogenesis, stromal-epithelial interactions, zonal anatomy, and quantitative morphometry. In: Fitzpatrick JM, Krane RJ, eds. *The Prostate.* New York: Churchill Livingstone; 8-16, 1989.

Siegal JA, Brawer MK. Significance of neovascularity in human prostate carcinoma. In: Foster CS, Bostwick DG, eds. *Pathology of the Prostate.* Philadelphia: WB Saunders; 384-399, 1998.

Signoretti S, Waltregny D, Dilks J, et al. p63 Is a prostate basal cell marker and is required for prostate development. *Am J Pathol* 157:1769-1775, 2000.

Sinha AA, Gleason DF, Deleon OF, et al. Localization of a biotinylated cathepsin B oligonucleotide probe in human prostate including invasive cells and invasive edges by in situ hybridization. *Anat Rec* 235:233-240, 1993.

Sinha AA, Gleason DF, Wilson MJ, et al. Immunohistochemical localization of laminin in the basement membranes of normal, hyperplastic, and neoplastic human prostate. *Prostate* 15:299-313, 1989.

Sloboda J, Zaviacic M, Jakubovsky J, et al. Metastasizing adenocarcinoma of the female prostate (Skene's paraurethral glands). Histological and immunohistochemical prostate marker studies and first ultrastructural observation. *Pathol Res Pract* 194:129-136, 1998.

Smith CET, Toplis PJ, Nogales FF. Ovarian prostatic tissue originating from hilar mesonephric nests. *Am J Surg Pathol* 23:232-236, 1999.

Soh S, Kawakami T, Egawa S, et al. Use of ultrasonography in the diagnosis of cystic lesions in seminal vesicles and prostate. *Hinyokiha Kiyo* 41:33-37, 1995.

Sokoll LJ, Chan DW. Prostate-specific antigen. Its discovery and biochemical characteristics. *Urol Clin North Am* 24:253-259, 1997.

Spencer JR, Brodin AG, Ignatoff JM. Clear cell adenocarcinoma of the urethra: evidence for origin within paraurethral ducts. *J Urol* 143:122-125, 1990.

Spiro LH, Levine B. Ectopic subvesical prostatic tissue. *J Urol* 112:631-633, 1994.

Srigley JR, Dardick I, Hartwick RWJ, et al. Basal epithelial cells of human prostate gland are not myoepithelial cells. *Am J Pathol* 136:957-968, 1990.

Srigley JR, Amin MB, Kapusta L, Cohen C. An immunohistochemical study of the prostatic central zone (CZ) with histogenetic and diagnostic considerations [abstract]. *Mod Pathol* 13: 115A, 2000.

Srodon M, Epstein JI. Central zone (CZ) histology of the prostate: a mimicker of high-grade prostatic intraepithelial neoplasia. *Hum Pathol* 33:518-523, 2002.

Stephens FD, Gupta D. Pathogenesis of the prune belly syndrome. *J Urol* 152:2328-2331, 1994.

Szemes GC, Rubin DJ. Squamous cell carcinoma in a müllerian duct cyst. *J Urol* 100:40-43, 1968.

Tepper S, Jagirdar J, Heath D, et al. Homology between the female paraurethral (Skene's) glands and the prostate. *Arch Pathol Lab Med* 108:423-425, 1984.

Timms BG, Lee CW, Aumüller G, et al. Instructive induction of prostate growth and differentiation by a defined urogenital sinus mesenchyme. *Micro Res Tech* 30:319-332, 1995.

Timms BG. Anatomical perspectives of prostate development. In: Naz RK, ed. *Prostate: Basic and Clinical Aspects.* New York: CRC Press; 30-32, 1997.

Tokumitsu S, Tokumitsu K, Takeya M, et al. Developmentally heterotopic urogenital tissues in a retroperitoneal lipoma with hematopoiesis. *Acta Pathol Jpn* 31:289-297, 1981.

Unger PD, Cohen EL, Talerman A. Mixed germ cell tumor of the testis. *J Urol Pathol* 9:257-263, 1998.

Uzoaru I, Akang EEU, Aghadiuno PU, et al. Benign cystic teratomas with prostatic tissue: a report of two cases. *Teratology* 45:235-239, 1992.

Vaalasti A, Hervonen A. Autonomic innervation of the human prostate. *Invest Urol* 17:293-297, 1980.

Vadmal M, Hajdu SI. Prostatic tissue in benign cystic ovarian teratomas. *Hum Pathol* 27:428-429, 1996.

Val-Bernal JF, Gómez-Ortega J. Hyperplasia of prostatic mesonephric remnants: a potential pitfall in the evaluation of prostate gland biopsy. *J Urol* 154:1138-1139, 1995.

van Leenders G, Dijkman H, Hulsbergen-von de Kaa C, et al. Demonstration of intermediate cells during human prostate epithelial differentiation in situ and in vitro using triple-staining confocal scanning microscopy. *Lab Invest* 80: 1251-1258, 2000.

van Poppel H, Vereecken R, de Getter P, et al. Hemospermia owing to utricular cyst: embryological summary and surgical review. *J Urol* 129:608-609, 1983.

Varlet F, Coupris L, Laumonier F, et al. Congenital dilatation of the prostatic utricle. Embryologic review, diagnosis and treatment. Apropos of 2 pseudo-tumoral cases, without hypospadias. *Ann Urol* 26:39-48, 1992.

Varma M, Lee MW, Tamboli P, et al. Morphologic criteria for the diagnosis of prostatic adenocarcinoma in needle biopsy specimens. A study of 250 consecutive cases in a routine surgical pathology practice. *Arch Pathol Lab Med* 126: 554-561, 2002.

Verhagan AP, Ramaekers FC, Aalders TW, et al. Colocalization of basal and luminal cell-type cytokeratins in human prostate cancer. *Cancer Res* 52:6182-6187, 1992.

Villers A, Terris MK, McNeal JE, et al. Ultrasound anatomy of the prostate: the normal gland and anatomical variations. *J Urol* 143:732-738, 1990.

Villers A, McNeal JE, Freiha FS, et al. Invasion of Denonvilliers' fascia in radical prostatectomy specimens. *J Urol* 149:793-798, 1993.

Vogel U, Negri G, Bültmann B. Ectopic prostatic tissue in the spleen. *Virchows Arch* 427:543-545, 1996.

Wallace C, Creager AJ, Cappellari JO, et al. Ectopic prostatic tissue in the uterine cervix. *Am J Surg Pathol* 25: 1215-1216, 2001.

Walsh PC, Madden JD, Harrod MJ, et al. Familial incomplete male pseudo-hermaphroditism, type 2: decreased dihydrotestosterone formation in pseudovaginal perineoscrotal hypospadias. *N Engl J Med* 291:944-949, 1974.

Walsh PC, Donker PJ. Impotence following radical prostatectomy: insight into etiology and prevention. *J Urol* 128:492-497, 1982.

Walsh PC, Lepor H, Eggleston JC. Radical prostatectomy with preservation of sexual function: anatomical and pathological considerations. *Prostate* 4:473-485, 1983.

Walsh PC. Anatomic radical retropubic prostatectomy. In: Walsh PC, Retik AB, Vaughan ED Jr, et al, eds. *Campbell's Urology.* 7th ed. Philadelphia: WB Saunders; 2568, 1998.

Wang Y, Hayward S, Cao M, et al. Cell differentiation lineage in the prostate. *Differentiation* 68:270-279, 2001.

Warren MM, Greene LF. Calculus in the prostatic utricle. *J Urol* 107:82-84, 1972.

Weaver MG, Abdul-Karim FW, Srigley J, et al. Paneth cell–like change of the prostate gland. A histological, immunohistochemical, and electron microscopic study. *Am J Surg Pathol* 16:62-28, 1992.

Wernert N, Seitz G, Achtstätter T. Immunohistochemical investigation of different cytokeratins and vimentin in the prostate from the fetal period up to adulthood and in prostate carcinoma. *Pathol Res Pract* 182:617-626, 1987.

Wernert N, Gerdes J, Loy V, et al. Investigations of the estrogen (ER-ICA-test) and the progesterone receptor in the prostate and prostatic carcinoma on immunohistochemical basis. *Virchows Arch* [A] 412:387-391, 1988.

Wernert N, Albrech M, Sesterhenn I, et al. The "female prostate": location, morphology, immunohistochemical characteristics and significance. *Eur Urol* 22:64-69, 1992.

Wigger HJ, Blanc WA. The prune belly syndrome. *Pathol Annu* 12:17-79, 1977.

Wilson JD, Griffin JE, Leshin M, et al. Role of gonadal hormones in development of the sexual phenotypes. *Hum Genet* 58:78-84, 1981.

Wojno KJ, Epstein JI. The utility of basal cell-specific anti-cytokeratin antibody (34βE12) in the diagnosis of prostate cancer. *Am J Surg Pathol* 19:251-260, 1995.

Woods JE, Soh S, Wheeler TM. Distribution and significance of microcalcifications in the neoplastic and nonneoplastic prostate. *Arch Pathol Lab Med* 122:152-155, 1998.

Workman C, Porch P, Rhamy RK. The congenitally dilated prostatic utricle. *J Urol* 120:508-510, 1978.

Xia T, Blackburn WR, Gardner WA Jr. Fetal prostate growth and development. *Pediatr Pathol* 10:527-537, 1990.

Xue Y, Verhofstad A, Lange W, et al. Prostatic neuroendocrine cells have a unique keratin expression pattern and do not express bcl-2. *Am J Pathol* 151:1759-1765, 1997.

Yang Y, Hao J, Liu X, et al. Differential expression of cytokeratin mRNA and protein in normal prostate, prostatic intraepithelial neoplasia, and invasive carcinoma. *Am J Pathol* 150:693-704, 1997.

Yantiss RK, Young RH. Transitional cell "metaplasia" in the prostate gland. A survey of its frequency and features based on 103 consecutive prostatic biopsy specimens. *J Urol Pathol* 7:71-80, 1997.

Yasukawa S, Aoshi H, Takamatsu M. Ectopic prostatic adenoma in retrovesical space. *J Urol* 137:998-999, 1987.

Young RH. Pseudoneoplastic lesions of the prostate gland. *Pathol Annu* 23:105-128, 1988.

Zaviacic M. The adult human female prostatic homologue and male prostate gland: a comparative enzyme-histochemical study. *Acta Histochem* 77:19-31, 1985

Zaviacic M, Ablin RJ. The female prostate and prostate-specific antigen. Immunohistochemical localization, implication of this prostate marker in women and reasons for using the term "prostate" in the human female. *Histol Histopathol* 15:131-142, 2000A.

Zaviacic M, Jakubovska V, Belosovic M, et al. Ultrastructure of the normal adult human female prostate gland (Skene's gland). *Anat Embryol* 201:51-61, 2000B.

CHAPTER 2

Prostatic Tissue Handling and Sampling

[2.1] Cytologic Specimens **32**

[2.2] Core Needle Biopsy **32**

[2.3] Transurethral Prostatectomy (TURP) **40**

[2.4] Open Suprapubic or Retropubic Simple Prostatectomy (Enucleation) Tissue **44**

[2.5] Radical Perineal and Retropubic Prostatectomy **44**

[2.6] Cystoprostatectomy **51**

[2.7] Postmortem Examination of the Prostate **51**

The most common prostatic parenchymal tissue samples examined in surgical pathology laboratories in the United States are, in order, 18-gauge needle cores, transurethral resections, radical prostatectomy specimens, open prostatectomy specimens, and fine needle aspirates. The estimated number of these procedures performed in the United States in 1997 is given in **t2.1**.

By far the most common type of prostatic tissue specimen currently encountered in surgical pathology laboratories in the United States is the 18-gauge needle core biopsy. Over the last 16 years there has been a remarkable increase in the number of prostate core needle biopsies performed, and this is reflected in the numbers of new prostate cancer cases diagnosed in 1985 and 1997. In 1985, 86 000 new prostate cancer cases were diagnosed in the United States (Steele 1994), increasing to 317 000 cases in 1996 (Parker 1996) and then declining to an estimated 189 000 new cases in 2002 (Jemal 2002). (This pattern of incidence increase and subsequent decline probably results from prostate-specific antigen [PSA] screening [Gann 1997]). Based on an estimate of 4 men biopsied for each positive biopsy (Catalona 1994), roughly 189 000 × 4 = 756 000 men were biopsied in 2002.

The second most common type of tissue specimen is prostatic chips from transurethral resection of the prostate (TURP), also known as transurethral prostatectomy. The number of TURPs has declined over the last decade, from a peak of 258 000 in 1987 to 168 000 in 1993 (Holtgrewe 1995). This operation is still common in American urology and is considered the gold standard for the surgical management of benign prostatic hyperplasia (BPH) (Fitzpatrick 2002). The decline in use of the operation has resulted from development of alternative therapies including medical therapy and minimally invasive treatment of BPH (Holtgrewe 1995, Fitzpatrick 2002) and increased awareness of watchful waiting (Holtgrewe 1995). The minimally invasive methods, including laser therapy, transurethral balloon dilation, hyperthermia and thermotherapy, transurethral electrovaporization, intraurethral stents, and transurethral needle ablation of the prostate, do not provide tissue for histologic examination (Fitzpatrick 2002).

Radical prostatectomy specimens are the third most common tissue sample type. A 6-fold increase in performance of the radical prostatectomy operation was observed from 1984 to 1990 (Lu-Yao 1993, 1994), with an apparent peak in 1992, at least in one patient population (Xia 1998). Increased use of radical prostatectomy has resulted from the vast increase in prostate cancer incidence, the increase in cases being detected as clinically localized disease (Mettlin 1996, 1997A), and advances in surgical techniques, particularly nerve-sparing approaches, which decrease the risk of impotence (Lu-Yao 1993, Walsh 2002). The use of this form of treatment varies according to geographic region of the country (Mettlin 1997B). From 1992 to 1994, 28.3% of patients diagnosed with prostate were treated with this modality. For the 189 000 men newly diagnosed with prostate cancer in 2002, this would translate into about 53 000 radical prostatectomy procedures in the United States in 2002.

Open prostatectomy for treatment of BPH is uncommon and is typically reserved for men with large prostate glands greater than 75 g (Han 2002). This procedure, which may be performed via a retropubic or suprapubic approach and entails enucleation of BPH nodules, is also indicated for men with a symptomatic bladder diverticulum, urethral stricture or previous hypospadias repair, a large bladder stone, a coexisting unilateral or bilateral inguinal hernia, and marked hip ankylosis (Han 2002).

■ **t2.1 Number of Prostatic Tissue Specimens Examined in the United States in 2002**

Tissue Type	Estimated Number
Fine needle aspirate	Rare
18-gauge core needle biopsy	756,000
Transurethral resectate (TURP chips)	168,000 [a]
Open (simple) prostatectomy	Uncommon
Radical prostatectomy	53,000

[a]1993 Medicare estimate

■ **t2.2 Clinical Goals of Prostate Tissue Sampling by Needle Biopsy**

To maximize the opportunity to recognize the presence of clinically significant carcinoma of the prostate
To provide reliable information regarding histologic grade
To document extent of intraprostatic tumor
To accomplish the sampling procedure with minimal risk, anxiety, inconvenience, and expense

Modified after Koslowski and Grayhack 1996

Cytologic sampling of the prostate may be achieved by expression of prostatic secretions, by acquisition of voided urine with prostate secretions, by fine needle aspiration (FNA) biopsy of the prostate, and by washings or touch preparation of radical prostatectomy specimens for margin evaluation. Microscopic examination of expressed prostatic secretions usually is performed by clinicians in evaluation for leukocytes and lipid-laden macrophages that are found in prostatitis (Nickel 2002). Prostate cancer can be detected in prostatic secretions after massage (DeMay 1996B), but these exfoliative cytology studies are not useful because of the low sensitivity and high unsatisfactory rate (Guinan 1980). Prostatic cells are rarely shed spontaneously into voided urine (DeMay 1996C, Krishnan 2000), and so exfoliative cytologic examination of urine is not indicated for diagnosing prostate cancer. FNA biopsy of the prostate is rarely performed in the United States (Wojcik 1997) because of widespread use of the 18-gauge needle biopsy mounted on a biopsy gun. FNA prostatic biopsy has been widely used in Scandinavia (Ekman 1967, Esposti 1966, Hostetter 1990). Also, touch imprints and washings from radical prostatectomy specimens have been used in an effort to assess surgical margin status (Pearle 1994), but these are experimental tools and not standard of practice. Lastly, metastatic prostate cancer can rarely present in a malignant effusion, with a cytologic diagnosis (Renshaw 1997B).

Sampling and handling of these different types of prostatic tissue specimens may be examined at several different levels. In this chapter, we explore methods of clinical sampling, gross (macroscopic) sampling, and histologic sampling.

The first two sections are on sampling of the prostate gland by FNA biopsy and needle core biopsy. The clinical indication for performing these biopsies usually is to rule out prostate cancer in the clinical setting of an abnormal digital rectal examination (DRE) or elevated serum PSA (above 4 ng/mL; see Chapter 13). Therefore, guiding principles for this clinical sampling have been devised **t2.2** (Kozlowski 1996).

[2.1] Cytologic Specimens

The focus of this sampling section is on comparison and contrast of FNA biopsy and core needle biopsy. FNA biopsy is "the removal of a sample of cells, using a fine needle, from a suspicious mass for diagnostic purposes" (DeMay 1996A). The needle used for FNA of the prostate may be a fine needle of 22 gauge or an intermediate gauge of 20 (Kline 1977), although intermediate 18-gauge needles have also been used (Ferguson 1930, Kline 1982). An excellent overview of the FNA technique has been published (DeMay 1996A,B), and FNA diagnosis of prostate disease is presented in Chapter 3.

FNA of the prostate may have utility when there is a mass palpable by DRE, but in this PSA-screening era, many patients have nonpalpable prostate cancers detected solely by an increase in serum PSA (stage T1c cancers) (Amling 1998, Humphrey 1998). Indeed, in our screened population, 78% of men had T1c cancers and did not have a suspicious mass by DRE (Humphrey 1996). Additional clinical sampling disadvantages of FNA include a lack of ultrasound guidance and inability to evaluate tumor distribution and extent, as may be done using 6 or more systematic needle core biopsies. A potential advantage of the FNA technique is that the prostate gland may be well sampled by multiple passes of the fine needle within the gland. However, the clinical acquisition of multiple (usually 6 or more core biopsies) is already standard of practice in the United States.

The degree of clinical sampling clearly contributes to the sensitivity of a given biopsy technique. There are few comparative data available on the sensitivity of prostate cancer detection using FNA biopsy and contemporary 18-gauge systematic core biopsy methods. In one comparative study (Wojcik 1997), it was concluded that FNA of the prostate has a low sensitivity (56%) and should not be used as a screening procedure. Overall, FNA biopsy of the prostate has been reported to have a sensitivity of 68% to 99% (Kline 1985). Diagnostic experience also clearly relates to sensitivity of FNA for detection of prostate cancer.

Currently, in the United States, standard of practice for clinical sampling of the prostate gland by needle biopsy is the systematic transrectal 18-gauge core needle biopsy.

A review on the performance and laboratory processing of prostate aspiration biopsies has been published recently (Maksem 1995).

[2.2] Core Needle Biopsy

14-Gauge Biopsy

Core needle biopsy of the prostate was performed by transrectal digital guidance of a 14-gauge needle into a palpable mass. Examples of this type of "cutting" large-gauge needle biopsy include the Franklin modification of the Vim Silverman and Tru Cut needles (Kozlowski 1996). Transperineal punch biopsies have also been performed in the past (Bianchi 1956, Müller 1980).

Clinical disadvantages of the 14-gauge needle biopsy compared with the sextant 18-gauge needle biopsy of the prostate relate to goals 1, 3, and 4 in **t2.2**. First, because the 14-gauge needle is directed toward a palpable mass, only this portion of the prostate is sampled (along with a blind biopsy of the other side or "lobe" in some cases). More biopsies of more regions of the prostate are taken with the 18-gauge systematic biopsy approach and these can be guided by transrectal ultrasound (TRUS). It has been clearly shown that the TRUS-guided systematic sextant 18-gauge biopsy method is superior to DRE-guided biopsy in detecting prostate cancer (Narayan 1998). Second, given the directed nature of the digitally guided 14-gauge needle biopsy, mapping of the distribution and extent of intraprostatic tumor is not performed. Lastly, the complications of hemorrhage, infection, urinary retention, and needle track seeding by carcinoma are more common with 14-gauge needle biopsy (Kozlowski 1996). Significant bleeding can occur in 1% to 2% of patients after digitally guided transrectal and transperineal needle biopsy and has been severe in a few cases (Dauleh 1996, Wendel 1967). An infection rate of 16% to 48% after the digitally guided transrectal biopsy (Catalona 1984) has been improved with prebiopsy antimicrobial prophylaxis. (The need for such prophylaxis is underscored by a study that reported bacteremia in 76% of patients after transrectal biopsy [Ashby 1978]). Urinary retention has been reported in up to 10% of patients after transrectal biopsy (Kozlowski 1996). Needle track seeding after use of the 14-gauge needle biopsy has been reported for about 27 patients (reviewed in DeMay 1996A and Moul 1998), whereas only 5 patients have had seeding after use of the transrectal 18-gauge needle biopsy (Bastacky 1991). The incidence of needle tracking for the 14-gauge needle biopsy of tumor is low, at 0.2% to 0.4% (Haddad 1990), whereas the incidence of tracking after 18-gauge needle biopsy has not been quantified; in one series (Bostwick 1994), no example of tracking was identified in 311 whole prostate glands that had been previously biopsied using 18-gauge needles. All but 2 of the patients with needle track seeding after 14-gauge needle biopsy had biopsies performed via the transperineal approach. Clinically, these patients presented with a palpable perineal nodule of 0.3cm to 5cm after an average interval of 16 months (Moul 1989) but with range of 1 month to 7 years. Risk factors for developing such local masses secondary to tumor tracking include high clinical stage and high-grade (poorly differentiated) carcinoma (Moul 1989), although intermediate-grade tumors can also implant along the needle tract (Bastacky 1991, Kozlowski 1996), with periprostatic tumor extension (Bastacky 1991). Even benign glands can be found along these needle tracks (Bastacky 1991). One case of prostatic leiomyosarcoma tracking along the 14-gauge needle pathway has been reported (Fortunoff 1962).

An advantage of the 14-gauge biopsy is that it provides more than twice as much tissue per needle core as the 18-gauge needle biopsy specimen **i2.1A,B**.

18-Gauge Biopsy

Clinical sampling of the prostate gland to assess for prostate cancer is now most often accomplished using an ultrasound-guided transrectal systematic biopsy procedure (Terris 2002), with an 18-gauge needle mounted on a spring-loaded biopsy gun **i2.2A-D**. After administration of oral antibiotics and performance of a DRE and cleansing enema, the ultrasound probe is inserted into the rectum, with the patient in a left lateral decubitus position (Terris 2002). The sonographic images are used to guide the needle into regions of the prostate. Also, any peripheral zone hypoechoic areas are targeted for maximal sampling **i2.3A-D**. These hypoechoic foci suggest prostate cancer but are not specific, and 30% to 80% of prostate cancers are not visible by ultrasound (Terris 2002); that is, they are isoechoic.

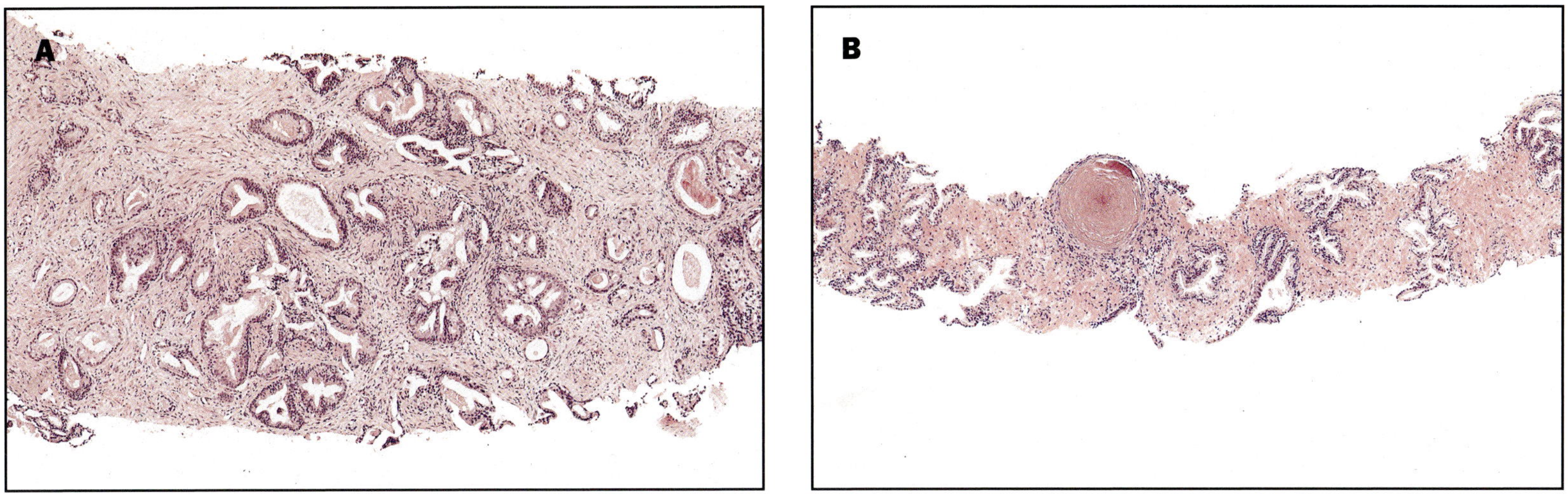

■ **i2.1** *Thickness of 14-gauge prostate needle biopsy core (A) vs 18-gauge needle biopsy core (B).*

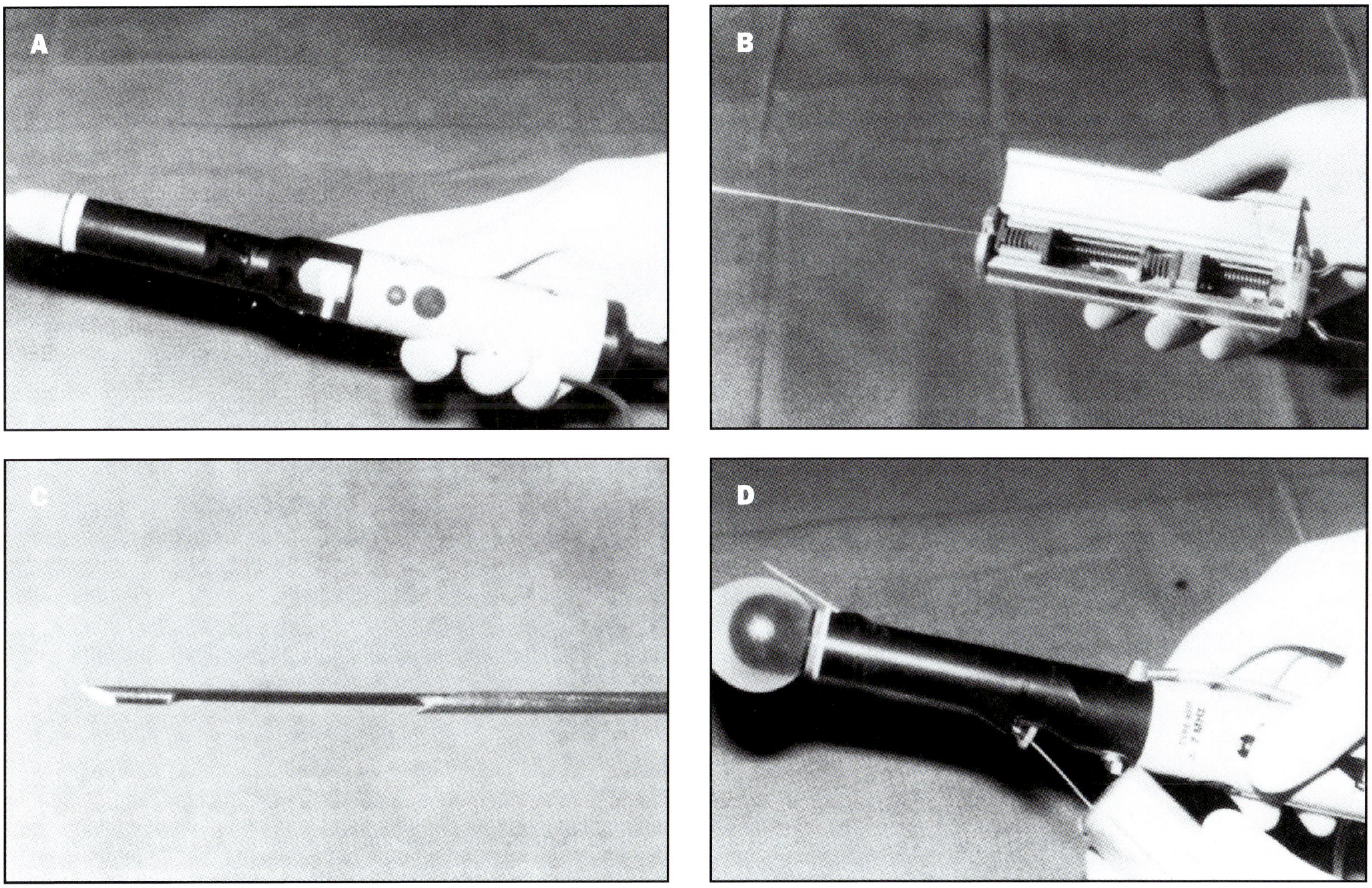

■ **i2.2** *Prostate biopsy needle and gun (Bard Biopty Needle and Gun, Bard Urological Division, Covington, Georgia). A: Multiplanar 7-MHz probe. B: Spring-loaded Biopty gun and needle. C: Inner needle is "fired" into prostate and outer sheath is then advanced to capture tissue core. D: Biopsy needle can be directed by ultrasound guidance, with needle in probe sleeve. (Reproduced from* Campbell's Urology, *6th ed, p 362, with permission of WB Saunders).*

In 1989 a sextant biopsy approach was introduced, with procurement of 6 cores of tissue. The intent of this biopsy technique is to widely sample for prostate cancer, to map carcinoma distribution within the gland, and to provide information for pretreatment staging based on tumor characteristics in needle biopsy, such as Gleason grade and amount of tumor in needle biopsy tissue. This sextant sampling is accomplished by biopsy of 6 separate sectors (Hodge 1989, Narayan 1998, Stamey 1995), with the biopsy sites about 1cm apart (Hodge 1989). Usually these biopsies are directed toward the peripheral zone; as originally described (Hodge 1989), laterally placed biopsies from the base, midgland, and apex of both sides of the prostate are performed. Lateral placement of the needles has been emphasized (Terris 1997A). Additional cores may be submitted based on DRE and ultrasound findings, so additional cores may be obtained from any palpable or sonographic abnormality. The transition zone may also be targeted for biopsy, but the yield of carcinoma with such

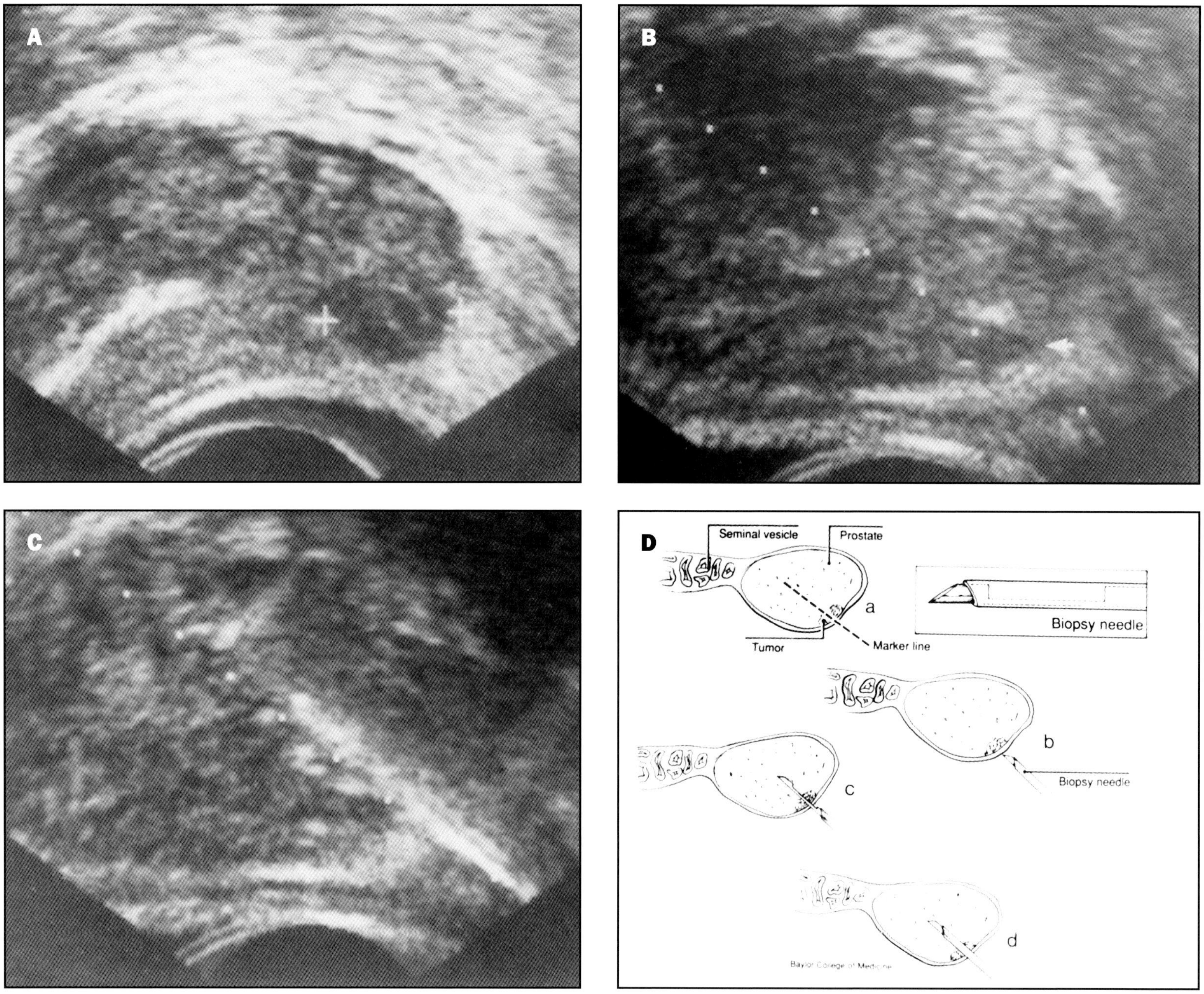

■ **i2.3** *A: Ultrasound appearance (transverse plane) of hypoechoic prostate lesion (between cursors). B: Longitudinal view showing planned path of needle. Hypoechoic lesion is at arrow. C: Hyperechoic line indicates path of needle after firing. D: Representation of this sequence of events. (Reproduced from* Campbell's Urology, *6th ed, p. 364, with permission).*

biopsies is low (Bazinet 1996, Egawa 1998, Epstein 1997, Fleshner 1997, Keetch 1995, Lui 1995, Onder 1998, Terris 1997C). Adding transition zone biopsies to the standard peripheral zone sextant biopsies has increased the detection of carcinoma by only 2% (Bazinet 1996, Epstein 1997, Terris 1997C).

Although submitting 6 biopsy cores per patient biopsy session has been a common practice, recently more extensive sampling protocols have been used. In these protocols, 8 to 13 biopsy cores are taken per biopsy session (Babaian 2000, Eskew 1997, 1998, Gore 2001, Levine 1998, Presti 2000, Ravery 2000). Using a saturation biopsy technique, one group obtained a mean of 23 biopsy cores (range 14 to 45) per patient (Stewart 2001). Procurement of 8-13 cores is currently favored because of increased cancer detection rate. Recent data suggest that a systematic 5-region biopsy approach (with 13 needle cores procured) increases the cancer detection rate by 35% (Eskew 1997, 1998). Two consecutive sets of sextant biopsies (12 total biopsy cores) at the same office visit also increased the number of cancers detected by 30% (Levine 1998). In our experience, men who were older, with higher serum PSA levels and larger prostates (greater than 30cm^3 by TRUS), needed more biopsies to detect prostate cancer (Naughton 1998). The postbiopsy incidence of hematospermia and hematochezia was higher in the 12-core than in the 6-core biopsy approach, but overall there was no significant difference between the 2 procedures in pain or morbidity (Naughton 2000). Increased sampling of the prostate does not appear to increase detection of pathologically insignificant tumors (Chan 2001, Levine 1998), although clinical outcome data are not yet available.

Data on repeat sextant biopsy after an initial set of 6 biopsies also demonstrate the clinical sampling error inherent in the sextant biopsy approach to prostate cancer detection. In patients with histopathologically diagnosed prostate cancer on a first set of sextant biopsies, 20% to 46% of patients had a false-negative second set of sextant biopsies (Epstein 1997, Stroumbakis 1997, Svetec 1998). This high false-negative rate is not surprising, given that an 18-gauge needle biopsy samples only 0.03% of all tissue in the prostate gland (Humphrey 1995).

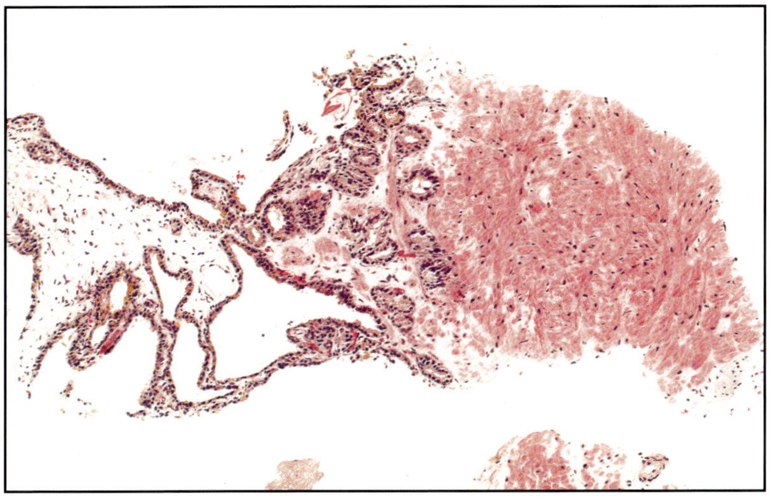

■ **i2.4** *Intentional seminal vesicle sampling by needle biopsy. Note more dilated glands surrounded by smaller glands.*

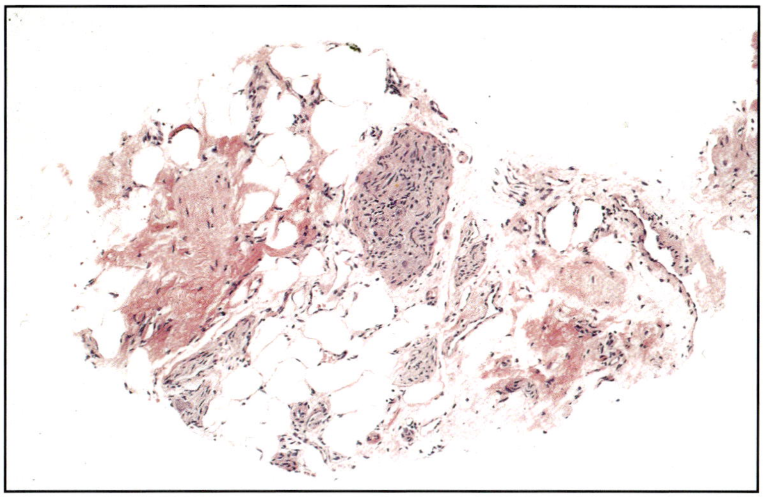

■ **i2.5** *Periprostatic adipose tissue sampled by prostate needle biopsy. This fat is most often found at the needle core tips (ends).*

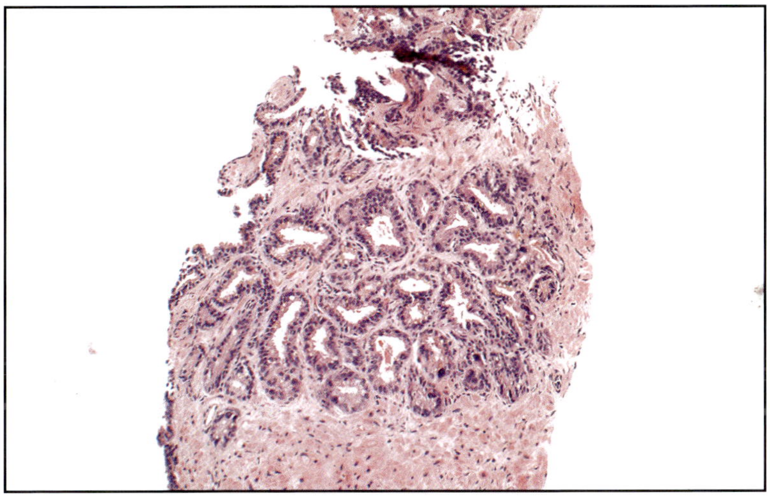

■ **i2.6** *Incidentally sampled seminal vesicle is often found at the tip of the needle.*

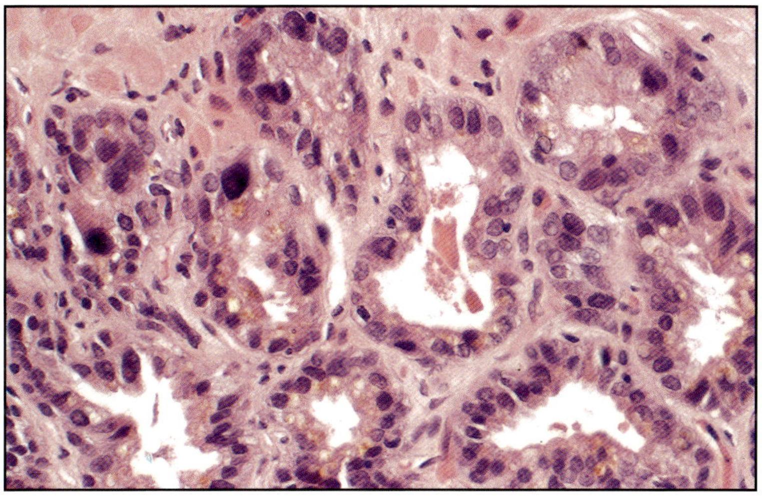

■ **i2.7** *Characteristic irregularly dispersed large, hyperchromatic "smudge" cells of seminal vesicle.*

Recently, models, including computer-generated ones, have been developed in an effort to determine the optimal number of core biopsies needed to detect prostate cancer (Aus 1997, Chen 1997, Daneshgari 1995, Karakiewicz 1998, Vashi 1998). These models take into account one or more factors that influence cancer detection rate, such as serum PSA level, DRE findings, patient age, gland size, and tumor location (in the transition zone, midline peripheral zone, and inferior portion of the anterior horn of the peripheral zone) (Aus 1997, Chen 1997, Daneshgari 1995, Karakiewicz 1998, Vashi 1998). Recent models indicate that a 10- to 12-core biopsy protocol detects substantially more cancers than a sextant approach (Bauer 1999, Chen 1999). Laterally placed needle biopsies also increased the detection rate.

Clinical sampling of extraprostatic tissues may represent a specific clinical attempt at staging (Allepuz Losa 1995, Norberg 1996B, Stone 1995, Terris 1997C, Vallancien 1994) or may represent an incidental histologic finding. In general, because of the low yield rate, directed routine seminal vesicle biopsies are not indicated (Terris 1997C). This is particularly true in this serum PSA screening era, where only 3% to 9% of screen-detected prostate cancers invade the seminal vesicle (Humphrey 1996). Nevertheless, some have advocated performance of seminal vesicle biopsy when detection of seminal vesicle invasion would change treatment (Terris 1997C), when the seminal vesicles are enlarged by palpation or ultrasound (Terris 1997C), when the serum PSA is greater than 10 ng/mL (Stone 1995, Terris 1997C, Vallancien 1994), when the clinical stage is T2b or greater (Allepuz Losa 1995, Stone 1995), or when the Gleason score in needle biopsy is greater than 4 (Stone 1995) or 7 (Allepuz Losa 1995). Seminal vesicle biopsies are rarely performed in our hospital and in the Washington University Medical Center prostate cancer screening program. It is possible to specifically capture seminal vesicle tissue by TRUS-guided biopsy **i2.4** in 83% of cases (Lane 1998A). Other periprostatic sites that can be targets for local staging biopsies include neurovascular bundle, extraprostatic tissue, and invaginated extraprostatic space (Lane 1998A). However, because local spread into these tissues does not necessarily equate with disease that is incurable by local therapy, these staging biopsies may or may not influence treatment strategy.

Incidental sampling of periprostatic adipose tissue is common in prostate needle biopsies **i2.5**, with 77% of cases with identifiable periprostatic tissue in one series (Ravery 1994). Seminal vesicle or ejaculatory duct tissue is found in up to 20% of needle biopsies as an incidental finding **i2.6, i2.7** (Bostwick 1997B). Extraprostatic spread of carcinoma can be diagnosed if one identifies carcinoma in adipose tissue, but as noted earlier, this discovery does not preclude use of local therapies (such as surgery or radiation). One should be cautious in diagnosing extraprostatic carcinoma in needle biopsy based on apparent seminal vesicle invasion by carcinoma because

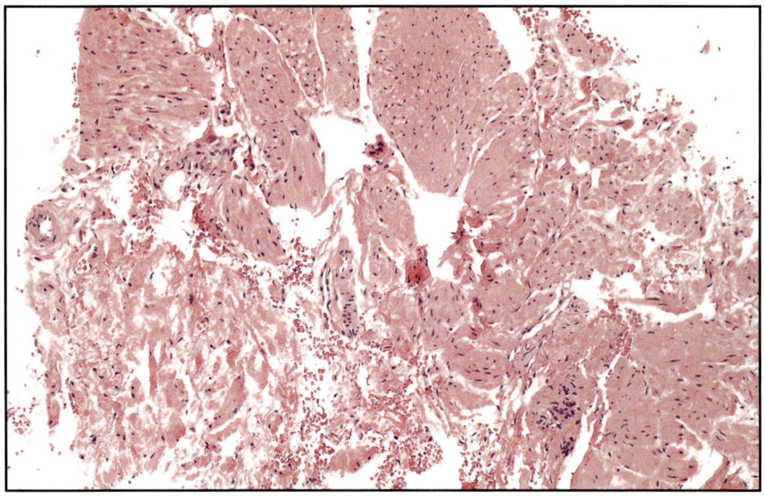

■ **i2.8** *Incidentally sampled smooth muscle bundles of bladder neck.*

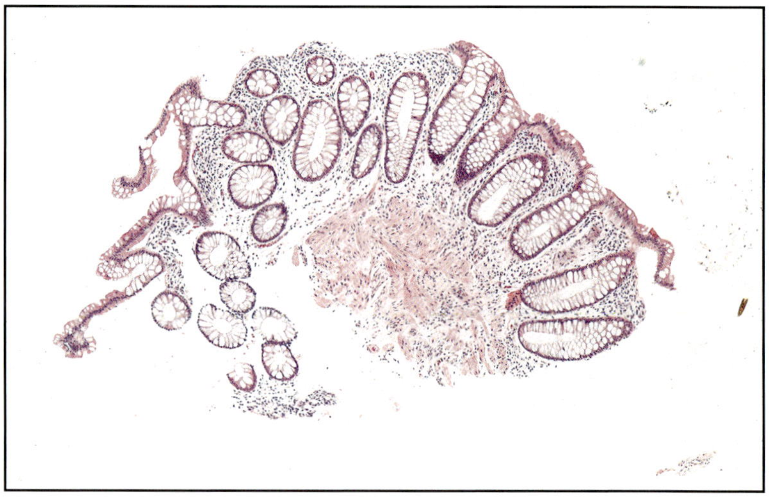

■ **i2.9** *Due to the transrectal approach of the needle biopsy, fragments of rectum or colon are often seen along with prostate needle biopsy tissue. This colorectal tissue is usually of colonic type.*

ejaculatory duct epithelium is identical and carcinoma surrounding ejaculatory duct epithelium is still intraprostatic. The seminal vesicle smooth muscle wall is thicker than the ejaculatory duct wall, but this difference can be difficult or impossible to ascertain in needle biopsy if sampling of the ejaculatory duct and seminal vesicle is incomplete. Additional nonprostatic tissues that can be incidentally sampled include smooth muscle bundles of the bladder neck **i2.8** and rectal tissue **i2.9, i2.10**. In the former case, the biopsy should be interpreted as inadequate if no prostatic epithelium is identified (after thorough histologic sampling, including additional levels). Small fragments of colorectal tissue are commonly seen in the transrectal biopsy approach, but this author has not yet appreciated disease involving this incidentally sampled tissue.

Major clinical complications of the 18-gauge sextant biopsy sampling method are uncommon, at 1% to 6% (Gustafsson 1990, Kapoor 1998, Norberg 1996A, Terris 2002). These major complications include infection (including bacteremia and bacteriuria), bleeding, and urinary retention. The minor complications such as transient, self-limited hematuria and hemospermia are extremely common, occurring in up to 78% of patients (Norberg 1996A).

Additional complications of 18-gauge transrectal needle biopsy include needle track seeding and release of prostatic epithelial cells into the bloodstream circulation. As noted earlier, needle track seeding with extraprostatic carcinoma extension due to biopsy with this thin needle appears to be rare (Bastacky 1991, Bostwick 1994). Higher histologic grade and higher clinical stage seem to be general risk factors for needle track seeding after prostate biopsy, but clinically prostate confined and intermediate-grade cancers can also exhibit tracking. Such tracking should be specifically sought when needle tracks are identified in radical prostatectomy specimens **i2.11-i2.16**. Tracks at least 2mm long can be identified in only about 12% of completely embedded radical prostatectomy specimens (Bostwick 1994). More commonly, one can see focal scarring that could be caused by needle biopsy, but without detection of a long, linear scar it is difficult to be certain that this is a biopsy track. The longer tracks are characterized by "a straight narrow path of granulation tissue or fibrosis with hemosiderin and red blood cells, usually with cavity formation" (Bostwick 1994) **i2.11-i2.14**. There is a peripheral rim of a mixed acute and chronic inflammatory cell infiltrate (Bostwick 1994) **i2.13**. I also have seen hemorrhage, cellular debris, and inflammatory cells in cystic cavities created by biopsy **i2.14**. The benign epithelium

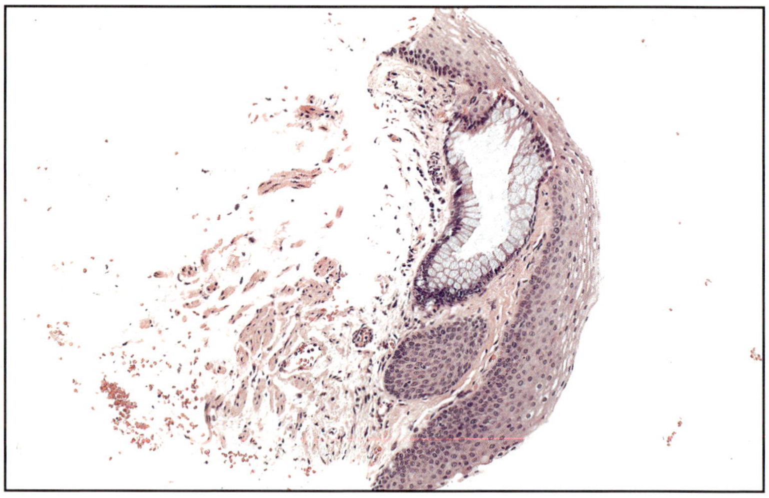

■ **i2.10** *Squamous epithelium in incidentally sampled rectal tissue in prostate needle biopsy sample.*

adjacent to the biopsy track can exhibit basal cell prominence **i2.14**, and squamous metaplasia **i2.15** can be found in disrupted glands. Nuclear atypia can be seen in these foci of squamous metaplasia. Carcinoma can be often noted within the fibrous tissue of a needle track scar (Bostwick 1994). An atrophic appearance, with cytoplasmic volume loss, can be assumed by these entrapped malignant glands **i2.16**. It is important to follow the tracks out to the periprostatic soft tissue and peripheral inked margin to assess for possible extension of tumor along the biopsy track.

Another complication of needle biopsy is release of benign prostatic epithelial cells and tumor cells into the bloodstream circulation (Price 1998). In one study (Price 1998), 22% of patients with a carcinoma and 19% of patients without carcinoma converted their reverse transcriptive-polymerase chain reaction (RT-PCR) assay for PSA and prostate-specific membrane antigen in serum (presumably reflecting circulatory prostatic epithelial cells) to positive at 30 minutes after biopsy. By 1 month most (but not all) patients had cleared these circulating cells, as indicated by a negative RT-PCR assay. In other studies targeting PSA only by RT-PCR, conversion rates were 2.6% to 9.5% (Cama 1997, Goldman 1998, Moreno 1997). There are no data to suggest that these transiently circulating cells have an adverse impact on patient outcome.

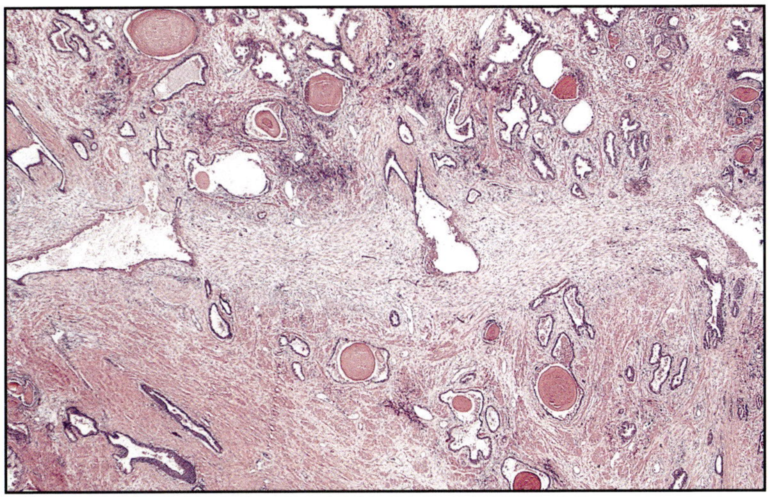

■ **i2.11** *Linear fibrous scar of a needle biopsy track.*

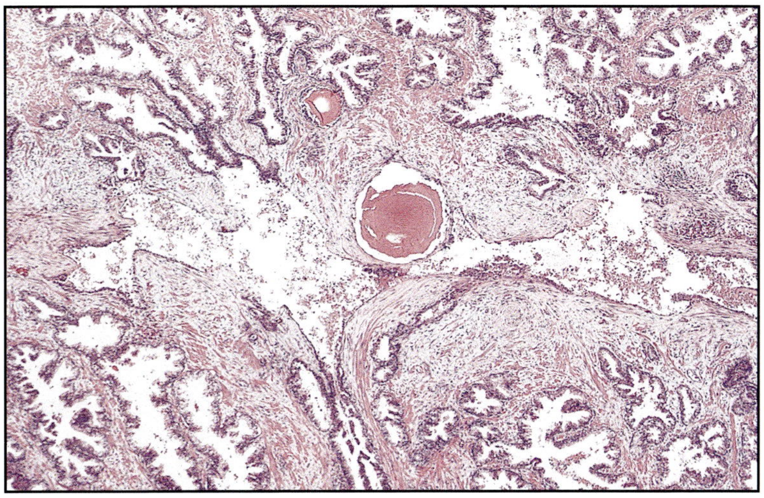

■ **i2.12** *Needle biopsy track with scar, and benign glands with disruption, cystic change, and flat atrophic lining.*

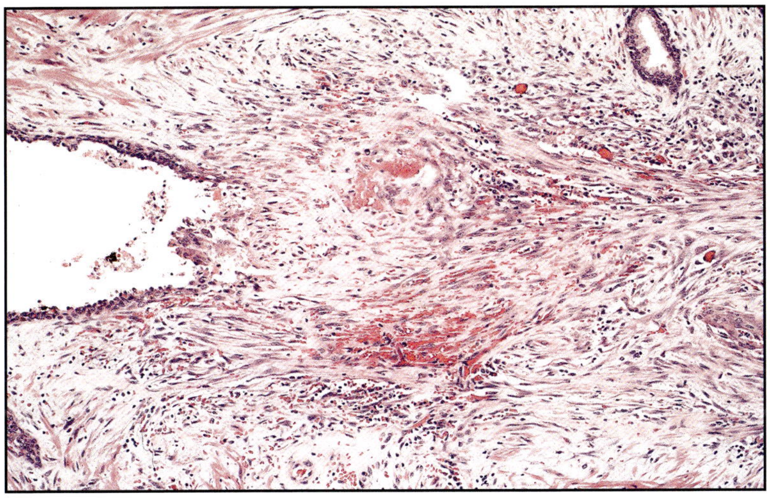

■ **i2.13** *Acute and chronic inflammatory cell infiltrates are commonly seen around needle tracks.*

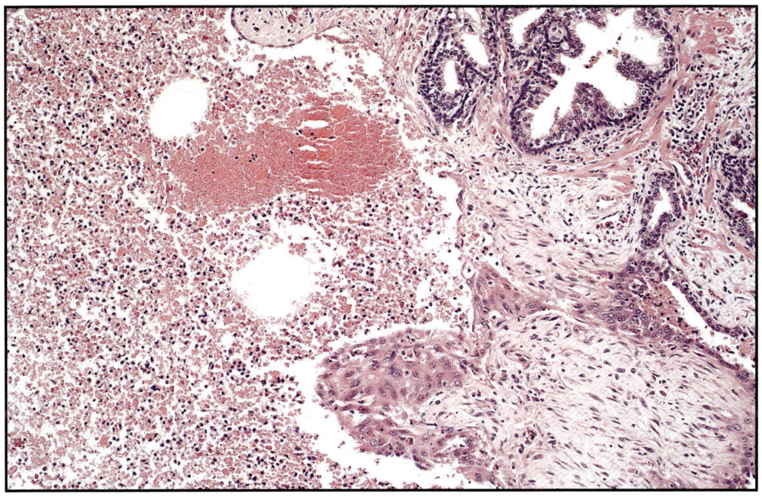

■ **i2.14** *Cystic glandular change induced by needle biopsy, with intracystic cellular debris and blood. Basal cell prominence is present in a few glands (upper right).*

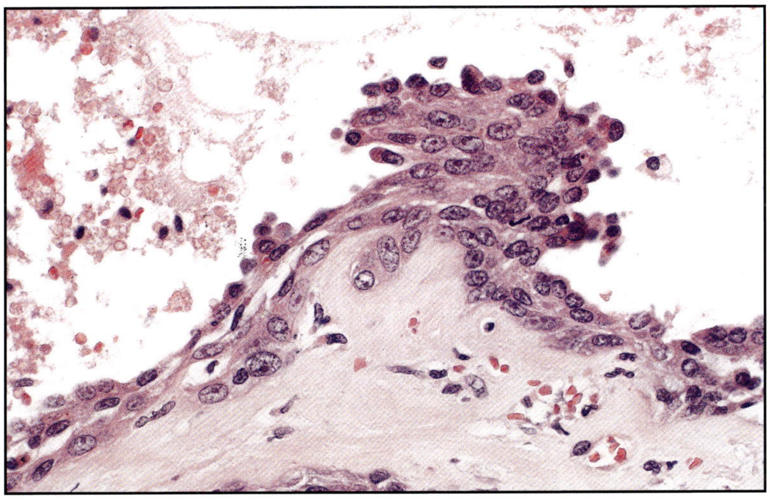

■ **i2.15** *Gland along biopsy track with mound of squamous metaplastic cells surrounded by flattened metaplastic lining layer.*

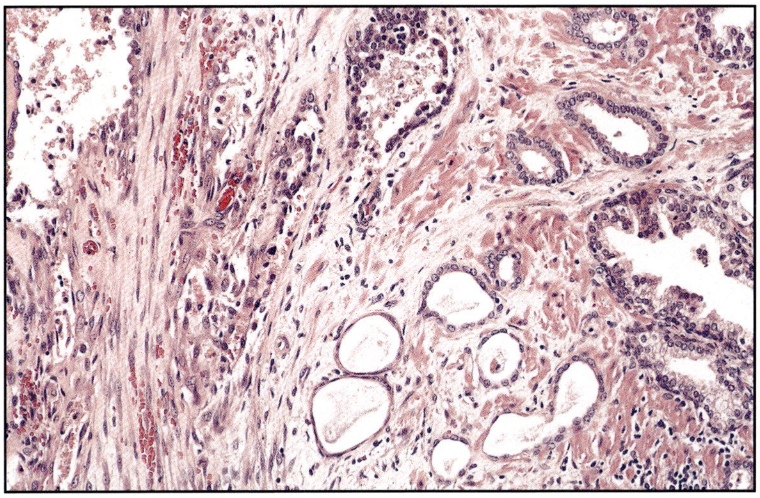

■ **i2.16** *Atrophic appearance of prostatic adenocarcinoma next to biopsy track.*

Handling and processing of the needle biopsy tissue begins in the office or room where the biopsy is performed. In the biopsy suite, the needle biopsy tissue should be gently placed immediately into a container with fixative. Stretching and orientation of the cores between 2 meshes in tissue cassettes before biopsy fixation appears to enhance diagnostic yield (Rogatsch 2000). The fixative usually is 10% neutral buffered formalin, although some laboratories prefer Bouin's solution, which is a picric acid fixative. Hollande's solution is another

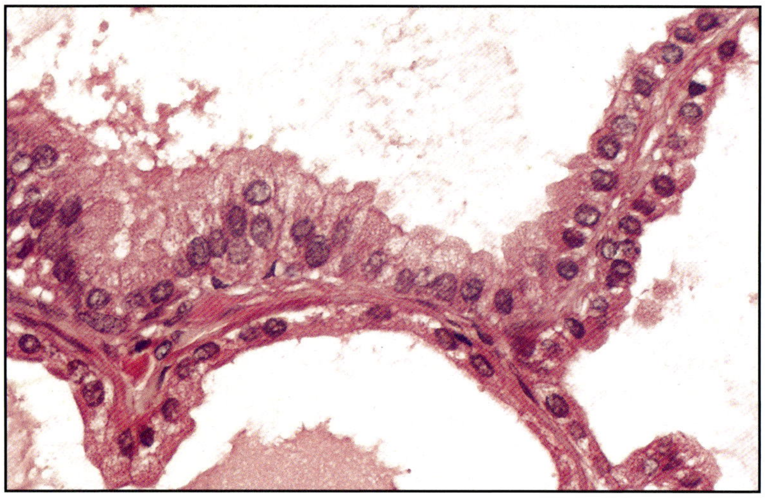

■ **i2.17** *Nuclear detail in cells of a benign prostate gland fixed in Bouin's fluid.*

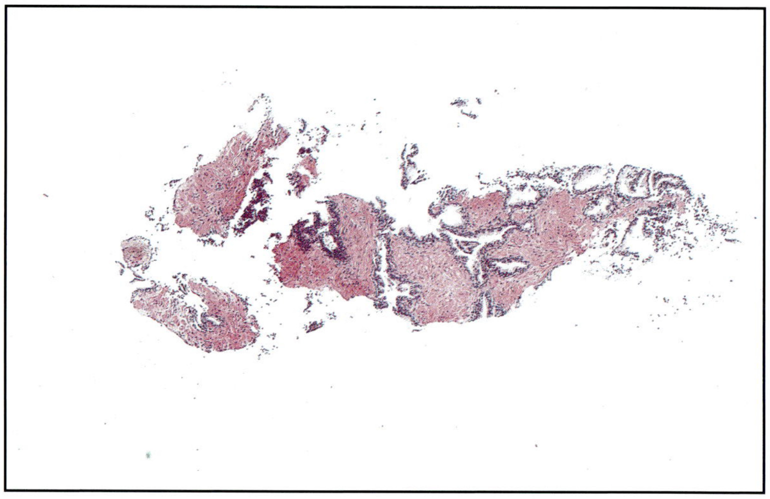

■ **i2.18** *Fragmented prostate needle cores.*

picric acid–based fixative that has been forwarded as an alternative to formalin fixation for prostate biopsies (Murphy 1993). Both Bouin's and Hollande's solutions provide superior nuclear preservation and detail compared with formalin **i2.17**, but picric acid is a strong oxidizing agent that reacts violently with combustible materials and reducing agents (Woods 1994). It is also a neurotoxin. The powder form is explosive when dry (Woods 1994). For these reasons, many laboratories choose not to work with picric acid–based fixatives.

Formalin fixation of core needle biopsies should be for 4 to 8 hours, with a goal of at least 6 hours, to minimize tissue fragmentation **i2.18** and to optimize preservation of nuclear detail (Delahunt 1998, Feldman 1995). Because of shearing forces generated by the firing of the biopsy needle into the gland, a degree of nuclear distortion may be unavoidable in needle biopsy (McNeal 1988), particularly at the edges of the needle biopsy tissue.

The number of needle cores placed into an individual container with fixative is highly variable. For sextant biopsies, the doctor performing the biopsy may place a single needle core in each of 6 separate containers, 3 biopsies from each side in 1 container, or all 6 or more biopsies in a single container **i2.19**. We render a separate diagnosis for each separately submitted container, using the site designation for that container. We have been asked in the past to render separate diagnoses on color-coded needle biopsies (with different color ink applied to different needle cores from different sites) submitted in the same container, but we have not agreed to this because prostate needle biopsies may fragment, thereby rendering assignment of a specific needle biopsy fragment to a specific site difficult or impossible.

Most prostate needle biopsy cores are received in the laboratory in containers with fixative. Rarely, the attending physician may request a frozen section on a prostate needle biopsy. There are specific clinical indications for performing a frozen section on prostate needle core tissue **t2.3**. Only patients with

■ **t 2.3 Clinical Indications for Frozen Section of Prostate Needle Biopsy**

Confirmation of a clinical diagnosis of metastatic prostate cancer, which is to be treated by immediate orchiectomy
Not indicated in clinically localized prostate cancer

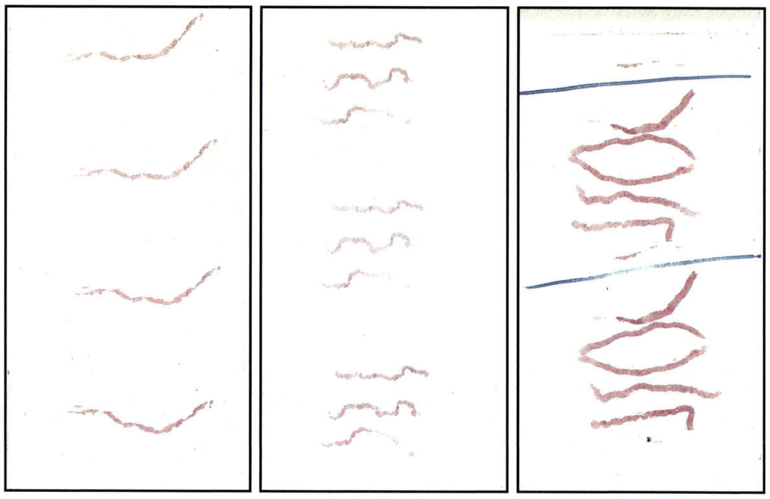

■ **i2.19** *Sections from blocks with one (left slide), three (middle slide), and six (right slide) needle cores. One of the cores from the six core slide is only partially sampled. A potential difficulty with embedding more than 3 cores in a single block is alignment of all cores in a single plane so that all cores are well-sampled when histologic sections are taken.*

substantial clinical evidence of metastatic prostate cancer who are to undergo immediate orchiectomy (usually for pain relief) are candidates for frozen section preparations of prostate needle biopsies. The few prostate needle biopsy frozen sections I have seen in this setting have been diagnostically straightforward, with high-grade carcinoma involving much of the needle core. We refuse frozen section requests on prostate needle biopsies from patients with clinically localized disease.

Gross handling and sampling of prostate needle biopsies received in containers with fixative are the second level of processing. Recommendations for gross examination and description of prostate needle biopsies have been generated (ADASP 1996, Delahunt 1998, Harden 1995, Henson 1994, Srigley 2000) **t2.4**. The gross or macroscopic examination of the needle cores is not diagnostic but is important for correlation with amount of tissue seen in histologic sections. Therefore, it is particularly important to record size and number of tissue cores or fragments (using a no-touch technique). Color of the cores should be described, and, specifically, the presence and extent of yellow coloration, which could suggest adipose tissue (if at the tips of a core) or malignancy (Delahunt 1998),

■ t2.4 Recommendations for Gross Examination and Reporting for Prostate Needle Biopsies

How container is labeled	Patient name, birthdate, identification number, container number, anatomic site
Specimen fresh or in fixative (specify type)	
Size, number of pieces, and orientation (if designated)	
Recognizable gross features	
Amount submitted for histologic precessing	
Total	
Selected sample	
Submitted for special studies (name)	
Paraffin block key	

From checklists in ADASP 1996, Henson 1994, Srigley 2000

■ t2.5 Indications for Additional Sections of Prostate Needle Biopsies

Small amount of tissue on the slide compared with tissue remaining in the block
No prostate epithelium identified
Focal glandular atypia
Evaluation of necrosis
Evaluation of crush artifact
Initial sections too thick and/or poorly stained
Performance of histochemical stains
Performance of immunohistochemical stain (usually 34βE12 stain)

should be mentioned. This finding of yellow coloration in needle biopsy has not been proven to be a specific finding. If the cores have been inked before receipt in the laboratory, this should be noted. Inking may be performed to indicate location of a particular core (although as previously mentioned, such a practice is to be discouraged) or to indicate orientation of the needle (deep vs superficial and capsular). There is no known clinical or histopathologic advantage in demonstrating this orientation. The only definitive method of detecting periprostatic tissue in needle biopsy is identification of adipose tissue or seminal vesicle tissue under the light microscope, and so orienting the needle cores as to which is the capsular end is not necessary. Orientation of cores by placement on labeled blotting paper (in the biopsy suite), with subsequent pre-embedding in agar and use of colored agar markers, has been reported (Shaw 1996), but such orientation is not of proven utility.

Submission of prostate needle cores for processing and embedding is driven by container number and number of cores per container. We submit cores from separate containers, which usually represent different biopsy sites, into separate cassettes for processing. To reiterate, if the referring and attending physician wants a separate diagnosis for different biopsy sites, those biopsies should be submitted in separate, site-designated containers. Any number of cores may be received in a single container. When we receive 1 to 3 cores, they are placed (between sponges) into a single cassette. If more than 3 cores are received in a single container, the cores are placed in separate cassettes, with no more than 3 per cassette. It is possible to process and embed more than 3 cores per cassette, but this is not desirable because of the likelihood of fragmentation, the difficulty in even histologic sampling of 4 or more cores, and the ability to mount only 2 sections per slide rather than a mean of 4, which is the average in our laboratory (Reyes 1998). Embedding 1 core per block seems to optimize surface representation (Kao 2002) and diagnostic yield (Srigley 2001), but this may be costly in terms of block and slide generation when 12 or more cores are submitted for each case.

Prostate needle biopsies should be submitted in toto for processing and embedding. The cores can be marked with ink; this facilitates identification and correct orientation of the cores during embedding (Winsor 1994) and enhances the ability to see the cores in the paraffin blocks. The cores should be placed into a cassette after being put into a fine mesh envelope, wrapped in lens paper, sandwiched between sponge biopsy pads, or double-embedded in agar-paraffin wax (Winsor 1994). Biopsy bags or envelopes probably should be avoided because tissue defects ("biopsy bag artifact") may result (Niemann 1998). After processing (Winsor 1994), the cores should be embedded in the same plane to ensure even sampling of all cores upon sectioning of the block. Also, ease of microscopic examination is enhanced by orienting the cores in the same direction along the long axis of the mold (Winsor 1994), with the cores evenly spaced and parallel to one another **i2.19**. If fragmented, the core fragments should be placed in a row along the long axis of the mold (Winsor 1994).

The third level of sampling is at the step of procurement of sections from the paraffin block. There is little standardization of sampling at this step (Delahunt 1998, Humphrey 1993A). Until recently, there were few data on methods of block sectioning and slide preparation that would optimize cancer detection. Emerging data suggest that preparing 3 hematoxylin and eosin (H&E)-stained slides, each with several 4µm sections (usually 3 to 4 serial sections) on each slide, is an optimal initial approach (Brat 1999, Lane 1998B, Renshaw 1997A). This is also our standard approach (Humphrey 1993A). There are many variations of this approach, with most involving the retention of interval, unstained sections on coated slides for special studies such as 34βE12 immunohistochemical staining for basal cells (Abboud 1998, Green 1999) or retaining additional slides beyond the first slide for additional H&E or immunohistochemical staining (Delahunt 1998). In our experience, preparing 3 H&E slides (levels) with 3 or 4 5µm serial sections per slide has been the method of choice. If immunohistochemistry for basal cells is necessary (and we uncommonly use this immunostain [Reyes 1998, Thorson 1998]), we perform the immunostain on additional sections of the block or on one of the initial H&E-stained sections after destaining.

There are numerous indications for obtaining additional sections of prostate needle biopsies in the paraffin block, beyond the initial set of 3 slides **t2.5** (Humphrey 1993A). First, if the dimensions of the histologic sections of tissue on the glass slide are less than the dictated gross description or if the amount of tissue sampled is increasing from slide 1 to 3, the block should be examined and additional levels ordered. Second, if no prostatic epithelium is identified and the targeted biopsy site is prostatic parenchyma (rather than seminal vesicle, for example), then additional levels should be requested. A typical problem here is that bladder neck tissue is sampled rather than prostatic parenchyma, and sections show abundant smooth muscle bundles, without prostatic epithelium **i2.8**. If prostatic parenchyma is not represented on the glass slides despite additional levels, one should report the specific tissue components identified (such as smooth muscle or seminal vesicle) rather than rendering a diagnosis of "inadequate." Third, if the initial 3 sections are remarkable for a focal atypical glandular or atypical small acinar proliferation that is worrisome but not diagnostic for carcinoma, then additional sections on an

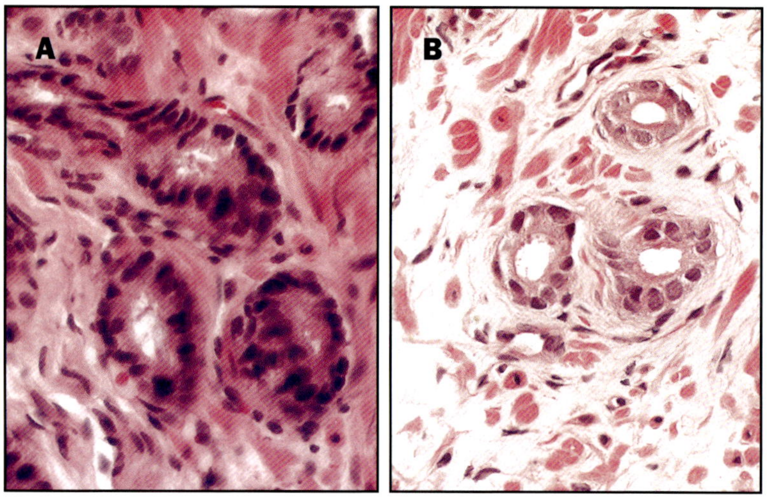

■ **i2.20** *Initial thick section of adenocarcinoma (A), with thin 3μm additional section procured in levels (B).*

additional slide should be cut and stained with H&E. We found that when we completely sectioned through prostate needle biopsy cases of focal glandular atypia (FGA), a definitive diagnosis of carcinoma could be rendered in 10% of cases (Reyes 1998) because sampling of the atypical glands was more extensive. Complete histologic sampling of prostate needle biopsies entailed an average of 30 slides (with an average of 4 5-μm sections per slide), but because diagnostic carcinoma was identified in sections on slide number 4 after an initial diagnosis of FGA was given on the initial 3 slides, our current practice is to obtain a single additional level (single slide with several sections), with H&E staining or 34βE12 immunostaining, or several levels after an initial diagnosis of FGA. Of significance, no carcinoma was identified in the completely sectioned prostate needle biopsy tissue after a diagnosis of benign prostatic tissue or high-grade prostatic intraepithelial neoplasia (PIN) was rendered on the initial set of 3 slides. Therefore, we do not currently obtain levels after a diagnosis of high-grade PIN in the initial 3 slides. Additional findings in the first 3 slides that might prompt ordering of levels include further evaluation of atypical features such as intraluminal wispy blue mucin or crystalloids, although the yield rate of diagnostic carcinoma from such additional levels is not known. Necrosis in prostate needle biopsies should be thoroughly studied, and if the nature of the process associated with necrosis (eg, bacille Calmette-Guérin granulomas vs infarct vs tumoral necrosis) is not clear, levels may be helpful. If there is crush artifact and distortion of cells, levels may be productive in clarifying the nature of the cells. Also, if the initial sections are technically suboptimal because they were poorly stained, folded, or too thick **i2.20A**, thin 3μm levels **i2.20B** may be helpful. Additional sections for performing histochemical stains rarely are needed. Fungal prostatitis, mycobacterial prostatitis, and malakoplakia of the prostate necessitate use of appropriate histochemical stains for diagnosis. Finally, as noted earlier, interval levels or additional levels may be necessary for applying a 34βE12 immunohistochemical stain for basal cells. Other situations in which levels for immunohistochemical staining are important include the differential diagnosis of granulomatous prostatitis and carcinoma, of poorly differentiated prostatic carcinoma and poorly differentiated transitional cell carcinoma, and of poorly differentiated prostatic adenocarcinoma, lymphoma, and small cell carcinoma (Humphrey 1993A).

[2.3] Transurethral Prostatectomy (TURP)

The most common clinical indication for endoscopic TURP is as treatment for prostatism symptoms (eg, decrease in force and caliber of stream, urinary frequency, urgency, and nocturia) in patients with obstructing BPH (Holtgrewe 1995, Mebust 1989, Fitzpatrick 2002). TURP can also be performed to relieve obstruction in patients with known carcinoma; this procedure accounted for 10% of TURPs in one series (Mebust 1989). Loop resection to encompass both prostatic urethral mucosa and prostatic parenchyma is also performed in the setting of selected site mucosal mapping and sampling in patients with bladder cancer (Hudson 1996). What is not a clinical practice is to sample the prostate with an intent to detect prostate cancer by TURP for persistently elevated serum PSA after multiple negative transrectal biopsies (Rovner 1997) because there is a negligible yield rate.

The amount of prostate tissue sampled by TURP is variable, with a range of 5 to more than 75g of resected tissue (Green 1996). The mean weight of resected tissue was 22 to 26g in two large series (Green 1996, Mebust 1989). Patients with larger glands had more tissue resected and a greater percentage of the gland resected (Green 1996). Therefore, the number of TURP chips received by the laboratory is highly variable. Tissues sampled by TURP include transition zone **i2.21**, urethral and periurethral tissues **i2.22**, bladder neck fragments **i2.23**, and anterior fibromuscular stroma (McNeal 1988). Apical skeletal muscle and adipose tissue can also be seen **i2.24, i2.25**, as well as seminal vesicle tissue in 3% to 23% of cases (Jensen 1983, Tsuang 1981). Although the intent of the surgery is to remove transition zone hyperplastic nodules, complete removal of the transition zone does not occur (McNeal 1988). The histologic composition of the resected tissue depends on the size of the specimen: in the smallest resections (6g of tissue), mainly bladder neck and anterior fibromuscular tissue is removed, and in the largest specimens (43g) normal transition zone tissue and hyperplastic nodules are the principal sampled tissues (Price 1990). Almost always the TURP chips are received in containers with fixative, usually formalin. No established indicators exist for performing frozen section of TURP chips.

The gross description **t2.6** should include, most importantly, the weight of all chips (ADASP 1996, Henson 1994, Srigley 2000). The 3-dimensional aggregate size can also be measured, but it is not necessary to grossly count the number of chips unless only a few are submitted.

■ **t2.6 Recommendations for Gross Examination and Reporting for TURP Chips**

How container is labeled
- Patient name, birthdate, identification number, container number, anatomic site

Specimen fresh or in fixative (Specify type and volume of fixative)
Weight of chips (In grams)
Recognizable gross features: Size, color and shape of chips
Amount submitted for histologic processing
- Total
- Partial
- Submitted for special studies (name)

Paraffin block key

Modified from checklists in ADASP 1996, Henson 1994, Srigley 2000

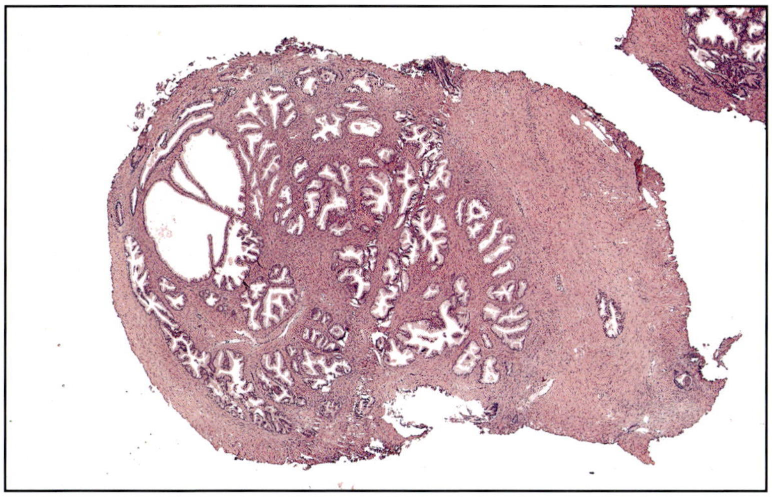

■ **i2.21** *Transition zone nodule of glandular and stromal hyperplasia (BPH) sampled by TURP.*

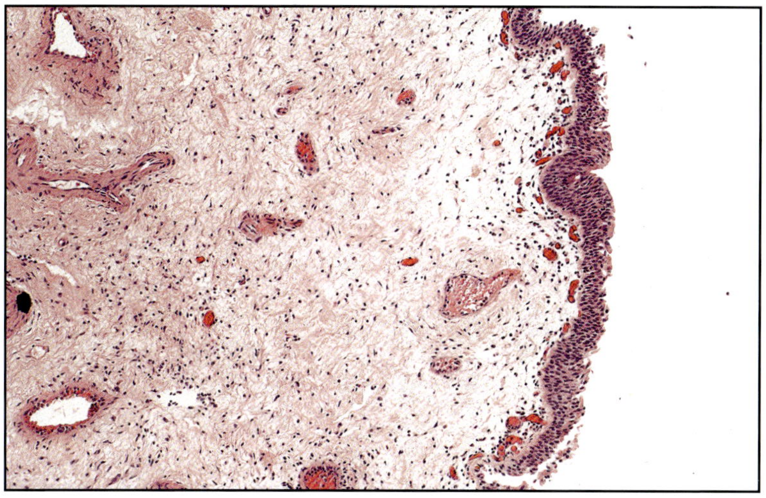

■ **i2.22** *Urothelium of prostatic urethral and periurethral tissues sampled by TURP.*

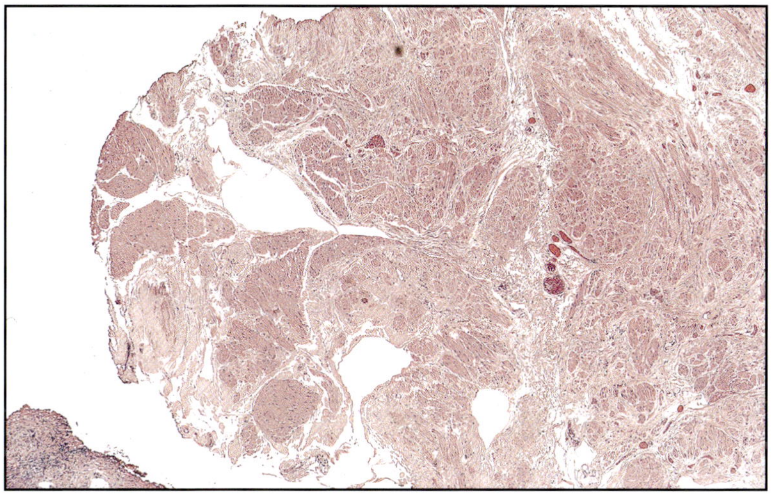

■ **i2.23** *Thick smooth muscle bundles sampled by TURP.*

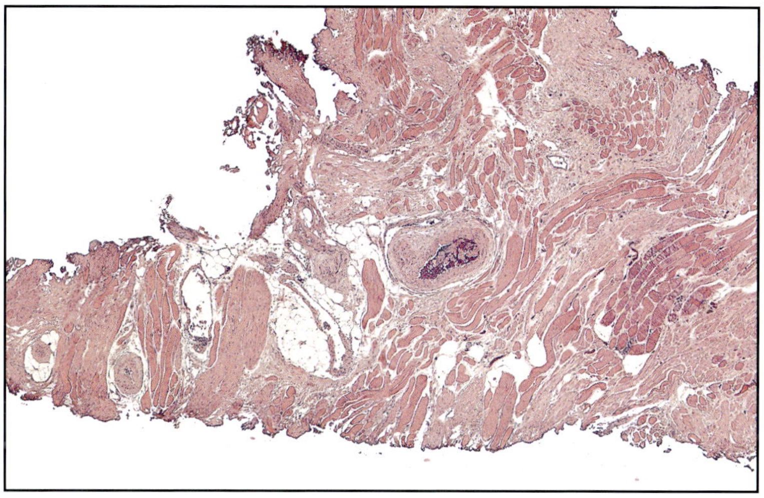

■ **i2.24** *Skeletal muscle and adipose tissue from apex, sampled by TURP: Low magnification.*

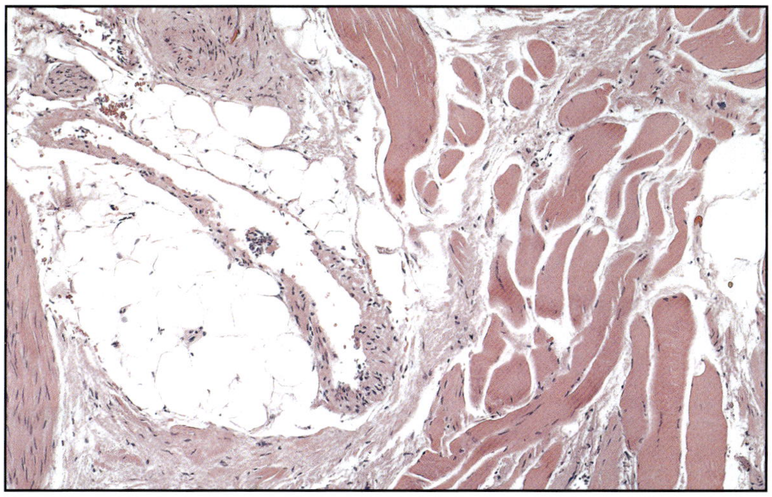

■ **i2.25** *Skeletal muscle and adipose tissue from apex, sampled by TURP: High magnification.*

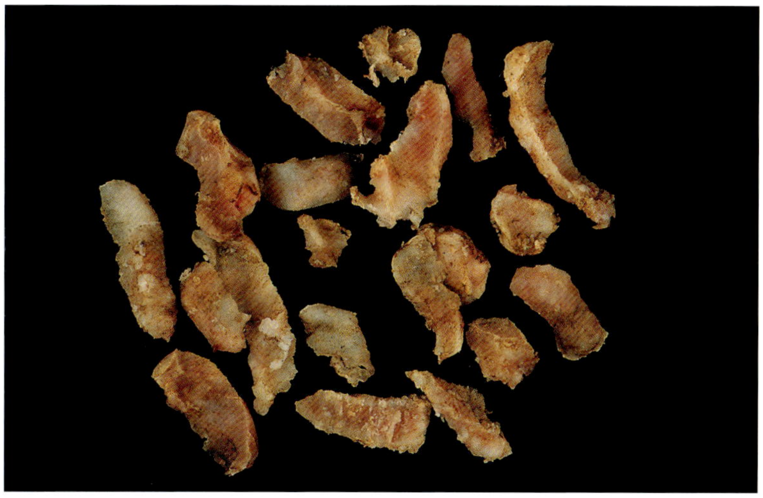

■ **i2.26** *Variable size, shape and coloration of TURP chips.*

"Recognizable gross features" (Henson 1994) should be recorded, but the gross features of TURP chips generally are not of value in identifying chips with carcinoma **i2.26** (Mills 1990, Murphy 1989). Yellow and indurated chips may be grossly suggestive of carcinoma, but this coloration correlates microscopically with cellular and epithelial proliferation in general, not carcinoma specifically (Mills 1990). Furthermore, palpable abnormalities in prostatic chips with adenocarcinoma usually are not evident. However, some recommendations have been made regarding the selection of chips for sampling. It has been recommended that the pathologist ask the urologist to place firmer chips and chips from more peripheral areas into a different container and to embed all these tissues while partially sampling the other chips and also to select yellow to

■ **t2.7 Clinical Stage T1a & T1b Cancer Defined by Percentage of TURP Tissue Involved by Tumor**

TNM	Whitmore-Jewett	Description
T1	A	Clinically inapparent tumor Not palpable or visible by imaging
T1a	A1	Tumor found incidentally in 5% or less of TURP chip tissue
T1b	A2	Tumor found incidentally in more than 5% of TURP chip or tissue

Histologic grade is also used in the distinction between T1a and T1b where T1a is considered low-grade and T1b high-grade carcinoma. Variable definitions of "low-grade" carcinoma have been used, though, with some considering Gleason score 2-4 low-grade and others viewing Gleason score 2-6 as low-grade (Humphrey 1993C), and Gleason score 2-7 as low to moderate grade (Monda 1994)

yellow-gray and firm to solid chips (Mostofi 1986). Selecting smaller chips, which may represent peripheral resections that may be more likely to harbor carcinoma, has also been advised (Schmidt 1983). However, the peripheral zone usually is not sampled by TURP (McNeal 1988). Furthermore, the selection of medium-sized chips has also been recommended (Moore 1986). Because a rigorous, controlled study of the value of chip selection based on chip color and size has not been performed, we suggest random chip selection if chips are to be partially submitted.

Gross sampling of prostatic chips in the pathology laboratory is important because the degree of sampling is related to the frequency of detection of incidental carcinoma (stage A or T1 carcinoma). These clinical stage T1 carcinomas are defined as those that are not palpable or visible by imaging (Greene 2002) **t2.7**. (Histologic grade is also used in the definition of T1 substages [Eble 1990]). Such clinically unsuspected carcinoma is diagnosed by histologic examination in about 12% to 16% of TURP cases (Humphrey 1993A, Mebust 1989). The critical issue is how many chips should be grossly submitted to identify, in a cost-effective manner, clinically significant prostate cancer. Many of these incidentally detected prostate cancers are of transition zone origin and are small, involving 5% or less of chip tissue (stage A1 or T1a), but some tumors are of higher volume (greater than 5% involvement). T1a cancers are clearly of lower biologic aggressiveness than T1b tumors. At radical prostatectomy, 94% of T1a patients have organ-confined tumors compared with 68% of T1b patients (Catalona 1990, Partin 1993, Zincke 1994). Moreover, the clinical progression rate for T1a disease, at 8% to 27% (Blute 1986, Cheng 1998, Epstein 1986B, Lowe 1988, Roy 1990, Thompson 1989), is less than that for T1b disease, at 33% (Epstein 1986B). Therefore, it is desirable to detect as many T1b cancers as possible because those patients should be treated (van Andel 1995), whereas the need to detect all T1a cancers is not as clear because aggressive treatment is not necessary for most T1a patients, except those who are less than 60 years old (Lowe 1996).

The number of prostatic chips to submit for microscopic examination is controversial (Eble 1990, Harden 1995, Mills 1990, Vollmer 1989). It is clear that unless all prostatic chip tissue is submitted, with generation of a single section from each block, some carcinomas will be missed. However, it is not currently the standard of practice in pathology to submit all prostatic chip tissue when more than 10g of chips is received (Golimbu 1981). Only 11% of pathologists entirely embed all TURP chips regardless of weight (True 1994). Also not standardized is how many chips to place in a single tissue cassette; recommendations range from only a few chips per block to crowding of chips into each cassette. Such crowding translates into about 2.5g per block **i2.27A,B**. The correct number of chips that should be placed in each cassette has not been rigorously studied, but Vollmer, in his review (Vollmer 1989), did not ascribe critical significance to the amount of tissue per block. Like others (Mills 1990, Murphy 1989, Vollmer 1989), we recommend that 1 to 2g of

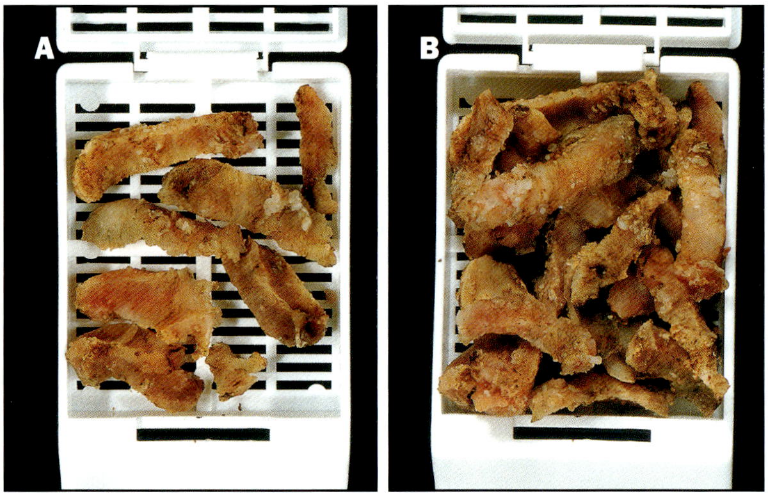

■ **i2.27** *Tissue cassette loaded with (A) 1g of TURP chips, and (B) 2.5g of TURP chips.*

prostatic chips be placed in each cassette. The chips should not be so tightly packed that some lie on top of others **i2.27B**, such that only some of the chips are sampled on sectioning (Mostofi 1982).

Should all prostatic chips be submitted, with generation of a single histologic section from each block? For detection of 90% of incidental stage T1a (A1) carcinomas and detection of all stage T1b (A2) tumors, 12g or 5 to 8 blocks of tissue should be submitted (Murphy 1986, Rohr 1987, Vollmer 1986). If one uses these guidelines, 10% of stage A1 carcinomas will be missed. Will this nondetection rate affect these patients? Usually not, because T1a (A1) carcinomas are small and of low histologic grade, but as noted, 8% to 27% of these patients experience clinical progression. Additionally, 20% to 30% of stage T1a (A1) patients have a significant amount of residual tumor in the prostate gland (Greene 1991, Larsen 1991). Based on these data, one approach would be to submit all prostatic chip tissue from younger patients (under 60 years of age) in whom clinical tumor progression of a stage T1a (A1) carcinoma may affect lifespan, whereas partial sampling to entail submission of 12g or 5 to 8 blocks may be sufficient for older patients (Vollmer 1989). A potential difficulty with this approach is that some older patients live beyond the average lifespan and then may be affected by clinical progression of a stage T1a (A1) carcinoma. Some therefore advocate complete submission of chips for all patients. The issue of whether to partially or completely submit TURP chips is likely to remain controversial.

The indications for submitting additional tissue after microscopic examination of partially submitted chips also are not standardized. Some favor submitting the remainder of the tissue if an incidental carcinoma is detected by histologic examination of the partially submitted chips (Henson 1994, Mills 1990, Schmidt 1983), whereas others do not (Mills 1990). One study (Fan 1983) did not find a significant difference in

■ t2.8 Recommendations for Gross TURP Chip Sampling

Initially submit 12g of tissue or 5-8 cassettes
If patient is younger than 60, submit all tissue
If high-grade prostatic intraepithelial neoplasia, atypical adenomatous hyperplasia (adenosis), or focal glandular atypia suspicious for malignancy, is found in initial sections of partially submitted chips, submit remaining chips

percentage carcinoma in TURP chips that were partially submitted when compared with complete submission of the same cases, and in no case was the patient classified up or down into the next stage subgroup of T1a versus T1b. Yet another investigation recommended complete submission after discovery of T1a but not T1b carcinoma on the initial slides, but this was based on upstaging of only 1 case (McDowell 1994). One should also consider embedding more tissue after detecting high-grade PIN, atypical adenomatous hyperplasia (adenosis), or FGA in the initial sections of a case of partially submitted chips, but no data exist to provide definitive guidance on this issue. Because PIN, adenosis, and FGA have been associated with malignancy (although adenosis is controversial in this regard), submitting the remaining tissue seems reasonable. The recommendations of this author for TURP chip sampling are in **t2.8**. The costs of submitting additional tissue beyond partial sampling have been studied (Eble 1986, Vollmer 1986, 1989) and should be a minor consideration in this debate of partial versus complete sampling and complete sampling after initial partial sampling.

Typically, only 1 H&E-stained slide with 1 or 2 sections is prepared from each paraffin block of TURP chips **i2.28**. The indications for obtaining additional histologic sections or levels from paraffin blocks with embedded TURP chips are similar but not identical to indications for levels of needle biopsies. One should first consider differences in the feasibility of serially sectioning TURP chips rather than needle biopsies. Serial sectioning of paraffin blocks with TURP chips increases the detection rate of incidental carcinomas (Suzuki 1988), but complete serial sectioning is a difficult undertaking and is clearly not practical. Consider that for a 3mm block with TURP chips, complete sectioning through the block would theoretically require 600 5μm histologic sections and slides. For a case with 5 blocks, this would mean that 3000 slides would need to be examined under the microscope. The true incidence of incidental carcinoma in TURP chips will not be known until such a sampling method is applied to a large series of cases; such a study, if ever performed, would require hundreds of thousands of slides. Therefore, TURP specimens differ from needle biopsies in that it is easy to serially section through a paraffin block with a needle biopsy, whereas it is not practical to serially section through any block with TURP chips. The issue of whether obtaining additional levels of TURP chips will result in detection of clinically significant prostate cancers has not been addressed. The indications for obtaining additional levels of needle biopsies, as listed in **t2.5**, may also be considered to be valid indications for TURP chips, with the following qualifiers. First, some pathologists do not obtain levels to address the differential diagnosis of atypical adenomatous hyperplasia (adenosis) and well-differentiated adenocarcinoma. This relates in part to the controversy surrounding the premalignant potential of adenosis; some investigators consider adenosis to be a marker for carcinoma, like PIN, whereas others do not favor this concept. Second, infarction with coagulative necrosis is more likely to be encountered in TURP chips than in needle biopsies because nodular hyperplasia often undergoes infarction and occurs within the transition zone, which is the zone most prominently

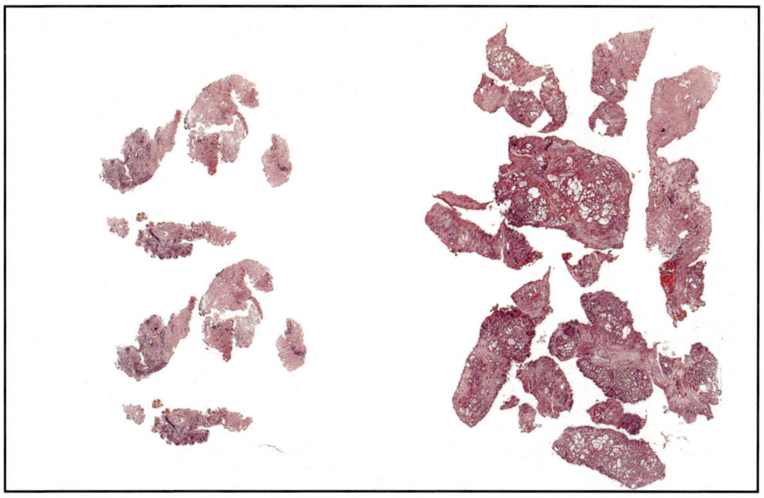

■ i2.28 *Several sections may be placed on a glass slide if only a few chips are embedded (left), but often only a single section per slide is possible (right).*

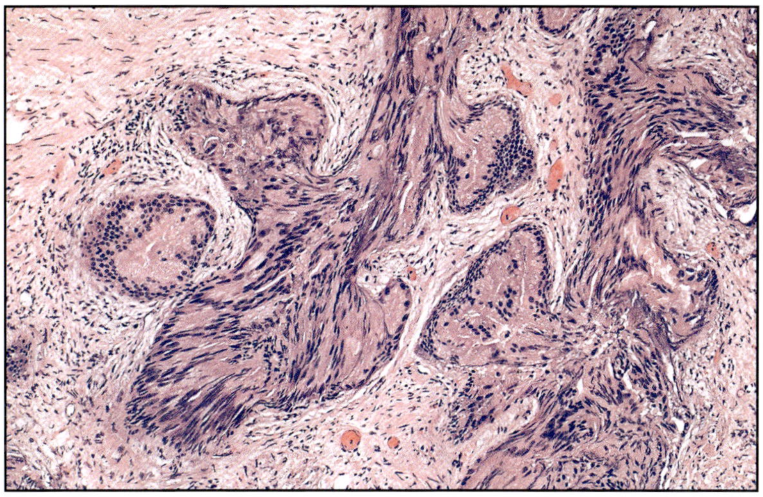

■ i2.29 *Cauterized high-grade PIN in TURP chip.*

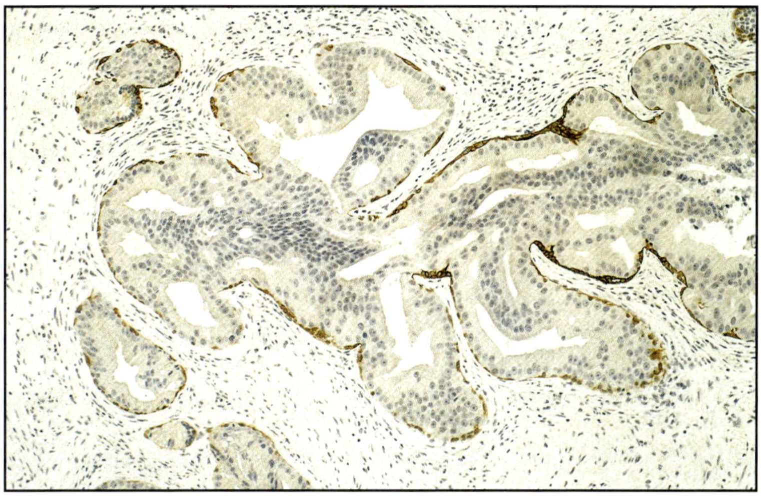

■ i2.30 *Absence of cautery artifact in deeper section from block with cauterized PIN in TURP chip depicted in* **i2.29**. *(34βE12 immunostain highlights basal cells in PIN glands.)*

sampled by TURP. One should always attempt to ascertain what type of tissue is necrotic because both hyperplastic and carcinomatous tissue may infarct. Third, an artifact that is unique to TURP chip tissue as compared with needle biopsy is cautery artifact. This artifact may be extensive and obscure a focus of concern **i2.29**; levels may then identify a diagnostic noncauterized area **i2.30**. Smooth muscle of the bladder

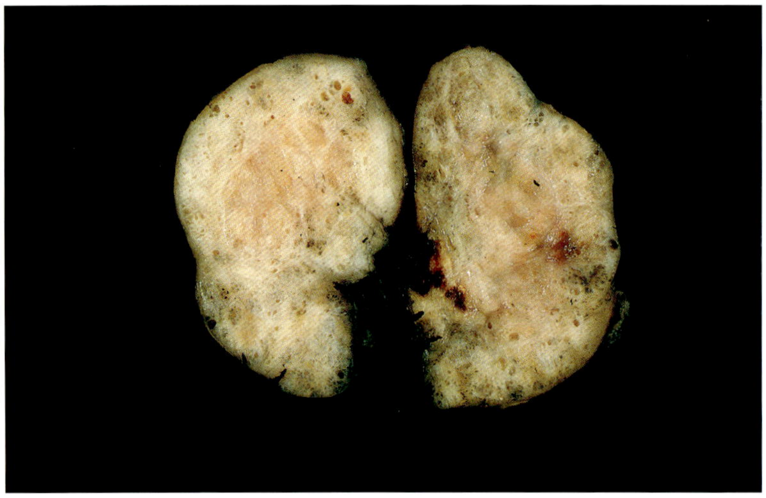

■ **i2.31** *Cut surfaces of a bivalved 263g simple prostatectomy specimen. Extensive nodular hyperplasia, but no carcinoma, was detected on H&E-stained sections.*

■ t2.9	Recommendations for Gross Examination & Reporting for Suprapubic or Retropubic Simple (Enucleation) Prostatectomy

How container is labeled:
- Patient name, birthdate, identification number, container number, anatomic site

Specimen fresh or in fixative (Specify type & volume of fixative)
Number of tissue pieces
Size in three dimensions
Weight of chips (In grams)
Recognizable gross features: Size, color and shape
Amount submitted for histologic processing
- Total
- Partial
- Submitted for special studies (none)

Paraffin block key

Modified from checklists in ADASP 1996, Henson 1994, Srigley 2000

■ t2.10	Recommendations for Gross (Enucleation) Prostatectomy Sampling

Initially submit one cassette for each 5g of tissue or eight cassettes total
Submit additional tissue if carcinoma is detected in initial sections

neck is more likely to be found in TURP specimens than in needle biopsies **i2.23**. If atypical glands are identified in this tissue, additional levels are indicated to rule out carcinoma, even if carcinoma is present elsewhere in the TURP chips, because carcinoma in bladder neck tissue usually signals extensive carcinoma.

[2.4] Open Suprapubic or Retropubic Simple Prostatectomy (Enucleation) Tissue

In about 10% of men with clinically evident BPH, an open or simple prostatectomy is performed rather than TURP (Stutzman 1992). In this operation the hyperplastic mass (often incorrectly called an adenoma) is enucleated by a direct incision through the anterior prostate (in the retropubic approach) or by an extraperitoneal incision of the lower anterior bladder wall (Oesterling 1998). The peripheral zone is not removed and may be the soil for subsequent development of carcinoma.

A single mass **i2.31** or 2 masses (lobes) or pieces are received in the surgical pathology laboratory in fixative. No attached seminal vesicles are present, as in radical prostatectomy specimens. Even though this is not a cancer operation, and the operation is contraindicated if the patient has prostate cancer, we prefer to ink the periphery of the surgical specimen (with India ink) because incidental (stage T1) carcinoma has been detected in 4% to 13% of open prostatectomy cases (Bauer 1960, Delides 1976, Labess 1952, Stillwell 1989, Trieger 1948). The India ink can be fixed in place with acetone or Bouin's solution and blotted dry.

Grossly, areas of carcinomas may be yellow and firmer when compared with hyperplastic tissue but, as with TURP chips, this is not completely reliable (Murphy 1989). Each piece of prostatectomy tissue should be weighed and sectioned at 3mm to 5mm intervals. The gross description for each piece should also include size in 3 dimensions, weight (in grams), firmness, coloration, and texture (Schmidt 1983) **t2.9**.

No consensus exists on sampling of open prostatectomy tissue (Golimbu 1981). Submission of specific sections (including urethral mucosa, verumontanum, capsule, hard nodules, median bar, lateral lobes, nodules adjacent to normal tissue, and regions differing in color and texture) (Schmidt 1983) and random sections, with preferential sampling of peripheral areas (Murphy 1989), has been recommended. The optimum number of blocks to submit has not been studied in detail, but a minimum of 1 cassette for each 5g of tissue (Schmidt 1983) or 8 cassettes (Henson 1994) has been recommended **t2.10**.

It is not clear whether additional tissue should be submitted after detection of carcinoma in initial sections, although this has been recommended (ADASP 1996, Henson 1994). These recommendations do not specify exactly how many additional cassettes should be submitted. It also has not been established whether additional cassettes of tissue should be submitted after a diagnosis of high-grade PIN, atypical adenomatous hyperplasia (adenosis), or FGA in initial sections.

A single H&E slide should be prepared from each block. No study on serial sectioning of paraffin blocks with open prostatectomy tissue has been performed; the indications for levels are essentially the same as those described earlier for TURP chips.

[2.5] Radical Perineal and Retropubic Prostatectomy

The entire prostate gland is excised in cancer surgery for prostate cancer (radical prostatectomy) or for bladder cancer (radical cysto-prostatectomy).

Radical prostatectomy to treat prostate cancer may be performed via a perineal (Gibbons 2002) or, more commonly, a retropubic (Walsh 2002) approach. These 2 surgical approaches seem to yield similar outcomes in terms of preservation of potency, positive surgical margins, and biochemical failure (elevated postoperative serum PSA) rates (Boccon-Gibod 1998, Gibbons 2002). However, the perineal approach may be associated with a higher

■ **t2.11 Pretreatment Prediction of Pelvic Lymph Node Metastasis**

Study	Model	Comment
Ackerman 1993	PSA density, number of positive cases	Formula devised that had 70% accuracy in predicting lymph node status
Sands 1994	PSA, histologic grade, clinical stage	Probability tables developed based on all three parameters
Kleer 1993	Probability plots generated from local clinical stage (determined by DRE), histologic grade, & serum PSA	Predicted probability curve for lymph node involvement was presented
Arai 1990	Group A: Serum PSA <10 ng/mL and Gleason score 2-7	Only 1/18 patients (6%) in group A had lymph node metastasis versus 12/17 (71%) in group B
	Group B: Serum PSA>10 ng/mL and Gleason score 8-10	
Bishoff 1995	Combination of serum PSA, clinical stage, & biopsy Gleason score	It is proposed that, by using these predictive parameters, pelvic lymph node dissection could be avoided in up to 50% of patients with clinically localized prostate cancer
Bluestein 1994	Combination of local stage, primary Gleason grade, and serum PSA	Table generated showing probabilities that a patient will have positive lymph nodes
Danella 1993	Serum PSA >15 ng/mL and Gleason score >7	Routine laparoscopic node dissection deemed unnecessary unless PSA >40 ng/mL or PSA >15 ng/mL *and* Gleason score >7
Narayan 1994	PSA <10 ng/mL & Gleason score <6	In this setting, staging pelvic lymphadenectomy may be unnecessary
Roach 1994	Risk of positive lymph nodes (N+): N+ = 2/3 (PSA) +(Gleason score - 6) x 10	Low-risk group with calculated risk of positive nodes <15% had 6% observed incidence; high-risk group with calculated risk of >15% had 40% observed incidence
Stone 1998	Perineural invasion & positive seminal vesicle biopsy	28% of men with both had positive nodes vs 2% without both
Rogers 1996	PSA & biopsy Gleason score	Not sufficiently sensitive; lymphadenectomy recommended
Alagiri 1997	PSA & biopsy Gleason score	PSA <20 & Gleason score <8: lymph node metastasis unlikely
Hoenig 1997	PSA, Gleason score, clinical stage	Laparoscopic pelvic lymph node dissection indicated for any patient with Gleason score > 7, PSA >20 ng/mL and/or advanced clinical stage
Puppo 1997	PSA, Gleason grade, clinical stage	Nomograms developed based on 1,738 patients
Partin 1997	PSA, Gleason score, clinical stage	Nomograms developed based on 4,133 men; 83% accuracy in predicting lymph node involvement
Bangma 1995B	PSA, Anderson grade, clinical stage	Attempt to predict pelvic lymph node frozen section diagnosis
Conrad 1998	Gleason grade, number of positive biopsies, PSA	Presence & amount of poorly differentiated Gleason pattern 4 or 5 best predictors of positive nodes
Tewari 1998	Neural network using PSA, number of positive cores, Gleason grade, clinical stage; perineural invasion, age, race	73% accuracy in predicting lymph node status
Haese 2002	High risk: More than 3/6 cores with Gleason pattern 4; intermediate risk: 1-3/6 cores with dominant pattern 4; low risk: all others	Frequency of lymph node metastasis: 44% of patients in high-risk group, 20% of intermediate risk patients, and 2% of low-risk patients

rate of surgical incision into the gland, with surgically induced positive margins (Boccon-Gibod 1998). Also, for patients undergoing radical perineal prostatectomy, pelvic lymphadenectomy must be performed as a separate procedure, unlike the retropubic radial prostatectomy, where pelvic lymph nodes may be excised at the same time as the prostate. Clinical advantages to the perineal procedure include less blood loss, a shorter hospital stay, access to the prostate apex, and ease of performance of the vesicourethral anastomosis (Boccon-Gibod 1998, Gibbons 2002).

Clinical tissue sampling differences between the 2 procedures have not been quantitatively delineated, but personal experience of this author suggests that a greater amount of periprostatic soft tissue is excised in the retropubic approach. In contrast, a recent study found an equivalent amount of extracapsular tissue excised in specimens from the 2 approaches (Korman 2002). Tissues sampled as part of the radical prostatectomy procedure include pelvic lymph nodes and the prostate gland with attached seminal vesicles and vasa deferentia stumps.

Recently, laparoscopic radical prostatectomy has been performed (Cadeddu 2001, Guillonneau 2000, Rassweiler 2001). Tissue sampling, complications, and outcome are being addressed for this new procedure.

Pelvic Lymph Nodes

Pelvic lymphadenectomy provides important staging information and has been used to guide the intraoperative decision to perform the radical prostatectomy. In the 1970s the incidence of metastatic prostate carcinoma in pelvic lymph nodes was 20% to 40%, whereas with PSA screening 1% to 6% of patients are found to have metastatic tumor in lymph nodes (Humphrey 1996, Petros 1992). Before the 1990s, frozen section analysis of pelvic lymph nodes was routine before radical prostatectomy, and the prostate gland was not usually removed if the pelvic lymph nodes were positive because radical prostatectomy would be of little benefit to the patient in the face of metastatic disease. With the now infrequent involvement of pelvic lymph nodes by carcinoma, some urologists do not request frozen sections of lymph nodes at all, and some urologists select patients for pelvic lymphadenectomy for frozen section analysis based on the presurgical parameters of total serum PSA, needle biopsy histologic grade, and clinical stage **t2.11** (Alagiri 1997, Bangma 1995B, Conrad 1998, Danella 1993, Hause 2002, Hoenig 1997, Narayan 1994, Partin 1997, Puppo 1997, Roach 1988, Rogers 1996, Stone 1998, Tewari 1998). None of these models is completely accurate, however, and few have been validated using separate independent patient populations (Kattan 1997, Spevack 1996). In rare cases, I have seen positive pelvic lymph nodes that were not submitted for frozen section.

Clinical pelvic lymph node sampling must be performed as a separate procedure for patients undergoing a radical perineal prostatectomy. The lymph nodes can be clinically identified and dissected using either open surgery or laparoscopy (Cadeddu 1997, Herrell 1997, Kava 1998). In a few cases, sentinel lymph node sampling has been performed (Wawroschek 1999), but this is not an established procedure. For laparoscopic sampling, a variable number of pelvic nodes are obtained, with a range of 2 to 52 in one series (Cadeddu 1997). Laparoscopy, minilaparotomy, and modified open lymphadenectomy were equivalent in the number of nodes dissected, with a mean of 9 lymph nodes for each procedure (Herrell 1997). A single case of abdominal wall tumor implantation at the trocar site has been reported for laparoscopic pelvic lymph node dissection in patients with prostate cancer (Bangma 1995A), but this seems to be quite rare. Clinical pelvic lymph node sampling in the setting of radical retropubic prostatectomy is performed during the radical prostatectomy operation but before the prostate is removed (Walsh 2002).

The gross description of pelvic lymph nodes should include number, location, and size (Harden 1995, Henson 1994). This size measurement should include the overall size of the received lymph node "packet" with associated adipose tissue and the size of grossly identifiable lymph nodes. Palpable abnormalities should be noted before sectioning. After sectioning, any abnormalities, including gross metastatic deposits, should be described. Sampling of pelvic lymph nodes as part of an intraoperative consultation can involve either frozen section preparation alone or frozen section and generation of touch imprints (smears). Because the pelvic lymph node dissections are limited, these are usually only a few nodes to be sampled. In one study, the mean number of lymph nodes frozen per unilateral lymphadenectomy was 1.7 (Epstein 1986A). It is desirable to freeze all grossly recognizable lymph nodes because gross diagnosis of metastatic prostate cancer in pelvic lymph nodes is possible only in a minority of cases (32% in one series) (Sgrignoli 1994). Technically, these are challenging frozen section slides to make because of the fat content of these pelvic lymph nodes. Cytologic touch imprints or smears can be useful for larger lymph nodes but are insensitive (Bastacky 1994) and should not be used in place of frozen sections. It should be recognized that frozen sections are highly specific but somewhat insensitive in detecting pelvic lymph node metastases because of the small size of many metastatic deposits (so-called micrometastases). The sensitivity is 58% to 73% (Catalona 1982, Davis 1995, Epstein 1986A, Fowler 1981, Kramolowsky 1984, Saltzstein 1977, Sgrignoli 1994), where this low sensitivity results from sampling error. That is, there are micrometastases diagnosed in the permanent sections of the tissue used for frozen section and in additionally submitted tissue that did not contain grossly evident lymph nodes. It is likely that preparation of additional slides and levels at frozen section would increase the detection rate, but this is not really a practical option because of the increase in operative time that would result. Accordingly, the current frozen section standard remains preparation of a single H&E slide from all grossly seen pelvic lymph nodes.

Gross sampling of tissue after frozen section and of lymph node tissue not submitted for frozen section should entail submission of all grossly identifiable lymph node tissue and wide sampling of associated adipose tissue without macroscopically identified lymph nodes. If feasible, all the tissue should be submitted. The reason for this is that in a significant minority of patients (10% in one series) (Bastacky 1994), micrometastases are found in small, not grossly visible lymph nodes and soft tissue.

Histologic sampling of the paraffin blocks of pelvic lymph nodes typically is accomplished using 1 H&E slide. The diagnostic effect of H&E levels in the detection of micrometastatic disease is unknown (Humphrey 1993A). Additional sampling of the paraffin blocks may be performed for immunohistochemical studies in the rare event that there is concern that the metastatic deposit of carcinoma is not prostatic in origin or if there is a concern for a lymphoproliferative disorder. As an incidental finding, 13 of 1092 patients (1.2%) were found to have a hematolymphoid malignancy in pelvic lymph nodes removed during radical prostatectomy (Terris 1997B). The histologic types of incidentally discovered hematolymphoid malignancy, in order from most to least common, were small lymphocytic lymphoma (6 patients), chronic lymphocytic leukemia (3 patients), Hodgkin lymphoma (3 patients), and hairy cell leukemia (1 patient). In these cases, immunohistochemical studies on additional sections are indicated. Investigational approaches that necessitate additional pelvic lymph node tissue sampling include immunohistochemical stains for occult lymph node metastases (Freeman 1995, Gomella 1993, Moul 1994), immunoassay for PSA protein in homogenates of fresh frozen pelvic lymph nodes (Shoskes 1993), and RT-PCR for PSA RNA extracted from pelvic lymph node tissue (Deguchi 1993, Mao 1998). The goal of these procedures is to diagnose metastatic prostatic cancer and to attempt to provide greater sensitivity than morphologic diagnosis. Greater sensitivity has been claimed, but these studies are flawed because they used additional tissue to detect more tumor cells. The only reliable means of directly determining whether a new test improves diagnostic sensitivity is to use the very H&E section interpreted as negative for further testing. Currently, this additional pelvic lymph node testing for occult metastatic disease is experimental.

Prostate Gland and Seminal Vesicles

The whole prostate gland with seminal vesicles **i2.32, i2.33** may be received fresh or in fixative. It is uncommon for the prostate gland to be received fresh, with a request for a frozen section from the gland itself. The most common clinical reason for frozen section sampling is to evaluate margin status, particularly in the region of the neurovascular bundles (Cangiano 1999, Epstein 1996). Here, in a nerve-sparing radical prostatectomy operation, the intraoperative question is whether a frozen section of the excised prostate gland will help in the decision to excise the neurovascular bundle left in the patient. The argument has been made that this decision should be based on clinical judgment, with consideration of preoperative potency, serum PSA level, size and grade of the tumor, and whether on palpation it appears that the tumor may have spread outside the gland (Epstein 1996). This seems to be a reasonable approach; we do not perform frozen sections to evaluate margins of radical prostatectomy specimens.

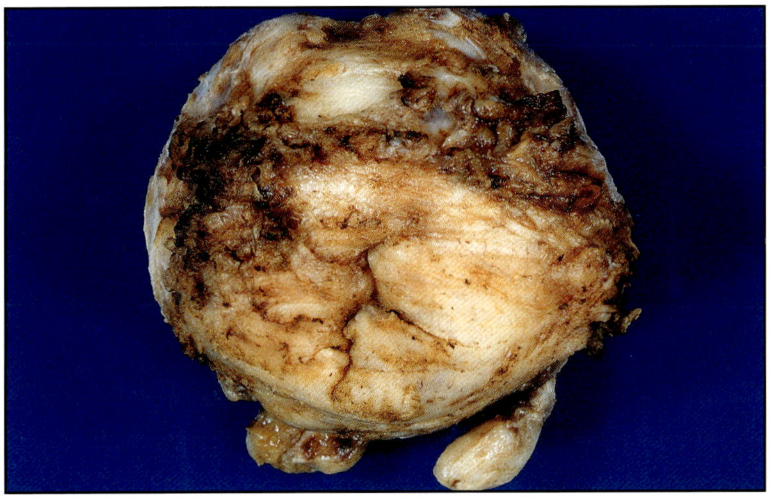

■ **i2.32** *View of superior aspect of radical prostatectomy specimen, showing bladder neck and seminal vesicles.*

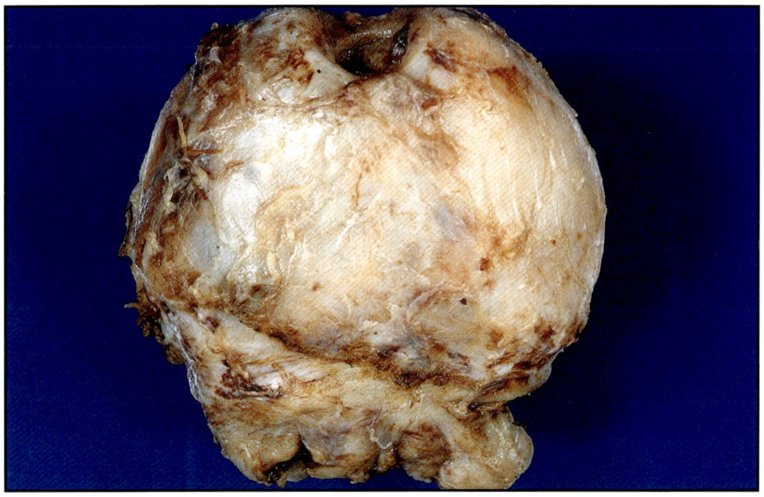

■ **i2.33** *Inferior view of radical prostatectomy specimen, with distal urethral margin at top. This is a large specimen at 95g. The mean weight of radical prostatectomy specimens is around 48g, with a wide range of 6g to 204g* (Naughton 1998).

The histopathologic assessment of the whole prostate gland is critical for prognostication and for determination of whether adjuvant postoperative therapy should be administered. Therefore, the gland should be handled and sampled in such a way as to allow accurate reporting of the important pathologic features. These features include confirmation of carcinoma presence, tumor size (intraglandular tumor extent), carcinoma histologic grade, pathologic stage, and margin status (Humphrey 1993A, 1993B). Sampling for other markers of biologic behavior of prostatic carcinoma should be considered experimental (Bostwick 2000, Humphrey 1993C).

Numerous protocols have been published on gross examination and sampling of radical prostatectomy specimens (ADASP 1996, Bostwick 1997A, Egevad 1998, Epstein 2001, Furman 1998, Harden 1995, Hoedemaeker 1998, Renshaw 1996, Sakr 1996, 1999, Sehdev 2001, Srigley 2000). The protocols describe sampling of the prostate gland for tissue banking and research purposes (Bova 1993, Egevad 1998, Furman 1998, Sakr 1995, Wheeler 1994), partial versus complete sampling (Bostwick 1997A, Cohen 1994, Epstein 1991, Hall 1992, Renshaw 1996, Schmid 1992, Sakr 1996), and whole-mount versus standard section embedding (Bostwick 1997A, Epstein 1991, Furman 1998, Sakr 1996). Recommended guidelines (ADASP 1996, Cohen 1994, Hall 1992, Henson 1994, Srigley 2000) for gross examination and description of the radical prostatectomy specimen are summarized in **t2.12**. After recording container labeling information, fixative information, and type of specimen, the first task is to measure the size of the prostate in 3 dimensions and the weight in grams. Prostate shapes vary and often do not conform to the shape of a truncated cone, a top laying on its side, or a prolate ellipsoid, which is the shape often used to measure prostate volume in vivo by ultrasound (Terris 2002). (Sometimes, the prostate can even assume the shape of a cylinder when it is forced into a small vial.) The entire outer surface of the specimen should then be inked to allow microscopic evaluation of margin status. Some protocols suggest the use of different-colored inks for different sides or regions of the prostate (Bostwick 1997A, Furman 1998, Sakr 1995, 1996), but we have not found

■ **t2.12 Recommendations for Gross Examination & Reporting for Radical Prostatectomy Specimens**

How container is labeled	Patient name, birthdate, identification number, container number, anatomic site
Specimen fresh or in fixative	If in fixative, specify type and volume
Structures in specimen	Prostate Seminal vesicles Segments of vasa deferentia Bladder (cystoprostatectomy) Urethra
Description	Size in three dimensions Weight Palpable abnormalities Size, color, shape, zonal location of mass(es)
Sections submitted	
Partial embedding	Sections of each grossly recognizable tumor, followed by alternate sections For grossly normal glands, alternate sections Sections of base of each seminal vesicle to include prostate-seminal vesicle junction and periprostatic soft tissue Bladder neck shave margin Conization of distal apical margin
Complete embedding	Sections of all prostate tissue Sections of base of each seminal vesicle junction and periprostatic soft tissue Bladder neck shave margin Conization of distal apical margin

Modified from ADASP 1996, Henson 1994, Srigley 2000, Hall 1992, Cohen 1994, Epstein 2001

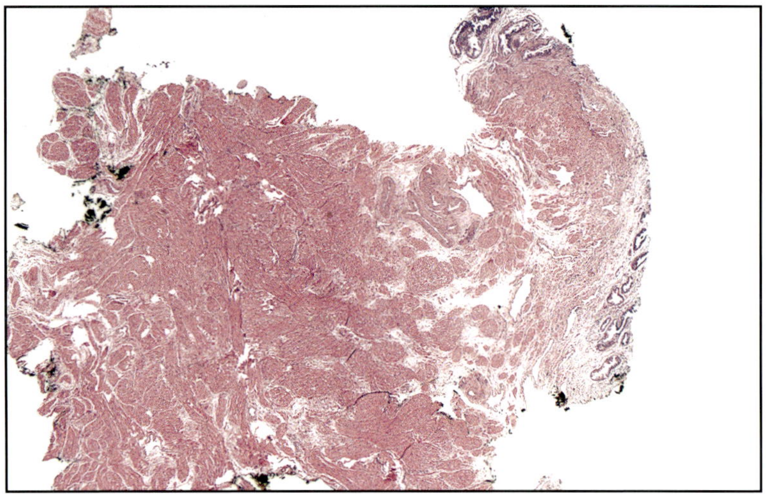

■ **i2.34** *Thin shave section of bladder neck margin margin.*

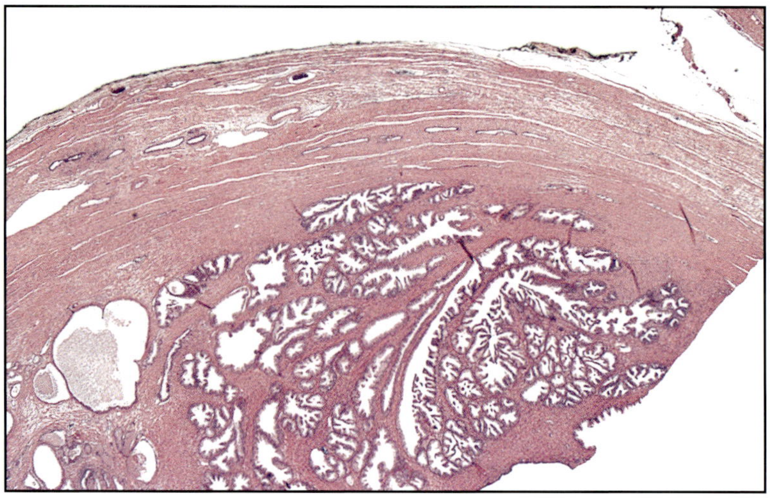

■ **i2.35** *Radial section from a "cone" with the distal apical margin.*

this to be necessary. We designate anatomic site of sections by quadrant (right base, right apex, left base, left apex), thereby eliminating the need for different-colored inks (Epstein 1991). After inking, the entire specimen can be briefly immersed in acetone or Bouin's fixative and air dried or blotted dry (Bostwick 1997A).

Harvest of fresh tissue for tissue banking or research purposes may be performed, if desired, at this stage. The procurement of prostatic tissues for research purposes should be closely coordinated with the operating urologist and the collaborating research laboratories. This process should entail an established, human studies committee–approved, written protocol and funding agreements before initiation of harvest and agreements as to the plan for procurement, histologic analysis, tissue preparation for storage, and physical storage. The ideal case for distributing tissue for research studies is a grossly obvious, large tumor. However, in the PSA screening era, the detected cancers often are quite small (Humphrey 1996, 1998). Another complicating factor is that prostate cancer can be quite difficult to grossly visualize, so many glands must be sampled without gross evidence of a suspicious mass. The method of tissue procurement varies among the published studies, but most describe sectioning the entire gland while fresh before (Wheeler 1994) or after inking. Here, the whole gland is sectioned with a large, sharp knife from apex to base at 3mm to 4mm intervals perpendicular to the posterior surface (Sakr 1995). The resulting tissue slices are inspected and palpated to aid in gross identification of prostatic carcinoma, which can present as a nodule or asymmetry, with solid yellow to white coloration. These suspicious areas can be sampled by imprints, scrapes, core biopsy, or small wedge sections. The type, location, and size of each sample removed for banking should be recorded in the gross description. It is critical that the sample be obtained from within the prostate so that the "capsule" and peripheral margins are not altered by the procurement. This is vital so that accurate staging and margin status information can still be provided in this setting. Because some macromolecules are labile, the procurement should be performed as soon as possible after removal of the gland, and the tissue samples should be snap-frozen in liquid nitrogen as soon as possible. For the research performed on the tissue samples to be of any meaning, the histologic and cellular composition of the banked tissue must be documented. After tissue harvest, the prostate gland slices should be fixed and sectioned as detailed later in this chapter for whole glands received in a fixative.

The amount of time, effort, and expense to harvest tissue for research in a rigorous manner should not be underestimated. For our prostate cancer procurement program, a full-time individual was hired to be on call to pick up the gland in the operating room immediately after its removal. A dedicated freezing microtome was purchased for the program. The interpretation of the frozen sections, storing of the tissue samples in -70° freezers, and the creation of databases linking the frozen section results to the radical prostatectomy findings to the clinical database take substantial planning, funding, and effort. The reader is referred to the published protocols for comparison of the details of prostate cancer tissue banking and harvesting methods (Bova 1993, Egevad 1998, Furman 1998, Sakr 1995, Wheeler 1994).

For cases where tissue banking is not needed, the radical prostatectomy specimen should be inked (as described earlier) and well fixed before sectioning. Some have suggested cannulation of the urethra with instillation of formalin into the urethra or needle injection of formalin into the gland (True 1994), but these maneuvers are rarely performed. Instead, overnight immersion at room temperature in 10% neutral buffered formalin at 10 times the volume of the specimen is preferable. (Volume of the specimen can be assumed to be nearly equivalent to specimen weight because prostate specific gravity is close to 1.0 g/cm^3.) Longer fixation times of 24 hours (Schmid 1992) to 2 days or more (Cohen 1994, Wheeler 1989) have been used, but overnight fixation is generally sufficient and is more timely for reporting. Longer than overnight fixation times may be necessary if whole-mount sections are to be generated (Epstein 1991).

The next day the gland should be grossly examined and sectioned. Any palpable abnormalities of the whole gland, including their size, shape, location, color, and character (eg, firm or hard) should be recorded. Care should be taken during palpation to avoid disrupting the outer soft tissue and peripheral margin. If the distal apical (urethral) and proximal bladder neck margins have not been submitted separately, these sections should be taken. The most cost-effective and practical approach to sampling the bladder neck margin is to take a thin shave margin of 2mm (Ayala 1989, Epstein 1991) **i2.34**. Tumor anywhere in this shave margin tissue represents a positive margin. The best way to sample the distal apical or so-called distal urethral margin is by conization (Epstein 2001). This can be accomplished by taking radial sections from the amputated distal 5mm to 10mm apex of the prostate gland (ADASP 1996, Ayala 1989, Epstein 2001, Schmid 1992) **i2.35**. Here, ink on tumor cells indicates a positive

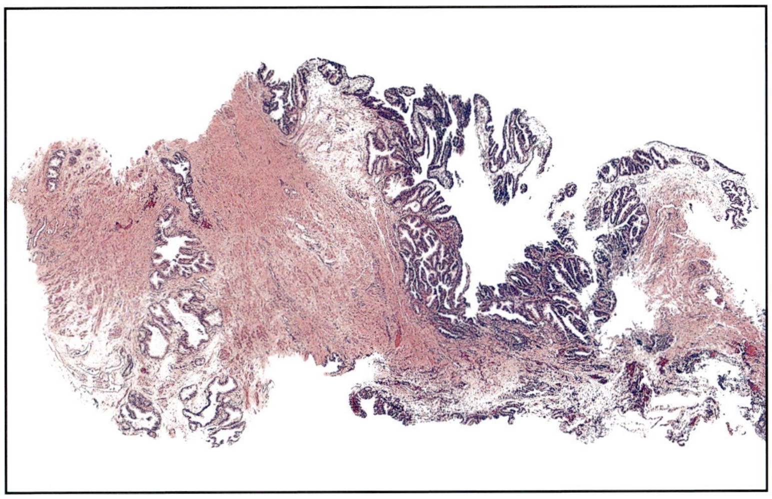

■ **i2.36** *Thin shave section of distal "urethral" margin.*

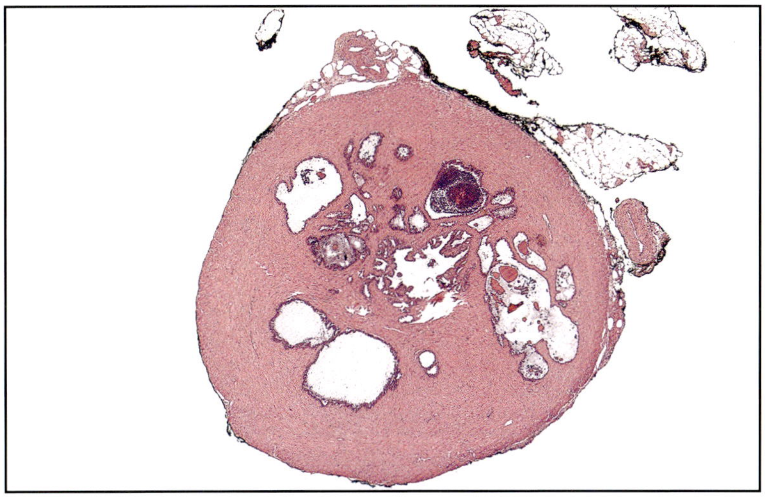

■ **i2.37** *Vas deferens stump margin.*

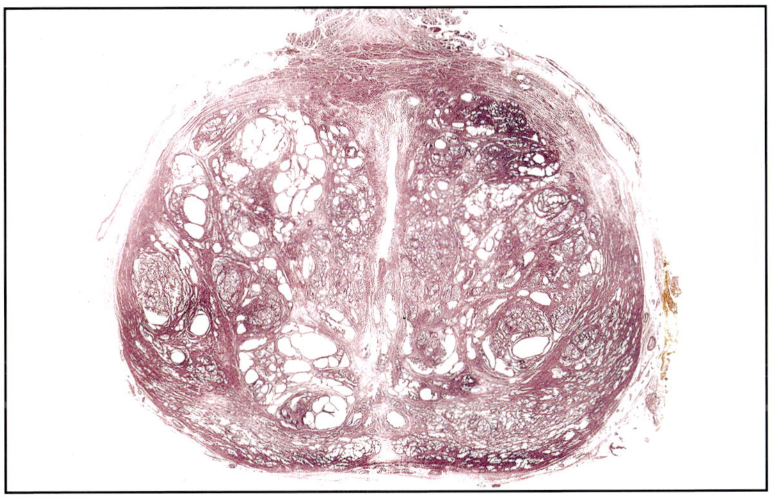

■ **i2.38** *Whole-mount section of radical prostatectomy specimen. (Courtesy of Dr. Pat Troncoso).*

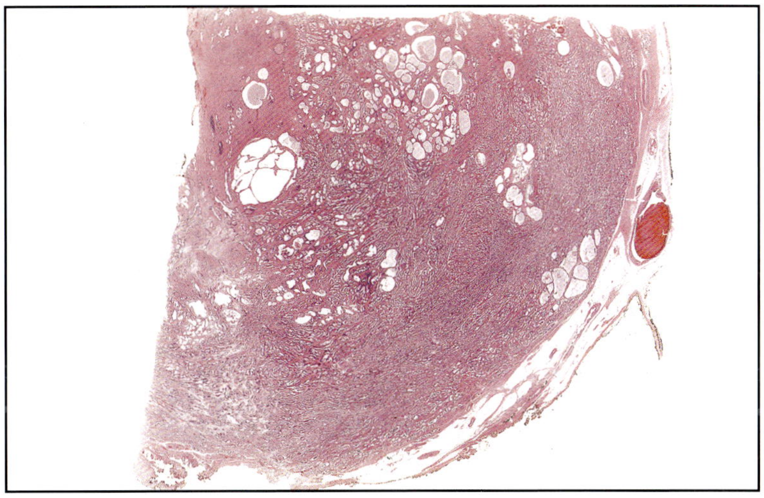

■ **i2.39** *Section of quarter of prostate gland on standard 1- × 3-inch slide.*

margin. Shave margins of the distal apex, sometimes called the distal urethral margin, are submitted separately by some surgeons **i2.36**. Here one should not view the urethral mucosa or urothelium as the sole marginal tissue; the distal "urethral" margin is a misnomer in that the urethra is only one component of the marginal tissue. Indeed, the urethra itself is uncommonly involved in a positive distal margin because the tumor usually is periurethral. Failure to identify urothelium in a distal urethral margin should not prompt ordering of levels or additional sampling because sometimes the urethral mucosa retracts into the prostate after its surgical transection. Carcinoma anywhere in the distal apical or urethral shave margin should be interpreted as a positive margin. There are advantages and disadvantages to sampling with tangential (shave margin) and perpendicular (conization) techniques. Tangential shave margins sample a wide surface area, but if the shaved section is too thick, then the prostate gland proper may be sampled. In contrast, whereas the true inked distal margin is clearly visualized with the conization approach, only a small region of the margin is assessed because only 5µm of tissue is on each slide out of each 3mm perpendicular section. We prefer the conization approach for the distal apical margin and a shaved margin for the bladder neck.

At this point the seminal vesicles should be amputated with a small portion of soft tissue and prostatic tissue at the base of the seminal vesicles. This type of sectioning is important because seminal vesicle invasion by prostatic carcinoma commonly occurs by direct extension into soft tissue after extraprostatic extension near the seminal vesicle base (Ohori 1993). Gross involvement of the seminal vesicle by carcinoma should be reported, but such involvement in this PSA screening era typically is microscopic, and the current incidence of positive seminal vesicles is only about 5% (Humphrey 1996).

Vasa deferentia stumps may be sampled using en face sections **i2.37**, but this is not routinely done.

Before complete sectioning of the prostate gland, consideration should be given as to whether whole-mount slides **i2.38** or standard 1 inch × 3 inch slides will be prepared. Although they are more aesthetically pleasing, whole mounts do not provide additional morphologic information (Cohen 1994, Epstein 1991, Hollenbeck 2000). Moreover, they are more expensive and time-consuming to prepare. With some glands it is possible to fit sections of one quarter **i2.39** or one half of the prostate on the standard 1 inch × 3 inch glass slides.

Coronal sectioning of the gland in a plane perpendicular to the urethra should be performed at 3mm to 5mm intervals using a knife with a long, sharp blade, a commercial meat slicer (Ayala 1989), or a prostate slicing device (Schmid 1992). These cross-sections **i2.40** should then be assessed for gross evidence of hyperplasia and carcinoma.

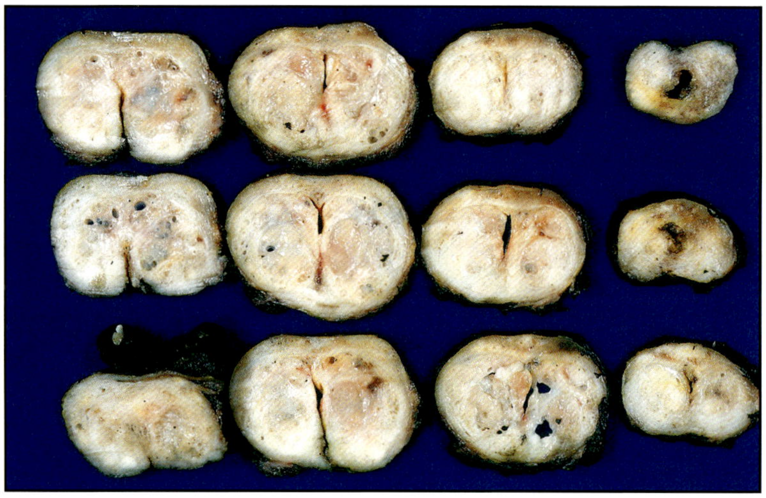

■ **i2.40** *Serial cross-sections of prostate gland corresponding to intact gland depicted in* **i2.33**.

Prostatic adenocarcinoma in radical prostatectomy specimens may be difficult to recognize grossly, but a recent report (Hall 1992) claims that most stage A (T1) and B (T2) tumors can be identified at the macroscopic level. In a second report, carcinoma was grossly visualized in 63% of radical prostatectomy specimens (Renshaw 1998). Many or most smaller carcinomas that are detected in this PSA screening era are difficult or impossible to see on cut surfaces of radical prostatectomy tissues. When grossly evident, carcinomas in whole cross-sections of radical prostatectomy specimens appear as solid gray to yellow-white masses, with wide variation in gross appearance (Hall 1992). Grossly, it is unusual for carcinomas to be discrete masses that are clearly defined from surrounding prostatic tissue. Rather, asymmetry with slightly greater yellow coloration is more common (Renshaw 1998). Palpation of fixed tissue generally is not helpful in defining carcinoma from benign tissue. It may be useful to photograph or to generate an image of the cross-sections by photocopy machine to document the location and gross appearance of tissue in submitted cassettes. Alternatively, diagrams or pictorial maps may be used to indicate location of sections and any gross abnormality (Henson 1994, Sakr 1995, 1996, Wheeler 1994). Some also use the diagrams to indicate microscopic findings. Such photographs, photocopy images, and diagrams are not absolutely necessary if an accurate gross description of gross abnormalities and sites of sampling are provided.

The number of sections to submit from a radical prostatectomy specimen is not standardized, but data suggest that partial submission of the gland may provide most of the important prognostic information (Cohen 1994, Hall 1992, Schmid 1992). Sections of all grossly suspicious lesions should be submitted (Henson 1994). For these cases, if one also submits standard sections of proximal and distal margins, base of seminal vesicles, and an apical section, 91% of foci of extraprostatic extension and 96% of positive margins will be identified (Hall 1992). This sampling method required an average of 13 blocks (range 7 to 36) compared with an average of 42 (range 21 to 81) for completely embedded glands. Given the difficulty of recognizing prostate cancer grossly, another approach would be to sample all grossly suspicious lesions, followed by submission of alternate sections **t2.12**. For grossly normal glands, alternate sections are recommended. Using the alternate section method, 85% of examples of extraprostatic extension would have been detected (Cohen 1994). The annual estimated cost savings in the United States if alternate sections rather than complete embedding were done on 60 000 radical prostatectomies, based solely on cost of reagents, slides, and technical time, would be $1.7 to $3.5 million (Cohen 1994, Humphrey 1994). Also, the professional time needed to review slides from completely embedded glands can be substantial because complete embedding takes a mean of 26 to 42 blocks (Hall 1992, Humphrey 1996, Schmid 1992) and can range up to 118 blocks per case (Humphrey 1996). Finally, complete embedding of all prostatic tissue is performed by only 12% of all pathologists (True 1994) and should not be considered standard or routine practice. Complete embedding of all prostatic tissue from radical prostatectomy specimens will continue to be a critical research tool that provides a high degree of accuracy on morphologic prognosticators, particularly tumor volume. Also, classifications of prostatic carcinoma into categories such as "clinically insignificant," "minimal," "moderate," or "advanced" (Epstein 1994), "clinically unimportant," "curable," or "advanced" (Ohori 1994), or "clinically potentially harmless" (Humphrey 1996) entail complete embedding and tumor volume measurement.

It is occasionally essential to submit more tissue or to completely embed all prostatic tissue after initially embedding only part of the gland. Most often additional gross sampling is dictated by identification of minimal or no carcinoma in the initial sections. This has been called "minimal residual cancer" or "vanishing cancer phenomenon" (Di Giuseppe 1997, Goldstein 1995). These small foci of cancer usually are less than 0.1cm^3 in volume (range 0.01cm^3 to 0.13cm^3) **i2.41**. Because of increased PSA screening, these tiny cancers have been increasing in incidence, from 0.5% in 1988 to a current level of 3% to 4% (Di Giuseppe 1997). These minute tumors would be easy to miss in an alternate-section protocol, and additional sections would be necessary. Additional indications for submitting additional sections for microscopy include evaluation of indeterminate surgical margins, extraprostatic extension by carcinoma, or histologic grade.

Histologic sampling of paraffin blocks from a radical prostatectomy specimen usually is straightforward, with generation of a single H&E-stained slide per block. Additional sections from the block may be requested if there are indeterminate findings on margin status, extraprostatic extension by carcinoma, or histologic grade or if there is minimal or no carcinoma in initial sections.

In the uncommon event that no tumor is seen in initial sections of a completely embedded gland, one should recheck patient identification of the diagnostic needle biopsy or TURP specimen and radical prostatectomy and confirm the diagnosis of malignancy in the needle biopsy or TURP chips. If there is concern about specimen misidentification, the most definitive means of verifying identity is by polymerase chain reaction genotyping using human leukocyte antigen alleles (Bateman 1997, Shibata 1993) or short tandem repeat sequences (microsatellites) (O'Briain 1996). If patient misidentification is not a concern, then a single H&E deep recut should be taken from each block, and if these slides do not harbor tumor, then no further sampling is needed; the patient should be considered to have a minute cancer, with a very high likelihood of cure. Complete histologic sampling of radical prostatectomy blocks is not practical in detecting such prostatic carcinomas because several thousand slides are needed to serially section a completely embedded prostate gland (Benoit 1994, Humphrey 1993C). We completely embedded and serially sectioned a 37.7-g prostate, and this took 2678 slides (Humphrey 1993C). Even if one serially sectioned an entire prostate gland in this manner to find a minute prostatic carcinoma, a negative result does not mean that carcinoma was not in the radical prostatectomy because the tumor could have lost in facing off the block.

[2.6] Cystoprostatectomy

Radical cystoprostatectomy, which is performed primarily for bladder muscle wall–invasive transitional cell carcinoma, is another major operation in which the entire prostate gland is removed. There is no standardization of gross sampling of the prostate in radical cystoprostatectomy specimens. An increased extent of prostate sampling results in increased detection of bladder cancer involvement of the prostate, which can be as high as 50% (see Chapter 23 and **t23.12**). Similarly, the detection rate of incidental (latent or autopsy) prostatic adenocarcinomas in radical cystoprostatectomy specimens depends on the extent of sampling (Abbas 1996, Arakawa 1997, Babaian 1991, Kabalin 1989, Montie 1989, Pritchett 1988, Winfield 1987). In completely embedded prostate glands from cystoprostatectomy specimens from men with mean age of 62 to 64, 45% to 68% (Abbas 1996, Arakawa 1997, Kabalin 1989, Montie 1989) of patients have prostate cancer. Most of these cancers are extremely small (median volume = 0.04cm^3), and almost all (90% to 97%) are organ-confined (Kabalin 1989, Ohori 1994). However, a minority (17%) of patients have tumors larger than 0.5cm^3, and 11% have high-grade Gleason pattern 4 or 5 (Ohori 1994), suggesting potential clinical significance. A gross sampling protocol that will catch all of these potentially clinically significant cancers has not been devised. Currently, complete embedding of all prostatic tissue from radical cystoprostatectomy specimens is not standard practice. Recommendations include sampling of the verumontanum, any gross lesions, and at least 1 block from the periphery of each side (Murphy 1997).

[2.7] Postmortem Examination of the Prostate

At autopsy, the prostate usually is not widely sampled unless there is a clinical history of prostate cancer or unless there are striking gross abnormalities of the prostate. For 60 years it has been recognized that there is a high incidence of latent or occult carcinomas incidentally detected at autopsy (Andrews 1949, Baron 1941, Brawn 1995, Breslow 1977, Edwards 1952, Hirst 1954, Lundberg 1970, Moore 1935, Rich 1935, Sakr 1994, Scott 1969). As with cystoprostatectomy specimens, the detection rate depends on the extent of sampling. Most of these incidental autopsy cancers are exceedingly small and are not detected unless the gland is completely embedded. The detection rate also depends on patient age **t2.13**), with up to 80% of men in the 10th decade diagnosed with prostatic carcinoma at autopsy (Hirst 1954). The number of sections to routinely take from the prostate gland at autopsy is not standardized. For patients with a clinical history of prostatic carcinoma, the prosector should consider a greater degree of sampling than just a section or two. For research purposes, completely embedded autopsy prostate glands will remain an important resource.

■ t2.13 Age-Dependent Incidence of Detection of Prostatic Carcinoma at Autopsy

Age	Incidence
20-29	2%
30-39	29%
40-49	32%
50-59	55%
60-69	63%
80-89	52%
90-100	80%

Data from Hirst 1954, Sakr 1994

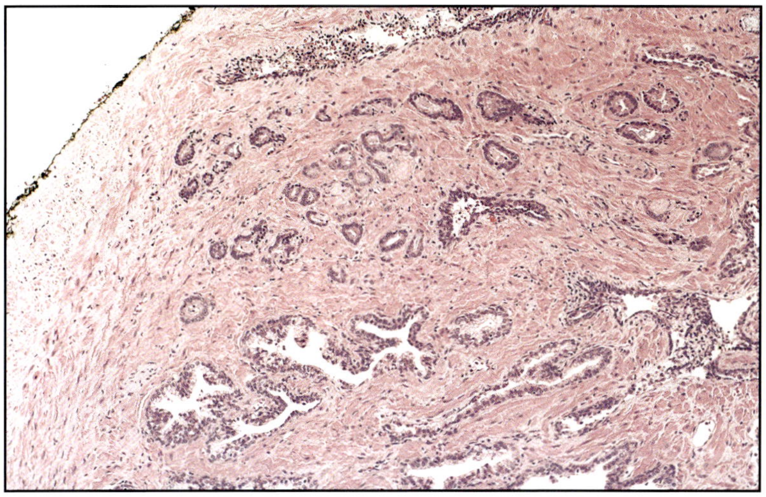

■ i2.41 *Small focus of minimal adenocarcinoma in a radical prostatectomy case. This was the only area of malignancy in the entire gland.*

References

Abbas F, Hochberg D, Civantos F, et al. Incidental prostatic adenocarcinoma in patients undergoing radical cystoprostatectomy for bladder cancer. *Eur Urol* 30:322-326, 1996.

Abboud E, Rhone D, August C. Optimizing preparation of prostatic needle biopsies [abstract]. *Mod Pathol* 11:74A, 1998.

Ackerman DA, Barry JM, Wicklund RA, et al. Analysis of risk factors associated with prostate cancer extension to the surgical margin and pelvic node metastasis at radical prostatectomy. *J Urol* 150:1845-1850, 1993.

ADASP (Association of Directors of Anatomic and Surgical Pathology). Recommendations for the reporting of resected prostate carcinomas. *Am J Clin Pathol* 105:667-670, 1996.

Alagiri M, Colton MD, Seidmon EJ, et al. The staging of pelvic lymphadenectomy: implications as an adjunctive procedure for clinically localized prostate cancer. *Br J Urol* 80:243-246, 1997.

Allepuz Losa CA, Sanz Velez JI, Gil Sanz MJ, et al. Seminal vesicle biopsy in prostate cancer staging. *J Urol* 154:1407-1411, 1995.

Amling CL, Blute ML, Lerner SE, et al. Influence of prostate-specific antigen testing on the spectrum of patients with prostate cancer undergoing radical prostatectomy at a large referral practice. *Mayo Clin Proc* 73:401-406, 1998.

Andrews GS. Latent carcinoma of the prostate. *J Clin Pathol* 2:197-208, 1949.

Arai Y, Yoshiki T, Yamabe H, et al. Value of prostate-specific antigen measurements in predicting lymph node involvement in prostate cancer. *Urol Int* 45:356-360, 1990.

Arakawa A, Soh S, Wheeler TM. High-grade prostatic intraepithelial neoplasia in cystoprostatectomy specimens. *J Urol Pathol* 7:1-8, 1997.

Ashby EC, Rees M, Dowding CH. Prophylaxis against systemic infection after transrectal biopsy for suspected prostatic carcinoma. *BMJ* 2:1263-1264, 1978.

Aus G, Ahlgren G, Hugosson J, et al. Diagnosis of prostate cancer: optimal number of prostate biopsies related to serum prostate-specific antigen and findings on digital rectal examination. *Scand J Urol Nephrol* 31:541-544, 1997.

Ayala AG, Ro JY, Babaian R, et al. The prostatic capsule: does it exist? *Am J Surg Pathol* 13:21-27, 1989.

Babaian RJ, Troncoso P, Ayala A. Transurethral-resection zone prostate cancer detected at cystoprostatectomy. A detailed histologic analysis and clinical implications. *Cancer* 67:1418-1422, 1991.

Babaian RJ, Toi A, Kamoi K, et al. A comparative analysis of sextant and an extended 11-core multisite directed biopsy strategy. *J Urol* 163:152-157, 2000.

Bangma CH, Kirkels WJ, Chadha S, et al. Cutaneous metastasis following pelvic lymphadenectomy for prostatic carcinoma. *J Urol* 153:1635-1636, 1995A.

Bangma CH, Hop WC, Schroder FH. Eliminating the need for preoperative frozen section analysis of pelvic lymph nodes during radical prostatectomy. *Br J Urol* 76:595-599, 1995B.

Baron E, Angrist A. Incidence of occult adenocarcinoma of the prostate. After fifty years of age. *Arch Pathol* 32:787-793, 1941.

Bastacky SS, Walsh PC, Epstein JI. Needle biopsy associated tumor tracking of adenocarcinoma of the prostate. *J Urol* 145:1003-1007, 1991.

Bastacky S, Silver SA, Epstein JI. Composite cytological smears of pelvic lymph nodes at the time of radical prostatectomy to identify nodal metastases. *Hum Pathol* 25:1352-1359, 1994.

Bateman AC, Hemmatpour SK, Theaker JM, et al. Nested polymerase chain reaction-based HLA class II typing for the unique identification of formalin-fixed and paraffin-embedded tissue. *J Pathol* 181:228-234, 1997.

Bauer JJ, Zeng J, Weir J, Zhang W, et al. Three-dimensional computer-simulated prostate models: lateral prostate biopsies increase the detection rate of prostate cancer. *Urology* 53:961-967, 1999.

Bauer WC, McGavran MH, Carlin MR. Unsuspected carcinoma of the prostate in suprapubic prostatectomy specimens: a clinicopathological study of 55 consecutive cases. *Cancer* 13:370-378, 1960.

Bazinet M, Karakiewicz PI, Aprikian AG, et al. Value of systematic transition zone biopsies in the early detection of prostate cancer. *J Urol* 155:605-606, 1996.

Benoit G, Merlaud L, Meduri G, et al. Anatomy of the prostatic nerves. *Surg Radiol Anat* 16:23-29, 1994.

Bianchi F. Practical advantages of the perineal biopsy of the prostate. *J Urol* 76:645-650, 1956.

Bishoff JT, Reyes A, Thompson IM, et al. Pelvic lymphadenectomy can be omitted in selected patients with carcinoma of the prostate: development of a system of patient selection. *Urology* 45:270-274, 1995.

Bluestein DL, Bostwick DG, Bergstralh JE, et al. Eliminating the need for bilateral pelvic lymphadenectomy in select patients with prostate cancer. *J Urol* 151:1315-1320, 1994.

Blute ML, Zincke H, Farrow GM. Long-term follow up of young patients with stage A adenocarcinomas of the prostate. *J Urol* 136:840-843, 1986.

Boccon-Gibod L, Ravery V, Vordos D, et al. Radical prostatectomy for prostate cancer: the perineal approach increases the risk of surgically induced positive margins and capsular incisions. *J Urol* 160:1383-1385, 1998.

Bostwick DG, Vonk JB, Picado A. Pathologic changes in the prostate following contemporary 18-gauge needle biopsy. No apparent risk of local cancer seeding. *J Urol Pathol* 2:203-211, 1994.

Bostwick DG, Montironi R. Evaluating radical prostatectomy specimens: therapeutic and prognostic importance. *Virchows Arch* 430:1-6, 1997A.

Bostwick DG, Dundore PA. Normal anatomy and histology. In: *Biopsy Pathology of the Prostate.* London: Chapman & Hall Medical; 12, 1997B.

Bostwick DG, Grignon DJ, Hammond EH, et al. Prognostic factors in prostate cancer. College of American Pathologists Concensus Statement 1999. *Arch Pathol Lab Med* 124:995-1000, 2000.

Bova GS, Fox WM, Epstein JI. Methods of radical prostatectomy specimen processing: a novel technique for harvesting fresh prostate cancer tissue and review of processing techniques. *Mod Pathol* 6:201-207, 1993.

Brat DJ, Wills ML, Lecksell KL, et al. How often are diagnostic features missed with less extensive sampling of prostate needle biopsy specimens? *Am J Surg Pathol* 23:257-262, 1999.

Brawn PN, Kuhl D, Speights VO, et al. The incidence of unsuspected metastases from clinically benign prostate glands with latent prostate carcinoma. *Arch Pathol Lab Med* 119:731-733, 1995.

Breslow N, Chan CW, Dhom G, et al. Latent carcinoma of the prostate at autopsy in seven areas. *Int J Cancer* 20:680-688, 1977.

Cadeddu JA, Elashry OM, Snyder O, et al. Effect of laparoscopic pelvic lymph node dissection on the natural history of D1 (T1-3, N1-3, MO) prostate cancer. *Urology* 50:391-394, 1997.

Cadeddu JA, Kavoussi LR. Laparoscopic radical prostatectomy: is it feasible and reasonable? *Urol Clin North Am* 28:655-661, 2001.

Cama C, Olsson CA, Buttyan R, et al. Molecular staging of prostate cancer. III. Effects of cystoscopy and needle biopsy on the enhanced reverse transcriptase polymerase chain reaction assay. *J Urol* 157:1748-1751, 1997.

Cangiano TG, Litwin MS, Naitoh J, et al. Intraoperative frozen section monitoring of nerve sparing radical retropubic prostatectomy. *J Urol* 162:655-658, 1999.

Catalona WJ, Stein AJ. Accuracy of frozen section detection of lymph node metastases in prostatic adenocarcinomas. *J Urol* 127:460-461, 1982.

Catalona WJ: Diagnosis. In: *Prostate Cancer.* New York: Grune & Stratton, 1984:48-56.

Catalona WJ, Bigg SW. Nerve-sparing radical prostatectomy: evaluation of results after 250 patients. *J Urol* 143:538-544, 1990.

Catalona WJ, Richie JP, Ahmann FR, et al. Comparison of digital rectal examination and serum prostate specific antigen in the early detection of prostate cancer: results of a multicenter trial of 6,630 men. *J Urol* 151:1283-1290, 1994.

Chan TY, Chan DY, Stutzman KL, et al. Does increased needle biopsy sampling of the prostate detect a higher number of potentially insignificant tumors? *J Urol* 166:2181-2184, 2001.

Chen ME, Troncoso P, Johnston DA, et al. Optimization of prostate biopsy strategy using computer based analysis. *J Urol* 158:2168-2175, 1997.

Chen ME, Troncoso P, Tang K, et al. Comparison of prostate biopsy schemes by computer simulation. *Urology* 53: 951-960, 1999.

Cheng L, Neumann RM, Blute ML, et al. Long-term follow-up of untreated stage T1a prostate cancer [letter]. *J Natl Cancer Inst* 90:1105-1107, 1998.

Cohen MB, Soloway MS, Murphy WM. Sampling of radical prostatectomy specimens. How much is adequate? *Am J Clin Pathol* 101:250-252, 1994.

Conrad S, Graefen M, Pichlmeier U, et al. Systematic sextant biopsies improve preoperative prediction of pelvic lymph node metastases in patients with clinically localized prostatic carcinoma. *J Urol* 159:2023-2029, 1998.

Danella JF, deKernion JB, Smith RB, et al. The contemporary incidence of lymph node metastases in prostate cancer: implications for laparoscopic lymph node dissection. *J Urol* 149:1488-1491, 1993.

Daneshgari F, Taylor GD, Miller GJ, et al. Computer simulation of the probability of detecting low volume carcinoma of the prostate with six random systematic core biopsies. *Urology* 45:604-609, 1995.

Dauleh MI, Byrne DJ. Severe bleeding following transrectal Tru-cut prostatic biopsy. *Scand J Urol Nephrol* 30:153-154, 1996.

Davis G. Sensitivity of frozen section examination of pelvic lymph node for metastatic prostate carcinoma. *Cancer* 76:661-668, 1995.

Deguchi T, Doi T, Ehara H, et al. Detection of micrometastatic prostate cancer cells in lymph nodes by reverse transcriptase-polymerase chain reaction. *Cancer Res* 53:5350-5354, 1993.

Delahunt B, Nacey JN. Broadsheet number 45: thin core biopsy of prostate. *Pathology* 30:247-256, 1998.

Delides GS, Baltopoulos G, Papaharalampous NX. Latent carcinoma of the prostate: the probability of identifying small lesions in routine histology. *Br J Urol* 48:207-209, 1976.

DeMay RM. Fine needle aspiration biopsy. In: *The Art and Science of Cytopathology. Aspiration Cytology.* Chicago: ASCP Press; 464-492, 1996A.

DeMay RM. Prostate. In: *The Art and Science of Cytopathology. Aspiration Cytology.* Chicago: ASCP Press; 1135-1155, 1996B.

DeMay RM. Urine. In: *The Art and Science of Cytopathology. Exfoliative Cytology.* Chicago: ASCP Press; 385-426, 1996C.

Di Giuseppe JA, Sauvageot J, Epstein JI. Increasing incidence of minimal residual cancer in radical prostatectomy specimens. *Am J Surg Pathol* 21:174-178, 1997.

Eble JN, Tejada E. Cost implications of sampling strategies for prostatic transurethral resection specimens: analysis of 549 cases [abstract]. *Am J Clin Pathol* 85:382-383, 1986.

Eble JN, Epstein JI. Stage A carcinoma of the prostate. In: Bostwick DG, ed. *Pathology of the Prostate.* New York: Churchill Livingstone; 61-82, 1990.

Edwards CN, Steinthorsson E, Nicholson D. An autopsy study of latent prostatic cancer. *Cancer* 6:531-554, 1952.

Egawa S, Matsumoto K, Shitara T, et al. Zonal biopsy in the detection of prostate cancer in Japanese men. *Jpn J Clin Oncol* 28:20-26, 1998.

Egevad L, Engström K, Busch C. A new method for handling radical prostatectomies enabling fresh tissue harvesting, whole mount sections, and landmarks for alignment of sections. *J Urol Pathol* 9:17-29, 1998.

Ekman H, Hedberg K, Persson PS. Cytological versus histological examination of needle biopsy specimens in the diagnosis of prostatic cancer. *Br J Urol* 39:544-548, 1967.

Epstein JI, Oesterling JE, Eggleston JC, et al. Frozen section detection of lymph node metastases in prostatic carcinoma: accuracy in grossly uninvolved pelvic lymphadenectomy specimens. *J Urol* 136:1234-1237, 1986A.

Epstein JI, Paull G, Eggleston JC, et al. Prognosis of untreated stage A1 prostatic carcinoma: a study of 94 cases with extended follow-up. *J Urol* 136:837-839, 1986B.

Epstein JI. The evaluation of radical prostatectomy specimens. Therapeutic and prognostic implications. *Pathol Annu* 26:159-210, 1991.

Epstein JI, Walsh PC, Carmichael M, et al. Pathologic and clinical findings to predict tumor extent of nonpalpable (stage T1c) prostate cancer. *JAMA* 271:368-374, 1994.

Epstein JI. Incidence and significance of positive margins in radial prostatectomy specimens. *Urol Clin North Am* 23:651-663, 1996.

Epstein JI, Walsh PC, Sauvageot J, et al. Use of repeat sextant and transition zone biopsies for assessing extent of prostate cancer. *J Urol* 159:1886-1890, 1997.

Epstein JI. Pathologic assessment of the surgical specimen. *Urol Clin North Am* 28:567-594, 2001.

Eskew LA, Bare RL, McCullough DL. Systematic 5 region prostate biopsy is superior to sextant method for diagnosing carcinoma of the prostate. *J Urol* 157:199-203, 1997.

Eskew LA, Woodruff RD, Bare RL, et al. Prostate cancer diagnosed by the 5 region biopsy method is significant disease. *J Urol* 160:794-796, 1998.

Esposti PL. Cytology diagnosis of prostatic tumors with aid of transrectal aspiration biopsy. A critical review of 1110 cases and a report of morphologic and cytochemical studies. *Acta Cytol* 10:182-186, 1966.

Fan K, Peng CF. Predicting the probability of bone metastases through histologic grading of prostate carcinoma: a retrospective analysis of 81 autopsy cases with antemortem transurethral resection specimen. *J Urol* 130:708-711, 1983.

Feldman AT. The new goal: Blurry nuclei and hazy cytoplasm. *J Histotechnol* 18:289-290, 1995.

Ferguson RS. Prostatic neoplasms. Their diagnosis by needle puncture and aspiration. *Am J Surg* 9:507-511, 1930.

Fitzpatrick JM, Mebust WK. Minimally invasive and endoscopic management of binign prostatic hyperplasia. In: Walsh PC, Retik AB, Vaughn ED Jr, et al, eds. *Campbell's Urology*. 8th ed. Philadelphia: Saunders; 1379-1422, 2002.

Fleshner NE, Fair WR. Indications for transition zone biopsy in the detection of prostatic carcinoma. *J Urol* 157:556-558, 1997.

Fortunoff S. Needle biopsy of the prostate: a review of 346 biopsies. *J Urol* 87:159-163, 1962.

Fowler JE Jr, Torgerson L, McLeod DG, et al. Radical prostatectomy with pelvic lymphadenectomy: observations on the accuracy of staging with lymph node frozen sections. *J Urol* 126:618-619, 1981.

Freeman JA, Esrig D, Grossfeld GD, et al. Incidence of occult lymph node metastasis in pathological stage C (pT3NO) prostate cancer. *J Urol* 154:474-478, 1995.

Furman J, Murphy WM, Rice L, et al. Prostatectomy tissue for research. Balancing patient care and discovery. *Am J Clin Pathol* 110:4-9, 1998.

Gann PH. Interpreting recent trends in prostate cancer incidence and mortality [editorial]. *Epidemiology* 8:117-120, 1997.

Gibbons RP. Radical perineal prostatectomy. In: Walsh PC, Retik AB, Vaughan ED Jr, et al, eds. *Campbell's Urology.* 8th ed. Philadelphia: Saunders; 3131-3146, 2002.

Goldman HB, Israeli RS, Lerner JL, et al. Effect of prostate biopsy on results of the PSA RT-PCR test. *Urology* 52:1073-1078, 1998.

Goldstein NS, Bégin LR, Grody WW, et al. Minimal or no cancer in radical prostatectomy specimens: report of 13 cases of the "vanishing cancer phenomenon." *Am J Surg Pathol* 19:1002-1009, 1995.

Golimbu M, Glasser J, Schinella R, et al. Stage A prostatic cancer from pathologist's viewpoint. *Urology* 18:134-136, 1981.

Gomella LG, White JL, McCue PA, et al. Screening for occult nodal metastasis in localized carcinoma of the prostate. *J Urol* 149:776-778, 1993.

Gore JL, Shariat SF, Miles BJ, et al. Optimal combinations of systematic sextant and laterally directed biopsies for the detection of prostate cancer. *J Urol* 165:1554-1559, 2001.

Green JSA, Bose P, Thomas DP, et al. How complete is a transurethral resection of the prostate? *Br J Urol* 97:398-400, 1996.

Green R, Epstein JI. Use of intervening unstained slides for immunohistochemical stains for high molecular weight cytokeratin on prostate needle biopsies. *Am J Surg Pathol* 23:567-570, 1999.

Greene DR, Egawa S, Neerhut G, et al. The distribution of residual cancer in radical prostatectomy specimens in stage A prostate cancer. *J Urol* 45:324-329, 1991.

Greene FL, Page DL, Fleming ID, et al. Prostate. In: *AJCC Cancer Staging Manual.* 6th ed. New York: Springer-Verlag; 309-316, 2002.

Guillonneau B, Vallancien G. Laparoscopic radical prostatectomy: the Montsouris Technique. *J Urol* 163:1643-1649, 2000.

Guinan P, Bush I, Ray V, et al. The accuracy of the rectal examination in the diagnosis of prostate carcinoma. *N Engl J Med* 303:499-503, 1980.

Gustafsson O, Norming V, Nyman CR, et al. Complications following combined transrectal aspiration and core biopsy of the prostate. *Scand J Urol Nephrol* 24:249-251, 1990.

Haddad FS. Risk factors for perineal seeding of prostate cancer after needle biopsy [letter]. *J Urol* 143:587-588, 1990.

Haese A, Epstein JI, Huland H, et al. Validation of a biopsy-based algorithm for predicting lymph node metastasis in patients with clinically localized prostate carcinoma. *Cancer* 95:1016-1021, 2002.

Hall GS, Kramer CE, Epstein JI. Evaluation of radical prostatectomy specimens. A comparative analysis of sampling methods. *Am J Surg Pathol* 16:315-324, 1992.

Han M, Alfert HJ, Partin AW. Retropubic and suprapubic open prostatectomy. In: Walsh PC, Retik AB, Vaughn ED Jr, et al, eds. *Campbell's Urology.* 8th ed. Philadelphia: Saunders; 1423-1434, 2002.

Harden P, Parkinson MC. Macroscopic examination of prostatic specimens. *J Clin Pathol* 48:693-700, 1995.

Henson DE, Hutter RVP, Farrow G, for the Members of the Cancer Committee, College of American Pathologists, and the Task Force on the Examination of Specimens Removed From Patients With Prostate Cancer. Practice protocol for the examination of specimens removed from patients with carcinoma of the prostate gland. *Arch Pathol Lab Med* 118:779-783, 1994.

Herrell DS, Trachtenberg J, Theodorescu D. Staging pelvic lymphadenectomy for localized carcinoma of the prostate: a comparison of 3 surgical techniques. *J Urol* 157:1337-1339, 1997.

Hirst AE Jr, Bergman RT. Carcinoma of the prostate in men 80 or more years old. *Cancer* 7:136-141, 1954.

Hodge KK, McNeal JE, Terris MK, et al. Random systematic versus directed ultrasound guided transrectal core biopsies of the prostate. *J Urol* 142:71-75, 1989.

Hoedemaeker RF, Ruijter ETG, Ruizeveld-de Winter JA, et al. Processing radical prostatectomy specimens: a comprehensive and standardized protocol. *J Urol Pathol* 9:211-222, 1998.

Hoenig DM, Chi S, Porter C, et al. Risk of nodal metastases at laparoscopic pelvic lymphadenectomy using PSA, Gleason score, and clinical stage in men with localized prostate cancer. *J Endourol* 11:263-265, 1997.

Hollenbeck BK, Bassily N, Wei JT, et al. Whole mounted radical prostatectomy specimens do not increase detection of adverse pathological features. *J Urol* 164:1583-1586, 2000.

Holtgrewe HL. Transurethral prostatectomy. *Urol Clin North Am* 22:357-368, 1995.

Hostetter AL, Pedersen DV, Gustafsson BL, et al. Diagnosis and localization of prostate carcinoma by fine-needle aspiration cytology and correlation with histologic whole-organ sections after radical prostatectomy. *Am J Clin Pathol* 94:693-697, 1990.

Hudson MA, Catalona WJ. Urothelial tumors of the bladder, upper tracts, and prostate. In: Gillenwater JY, Grayhack JT, Howards SS, et al, eds. *Adult and Pediatric Urology.* 3rd ed. St Louis, Mo: Mosby, 1996:1405-1406.

Humphrey PA, Walther PJ. Adenocarcinoma of the prostate. Part I. Tissue sampling considerations. *Am J Clin Pathol* 99:746-759, 1993A.

Humphrey PA, Walther PJ. Adenocarcinoma of the prostate. Part II. Tissue prognosticators. *Am J Clin Pathol* 100:256-269, 1993B.

Humphrey PA. Complete histologic serial sectioning of a prostate gland with adenocarcinoma. *Am J Surg Pathol* 17:468-472, 1993C.

Humphrey PA. Tissue sampling in the era of cost constraints. *Am J Clin Pathol* 101:247-248, 1994.

Humphrey PA, Baty J, Keetch DW. Relationship between serum prostate-specific antigen, needle biopsy findings, and histopathologic features of prostate carcinoma in radical prostatectomy tissue. *Cancer* 75:1842-1849, 1995.

Humphrey PA, Keetch DW, Smith DS, et al. Prospective characterization of pathologic features of prostatic carcinomas detected via serum prostate specific antigen-based screening. *J Urol* 155:816-820, 1996.

Humphrey PA. Prostate cancer in the serum prostate-specific antigen era [editorial]. *Mayo Clin Proc* 73:489-496, 1998.

Jemal A, Thomas A, Murray T, et al. Cancer statistics, 2002. *CA Cancer J Clin* 52:23-47, 2002.

Jensen KME, Sonneland P, Madsen PO. Seminal vesicle tissue in "resectate" of transurethral resection of prostate. *Urology* 22:20-33, 1983.

Kabalin JN, McNeal JE, Price HM, et al. Unsuspected adenocarcinoma of the prostate in patients undergoing cystoprostatectomy for other causes: incidence, histology and morphometric observations. *J Urol* 141:1091-1094, 1989.

Kao J, Upton M, Zhang P, et al. Individual prostate biopsy core (Bc) embedding facilitates maximal tissue representation. *J Urol* 168:496-499, 2002.

Kapoor DA, Klimberg IW, Malek GH, et al. Single-dose oral ciprofloxacin versus placebo for prophylaxis during transrectal prostate biopsy. *Urology* 52:552-558, 1998.

Karakiewicz PI, Hanley JA, Bazinet M. Three-dimensional computer-assisted analysis of sector biopsy of the prostate. *Urology* 52:208-212, 1998.

Kattan MW, Stapleton AM, Wheeler TM, et al. Evaluation of a nomogram to predict the pathologic stage of clinically localized prostate carcinoma. *Cancer* 79:528-537, 1997.

Kava BR, Dalbagni G, Conlon KC, et al. Results of laparoscopic pelvic lymphadenectomy in patients at high risk for nodal metastases from prostate cancer. *Ann Surg Oncol* 5:173-180, 1998.

Keetch DW, Catalona WJ. Prostatic transition zone biopsies in men with previous negative biopsies and persistently elevated serum prostate specific antigen values. *J Urol* 154:1795-1797, 1995.

Kleer E, Larson-Keller JJ, Zincke H, et al. Ability of preoperative serum prostate-specific antigen value to predict pathologic stage and DNA ploidy. Influence of clinical stage and tumor grade. *Urology* 41:207-216, 1993.

Kline TS, Kelsey DM, Kohler FP. Prostatic carcinoma and needle aspiration biopsy. *Am J Clin Pathol* 67:131-133, 1977.

Kline TS, Kohler FP, Kelsey DM. Aspiration biopsy cytology (ABC). Its use in diagnosis of lesions of the prostate gland. *Arch Pathol Lab Med* 106:136-139, 1982.

Kline TS, Kannan V. Prostatic aspirates. A cytomorphologic analysis with emphasis on well-differentiated carcinoma. *Diagn Cytopathol* 1:13-17, 1985.

Korman HJ, Leu PB, Huang RR, et al. A centralized comparison of radical perineal and retropubic prostatectomy specimens: is there a difference according to the surgical approach? *J Urol* 168:991-994, 2002.

Kozlowski JM, Grayhack JT. Carcinoma of the prostate. In: Gillenwater JT, Howards SS, Duckett JW, eds. *Adult and Pediatric Urology.* 3rd ed. St Louis: Mosby; 1604-1607, 1996.

Kramolowsky EV, Narayana AS, Platz CE, et al. The frozen section in lymphadenectomy for carcinoma of the prostate. *J Urol* 131:899-900, 1984.

Krishnan B, Truong LD. Prostatic adenocarcinoma diagnosed by urinary cytology. *Am J Clin Pathol* 113:29-34, 2000.

Labess M. Occult carcinoma in clinically benign hypertrophy of the prostate: a pathological and clinical study. *J Urol* 68:893-896, 1952.

Lane RB Jr, Babaian RJ, Troncoso P. Accuracy of staging biopsies for prostatic carcinoma [abstract]. *Mod Pathol* 11:87A, 1998A.

Lane RB Jr, Lane CG, Mangold KA, et al. Needle biopsies of the prostate. What constitutes adequate histologic sampling? *Arch Pathol Lab Med* 122:833-835, 1998B.

Larsen MP, Carter HB, Epstein JI. Can stage A1 tumor extent be predicted by transurethral resection tumor volume, percent or grade? A study of 64 stage A1 radical prostatectomies with comparison to prostates removed for stages A2 and B disease. *J Urol* 146:1059-1063, 1991.

Levine MA, Ittman M, Melamed J, et al. Two consecutive sets of transrectal ultrasound guided sextant biopsies of the prostate for detection of prostate cancer. *J Urol* 159:471-476, 1998.

Lui PD, Terris MK, McNeal JE, et al. Indications for ultrasound guided transition zone biopsies in the detection of prostate cancer. *J Urol* 153:1000-1003, 1995.

Lowe BA, Listrom MB. Incidental carcinomas of the prostate: an analysis of the predictors of progression. *J Urol* 140:1341-1347, 1988.

Lowe BA. Management of stage T1a prostate cancer. *Semin Urol Oncol* 14:178-182, 1996.

Lu-Yao GL, Greenberg ER. Changes in prostate cancer incidence and treatment in USA. *Lancet* 343:251-254, 1994.

Lu-Yao GL, McLerran D, Wasson J, et al, for the Prostate Patient Outcomes Research Team. An assessment of radical prostatectomy. Time trends, geographic variation, and outcomes. *JAMA* 269:2633-2636, 1993.

Lundberg S, Berge T. Prostatic carcinoma: an autopsy study of latent prostatic cancer. *Scand J Urol Nephrol* 4:93-103, 1970.

Maksem JA. Performance and processing of prostate aspiration biopsies. A strategy to ensure optimum cellularity and fixation. *J Urol Pathol* 3:347-353, 1995.

Mao H, Hoshi S, Takahashi T, et al. Detection of PSA mRNA from the peripheral blood and pelvic lymph nodes in patients with prostatic cancer by means of reverse transcription-polymerase chain reaction (RT-PCR) [in Japanese]. *Jpn J Urol* 84:596-603, 1998.

McDowell PR, Fox WM, Epstein JI. Is submission of remaining tissue necessary when incidental carcinoma of the prostate is found on transurethral resection? *Hum Pathol* 25:493-497, 1994.

McNeal JE. Normal histology of the prostate. *Am J Surg Pathol* 12:619-633, 1988.

Mebust WK, Holtgrewe HL, Cockett ATK, et al. Transurethral prostatectomy: immediate and postoperative complications. A cooperative study of 13 participating institutions evaluating 3,885 patients. *J Urol* 141:243-247, 1989.

Mettlin CJ, Murphy GP, Ho R, et al. The National Cancer Data Base Report on longitudinal observations on prostate cancer. *Cancer* 77:2162-2166, 1996.

Mettlin C. Changes in patterns of prostate cancer case in the United States: results of the American College of Surgeons Commission on Cancer Studies, 1974-1993. *Prostate* 32:221-226, 1997A.

Mettlin CJ, Murphy GP, Cunningham MP, et al. The National Cancer Data Base Report on race, age, and region variations in prostate cancer treatment. *Cancer* 80:1261-1266, 1997B.

Mills SE, Bostwick DG, Murphy WM, et al. A symposium on the surgical pathology of the prostate. *Pathol Annu* 25:109-158, 1990.

Monda JM, Barry MJ, Oesterling JE. Prostate specific antigen cannot distinguish stage T1a (A1) prostate cancer from benign prostatic hyperplasia. *J Urol* 151:1291-1295, 1994.

Montie JE, Wood DP Jr, Pontes JE, et al. Adenocarcinoma of the prostate in cystoprostatectomy specimens removed for bladder cancer. *Cancer* 63:381-385, 1989.

Moore GH, Lawshe B, Murphy J. Diagnosis of adenocarcinoma in transurethral resectates of the prostate gland. *Am J Surg Pathol* 10:165-169, 1986.

Moore RA. The morphology of small prostatic carcinoma. *J Urol* 33:224-230, 1935.

Morena JG, O'Hara SM, Long JP, et al. Transrectal ultrasound-guided biopsy causes hematogenous dissemination of prostate cells as determined by RT-PCR. *Urology* 49:515-520, 1997.

Mostofi FK. Editorial comments. *J Urol* 128:950, 1982.

Mostofi FK. Prostate sampling [editorial]. *Am J Surg Pathol* 10:175, 1986.

Moul JW, Miles BJ, Skoog SJ, et al. Risk factors for perineal seeding of prostate cancer after needle biopsy. *J Urol* 142:86-88, 1989.

Moul JW, Lewis DJ, Ross AA, et al. Immunohistologic detection of prostate cancer pelvic lymph node micrometastases: correlation to preoperative serum prostate-specific antigen. *Urology* 43:68-73, 1994.

Moul JW, Bauer JJ, Srivastava S, et al. Perineal seeding of prostate cancer as the only evidence of clinical recurrence 14 years after needle biopsy and radical prostatectomy: molecular correlation. *Urology* 51:158-160, 1998.

Müller H-A, Ackerman R, Frohmüller HG. The value of perineal punch biopsy in estimating the histological grade of carcinoma of the prostate. *Prostate* 1:303-309, 1980.

Murphy WM, Dean PJ, Brasfield JA, et al. Incidental carcinoma of the prostate: how much sampling is adequate? *Am J Surg Pathol* 10:170-174, 1986.

Murphy WM, Gaeta JF. Diseases of the prostate gland and seminal vesicles. In: Murphy WM, ed. *Urological Pathology.* Philadelphia: Saunders; 170-202, 1989.

Murphy WM, Ramsey J, Soloway MS. A better nuclear fixative for diagnostic bladder and prostate biopsies. *J Urol Pathol* 1:79-87, 1993.

Murphy WM. Diseases of the urinary bladder, urethra, ureters, and renal pelves. In: Murphy WM, ed. *Urological Pathology.* 2nd ed. Philadelphia: Saunders; 72, 1997.

Narayan P, Fournier G, Gajendran V, et al. Utility of preoperative serum prostate-specific antigen concentration and biopsy Gleason score in predicting risk of pelvic lymph node metastases in prostate cancer. *Urology* 44:519-524, 1994.

Narayan P, Tewari A. Systematic biopsy-based staging of prostate cancer: scientific background, individual variables, combination of parameters, and current integrative models. *Semin Urol Oncol* 16:172-181, 1998.

Naughton CK, Smith DS, Humphrey PA, et al. Clinical and pathologic tumor characteristics of prostate cancer as a function of the number of biopsy cores. A retrospective study. *Urology* 52:808-813, 1998.

Naughton CK, Ornstein DK, Smith DS, et al. Pain and morbidity of transrectal ultrasound guided prostate biopsy: a prospective randomized trial of 6 versus 12 cores. *J Urol* 163:168-171, 2000.

Nickel JC. Prostatitis and related conditions. In: Walsh PC, Retik AB, Vaughn ED Jr, et al, eds. *Campbell's Urology.* 8th ed. Philadelphia: Saunders; 603-630, 2002.

Niemann TH, Tranovich JG, De Young BR. Biopsy bag artifact. *Am J Clin Pathol* 110:224-226, 1998.

Norberg M, Holmberg L, Häggman M, et al. Determinants of complications after multiple transrectal core biopsies of the prostate. *Eur Radiol* 6:457-461, 1996A.

Norberg M, Holmberg L, Busch C, et al. Multiple transrectal ultrasound-guided biopsies for the detection of prostate cancer and the determination of tumor volume, grade, and seminal vesicle invasion. *Eur Radiol* 6:56-61, 1996B.

O'Briain DS, Sheils O, McElwaine S, et al. Sorting out mix-ups: the provenance of tissue sections may be confirmed by PCR using microsatellite markers. *Am J Clin Pathol* 106:758-764, 1996.

Ohori M, Scardino PT, Lapin SL, et al. The mechanisms and prognostic significance of seminal vesicle involvement by prostate cancer. *Am J Surg Pathol* 17:1252-1259, 1993.

Ohori M, Wheeler TM, Dunn JK, et al. The pathological features and prognosis of prostate cancer detectable with current diagnostic tests. *J Urol* 152:1714-1720, 1994.

Onder AU, Yalcin V, Arar O, et al. Impact of transition zone biopsies in detection and evaluation of prostate cancer. *Eur Urol* 33:542-548, 1998.

Parker SL, Tong T, Bolden S, et al. Cancer statistics, 1996. *CA Cancer J Clin* 46:5-27, 1996.

Partin AW, Yoo JK, Carter HB, et al. The use of prostate-specific antigen clinical stage and Gleason score to predict pathologic stage in men with localized prostate cancer. *J Urol* 150:110-114, 1993.

Partin AW, Subong ENP, Walsh PC, et al. Combination of prostate-specific antigen, clinical stage, and Gleason score to predict pathological stage of localized prostate cancer: a multi-institutional update. *JAMA* 277:1445-1451, 1997.

Pearle MS, Oyasu R, Hidvegi D, et al. Touch preparation cytological evaluation of radical prostatectomy specimens. *J Urol* 152:124-128, 1994.

Petros JA, Catalona WJ. Lower incidence of unsuspected lymph node metastases in 521 consecutive patients with clinically localized prostate cancer. *J Urol* 147:1574-1575, 1992.

Presti JC, Chang JJ, Bhargava V, et al. The optimal systematic prostate biopsy scheme should include 8 rather than 6 biopsies: results of a prospective clinical trial. *J Urol* 163:163-167, 2000.

Price DK, Clontz DR, Woodard WL III, et al. Detection and clearance of prostate cells subsequent to ultrasound-guided needle biopsy as determined by multiplex nested reverse transcription polymerase chain reaction assay. *Urology* 52:261-267, 1998.

Price H, McNeal JE, Stamey TA. Evolving patterns of tissue composition in benign prostatic hyperplasia as a function of specimen size. *Hum Pathol* 21:578-585, 1990.

Pritchett TR, Moreno J, Warner NE, et al. Unsuspected prostatic adenocarcinoma in patients who have undergone radical cystoprostatectomy for transitional cell carcinoma of the bladder. *J Urol* 139:1214-1216, 1988.

Puppo P, Perachino M. Clinical stage, prostate-specific antigen and Gleason grade to predict extracapsular disease or nodal metastasis in men with newly diagnosed, previously untreated prostate cancer. A multicenter study. *Eur Urol* 32:273-279, 1997.

Rassweiler J, Sentker L, Seeman O, et al. Laparoscopic radical prostatectomy with the Heilbronn technique: an analysis of the first 180 cases. *J Urol* 166:2101-2108, 2001.

Ravery V, Boccon-Gibod LA, Dauge-Geffroy MC, et al. Systematic biopsies accurately predict extracapsular extension of prostate cancer and persistent/recurrent detectable PSA after radical prostatectomy. *Urology* 44:371-376, 1994.

Ravery V, Goldblatt L, Royer B, et al. Extensive biopsy protocol improves the detection rate of prostate cancer. *J Urol* 164:393-396, 2000.

Renshaw AA, Chang H, D'Amico AV. An abbreviated protocol for processing radical prostatectomy specimens. Analysis of tumor grade, stage, margin status, and volume. *J Urol Pathol* 5:183-192, 1996.

Renshaw AA. Adequate tissue sampling of prostate core needle biopsies. *Am J Clin Pathol* 107:26-29, 1997A.

Renshaw AA, Nappi D, Cibas ES. Cytology of metastatic adenocarcinoma of the prostate in pleural effusions. *Diagn Cytopathol* 15:103-107, 1997B.

Renshaw AA. Correlation of gross morphologic features with histologic features in radical prostatectomy specimens. *Am J Clin Pathol* 110:38-42, 1998.

Reyes AO, Humphrey PA. Diagnostic effect of complete histologic sampling of prostate needle biopsy specimens. *Am J Clin Pathol* 109:416-422, 1998.

Rich AR. On the frequency of occurrence of occult carcinoma of the prostate. *J Urol* 33:215-223, 1935.

Roach M, Marquez C, Yuo HS, et al. Predicting the risk of lymph node involvement using the pre-treatment prostate-specific antigen and Gleason score in men with clinically localized prostate cancer. *Int J Radiat Oncol Biol Phys* 28:33-37, 1994.

Rogatsch H, Moser P, Volgger H, et al. Diagnostic effect of an improved preembedding method of prostate needle biopsy specimens. *Hum Pathol* 31:1102-1107, 2000.

Rogers E, Gurpinar T, Dillioglugil O, et al. The role of rectal examination, biopsy Gleason sum, and prostate-specific antigen in selecting patients who require pelvic lymph node dissections for prostate cancer. *Br J Urol* 78:419-425, 1996.

Rohr LR. Incidental adenocarcinoma in transurethral resections of the prostate: partial versus complete microscopic examination. *Am J Surg Pathol* 11:53-58, 1987.

Rovner ES, Schanne FJ, Malkowicz SB, et al. Transurethral biopsy of the prostate for persistently elevated or increasing prostate specific antigen following multiple negative transrectal biopsies. *J Urol* 158:138-142, 1997.

Roy CR, Horne D, Raife M, et al. Incidental carcinoma of the prostate: long-term follow-up. *Urology* 36:210-213, 1990.

Sakr WA, Grignon DJ, Crissman JD, et al. High-grade prostatic intraepithelial neoplasia (HGPIN) and prostatic adenocarcinoma between the ages of 20-69: an autopsy study of 249 cases. *In Vivo* 8:439-444, 1994.

Sakr WA, Grignon DJ, Visscher DW, et al. Evaluating the radical prostatectomy specimen, part I. *J Urol Pathol* 3:355-364, 1995.

Sakr WA, Wheeler TM, Blute M, et al. Workgroup 2. Staging and reporting of prostate cancer-sampling of the radical prostatectomy specimen. *Cancer* 78:366-368, 1996.

Sakr WA, Grignon DJ. Prostate. Practice parameters, pathologic staging, and handling radical prostatectomy specimens. *Urol Clin North Am* 26:453-463, 1999.

Saltzstein SL, McLaughlin AP. Clinicopathologic features of unsuspected regional lymph node metastases in prostatic adenocarcinoma. *Cancer* 40:1212-1221, 1977.

Sands ME, Zagars GK, Pollack A, et al. Serum prostate-specific antigen, clinical stage, pathologic grade, and the incidence of nodal metastases in prostate cancer. *Urology* 44:215-220, 1994.

Schmid HP, McNeal JE. An abbreviated standard procedure for accurate tumor volume estimation in prostate cancer. *Am J Surg Pathol* 16:184-191, 1992.

Schmidt WA. Urinary and male genital systems. In: *Principles and Techniques of Surgical Pathology.* Menlo Park, Ca: Addison-Wesley; 537-548, 1983.

Scott R Jr, Mutchnik DL, Laskowski TZ, et al. Carcinoma of the prostate in elderly men. *J Urol* 101:602-607, 1969.

Sehdev AE, Pan CC, Epstein JI. Comparative analysis of sampling methods for grossing radical prostatectomy specimens performed for nonpalpable (stage T1c) prostatic adenocarcinoma. *Hum Pathol* 32:494-499, 2001.

Sgrignoli AR, Walsh PC, Steinberg GD, et al. Prognostic factors in men with stage D1 prostate cancer: Identification of patients less likely to have prolonged survival after radical prostatectomy. *J Urol* 152:1077-1081, 1994.

Shaw EB, Daniel BW, Wofford ED, et al. Prostate biopsies: optimized cancer detection and staging. *J S C Med Assoc* 92:261-266, 1996.

Shibata D. Identification of mismatched fixed specimens with a commercially available kit based on the polymerase chain reaction. *Am J Clin Pathol* 100:666-670, 1993.

Shoskes DA, Trachtenberg J. The value of prostate-specific antigen levels in pelvic lymph nodes for diagnosing metastatic spread of prostate cancer. *Can J Surg* 36:33-36, 1993.

Spevack L, Killion LT, West JC Jr, et al. Predicting the patient at low risk for lymph node metastasis with localized prostate cancer: an analysis of four statistical models. *Int J Radiat Oncol Biol Phys* 34:543-547, 1996.

Srigley JR, Amin MB, Bostwick DG, et al, Members of Cancer Committee, College of American Pathologists: Updated protocol for examination of specimens from patients with carcinomas of the prostate gland. A basis for checklists. *Arch Pathol Lab Med* 124:1034-1039, 2000.

Srigley JR, Jones B, Kapusta L. The effect of specimen submission protocols on the detection rate of histologic abnormalities in sextant prostate biopsies [abstract]. *Mod Pathol* 14:123A, 2001.

Stamey TA. Making the most out of six systematic sextant biopsies. *Urology* 45:2-12, 1995.

Steele GD Jr, Osteen RT, Winchester DP, et al. Clinical highlights from the National Cancer Data Base: 1994. *CA Cancer J Clin* 44:71-80, 1994.

Stewart CS, Leibovich BC, Weaver AL, et al. Prostate cancer diagnosis using a saturation needle biopsy technique after previous negative sextant biopsies. *J Urol* 166:86-92, 2001.

Stillwell TJ, Malek RS, Engen DE, et al. Incidental adenocarcinomas after open prostatic adenectomy. *J Urol* 141:76-78, 1989.

Stone NN, Stock RG, Unger P. Indications for seminal vesicle biopsy and laparoscopic pelvic lymph node dissection in men with localized carcinoma of prostate. *J Urol* 154:1392-1396, 1995.

Stone NN, Stock RG, Parikh D, et al. Perineural invasion and seminal vesicle involvement predict pelvic lymph node metastasis in men with localized carcinoma of the prostate. *J Urol* 160:1722-1726, 1998.

Stroumbakis N, Cookson MS, Reuter VE, et al. Clinical significance of repeat sextant biopsies in prostate cancer patients. *Urology* 49:(suppl 3A):113-118, 1997.

Suzuki T, Jinho S, Imui K. Histopathological study of incidental carcinoma of the prostate. *Jpn J Urol* 79:1529-1534, 1988.

Svetec D, McCabe K, Peretsman S, et al. Prostate rebiopsy is a poor surrogate of treatment efficacy in localized prostate cancer. *J Urol* 159:1606-1608, 1998.

Terris MK, Wallen EM, Stamey TA. Comparison of mid-lobe versus lateral systematic sextant biopsies in the detection of prostate cancer. *Urol Int* 59:239-242, 1997A.

Terris MK, Hausdorff J, Freiha FS. Hematolymphoid malignancies diagnosed at the time of radical prostatectomy. *J Urol* 158:1457-1459, 1997B.

Terris MK, Pham TQ, Issa MM, et al. Routine transition zone and seminal vesicle biopsies in all patients undergoing transrectal ultrasound guided prostate biopsies are not indicated. *J Urol* 157:204-206, 1997C.

Terris MK. Ultrasonography and biopsy of the prostate. In: Walsh PC, Retik AB, Vaughn ED Jr, et al, eds. *Campbell's Urology.* 8th ed. Philadelphia: Saunders; 3038-3054, 2002.

Tewari A, Narayan P. Novel staging tool for localized prostate cancer: a pilot study using genetic adaptive neural networks. *J Urol* 160:430-436, 1998.

Thompson IM, Zeidman EJ. Extended follow-up of stage A1 carcinoma of the prostate. *Urology* 33:455-458, 1989.

Thorson P, Vollmer RT, Arcangeli C, et al. Minimal carcinoma in prostate needle biopsy specimens: diagnostic features and radical prostatectomy follow-up. *Mod Pathol* 11:543-551, 1998.

Trieger P, Welfeld J, Marx J. Suprapubic prostatectomy: a review of 108 cases. *Urol Cutan Rev* 52:8-9, 1948.

True LD. Surgical pathology examination of the prostate gland. Practice survey by American Society of Clinical Pathologists. *Am J Clin Pathol* 102:572-579, 1994.

Tsuang MT, Weiss MA, Evans AT. Transurethral resection of the prostate with partial resection of the seminal vesicle. *J Urol* 126:615-617, 1981.

Vallancien G, Bochereau G, Wetzel O, et al. Influence of preoperative positive seminal vesicle biopsy on the staging of prostatic cancer. *J Urol* 152:1152-1156, 1994.

van Andel G, Vleeming R, Kurth K, et al. Incidental carcinoma of the prostate. *Semin Surg Oncol* 11:36-45, 1995.

Vashi AR, Wojno KT, Gillespie B, et al. A model for the number of cores per prostate biopsy based on patient age and prostate gland volume. *J Urol* 159:920-924, 1998.

Vollmer RT. Prostate cancer and chip specimens: complete versus partial sampling. *Hum Pathol* 17:285-290, 1986.

Vollmer RT. Tissue sampling to detect incidental carcinoma of the prostate: In: *Progress in Reproductive and Urinary Tract Pathology.* Vol 1. 91-100, 1989.

Walsh PC. Anatomic radical retropubic prostatectomy. In: Walsh PC, Retik AB, Vaughan ED Jr, et al, eds. *Campbell's Urology.* 8th ed. Philadelphia: Saunders; 3107-3129, 2002.

Wawroschek F, Vogt H, Weckermann D, et al. The sentinel lymph node concept in prostate cancer: first results of gamma probe-guided sentinel lymph node identification. *Eur Urol* 36:595-600, 1999.

Wendel RG, Evans AT. Complications of punch biopsy of the prostate gland. *J Urol* 97:122-126, 1967.

Wheeler TM. Anatomic considerations in carcinoma of the prostate. *Urol Clin North Am* 16:623-634, 1989.

Wheeler TM, Lebovitz RM. Fresh tissue harvest for research from prostatectomy specimens. *Prostate* 25:274-279, 1994.

Winfield HW, Reddy PK, Lange PH. Coexisting adenocarcinoma of prostate in patients undergoing cystoprostatectomy for bladder cancer. *Urology* 30:100-101, 1987.

Winsor L. Tissue processing. In: Woods AE, Ellis RC, eds. *Laboratory Histopathology: A Complete Reference.* New York: Churchill Livingstone; 4.2-1 to 4.2-42, 1994.

Wojcik EM, Orozco R, O'Dowd GJ. The role of fine needle aspiration of the prostate in the era of an automated thin needle biopsy gun. *J Urol Pathol* 7:87-97, 1997.

Woods AE, Ellis RC. Tissue and section preparation-safely data. In: Woods AE, Ellis RC, eds. *Laboratory Histopathology: A Complete Reference.* Vol 1. New York: Churchill Livingstone; 4.7, 1994.

Xia Z, Jacobsen SJ, Bergstralh EJ, et al. Secular changes in radical prostatectomy utilization rates in Olmstead County, Minnesota 1980 to 1995. *J Urol* 159:904-908, 1998.

Zincke H, Oesterling JE, Blute ML, et al. Long-term (15 years) results after radical prostatectomy for clinically localized (stage T2c or lower) prostate cancer. *J Urol* 152:1850-1857, 1994.

Fine Needle Aspiration Biopsy of the Prostate

[3.1] The Cells **59**

[3.2] Benign Diseases of the Prostate **62**

[3.3] Malignant Diseases of the Prostate **64**

[3.4] Variants of Prostatic Carcinoma **68**

CHAPTER 3

Needle aspiration biopsy in the diagnosis of prostatic neoplasms has been practiced since at least 1930 (Ferguson 1930), but its use became widespread only after the description of the Franzén needle guide in 1960 (Franzén 1960). Although transrectal ultrasound–guided core needle biopsy is currently popular, fine needle aspiration (FNA) biopsy of the prostate may still find a place in clinical practice. FNA biopsy of the prostate is a safe, easy, and highly accurate diagnostic technique (Adolfsson 1991, Ajzen 1989, Alfthan 1970, Andersson 1967, M Benson 1988, Brenner 1990, Carter 1986, Chodak 1984, 1986, Dejter 1988, Ekman 1967, Engelstein 1994, N Epstein 1976A, Graham 1988, Hosking 1983, Ito 1995, Kaufman 1982, Kelsey 1976, Kline 1977, Klotz 1989, Melograna 1982, Narayan 1989, 1991, Polito 1990, Walsh 1986). Unfortunately, FNA biopsy of the prostate cannot currently be recommended as a screening test for prostatic cancer in asymptomatic men (Agatstein 1987, Breda 1994, Conrad 2001, Hautmann 2000, Juusela 1992, Palmer 1995, Stege 1999). However, FNA biopsy can be used to obtain material for sophisticated diagnostic and prognostic testing, such as DNA analysis, molecular diagnostics, cytogenetic studies, and biochemical and immunochemical analysis (Buhmeida 2001a, Maffini 2001, Muñoz de Toro 1998, Pousette 1997).

The diagnostic accuracy correlates with the grade and stage of the tumor: the more advanced, the more accurate. The sensitivity of FNA biopsy (to the presence of cancer) is about 90% (Al-Abadi 1997, M Benson 1988, Bentley 1988, Ljung 1986, Niejadlik 1990, Singh 1997). This compares favorably with core biopsy.

False-negative diagnostic results are difficult to prove because lesions thought to be benign are likely to be treated conservatively, and many patients are lost to follow-up evaluation or die of an unrelated illness. False-negative results usually are related to sampling error, underdiagnosis of a well-differentiated adenocarcinoma, or tumor sclerosis, yielding few diagnostic cells (Willems 1981). Sampling not only the nodule but also other areas of the gland may increase the diagnostic yield (Maksem 1988A). The unsatisfactory rate depends greatly on the experience of the operator but is generally in the range of 2% to 10% (Bishop 1977, Brenner 1990, Denton 1967, Eble 1992, Esposti 1966, 1980, Jocham 1983, Lin 1979, Melograna 1982, Suhrland 1988).

False-positive results are rare, less than 1% of cases (Eble 1992). Be cautious making an unequivocally malignant diagnosis based on only a few atypical cells or in the presence of inflammation (Ljung 1985). Most false-positive results represent errors of interpretation of inflammatory changes. False-positive diagnoses can also be related to atypical hyperplasia and dysplasia (prostatic intraepithelial neoplasia [PIN]), squamous metaplasia, granulomatous prostatitis, and seminal vesicle or other atypical but benign cells (Tannenbaum 1983A, Willems 1981). However, a positive result on FNA biopsy in the face of a negative core biopsy result or transurethral resection specimen cannot be simply dismissed as a false-positive cytologic diagnosis; these patients need careful follow-up (Polito 1990). Most patients who have contradictory tissue and cytologic biopsy results ultimately are found to have cancer (Anandan 1983). Moreover, patients with aspirates diagnosed as suspicious subsequently are proven to have prostatic carcinoma in up to three quarters of cases (Ritchie 1988, Smith 1988, Stilmant 1989). False-positive diagnostic results could be proven only by meticulous examination of the entire gland (prostatectomy, autopsy) (M Benson 1988, Maksem 1988A).

FNA biopsy of the prostate is generally safe. Serious complications are rare (<1% to 2%) and mostly infectious in nature (Ito 1995). Fever and septicemia (which has proven fatal in at least 1 case) have been reported after FNA biopsy of active prostatitis (Esposti 1975). Therefore, patients with evidence of clinical prostatitis should be evaluated with utmost caution. Clinically active prostatitis (with pain and fever) is a contraindication to biopsy and should be treated before prostate biopsy is performed. FNA biopsy should be performed to diagnose only cancer, not prostatitis. However, a history of prostatitis is not in itself a contraindication to FNA biopsy. Prostatic cancer and prostatitis coexist in a significant number of patients (Maksem 1988A).

Prophylactic antibiotic administration for asymptomatic patients may be considered, particularly for diabetic or other high-risk (ie, immunodeficient) patients (deKernion 1983, Ljung 1986). If antibiotics are given, they should be administered before the procedure to be effective (Bissa 1977). It has been recommended that urine cultures be checked—and be sterile—before performing the biopsy, as with other urologic procedures (M Benson 1988). Because of the small risk of serious infection, patients should be instructed to seek immediate medical attention if they develop a fever within a few days of the procedure.

No other special preparation (eg, diets, enemas) is necessary. Transient hematuria or hematospermia and minor rectal bleeding may occur; although benign, these can be frightening to the patient, who should therefore be forewarned (deKernion 1983, Gustafsson 1990). Significant bleeding is extremely rare with FNA biopsy of the prostate but has been reported (Narayan 1989).

The procedure can be performed with the patient in the knee-chest position, in the dorsal lithotomy position, bent over an examining table, or lying on his side with his knees pulled toward his head. Anesthesia usually is not necessary, but adequate lubrication should be used. The prostate is examined; the lesion is located and mentally visualized. The biopsy specimen is then obtained by direct palpation with a Franzén needle guide or other similar device (which can even be constructed from the plastic sleeve the biopsy needle comes in or from a plastic syringe [Lal 1998, Maksem 1990]). Except for the guiding device, the biopsy procedure is quite similar to aspiration of a superficial target (Ljung 1985, Wajsman 1987, Willems 1981).

[3.1] The Cells

The prostate gland is composed of ducts and acini set in a fibromuscular stroma. The walls of the ducts and acini have corrugations that are distensible, providing a reservoir for prostatic secretions. Except for the main excretory ducts near the urethra, the duct and acinar cells are identical. The ductal-acinar units are lined by 2 layers of cells—basal cells and epithelial (secretory) cells—analogous to the arrangement of myoepithelial and epithelial cells seen in the breast. However, the prostatic basal cells lack muscle filaments of breast myoepithelial cells (Brandes 1964, Fisher 1965). The epithelial cells secrete a variety of substances into the seminal fluid. In addition, scattered neuroendocrine cells are present, but special stains are needed to distinguish them (Di Sant'Agnese 1992). Transitional epithelium (urothelium) lines the prostatic urethra and extends for variable distances into the main excretory ducts.

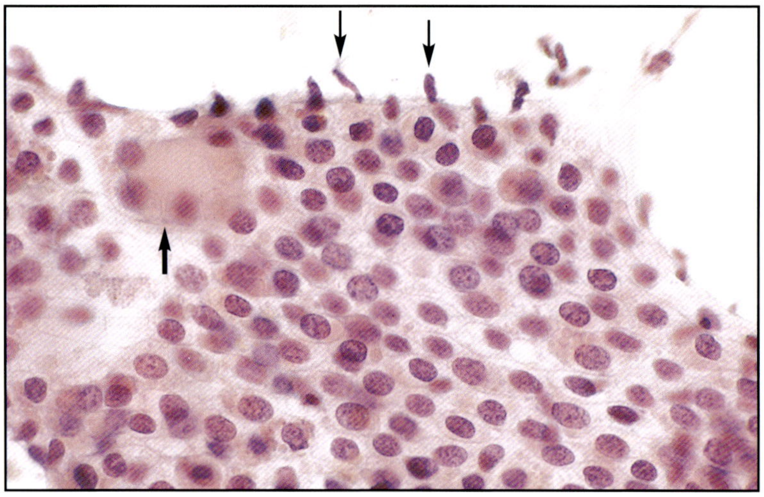

■ **i3.1** *Prostatic secretory cells. Reminiscent of endocervical cells. The cells are uniform, with smooth, round nuclei, fine chromatin, and inconspicuous or invisible nucleoli, in cohesive flat, honeycombed sheets. Monolayered sheets of these cells, with bland nuclei, are characteristic of benign prostatic aspirates. Note basal cells attached at the periphery (light arrows) and small corpus amylaceum (heavy arrow). (Pap)*

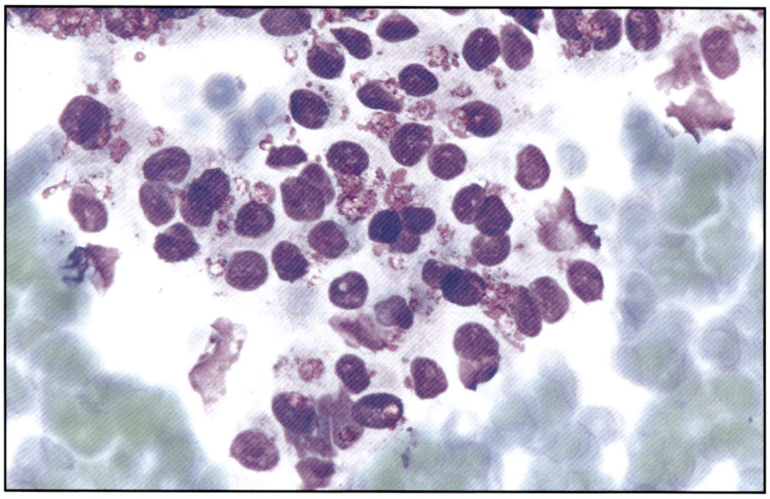

■ **i3.2** *Prostatic secretory cells. The presence of coarse red (metachromatic) granules in the cytoplasm is a clue to a benign diagnosis. Be cautious diagnosing malignancy when red granules are seen in the cells. (Diff-Quik)*

Secretory Epithelial Cells

The secretory epithelial cells of the prostate are reminiscent of endocervical cells **i3.1, i3.2**. They occur in aspirates as cohesive, flat, orderly sheets of variable size (Koss 1984). The cells are uniform and arranged in orderly ranks and files with few or no microacinar formations; microacinar complexes suggest malignancy. Single cells are normally sparse. Prostate aspirates from younger men (<40 years old) tend to be more cellular, the cells are more columnar in shape, and occasional microacinar groups may be seen (Howell 1990).

The nuclei are particularly important diagnostically and lack any significant atypia in benign, noninflamed aspirate specimens. The normal nucleus is about the size of a red blood cell; larger nuclei are suspicious for malignancy (Kline 1985, Maksem 1988A). The nuclear membrane is smooth and uniform, the chromatin is fine and evenly distributed, and nucleoli are inconspicuous or invisible in normal prostatic cells. In the absence of inflammation, numerous prominent nucleoli strongly suggest malignancy.

The cytoplasm is delicate and vacuolated, and the cell borders are distinctly visualized (forming well-defined honeycombs) (Faul 1973). Coarse cytoplasmic granules, or “freckles” (golden-brown, Papanicolaou; red-purple, Diff-Quik®) (Koizumi 1990), are common in benign aspirates and absent or rare in cancer **i3.2**.

Basal Cells

Basal cells are small, with scant cytoplasm, and have uniform ovoid or bipolar, slightly hyperchromatic nuclei. Like myoepithelial cells of the breast, basal cells often are attached to sheets of epithelial cells at the periphery or half a plane above **i3.1**, and may also be dispersed in the background of the smear as naked oval nuclei. In hyperplasia, basal cells are increased in number, may aggregate, and appear larger and plumper **i3.3** (Maksem 1988A). There are fewer basal cells in prostatic atrophy. Keratin staining, using a basal cell–specific antibody, may be helpful in distinguishing benign lesions, which highlight intermingled basal cells, from well-differentiated adenocarcinoma, which lacks basal cells (Ostrzega 1988).

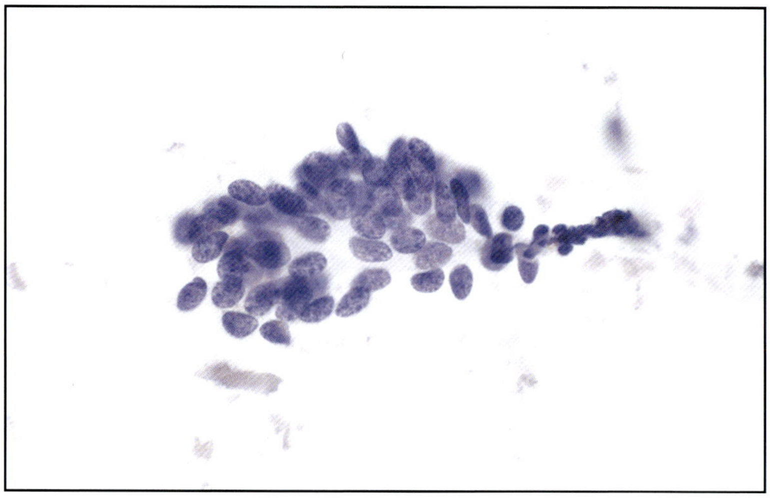

■ **i3.3** *Basal cells. Spindle-shaped cells that are the equivalent of myoepithelial cells in the breast. In hyperplasia (illustrated), basal cells are increased in number, form cohesive groups, and appear larger and plumper. (Pap)*

Bizarre Benign Cells

Occasionally, bizarre epithelial cells deriving from seminal vesicle (Arias-Stella 1958, Ibarrola de Andrés 2000, Singh 1997), epididymis (Kuo 1981), or ejaculatory ducts (Mesonero 1991) may be sampled during prostatic FNA biopsy (Koivuniemi 1976). Such atypical cells are more common in older men **i3.4, i3.5**.

The appearance of these bizarre cells can be quite alarming, possibly leading to a mistaken diagnosis of malignancy (Ibarrola de Andrés 2000, Koizumi 1990, Koss 1984, Kuo 1981, Melograna 1982). However, the changes are degenerative, and highly atypical cells usually are not numerous. The atypical cells can have markedly enlarged, pleomorphic, hyperchromatic (polyploid), occasionally even monstrous nuclei; high nuclear-cytoplasmic ratios; macronucleoli; and intranuclear cytoplasmic invaginations. Seminal vesicle cells can form microacinar structures (Droese 1976). The chromatin usually is smudgy (suggesting degeneration) but can vary from fine to very coarse.

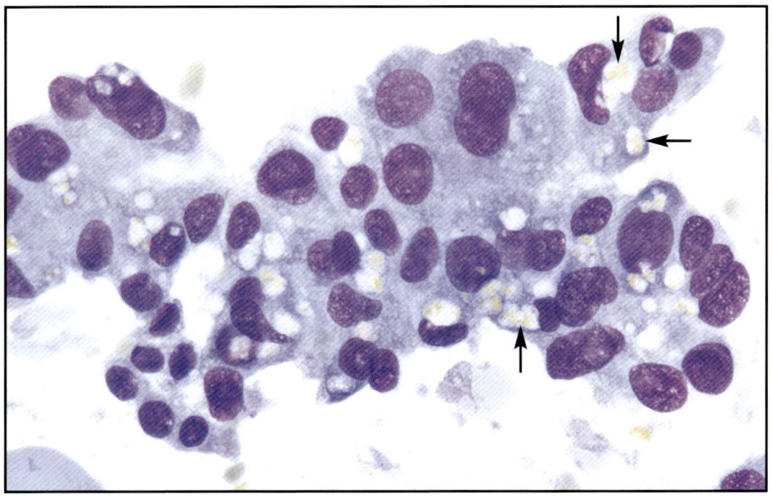

■ **i3.4** *Seminal vesicle cells. Often have an atypical appearance, with enlarged, pleomorphic nuclei. A clue to the proper diagnosis is presence of golden brown cytoplasmic lipochrome pigment (arrows). Sperm are often present in the background. (Diff-Quik)*

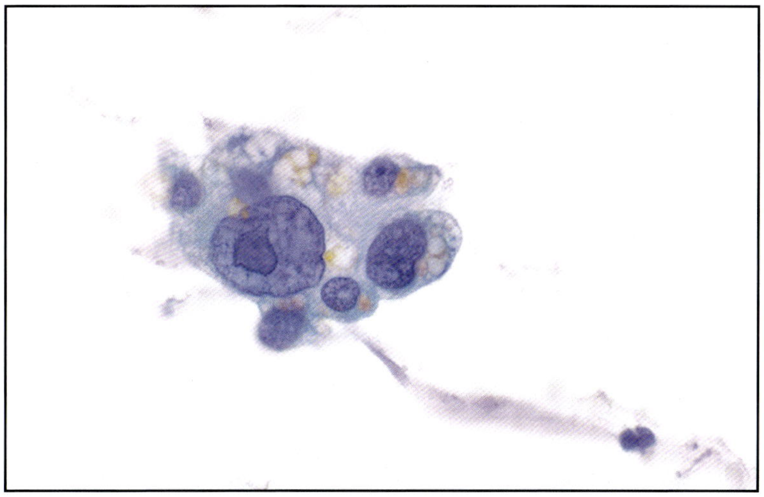

■ **i3.5** *Seminal vesicle cells. Occasionally, bizarre cells are present, with macronucleoli or intranuclear cytoplasmic invaginations. Note golden brown cytoplasmic pigment. (Pap)*

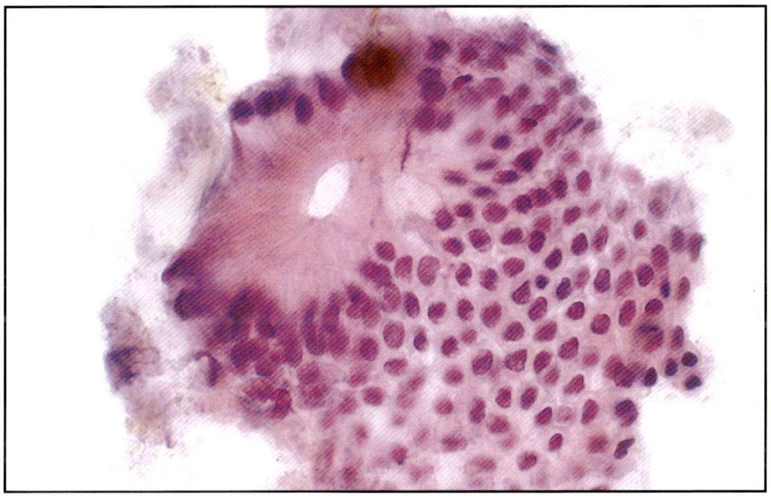

■ **i3.6** *Rectal mucosa. Rectal mucosa is commonly aspirated. Rectal cells normally form acinar structures and may have reactive atypia, including prominent nucleoli, mimicking prostatic adenocarcinoma. (Pap)*

Two helpful clues to the proper recognition of these cells are cytoplasmic pigment and sperm. The pigment is golden-brown in Papanicolaou and dark blue-green in Diff-Quik; it is usually present but may be sparse. Sperm usually are numerous but may be rare or absent in older or azoospermatic men. Degenerated cells and histiocytes are also present in a dirty or mucoid background, which may exhibit "crack artifact" similar to thyroid colloid (Droese 1976, Melograna 1982). Seminal vesicle and ejaculatory duct cells are prostate-specific antigen (PSA) and prostatic acid phosphatase (PAP) negative (Mostofi 1992B). Of course, the presence of seminal vesicle cells does not exclude the possibility of a coexisting prostatic carcinoma (Koivuniemi 1976). Although extremely rare, seminal vesicle carcinoma also occurs (R Benson 1984).

Other possible sources of atypical but benign cells include prostatic stromal hyperplasia with bizarre nuclei, akin to those occurring in symplastic leiomyoma (Eble 1991); megakaryocytes (and other bone marrow elements obtained from accidental penetration of the ischium); and ganglion cells (accompanied by strands of wavy neural tissue) (Greenebaum 1988). Paucity of atypical cells is a clue to a benign diagnosis.

Rectal Contaminants

Rectal mucosa can be aspirated inadvertently. It occurs as sheets of cells that, in contrast with benign prostate, normally form acinar structures (ie, crypts) and often display reactive nuclear atypia, including nucleoli, nuclear grooves, and some degree of pleomorphism **i3.6**. These features could be mistaken for prostate cancer. Clues to benign rectal cells include overall uniformity and cohesion of the cells, larger cell size, tall columnar shape, cytoplasmic mucin (goblet cells), thick mucus in the background, and lack of frankly malignant criteria (Koss 1984). Other elements found in the rectum, including granular debris and vegetable matter, may also be seen.

Squamous Cells

Squamous cells can be found in prostatic aspirates either as contaminants from the anus or as a result of squamous metaplasia of the prostatic glandular epithelium. Squamous metaplasia is common and associated with prostatic hyperplasia, infarcts, infection, surgery, and long-term catheterization and in estrogen therapy used to treat prostate cancer (Koss 1984, Singh 1997). Prostatic squamous cells usually resemble immature or mature metaplasia, as seen in the Pap test, but may show reactive/reparative changes (Miralles 1988).

Miscellaneous Findings

A variety of miscellaneous cell types can occasionally be seen in prostatic aspirates (N Epstein 1976A). Transitional (urothelial) cells can be sampled from the prostatic urethra or, in some cases, the bladder. Smooth muscle cells, although abundant in the prostate, usually are inconspicuous in FNA biopsy specimens of the gland.

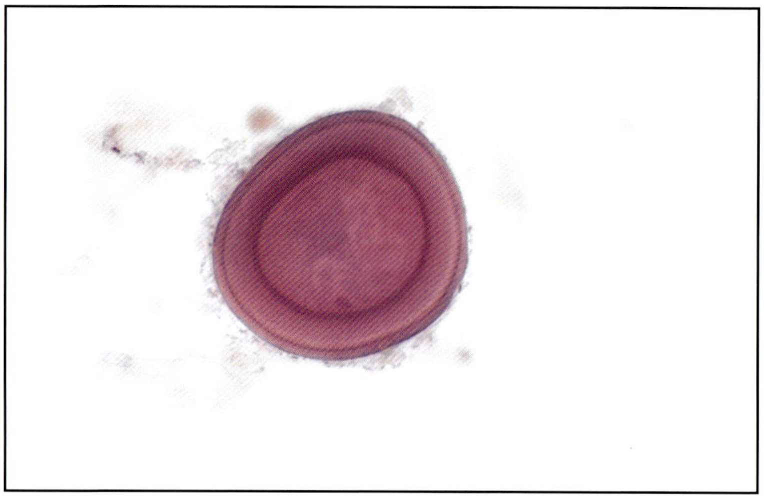

■ **i3.7** *Corpus amylaceum. Also known as prostatic concretions. These are concentrically laminated spherules of inspissated secretory product and are a relatively common finding that increases with age. (Pap)*

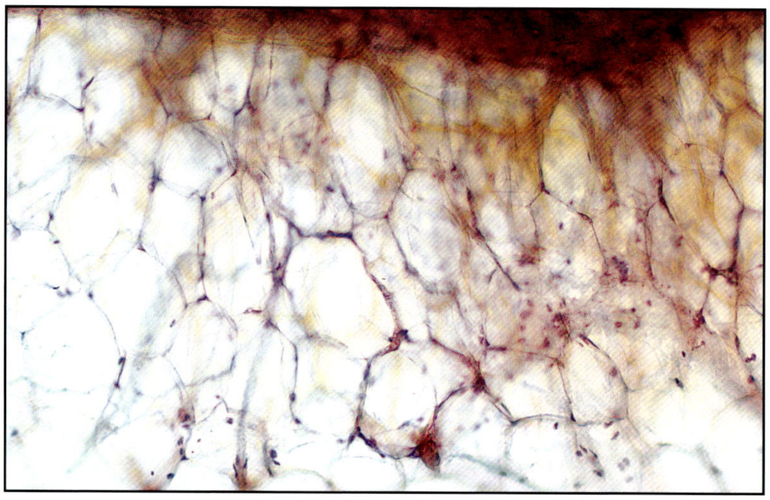

■ **i3.8** *Other contaminants. Squamous cells from the anus, urothelial cells from the urethra or bladder, megakaryocytes and ganglion cells, and perirectal adipose tissue (illustrated) may occasionally be aspirated. (Pap)*

Corpora amylacea, or prostatic concretions, are common and increase with age. They are concentrically laminated, slightly faceted spherules of inspissated secretory product, which may calcify **i3.7**. Occasionally, perirectal adipose tissue is aspirated **i3.8**.

[3.2] Benign Diseases of the Prostate

A variety of benign diseases, including cysts (Hessel 1993, Stricker 1993), inflammations, and hyperplasias, can affect the prostate.

Prostatitis

Although FNA biopsy is contraindicated in the presence of known active prostatitis (Esposti 1975, Maksem 1988C), it can sometimes be difficult to distinguish prostatitis from carcinoma clinically (Leistenschneider 1979, Maksem 1988C). Moreover, because of epithelial atypia associated with inflammation, the cytologic distinction can also be difficult in some cases. Furthermore, prostatitis can coexist with carcinoma (Esposti 1975, Maksem 1988C).

Acute Prostatitis

Acute prostatitis usually is bacterial in origin. It can present dramatically, with fever, chills, and signs of lower urinary tract disease (frequency, urgency, dysuria). The digital rectal examination reveals a swollen, tender prostate gland. There is no reason to obtain a biopsy of the prostate in this clinical setting; in fact, biopsy is contraindicated when active prostatitis is suspected. However, typical clinical findings are not always present (Maksem 1988C). An indurated area of the prostate gland may suggest carcinoma.

The FNA biopsy of acute prostatitis yields a cellular smear and may include various forms of atypical epithelium (ie, reactive or metaplastic cells) **i3.9** (Maksem 1988C). The cytologic picture is one of acute inflammation or abscess, consisting of abundant neutrophils, macrophages, cellular debris, and a few small sheets of degenerative or regenerative epithelial cells (Koizumi 1990, Maksem 1988C, Rørvik 1989). Bacteria may be seen (Maksem 1988A, 1988C). Culture and sensitivity studies on a portion of aspirated material facilitate diagnosis and treatment.

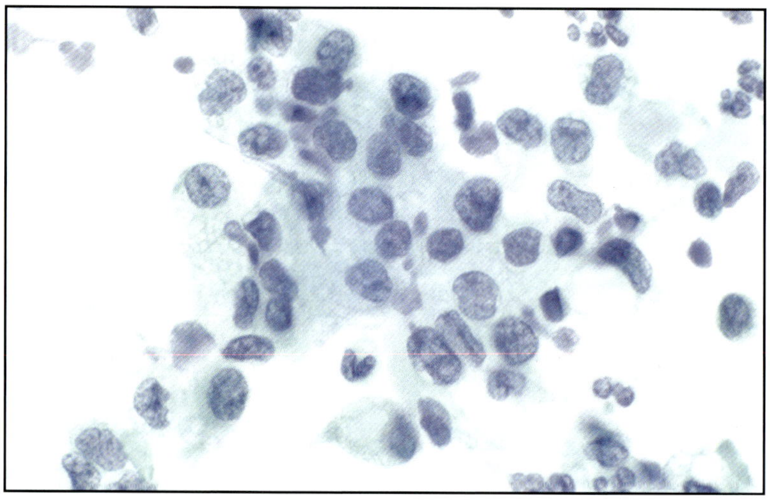

■ **i3.9** *Active prostatitis. FNA biopsy is contraindicated in suspected active prostatitis; however, occasionally, a focus of prostatitis is aspirated and the cytologic changes, including loss of orderly arrangements, prominent nuclear pleomorphism, and conspicuous nucleoli, must be distinguished from malignancy. Be extremely cautious diagnosing malignancy in the presence of significant inflammation. (Pap)*

Be cautious in diagnosing cancer in the presence of inflammation (Koss 1984). Reactive or reparative prostatic cells can show several features suggesting malignancy, including crowding, overlapping, and occasional microacinar structures; mild to moderate nuclear size variation and prominent nucleoli; and loss of both cytoplasmic pigment and distinct cell borders (honeycombing) **i3.10** (Kline 1985, Maksem 1988A, Ritchie 1988). Cytoplasmic vacuoles, including apparent intracytoplasmic lumens, may be seen in acute prostatitis (Maksem 1988C). With resolution, the atypical epithelium may be replaced by immature and mature squamous metaplastic cells (Maksem 1988C).

Chronic Prostatitis

The symptoms of chronic prostatitis can be vague. Digital rectal examination may disclose a firm, enlarged, nodular prostate that can mimic malignancy (Maksem 1988A). Although cancer and chronic prostatitis often coexist, inflammation can cause reactive changes that mimic cancer cytologically (N Epstein 1976B). Therefore, one must sail a course between the Scylla of overdiagnosing malignancy in the

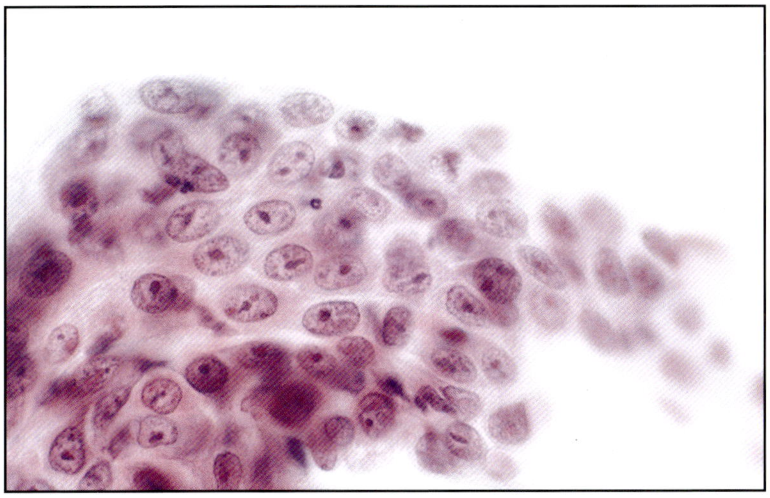

■ **i3.10** *Active prostatitis. Occasionally, more marked atypia, akin to reparative changes described in the Pap smear, are seen in association with prostatitis. The presence of prominent nucleoli may lead to a mistaken diagnosis of malignancy. However, note orderly arrangements, good intercellular cohesion, and fine chromatin—the usual cytologic features of repair. (Pap)*

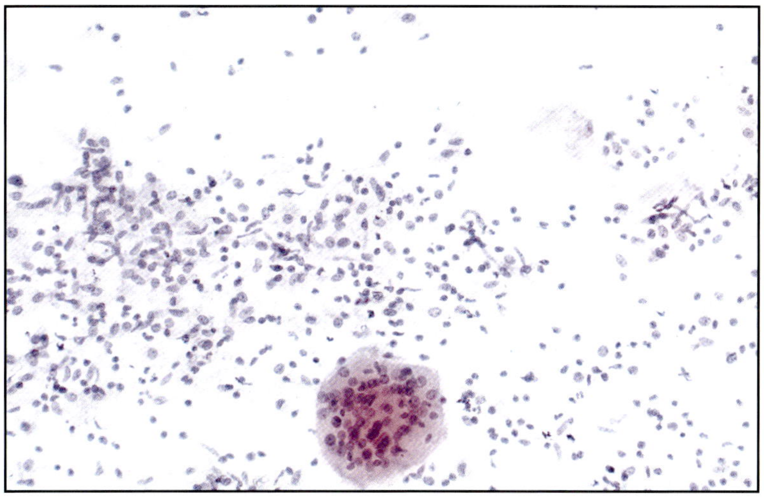

■ **i3.11** *Granulomatous prostatitis. An uncommon lesion, usually a nonspecific reaction to prostatic secretions. However, occasionally, there may be a more specific cause, such as infection, bacillus Calmette-Guérin therapy of bladder cancer, or consequence of prior surgery. Note epithelioid histiocytes with oval- to spindle-shaped nuclei and giant cells. (Pap)*

face of inflammation and the Charybdis of overlooking cancer merely because inflammation is present (Maksem 1988A).

The FNA biopsy of chronic prostatitis characteristically yields a cellular sample composed of a mixture of epithelial and inflammatory cells in a dirty, inflammatory background (Matsumoto 1992). Histiocytes, often containing pigment or phagocytosed material, may be the predominant finding in severe cases (Maksem 1988A, 1988C).

The epithelial cells form either small, crowded sheets or dissociated groups with increased single cells. However, microacinar groups are not prominent, if present at all. Degenerative and regenerative changes can occur in the prostatic cells. Reactive cells can show mild but not marked pleomorphism and nuclear enlargement. Small nucleoli may be present, but numerous prominent nucleoli are worrisome. Cytoplasmic pigment granules are a benign feature usually present in chronic prostatitis. Cytoplasmic vacuolization may be seen. Squamous metaplasia, transitional cell (urothelial) metaplasia, or basal cell hyperplasia can also occur (Maksem 1988A).

Granulomatous Prostatitis

Granulomatous prostatitis is uncommon, seen in only about 1% to 2% of prostatic FNA biopsies (Tuero 1988). Granulomatous prostatitis usually represents a nonspecific reaction, possibly to prostatic secretions. Specific causes of granulomatous prostatitis include tuberculosis, syphilis, fungal, or viral infections; sarcoid; hypersensitivity or autoimmune disease; bacille Calmette-Guérin therapy of bladder cancer (Oates 1988, Stilmant 1985); and reaction to prior prostate surgery (Maksem 1988A, Schmidt 1965, Tuero 1988). Granulomatous prostatitis can mimic prostatic cancer clinically, and FNA biopsy can be helpful in the differential diagnosis (Koizumi 1990, Stanley 1991).

The FNA biopsy shows characteristic granulomas, consisting of aggregates of epithelioid histiocytes and, sometimes, giant cells **i3.11** (Maksem 1988A, Miralles 1990). Other inflammatory cells, such as neutrophils, lymphocytes, and plasma cells, as well as eosinophils (eosinophilic prostatitis [J Epstein 1984, Miralles 1990]) can also be seen. Necrotic material may be identified in some cases, such as caseous necrosis in tuberculous prostatitis (Koss 1984). Special stains or culture may reveal an organism (Maksem 1988C, Miralles 1990). Reactive and degenerative changes in the epithelial cells, as previously described, can also occur. Marked proliferation of epithelioid cells with a spindly configuration may suggest a spindle cell tumor of the prostate (Stanley 1991). Giant cells are rare in prostatic carcinomas, except for high-grade tumors, which show obvious malignant features.

Malacoplakia

Malacoplakia is a rare chronic granulomatous disease that usually occurs in the bladder but has been described in many other tissues, including the prostate. The FNA biopsy specimen is cellular and characterized by mixed inflammation, including neutrophils, lymphocytes, and plasma cells. Intermingled are isolated (von Hansemann) histiocytes, with abundant foamy cytoplasm, that may contain characteristic targetoid Michaelis-Gutmann (MG) bodies (Cazzaniga 1987, Pérez-Barrios 1992). MG bodies are round, basophilic, and often laminated. MG bodies can also be free in the background. MG bodies react with periodic acid-Schiff, iron, and Von Kossa (calcium) stains. Other elements of granulomatous inflammation, as previously described, may be present.

Benign Prostatic Hyperplasia

Benign enlargement of the prostate gland (benign prostatic hyperplasia [BPH]) is so common as to be considered an almost normal part of aging. However, there is no question that BPH can cause disease (urinary obstruction and its consequences) in some patients.

BPH involves hyperplasia of the glands and stroma of the prostate in variable proportions. Hormonal imbalance (ratio of estrogen to androgen [Wilson 1980]) is thought to be involved in the pathogenesis. BPH affects primarily the central area of the prostate gland (specifically, periurethral ducts in the preprostatic region). Benign enlargement of the prostate can sometimes be difficult to distinguish from malignancy clinically, thus necessitating biopsy. Although no causal relationship between BPH and prostate cancer has been proven, there are a number of similarities that suggest a link (prevalence increases with age, cancer usually occurs in a hyperplastic gland, and both need androgens for growth) (Bostwick 1992).

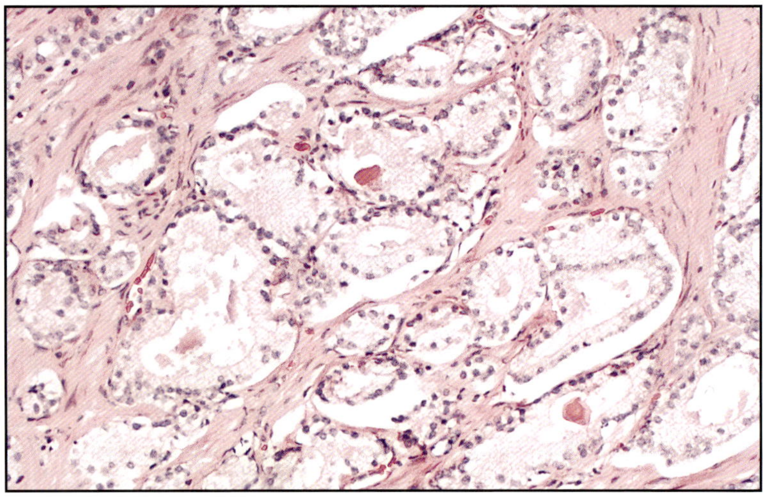

■ **i3.12** *Adenocarcinoma. Tissue showing infiltration of fibromuscular stroma by relatively well-differentiated malignant glands. Note intraluminal crystalloids.*

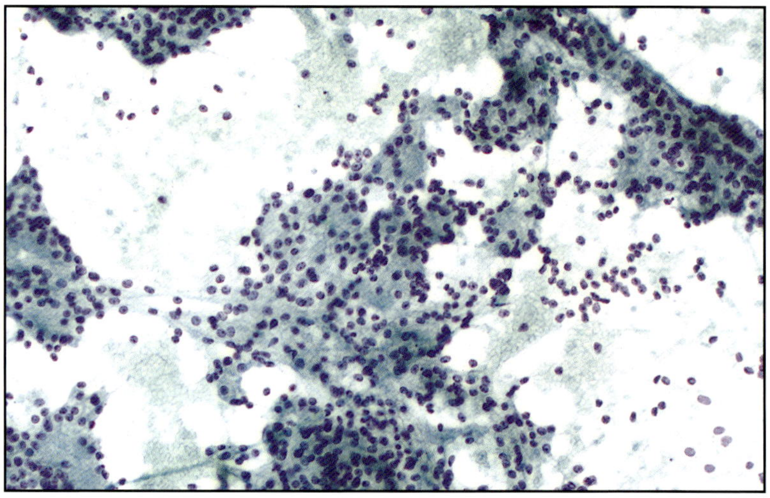

■ **i3.13** *Adenocarcinoma. Adenocarcinoma is characterized by abnormal groupings (including microacinar complexes and increased single cells) and nuclear abnormalities (including nuclear enlargement and prominent nucleoli). Cytoplasmic pigment and basal cells are usually absent. (Pap)*

The FNA biopsy of BPH yields a blood-tinged or milky fluid. The cellularity is variable, depending on the ratio of glandular to stromal hyperplasia, but usually is not marked. Large sheets of cells in a honeycomb arrangement with good intercellular cohesion characterize benign aspirate specimens (Kline 1985, Koss 1984, Mostofi 1993). Occasionally, papillary groups are seen. However, repeated or numerous microacini (microacinar complexes) are not a feature of benign prostatic aspirates (Kline 1985).

The nuclei are uniform, and the nuclear membranes are smooth. The chromatin is fine and even, and the nucleoli are absent or tiny and inconspicuous (Mostofi 1993). Prominent nucleoli are rare (Kline 1985). The cytoplasm often contains granules.

Basal cells, reminiscent of myoepithelial cells in benign breast aspirates, are seen associated with the epithelial sheets or scattered in the background of the smear (often as naked oval nuclei). A few small fragments of prostatic stroma, composed of spindle cells with elongated nuclei, may be seen occasionally, but the stroma usually does not aspirate well (Koss 1984). Corpora amylacea, squamous metaplasia, inflammation, or contaminants from the rectum or seminal vesicles may also be present. In atrophy, small clusters of atypical cells with increased nuclear-cytoplasmic ratios and occasional prominent nucleoli may be seen (Ritchie 1988).

Basal Cell Hyperplasia

Basal cell hyperplasia usually occurs in the setting of benign prostatic hyperplasia. It can also result from inflammation or ischemia.

The FNA biopsy specimen shows clusters of epithelial and basal cells. The basal cells form disorderly, tightly cohesive groups of fairly uniform cells, with scant cytoplasm. The nuclei are regular, round to oval, and hyperchromatic and have distinct nucleoli **i3.3** (Jacobs 1987). Nuclear palisading at the edge of cell groups, similar to other basal cell lesions occurring in the skin, salivary gland, or breast, is a characteristic feature.

Disorderly clusters of small cells, with little cytoplasm and prominent nucleoli, can mimic prostatic adenocarcinoma (J Epstein 1992). There may even be a suggestion of microacinar formation. However, in contrast with adenocarcinoma, single intact cells are rare. Also, benign basal cells are too uniform for high-grade carcinoma, and microacini are too few for low-grade carcinoma. Basal cells do not express PAP, whereas prostatic epithelial cells, whether benign or malignant, usually do (Jacobs 1987). Basal cell carcinoma also occurs rarely.

[3.3] Malignant Diseases of the Prostate

Prostatic carcinoma is the single most common human malignancy, second only to lung cancer as a cause of cancer-related deaths in men. It is rare before 40 years of age and unusual before 50, although it has been described rarely in infants and children (Shimada 1980). The cause is unknown.

Most cancers of the prostate are adenocarcinomas **i3.12**. Grading of prostatic adenocarcinoma correlates with stage and prognosis and therefore is important in therapeutic decisions. FNA biopsy can be helpful in the diagnosis, grading, and staging of the tumor (Efremidis 1979, 1981, Göthlin 1981, Hasenson 1989, Honig 1992, Mestitz 1989, Van Poppel 1994).

Prostatic carcinoma may present with metastases, particularly to bone or lymph node. Osteoblastic metastases in older men should be considered prostate cancer until proven otherwise. Pulmonary metastases can mimic primary lung cancer (Gentile 1988). Small prostatic primaries (<1 mL) are rarely the source of widespread metastases (Brawn 1992).

Elevations of serum PSA or PAP are found in about 80% of cases of prostatic carcinoma (Catalona 1991, G Murphy 1981). BPH, prostatic infarction, prostatitis, vigorous massage, and biopsy can all cause PSA elevations (Charrie 1986, Schmidt 1992). Immunocytochemical demonstration of these antigens in the aspirated material may help identify the prostatic origin of metastases when the primary lesion is occult (Hasenson 1989, Jöbsis 1978, Katz 1985, Keshgegian 1984, Rockey 1990, Tell 1985). However, negative staining does not completely eliminate the possibility of a prostatic primary, particularly when the tumor is high-grade or sarcomatoid (Brawn 1992, Renshaw 2000).

Adenocarcinoma

The FNA biopsy of prostatic adenocarcinoma usually obtains a highly cellular specimen, which may be the first clue to malignancy **i3.13** (Kline 1985). Mixtures of benign and malignant cells are more

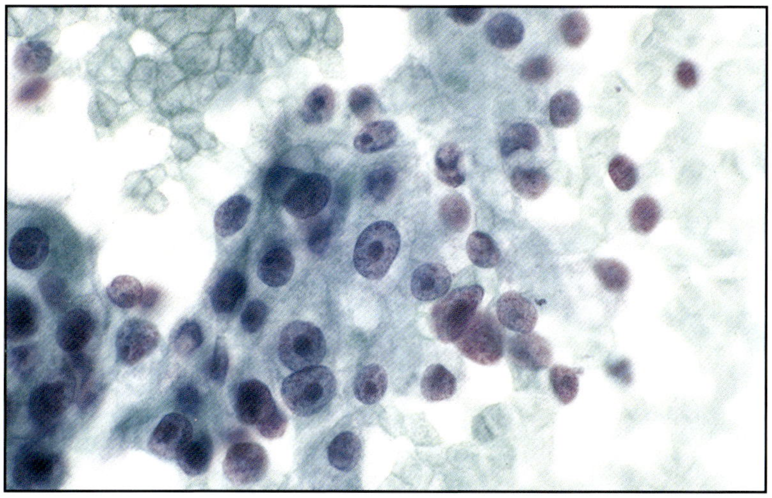

■ **i3.14** *Adenocarcinoma. Note microacini and prominent nucleoli. Cytoplasm is delicate and finely vacuolated. (Pap)*

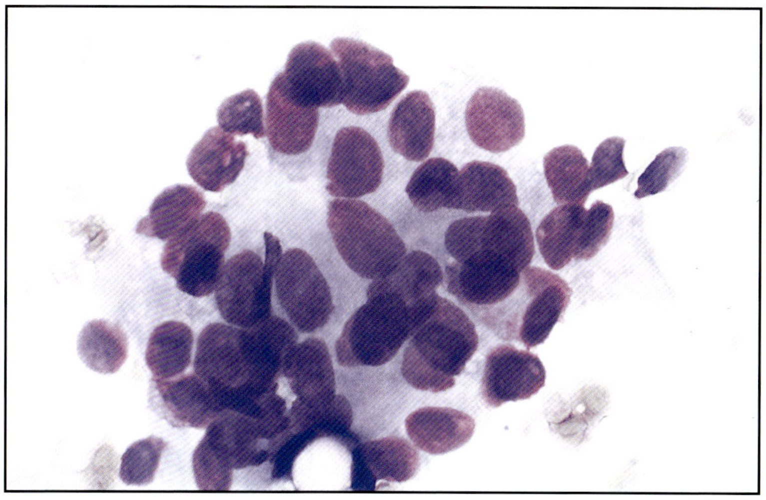

■ **i3.15** *Adenocarcinoma. Microacini may be easier to appreciate in Diff-Quik, but nucleoli are more difficult to see.*

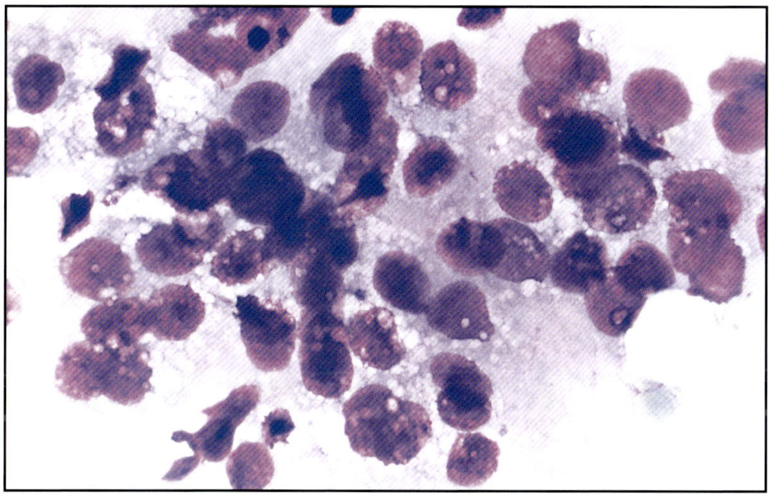

■ **i3.16** *Adenocarcinoma. Cytoplasmic lipid accumulation, best appreciated in Diff-Quik as myriads of tiny cytoplasmic vacuoles, is common and can be marked.*

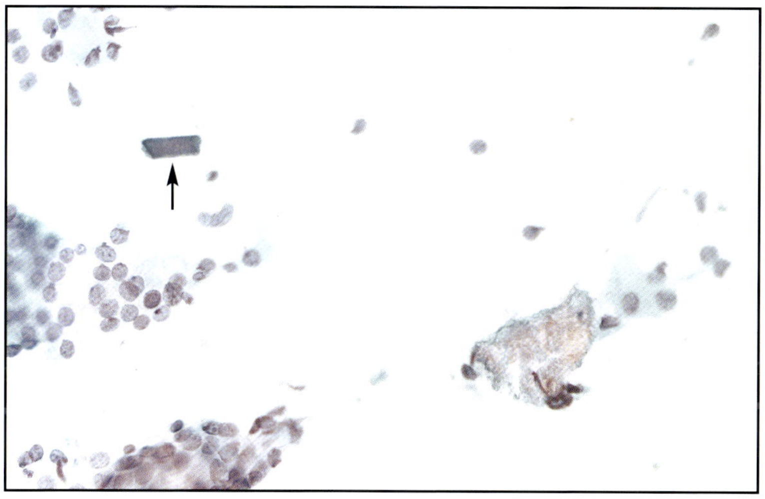

■ **i3.17** *Adenocarcinoma. Extracellular crystalloids (blue-staining body [arrow], Pap) are occasionally found in adenocarcinoma, but are rarely, if ever, found in benign prostate. (Courtesy of Fred Worsham, MD)*

common than in tumors of other organs (although if malignant-appearing cells are sparse, be careful). An admixture of benign cells provides an internal control for assessing nuclear size, nuclear-cytoplasmic ratio, and cellular arrangements and can make the malignant cells stand out conspicuously in some cases. The architectural arrangements and appearance of the tumor cells depend on the grade of the tumor. Mixtures of grades of malignancy are also common.

As usual, nuclear features, such as nuclear enlargement, pleomorphism, nucleoli, loss of polarity, and crowding, are critical in the diagnosis of malignancy (Polito 1990, Singh 1997). Nuclear and, particularly, nucleolar enlargement are particularly important diagnostic criteria (Gleason 1985, Kelemen 1990, Koizumi 1990). Nuclei less than 35 μm^2 (the area of an intermediate squamous cell nucleus, or about the size of a red blood cell) usually are benign; those greater than 60 μm^2 usually are malignant (Buhmeida 2000, 2001B). The presence of large nucleoli (in secretory epithelial cells) is perhaps the single most important diagnostic criterion for prostatic adenocarcinoma **i3.14** (Mostofi 1992A, 1992B). The larger the nucleoli, the more likely the lesion is to be malignant and the worse the prognosis (Buhmeida 2001A, Tannenbaum 1982). However, nucleoli are not perfect markers of malignancy (Kramer 1993). Some cancers have small or absent nucleoli (particularly in a biopsy), and some benign cells have prominent nucleoli (from the prostate, eg, inflammation, infarction, adenosis, basal cell hyperplasia, and from outside the prostate, such as seminal vesicle or colonic epithelium) (Kramer 1993).

The formation of numerous, repeated microacinar structures (microacinar complexes) is a hallmark of prostatic malignancy (Ljung 1985). They are common in prostatic adenocarcinomas but not in benign aspirate specimens **i3.14, i3.15** (Kline 1985). Cellular crowding and disorder, dyshesion with increased single cells, and loss of the honeycomb appearance (with inconspicuous cell membranes) also suggest cancer (N Epstein 1976A, Koss 1984). The degree of cellular disaggregation correlates with the grade of the tumor (ie, more single cells, higher grade).

The cytoplasm is delicate and finely vacuolated. Lipid accumulation of the cytoplasm is common in prostatic carcinoma and in some cases is marked **i3.16** (Stanley 1989). (Lipid-rich, retroperitoneal lymph node metastases can even mimic liposarcoma.) Cytoplasmic pigment granules usually are absent in cancer cells; pigment granules favor a benign diagnosis. Despite some teachings, epithelial mucin may be)present in prostatic carcinoma (Allsbrook 1992). Clear cell (Cantrell 1981) or oncocytic (Ordóñez 1992) change can occur rarely.

Extracellular crystalloids, distinct from corpora amylacea or Bence Jones crystals, are found in about 10% of prostatic carcinomas but rarely, if ever, in benign prostates **i3.17** (Ro 1986). The

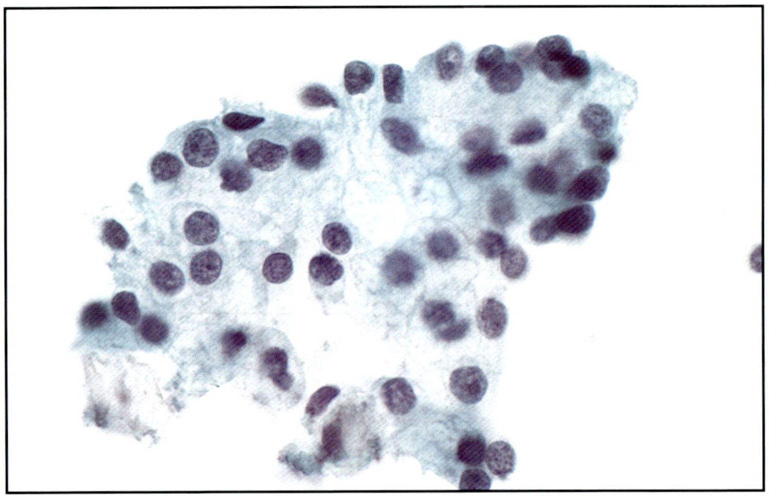

■ **i3.18** *Adenocarcinoma. Well-differentiated tumors are characterized by an overall uniformity of the cells, bland chromatin, small nucleoli, and relatively maintained intercellular cohesion, which can make the diagnosis of malignancy difficult. (Pap)*

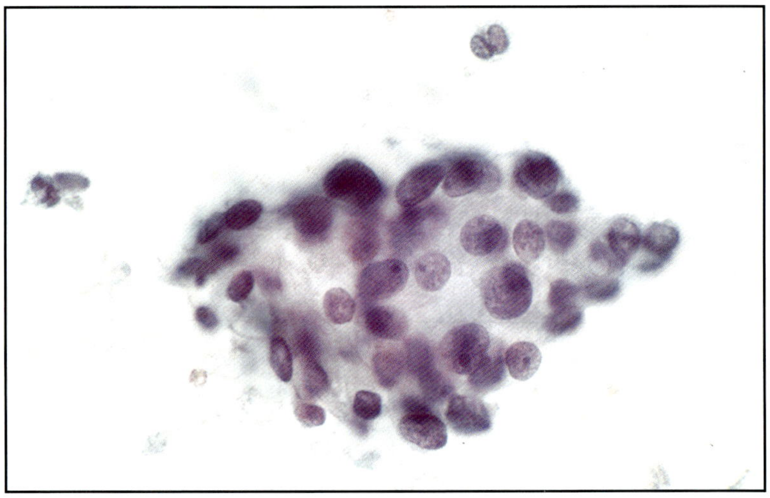

■ **i3.19** *Adenocarcinoma. Moderately differentiated tumors, the most common type, are characterized by increasingly obvious malignant features, including nuclear enlargement and pleomorphism, prominent nucleoli, and decreased intercellular cohesion. (Pap)*

small, dark nuclei of basal cells are almost never associated with clusters of cancer cells (Koss 1984).

Well-differentiated cancers show an overall uniformity of the cells, bland chromatin, and maintained intercellular cohesion, which may make the diagnosis of malignancy difficult **i3.18**. As the grade of the tumor increases, the features of malignancy become more obvious **i3.19**. Poorly differentiated cancers are characterized by a highly dissociated pattern of obviously malignant cells with large, irregular nuclei; abnormal coarse, dark chromatin; and prominent nucleoli **i3.20**.

In summary, the 2 key features of malignancy pertain to nuclear abnormalities and abnormal groups. Nuclear abnormalities include nuclear enlargement, hyperchromasia, membrane irregularity, and, especially, prominent nucleoli. Abnormal groups include disorderly aggregates, with nuclear crowding and loss of polarity, loss of prominent honeycomb cell membranes, absence of associated basal cells, increased single cells, and, especially, microacinar complexes.

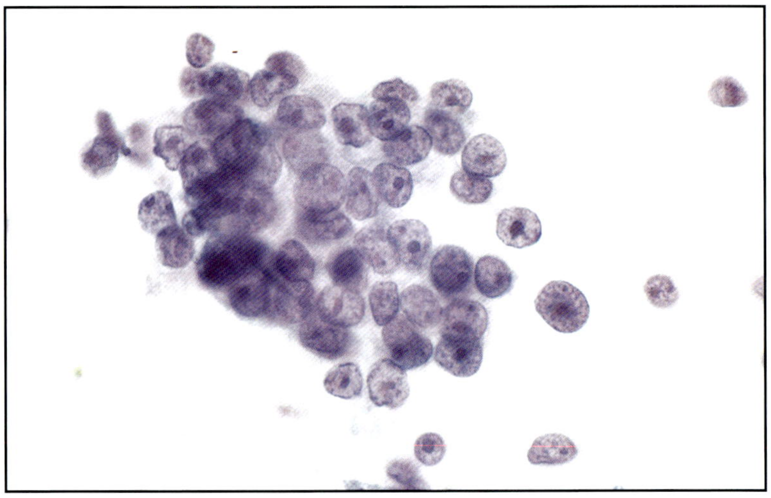

■ **i3.20** *Adenocarcinoma. Poorly differentiated tumors are characterized by obviously malignant cells with large, irregular nuclei, coarse, dark chromatin, and large nucleoli. Many single cells are usually present. (Pap)*

Grading of Prostatic Carcinoma

Grading of prostate cancer is clinically useful; in general, the prognosis and response to therapy are related to stage and grade of the tumor (Maksem 1990). All grading systems are subjective and difficult to reproduce (Mostofi 1992B). Gleason grading is currently the most widely used in histologic studies (Gleason 1974, 1992, Tannenbaum 1983B). It is fundamentally an architectural rather than a cytologic system, making it difficult to apply directly to FNA biopsy (Jacobs 1989, Layfield 1987, Maksem 1987, 1988B, 1990). The Gleason system may also be difficult to apply to core biopsy samples in some cases, and, of course, sampling is a potential problem in any biopsy (Mostofi 1992B).

Traditional cytologic grading (ie, well, moderate, and poorly differentiated, or grades I, II, and III) correlates well with prognosis (Esposti 1971). In fact, as stated by Mostofi, "since the behavior of a tumor in an individual patient is based almost entirely on the interplay between the neoplastic cell and the host, the most productive line of approach would seem to be the study of tumor cells: the nucleus, the nucleolus, the cytoplasm, the nuclear and cell membrane (all cytologic features), and the epithelial and stromal interaction" (Mostofi 1992B).

For cytologic grading, 6 factors, each with 3 degrees of magnitude, have been proposed by the Uropathology Study Group on prostatic carcinoma for cytologic grading of prostatic adenocarcinoma (Maksem 1988A, 1990): average nuclear size, variability in nuclear size, average nucleolar size, nucleolar variability (size, shape, number), disturbance of nuclear arrangement, and cellular and nuclear distortion. The lowest possible score is 6 (1×6), and the highest is 18 (3×6). Scores of 10 or less are considered grade I (well differentiated), 11 to 14 are grade II (moderately differentiated), and 15 or higher are grade III (poorly differentiated).

The cytologic grade is assigned according to the worst component of the tumor (Willems 1981). In general, the grading is based on nuclear features, but numerous microacinar arrangements are characteristic of well-differentiated cancer, whereas a highly dissociated cell pattern may be seen in poorly differentiated cancer (Linsk 1972, Maksem 1990).

Cytologic grading has been shown to correlate reasonably well with survival, stage, and response to therapy (M Benson 1988, Esposti 1971, Faul 1980, Willems 1981). Cytologic grading also correlates reasonably well with grading based on simultaneously obtained core tissue biopsies, although there may be a tendency for cytology to undergrade (Adolfsson 1991). Exact correlation is possible in at least three quarters of cases, with few cases missed by more than 1 grade (M Benson 1988, Ekman 1967, Faul

1973, Waisman 1991, Willems 1981, Yatani 1985, Zattoni 1983). There is a similar degree of correlation (ie, about 75%) between cytologic grades (I to III) and the histologic Gleason grade, when the Gleason score is divided into 3 categories (2-4, 5-7, and 8-10) (M Benson 1988, Carter 1986, Jacobs 1989, Layfield 1987, Maksem 1988B). However, when the results of either FNA or core tissue biopsy are compared with the grading of the radical prostatectomy specimen, disagreement (usually undergrading) occurs in about half of cases (Catalona 1982, Eble 1992, Hostetter 1990, Lange 1983, Mills 1986, Narayan 1989, 1991).

The availability of DNA analysis, or other advanced techniques such as morphometry or monoclonal antibodies (which can be performed on aspirated material), may provide a quantitative guide to diagnosis and prognosis of prostatic carcinoma (Adolfsson 1990A, 1990B, Bichel 1977, Böcking 1988, Chodak 1984, Clar-Branch 1992, Forsslund 1992, Frederiksen 1978, Hasenson 1989, Helpap 1981, Jones 1990, Koss 1988, Mostofi 1993, Oomens 1991, Rönström 1981, Sprenger 1974, Stege 1990, 1992, Stenkvist 1990, Tribukait 1980, 1991, Zetterberg 1976, 1980, 1991).

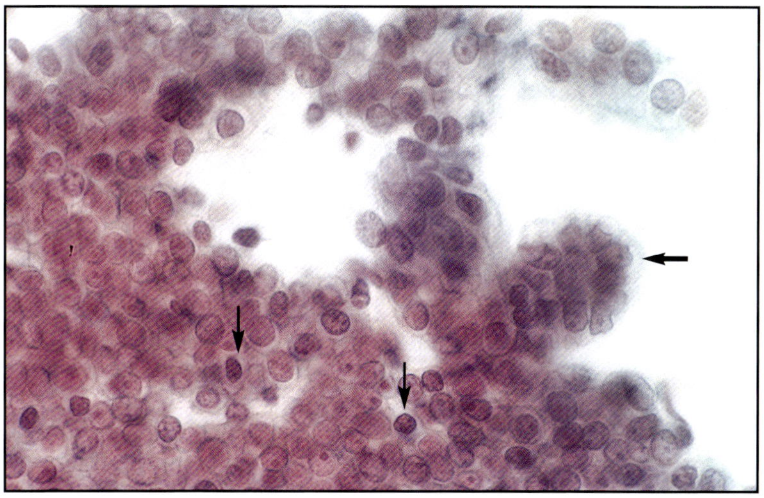

■ **i3.21** *Dysplasia (PIN). Cohesive but crowded aggregates of cells with nuclear enlargement, hyperchromasia, and conspicuous nucleoli. Atypical groups, microacini, and single cells are sparse, but basal cells are present (dark cells at light arrows). Note tuft of cells extending into acinar spaces (heavy arrow). Low-grade dysplasia may be difficult to distinguish from reactive changes, while high-grade dysplasia/CIS may be difficult to distinguish from invasive carcinoma.*

Monitoring Response to Therapy

FNA biopsy can be useful in the follow-up of patients treated for prostatic cancer (Jocham 1983, Maksem 1988A). Disease progression can be predicted with FNA biopsy before it becomes clinically manifest. FNA biopsy also offers the advantage over tissue biopsies of being able to sample a large area of the gland, although false-negative results may still occur (Hedlund 1989).

The effect of therapy on tumor cells includes cytoplasmic vacuolization and nuclear degeneration (pyknosis, lysis, and giant forms). The degree of cytologic change correlates directly with a favorable therapeutic effect (the more change, the better the response) (Spieler 1976). The presence of unaltered cancer cells indicates a poor therapeutic response.

Hormone Therapy

The effects (ie, regressive changes) of estrogen therapy include atrophic cells, shrunken or pyknotic nuclei, reduction or loss of nucleoli, squamous metaplasia, cytoplasmic vacuolization, and glycogenation (Böcking 1987, Das 1990, 1991, Hedlund 1989, Kline 1982, Koss 1984, Spieler 1976, Tomic 1985, Williams 1967). Glycogenated squamous cells are reminiscent of navicular cells (as seen in Pap tests from pregnant women). Failure to convert to glycogenated cells is a sign that the tumor is not hormonally responsive (Tannenbaum 1983A). Survival in patients showing signs of tumor regression is longer than in those who do not show regressive changes.

Radiation Therapy

Patients can be assessed after radiation therapy with FNA biopsy (Kurth 1977). The effects of radiation include enlargement of nuclei, chromatin clumping and pyknosis, cytoplasmic and nuclear vacuolization, and bizarre cells (Mostofi 1992A, Spieler 1976). Radiation changes can be difficult to evaluate, and a combination of clinical and pathologic parameters must be used to assess the effects of radiation therapy (Cox 1977, Herr 1982, Phillips 1972).

Premalignant Lesions of the Prostate

Premalignant lesions of the prostate are grouped into 2 categories: those with new gland formation (atypical adenomatous hyperplasia, or adenosis) and those in which the epithelium in preexisting glands undergoes neoplastic change (dysplasia or PIN). In adenosis, nuclear changes are insufficient to qualify as dysplastic (PIN). In dysplasia (PIN), there is no new gland formation and no invasion. Although either type of lesion may be associated with subsequent development of cancer, the malignant potential of dysplasia (PIN) apparently is greater than that of adenosis.

Prostatic Intraepithelial Neoplasia (Dysplasia)

Dysplasia of the ductal or acinar epithelium is a primary proliferation of abnormal epithelium, not a transient, reactive condition related to injury and repair or metaplasia (Maksem 1988A). Dysplasia (PIN [Bostwick 1989]) is considered a premalignant lesion (Brawer 1992, McNeal 1986). The presence of this lesion is strongly associated with and apparently progresses to prostatic adenocarcinoma (Bostwick 1989, McNeal 1986). Invasion is associated with high-grade PIN (Bostwick 1987). Patients with high-grade PIN on biopsy have a high likelihood of having concomitant carcinoma, which usually merits very close, vigorous follow-up. However, radical surgery or radiation therapy is not indicated for PIN alone (Weinstein 1993).

The premalignant lesions are microscopic and nonpalpable. However, the lesion may be seen in a biopsy of a gland that was obtained for some other reason.

PIN is characterized cytologically by the presence of a few crowded groups of cells with increased nuclear-cytoplasmic ratios, indistinct cell borders, and dark nuclei **i3.21, t3.1**.

In low-grade PIN, intercellular cohesion is maintained, nuclear enlargement is not marked, the chromatin is bland, and nucleoli are inconspicuous. There are few groups of atypical cells, rare or no single atypical cells, and little or no tendency to microacinar formation. Cytoplasmic pigment granules and basal cells are maintained. Low-grade dysplasia can be difficult to distinguish from reactive changes.

As grade increases, the cytologic changes become more marked, including more nuclear enlargement, hyperchromasia, crowding, and prominent nucleoli. Groups are multilayered, with loss of nuclear polarity, and microacini may form. Intercellular cohesion,

■ t3.1 **Grading Dysplasia (PIN) of the Prostatic Epithelium**

PIN	Groups	Basal Cells	Cytoplasmic Granules	Nuclear Enlargement and Pleomorphism	Chromatin	Nucleoli
I	Crowded	Present	May be present	Slight–moderate	Fine	Few
II	Increased crowding	Mild decrease	Absent	Moderate	Granular	Conspicuous
III	Microacini may be present	Marked decrease	Absent	Moderate–marked	Coarse	Prominent

(Bostwick 1987,1989a,b, Brawer 1992, De Gaetani 1978, Markham 1989, McNeal 1986a)

cytoplasmic granules, and the presence of basal cells diminish. High-grade PIN may be cytologically indistinguishable from frankly invasive well-differentiated carcinoma (De Gaetani 1978, W Murphy 1991).

In theory, the cytologic findings in PIN are more than benign reactive changes but less than frankly malignant. In practice, however, a cytodiagnosis of PIN is difficult. The diagnosis may be suggested when the aspirate shows a few dyshesive groups of cells with nuclear abnormalities, without evidence of prostatitis or a history of radiation therapy or chemotherapy (Kline 1988). Of great importance is that patients with cytologic atypia on FNA biopsy are at high risk of having or developing prostatic carcinoma (Oyasu 1986, Ritchie 1988, Smith 1988, Stilmant 1989). These patients must be monitored closely (Markham 1989).

Atypical Adenomatous Hyperplasia, or Adenosis

Atypical adenomatous hyperplasia, or adenosis, may be a precursor of prostate cancer, but the association is certainly weaker than that between PIN and cancer (Kovi 1989). Histologically, adenosis consists of tightly packed clusters of small glands, lined by more normal-appearing cells, which may show mild nuclear pleomorphism and hyperchromasia (Bostwick 1989, Koss 1984). Prominent nucleoli can be seen in some cases of adenosis (Kramer 1993). Atypia in the absence of microacinar formation is insufficient for a diagnosis of frank cancer (Tannenbaum 1983A), although follow-up is indicated (Koss 1984). Features that are more common in adenocarcinoma than in adenosis include prostatic crystalloids, mitotic figures, and basophilic mucinous secretions. On the other hand, clear cytoplasm and corpora amylacea are more common in adenosis than in adenocarcinoma (Kramer 1993).

[3.4] Variants of Prostatic Carcinoma

Prostatic Duct Adenocarcinoma

Most prostatic adenocarcinomas show acinar differentiation; however, a few (<1% of cases) show prostatic duct differentiation, and some are mixed acinar-ductal carcinoma (about 5%). Prostatic duct carcinoma was formerly known as endometrioid carcinoma because of its histologic resemblance to uterine endometrial carcinoma and because of its tendency to arise near the verumontanum, a müllerian remnant. Serum PSA may be normal in patients with this cancer. Fewer patients respond well to hormonal therapy.

The FNA biopsy obtains atypical glandular cells. Some tumors are well differentiated with subtle malignant features (Howell 1989, Stilmant 1989). In other cases, the tumor cells are obviously malignant, with hyperchromatic nuclei and prominent nucleoli. Papillae, tall columnar cells, and grooved nuclear membranes are characteristic but variable from case to case (N Epstein 1977, Howell 1989, Masood 1991). The differential diagnosis includes villous adenoma and papillary transitional cell carcinoma (Stilmant 1989).

Mucinous Adenocarcinoma or Signet-Ring Carcinoma

Mucinous adenocarcinoma is one of the least common prostate cancers; it can show either a colloid pattern (rare) (J Epstein 1985) or signet-ring cell pattern (rarer still) (Alline 1992). This tumor may be difficult to distinguish from bowel or bladder cancer.

Transitional Cell (Urothelial) Carcinoma

Transitional cell (urothelial) carcinoma can occur in the prostate as either a primary tumor arising in the transitional epithelium of the prostatic urethra or by secondary invasion of a bladder tumor into the prostate (Stilmant 1989). Although FNA biopsy is not highly sensitive in diagnosing prostatic involvement by urothelial carcinoma, and stromal invasion cannot be assessed cytologically, the prostate FNA biopsy may be positive when other biopsy results are negative (Wood 1989).

The FNA biopsy specimen shows loose clusters and single malignant urothelial cells with dense cytoplasm and distinct cell borders **i3.22**. When involving the prostate, the tumor usually is high grade. Squamous or glandular differentiation can be seen.

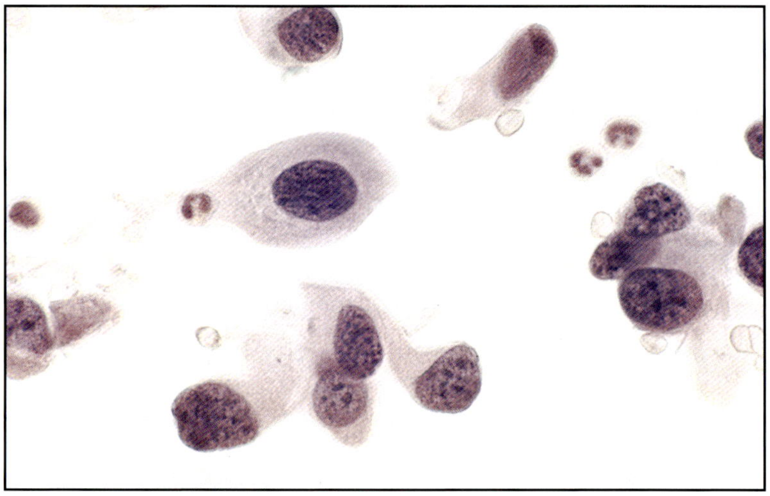

■ **i3.22** *Transitional cell (urothelial) carcinoma. Can involve the prostate either as a primary tumor arising in the prostatic urethra or as a bladder tumor invading the prostate. Cytologic studies show loose clusters and single malignant transitional cells with dense cytoplasm. Squamous or glandular differentiation can occur, particularly in high-grade tumors. Rarely, squamous cell carcinomas, adenosquamous carcinomas, or mucinous carcinomas arise in the prostate.*

PSA staining can be helpful in differentiating urothelial carcinoma from prostatic carcinoma. Note also that because both cancers are common, they can coexist. Occasionally, prostatic carcinoma exfoliates malignant cells in urine (Varma 1988); however, benign prostatic hyperplasia is a potential cause of atypical (reactive) urothelial cells in urine cytology (Krishnan 2000).

Squamous Cell Carcinoma

Although squamous metaplasia is common in the prostate, squamous cell carcinoma (Gray 1975) and adenosquamous carcinoma (Devaney 1991) are rare. However, hormonal manipulation of ordinary adenocarcinoma of the prostate can induce squamous changes in the cancer. Interestingly, the squamous epithelium derived from the prostatic adenocarcinoma can express prostate antigens on immunostain (Accetta 1982), although expression may be lost or reduced (Lager 1988).

Neuroendocrine Carcinoma

Primary small cell carcinoma (Bleichner 1986) and carcinoid tumors (Wasserstein 1981) have been described rarely in the prostate. Also, conventional adenocarcinomas commonly exhibit focal neuroendocrine differentiation (Di Sant'Agnese 1992). Islet cell tumors and carcinoids, particularly of hindgut origin, commonly express prostate-specific acid phosphatase (Kimura 1986).

Mesenchymal Tumors

Benign mesenchymal tumors of the prostate are rare; most are leiomyomas. Less than 1% of malignant prostate tumors are sarcomas **i3.23**, and many of these, particularly rhabdomyosarcomas (Henkes 1987, Moroz 1995, Yao 1988), usually occur in the first decade of life.

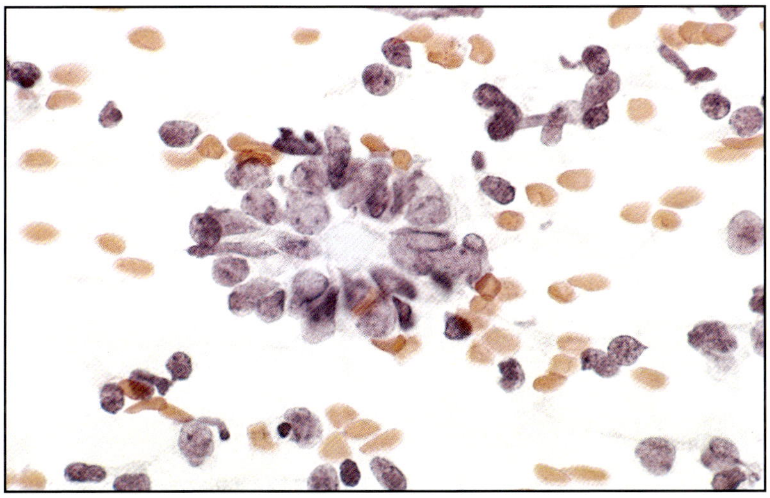

■ **i3.23** *Sarcoma. Sarcomas arising in the prostate are rare; many are rhabdomyosarcomas occurring in children. Illustrated is a rare primary Wilms' tumor of the prostate gland in an adult. Sarcomatoid carcinomas also occur, rarely, and could be difficult to distinguish from a sarcoma. Other tumors, such as neuroendocrine carcinoma and lymphoma, can also occur rarely in the prostate gland.*

Other sarcomas, including osteosarcoma, leiomyosarcoma, and fibrosarcoma, also occur, more often in later life (Cookingham 1985, Müller 1981). Sarcomatoid carcinoma of the prostate (ie, adenocarcinoma with spindle and pleomorphic areas) is a rare tumor that may be difficult to distinguish from a true sarcoma (Shannon 1992).

Malignant Lymphoma

Primary malignant lymphoma, without lymph node involvement, is rare; secondary involvement of the prostate by a wide variety of hematologic malignancies is more common. Briefly, malignant lymphomas are characterized cytologically by absence of true tissue aggregates, typical lymphoid morphology (best appreciated in Diff-Quik), and presence of lymphoglandular bodies. Florid lymphocytic chronic prostatitis is a differential diagnosis (look for range of maturation, predominance of small lymphocytes, and tingible body macrophages).

Metastatic Malignancy

The prostate is rarely involved in metastatic disease. The diagnosis of metastatic malignancy is suggested by identification of malignant tumor cells different from those of the usually recognized types of prostatic carcinoma. Lung cancer and malignant melanoma are the most common sources. Also, consider aspiration of a contiguous rectal carcinoma in the differential diagnosis (Stilmant 1989).

References

Accetta PA, Gardner WA Jr. Squamous metastases from prostatic adenocarcinoma. *Lab Invest* 46:2A, 1982.

Adolfsson J, Tribukait B. Evaluation of tumor progression by repeated fine needle biopsies in prostate adenocarcinoma: modal deoxyribonucleic acid value and cytological differentiation. *J Urol* 144:1408-1410, 1990A.

Adolfsson J, Rönström L, Hedlund PO, et al. The prognostic value of modal deoxyribonucleic acid in low grade, low stage untreated prostate cancer. *J Urol* 144:1404-1407, 1990B.

Adolfsson J, Skoog L, Löwhagen T, et al. Franzen transrectal fine-needle biopsy versus ultrasound-guided transrectal core biopsy of the prostate gland. *Acta Oncol* 30:159-160, 1991.

Agatstein EH, Hernandez FJ, Layfield LJ, et al. Use of fine needle aspiration for detection of stage a prostatic carcinoma before transurethral resection of the prostate: a clinical trial. *J Urol* 138:551-553, 1987.

Ajzen SA, Goldenberg SL, Allen GJ, et al. Palpable prostatic nodules: comparison of US and digital guidance for fine-needle aspiration biopsy. *Radiology* 171:521-523, 1989.

Al-Abadi H. Fine needle aspiration biopsy vs. ultrasound-guided transrectal random core biopsy of the prostate: comparative investigations in 246 cases. *Acta Cytol* 41:981-986, 1997.

Alfthan O, Klintrup HE, Koivuniemi A, et al. Cytological aspiration biopsy and VIM-Silverman biopsy in the diagnosis of prostatic carcinoma. *Ann Chir Gynaecol Fenn* 59:226-229, 1970.

Alline KM, Cohen MB. Signet-ring cell carcinoma of the prostate. *Arch Pathol Lab Med* 116:99-102, 1992.

Allsbrook WC Jr, Simms WW. Histochemistry of the prostate. *Hum Pathol* 23:297-305, 1992.

Anandan N, MacKenzie E, Gingell JC, et al. Role of Franzen needle aspiration biopsy in carcinoma of the prostate. *J R Soc Med* 76:828-830, 1983.

Andersson L, Jönsson G, Brunk U. Puncture biopsy of the prostate in the diagnosis of prostatic cancer. *Scand J Urol Nephrol* 1:227-234, 1967.

Arias-Stella J, Takano-Moron J. Atypical epithelial changes in the seminal vesicle. *Arch Pathol* 66:761-766, 1958.

Benson MC. Fine-needle aspiration of the prostate. *NCI Monogr* 7:19-24, 1988.

Benson RC, Clark WR, Farrow GM. Carcinoma of the seminal vesicle. *J Urol* 132:483-485, 1984.

Bentley EM, Mallery WR, Mueller JJ, et al. Fine needle aspiration of the prostate gland in the community hospital: a predictive value analysis. *Acta Cytol* 32:499-503, 1988.

Bichel P, Frederiksen P, Kjær TB, et al. Flow microfluorometry and transrectal fine-needle biopsy in the classification of human prostatic carcinoma. *Cancer* 40:1206-1211, 1977.

Bishop D, Oliver JA. A study of transrectal aspiration biopsies of the prostate, with particular regard to prognostic evaluation. *J Urol* 117:313-315, 1977.

Bissa NK, Rountree GA, Sulieman JS. Factors affecting accuracy and morbidity in transrectal biopsy of the prostate. *Surg Gynecol Obstet* 145:869-872, 1977.

Bleichner JC, Chun B, Klappenbach RS. Pure small-cell carcinoma of the prostate with fatal liver metastasis. *Arch Pathol Lab Med* 110:1041-1044, 1986.

Böcking A, Auffermann W. Cytological grading of therapy-induced tumor regression in prostatic carcinoma: proposal of a new system. *Diagn Cytopathol* 3:108-111, 1987.

Böcking A, Chatelain R, Orthen U, et al. DNA-grading of prostatic carcinoma: prognostic validity and reproducibility. *Anticancer Res* 8:129-136, 1988.

Bostwick DG, Brawer MK. Prostatic intra-epithelial neoplasia and early invasion in prostate cancer. *Cancer* 59:788-794, 1987.

Bostwick DG. The pathology of early prostate cancer. *CA Cancer J Clin* 39:376-393, 1989.

Bostwick DG, Cooner WH, Denis L, et al. The association of benign prostatic hyperplasia and cancer of the prostate. *Cancer* 70:291-301, 1992.

Brandes D, Kirchheim D, Scott WW. Ultrastructure of the human prostate: normal and neoplastic. *Lab Invest* 13:1541-1560, 1964.

Brawer MK. Prostatic intraepithelial neoplasia: a premalignant lesion. *Hum Pathol* 23:242-248, 1992.

Brawn P. Histologic features of metastatic prostate cancer. *Hum Pathol* 23:267-272, 1992.

Breda G, Silvestre P, Giunta A, et al. Stage A1 prostate cancer: follow-up with digital rectal exploration, prostate markers, fine-needle aspiration, ultrasonographically guided needle biopsy and biopsies of the residual prostate with resectoscope. *Eur Urol* 25:116-118, 1994.

Brenner DW, Ladaga LE, Fillion MB, et al. Comparison of transrectal fine-needle aspiration cytology and core needle biopsy in diagnosis of prostate cancer. *Urology* 35:381-384, 1990.

Buhmeida AB, Kuopio T, Collan Y. Nuclear size and shape in fine needle aspiration biopsy samples of the prostate. *Analyt Quant Cytol Histol* 22:291-298, 2000.

Buhmeida AB, Collan Y: Improving the value of fine needle aspiration biopsy of the prostate. *Pathologica* 93:242-243, 2001A.

Buhmeida AB, Kujari H, Collan Y: Nucleolar morphometry in fine needle biopsies of the prostate. *Analyt Quant Cytol Histol* 23:185-192, 2001B.

Cantrell BB, Leifer G, DeKlerk DP, et al. Papillary adenocarcinoma of the prostatic urethra with clear-cell appearance. *Cancer* 48:2661-2667, 1981.

Carter HB, Riehle RA, Koizumi JH, et al. Fine needle aspiration of the abnormal prostate: a cytohistological correlation. *J Urol* 135:294-298, 1986.

Catalona WJ, Stein AJ, Fair WR. Grading errors in prostatic needle biopsies: relation to the accuracy of tumor grade in predicting pelvic lymph node metastases. *J Urol* 127:919-922, 1982.

Catalona WJ, Smith DS, Ratliff TL, et al. Measurement of prostate-specific antigen in serum as a screening test for prostate cancer. *N Engl J Med* 324:1156-1161, 1991.

Cazzaniga MG, Tommasini-Degna A, Negri R, et al. Cytologic diagnosis of prostatic malakoplakia: report of three cases. *Acta Cytol* 31:48-52, 1987.

Charrie A, Fleury-Goyon MC, Dutey P, et al. The effect of prostate aspiration biopsy on serum levels of prostatic acid phosphatase and prostate-specific antigen. *JAMA* 256:474, 1986.

Chodak GW, Bibbo M, Straus FH III, et al. Transrectal aspiration biopsy versus transperineal core biopsy for the diagnosis of carcinoma of the prostate. *J Urol* 132:480-482, 1984.

Chodak GW, Steinberg GD, Bibbo M, et al. The role of transrectal aspiration biopsy in the diagnosis of prostatic cancer. *J Urol* 135:299-302, 1986.

Clar-Branch F, Morell-Quadreny L, Fenollosa-Entrena B, et al. Correlation between serum values of prostatic acid phosphatase and morphometric analysis in the cytologic diagnosis of prostatic carcinoma. *Eur Urol* 21(suppl 1):75-78, 1992.

Conrad S, Hautmann SH, Henke RP, et al. Detection and characterization of early prostate cancer by six systematic biopsies and fine needle aspiration cytology in prostates from bladder cancer patients. *Eur Urol* 39(suppl 4):25-29, 2001.

Cookingham CL, Kumar NB. Diagnosis of prostatic leiomyosarcoma with fine needle aspiration cytology. *Acta Cytol* 29:170-172, 1985.

Cox JD, Stoffel TJ: The significance of needle biopsy after irradiation for stage C adenocarcinoma of the prostate. *Cancer* 40:156-160, 1977.

Das DK, Hedlund PO, Löwhagen T, et al. Improved early detection of recurrence in prostatic carcinoma following hormonal therapy. *Urology* 36:341-345, 1990.

Das DK, Hedlund PO, Löwhagen T, et al. Squamous metaplasia in hormonally treated prostatic cancer: significance during follow-up. *Urology* 38:70-75, 1991.

De Gaetani CF, Trentini GP. Atypical hyperplasia of the prostate: a pitfall in the cytologic diagnosis of carcinoma. *Acta Cytol* 22:483-486, 1978.

Dejter SW Jr, Constantinople NL, Bresette JF, et al. Cytologic diagnosis of prostatic carcinoma by fine-needle aspiration biopsy: community hospital experience. *Urology* 31:255-259, 1988.

deKernion JB. Aspiration biopsy of the prostate: the urologist's viewpoint. *Semin Urol* 1:166-171, 1983.

Denton SE, Valk WL, Jacobson JM, et al. Comparison of the perineal needle biopsy and the transurethral prostatectomy in the diagnosis of prostatic carcinoma: an analysis of 300 cases. *J Urol* 97:127-129, 1967.

Devaney DM, Dorman A, Leader M. Adenosquamous carcinoma of the prostate: a case report. *Hum Pathol* 22:1046-1050, 1991.

Di Sant'Agnese PA. Neuroendocrine differentiation in human prostatic carcinoma. *Hum Pathol* 23:287-296, 1992.

Droese M, Voeth C. Cytologic features of seminal vesicle epithelium in aspiration biopsy smears of the prostate. *Acta Cytol* 20:120-125, 1976.

Eble JN, Tejada E. Prostatic stromal hyperplasia with bizarre nuclei. *Arch Pathol Lab Med* 115:87-89, 1991.

Eble JN, Angermeier PA. The roles of fine needle aspiration and needle core biopsies in the diagnosis of primary prostatic cancer. *Hum Pathol* 23:249-257, 1992.

Efremidis SC, Pagliarulo A, Dan SJ, et al. Post-lymphangiography fine needle aspiration lymph node biopsy in staging carcinoma of the prostate: preliminary report. *J Urol* 122:495-497, 1979.

Efremidis SC, Dan SJ, Nieburgs H, et al. Carcinoma of the prostate: lymph node aspiration for staging. *AJR Am J Roentgenol* 136:489-492, 1981.

Ekman H, Hedberg K, Persson PS. Cytological versus histological examination of needle biopsy specimens in the diagnosis of prostatic cancer. *Br J Urol* 39:544-548, 1967.

Engelstein D, Mukamel E, Cytron S, et al. A comparison between digitally-guided fine needle aspiration and ultrasound-guided transperineal core needle biopsy of the prostate for the detection of prostate cancer. *Br J Urol* 74:210-213, 1994.

Epstein JI, Hutchins GM. Granulomatous prostatitis: distinction among allergic, nonspecific, and posttransurethral resection lesions. *Hum Pathol* 15:818-825, 1984.

Epstein JI, Lieberman PH. Mucinous adenocarcinoma of the prostate gland. *Am J Surg Pathol* 9:299-308, 1985.

Epstein JI, Armas OA. Atypical basal cell hyperplasia of the prostate. *Am J Surg Pathol* 16:1205-1214, 1992.

Epstein NA. Prostatic biopsy: a morphologic correlation of aspiration cytology with needle biopsy histology. *Cancer* 38:2078-2087, 1976A.

Epstein NA. Prostatic carcinoma: correlation of histologic features of prognostic value with cytomorphology. *Cancer* 38:2071-2077, 1976B.

Epstein NA. Primary papillary carcinoma of the prostate: report of a histopathologic, cytologic and electron microscopic study on one case. *Acta Cytol* 21:543-546, 1977.

Esposti PL: Cytologic diagnosis of prostatic tumors with the aid of transrectal aspiration biopsy: a critical review of 1,110 cases and a report of morphologic and cytochemical studies. *Acta Cytol* 10:182-186, 1966.

Esposti PL. Cytologic malignancy grading of prostatic carcinoma by transrectal aspiration biopsy. *Scand J Urol Nephrol* 5:199-209, 1971.

Esposti PL, Elman A, Norlén H. Complications of transrectal aspiration biopsy of the prostate. *Scand J Urol Nephrol* 9:208-213, 1975.

Esposti PL, Franzén S. Transrectal aspiration biopsy of the prostate. *Scand J Urol Nephrol* 55:49-52, 1980.

Faul P, Schmiedt E. Cytologic aspects of diseases of the prostate. *Int Urol Nephrol* 5:297-310, 1973.

Faul P, Schmiedt E, Kern R. Prognostic significance of cytological differentiation grading in estrogen-treated prostatic carcinoma diagnosed by fine-needle aspiration biopsy: (five-year follow-up of 496 patients). *Int Urol Nephrol* 12:347-354, 1980.

Ferguson RS. Prostatic neoplasms: their diagnosis by needle puncture and aspiration. *Am J Surg* 9:507-511, 1930.

Fisher ER, Jeffrey W. Ultrastructure of human normal and neoplastic prostate: with comments relative to prostatic effects of hormonal stimulation in the rabbit. *Am J Clin Pathol* 44:119-134, 1965.

Forsslund G, Esposti PL, Nilsson B, et al. The prognostic significance of nuclear DNA content in prostatic carcinoma. *Cancer* 69:1432-1439, 1992.

Franzén S, Giertz G, Zajicek J. Cytological diagnosis of prostatic tumours by transrectal aspiration biopsy: a preliminary report. *Br J Urol* 32:193-196, 1960.

Frederiksen P, Thommesen P, Kjær TB, et al. Flow cytometric DNA analysis in fine needle aspiration biopsies from patients with prostatic lesions: diagnostic value and relation to clinical stages. *Acta Pathol Microbiol Scand Sect* 86:461-464, 1978.

Gentile PS, Carloss HW, Huang TY, et al. Disseminated prostatic carcinoma simulating primary lung cancer: indications for immunodiagnostic studies. *Cancer* 62:711-715, 1988.

Gleason DF, Mellinger GT, Veterans Administration Cooperative Urological Research Group. Prediction of prognosis for prostatic adenocarcinoma by combined histological grading and clinical staging. *J Urol* 111:58-64, 1974.

Gleason DF. Atypical hyperplasia, benign hyperplasia, and well-differentiated adenocarcinoma of the prostate. *Am J Surg Pathol* 9:53-67, 1985.

Gleason DF. Histologic grading of prostatic cancer: a perspective. *Hum Pathol* 23:273-279, 1992.

Göthlin JH, Hölem L. Percutaneous fine-needle biopsy of radiographically normal lymph nodes in the staging of prostatic carcinoma. *Radiology* 141:351-354, 1981.

Graham JB, Ignatoff JM, Holland JM, et al. Prostatic aspiration biopsy: an assessment of accuracy based on long-term observations. *J Urol* 139:971-974, 1988.

Gray GF Jr, Marshall VF. Squamous carcinoma of the prostate. *J Urol* 113:736-738, 1975.

Greenebaum E. Megakaryocytes and ganglion cells mimicking cancer in fine needle aspiration of the prostate. *Acta Cytol* 32:504-508, 1988.

Gustafsson O, Norming U, Nyman CR, et al. Complications following combined transrectal aspiration and core biopsy of the prostate. *Scand J Urol Nephrol* 24:249-251, 1990.

Hasenson M, Lundh B, Stege R, et al. PAP and PSA in prostatic carcinoma cell lines and aspiration biopsies. *Prostate* 14:83-90, 1989.

Hautmann SH, Conrad S, Henke RP, et al. Detection rate of histologically insignificant prostate cancer with systematic sextant biopsies and fine needle aspiration cytology. *J Urol* 163:1734-1738, 2000.

Hedlund PO, Das D, Löwhagen T, et al. Rectal palpation and transrectal fine needle aspiration of the prostate in the monitoring of prostate cancer: a study of 59 patients during treatment with estramustine phosphate or estrogens. *Prostate* 15:327-333, 1989.

Helpap B. Cell kinetic and cytological grading of prostatic carcinoma. *Virchows Arch Pathol Anat* 393:205-214, 1981.

Henkes DN, Stein N. Fine-needle aspiration cytology of prostatic embryonal rhabdomyosarcoma: a case report. *Diagn Cytopathol* 3:163-165, 1987.

Herr HW, Whitmore WF Jr. Significance of prostatic biopsies after radiation therapy for carcinoma of the prostate. *Prostate* 3:339-350, 1982.

Hessel RG, Reyes CV, Jensen J, et al. Malignant cystic epithelial-stromal tumor of the prostate. *Diagn Cytopathol* 9:314-317, 1993.

Honig SC, Stilmant MM, Klavans MS, et al. The role of fine-needle aspiration biopsy of the prostate in staging adenocarcinoma. *Cancer* 69:2978-2982, 1992.

Hosking DH, Paraskevas M, Hellsten OR, et al. The cytological diagnosis of prostatic carcinoma by transrectal fine needle aspiration. *J Urol* 129:998-1000, 1983.

Hostetter AL, Pedersen KV, Gustafsson BL, et al. Diagnosis and localization of prostate carcinoma by fine-needle aspiration cytology and correlation with histologic whole-organ sections after radical prostatectomy. *Am J Clin Pathol* 94:693-697, 1990.

Howell LP, Teplitz RL. Papillary carcinoma of prostatic ductal origin: a cytologic case report with immunohistochemical and quantitative DNA correlation. *Diagn Cytopathol* 5:211-216, 1989.

Howell LP, Amott TR, deVere-White R. Aspiration biopsy cytology of the prostate in young adult men. *Diagn Cytopathol* 6:89-94, 1990.

Ibarrola de Andrés C, Megías VMC, Barrios AP, et al. Seminal vesicle epithelium as a potential pitfall in the cytodiagnosis of presacral masses: a report of two cases. *Acta Cytol* 44:399-402, 2000.

Ito H, Yamaguchi K, Kotake T, et al. Usefulness of aspiration cytology in prostate cancer detection. *Int Urol Nephrol* 27:93-100, 1995.

Jacobs DM, Weiss MA. Basal cells of prostate in fine-needle aspiration. *Am J Clin Pathol* 88:503-506, 1987.

Jacobs DM, Vago JF, Weiss MA. Gleason grading of prostatic adenocarcinoma on fine-needle aspiration. *Diagn Cytopathol* 5:126-133, 1989.

Jöbsis AC, De Vriess GP, Anholt RRH, et al. Demonstration of the prostatic origin of metastases: an immunohistochemical method for formalin-fixed embedded tissue. *Cancer* 41:1788-1793, 1978.

Jocham D, Schmiedt E, Göttinger H, et al. Die Prostatazytologie: zwölf Jahre Erfahrungen mit der transrektalen Feinnadelbiopsies. *Urologe (A)* 22:120-126, 1983.

Jones EC, McNeal J, Bruchovsky N, et al. DNA content in prostatic adenocarcinoma: a flow cytometry study of the predictive value of aneuploidy for tumor volume, percentage Gleason grade 4 and 5, and lymph node metastases. *Cancer* 66:752-757, 1990.

Juusela H, Ruutu M, Permi J, et al. Can fine needle aspiration biopsy detect incidental prostatic carcinoma (TI) prior to TUR? *Eur Urol* 21:131-133, 1992.

Katz RL, Raval P, Brooks TE, et al. Role of immunocytochemistry in diagnosis of prostatic neoplasia by fine needle aspiration biopsy. *Diagn Cytopathol* 1:28-32, 1985.

Kaufman JJ, Ljung BM, Walther P, et al. Aspiration biopsy of prostate. *Urology* 19:587-591, 1982.

Kelemen PR, Buschman RJ, Weisz-Carrington P. Nucleolar prominence as a diagnostic variable in prostatic carcinoma. *Cancer* 65:1017-1020, 1990.

Kelsey DM, Kohler FP, Mackinney CC, et al. Outpatient needle aspiration biopsy of the prostate. *J Urol* 116:327-328, 1976.

Keshgegian AA, Kline TS. Immunoperoxidase of prostatic acid phosphatase in aspiration biopsy cytology (ABC). *Am J Clin Pathol* 82:586-589, 1984.

Kimura N, Sasano N. Prostate-specific acid phosphatase in carcinoid tumors. *Virchows Arch A* 410:247-251, 1986.

Kline TS, Kelsey DM, Kohler FP. Prostatic carcinoma and needle aspiration biopsy. *Am J Clin Pathol* 67:131-133, 1977.

Kline TS, Kohler FP, Kelsey DM. Aspiration biopsy cytology (ABC): its use in diagnosis of lesions of the prostate gland. *Arch Pathol Lab Med* 106:136-139, 1982.

Kline TS, Kannan V. Prostatic aspirates: a cytomorphologic analysis with emphasis on well-differentiated carcinoma. *Diagn Cytopathol* 1:13-17, 1985.

Kline TS. Aspiration biopsy cytology of the prostate: theme and variations. *J Urol* 140:802, 1988.

Klotz LH, Shaw PA, Srigley JR. Transrectal fine-needle aspiration and Truecut (sic) needle biopsy of the prostate: a blinded comparison of accuracy. *Can J Surg* 32:287-289, 1989.

Koivuniemi A, Tyrkkö J. Seminal vesicle epithelium in fine-needle aspiration biopsies of the prostate as a pitfall in the cytologic diagnosis of carcinoma. *Acta Cytol* 20:116-119, 1976.

Koizumi JH. Fine-needle aspiration biopsy in prostate cancer. *Semin Urol* 8:19-30, 1990.

Koss LG, Woyke S, Schreiber K, et al. Thin-needle aspiration biopsy of the prostate. *Urol Clin North Am* 11:237-251, 1984.

Koss LG. The puzzle of prostatic carcinoma. *Mayo Clin Proc* 63:193-197, 1988.

Kovi J, Mostofi FK. Atypical hyperplasia of prostate. *Urology* 34(suppl 6):23-27, 1989.

Kramer CE, Epstein JI. Nucleoli in low-grade prostate adenocarcinoma and adenosis. *Hum Pathol* 24:618-623, 1993.

Krishnan B, Truong LD. Prostatic adenocarcinoma diagnosed by urinary cytology. *Am J Clin Pathol* 113:29-34, 2000.

Kuo TT, Gomez LG. Monstrous epithelial cells in human epididymis and seminal vesicles: a pseudomalignant change. *Am J Surg Pathol* 5:483-490, 1981.

Kurth KH, Altwein JE, Skoluda D, et al. Followup of irradiated prostatic carcinoma by aspiration biopsy. *J Urol* 117:615-617, 1977.

Lager DJ, Goeken JA, Kemp JD, et al. Squamous metaplasia of the prostate. *Am J Clin Pathol* 90:597-601, 1988.

Lal P, Gupta A, Minocha VR. Prostatic aspiration cytology using lumbar puncture needle. *J Surg Oncol* 67:192-193, 1998.

Lange PH, Narayan P. Understaging and undergrading of prostate cancer: argument for postoperative radiation as adjuvant therapy. *Urology* 21:113-118, 1983.

Layfield LJ, Mukamel E, Hilborne LH, et al. Cytological grading of prostatic aspiration biopsy: a comparison with the Gleason grading system. *J Urol* 138:798-800, 1987.

Leistenschneider W, Nagel R. Die zytologische Differenzierung der Prostatitis [The cytologic differentiation of prostatitis]. *Pathol Res Pract* 165:429-444, 1979.

Lin BPC, Davies WEL, Harmata PA. Prostatic aspiration cytology. *Pathology* 11:607-614, 1979.

Linsk JA, Axilrod HD, Solyn R, et al. Transrectal cytologic aspiration in the diagnosis of prostatic carcinoma. *J Urol* 108:455-459, 1972.

Ljung BM. Fine-needle aspiration biopsy of the prostate gland: technique and review of the literature. *Semin Urol* 3:18-26, 1985.

Ljung BM, Cherrie R, Kaufman JJ. Fine needle aspiration biopsy of the prostate gland: a study of 103 cases with histological followup. *J Urol* 135:955-958, 1986.

Maffini M, Ortega HH, Stoker C, et al. Bcl-2 correlates with tumor ploidy and nuclear morphology in early stage prostate carcinoma: a fine needle aspiration biopsy study. *Pathol Res Pract* 197:487-492, 2001.

Maksem JA, Resnick MI, Johenning PW. Can a cytological grading system be predictive of Gleason's scores in aspiration biopsy cytology specimens of prostate carcinoma. *World J Urol* 5:99-102, 1987.

Maksem JA, Park CH, Johenning PW, et al. Aspiration biopsy of the prostate gland. *Urol Clin North Am* 15:555-575, 1988A.

Maksem JA, Johenning PW. Is cytology capable of adequately grading prostate carcinoma? Matched series of 50 cases comparing cytologic and histologic pattern diagnoses. *Urology* 31:437-444, 1988B.

Maksem JA, Johenning PW, Galang CF. Prostatitis and aspiration biopsy cytology of prostate. *Urology* 32:263-268, 1988C.

Maksem JA, Galang CF, Johenning PW, et al. Aspiration biopsy of the prostate gland: a brief review of collection, fixation, and pattern recognition with special attention to benign and malignant prostatic epithelium. *Diagn Cytopathol* 6:258-266, 1990.

Markham CW. Prostatic intraepithelial neoplasia: detection and correlation with invasive cancer in fine-needle biopsy. *Urology* 34(suppl 6):57-61, 1989.

Masood S, Swartz DA, Meneses M, et al. Fine needle aspiration cytology of papillary endometrioid carcinoma of the prostate: the grooved nucleus as a cytologic marker. *Acta Cytol* 35:451-455, 1991.

Matsumoto T, Soejima T, Tanaka M, et al. Cytologic findings of fine needle aspirates in chronic prostatitis. *Int Urol Nephrol* 24:43-47, 1992.

McNeal JE, Bostwick DG. Intraductal dysplasia: a premalignant lesion of the prostate. *Hum Pathol* 17:64-71, 1986.

Melograna F, Oertel YC, Kwart AM. Prospective controlled assessment of fine-needle prostatic aspiration. *Urology* 19:47-51, 1982.

Mesonero CE, Oertel YC. Cells from ejaculatory ducts and seminal vesicles and diagnostic difficulties in prostatic aspirates. *Mod Pathol* 4:723-726, 1991.

Mestitz H, Pierce RJ, Holmes PW. Intrathoracic manifestations of disseminated prostatic adenocarcinoma. *Respir Med* 83:161-166, 1989.

Mills SE, Fowler JE Jr. Gleason histologic grading of prostatic carcinoma: correlations between biopsy and prostatectomy specimens. *Cancer* 57:346-349, 1986.

Miralles TG, Rodriguez-Perez JA, de la Campa JMA. Squamous metaplasia of the prostate: a potential pitfall in fine needle aspiration cytology. *Acta Cytol* 32:272-274, 1988.

Miralles TG, Gosalbez F, Menendez P, et al. Fine needle aspiration cytology of granulomatous prostatitis. *Acta Cytol* 34:57-62, 1990.

Moroz K, Crespo P, de las Morenas A. Fine needle aspiration of prostatic rhabdomyosarcoma. *Acta Cytol* 39:785-790, 1995.

Mostofi FK, Davis CJ Jr, Sesterhenn IA: Pathology of carcinoma of the prostate. *Cancer* 70:235-253, 1992A.

Mostofi FK, Sesterhenn IA, Davis CJ Jr. Prostatic carcinoma: problems in the interpretation of prostatic biopsies. *Hum Pathol* 23:223-241, 1992B.

Mostofi FK, Sesterhenn IA, Davis CJ Jr. A pathologist's view of prostatic carcinoma. *Cancer* 71:906-932, 1993.

Müller HA, Wünsch PH. Features of prostatic sarcomas in combined aspiration and punch biopsies. *Acta Cytol* 25:480-484, 1981.

Muñoz de Toro M, Maffini MV, Giardina RH, et al. Processing fine needle aspirates of prostate carcinomas for standard immunocytochemical studies and *in situ* apoptosis detection. *Pathol Res Pract* 194:631-636, 1998.

Murphy GP. The diagnosis and detection of urogenital cancers. *Cancer* 47:1193-1199, 1981.

Murphy WM. Atypical intraepithelial lesions of the prostate gland. *Am J Clin Pathol* 96:561-563, 1991.

Narayan P, Jajodia P, Stein R, et al. A comparison of fine needle aspiration and core biopsy in diagnosis and preoperative grading of prostate cancer. *J Urol* 141:560-563, 1989.

Narayan P, Jajodia P, Stein R. Core biopsy instrument in the diagnosis of prostate cancer: superior accuracy to fine needle aspiration. *J Urol* 145:795-797, 1991.

Niejadlik DC, Dwyer RD, Rousseau D. Aspiration biopsy of the prostate: a community hospital's experience. *Conn Med* 54:243-245, 1990.

Oates RD, Stilmant MM, Freedlund MC, et al. Granulomatous prostatitis following bacillus Calmette-Guérin immunotherapy of bladder cancer. *J Urol* 140:751-754, 1988.

Oomens EHGM, Van Steenbrugge GJ, Van Der Kwast TH, et al. Application of the monoclonal antibody Ki-67 on prostate biopsies to assess the fraction of human prostatic carcinoma. *J Urol* 145:81-85, 1991.

Ordóñez NG, Ro JY, Ayala AG. Metastatic prostatic carcinoma presenting as an oncocytic tumor. *Am J Surg Pathol* 16:1007-1012, 1992.

Ostrzega N, Cheng L, Layfield LJ. Keratin immunoreactivity in fine-needle aspiration of the prostate: an aid in the differentiation of benign epithelium from well-differentiated adenocarcinoma. *Diagn Cytopathol* 4:38-41, 1988.

Oyasu R, Bahnson RR, Nowels K, et al. Cytological atypia in the prostate gland: frequency, distribution and possible relevance to carcinoma. *J Urol* 135:959-962, 1986.

Palmer LS, Laor E, Skinner WK, et al. Prostate cancer screening using fine-needle aspiration cytology prior to open prostatectomy. *Eur Urol* 27:96-98, 1995.

Pérez-Barrios A, Rodrigue-Peralto JL, Martinez-Gonzalez MA, et al. Malacoplakia of the pelvis: report of a case with cytologic and ultrastructural findings obtained by fine needle aspiration. *Acta Cytol* 36:377-380, 1992.

Phillips NB, Lattimer JK. Complications and regression of primary tumor size with radiotherapy in prostatic cancer. *J Urol* 108:921-923, 1972.

Polito M, Alberti R, Muzzonigro G, et al. Fine needle aspiration biopsy of the prostate gland: our experience concerning 101 cases with histological follow-up. *Prostate* 17:85-94, 1990.

Pousette A, Carlström, Tribukait B, et al. Prostate-specific antigen in tissue from fine-needle aspiration biopsies. *Br J Urol* 79(suppl 1):104-106, 1997.

Renshaw AA, Granter SR. Metastatic, sarcomatoid, and PSA- and PAP-negative prostatic carcinoma: diagnosis by fine-needle aspiration. *Diagn Cytopathol* 23:199-201, 2000.

Ritchie AWS, Layfield LJ, Turcillo P, et al. The significance of atypia in fine needle aspiration cytology of the prostate. *J Urol* 140:761-765, 1988.

Ro JY, Ayala AG, Ordonez NG, et al. Intraluminal crystalloids in prostatic adenocarcinoma: immunohistochemical, electron microscopic, and x-ray microanalytic studies. *Cancer* 57:2397-2407, 1986.

Rockey KE, Graham TE. Prostate adenocarcinoma metastatic to the lung. *Postgrad Med* 87:199-208, 1990.

Rönström L, Tribukait B, Esposti PL. DNA pattern and cytological findings in fine-needle aspirates of untreated prostatic tumors: a flow-cytofluorimetric study. *Prostate* 2:79-88, 1981.

Rørvik J, Dæhlin L. Prostatic abscess: imaging with transrectal ultrasound: case report. *Scand J Urol Nephrol* 23:307-308, 1989.

Schmidt JD. Non-specific granulomatous prostatitis: classification, review and report of cases. *J Urol* 94:607-615, 1965.

Schmidt JD. Clinical diagnosis of prostate cancer. *Cancer* 70(suppl 1):221-224, 1992.

Shannon RL, Ro JY, Grignon DJ, et al. Sarcomatoid carcinoma of the prostate: a clinicopathologic study of 12 patients. *Cancer* 69:2676-2682, 1992.

Shimada H, Misugi K, Sasaki Y, et al. Carcinoma of the prostate in childhood and adolescence: report of a case and review of the literature. *Cancer* 46:2534-2542, 1980.

Singh N, Shenoi UD, Raghuveer CV. FNAC and transabdominal ultrasonography in the diagnosis of prostatomegaly. *Ind J Pathol Microbiol* 40:473-479, 1997.

Smith FL, Bibbo M, Schoenberg HW, et al. Transrectal aspiration biopsy of the prostate: the importance of atypia. *J Urol* 140:766-768, 1988.

Spieler P, Gloor F, Egle N, et al. Cytological findings in transrectal aspiration biopsy on hormone-and radio-treated carcinoma of the prostate. *Virchows Arch A Pathol Anat Histol* 372:149-159, 1976.

Sprenger E, Volk L, Michaelis WE. Die Aussagekraft der zellkern-DNS-Bestimmung bei der Diagnostik des Prostatakarzinoms [the significance of nuclear DNA measurement in the diagnosis of prostatic carcinomas]. *Beitr Pathol Bd* 153:370-378, 1974.

Stanley MW, Hedlund PO, Rönstrom L, et al. Determination of false negative rate in fine-needle aspiration of prostate. *Urology* 34:73-75, 1989.

Stanley MW, Horwitz CA, Sharer W, et al. Granulomatous prostatitis: a spectrum including nonspecific, infectious, and spindle cell lesions. *Diagn Cytopathol* 7:508-512, 1991.

Stege R, Lundh B, Tribukait B, et al. Deoxyribonucleic acid ploidy and the direct assay of prostatic acid phosphate and prostate specific antigen in fine needle aspiration biopsies as diagnostic methods in prostatic carcinoma. *J Urol* 144:299-302, 1990.

Stege R, Tribukait B, Lundh B, et al. Quantitative estimation of tissue prostate specific antigen, deoxyribonucleic acid ploidy and cytological grade in fine needle aspiration biopsies for prognosis of hormonally treated prostatic carcinoma. *J Urol* 148:833-837, 1992.

Stege RH, Tribukait B, Carlström KAM, et al. Tissue PSA from fine-needle biopsies of prostatic carcinoma as related to serum PSA, clinical state, cytological grade, and DNA ploidy. *Prostate* 38:183-188, 1999.

Stenkvist B, Olding-Stenkvist E. Cytological and DNA characteristics of hyperplasia/inflammation and cancer of the prostate. *Eur J Cancer* 26:261-267, 1990.

Stilmant M, Siroky MB, Johnson KB. Fine needle aspiration cytology of granulomatous prostatitis induced by BCG immunotherapy of bladder cancer. *Acta Cytol* 29:961-966, 1985.

Stilmant MM, Freedlund MC, de las Morenas A, et al. Expanded role for fine needle aspiration of the prostate. *Cancer* 63:583-592, 1989.

Stricker HJ, Kunin JR, Faerber GJ. Congenital prostatic cyst causing ejaculatory duct obstruction: management by transrectal cyst aspiration. *J Urol* 149:1141-1143, 1993.

Suhrland MJ, Deitch D, Schreiber K, et al. Assessment of fine needle aspiration as a screening test for occult prostatic carcinoma. *Acta Cytol* 32:495-498, 1988.

Tannenbaum M, Tannenbaum S, DeSanctis PN, et al. Prognostic significance of nucleolar surface area in prostate cancer. *Urology* 19:546-551, 1982.

Tannenbaum M. Aspiration biopsy of the prostate: the pathologist's viewpoint. *Semin Urol* 1:172-175, 1983A.

Tannenbaum M. Prostate cancer grading: light and electron microscopy. *Semin Urol* 1:186-192, 1983B.

Tell DT, Khoury JM, Taylor HG, et al. Atypical metastasis from prostate cancer: clinical utility of the immunoperoxidase technique for prostate-specific antigen. *JAMA* 253:3574-3575, 1985.

Tomic R, Bergman B, Hietala SO, et al. Prognostic significance of transrectal fine-needle aspiration biopsy findings after orchiectomy for carcinoma of the prostate. *Eur Urol* 11:378-381, 1985.

Tribukait B, Esposti PL, Rönström L. Tumour ploidy for characterization of prostatic carcinoma: flow-cytofluorometric DNA studies using aspiration biopsy material. *Scand J Urol Nephrol* 55:59-64, 1980.

Tribukait B. DNA flow cytometry in carcinoma of the prostate for diagnosis, prognosis and study of tumor biology. *Acta Oncol* 30:187-192, 1991.

Tuero JG, de la Campa JA, Lacort LP, et al. Granulomatous prostatitis. *Urol Int* 43:97-101, 1988.

Van Poppel H, Ameye F, Oyen R, et al. Accuracy of combined computerized tomography and fine needle aspiration cytology in lymph node staging of localized prostatic carcinoma. *J Urol* 151:1310-1314, 1994.

Varma VA, Fekete PS, Franks MJ, et al. Cytologic features of prostatic adenocarcinoma in urine: a clinicopathologic and immunocytochemical study. *Diagn Cytopathol* 4:300-305, 1988.

Waisman J, Adolfsson J, Löwhagen T, et al. Comparison of transrectal prostate digital aspiration and ultrasound-guided core biopsies in 99 men. *Urology* 37:301-307, 1991.

Wajsman Z, Klimberg I. Needle aspiration and needle biopsy procedures. *Urol Clin North Am* 14:103-113, 1987.

Walsh PC. Fine needle aspiration of the prostate: why has it taken so long to accept? *J Urol* 135:334-335, 1986.

Wasserstein PW, Goldman RL. Diffuse carcinoid of prostate. *Urology* 18:407-409, 1981.

Weinstein MH, Epstein JI. Significance of high-grade prostatic intraepithelial neoplasia on needle biopsy. *Hum Pathol* 24:624-629, 1993.

Willems JS, Löwhagen T. Transrectal fine-needle aspiration biopsy for cytologic diagnosis and grading of prostatic carcinoma. *Prostate* 2:381-395, 1981.

Williams JP, Still BM, Pugh RCB. The diagnosis of prostatic cancer: cytological and biochemical studies using the Franzen biopsy needle. *Br J Urol* 39:549-554, 1967.

Wilson JD. The pathogenesis of benign prostatic hyperplasia. *Am J Med* 68:745-756, 1980.

Wood DP Jr, Montie JE, Pontes JE, et al. Identification of transitional cell carcinoma of the prostate in bladder cancer patients: a prospective study. *J Urol* 141:83-85, 1989.

Yao JCT, Wang WCC, Tseng HH, et al. Primary rhabdomyosarcoma of the prostate: diagnosis by needle biopsy and immunocytochemistry. *Acta Cytol* 32:509-512, 1988.

Yatani R, Shiraishi T, Soga T, et al. Reliability of cytological grading of prostatic carcinoma compared with histological grading. *Pathol Res Pract* 180:68-73, 1985.

Zattoni F, Pagano F, Rebuffi A, et al. Transrectal thin-needle aspiration biopsy of prostate: four years' experience. *Urology* 22:69-72, 1983.

Zetterberg A, Esposti PL. Cytophotometric DNA-analysis of aspirated cells from prostatic carcinoma. *Acta Cytol* 20:46-57, 1976.

Zetterberg A, Esposti PL. Prognostic significance of nuclear DNA levels in prostatic carcinoma. *Scand J Urol Nephrol* 55:53-58, 1980.

Zetterberg A, Forsslund G. Ploidy level and tumor progression in prostatic carcinoma. *Acta Oncol* 30:193-199, 1991.

CHAPTER 4

Inflammation and Infection

[4.1] Clinical Prostatitis 77

[4.2] Clinical Bacterial Prostatitis 77

[4.3] Histologic Acute Inflammation 78

[4.4] Clinical Chronic Bacterial Prostatitis 80

[4.5] Clinical Chronic Abacterial Prostatitis (Inflammatory) 80

[4.6] Histologic Chronic Inflammation 80

[4.7] Clinical Chronic Abacterial Prostatitis (Noninflammatory), or Prostatodynia 86

[4.8] Granulomatous Prostatitis 86

[4.9] Vasculitis 94

[4.10] Infectious Prostatitis: Additional Types 94

I nflammation of the prostate (prostatitis) and infection of the prostate are common clinical problems. However, the definition and the etiologic basis of some forms of prostatitis continue to be a source of confusion. It is important for histopathologists to appreciate the clinical definition of prostatitis and to not necessarily equate histologic evidence of prostatic inflammation ("histologic prostatitis") with clinical prostatitis. Infections of the prostate are most often bacterial and are diagnosed clinically. Histopathologic detection of inflammatory cells in the prostate is common, but histologic identification of specific infectious agents in prostatic tissues is rare.

t4.1 Clinical Classification of Prostatitis

I	Drach et al (1978)		
	Acute and chronic bacterial prostatitis		
	Nonbacterial prostatitis		
	Prostatodynia		
II	NIH (CPW 1995)		
	Category I		Acute bacterial prostatitis
	Category II		Chronic bacterial prostatis
	Category III		Chronic abacterial prostatitis/chronic pelvic pain syndrome
		IIIA	Inflammatory chronic pelvic pain syndrome
		IIIB	Noninflammatory chronic pelvic pain syndrome
	Category IV		Asymptomatic inflammatory prostatitis
III	Roberts et al (1997)		
	Acute bacterial prostatitis		
	Chronic bacterial prostatitis		
	Chronic prostatitis (inflammatory)		
	Chronic prostatitis (noninflammatory)		
	Granulomatous prostatitis		

[4.1] Clinical Prostatitis

From a strict definitional standpoint, prostatitis is inflammation of the prostate. However, clinically, use of the term *prostatitis* is not confined to cases with inflammation (Roberts 1997). Conversely, when histopathologists see inflammation in, for example, a prostate needle biopsy, a diagnosis of prostatitis, although histologically correct, does not usually correlate with the clinical concept of prostatitis.

Prostatitis often is viewed as a clinically "confusing" (Roberts 1997) and "obscure and poorly understood" (Meares 1998) disorder. It can also be a difficult condition to treat (Nickel 2002, Roberts 1997). Clinical prostatitis is a major health problem and has been considered to be the third most important disease of the prostate gland (after benign prostatic hyperplasia [BPH] and cancer) (Roberts 1997). It accounts for 2 million annual doctor visits and 25% of all office visits for genitourinary-related complaints (NCHS 1993). The estimated community-based prevalence of clinical prostatitis is 10% to 16% (Collins 2002, Nickel 2001B, Roberts 1998), which is of a magnitude similar to that of diabetes and ischemic heart disease (Roberts 1998). Compared with BPH and prostate cancer, prostatitis is far more likely to affect younger men (18 to 50 years of age) (Collins 1998).

The most commonly used classification schemes for clinical prostatitis (CPW 1995, Drach 1978, Roberts 1997) are in **t4.1**. The etiology, pathogenesis, clinical features, clinical diagnosis, treatment, and sequelae have been used to define the different categories (Nickel 2002, Roberts 1997). Using the first classification scheme (Drach 1978), it was found that nonbacterial prostatitis is the most common type of clinical prostatitis at 64%, prostatodynia (literally "prostatic pain") was second most common at 31%, and 5% of patients had proven bacterial prostatitis.

This chapter mainly follows the National Institutes of Health (NIH) consensus classification of prostatitis (CPW 1995, Litwin 1999) **t4.1**. In these classification schemes, only NIH Category IV (CPW 1995) and the granulomatous prostatitis in the Roberts et al scheme (Roberts 1997) have a tissue-based component in the clinical diagnosis.

[4.2] Clinical Bacterial Prostatitis

The diagnosis of acute bacterial prostatitis is principally a clinical one, with a typical clinical presentation being of a young man with an abrupt onset of constitutional symptoms (fever, chills, malaise, and arthralgia), urinary tract symptoms (dysuria, frequency, nocturia, and urgency), and pain in the rectum, lower back, or perineum (Mears 1998, Roberts 1997). The urinary tract symptoms are related to concomitant urinary tract infection, most often due to *Escherichia coli;* other gram-negative bacteria have also been found, including *Proteus*, *Klebsiella*, *Enterobacter*, and *Serratia* (Nickel 2002, Roberts 1997). The bacterial infection in the prostate may be the direct result of reflux of infected urine into the major prostatic ducts. Other possible pathways for bacterial access into the prostate include urethral infection, direct or lymphatic spread of rectal bacteria, and hematogenous bacterial spread (Meares 1998). Digital rectal examination (DRE) reveals an enlarged, tender, warm, and firm prostate (Roberts 1997). Prostatic massage to yield expressed prostatic secretions for segmented cultures in the "4-glass test" (see section on clinical chronic bacterial prostatitis later in this chapter), urethral instrumentation, and prostatic biopsy are contraindicated in acute bacterial prostatitis because of the risk of septicemia. Most patients respond well to antibiotic therapy directed against the organism (or uncommonly, organisms) identified in urine cultures, but chronic prostatitis and prostatic abscess are potential complications.

Prostatic abscess formation has decreased in incidence with the use of antibiotics and is now rare. The type of causative organism has also changed. Before the antibiotic era, *Neisseria gonorrhoeae* was the most common cause, but now the most frequently isolated organisms are *E coli* and *Staphylococcus* (Granados 1992, Ludwig 1999, Nickel 2002, Weinberger 1988). Patients who are diabetic, immunocompromised, and on dialysis, who undergo urethral instrumentation, and who have indwelling urethral catheters are predisposed to prostatic abscess development (Granados 1992, Ludwig 1999, Nickel 2002, Weinberger 1988). Abscess tissue may be submitted to the surgical pathology laboratory in the form of transurethrally resected prostatic chips or a suprapubic prostatectomy specimen when these surgical treatments are pursued in addition to the mandatory antibiotic therapy (Granados 1992).

[4.3] Histologic Acute Inflammation

An acute inflammatory cell infiltrate made up of neutrophils is common in prostatic tissue samples acquired for reasons not related to clinical prostatitis. In needle core biopsies performed to rule out prostate cancer, we found that 109 (52%) of 209 patients had incidental acute inflammation (Nadler 1995). In the absence of prostate cancer, this subclinical acute prostatitis was associated with an elevated total serum prostate-specific antigen (PSA) (Nadler 1995, Okada 2000): 63% of patients with an elevated serum PSA (and no evidence of cancer on multiple biopsies) had acute inflammation compared with 27% of patients who had a normal PSA level and acute inflammation (Nadler 1995). A neutrophilic infiltrate does not appear to affect percentage free PSA levels (Ornstein 1998). In needle core biopsies with atrophy, 21% to 22% of needle biopsies harbor acute inflammation (Cheville 1995, Ruska 1998). Acute inflammation has been detected in 20% to 98% of transurethral and open prostatectomy specimens (Brawer 1989, Hasui 1994, Kohnen 1979). Acute inflammation in these tissues was associated with an elevated serum PSA (Brawer 1989). In whole prostate glands from autopsies, 14% (McNeal 1968) to 20% (Billis 1998) of cases have acute inflammatory infiltrates. This lower incidence of neutrophils in whole glands (where one would expect a higher incidence because more tissue is examined) probably results from a more restrictive definition of acute inflammation: In one of the whole gland studies (McNeal 1968), acute inflammation was defined not as the presence of any neutrophils but as an area where most of the gland lumina were filled with polymorphonuclear leukocytes.

The etiologic basis for such a high prevalence of acute inflammatory cell infiltrates in prostates is unclear. The neutrophils could be a response to a subclinical infectious prostatitis or to a "chemical" prostatitis related to urinary reflux into the prostate. In the setting of BPH, neutrophils in hyperplastic glands could be a reaction to obstruction.

Microscopically, acute inflammation in the prostate often is intraluminal **t4.2; i4.1-i4.3**. This intraluminal pattern of involvement can vary from a few scattered neutrophils **i4.1** to aggregates of neutrophils (essentially microabscesses) **i4.2, i4.3**. Cellular debris, including shed epithelial cells, can be admixed with the neutrophils **i4.3**. In prostate needle biopsies performed to rule out prostate cancer, there are usually only a few scattered neutrophils, with a minority of cases showing extensive acute inflammation. In prostatectomy specimens, the acute inflammation also tends to be focal and patchy. In one study of transurethral resection of the prostate (TURP) chips, less than 1% of all glands showed acute inflammation (Hasui 1994). Duct acinar glandular dilatation **i4.4** and rupture **i4.5** can be associated with severe neutrophilic infiltrates. Dark bluish necrotic debris can be seen in these distended or disrupted glands **i4.4, i4.5**. Such lesions typically are found in the transition zone in BPH nodules sampled in TURP chips or simple prostatectomy or radical prostatectomy specimens. Neutrophils in the prostate can also be found in intraepithelial and periglandular stromal locations **i4.1, i4.3**. In the stroma, they are often admixed with other inflammatory cell types, particularly lymphocytes and occasionally plasma cells.

■ t4.2 Acute Inflammation (Neutrophils) in the Prostate

Often intraluminal
Can form intraglandular microabscesses
Can be intraepithelial and periglandular
Often admixed with periglandular lymphocytes and plasma cells
Can be seen in dilated and ruptured glands

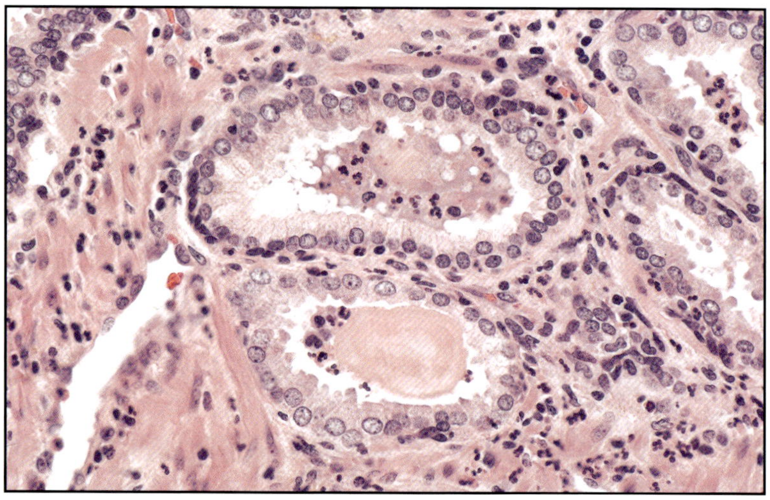

■ i4.1 *Scattered neutrophils in prostatic glands and stroma.*

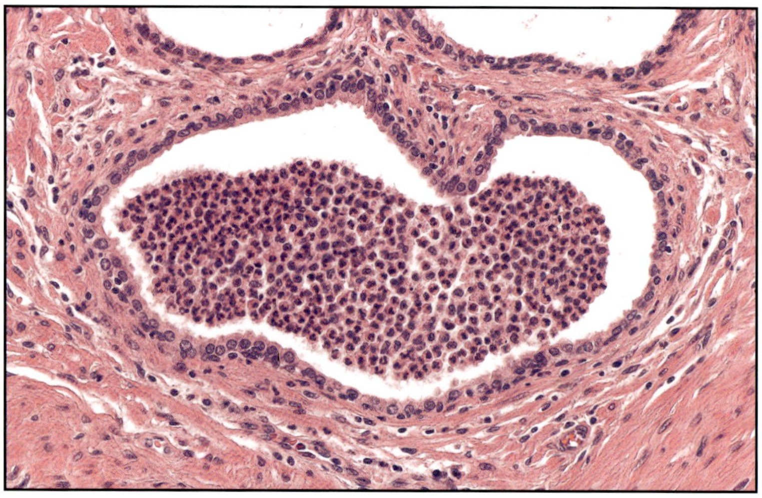

■ i4.2 *Intraluminal neutrophils in a prostatic gland, with microabscess formation.*

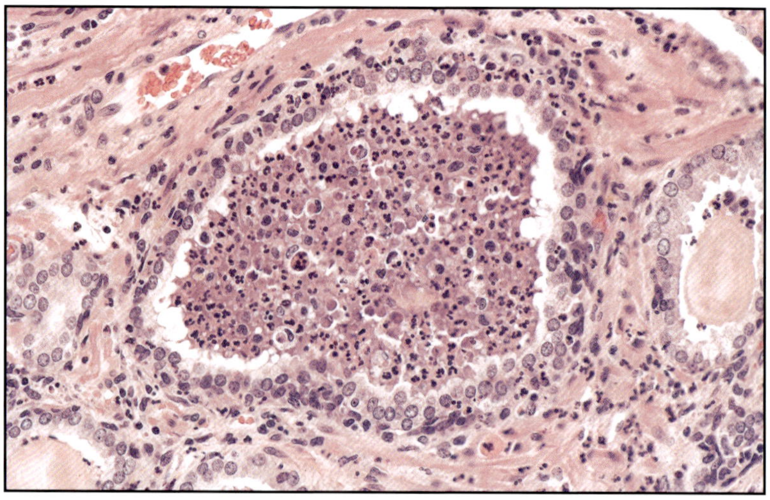

■ i4.3 *Distension of prostatic gland by neutrophils and cellular debris. Periglandular, stromal neutrophils are also present.*

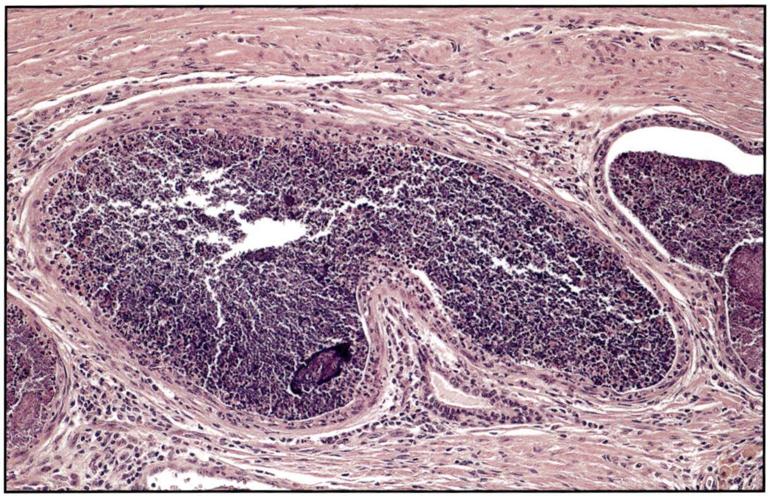

■ **i4.4** *Dark bluish acute inflammatory exudates in a dilated prostatic gland.*

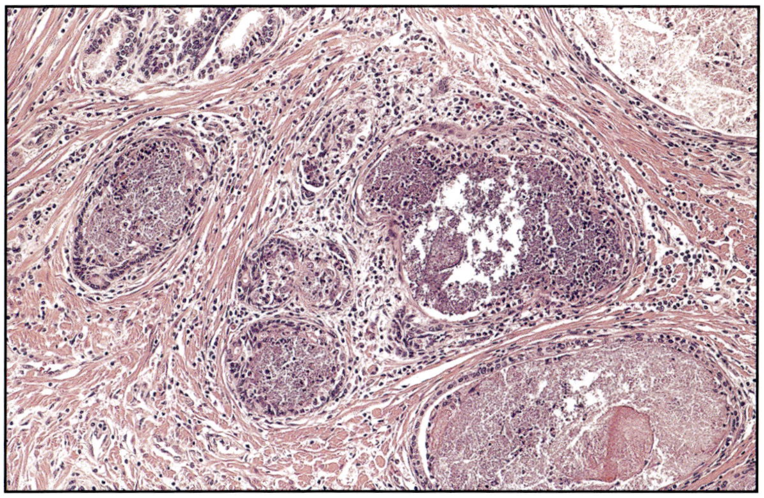

■ **i4.5** *Acute and chronic inflammatory cells in dilated and disrupted prostatic glands.*

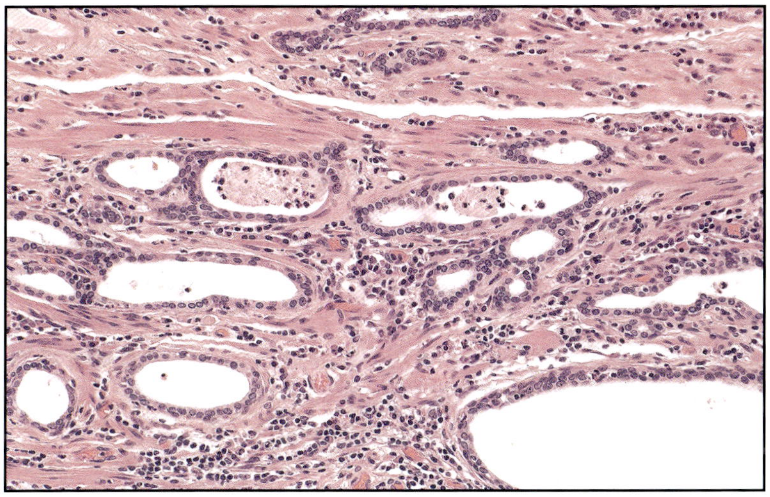

■ **i4.6** *A few intraluminal neutrophils and periglandular lymphocytes in peripheral zone atrophy.*

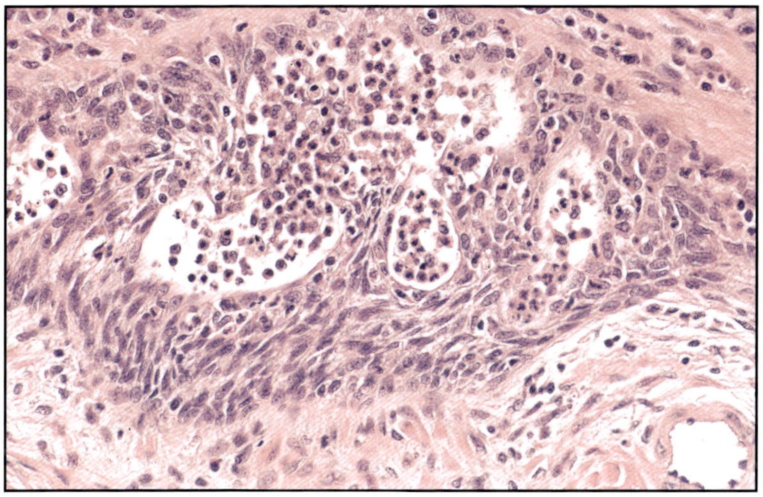

■ **i4.7** *Acutely inflamed squamous metaplasia in a prostatic gland.*

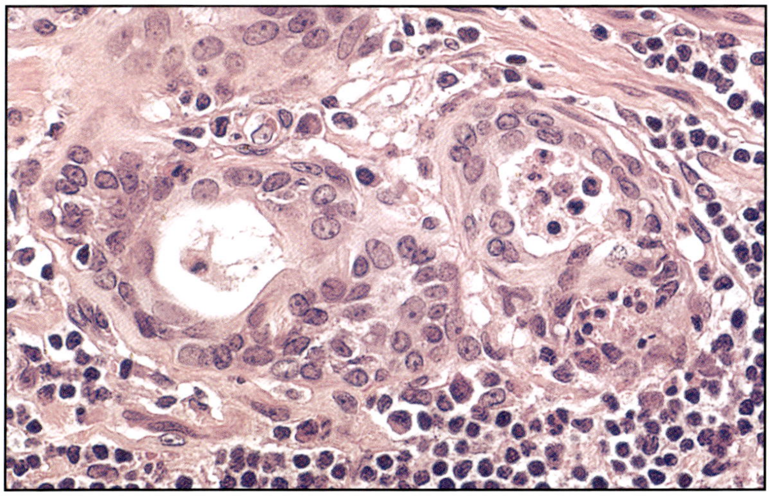

■ **i4.8** *Acutely and chronically inflamed prostatic glands, with reactive nuclear atypia, including pinpoint nucleoli.*

Acute inflammatory cell infiltrates in the prostate are associated with a variety of epithelial alterations, especially atrophy and hyperplasia (BPH). Needle biopsies of the prostate usually are directed toward the peripheral zone, where atrophy can be recognized in conjunction with acute inflammation **i4.6**. Metaplastic epithelium, including squamous cell metaplasia **i4.7** and transitional cell metaplasia, can be acutely inflamed. High-grade prostatic intraepithelial neoplasia (PIN) and prostatic carcinoma rarely exhibit neutrophilic infiltrates.

The main differential diagnostic difficulty in evaluating neutrophilic infiltrates in the prostate is the distinction of reactive nuclear atypia secondary to inflammation from prostatic adenocarcinoma. Although the nuclear atypia elicited by acute inflammation in prostatic glandular epithelium usually is manifested by nuclear enlargement with small pinpoint nucleoli **i4.8**, prominent nucleoli (larger than 1μm) are detectable in 45% of cases of acute inflamed atrophy (Ruska 1998). The most common trap is presented by postatrophic hyperplasia, in which fully 64% of needle biopsy cases had acute inflammation and prominent nucleoli in the atrophic epithelium, whereas only 13% of needle biopsy cases of simple atrophy had acute inflammation and prominent nucleoli in atrophic epithelium (Ruska 1998). A number of histologic features must be taken into account in separating atrophy, with or without inflammation, from atrophic prostatic carcinoma (Cina 1997, Egan 1997, Kaleem 1998) and usual prostatic carcinoma, which has a moderate amount of cytoplasm. Inflamed benign prostatic epithelium, even with nuclear atypia, harbors basal cells and lacks the disordered, infiltrative growth of prostatic adenocarcinoma. Another diagnostic hazard is interpretation of acutely inflamed squamous metaplastic epithelium as malignant. These reactive squamous cells in the prostate regularly contain nucleoli. The point that merits reiteration throughout this book is that large nucleoli in prostatic epithelial cell nuclei do not always indicate a neoplastic proliferation. Special studies generally are of limited value in assessing histologic acute inflammation of the prostate. The one special study that can be diagnostically beneficial is immunohistochemical staining to confirm basal cell presence (using antibody 34βE12) in acutely inflamed, reactive, benign glands, but this is not usually necessary. DNA content measurements are not of practical value in distinguishing reactive, inflammatory atypia from carcinoma because many prostatic carcinomas are diploid and because in some cases DNA ploidy measurements by image analysis cytometry demonstrate an overlap in DNA content between hyperplasia or inflammation and carcinoma (Stenkvist 1990). Also, a case of DNA aneuploidy in a prostate needle biopsy with acute inflammation has been reported (Lo 1996). One need not apply histochemical stains for organisms to sections of prostate with acute inflammation except when there is abscess formation with necrosis or when the patient is immunocompromised. Tissue Gram stains for bacteria in histologic sections almost always are negative.

Finally, an oft-posed question is whether it is necessary to report acute inflammation in prostatic tissue samples, particularly needle biopsies. If extensive, the inflammation should be reported, but if focal, the diagnosis of the acute inflammation should be considered optional. This is because, even though acute inflammation is associated with an elevated serum PSA, its presence does not provide reassurance that another process, such as prostate cancer, is absent, especially in a single set of biopsies. If over time there is persistence of acute inflammation in multiple sets of biopsies that are negative for cancer, then it may be worthwhile to report the acute inflammation as a possible cause of the patient's elevated serum PSA.

[4.4] Clinical Chronic Bacterial Prostatitis

The same bacteria that cause acute bacterial prostatitis are responsible for chronic bacterial prostatitis (Nickel 2002, Roberts 1997). Men with chronic bacterial prostatitis classically have recurrent urinary tract infections with the offending organism (usually *E coli*). These patients are older men who present with variable irritative voiding symptoms, including dysuria, urinary frequency and urgency, nocturia, and pelvic pain (Nickel 2002). The DRE can be normal, or the prostate can be swollen, tender, boggy, or firm (Roberts 1997). The clinical diagnosis may be established by the so-called 4-glass test to localize, by culture, the bacterial infection to prostatic secretions (Meares 1968). In practice, urologists rarely use this test (McNaughton-Collins 2000). The 4-glass test is performed by collecting the first 10 mL of voided urine in the first tube, midstream urine in the second tube for further culture, expressed prostatic secretions in the third tube, and the first voided 10 mL of urine after prostatic massage in the fourth tube. Numerous (>10) white blood cells per high-power field by light microscopy indicate prostatic inflammation. In men with bacterial prostatitis, lipid-laden macrophages are also common. If, by culture, the number of bacteria in the third tube is 10 times that of tubes 1 and 2, then a diagnosis of chronic bacterial prostatitis is rendered. If no bacteria are cultured in the prostatic secretions but increased white cells are present, the patient has chronic abacterial prostatitis (Nickel 2002, Roberts 1997). Treatment of chronic bacterial prostatitis often is ineffective because there is poor antibiotic penetration into the prostate (unlike in acute bacterial prostatitis) (Roberts 1997). Tissue is rarely obtained from these patients. Core needle biopsy is not indicated and has been performed in only a few cases (Schmidt 1966). In a few patients, transurethral prostatectomy can be curative but is often a last resort (Meares 1998, Roberts 1997). Unlike other prostatic tissue samples, it is important to document in the resection cases the type and extent of inflammation. It is also relevant to report whether calculi are present and, if so, their size and number because stones, particularly multiple large stones (Meares 1998), can be a source of entrapped bacteria that can seed the urine.

[4.5] Clinical Chronic Abacterial Prostatitis (Inflammatory)

Patients with chronic abacterial prostatitis present similarly to patients with chronic bacterial prostatitis. This clinical condition is diagnosed by finding prostatic inflammation but negative cultures in the 4-glass test. The cause is unknown, but *Chlamydia, Ureaplasma, Mycoplasma,* and *Trichomonas* organisms have been implicated; other possible causes include urinary reflux, autoimmune disease (Keetch 1994), estrogen (Robinette 1988, Stoker 1999), urethral obstruction (Takechi 1999), and viral infection (Meares 1998, Roberts 1997). Reflux is a favored theory (Meares 1998). Because the pathogenesis in humans is not established, treatment is empiric and difficult; antibiotics and α-blockers have been tried (Nickel 2002, Roberts 1997). Tissue is rarely procured from these patients. Core biopsies in a limited number of patients have demonstrated chronic inflammation in 50% to 88% of cases (Doble 1989, Nielsen 1973); in the largest series (N = 97 patients) to date, 33% of patients had any inflammation on biopsy, whereas fully 67% lacked inflammation (True 1999). The chronic inflammatory cell infiltrate was predominantly mononuclear, with only rare neutrophils and no eosinophils or granulomas. It was graded as mild in most cases. The pattern of tissue involvement was mainly one of diffuse stromal distribution, with only a minority of cases with intraglandular or periglandular localization of inflammatory cells (True 1999).

[4.6] Histologic Chronic Inflammation

Incidental detection of lymphocytes, histiocytes, and plasma cells is extremely common in prostatic tissue samples of all types. In needle biopsies of men without prostate cancer, almost all (99%) men with an elevated serum PSA had a lymphoplasmacytic infiltrate, whereas 77% of men without an elevated serum PSA had a lymphoplasmacytic infiltrate (Nadler 1995). A lower incidence of 46% was found in a second needle biopsy study (Blumenfeld 1992), but this study required well-defined 7- to 10-cell lymphoid aggregates to meet their definitional cutoff for chronic inflammation. Most (85% to 100%) of TURP, open prostatectomy, and radical prostatectomy specimens have evidence of chronic inflammation (Blumenfeld 1992, Hasui 1994, Kohnen 1979).

The etiologic basis for chronic histopathologic prostatitis is unknown but could relate, as in clinical chronic abacterial prostatitis, to undetected infection, autoimmune disease (Keetch 1994), or reflux. In BPH, the inflammation could be a consequence of obstruction and may itself contribute to the pathogenesis of BPH (Steiner 1994). Inflammation can also be induced in the prostate secondary to

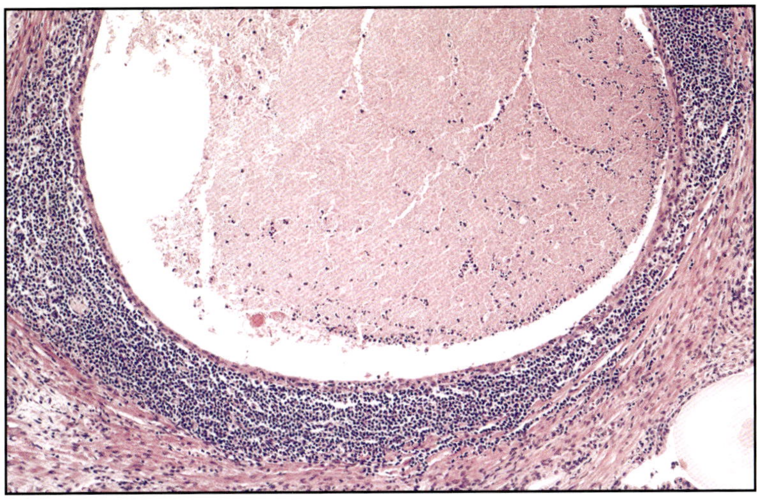

■ **i4.9** *Dilated prostatic gland with band-like ring of lymphocytes and plasma cells.*

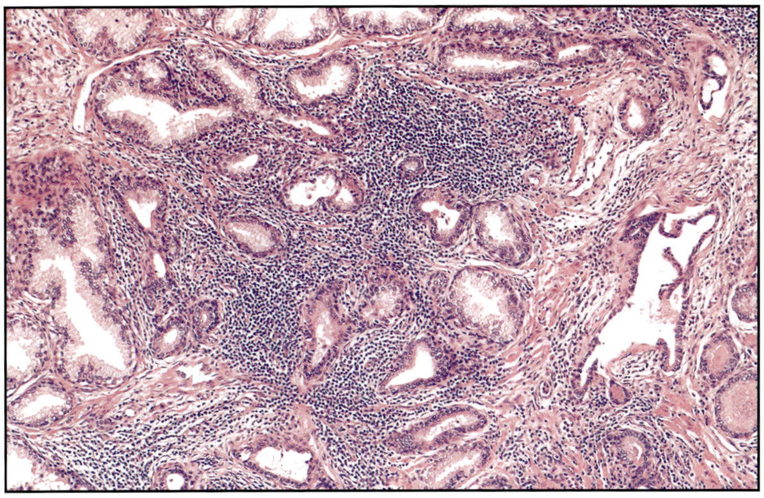

■ **i4.10** *Diffuse lymphoplasmacytic infiltrate in prostatic stroma.*

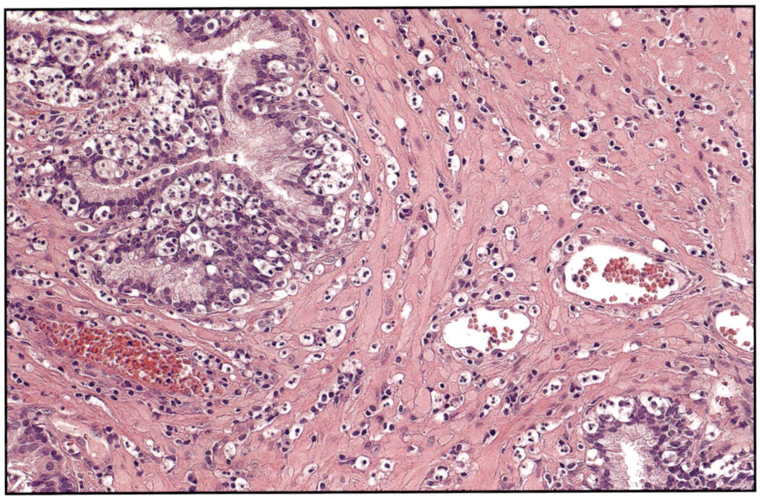

■ **i4.11** *Perinuclear clearing of stromal and intraepithelial lymphocytes.*

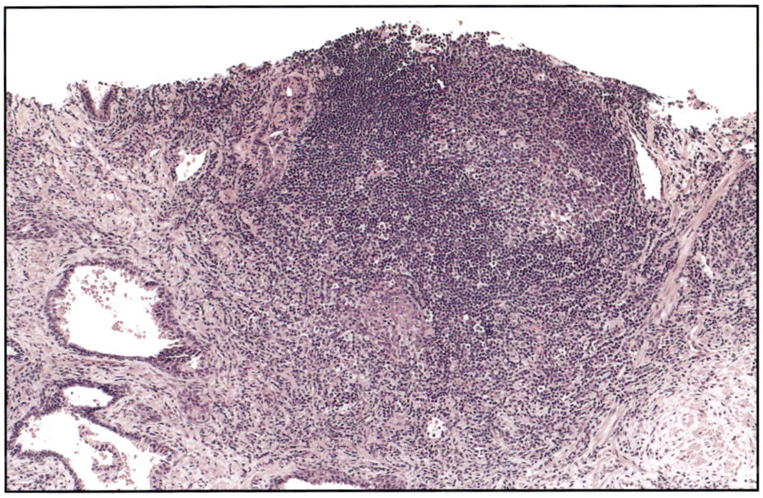

■ **i4.12** *Prostatic stromal lymphoid aggregate, with germinal center.*

biopsy, urethral instrumentation, and treatment, including transurethral and open prostatectomy, radiation therapy, and hormonal therapy.

Microscopically, several patterns of chronic inflammatory cell involvement of benign prostatic tissue have been described (Helpap 1994, Kohnen 1979, Steiner 1994) **t4.3**. Lymphocytic and plasmacytic chronic inflammatory cell infiltrates, in contrast to acute inflammation, tend to be stromal-based and periglandular. Admixture with other inflammatory cell types is common.

In hyperplastic TURP tissue, a very common pattern seen in 85% of TURP chips is dilated glands containing cell debris, foamy macrophages, neutrophils, and pink proteinaceous material, associated with a bandlike ring of periglandular lymphocytes and plasma cells (with an occasional neutrophil spotted) **i4.9** (Kohnen 1979). A second highly common arrangement (present in 89% of TURP chips) is a periglandular, lymphoplasmacytic infiltrate in the absence of intraluminal inflammatory cells. Another morphologic presentation is a more diffuse stromal extension by the lymphocytes and plasma cells **i4.10**. In these glandulocentric infiltrates of lymphocytes or plasma cells, direct extension of lymphocytes into benign prostatic epithelium commonly occurs, sometimes with perilymphocytic clearing that allows recognition of intraepithelial lymphocytes **i4.11**. Isolated stromal lymphoid nodules **i4.12** can also be seen in up to 62% of TURP chips. Scattered single lymphocytes can also be noted, especially in nodules of stromal hyperplasia (stromal nodules) **i4.13**. Additionally, perivenular lymphocytic cuffs can be observed **i4.14**; it is thought that these venules are an avenue of entry for the lymphocytes into the prostate gland (Blumenfeld 1992).

Similar patterns of chronic inflammation are observed in needle biopsy and whole prostate glands. One major difference compared with hyperplastic tissue is that in peripheral zone sampling, as accomplished by needle biopsies, chronic inflammation often is associated with atrophy **i4.6, i4.15**. In one series, about one third of cases of atrophy in needle biopsy had associated chronic inflammation (Ruska 1998). Indeed, atrophy in the prostate, which is extremely common, is viewed as a consequence of inflammation rather than aging (McNeal 1988).

■ **t4.3 Patterns of Chronic Inflammation in the Prostate**

Intraluminal neutrophils/macrophages and periglandular lymphocytes/plasma cells (so-called segregated glandular inflammation)
Periglandular inflammation (ring-like)
Diffuse stromal inflammation
Intraepithelial lymphocytes
Isolated stromal lymphoid nodules
Single scattered lymphocytes (especially in stromal nodules)

Modified from Kohnen 1979 and Blumenfeld 1992, with personal observations

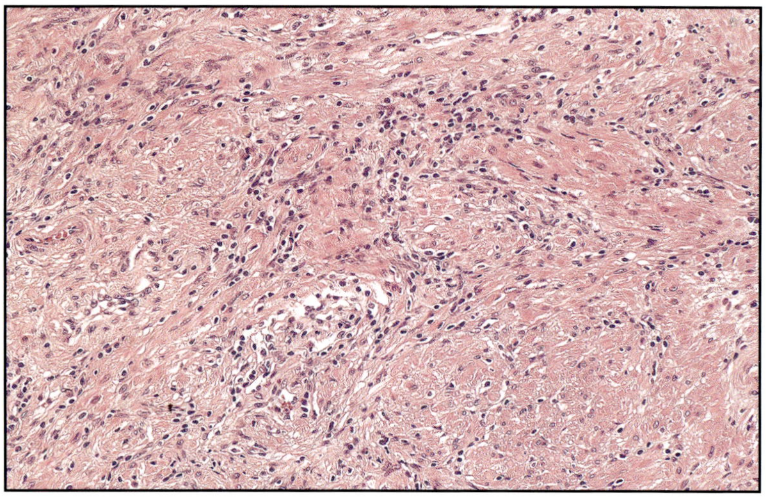

■ **i4.13** *Scattered lymphocytes in a stromal nodule.*

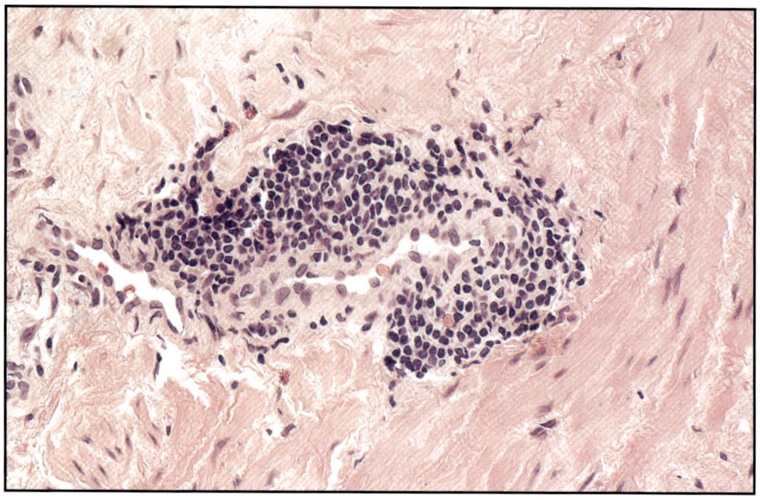

■ **i4.14** *Lymphocytes around a venule-portal of entry into the prostate.*

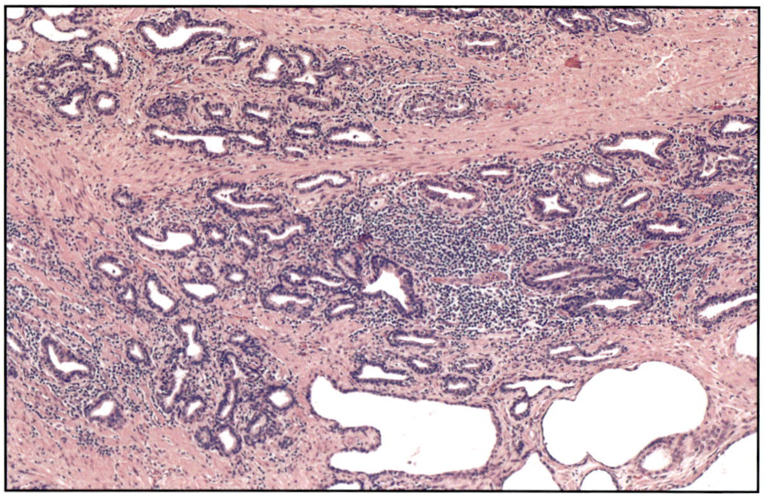

■ **i4.15** *Periglandular lymphocytic infiltrates in atrophy.*

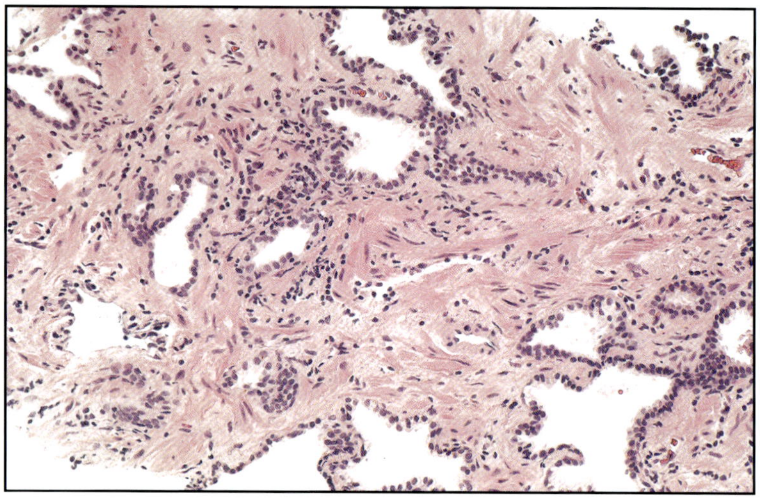

■ **i4.16** *Scattered stromal lymphocytes in needle biopsy of prostate—an extremely common finding.*

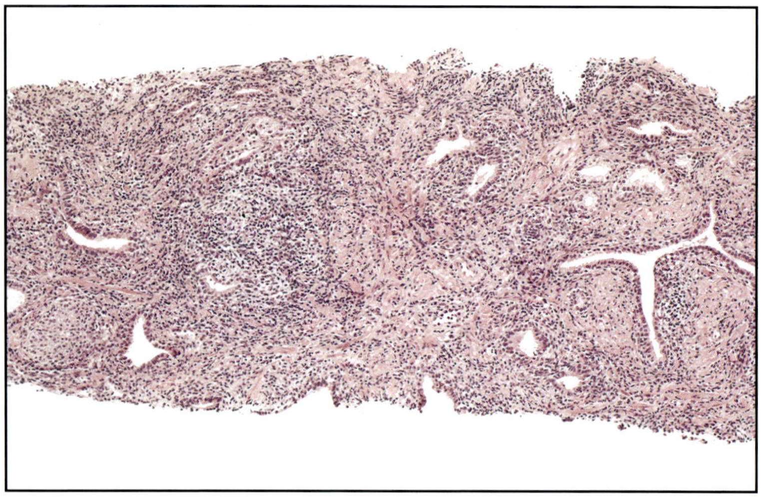

■ **i4.17** *Extensive chronic inflammation in prostate needle core biopsy.*

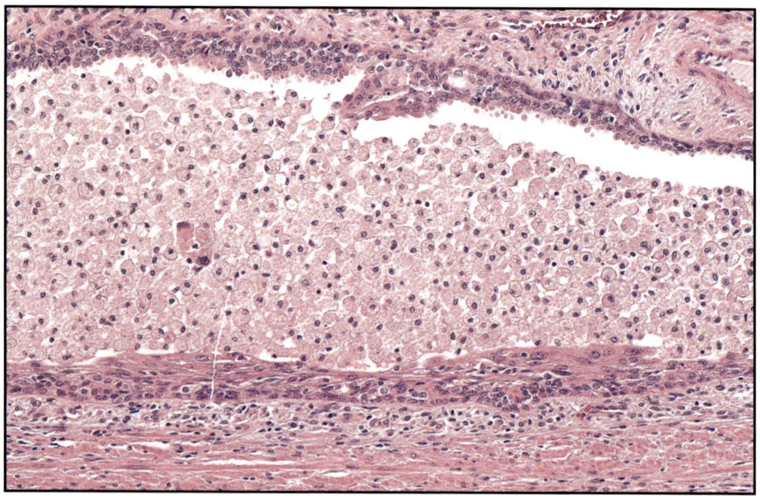

■ **i4.18** *Intraluminal macrophages in distended, inflamed prostatic duct, with associated, partial, squamous metaplasia of ductal lining cells.*

Chronic inflammation in the prostate usually is focal, patchy, and mild. In needle biopsies with chronic inflammation, we found that 88% of men had a low extent **i4.16**, and a minority (12%) had diffuse chronic inflammation **i4.17** (Nadler 1995). In TURP chips, a mean of about 5% of tissue was involved by chronic inflammation (Hasui 1994, Kohnen 1979). Overall, chronic histologic inflammation usually (90% of the time) is mild to moderate in prostatic tissues (Helpap 1994). Recently, a proposal was made to classify chronic prostatic inflammation, in standardized fashion, in terms of location (glandular, periglandular, stromal), extent (focal, multifocal, diffuse), and grade (mild, moderate, severe) (Nickel 2001A).

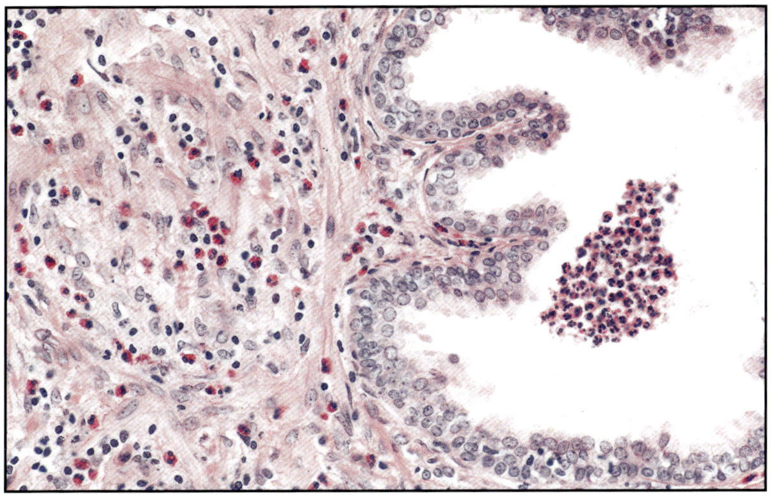

■ **i4.19** *Stromal eosinophils in a mixed acute (intraluminal) and chronic inflammatory cell infiltrate.*

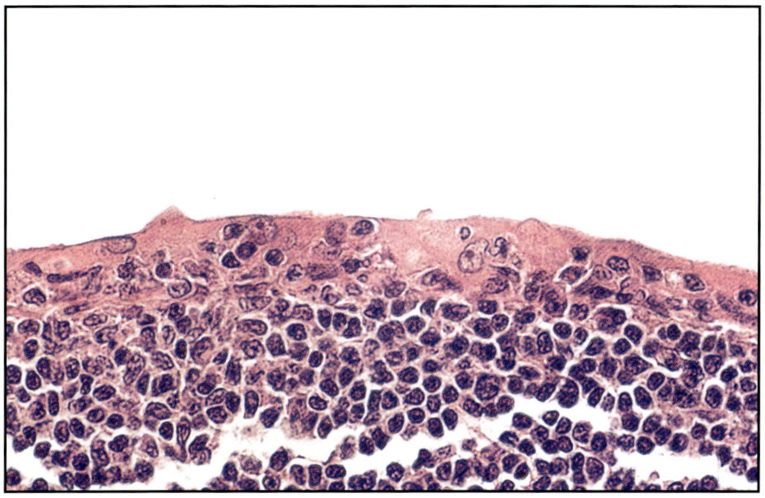

■ **i4.20** *Chronically inflamed, reactive, prostatic epithelium with cuboidal cell shape, dense eosinophilic cytoplasm, and reactive nuclear atypia, including a few nuclei with prominent nucleoli.*

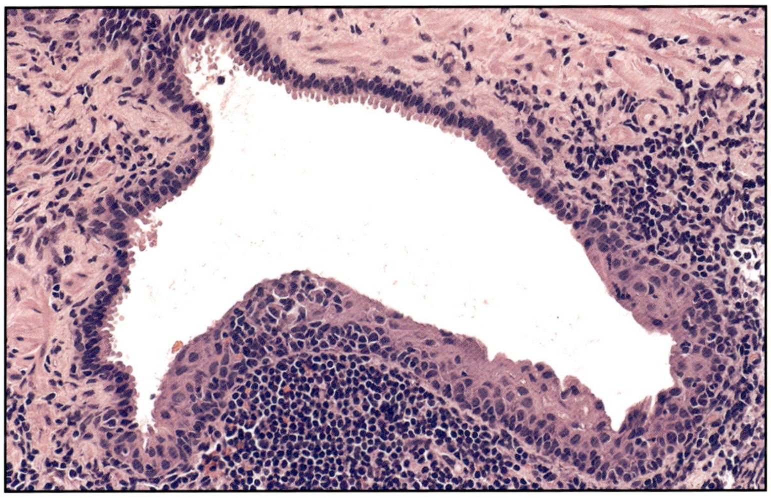

■ **i4.21** *Chronic inflammation associated with partial squamous metaplasia of a prostatic gland.*

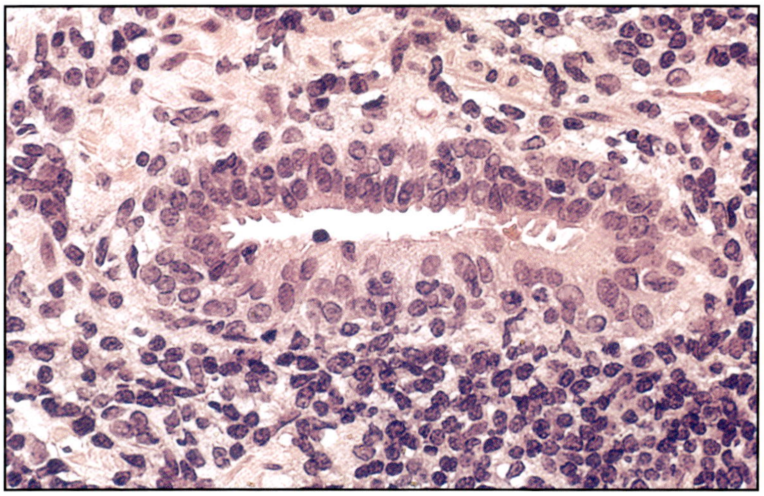

■ **i4.22** *Effect of chronic inflammation on prostatic glands—nuclear "jumbling" and reactive nuclear atypia with mild nuclear enlargement and pinpoint nucleoli.*

Cell types other than lymphocytes and plasma cells can be seen in chronic histologic prostatitis, including macrophages, mast cells, and eosinophils. Macrophages are commonly seen in distended, inflamed glandular lumina **i4.18** and in surrounding ruptured ducts and acini. (See section on granulomatous prostatitis later in this chapter.) By immunohistochemistry (for CD68), macrophages are commonly identified in benign prostatic tissues (Shepherd 1996) and in prostatic carcinoma (Shimura 2000). Mast cells are not often seen in prostatic tissues on hematoxylin and eosin–stained sections but can be detected by toluidine blue histochemical staining. They have been found to increase in number with age (Gupta 1970), but the mast cell counts in BPH and carcinoma are inconstant (del Rosario 1998, Gupta 1970). Mast cells are currently not of utility in differential diagnosis in the prostate. Eosinophils can nonspecifically accompany other inflammatory cells in histologic prostatitis **i4.19** or granulomatous prostatitis (Epstein 1984). The term *eosinophilic (allergic) prostatitis* should be reserved for the rare patients who have a history of a hypersensitivity disorder (such as asthma), peripheral eosinophilia, and significant numbers of eosinophils in the setting of prostatic granulomas (Epstein 1984, Kelalis 1964, Melicow 1951, Stewart 1954, Schmidt 1965, Towfighi 1972). This diagnosis is a clinicopathologic one; in the past a diagnosis of eosinophilic prostatitis has been inappropriately and broadly applied when prostatic tissue samples showed large numbers of eosinophils.

Benign prostatic epithelium in the setting of chronic histologic inflammation can display a range of reactive alterations **t4.4**. Secretory epithelial cells can lose cytoplasmic volume, some of the cells become cuboidal instead of columnar, and the cytoplasm becomes more dense and eosinophilic rather than cleared to granular **i4.20** (Blumenfeld 1992, Kohnen 1979). This lends an atrophic appearance to these glands. Basal cell hyperplasia of both ordinary and atypical types is often involved by lymphocytes (Epstein 1992, Thorson 1999). Transitional cell metaplasia, nephrogenic metaplasia (adenoma) (Allan 2001), and squamous cell metaplasia **i4.21** in the prostate also are often associated with inflammation. Reactive nuclear atypia in the chronically inflamed epithelium generally is mild (Helpap 1994) and is regularly manifested as crowded, enlarged nuclei with small nucleoli **i4.22** (Blumenfeld 1992, Helpap 1994, McNeal 1988). These nucleoli usually are less than 1μm, but in inflamed atypical

■ **t4.4 Reactive Benign Epithelial Changes Associated with Inflammation**

Atrophy
Basal cell prominence and hyperplasia
Transitional cell metaplasia
Squamous cell metaplasia
Small (less than 1μm usually) nucleoli but occasional macronucleoli

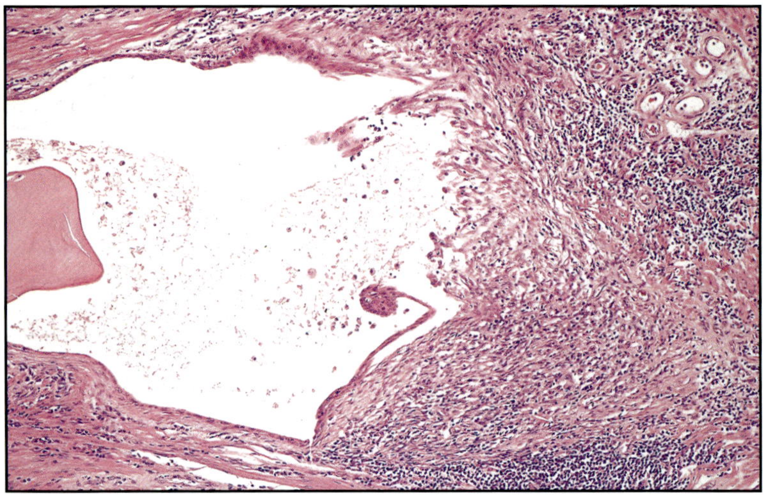

■ **i4.23** *Dilated and inflamed prostatic gland, with rupture and fibrotic response.*

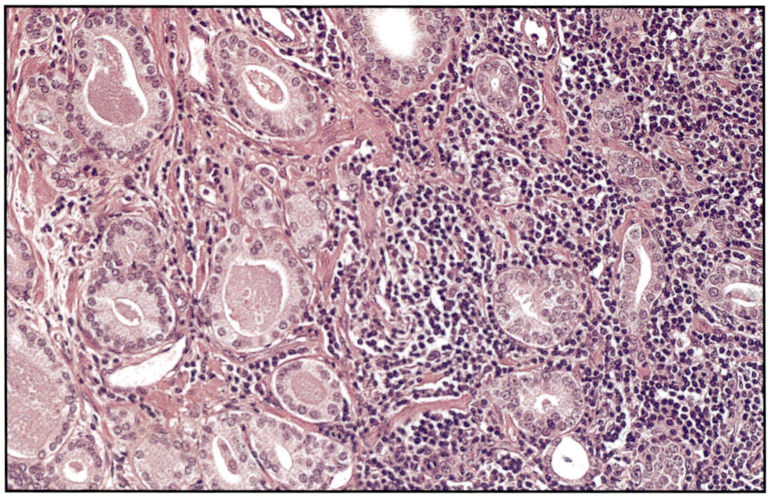

■ **i4.24** *Chronic inflammation in prostatic adenocarcinoma, ranging in intensity from mild (left) to marked (right).*

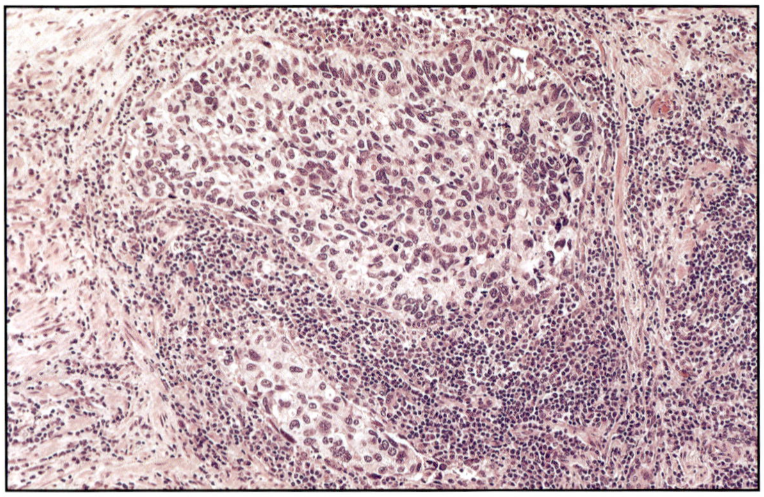

■ **i4.25** *Transitional cell carcinoma in the prostate with an exuberant peritumoral lymphocytic response.*

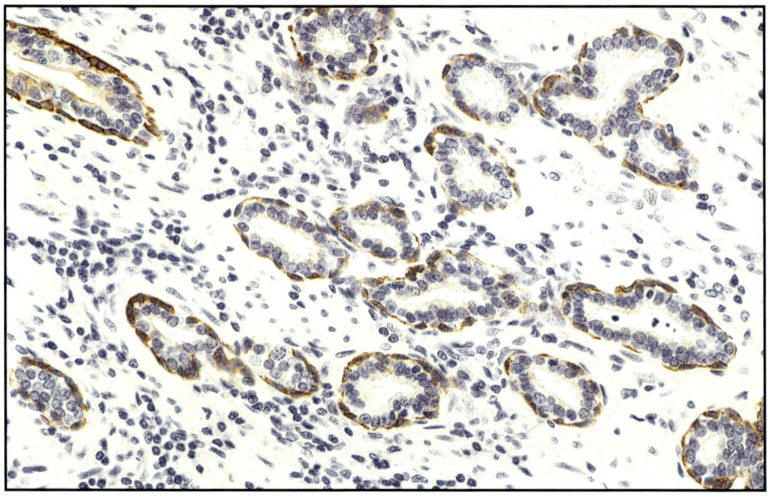

■ **i4.26** *Detection of basal cells in benign glands by 34βE12 immunostain is usually feasible.*

basal cell hyperplasia and in some inflamed atrophic or squamous metaplastic cells they can achieve true macronucleoli status.

Stromal alterations are less well-described in chronic prostatic inflammation, but stromal sclerosis can definitely occur (Helpap 1994), particularly in response to gland rupture **i4.23**.

Inflammation in the prostate involves neoplastic epithelium less often than benign epithelium (Blumenfeld 1992). Rarely is high-grade PIN involved by abundant inflammation (Bostwick 1993). A minor lymphocytic infiltrate is common in prostatic carcinoma (Shepherd 1996, Vesalainen 1994), but aggregates and extensive inflammation have been variably reported as rare (Blumenfeld 1992) or involving 26% of cases (Vesalainen 1994). In our experience (Shepherd 1996), only 11% of prostatic carcinomas had extensive lymphocytic aggregates, whereas most tumors were characterized by single-cell lymphocytic infiltrates in tumor stroma **i4.24**. Of note, when transitional cell carcinoma of urethra or bladder extends into the prostate, it can have an exuberant peritumoral inflammatory cell response **i4.25**. The difference in inflammation incidence in benign and malignant prostatic tissue is not sufficient to allow use of its presence or absence as a diagnostic tool.

It is of biologic interest that prostatic carcinoma usually does not elicit a significant inflammatory response. This may in part be caused by failure of the malignant epithelium to express HLA/DR (Blumenfeld 1993), with consequent escape from immune regulation. Most infiltrating inflammatory cells in prostatic carcinoma are T-lymphocytes (Blumenfeld 1992), along with a few macrophages (Shepherd 1996). (Most lymphocytes in chronic histologic inflammation of benign prostatic tissues are also T-lymphocytes [Blumenfeld 1992, 1993, Helpap 1994, Steiner 1994, Theyer 1992].) The degree of the tumor-infiltrating lymphocytic response to prostatic carcinoma may be related to patient survival (Lipponen 1996, Vesalainen 1994).

The differential diagnosis of chronic histologic inflammation in benign prostatic tissues encompasses high-grade PIN, inflamed carcinoma, and lymphoma or leukemia **t4.5**. Reactive nuclear atypia in inflamed benign prostatic epithelium can cause concern about neoplastic proliferations. This is particularly true for the benign entities that are most likely to be misdiagnosed as adenocarcinoma

■ **t4.5 Differential Diagnosis of Chronic Histologic Prostatitis**

Inflamed high-grade PIN*
Inflamed adenocarcinoma
Small cell carcinoma
Lymphoma/leukemia
High-grade adenocarcinoma with cord-like (Gleason pattern 4) and sheet-like (Gleason pattern 5) growth
Signet ring adenocarcinoma

*PIN = prostatic intraepithelial neoplasia

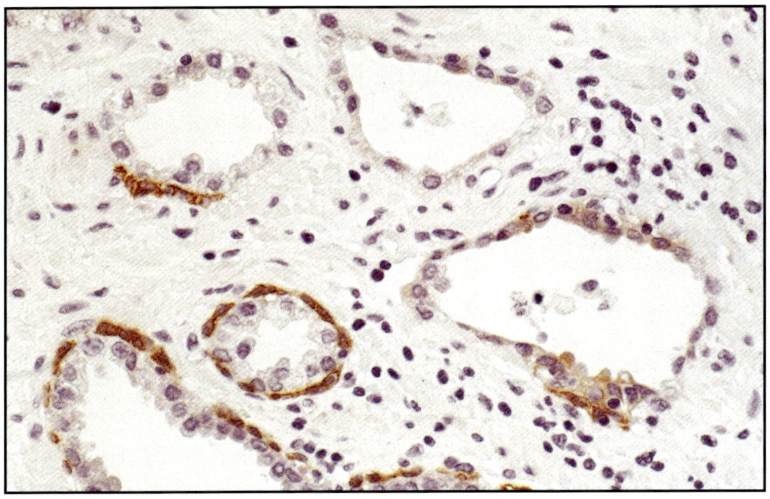

■ **i4.27** *Focal absence of basal cell labeling in benign, chronically inflamed, atrophic, prostatic glands: 34βE12 immunostain.*

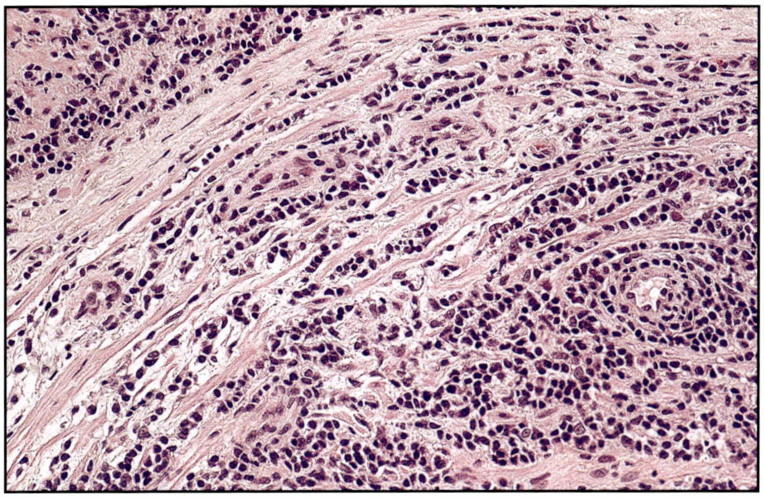

■ **i4.28** *Lymphocytes arranged in linear arrays, mimicking carcinoma.*

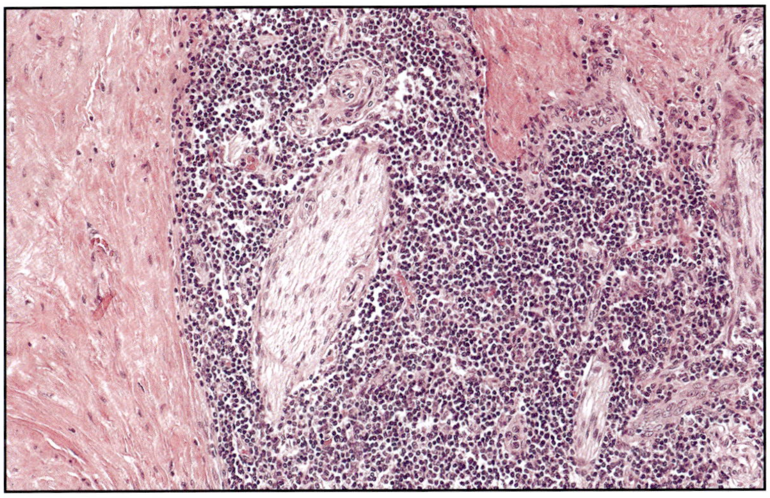

■ **i4.29** *Sheet of benign lymphocytes, with encirclement of nerves.*

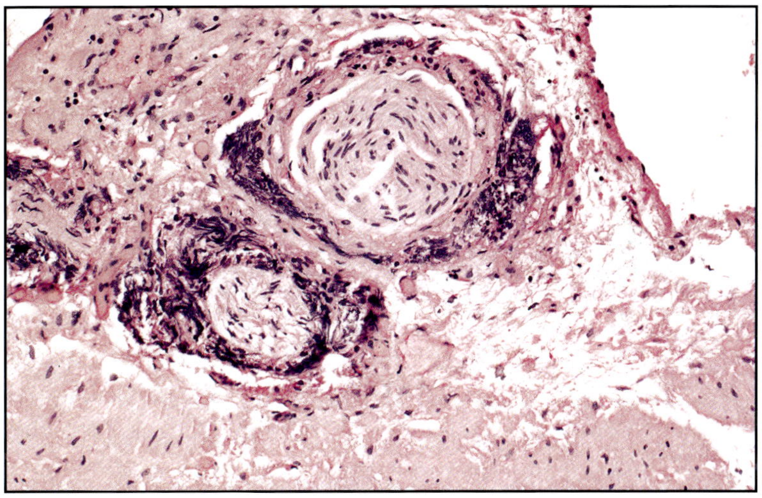

■ **i4.30** *Crushed lymphocytes around prostatic nerves can cause concern for perineural invasion by carcinoma.*

even in the absence of inflammation: atrophy and basal cell hyperplasia. As noted earlier for acute inflammation, chronically inflamed atrophic glands lack an infiltrative appearance (with the notable exception of sclerotic atrophy), possess basal cells **i4.26**, and typically do not have macronucleoli that are 2μm to 3μm in diameter. One caveat regarding basal cell detection is that in a small minority of chronically inflamed glands, 34βE12 immunohistochemical stains fail to identify basal cells **i4.27**. This failure to detect basal cell in a few inflamed glands should not be taken, in isolation, as a sign of malignancy. Chronically inflamed basal cell hyperplastic glands could be mistaken for PIN or adenocarcinoma, particularly if there are extremely large nucleoli, as seen in atypical basal cell hyperplasia (Epstein 1992, McNeal 1988). Inflamed, atypical basal cell hyperplasia can, on occasion, be difficult to distinguish from high-grade PIN because of overlap in nuclear cytology, yet basal cell hyperplasia does not grow as typical PIN, with its tufted and micropapillary architectures (Bostwick 1993). However, flat PIN can be difficult or impossible to distinguish from inflamed atypical basal cell hyperplasia. Here, a 34βE12 immunohistochemical stain may help resolve the question of whether the atypical cells are basal cells.

The benign lymphocytes and plasma cells of chronic histologic prostatitis may themselves be misinterpreted as malignant cells of either epithelial or hematopoietic types. If the lymphocytes are arranged in cords or linear arrays **i4.27** or sheets **i4.28**, misdiagnosis as high-grade Gleason pattern 4 or 5 carcinoma, respectively, could occur. This problem is readily resolved at high-power magnification, where bland, small lymphocytes are easily appreciated. Crushed lymphocytes around nerves **i4.30** can raise the specter of cancer, where perineural invasion by high-grade carcinoma is in the differential diagnosis. Here it is important to look for noncrushed areas (in levels, if necessary) or perform CD45 (leukocyte common antigen), PSA, and pan-cytokeratin immunohistochemistry to confirm cell type. Other artifacts that can potentially influence diagnosis include signet-ring change in lymphocytes (thought to be induced by heat during TURP) (Alguacil-Garcia 1986) **i4.31** and perinuclear clearing **i4.11**. Artifactual signet-ring change in lymphocytes can superficially resemble signet-ring carcinoma of the prostate, but the latter is a high-grade carcinoma, both cytologically and in infiltrative growth pattern. If doubt persists, CD45, PSA, and pan-cytokeratin immunostains will confirm the diagnosis. Perinuclear clearing can cause difficulty in recognizing infiltrating cells as lymphocytes. Lymphocytes can also create a conundrum in distinguishing the rare small cell carcinoma of the prostate. The small cell carcinoma cells are larger than the benign lymphocytes and show high mitotic and apoptotic body counts. Immunomarkers including CD45 for leukocytic differentiation, pan-cytokeratin for epithelial differentiation, and chromogranin and synaptophysin for neuroendocrine differentiation can be performed in difficult cases, but this is rarely necessary. Lastly, lymphoma or

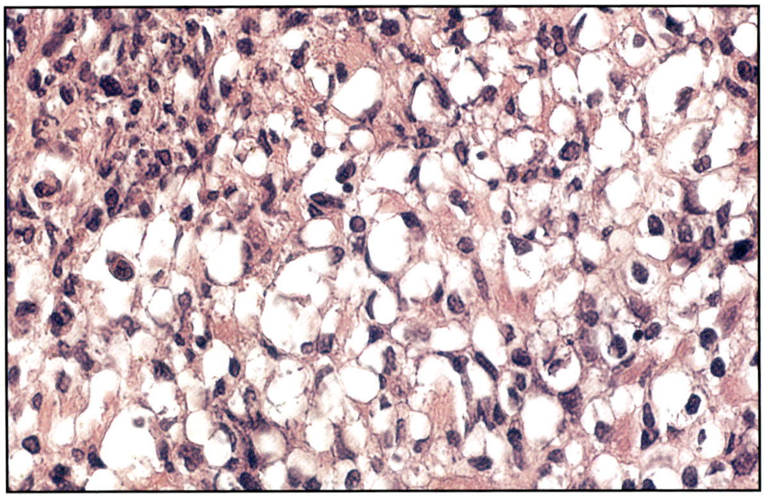

■ **i4.31** *Lymphocytes with signet-ring change, found at edge of cauterized TURP chip.*

leukemia involving the prostate (Bostwick 1998, Ferry 1997, Melchior 1974) is in the differential diagnosis with chronic histologic prostatitis. Lymphomatous infiltrates in the prostate can be patchy but still exhibit cytologic atypia. Dense, monomorphous, cytologically atypical lymphoid infiltrates favor lymphoma (Ferry 1997). A history of previous lymphoma can be helpful, but primary presentation of lymphoma in the prostate can occur. Immunohistochemical stains for B (CD20) and T (CD3, CD43) cells can be helpful because the most common types of lymphoma and leukemia to involve the prostate are B-cell chronic lymphocytic leukemia, small lymphocytic lymphoma, and diffuse large B-cell lymphoma (Bostwick 1998), whereas T cells predominate (and constitute 80% of all lymphocytes) in chronic histologic prostatitis (Blumenfeld 1992, 1993, Helpap 1994, Steiner 1994, Theyer 1992). If lymphoma or leukemia is suspected as a possibility before tissue acquisition, submitting additional tissue fresh for frozen section immunohistochemistry or flow cytometry can be helpful.

It is not established that chronic nongranulomatous inflammation in prostatic tissue samples should be reported. It is so common that it probably does not provide useful clinical information. For example, in needle biopsy, even though chronic inflammation is more common in men with an elevated serum PSA (99%) than in men with a normal PSA (77%) (Nadler 1995), this latter percentage is so high that chronic inflammation in needle biopsy should not be clinically interpreted as the reason for a patient's elevated serum PSA. If over time chronic inflammation is extensive and persistent in multiple needle biopsies, reporting it may be helpful. In hyperplastic tissues in TURP chips and simple prostatectomy specimens, inflammation so commonly accompanies BPH that we do not routinely report it. Finally, in radical prostatectomy specimens, we report inflammation in our synoptic report (see Chapter 14), but this is not an absolute necessity.

[4.7] Clinical Chronic Abacterial Prostatitis (Noninflammatory), or Prostatodynia

Patients with this clinical type of "prostatitis" have the same symptoms as patients with clinical chronic abacterial prostatitis (inflammatory), but no inflammation is seen microscopically in the expressed prostatic secretions. In these patients this "prostatitis" may not be due to inflammation at all, but rather the pain may be muscular (in muscle of bladder neck or pelvic floor) or even psychologic (Meares 1998, Roberts 1997). There is no indication to obtain prostatic tissue from these patients.

[4.8] Granulomatous Prostatitis

Granulomatous prostatitis is a distinctive form of prostatitis that can be mistaken for carcinoma clinically (Kelalis 1965, Taylor 1977, Thompson 1953), radiologically (by ultrasound) (Bude 1990, Rubenstein 1991), and histopathologically (Presti 1991). The incidence of granulomatous prostatitis in all prostatic tissue samples ranges from 0.4% to 4% (Helpap 1994, Kohnen 1979, Küehnelian 1964, Mbakop 1985, Oppenheimer 1997, Stillwell 1987A, Thybo 1973, Tuero 1988,), and it makes up 4% to 10% of all prostatitis cases (Helpap 1994, Kohnen 1979, Küehnelian 1964). The lowest incidence is in needle biopsy at less than 1% (Mbakop 1985, Oppenheimer 1997). Most patients are 50 to 70 years of age (mean = 62 years; range = 18 to 86 years) and present with irritative or obstructive voiding symptoms, fever, and chills. Consistent with this presentation, most patients had a urinary tract infection 1 to 8 weeks before diagnosis. Clinical concerns for malignancy are raised in granulomatous prostatitis because of an elevated total serum PSA, a low percentage free PSA, hypoechoic lesions on ultrasound, and a hard, fixed, indurated prostate gland on DRE (Bude 1990, O'Dowd 1999, Oppenheimer 1997, Roberts 1997, Rubenstein 1991, Speights 1996). Histopathologic examination is needed for a definitive diagnosis in patients with granulomatous prostatitis.

Granulomatous prostatitis can be classified based on cause **t4.6**. The most common cause of granulomatous prostatitis is so-called

■ **t4.6 Granulomatous Prostatitis: Classification**

I. Nonspecific (due to duct/acinar rupture)
  - Usual type
  - Xanthogranulomatous
  - Nodular histiocytic prostatitis
  - Xanthoma

II. Infectious
  - A. Bacterial
    - Tuberculosis
    - Brucellosis
  - B. Spirochetal
    - Syphilis
  - C. Fungal
    - Coccidioidomycosis
    - Cryptococcosis
    - Blastomycosis
    - Histoplasmosis
    - Paracoccidioidomycosis
    - Candidiasis
    - Aspergilliosis
  - D. Parasitic
    - Schistosomiasis
  - E. Viral
    - Herpes zoster

III. Post-biopsy/resection

IV. Malac)oplakia

V. Systemic granulomatous disease
  - Allergic (eosinophilic)
  - Sarcoidosis
  - Wegener's granulomatosis

VI. Foreign body
  - Teflon
  - Hair

Modified from Roberts 1997

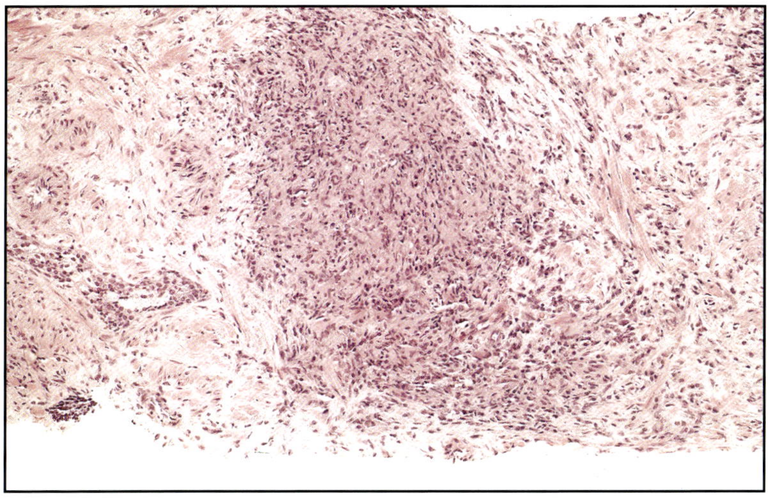

■ **i4.32** *Isolated, circumscribed, small, nonspecific granulomatous inflammatory nodule in prostate needle biopsy.*

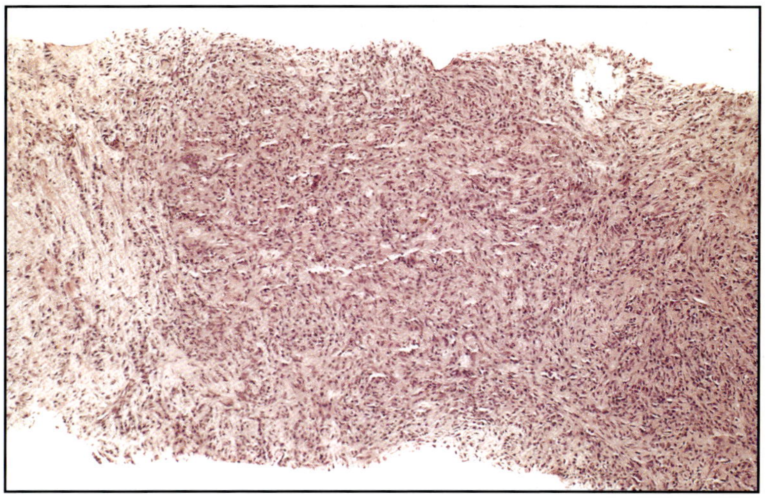

■ **i4.33** *Patternless sheet-like growth of nonspecific granulomatous inflammation in prostate needle biopsy.*

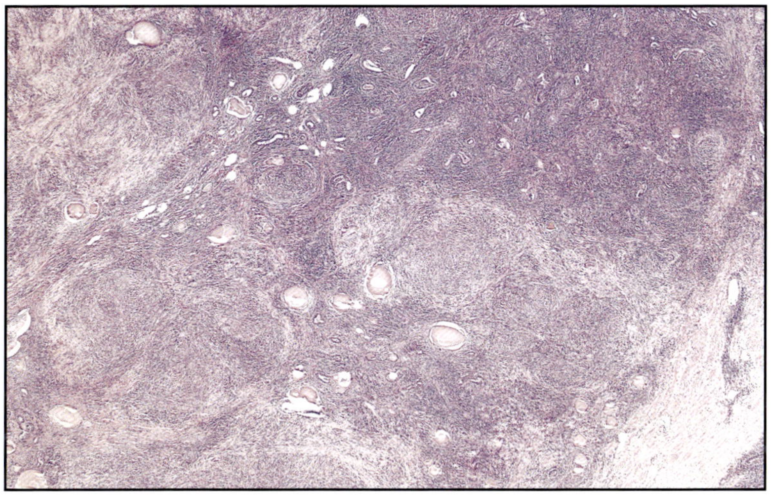

■ **i4.34** *Granulomatous nodules, with intervening lymphocytic sheets and gland loss.*

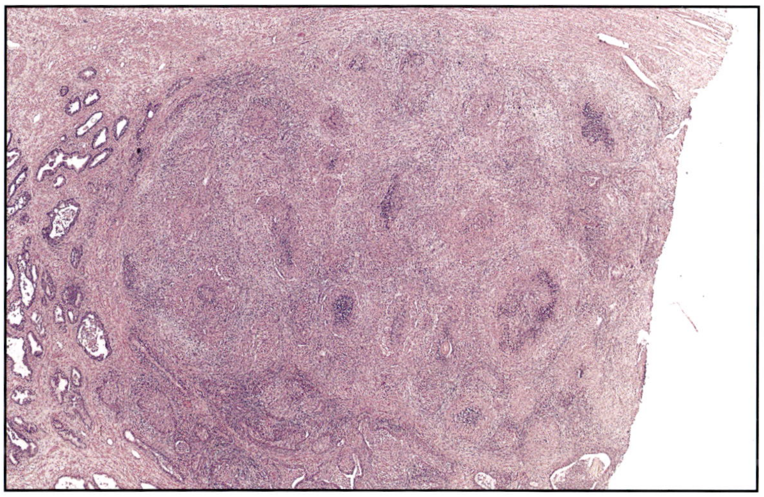

■ **i4.35** *Peripheral zone discrete mass representing multiple, fused nonspecific granulomas. Such a mass could be palpable by digital rectal examination.*

nonspecific granulomatous prostatitis, which accounts for about three quarters of granulomatous prostatitis cases. In needle biopsy, granulomatous prostatitis was categorized as nonspecific in 77% of cases, infectious in 18% of cases, and indeterminate in 4% of cases (Oppenheimer 1997). Infection here was caused by previous bacille Calmette-Guerin (BCG) therapy for transitional cell carcinoma. In larger tissue samples, postbiopsy and postresection granulomas are more common, being diagnosed in 25% of all granulomatous prostatitis cases (Stillwell 1987A). The other listed causes of granulomatous prostatitis in **t4.6** are uncommon to rare.

Nonspecific Granulomatous Prostatitis

Nonspecific granulomatous prostatitis is deemed nonspecific because it is not considered secondary to a specific agent but rather it is viewed as representing a foreign body–type response to prostatic secretions, with associated duct or acinar rupture (O'Dea 1977, Schmidt 1965, Tanner 1943). Yet some patients have positive urine cultures (mainly for *E coli*) (Meares 1998), such that some of this response may also be caused by bacterial products (Schmidt 1965). Impairment of drainage, perhaps secondary to BPH, and infection seem to be pathogenetic components (Kelalis 1965, O'Dea 1977).

Grossly, nonspecific granulomatous prostatitis appears as small, firm, yellow granular nodules (Kelalis 1965). Microscopically, the usual type of nonspecific granulomatous prostatitis is a lobulocentric noncaseating granulomatous inflammatory cell infiltrate **t4.7**. The inflammation is centered on ducts and glands, which exhibit a variable degree of destruction **i4.32-i4.39**. Liquefactive necrosis has been reported in the center of the inflammatory infiltrate (Epstein 1984), although other series do not allow necrosis (Stillwell 1987A). Necrosis raises the possibility of specific infectious granulomatous prostatitis and is not usually seen in nonspecific granulomatous prostatitis. The granulomas can be focal or diffuse. In needle biopsy, more than one core is involved in most cases (Oppenheimer 1997). The lobulocentricity of the granulomas can be appreciated in some needle biopsy cases,

■ **t4.7 Histologic Characteristics of Nonspecific Granulomatous Prostatitis**

Nodular granulomas centered around ducts and acini
Central ducts and acini disrupted/destroyed
Mixed granulomatous inflammation: epithelioid histiocytes, giant cells, lymphocytes, neutrophils, eosinophils
Caseous necrosis absent
Peripheral lymphocytes and sclerosis

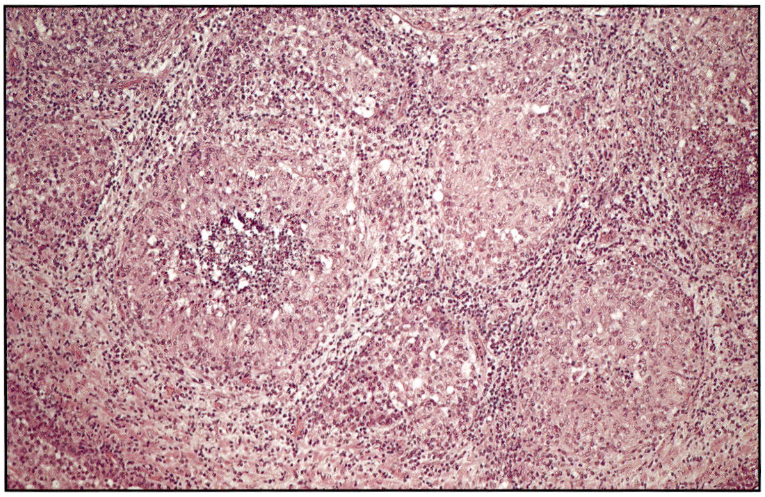

■ **i4.36** *Several, small, nonspecific granulomas, surrounded by lymphocytes. One of the granulomas has a prominent, central aggregate of neutrophils.*

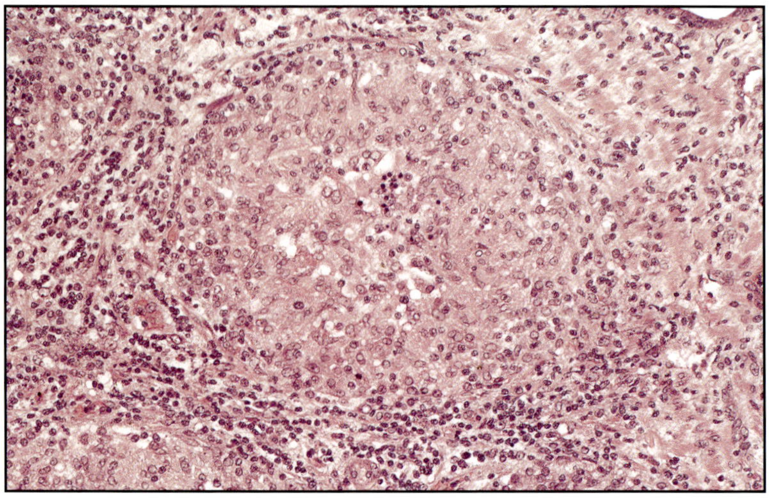

■ **i4.37** *Nonspecific granulomatous prostatitis: Granuloma comprising predominantly epithelioid histiocytes surrounded by lymphocytes and plasma cells.*

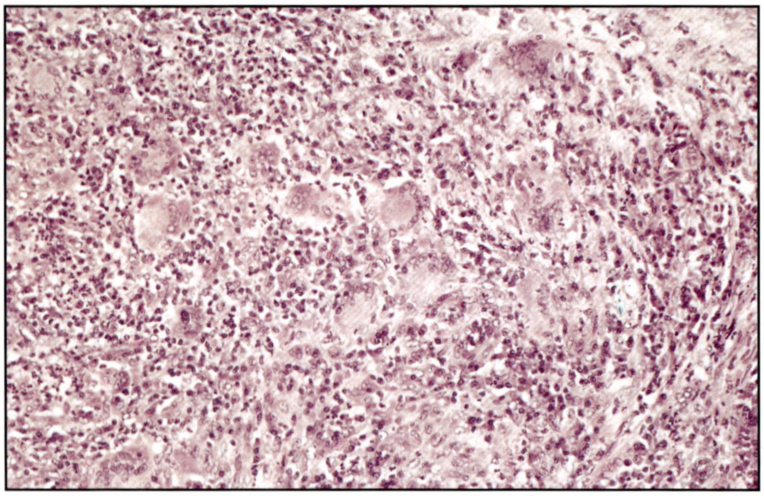

■ **i4.38** *A cluster of giant cells in nonspecific granulomatous prostatitis.*

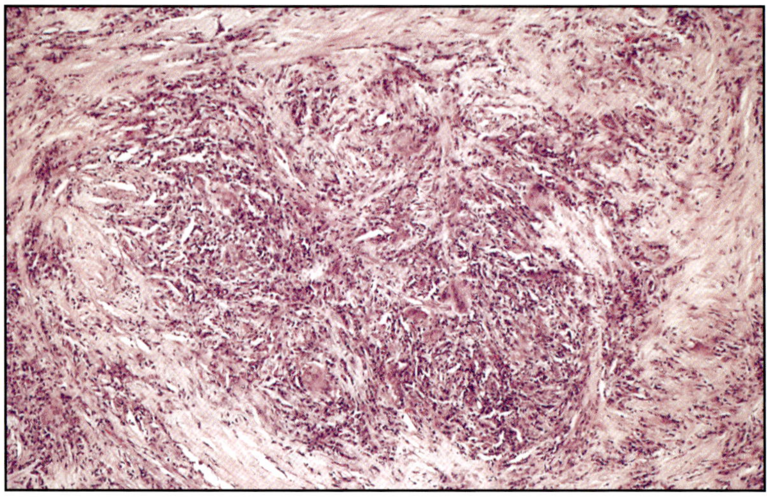

■ **i4.39** *Stromal sclerosis involving nonspecific granulomatous prostatitis.*

where smaller granulomas are present **i4.32**, but in other cases the granulomatous inflammation can appear more sheetlike **i4.33** because of partial sampling of larger granulomas. In TURP and simple prostatectomy specimens, only 1% of all tissue was involved (Kohnen 1979). In radical prostatectomy tissues, the granulomas can be extremely focal, can form a discrete mass **i4.35**, or can be a diffuse spread of fused nodules **i4.34**. The cellular infiltrate in usual nonspecific granulomatous prostatitis is mixed, with epithelioid histiocytes, lymphocytes, neutrophils, eosinophils, plasma cells, and multinucleated giant cells **i4.36-i4.38**. The giant cells can be of foreign body, Langhans, and Touton types (Bryan 1991). They can be difficult to detect in needle biopsies; giant cells were absent or rare in 69% of cases (Oppenheimer 1997). Lymphocytic infiltrates, sometimes with lymphoid follicle formation (Bryan 1991), surround the granulomatous nodules. The lymphocytes in the granulomas are mainly T cells (Bryan 1991, Helpap 1994) whereas those at the periphery tend to be B cells (Bryan 1991). Perinodular stromal fibrosis and scarring can ensue **i4.39** (Helpap 1994, Kelalis 1965).

The spectrum of morphologic abnormalities in nonspecific granulomatous prostatitis also includes "xanthogranulomatous prostatitis," "nodular histiocytic prostatitis," and "prostatic xanthoma." The first two designations have been applied when the epithelioid histiocytes possess a cleared to vacuolated cytoplasm (due to lipid accumulation [Kelalis 1965]) (Bryan 1991, Fox 1966, Matsumoto 1992, Miekos 1986, Scherrer 1951). In prostatic xanthoma there is a solitary, microscopic aggregate of foamy histiocytes (Redondo 1998, Sebo 1994). This is a rare entity that is usually an incidental finding in peripheral zone tissues removed to evaluate for BPH or carcinoma. Only one patient had hyperlipidemia.

Nonspecific granulomatous prostatitis can be associated with hyperplastic transition zone or peripheral zone epithelium. It can induce reactive atypia in disrupted glands in the center of the granuloma and in glands at the periphery of the nodules. Carcinoma has been found associated with nonspecific granulomatous prostatitis in a few cases (Helpap 1994, Sebo 1994) **i4.40**.

The differential diagnosis of nonspecific granulomatous prostatitis includes other types of granulomatous prostatitis **t4.6** and poorly differentiated carcinoma. Compared with specific granulomatous prostatitis, nonspecific granulomatous prostatitis lacks necrosis and is centered on ducts and acini, and the patients do not have a history of BCG treatment or previous biopsy or TURP. Necrosis in granulomatous prostatitis is worrisome for infectious prostatitis, but needle biopsy of BCG granulomatous prostatitis fails to show necrosis in one quarter of cases (Oppenheimer 1997), so in this situation one must also ask whether the patient has been treated for bladder carcinoma. Large numbers of eosinophils and neutrophils

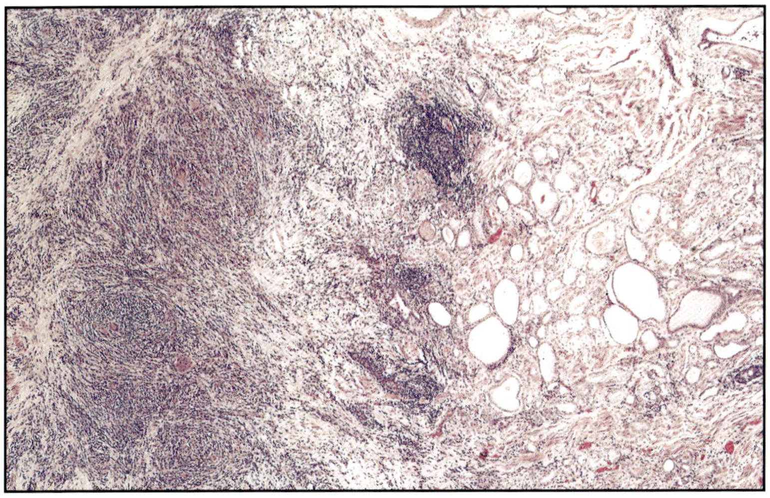

■ **i4.40** *Nonspecific granulomatous prostatitis, lymphocyte predominant (left) adjacent to prostatic adenocarcinoma (right).*

favor nonspecific granulomatous prostatitis over BCG granulomatous prostatitis (Oppenheimer 1997), but again, clinical history regarding BCG treatment is most helpful.

Sheets or cords of epithelioid histiocytes in nonspecific granulomatous prostatitis can masquerade as poorly differentiated carcinoma **i4.41, i4.42** (Dhundee 1991, Fox 1966, Gujral 1998, Oppenheimer 1997, Stillwell 1987A). This is particularly problematic when histiocytes predominate, without significant numbers of giant cells, plasma cells, lymphocytes, eosinophils, or neutrophils. Also, the epithelioid histiocytes can display prominent nucleoli, which can cause concern for malignancy **i4.42**. An immunohistochemical marker panel can be helpful in defining the differentiation status of the atypical epithelioid cells. Negative immunoreactions for pan-cytokeratin, PSA, and prostate specific acid phosphatase (PSAP), with immunopositivity for CD68 and lysozyme in the epithelioid cells, are useful in establishing a diagnosis of granulomatous prostatitis in this context (Dhundee 1991, Helpap 1994, Oppenheimer 1997, Presti 1991).

Infectious Granulomatous Prostatitis

Specific infectious types of granulomatous prostatitis include bacterial, fungal, parasitic, and viral prostatitis **t4.6**. Among these, the most common infectious type of granulomatous inflammation is that due to BCG therapy for transitional cell carcinoma (usually of the bladder). In fact, every case of infectious granulomatous prostatitis in one needle biopsy series was caused by BCG treatment (Oppenheimer 1997). Whereas only 10% of men treated with intravesical BCG for superficial bladder carcinoma develop clinically symptomatic BCG prostatitis (Lamm 1986), a substantial percentage (80% to 100%) of patients have histologic evidence of BCG granulomatous prostatitis (LaFontaine 1997, Lamm 1986, Miyashita 1992, Mukamel 1990, Oates 1988, Terris 1997). When palpable prostatic nodularity or induration developed after BCG treatment, the 100% figure was attained (Lamm 1986). Grossly, cut surfaces of prostate glands in radical cystoprostatectomies from patients treated with BCG show multiple, firm, white nodules or soft, yellowish-gray nodules with granular centers, central caseation, and focal cavitation (LaFontaine 1997). These large, confluent granulomas can measure up to 1.6cm in greatest dimension (LaFontaine 1997). Microscopically the granulomas, particularly the larger ones, are of the typical caseating, tuberculoid type **i4.43, i4.44**. Smaller (less than 1mm) granulomas composed predominantly of histiocytes can lack giant cells and caseous necrosis. Indeed, in needle biopsy up to one quarter of BCG granulomatous prostatitis cases lack caseous necrosis (Oppenheimer 1997). The smaller granulomas are periglandular **i4.45, i4.46**, often with intraluminal protrusion **i4.47**. BCG granulomas most often involve the peripheral zone, usually in combination with the central zone or transition zone (LaFontaine 1997). In needle biopsy, one to multiple cores can be involved (Oppenheimer 1997).

In the whole gland the number of BCG granulomas ranges from 1 to 7 (mean 2.7), and the greatest dimension is characteristically 4 to 10mm. With a history of previous BCG treatment, it is not necessary to stain sections with Ziehl-Neelsen for acid-fast organisms. If the stain is performed, 40% to 77% of cases demonstrate mycobacteria in the granulomas (LaFontaine 1997, Miyashita 1992).

Mycobacterial prostatitis due to *Mycobacterium tuberculosis* or atypical species is rare (Kostakopoulos 1998, Lee 1987, Meares 1998, Mikolich 1992, Moore 1937, O'Dea 1978, Scott 1924), with an incidence of 0.02% of benign prostatic tissue samples and 3% of all examples of granulomatous prostatitis (Stillwell 1987A). The spread to the prostate is hematogenous, usually from active pulmonary disease (Moore 1937, Scott 1924). The prostate is nodular to palpation. Grossly, yellow to grayish-yellow nodules are located in the peripheral zone (Moore 1937). Larger lesions

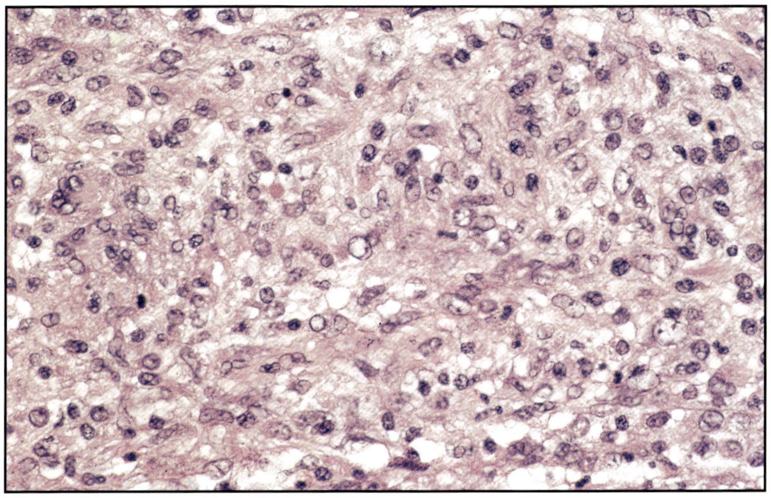

■ **i4.41** *Sheet of histiocytes, with a few scattered lymphocytes, in nonspecific granulomatous prostatitis.*

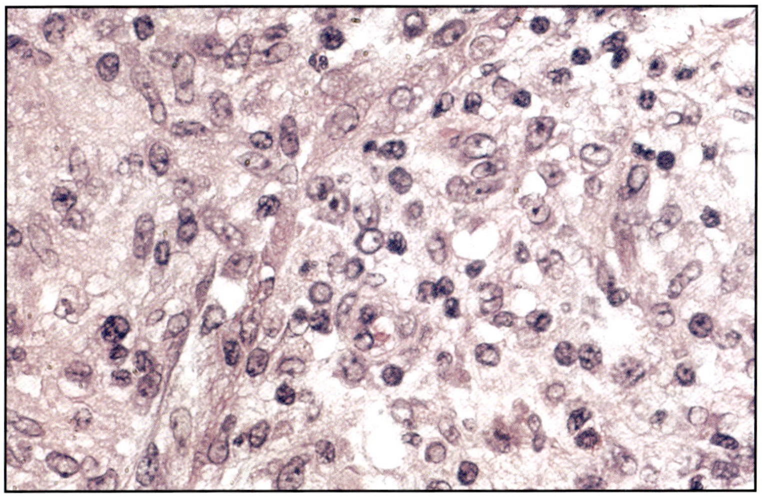

■ **i4.42** *Epithelioid histiocytes with nucleoli, including a few prominent ones, in nonspecific granulomatous prostatitis.*

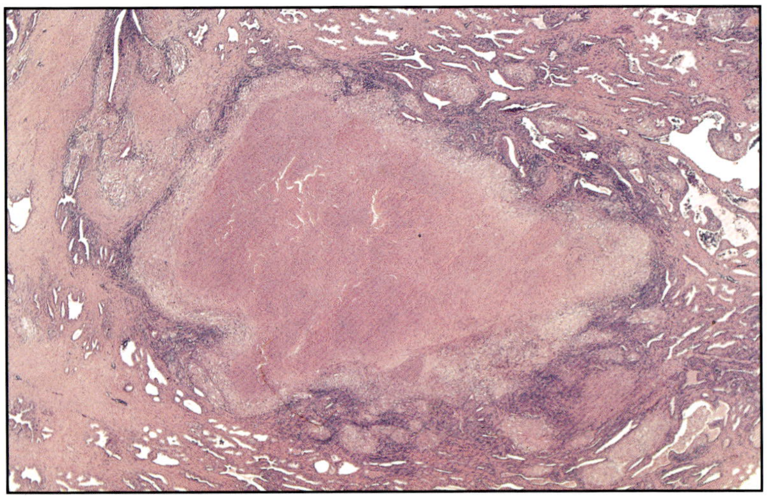

■ **i4.43** *BCG granulomatous prostatitis: Large caseating granuloma.*

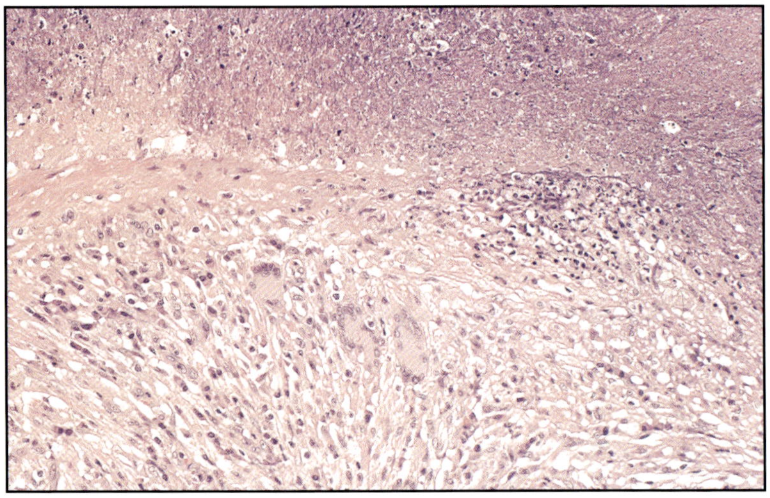

■ **i4.44** *BCG granuloma: Central necrosis (above) with rim of histiocytes and giant cells.*

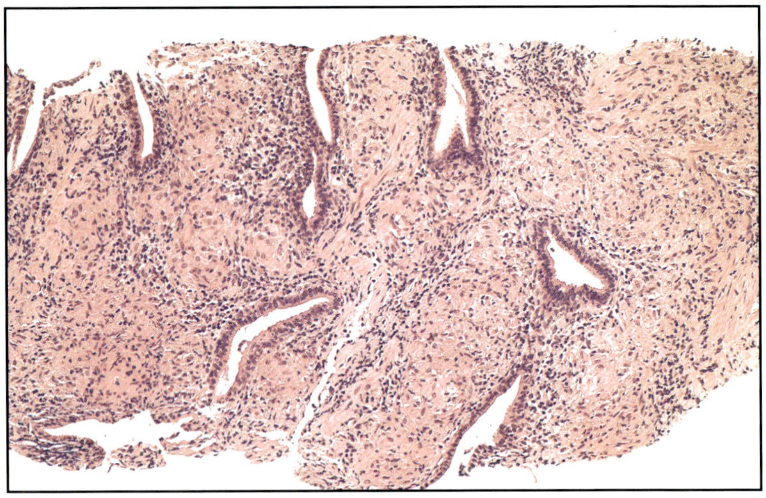

■ **i4.45** *Periglandular BCG granulomas without caseous necrosis, in needle biopsy.*

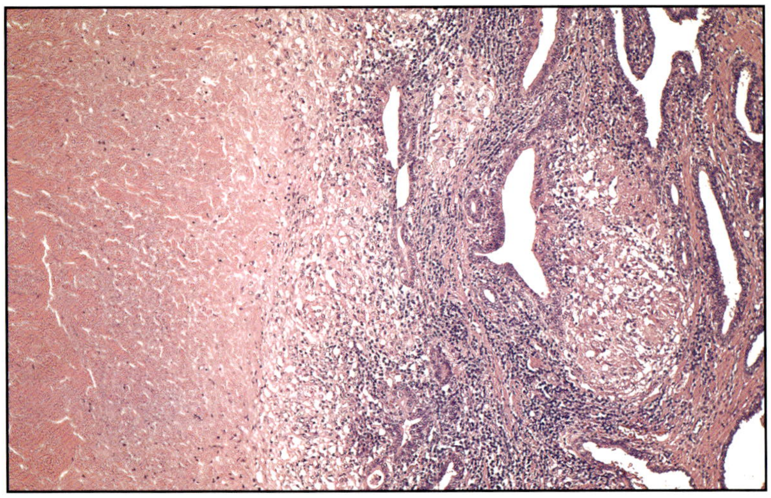

■ **i4.46** *BCG granulomas: The larger one on the left has extensive caseation, while the smaller periglandular one on the right does not.*

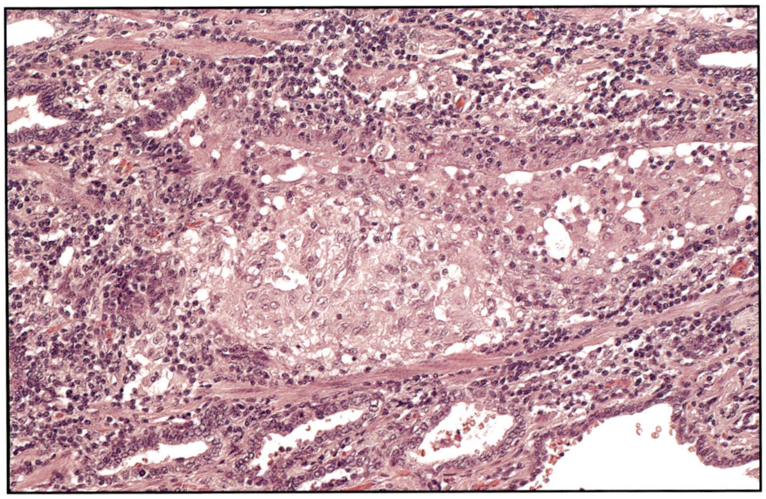

■ **i4.47** *Intraluminal localization of BCG granulomatous inflammation.*

exhibit caseation, but caseation is minimal in the "small yellow tubercle" granulomas (Moore 1937). The granulomas are similar to those in BCG granulomatous prostatitis, including lack of caseous necrosis in some examples in needle biopsy (O'Dea 1978). Presentation as an incidental finding in TURP chips has also been a mode of diagnosis (Kostakopoulos 1998, Meares 1998). For patients without a history of BCG treatment and those in whom tuberculosis is clinically suspected, special stains for acid-fast bacilli and fungi should be performed.

Isolated case reports of prostatic brucellosis (Kelalis 1962) and prostatic syphilis (Thompson 1920) indicate that these organisms can also elicit a granulomatous prostatitis.

Fungal, parasitic, and viral granulomatous prostatitis due to specific organisms are also rare (Bartkowski 1988, Bissada 1977, Chen 1985, Clason 1982, Gelfand 1970, Golz 1991, Gottesman 1974, Haas 1998, Indudhara 1994, Salyer 1973, Symmers 1997). Predisposing conditions for prostatic fungal infection include immunosuppression **i4.48-i4.51**, prolonged antibiotic use, diabetes mellitus, malignancy, and an indwelling bladder catheter (Abbas 1995, Campbell 1992, Cherasse 1997, Haas 1998, Wise 1998). Even in disseminated fungal infections, the prostate is uncommonly invaded. For example, in 6% of disseminated cases of coccidioidomycosis (Haddad 1996) and histoplasmosis (Rubin 1959) the prostate is affected, whereas the prostate is infected in 16% of cases of systemic blastomycosis (Eickenberg 1975). Additional fungi detected in the prostate include *Cryptococcus* (Caballes 1999, Hinchey 1981, Milchgrub 1990, Salyer 1973) **i4.50, i4.51**, *Paracoccidioides* (Melo 1992), *Candida* (Bartkowski 1988, Elert 2000, Golz 1991, Haas 1998, Indudhara 1994), and *Aspergillus* (Abbas 1995, Campbell 1992, Cherasse 1997). Among cases of granulomatous prostatitis,

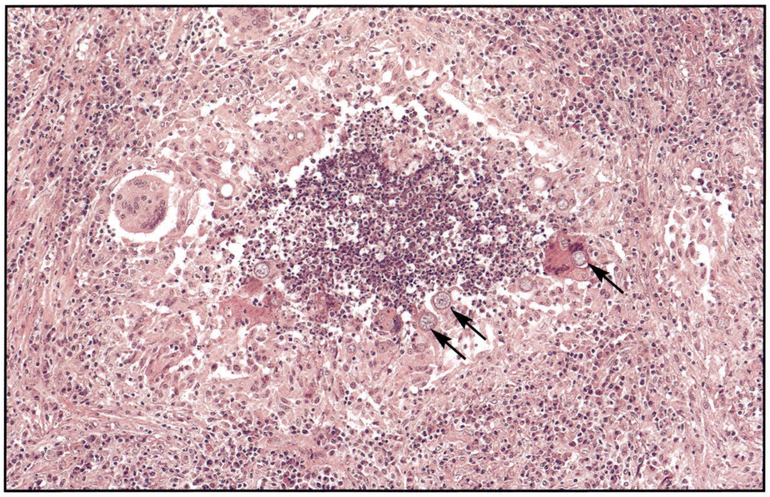

■ **i4.48** *Necrotizing granulomatous prostatitis due to* Coccidioides immitis *(arrows).*

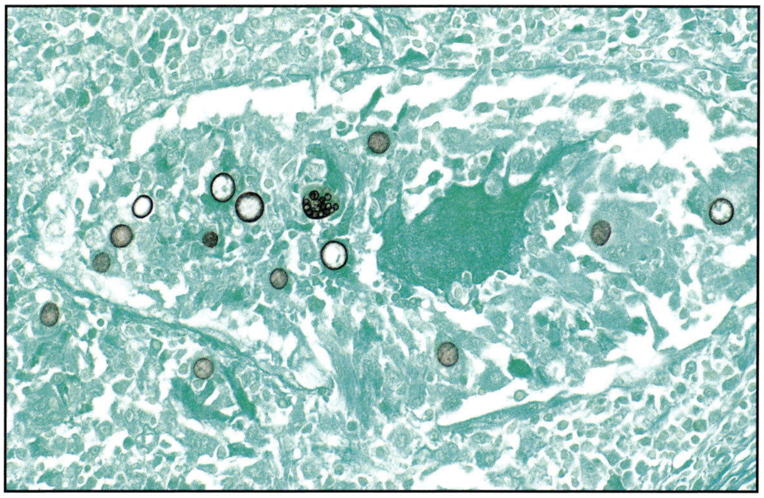

■ **i4.49** *Spherules of* Coccidioides immitis *highlighted by silver stain. The patient, a 54-year-old man, had been treated with prednisone for pneumonitis. (Courtesy of Dr. Daniel Niku, Dr. Gerald Dalgleish, and Dr. Ganesh Devendra* [Niku 1998]*).*

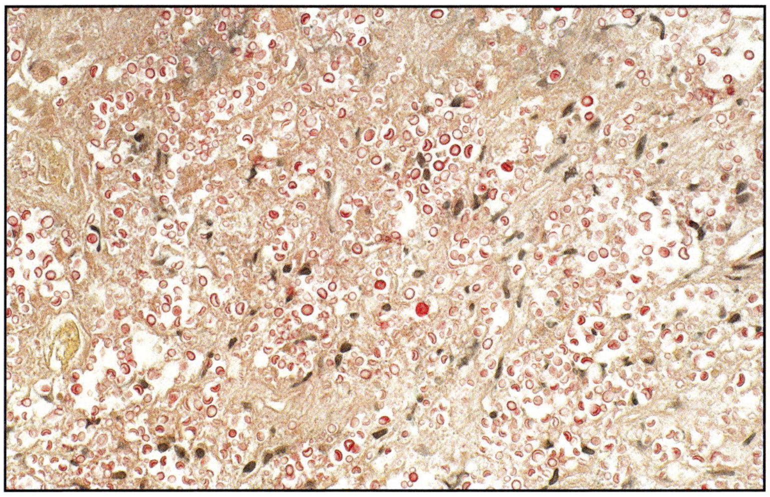

■ **i4.50** *Cryptococcal organisms in prostate of an immunosuppressed patient: Mucicarmine stain. (Courtesy of Dr. Hung Chiang)*

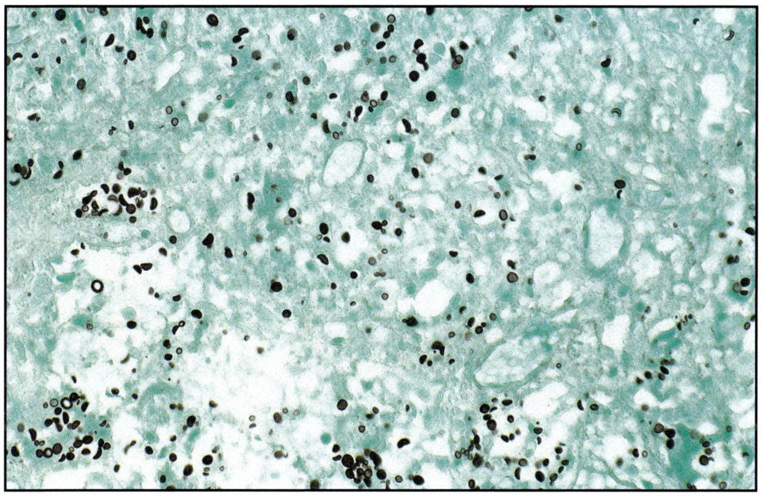

■ **i4.51** *Cryptococcal organisms in case illustrated in* **i4.50***: Silver stain.*

fungal (blastomycosis) granulomatous prostatitis accounted for 1 in 200 (0.5%) of cases (Stillwell 1987A). In patients with the aforementioned predisposing conditions and granulomatous prostatitis or necrotizing granulomas in the absence of BCG therapy, special stains for fungal organisms (eg, Gomori methenamine silver) and acid-fast bacilli should be performed.

Granulomatous prostatitis due to parasitic infection can occur in schistosomiasis. Eggs of *Schistosoma* (usually *haematobium*) are deposited in the prostate of about 20% of African men with schistosomiasis, but this rarely gives rise to prostate-related symptoms (Gelfand 1970).

Necrotizing, focally granulomatous prostatitis has been reported in 2 patients in association with herpes zoster infection (Clason 1982).

Postbiospy and Postresection Granulomatous Prostatitis

The incidence of this kind of granulomatous prostatitis is highly variable, depending on the type of tissue sample. Among cases of granulomatous prostatitis, the incidence in needle biopsy was 0% (Oppenheimer 1997), whereas in another series that included TURP chips, the incidence was 25% (Stillwell 1987A). This is so because this granulomatous process tends to be central, involving periurethral transition zone tissue, which is readily sampled by TURP, as opposed to involvement of the peripheral zone, which is most often the target of needle biopsies. Among all cases of prostatitis, it made up 7.1% (Helpap 1994). Patients were 51 to 87 years of age and 7 days to 3 years previously had undergone TURP (Epstein 1984, Hedelin 1981, Helpap 1986, Henry 1993, Kopolovic 1984, Mies 1984, Pieterse 1984) **t4.8**. Two patients had a history of needle biopsy only of the prostate (Mies 1984). The patients presented for repeat TURP (or initial TURP in the needle biopsy

■ **t4.8** **Features of Postbiopsy/Resection Granulomas**

Found 7 days to 3 years after TURP
Usually multiple but can be single
Round, ovoid, elongated, wedge-shaped
Communication with cauterized surface
Fibrinoid center
Palisading fibroblasts and histiocytes around center
Peripheral rim of lymphocytes, plasma cells and eosinophils
Eosinophils can be numerous if time interval from previous TURP < 2 months
Multinucleated giant cells in some cases*
Hyalinization of central zone and periphery occurs with time

TURP = transurethral resection of prostate
*Giant cells are usually foreign-body type but can be Touton or Langhan's types

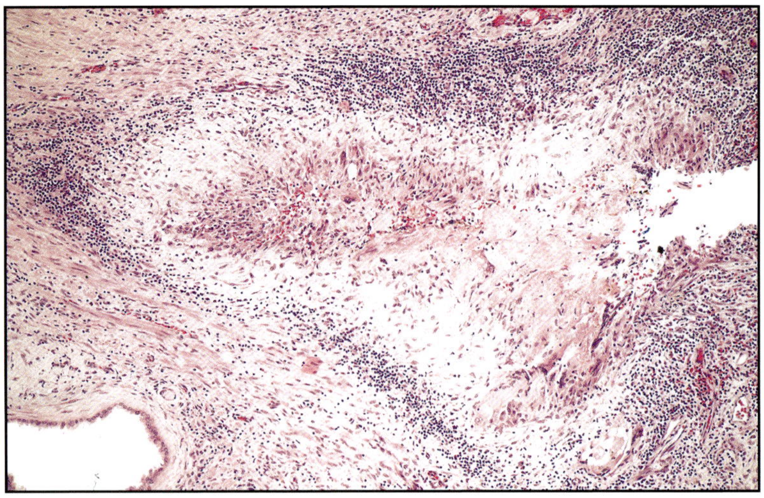

■ **i4.52** *Post-TURP granuloma with wedge-shaped, central necrosis and thin, peripheral lymphocytic cuff.*

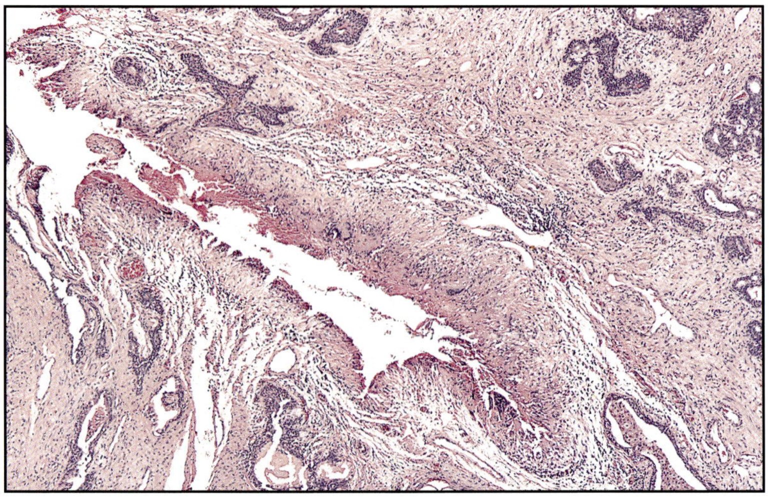

■ **i4.53** *Slit-like configuration of post-TURP granuloma, with central fibrinoid material and channel to TURP chip surface.*

patients) because of persistent prostatism, urinary obstruction or retention, and hematuria. It is noteworthy that TURP does not always seem to elicit such a granulomatous response, as 12 of 23 patients in one repeat TURP series (Pieterse 1984) did not have detectable granulomas, but the possibility remains that with additional chip sampling more granulomas might have been detected. The basis for the development of post-TURP granulomas appears to be a response to altered and cauterized prostatic epithelium and stroma, secretions, urine, or even metal from the diathermy instruments used for resection (Henry 1993). This response is not specific to the prostate; similar granulomas are seen in the bladder after transurethral resection of bladder tissue.

Grossly, no difference was recognized in chips with or without postbiopsy or postresection granulomas (Helpap 1986). Microscopically, the granulomas assume a variety of shapes; round, ovoid, elongated, stellate, serpiginous, triangular, slitlike, and rectangular forms have been described **i4.52, i4.53.** Almost all of the granulomas demonstrate a connection with a cauterized TURP chip surface **i4.53;** a common finding was the base of a wedge-shaped granuloma at the edge of a TURP chip (Epstein 1984). The granulomas measure 0.5mm to 2mm (Mies 1984) and are usually multiple, with an average of 4 to 5 per case, but can be single (Epstein 1984, Pieterse 1984). The granulomas are characterized by a fibrinoid central zone and surrounding, palisaded epithelioid histiocytes and fibroblasts. A rim of lymphocytes (which mark as T cells [Helpap 1994]) is present outside the palisaded cell layer. Admixed with the lymphocytes are occasional plasma cells and eosinophils. The eosinophils may be numerous if the previous TURP was performed earlier than 2 months ago (Epstein 1984, Hedelin 1981). Multinucleated giant cells are observed in some but not all cases and are usually of foreign body type but can also be of Touton or Langhans types (Pieterse 1984). Occasional giant cells contain brown pigment (iron), related to cautery-induced tissue carbonization (Helpap 1994). Older granulomas exhibit both central and peripheral hyalinization.

Reactive changes often are visualized in epithelium and stroma adjacent to postbiopsy TURP granulomas. Nearby prostatic glands to the granulomas may appear compressed (Helpap 1986) and reactive (Helpap 1994), with slight to moderate nuclear atypia and small nucleoli, but macronucleoli are generally absent. Squamous metaplasia can be seen in about one half of cases (Pieterse 1984). Postbiopsy and post-TURP granulomas have been found in chips with both BPH and carcinoma. Localized vasculitis confined to the prostate has been reported in association with a few cases of post-TURP granulomas (Bryan 1991, Kopolovic 1984).

Postbiopsy and post-TURP granulomas have been misdiagnosed as rheumatoid nodules and as tuberculous granulomatous prostatitis. A history of a previous procedure, in conjunction with the appearance of a palisading, fibrinoid granuloma, is most helpful in establishing the diagnosis of postbiopsy or post-TURP granulomatous prostatitis. In this setting it is not necessary to stain for organisms. Histochemical stains for organisms in these cases have been uniformly negative. Also invariably negative are examinations for birefringent material with polarized light. Other types of granulomas are also in the differential diagnosis, such as allergic (eosinophilic) granulomatous prostatitis and nonspecific granulomatous prostatitis (Epstein 1984). The former entity may overlap morphologically with early post-TURP granulomas in having numerous eosinophils, but allergic granulomatous prostatitis is seen in a different clinical context, with a clinical history of a hypersensitivity disorder (such as asthma) and a peripheral eosinophilia. Unlike nonspecific granulomatous prostatitis, postbiopsy and post-TURP granulomas are not centered on ducts and acini and also possess a striking fibrinoid central zone.

Malacoplakia

Malacoplakia is a specific variant of granulomatous prostatitis that could be categorized as an infectious type of inflammation because it is almost always associated with urinary tract infection due to *E coli*. However, it is distinctive in that the basic disease process is thought to be a macrophage defect in intraphagosomal bacterial digestion (Stanton 1981). Malacoplakia uncommonly involves the prostate, with only about 30 cases reported to date (Alpern 1991, Arena 2001, Cazzaniga 1987, Coup 1976, Ferreira 1976, Kerr 1972, Liu 1993, Rubenstein 1977, Sujka 1989, Thrasher 1992, Tisseau 2000). In one review of malacoplakia occurring at all sites, the prostate was primarily involved in 10% of all cases (Stanton 1981). Although uncommon, malacoplakia, like other forms of granulomatous prostatitis, can be misdiagnosed as carcinoma by DRE, transrectal ultrasound (TRUS) (Thrasher 1992), and histopathologic examination (Coup 1976, Ferreira 1976, Rubenstein 1977).

Patients with prostatic malacoplakia usually are in their 60s (range 49 to 85) and present with voiding symptoms (dysuria, frequency, urinary retention) and an enlarged, firm to hard prostate

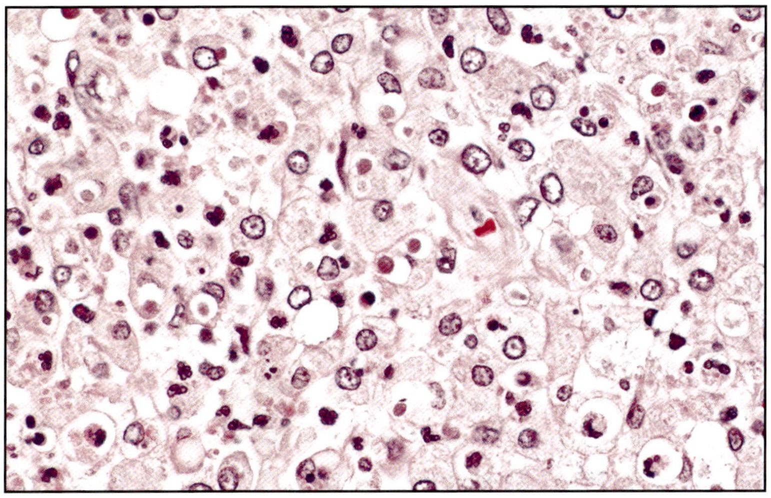

■ **i4.54** *Malacoplakia: Sheet of macrophages with targetoid Michaelis-Gutman bodies.*

by DRE. Hypoechoic regions on TRUS may further heighten the suspicion for carcinoma. Immunosuppression has been associated with malacoplakia in general (Stanton 1981), but only 2 patients with prostatic malacoplakia were known to be immunosuppressed (Konnak 1976, Sujka 1989).

The diagnosis of malacoplakia is definitely established by histopathologic examination, with core biopsy or transurethral resection being the typical means of tissue procurement. Malacoplakia can also be diagnosed by fine needle aspiration biopsy (Cazzaniga 1987). Grossly, the Greek meaning of *malacoplakia,* that is, "soft plaque," applies to urothelial surfaces rather than the prostate, where malacoplakia appears as soft, yellowish nodules (Andersen 1986). Resected prostatic chips involved by malacoplakia are soft and yellow-brown to gray (Ferreira 1976, Sterrett 1975). Microscopically, there are sheets of macrophages **i4.54** with smaller numbers of lymphocytes, plasma cells, eosinophils, and neutrophils. The macrophages (also known as von Hansemann cells [von Hansemann 1903]) contain round, often concentrically laminated, basophilic intracytoplasmic inclusions that are 2μm to 10μm in diameter. They look targetoid, with a central basophilic body surrounded by a clear zone. These are the characteristic Michaelis-Gutmann bodies (Michaelis 1902) **i4.54**, which represent calcified bacterial debris within phagolysosomes. These structures can also be extracellular. Although not absolutely necessary, special histochemical stains can be used to substantiate the presence of Michaelis-Gutmann bodies, which are typically periodic acid-Schiff–positive after diastase digestion, von Kossa or alizarin red S stain (for calcium) positive, with weak to negative staining with Perls Prussian blue stain (for iron). Tissue Gram stains for bacteria are negative. Not needed for diagnosis but of experimental interest are electron microscopy and roentgenogram microanalysis studies, which have demonstrated lysosomes with myelinlike membrane whorls and mineralized inclusions that contain calcium and phosphorus with only trace iron (Andersen 1986, Coup 1976, Shimizu 1981, Sterrett 1975, Thrasher 1992, Underwood 1982).

The essential differential diagnostic distinction is the separation of malacoplakia from poorly differentiated carcinoma. There are 3 published cases in which an initial diagnosis of carcinoma was rendered (Coup 1976, Ferreira 1976, Rubenstein 1977). As in other types of granulomatous prostatitis, the diffuse growth of epithelioid histiocytes creates diagnostic difficulty. In one case misdiagnosed as clear cell carcinoma, the malacoplakia was diffuse and extensive, involving 60% of the TURP chips (Ferreira 1976). The finding of Michaelis-Gutmann bodies excludes a diagnosis of high-grade carcinoma with clear cell features such as the hypernephromatoid pattern. The aforementioned immunohistochemical marker panel of pan-cytokeratin, PSA, PSAP, CD68, and lysozyme can also be diagnostically beneficial in selected cases, especially because malacoplakia and carcinoma can coexist in rare cases (Liu 1993, Sujka 1989). The presence of Michaelis-Gutmann bodies also distinguishes malacoplakia from other types of granulomatous prostatitis.

Treatment is directed toward control of the urinary tract infection (Stanton 1981). In one patient, failure of control resulted in a fatal prostate-rectal fistula (Andersen 1986). Overall, prognosis is related to extent of malacoplakia in the urinary tract and especially extent of renal involvement (Stanton 1981).

Systemic Granulomatous Disease Affecting the Prostate

Several systemic granulomatous diseases can involve the prostate and even present primarily as a prostatic disorder **t4.6**. All of these are uncommon to rare.

Allergic (eosinophilic) granulomatous prostatitis must be clearly defined and distinguished from other types of prostatitis that have eosinophils (Epstein 1984, Kelalis 1964, Melicow 1951, Oppenheimer 1997, Schmidt 1965, Stewart 1954, Stillwell 1987A, Towfighi 1972). The mere finding of eosinophils, even numerous eosinophils, does not equate with a diagnosis of allergic prostatitis. Rather, a histopathologic diagnosis of allergic (eosinophilic) granulomatous prostatitis should incorporate clinical findings of a hypersensitivity disorder (usually asthma or drug allergy), with or without peripheral eosinophilia. Peripheral eosinophilia without documented clinical hypersensitivity is not sufficient (Sugiura 1987). The diagnosis of "simple eosinophilic granulomatous prostatitis" (Redman 1984) should be avoided. Allergic (eosinophilic) granulomatous prostatitis is a rare condition, with an incidence of 0.06% in 3600 TURP chip cases (Michaelis 1902). Not a single case was diagnosed in 25 852 needle biopsies (Oppenheimer 1997). It accounts for 1% of all cases of granulomatous prostatitis (Stillwell 1987A). Only a handful of cases have been well documented (Epstein 1984). Microscopically, the prototypical case has central fibrinoid necrosis with surrounding, palisaded epithelioid histiocytes and numerous eosinophils. No Charcot-Leyden crystals are seen (Michaelis 1902). The differential diagnosis of allergic (eosinophilic) granulomatous prostatitis mainly includes other types of granulomatous prostatitis. Significant numbers of eosinophils can be seen in nonspecific granulomatous prostatitis (68% of cases), postbiopsy TURP cases, and less frequently in infectious granulomatous prostatitis (12% of cases) (Oppenheimer 1997). Patients with a clinicopathologic diagnosis of allergic (eosinophilic) prostatitis with accompanying vasculitis have a serious illness and should be treated with steroids (Sugiura 1987).

Sarcoidosis rarely involves the prostate, with only a few case reports (Morris 1993, Ricker 1949, Schaumann 1936). Two cases were autopsy-detected in the setting of widespread disease (Ricker 1949, Schaumann 1936). One 28-year-old man with bilateral hilar lymphadenopathy and nodular shadowing in both lung fields on chest roentgenogram had a prostatic biopsy with numerous granulomas and a negative acid-fast bacillus stain, consistent with prostatic sarcoidosis (Morris 1993).

Wegener granulomatosis usually involves the upper respiratory tract, lungs, and kidneys, but in 2.7% to 7.4% of patients, prostatic involvement can occur (Bray 1991, Huong 1995, Hussain 1990, Murty 1991, Stillwell 1987B, Vaught 1989, Walton 1958, Yalowitz 1966). Prostatic involvement at autopsy was seen in 7.4% of all Wegener cases (Yalowitz 1966), but only about 21 patients with Wegener granulomatosis have had symptoms referable to the prostate gland in the form of symptomatic prostatitis with urinary frequency, dysuria, hematuria, lower back pain, or acute urinary retention. Only a few patients ($n = 9$) had these prostatitis symptoms as their initial ones (Huong 1995). In a few patients localized induration on DRE has caused clinical concern for carcinoma (Huong 1995). Acute necrotizing granulomas have been detected in patients with prostatic Wegener granulomatosis in needle biopsy, in TURP chips, and at autopsy. An important microscopic finding is that of vasculitis, and this discovery, in conjunction with the necrotizing granulomas, should suggest a work-up for Wegener granulomatosis in these rare patients who present with Wegener granulomatosis in the prostate. As in other anatomic sites, it is important to exclude infectious granulomatous disease before diagnosing Wegener granulomatosis, and so performance of histochemical stains (acid-fast bacillus, Gomori methenamine-silver stain) for organisms is obligatory.

Foreign Body Granulomatous Prostatitis

A few examples each of specific foreign body granulomatous reaction to Teflon (polytetrafluoroethylene) (Orozco 1995) and hair (Day 1998, White 1994) have been described. Teflon injection has been used to treat urinary incontinence, and this can cause prostatic nodularity by DRE and elevated serum PSA (Orozco 1995). Prostate needle biopsy demonstrates an exuberant foreign body giant cell reaction to the refractile, irregular fragments of Teflon **i4.55A,B**. The degraded Teflon can appear purplish and mucinlike and thereby simulate mucin of a prostatic adenocarcinoma. With polarization, the Teflon is highly birefringent **i4.55B**. Detection of a Teflon granuloma does not rule out the coexistence of epithelial proliferative abnormalities. In one reported case, high-grade PIN was found, and in a second there was an associated Gleason score 7 adenocarcinoma (Orozco 1995). In a case we recently saw **i4.55A,B**, the sampled prostatic tissue was benign. Hair granulomas with prostatic hair implantation due to long-term catheterization (White 1994) or perineal prostatic biopsy (Day 1998) have also been seen.

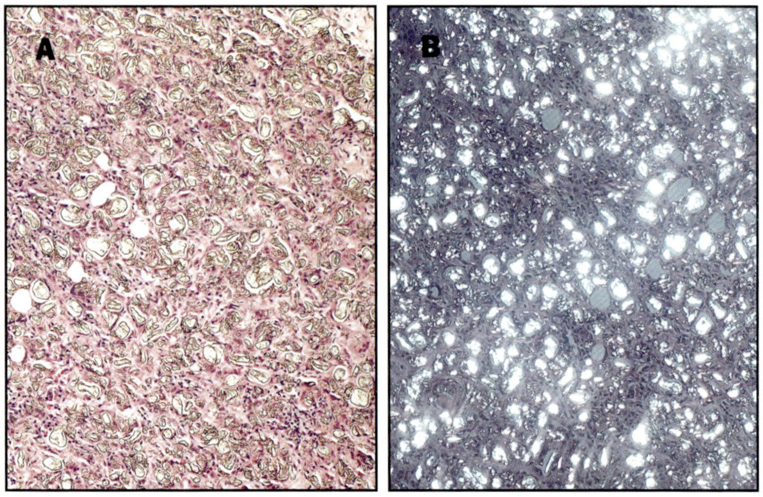

■ **i4.55** *Granulomatous reaction to Teflon injected into the prostate (A); Teflon particles are brightly birefringement (B).*

■ **t4.9 Prostatic Vasculitis: Classification**

Localized to prostate
Vasculitis in post-TURP granulomatous prostatitis
Giant cell arteritis
Isolated fibrinoid arteritis in BPH
Isolated non-fibrinoid arteritis in BPH
Not confined to prostate
Radiation-induced prostatic vasculitis
Systemic periarteritis nodosa
Vasculitis in Wegener's granulomtosis
Vasculitis in allergic (eosinophilic) granulomatous prostatitis

[4.9] Vasculitis

Inflammation of vessels in the prostate can represent a vasculitis confined to or isolated in the prostate or can represent a manifestation of systemic or nonprostatic confined vasculitis **t4.9**. As noted earlier, vasculitis has been found in Wegener granulomatosis, allergic (eosinophilic) granulomatous prostatitis, and a few cases of post-TURP granuloma. Prostatic vasculitis has also been found in localized polyarteritis nodosa–like vasculitis (Lopez-Beltran 1996, Val-Bernal 1997) and in systemic polyarteritis nodosa (including 2 patients in whom it was associated with hepatitis B infection) (Balague 1983, Cheatum 1981, Genesca 1984) as well as in isolated form as a giant cell arteritis limited to the prostate (Bretal-Laranga 1995). I have seen nonfibrinoid vasculitis in patients with BPH **i4.56**. The significance of vasculitis in this setting is unknown, but fibrinoid, necrotizing, or giant cell granulomatous vasculitis should prompt a clinical search for a systemic vasculitis. Also, irradiation can produce a prostatic vasculitis (Bostwick 1982, Sheaff 1997). Atherosclerotic changes, which are common in periprostatic vessels of older men **i4.57**, should not be classified as prostatic vasculitis.

[4.10] Infectious Prostatitis: Additional Types

Additional specific infections of the prostate have been reported for both immunocompetent and immunosuppressed patients. These include rare cases of prostatic actinomycosis (de Souza 1985), amebic prostatitis (Goff 1984), *Pseudomonas pseudomallei* prostatitis (Kan 1978), and prostatic echinococcus (Deklotz 1976, Houston 1975) in immunocompetent men. Microscopically, the prostatic response to these organisms was variable. For example, prostatic acute and chronic inflammation with fibrosis, granulation tissue, and abscess formation (with sulfur granules present) were evident in the patient with prostatic actinomycosis. A chronic, fibrosing prostatitis with eosinophils has been reported for echinococcal prostatic infection (Deklotz 1976). It is uncertain how often sexually transmitted infections of the prostate by *Neisseria gonorrhoeae* and human papillomavirus occur and whether this is a clinical problem (Meares 1998, Sarkar 1993).

In immunosuppressed patients, viral, bacterial, fungal, and parasitic prostatitis can occur. Most of these reports are of patients with acquired immunodeficiency syndrome (AIDS). In AIDS, patients can experience bacterial prostatitis, with progression toward abscess formation (Kwan 1995, Leport 1989). It has been estimated that 3%

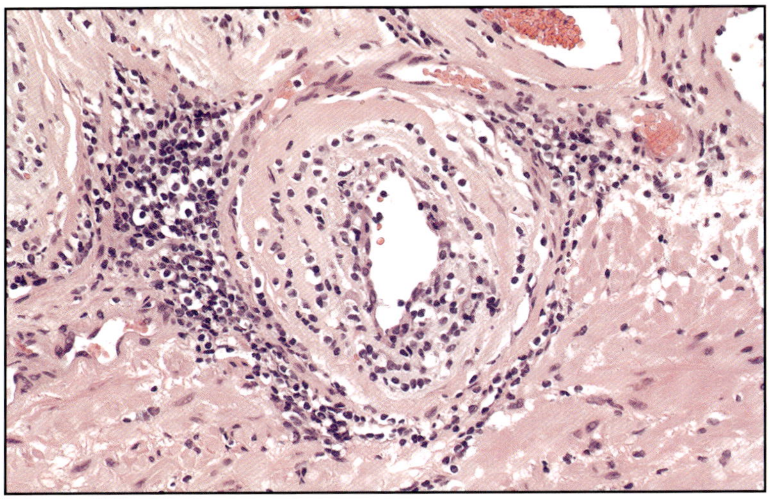

■ **i4.56** *Lymphocytic vasculitis in TURP chip from a patient with BPH.*

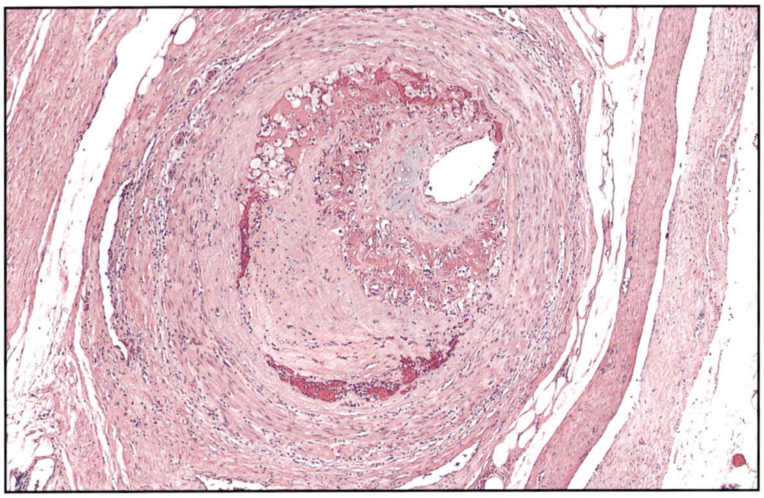

■ **i4.57** *Atherosclerotic narrowing of periprostatic vessel, with scattered lymphocytes and macrophages in vessel wall and atherosclerotic plaque.*

of asymptomatic patients with AIDS have a bacterial prostatitis, whereas 14% of symptomatic patients do (Leport 1989). Opportunistic infectious agents that have been reported in the prostates of patients with AIDS include cytomegalovirus (CMV) (Benson 1992, Mastroianni 1996, McKay 1994), *Mycobacterium* (Galbis 1997, Sevchuck 1989), *Histoplasma* (Marans 1991), *Candida* (Sevchuck 1989), *Pneumocystis* (Droste 1991), and *Cryptococcus* (Adams 1992, Larsen 1989, Lief 1986, Ndimbie 1994, Selzman 1994). Eight percent of patients with AIDS and systemic CMV infection had CMV involvement of the prostate, and 4% with systemic candidiasis had *Candida* in the prostate (Sevchuck 1989). Cryptococcal organisms may be sequestered in the prostate of patients with AIDS and thereby act as a reservoir for persistent infection (Larsen 1989, Ndimbie 1994). Microscopically, organisms can be identified in expressed prostatic secretions, prostate needle biopsy, or prostate glands from postmortem examination. The prostatic response to infection in patients with AIDS is variable and can be lacking (Benson 1992), or there can be necrosis or abscess formation (Marans 1991). A few cases of AIDS-related lymphoma involving the prostate have been reported (Sevchuck 1989). Another morphologic effect of human immunodeficiency virus (HIV) infection on the prostate is increased epithelial cell apoptosis, which could be related to the decreased testosterone levels seen in patients with AIDS (Dikov 1998). It is not clear whether the prostate can serve as a reservoir for HIV-infected cells because only a few HIV-infected macrophages and lymphocytes have been detected in the prostate of men with AIDS by in situ hybridization (Nuovo 1994, Pudney 1991).

References

Abbas F, Kamal MK, Talati J. Prostatic aspergillosis. *J Urol* 153:748-750, 1995.

Adams JR, Mata JA, Culkin DJ, et al. Acquired immunodeficiency syndrome manifesting as prostate nodule secondary to cryptococcal infection. *Urology* 39:289-291, 1992.

Alguacil-Garcia A. Artifactual changes mimicking signet ring cell carcinoma in transurethral prostatectomy specimens. *Am J Surg Pathol* 10:795-800, 1986.

Allan CH, Epstein JI. Nephrogenic adenoma of the prostatic urethra: a mimicker of prostate adenocarcinoma. *Am J Surg Pathol* 25: 802-808, 2001.

Alpern HD. Malakoplakia of the prostate. *Int Urol Nephrol* 23:257-259, 1991.

Altaffer LF III, Enghardt M. Malakoplakia of prostate gland. *Urology* 24:196-198, 1984.

Andersen T, Kristiansen W, Ruge S, et al. Malakoplakia of the prostate causing fatal fistula to rectum. *Scand J Urol Nephrol* 20:153-157, 1986.

Arena F, Fortunati C, di Stefano C, et al. Prostatic malacoplakia associated with prostatic abscess: diagnosis and treatment. *Urol Int* 66:212-215, 2001.

Balague F, Humair L, de Torrente A. Periarteritis nodosa in a patient carrying simultaneously HBs, HBc, and HBe antigens and anti-HBs antibodies [in French]. *Schweiz Med Wochenschr* 113:1201-1205, 1983.

Bartkowski DP, Lanesky JR. Emphysematous prostatitis and cystitis secondary to *Candida albicans*. *J Urol* 139:1063-1065, 1988.

Benson PJ, Smith CS. Cytomegalovirus prostatitis. *Urology* 40:165-167, 1992.

Billis A. Prostatic atrophy: an autopsy study of a histologic mimic of adenocarcinoma. *Mod Pathol* 11:47-54, 1998.

Bissada NK, Finkbeiner AE, Redman JF. Prostatic mycosis. Nonsurgical diagnosis and management. *Urology* 9:327-328, 1977.

Blumenfeld W, Tucci S, Narayan P. Incidental lymphocytic prostatitis. Selective involvement with nonmalignant glands. *Am J Surg Pathol* 16:975-981, 1992.

Blumenfeld W, Ye JQ, Dahiya R, et al. HLA expression by benign and malignant prostatic epithelium: augmentation by interferon-gamma. *J Urol* 150:1289-1292, 1993.

Boccon-Gibod L, Delmas V, Baron JC. Urologic manifestations of AIDS [in French]. *Ann Urol (Paris)* 23:173-177, 1989.

Bostwick DG, Egbert BM, Fajardo LF. Radiation injury of the normal and neoplastic prostate. *Am J Surg Pathol* 6:541-551, 1982.

Bostwick DG, Amin MB, Dundore P, et al. Architectural patterns of high-grade prostatic intraepithelial neoplasia. *Hum Pathol* 24:298-310, 1993.

Bostwick DG, Iczkowski KA, Amin MB, et al. Malignant lymphoma involving the prostate. Report of 62 cases. *Cancer* 83:732-738, 1998.

Brawer MK, Rennels MA, Nagle RB, et al. Serum prostate-specific antigen and prostate pathology in men having simple prostatectomy. *Am J Clin Pathol* 92:760-764, 1989.

Bray VJ, Hasbargen JA. Prostatic involvement in Wegener granulomatosis. *Am J Kidney Dis* 17:578-580, 1991.

Bretal-Laranga M, Insua-Vilarino S, Blanco-Rodriguez J, et al. Giant cell arteritis limited to the prostate. *J Rheumatol* 22:566-568, 1995.

Brock DJ, Greico MH. Cryptococcal prostatitis in a patient with sarcoidosis: response to 5-fluorocytosine. *J Urol* 107:1017-1021, 1972.

Brunner H, Weidner W, Schiefer HG. Studies of the role of *Ureaplasma urealyticum* and *Mycoplasma hominis* in prostatitis. *J Infect Dis* 147:807-813, 1983.

Bryan RL, Newman J, Campbell A, et al. Granulomatous prostatitis: a clinicopathologic study. *Histopathology* 19:453-457, 1991.

Bude R, Bree RL, Adler RS, et al. Transrectal ultrasound appearance of granulomatous prostatitis. *J Ultrasound Med* 9:677-680, 1990.

Caballes RL, Cabelles RA Jr. Primary cryptococcal prostatitis in an apparently uncompromised host. *Prostate* 39:119-122, 1999.

Campbell TB, Kaufman L, Cook JL. Aspergillosis of the prostate associated with an indwelling bladder catheter: case report and review. *Clin Infect Dis* 14:942-944, 1992.

Carruthers NC. Malakoplakia: report of a case. *Can J Surg* 2:213-214, 1959.

Cazzaniga MG, Tommasini-Degna A, Negri R, et al. Cytologic diagnosis of prostatic malakoplakia. Report of three cases. *Acta Cytol* 31:48-52, 1987.

Cheatum DE, Sowell DS, Dulany RB. Hepatitis B antigen associated periarteritis nodosa with prostatic vasculitis. *Arch Intern Med* 141:107-109, 1981.

Chen KT, Schiff JJ. Coccidioidomycosis of prostate. *Urology* 25:82-84, 1985.

Cherasse A, Herin M, Oana M, et al. Aspergillus prostatitis and prolonged corticotherapy. Apropos of a case report. [in French]. *Acta Urol Belg* 65:43-48, 1997.

Cheville JC, Bostwick DG. Postatrophic hyperplasia of the prostate. A histologic mimic of prostatic adenocarcinoma. *Am J Surg Pathol* 19:1068-1076, 1995.

Cina SJ, Epstein JI. Adenocarcinoma of the prostate with atrophic features. *Am J Surg Pathol* 21:289-295, 1997.

Clason AE, McGeorge A, Garland C, et al. Urinary retention and granulomatous prostatitis following sacral herpes zoster infection. A report of 2 cases with a review of the literature. *Br J Urol* 54:166-169, 1982.

Collins MM, Stafford RS, O'Leary MP, et al. How common is prostatitis? A national survey of physician visits. *J Urol* 159:1224-1228, 1998.

Collins MM, Meigs JB, Barry MJ, et al. Prevalence and correlates of prostatitis in the health professionals follow-up study cohort. *J Urol* 167:1362-1366, 2002.

Coup AJ: Malakoplakia of the prostate. *J Pathol* 119:119-121, 1976.

CPW (Chronic Prostatitis Workshop), National Institutes of Health, Bethesda, Md, Dec 7-8, 1995.

Day DS, Carpenter HD, Allsbrook WC Jr. Hair granuloma of the prostate. *Hum Pathol* 27:196-197, 1998.

de Souza E, Katz DA, Dworzack DL, et al. Actinomycosis of the prostate. *J Urol* 133:290-291, 1985.

Deklotz RJ. Echinococcal cyst involving the prostate and seminal vesicles: a case report. *J Urol* 115:116-117, 1976.

del Rosario AD, Ross JS. Stromal mast cell density (MCD) in benign and malignant prostatic lesions [abstract]. *Mod Pathol* 11:80A, 1998.

Devaraj LT, Bostwick DG. Atypical basal cell hyperplasia of the prostate. Immunophenotypic profile and proposed classification of basal cell proliferations. *Am J Surg Pathol* 17:645-659, 1993.

Dhundee J, Maciver AG. An immunohistochemical study of granulomatous prostatitis. *Histopathology* 18:435-441, 1991.

Dikov DI, Roland J, Chatelet FP, et al. An autopsy study of the prostate in acquired immunodeficiency syndrome. Evidence for excessive apoptosis and intracytoplasmic epithelial inclusions. *Arch Pathol Lab Med* 122:875-879, 1998.

Doble A, Carter S St C. Ultrasonographic findings in prostatitis. *Urol Clin North Am* 16:763-772, 1989.

Drach GW, Fair WR, Meares EM, et al. Classification of benign disease associated with prostatic pain: prostatitis or prostatodynia [letter]? *J Urol* 120:266, 1978.

Droste A, Grosse G, Niedobitek F. Extrapulmonary manifestations of *Pneumocystis carinii* infection in AIDS [in German]. *Verh Dtsch Ges Pathol* 75:158-162, 1991.

Egan AJM, Lopez-Beltran A, Bostwick DG. Prostatic adenocarcinoma with atrophic features: malignancy mimicking a benign process. *Am J Surg Pathol* 21:931-935, 1997.

Eickenberg HU, Amin M, Lich R Jr. Blastomycosis of the genitourinary tract. *J Urol* 113:650-652, 1975.

Elert A, von Knobloch R, Nusser R, et al. Isolated candidal prostatitis. *J Urol* 163:244, 2000.

Epstein JI, Hutchins GM. Granulomatous prostatitis: distinction among allergic, nonspecific, and posttransurethral resection lesions. *Hum Pathol* 15:818-825, 1984.

Epstein JI, Armas OA. Atypical basal cell hyperplasia of the prostate. *Am J Surg Pathol* 16:1205-1214, 1992.

Ferreira AA, Alvarenga M. Malacoplakia of the prostate confused with clear cell carcinoma. *J Urol* 116:828-829, 1976.

Ferry JA, Young RH. Malignant lymphoma of the genitourinary tract. *Curr Diagn Pathol* 4:145-169, 1997.

Fox H: Nodular histiocytic prostatitis. *J Urol* 96:372-374, 1966.

Galbis Sanjuan F, Jimenez Cidre M, Rodriguez Rodriguez R, et al. Tuberculous prostatic abscess in acquired immunodeficiency syndrome [in Spanish]. *Arch Esp Urol* 50:393-395, 1997.

Gelfand M, Ross CMD, Blair DM, et al. Schistosomiasis of the male pelvic organs. Severity of infection as determined by digestion of tissue and histologic methods in 300 cadavers. *Am J Trop Med Hyg* 19:779-784, 1970.

Genesca J, Esteban R, Cervantes M, et al. Prostatic vasculitis, an unusual beginning for panarteritis nodosa [in Spanish]. *Med Clin (Barc)* 83:545-546, 1984.

Goff DA, Davidson RA. Amebic prostatitis. *South Med J* 77:1053-1054, 1984.

Goldman RL. A case of malakoplakia with involvement of the prostate gland. *J Urol* 93:407-410, 1965.

Golz R, Mendling W. Candidosis of the prostate: a rare form of endomycosis. *Mycoses* 34:381-384, 1991.

Gottesman JE. Coccidioidomycosis of prostate and epididymis. With urethrocutaneous fistula. *Urology* 4:311-314, 1974.

Granados EA, Riley G, Salvador J, et al. Prostatic abscess: diagnosis and treatment. *J Urol* 148:80-82, 1992.

Gujral S, Gillatt DA. A peculiar case of granulomatous prostatitis: a cause for concern. *Br J Urol* 81:775, 1998.

Gupta RK. Mast cell variations in prostate and urinary bladder. *Arch Pathol* 89:302-305, 1970.

Haas CA, Bodner DR, Hampel N, et al. Systemic candidiasis presenting with prostatic abscess. *Br J Urol* 82:450-451, 1998.

Haddad FS. Coccidioidomycosis of the genitourinary tract with special emphasis on the epididymis and the prostate. *J Urol Pathol* 4:205-211, 1996.

Hasui Y, Marutsuka K, Asada Y, et al. Relationship between serum prostate specific antigen and histological prostatitis in patients with benign prostatic hyperplasia. *Prostate* 25:91-96, 1994.

Hedelin H, Johansson S, Nilsson S. Focal prostatic granulomas. A sequel to transurethral resection. *Scand J Urol Nephrol* 15:193-196, 1981.

Helpap B, Vogel J. TUR-prostatitis. Histological and immunohistochemical observations in a special type of granulomatous prostatitis. *Pathol Res Pract* 181:301-307, 1986.

Helpap B. Histological and immunohistochemical study of chronic prostatic inflammation with and without benign prostatic hyperplasia. *J Urol Pathol* 2:49-64, 1994.

Henry L, Wagner B, Faulkner MK, et al. Metal deposition in post-surgical granulomas of the urinary tract. *Histopathology* 22:457-465, 1993.

Hinchey WW, Someren A. Cryptococcal prostatitis. *Am J Clin Pathol* 75:257-260, 1981.

Hoffmann E, Garrido MW. Malakoplakia of the prostate: report of a case. *J Urol* 92:311-313, 1964.

Houston W. Primary hydatid cyst of the prostate gland. *J Urol* 113:732-733, 1975.

Huong DLT, Papo T, Piette JC, et al. Urogenital manifestations of Wegener granulomatosis. *Medicine* 74:152-161, 1995.

Hussain SF, Baker JT, De Bolla AR. Wegener's granulomatosis presenting as granulomatous prostatitis causing urinary retention. *Br J Urol* 65:104, 1990.

Ikemoto I, Ohishi Y, Onodera S, et al. A case of allergic granulomatous prostatitis [in Japanese]. *Hinyokika Kiyo* 30:1851-1859, 1984.

Indudhara R, Singh SK, Vaidyanathan S, et al. Isolated invasive candidal prostatitis. *Urol Int* 48:362-364, 1994.

Kaleem Z, Swanson PE, Vollmer RT, et al. Prostatic adenocarcinoma with atrophic features. A study of 202 consecutive completely embedded radical prostatectomy specimens. *Am J Clin Pathol* 109:695-703, 1998.

Kan SK, Kay RW. Melioidosis presenting as prostatitis: a case report from Sabah. *Trans R Soc Trop Med Hyg* 72:522-524, 1978.

Keetch DW, Humphrey P, Ratliff TL. Development of a mouse model for nonbacterial prostatitis. *J Urol* 152:247-250, 1994.

Kelalis PP, Greene LF, Weed LA. Brucellosis of the urogenital tract: a mimic of tuberculosis. *J Urol* 88:347-353, 1962.

Kelalis PP, Harrison EG Jr, Greene LF. Allergic granulomas of the prostate in asthmatics. *JAMA* 188:963-967, 1964.

Kelalis PP, Greene LF, Harrison EG Jr. Granulomatous prostatitis. A mimic of carcinoma of the prostate. *JAMA* 191:287-289, 1965.

Kerr JFR, Gaffney TJ, McGeary HM, et al. Malakoplakia: an electron-microscope and biochemical study. *J Pathol* 107:289-294, 1972.

Klaaborg KE, Bennedbaek J, Starklint H. Two cases of malakoplakia of the prostate. *Eur Urol* 11:137-138, 1985.

Kohnen PE, Drach GW. Patterns of inflammation in prostatic hyperplasia: a histologic and bacteriologic study. *J Urol* 121:755-760, 1979.

Konnak JW, Hart WR. Malacoplakia of the prostate in an immunosuppressed patient. *J Urol* 116:830-832, 1976.

Kopolovic J, Rivkind A, Sherman Y. Granulomatous prostatitis with vasculitis. A sequel to transurethral prostatic resection. *Arch Pathol Lab Med* 108:732-733, 1984.

Kostakopoulos A, Economou G, Pieramenos D, et al. Tuberculosis of the prostate. *Int Urol Nephrol* 30:153-157, 1998.

Küehnelian JG, Guida PM, Pearce JM, et al. Experiences with granulomatous prostatitis. *J Urol* 91:173-176, 1964.

Kwan DJ, Lowe FC. Genitourinary manifestations of the acquired immunodeficiency syndrome. *Urology* 45:13-27, 1995.

LaFontaine PD, Middleman BR, Graham SD Jr, et al. Incidence of granulomatous prostatitis and acid-fast bacilli after intravesical BCG therapy. *Urology* 49:363-366, 1997.

Lamm DL, Stogdill VD, Stogdill BJ, et al. Complications of bacillus Calmette-Guerin immunotherapy in 1,278 patients with bladder cancer. *J Urol* 135:272-274, 1986.

Larsen RA, Bozzette S, McCutchan JA, et al, and the California Collaborative Treatment Group. Persistent *Cryptococcus neoformans* infection of the prostate after successful treatment of meningitis. *Ann Int Med* 111:125-128, 1989.

Lee LW, Burgher LW, Price EB Jr, et al. Granulomatous prostatitis: association with isolation of *Mycobacterium kansasii* and *Mycobacterium fortuitum*. *JAMA* 237:2408-2409, 1987.

Leport C, Rousseau F, Perronne C, et al. Bacterial prostatitis in patients infected with the human immunodeficiency virus. *J Urol* 141:334-336, 1989.

Lief M, Sarfarazi F. Prostatic cryptococcosis in acquired immune deficiency syndrome. *Urology* 28:318-319, 1986.

Lipponen P, Vesalainen S, Kasurinen J, et al. A prognostic score for prostatic adenocarcinoma based on clinical, histological, biochemical and cytometric data from the primary tumor. *Anticancer Res* 16:2095-2100, 1996.

Litwin MS, McNaughton-Collins M, Fowler FJ Jr, et al. The National Institutes of Health chronic prostatitis symptom index : development and validation of a new outcome measure. Chronic Prostatitis Collaborative Research Network. *J Urol* 162:369-375, 1999.

Liu S, Christmas TJ, Kirby RS. Malakoplakia and carcinoma of the prostate. *Br J Urol* 72:120-121, 1993.

Lo J, Kerns BJ, Amling CL, et al. Correlation of DNA ploidy and histologic diagnosis from prostate core-needle biopsies: is DNA ploidy more sensitive than histology for the diagnosis of carcinoma in small specimens? *J Surg Oncol* 63:41-45, 1996.

Lopez-Beltran A. Vasculitis involving the prostate: report of two cases. *Pathol Case Rev* 1:70-73, 1996.

Ludwig M, Schroeder-Printzen I, Schiefer HG, et la. Diagnosis and therapeutic management of 18 patients with prostatitis abscess. *Urology* 53:340-345, 1999.

Marans HY, Mandell W, Kislak JW, et al. Prostatic abscess due to histoplasma capsulatum in acquired immunodeficiency syndrome. *J Urol* 145:1275-1276, 1991.

Mastroianni A, Coronado O, Manfredi R, et al. Acute cytomegalovirus prostatitis in AIDS. *Genitourin Med* 72:447-448, 1996.

Matsumoto T, Ih H, Yamada Y, et al. Prostatic malacoplakia. *Urol Int* 40:10-12, 1985.

Matsumoto T, Sakamoto N, Kimiya K, et al. Nonspecific granulomatous prostatitis. *Urology* 39:420-423, 1992.

McClure J: Malakoplakia of the prostate: a report of two cases and a review of the literature. *J Clin Pathol* 32:629-632, 1979.

McKay TC, Albala DM, Sendelbach K, et al. Cytomegalovirus prostatitis. Case report and review of the literature. *Int Urol Nephrol* 26:535-540, 1994.

McNaughton-Collins MM, Fowler FJ Jr, Elliott DB, et al. Diagnosing and treating chronic prostatitis: do urologists use the four-glass test? *Urology* 55:403-407, 2000.

McNeal JE. Regional morphology and pathology of the prostate. *Am J Clin Pathol* 49:347-357, 1968.

McNeal JE. Normal histology of the prostate. *Am J Surg Pathol* 12:619-633, 1988.

Meares EM, Stamey TA. Bacteriologic localization patterns in bacterial prostatitis and urethritis. *Invest Urol* 5:492-518, 1968.

Meares EM Jr. Prostatitis and related disorders. In: Walsh PC, Retik AB, Vaughan ED Jr, et al, eds. *Campbell's Urology*. 7th ed. Philadelphia: WB Saunders; 615-630, 1998.

Melchior J, Valk WL, Foret JD, et al. The prostate in leukemia: evaluation and review of the literature. *J Urol* 111:647-851, 1974.

Melicow MM. Allergic granulomas of the prostate. *J Urol* 65:288-296, 1951.

Melo CR, Melo JS, Cerski CT. Leukemic infiltration, paracoccidioidomycosis and nodular hyperplasia of the prostate. *Br J Urol* 70:329-330, 1992.

Mbakop A, Reverdin N, Cox JN. Nonspecific granulomatous prostatitis. Histopathological study of 53 cases with a review of the literature [in French]. *Schweiz Med Wochenschr* 115:522-525, 1985.

Michaelis L, Gutmann C. Über Einschlüsse in Blasentumoren. *Z Klin Med* 47:208, 1902.

Milchgrub S, Visconti E, Avellini J. Granulomatous prostatitis induced by capsule-deficient cryptococcal infection. *J Urol* 143:365-366, 1990.

Miekos E, Wlodarczyk W, Szram S. Xanthogranulomatous prostatitis. *Int Urol Nephrol* 18:433-437, 1986.

Mies C, Balogh K, Stadeker M. Palisading prostate granulomas following surgery. *Am J Surg Pathol* 8:217-221, 1984.

Mikolich DJ, Mates SM. Granulomatous prostatitis due to mycobacterium avium complex. *Clin Infect Dis* 14:589-591, 1992.

Miyashita H, Troncoso P, Babaian RJ. BCG-induced granulomatous prostatitis: a comparative ultrasound and pathologic study. *Urology* 39:364-367, 1992.

Moore RA: Tuberculosis of the prostate gland. *J Urol* 37:372-384, 1937.

Morris SB, Gordon EM, Corbishley CM. Prostatic sarcoidosis. A review of genitourinary sarcoidosis. *Br J Urol* 72:462-464, 1993.

Mukamel E, Konichezky M, Engelstein D, et al. Clinical and pathological findings in prostate following intravesical bacillus Calmette-Guerin instillations. *J Urol* 144:1399-1460, 1990.

Murty GE, Powell PH. Wegener's granulomatosis presenting as prostatitis. *Br J Urol* 67:107-108, 1991.

Nadler RB, Humphrey PA, Smith DS, et al. Effect of inflammation and benign prostatic hyperplasia on elevated serum prostate specific antigen levels. *J Urol* 154:407-413, 1995.

NCHS (National Center for Health Statistics). Advance data from vital and health statistics: Nos. 61-70 *Vital Health Stat* 16:1993.

Ndimbie OK, Dekker A, Martinez AJ, et al. Prostatic sequestration of *Cryptococcus neoformans* in immunocompromised persons treated for cryptococcal meningoencephalitis. *Histol Histopathol* 9:643-648, 1994.

Nickel JC, True LD, Krieger JN, et al, members of the North American Chronic Prostatitis Collaborative Research Network and the International Prostatitis Collaborative Network. Consensus development of a histopathological classification system for prostatic inflammation. *BJU Int* 87:797-805, 2001A.

Nickel JC, Downey J, Hunter D, et al. Prevalence of prostatitis-like symptoms in a population based study using the National Institutes of Health chronic prostatitis symptom index. *J Urol* 165:842-845, 2001B.

Nickel JC. Prostatitis and related conditions. In: Walsh PC, Retik AB, Vaughan ED Jr, et al, eds. *Campbell's Urology.* 8th ed. Philadelphia: Saunders; 603-630, 2002.

Nielsen ML, Asnaes S, Hattel T. Inflammatory changes in the non-infected prostate gland. A clinical, microbiological and histological investigation. *J Urol* 110:423-426, 1973.

Niku SD, Dalgleish G, Devendra G. Coccidioidomycosis of the prostate gland. *Urology* 52:127, 1998.

Nuovo GJ, Becker J, Simsir A, et al. HIV-1 nucleic acids localize to the spermatogonia and their progeny. A study by polymerase chain reaction in situ hybridization. *Am J Pathol* 144:1142-1148, 1994.

Oates RD, Stilmant MM, Freedlund MC, et al. Granulomatous prostatitis following bacillus Calmette-Guerin immunotherapy of bladder cancer. *J Urol* 140:751-754, 1988.

O'Bowd G, Bassler T, Holmboe MC, et al. Free/total prostate specific antigen ratio can differentiate nongranulomatous from granulomatous prostatitis [abstract]. *Mod Pathol* 12:102A, 1999.

O'Dea MJ, Hunting DB, Greene LF. Non-specific granulomatous prostatitis. *J Urol* 118:58-60, 1977.

O'Dea MJ, Moore SB, Greene LF. Tuberculous prostatitis. *Urology* 11:483-485, 1978.

Okada K, Kojima M, Naya Y, et al. Correlation of histological inflammation in needle biopsy specimens with serum prostate-specific antigen levels in men with negative biopsy for prostate cancer. *Urology* 55: 892-898, 2000.

Oppenheimer JR, Kahane H, Epstein JI. Granulomatous prostatitis on needle biopsy. *Arch Pathol Lab Med* 121:724-729, 1997.

Ornstein DK, Smith DS, Humphrey PA, et al. The effect of prostate volume, age, total prostate specific antigen level and acute inflammation on the percentage of free prostate specific antigen levels in men without clinically detectable prostate cancer. *J Urol* 159:1234-1237, 1998.

Orozco RE, Peters RL. Teflon granuloma of the prostate mimicking adenocarcinoma. *J Urol Pathol* 3:365-368, 1995.

Pieterse AS, Aarons I, Jose JS. Focal prostatic granulomas. Rheumatoid-like-probably iatrogenic in origin. *Pathology* 16:174-177, 1984.

Presti B, Weidner N. Granulomatous prostatitis and poorly differentiated prostate carcinoma. Their distinction with the use of immunohistochemical methods. *Am J Clin Pathol* 95:330-334, 1991.

Pudney J, Anderson D. Orchitis and human immunodeficiency virus type 1 infected cells in reproductive tissues from men with the acquired immune deficiency syndrome. *Am J Pathol* 139:149-160, 1991.

Redman JF, Downs RA. Simple eosinophilic granulomatous prostatitis. *J Urol* 132:358, 1984.

Redondo Martinez E, Rey Lopez A. Prostatic xanthoma [in Spanish]. *Arch Esp Urol* 51:188-190, 1998.

Rhodes RH, Wittmann AL. Malacoplakia of the prostate following chronic urinary tract infection. *J Urol* 117:808-810, 1977.

Ricker W, Clark M. Sarcoidosis. A clinicopathologic review of three hundred cases including twenty-two autopsies. *Am J Clin Pathol* 19:725-749, 1949.

Roberts RO, Lieber MM, Bostwick DG, et al. A review of clinical and pathological prostatitis syndromes. *Urology* 49:809-821, 1997.

Roberts RO, Lieber MM, Rhodes T, et al. Prevalence of a physician-assisted diagnosis of prostatitis: the Olmstead County study of urinary symptoms and health status among men. *Urology* 51:578-584, 1998.

Robinette CL. Sex-hormone-induced inflammation and fibromuscular proliferation in the rat lateral prostate. *Prostate* 12:271-286, 1988.

Rubenstein JB, Swayne LC, Magidson JG, et al. Granulomatous prostatitis: a hypoechoic lesion of the prostate. *Urol Radiol* 13:119-122, 1991.

Rubenstein M, Bucy JG. Malakoplakia of the prostate. *South Med J* 70:351-352, 1977.

Rubin H, Furcolow ML, Yates JL, et al. The course and prognosis of histoplasmosis. *Am J Med* 27:278-288, 1959.

Ruska KM, Sauvageot J, Epstein JI. Histology and cellular kinetics of prostate atrophy. *Am J Surg Pathol* 22:1073-1077, 1998.

Salyer WR, Salyer DC. Involvement of the kidney and prostate in cryptococcosis. *J Urol* 109:695-698, 1973.

Sarkar FH, Sakr WA, Li YW, et al. Detection of human papillomavirus (HPV) DNA in human prostatic tissues by polymerase chain reaction (PCR). *Prostate* 22:171-180, 1993.

Schaumann J. Lymphogranulomatous benigna in the light of prolonged clinical observations and autopsy findings. *Br J Dermatol Syph* 48:399-446, 1936.

Scherrer MP. Tumor-like proliferation of histiocytic phagocytes in chronic prostatitis. *Frankf Z Pathol* 62:155-166, 1951.

Schmidt JD. Non-specific granulomatous prostatitis: classification, review and report of cases. *J Urol* 94:607-615, 1965.

Schmidt JD, Patterson MC. Needle biopsy study of chronic prostatitis. *J Urol* 96:519-533, 1966.

Scott WW. Tuberculosis of the genitourinary tract confined to the prostate. *J Urol* 12:515-526, 1924.

Sebo TJ, Bostwick DG, Farrow GM, Eble JW. Prostatic xanthoma: a mimic of prostatic adenocarcinoma. *Hum Pathol* 25:386-389, 1994.

Selzman AA, Bennert KW, Kursh ED. Cryptococcal prostatitis causing urinary retention in an AIDS patient: a case report. *J Urol Pathol* 2:251-254, 1994.

Sevchuck M, de Silza MM, Armenakas NA, et al. The male genital tract in AIDS [abstract]. *J Urol* 141:354A, 1989.

Sheaff MT, Baithun SI. Effects of radiation on the normal prostate gland. *Histopathology* 30:341-348, 1997.

Shepherd DS, Humphrey PA, Swanson PE, et al. Tumor-infiltrating lymphocytes in prostatic carcinoma [abstract]. *Urology* 155:514A, 1996.

Shimizu S, Takimoto Y, Niimura T, et al. A case of prostatic malakoplakia. *J Urol* 126:277-279, 1981.

Shimura S, Yang G, Ebara S, et al. Reduced infiltration of tumor-associated macrophaes in human prostate cancer: association with cancer progression. *Cancer Res* 60:5857-5861, 2000.

Speights VO Jr, Brawn PN. Serum prostate specific antigen levels in non-specific granulomatous prostatitis. *Br J Urol* 77:408-410, 1996.

Stanton MJ, Maxted W. Malakoplakia: a study of the literature and current concepts of pathogenesis. *J Urol* 125:139-146, 1981.

Steiner G, Gessl A, Kramer G, et al. Phenotype and function of peripheral and prostatic lymphocytes in patients with benign prostatic hyperplasia. *J Urol* 151:480-484, 1994.

Stenkvist B, Olding-Stenkvist E. Cytological and DNA characteristics of hyperplasia/inflammation and cancer of the prostate. *Eur J Cancer* 26:261-267, 1990.

Sterrett GF, Heenan PJ, Wyche P, et al. Malakoplakia of the prostate: a morphological and biochemical study. *Pathology* 7:139-147, 1975.

Stewart MJ, Wray S, Hull M. Allergic prostatitis in asthmatics. *J Pathol Bacteriol* 67:423-430, 1954.

Stillwell TJ, Engen DE, Farrow GM. The clinical spectrum of granulomatous prostatitis: a report of 200 cases. *J Urol* 138:320-323, 1987A.

Stillwell TJ, DeRemee RA, McDonald TJ, et al. Prostatic involvement in Wegener's granulomatosis. *J Urol* 138:1251-1253, 1987B.

Stoker TE, Robinette CL, Cooper RL. Perinatal exposure to estrogenic compounds and the subsequent effects on the prostate of the adult rat: evaluation of inflammation in the ventral and lateral lobes. *Reprod Toxicol* 13:463-472, 1999.

Sugiura H, Hayashi M, Shimamura M, et al. Nonspecific simple eosinophilic granulomatous prostatitis with eosinophilia in peripheral blood. A case report. *Acta Pathol Jpn* 37:1973-1977, 1987.

Sujka SK, Malin BT, Asirwatham JE. Prostatic malakoplakia associated with prostatic adenocarcinoma and multiple prostatic abscesses. *Urology* 34:159-161, 1989.

Symmers WStC: Two cases of eosinophilic prostatitis due to metazoan infestation (with *Oxyuris vermicularis*, and with a larva of *Linguatula serrata*. *J Pathol Bact* 73:549-555, 1957.

Takechi S, Yokoyama M, Tanji N, et al. Nonbacterial prostatitis caused by partial urethral obstruction in the rat. *Urol Res* 27:346-350, 1999.

Tanner FH, McDonald JR. Granulomatous prostatitis. A histologic study of a group of granulomatous lesions collected from prostate glands. *Arch Pathol* 36:358-370, 1943.

Taylor EW, Wheelis RF, Correa RJ Jr, et al. Granulomatous prostatitis: confusion clinically with carcinoma of the prostate. *J Urol* 117:316-318, 1977.

Terris MK, Macy M, Freiha FS. Transrectal ultrasound appearance of prostatic granulomas secondary to bacillus Calmette-Guerin instillation. *J Urol* 158:126-127, 1997.

Theyer G, Kramer G, Assmann I, et al. Phenotypic characterization of infiltrating leukocytes in benign prostatic hyperplasia. *Lab Invest* 66:96-107, 1992.

Thompson GJ, Albers DO. Granulomatous prostatitis: condition which clinically may be confused with carcinoma of prostate. *J Urol* 69:530-538, 1953.

Thompson L. Syphilis of the prostate. *Am J Syph* 4:323-341, 1920.

Thorson P, Swanson PE, Humphrey PA. Basal cell proliferations in needle biopsies of the peripheral zone of the prostate gland [abstract]. *Mod Pathol* 12:108A, 1999.

Thrasher JB, Sutherland RS, Limoge JP, et al. Transrectal ultrasound in diagnosis of malakoplakia of prostate. *Urology* 39:262-265, 1992.

Thybo E, Zdravkovic D, Zdravkovic M. Granulomatous prostatitis. *Scand J Urol Nephrol* 7:111-114, 1973.

Tisseau L, Zini L, Lemaitre L, et al. Prostatic malacoplakia: report of 3 cases [in French]. *Prog Urol* 10:597-599, 2000.

Towfighi J, Sadeghee S, Wheeler JE, et al. Granulomatous prostatitis with emphasis on the eosinophilic variety. *Am J Clin Pathol* 58:630-641, 1972.

True LD, Berger RE, Rothman I, et al. Prostate histopathology and the chronic prostatitis/chronic pelvic pain syndrome: a prospective biopsy study. *J Urol* 162:2014-2018, 1999.

Tuero JG, de la Campa JA, Lacort LP, et al. Granulomatous prostatitis. *Urol Int* 43:97-101, 1988.

Underwood JCE, Durrant TE, Coup AJ. X-ray microanalysis of the Michaelis-Gutmann bodies of malakoplakia. *J Pathol* 138:41-48, 1982.

Val-Bernal JF, González-Vela C, Mayorga M, et al. Isolated fibrinoid arteritis of the prostate. *Int J Surg Pathol* 4:143-148, 1997.

Vaught WW, Wilson TM, Raife MJ, et al. Wegener granulomatosis: prostatic involvement and bladder outlet obstruction. *Urology* 34:43-45, 1989.

Vesalainen S, Lipponen P, Talja M, et al. Histological grade, perineural infiltration, tumor-infiltrating lymphocytes and apoptosis as determinants of long-term prognosis in prostatic adenocarcinoma. *Eur J Cancer* 30A:1797-1803, 1994.

von Hansemann D. Malakoplakia of the urinary tract [in German]. *Virchows Arch Pathol Anat* 173:302-308, 1903.

Walton EW. Giant-cell granuloma of the respiratory tract (Wegener's granulomatosis). *Br Med J* 2:265-270, 1958.

Weinberger M, Cytron S, Servadio C, et al. Prostatic abscess in the antibiotic era. *Rev Infect Dis* 10:239-249, 1988.

White J, Chan YF. Hair granuloma in the prostate. *Br J Urol* 74:260, 1994.

Wise GJ. Fungal infections of the urinary tract. In: Walsh PC, Retik AB, Vaughan ED Jr, et al, eds. *Campbell's Urology.* 7th ed. Philadelphia: WB Saunders; 779-806, 1998.

Yalowitz PA, Greene LF, Sheps SG, et al. Wegener's granulomatosis involving the prostate gland: report of a case. *J Urol* 96:801-804, 1966.

Atrophy

[5.1] Classification **101**

[5.2] Pathologic Features **101**

[5.3] Differential Diagnosis **109**

[5.4] Biological Significance **111**

CHAPTER 5

Atrophy in the prostate is a common, age-related process that represents the benign lesion most often misdiagnosed as carcinoma (Young 1997, Epstein 1996, Jones 1994). Surprisingly, prostatic atrophy begins at an early age **t5.1**. Although the common diseases benign prostatic hyperplasia (BPH) and carcinoma tend to affect men older than 50 years, atrophy is found in 67% of men 19 to 29 years of age (Gardner 1987). All men (100%) older than 40 years have atrophy in the whole prostate gland (Liavåg 1968, Billis 1998). Most men (63%) have marked atrophy; 27% have a moderate degree; and 10% have a slight amount of atrophy. There is an increase in incidence and extent of atrophy with age (Liavåg 1968, Billis 1998). In needle biopsy, atrophy is an extremely common finding, detectable in 90% of peripheral zone biopsies (Thorson 1999). Atrophy in transurethral resection of the prostate (TURP) chips usually represents cystic atrophy in nodular hyperplasia. In whole prostate glands, atrophy is principally localized to the peripheral zone (Billis 1998). The cause of age-related atrophy is unknown. Factors that have been invoked include compression by hyperplastic nodules, inflammation, hormones, obstruction, nutritional deficiency, and systemic or local ischemia, such as that induced by arteriosclerosis (Liavåg 1968, Billis 1998, Moore 1936, Franks 1954, McNeal 1988). Atrophy in the prostate can also be caused by treatment, including radiation therapy and androgen deprivation therapy (see Chapter 17). There are no clinical or radiologic findings that are specific for atrophy. This is exclusively a light microscopic diagnosis.

[5.1] Classification

Histologic classification of atrophy is useful for reasons of diagnostic awareness and differential diagnosis, but it is not absolutely necessary to subtype atrophy because there is currently no known clinical significance in doing so. In 1936, one of the earliest catalogues of atrophy separated it into simple acinar atrophy and sclerotic atrophy (Moore 1936). Subsequently, in 1954, Franks (Franks 1954) devised a scheme that included simple atrophy with or without cyst formation, sclerotic atrophy, and postatrophic hyperplasia. Partial atrophy has recently been defined (Oppenheimer 1998) and should also be incorporated into a codification of atrophy **t5.2**. These patterns are often admixed, which suggests that they represent a morphologic continuum (Billis 1998). Lastly, the term proliferative inflammatory atrophy (PIA) has been coined (De Marzo 1999). Most PIA lesions were simple atrophy, with a minority being postatrophic hyperplasia with or without admixed simple atrophy (De Marzo 1999). These atrophic foci displayed acute and/or chronic inflammatory cell infiltrates, with an increased proliferation index, as assessed by Ki-67 immunolabeling (De Marzo 1999).

t5.1 Incidence of Prostatic Atrophy: Relationship With Age

Age	Incidence in Whole Gland (%) *
19-29	67
40-49	84
50-59	89
60-69	92
70-79	98
80-89	98
90-99	100

*Data from Gardner 1987 and Liavåg 1968

[5.2] Pathologic Features

Generally speaking, atrophy is grossly visible only when there is cyst formation. Such cystic atrophy can occur in both the transition zone in BPH and in the peripheral zone. However, atrophy is only definable at the light microscopic level, and it is not possible to tell macroscopically whether prostatic cysts are atrophic or not. These cysts have been termed retention cysts (Emmett 1936) and impart a spongelike appearance. Their size can range up to 2cm in greatest diameter (Emmett 1936). Microscopically, atrophy is essentially characterized by a reduction in cytoplasmic volume of luminal epithelial cells (Moore 1936). A gradation of volume loss is possible, from minimal to partial to severe. The resultant increased nuclear/cytoplasmic volume ratio means that atrophic glands appear dark at scanning magnification. Stromal alterations, with fibrosis, accompany the epithelial cell shrinkage.

Simple atrophy can be found in the peripheral zone with or without cyst formation **t5.3**. This is the most common type of atrophy, occurring in 89% of prostates with atrophy, sometimes alone and sometimes in combination with other types of atrophy (Billis 1998). Simple atrophy is most often seen in combination with postatrophic hyperplasia (hyperplastic atrophy) and sclerotic atrophy (Billis 1998). Microscopically, atrophy can be focal, involving just a few such lobules, or it can involve virtually the entire peripheral zone. Simple acinar atrophy usually involves an entire lobule, with retention of a lobular

t5.2 Classification of Prostatic Atrophy

I. Simple atrophy
    A. Without cystic change
    B. With cystic change
II. Sclerotic atrophy
III. Partial atrophy
IV. Postatrophic hyperplasia (hyperplastic atrophy)

t5.3 Simple Atrophy

Noncystic Subtype
Lobular architecture
Rounded to angular small acini
Cuboidal to flattened epithelium
Lobular stroma with sclerosis
Inflammation common

Cystic Subtype
In peripheral zone: cystic dilatation of acini in lobules
In transition zone: cystic dilatation in nodular hyperplasia
Cysts of variable size
Flattened epithelium
Basal cells present but can be inconspicuous

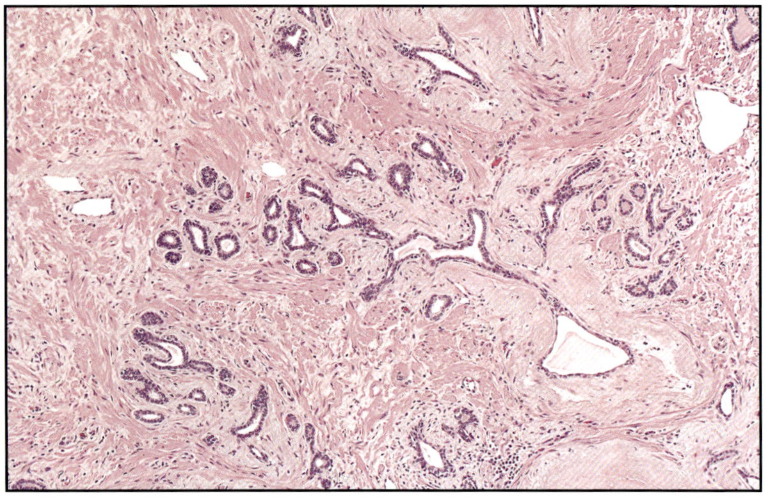

■ **i5.1** *Simple atrophy: Rounded, lobular grouping of peripheral small acini with central "feeder" duct.*

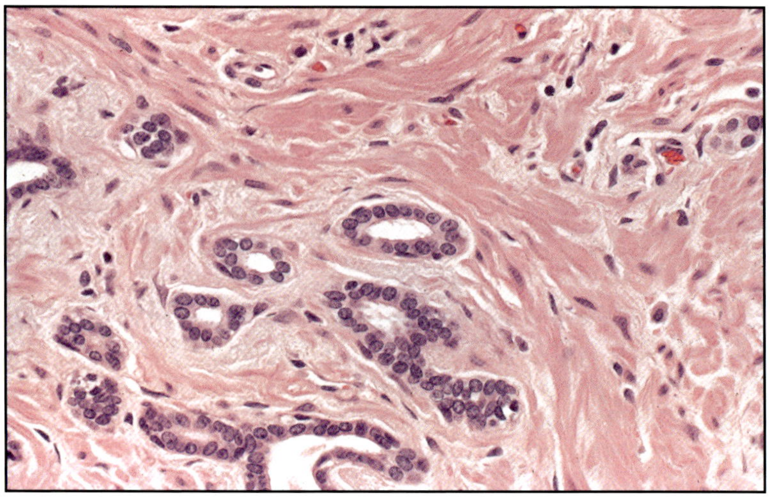

■ **i5.2** *Simple acinar atrophy: Small, dark acini with two cell layers. Note difference in fibrous stroma surrounding atrophic glands compared to smooth muscle outside the lobule.*

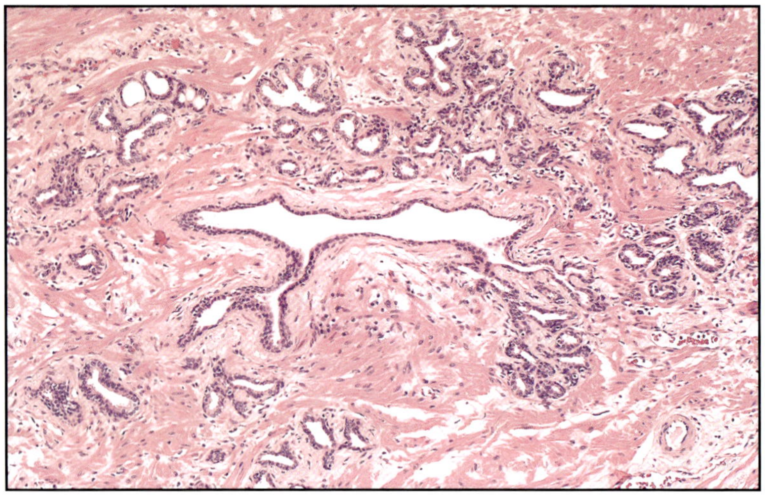

■ **i5.3** *Atrophy with central atrophic duct.*

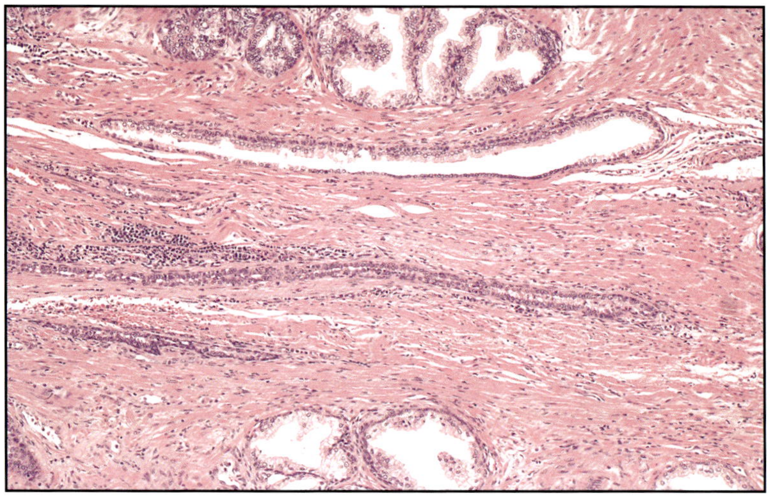

■ **i5.4** *Compressed atrophic duct found between BPH nodules.*

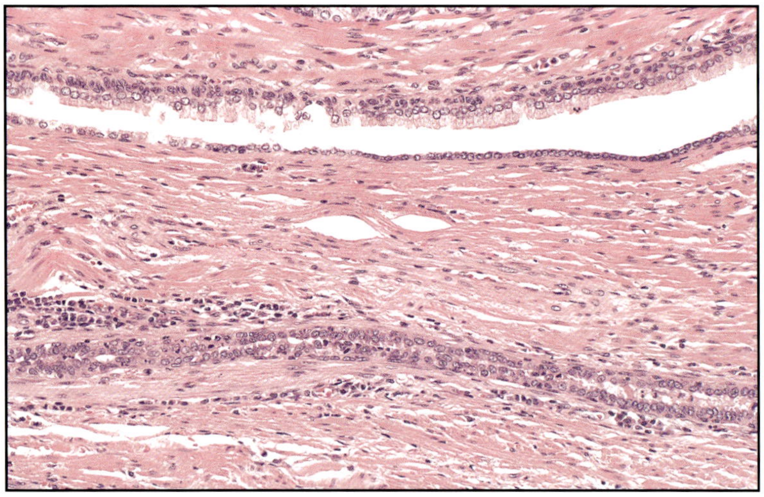

■ **i5.5** *Compressed duct found between BPH nodules: Higher-power view of* **i5.4**. *There is a second duct (above) with atrophic lining on one side only.*

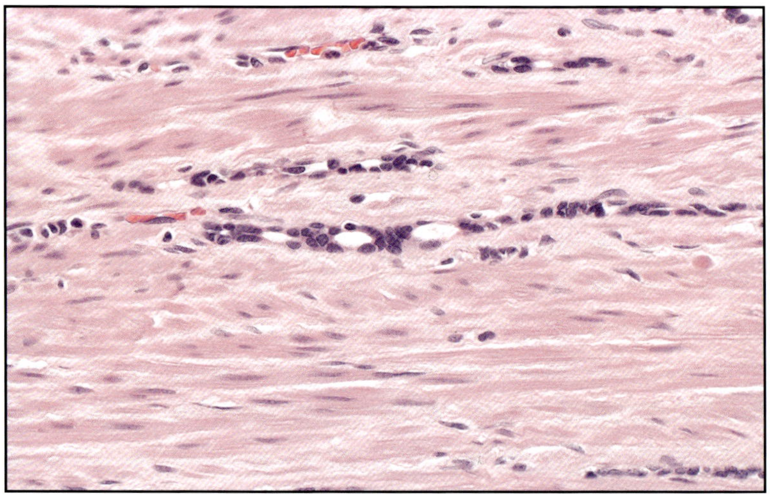

■ **i5.6** *Atrophic duct sectioned longitudinally, with minute glandular lumina.*

architecture **i5.1**. In noncystic atrophy, aggregates of small dark acini occur with open lumens **i5.2**. The acini are rounded to angular in shape and are not crowded. Atrophic ducts ramifying into atrophic acini can be noted **i5.1, i5.3**. Elongated, compressed, duct-like atrophic structures can be found between BPH nodules **i5.4, i5.5** or between BPH nodules and the peripheral zone. These atrophic structures can also be found in needle biopsies of the peripheral zone **i5.6**. Corpora amylacea are common in atrophic glands **i5.7, i5.8**, but crystalloids **i5.9** and

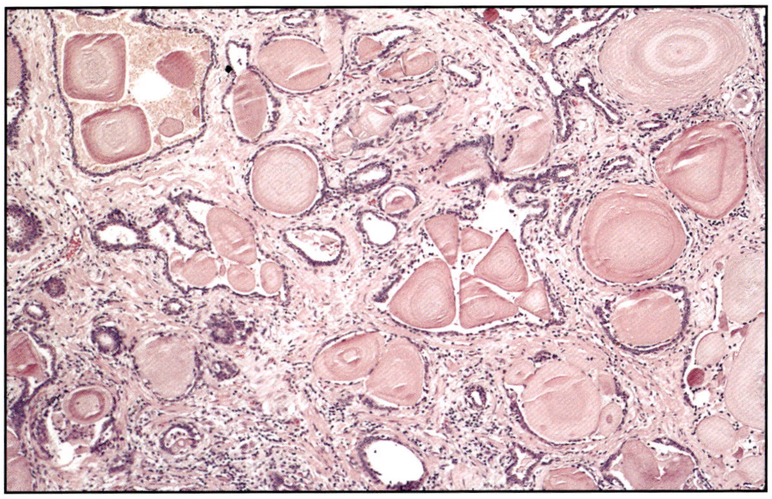

■ **i5.7** *Numerous intraluminal corpora amylacea in a field of atrophic glands.*

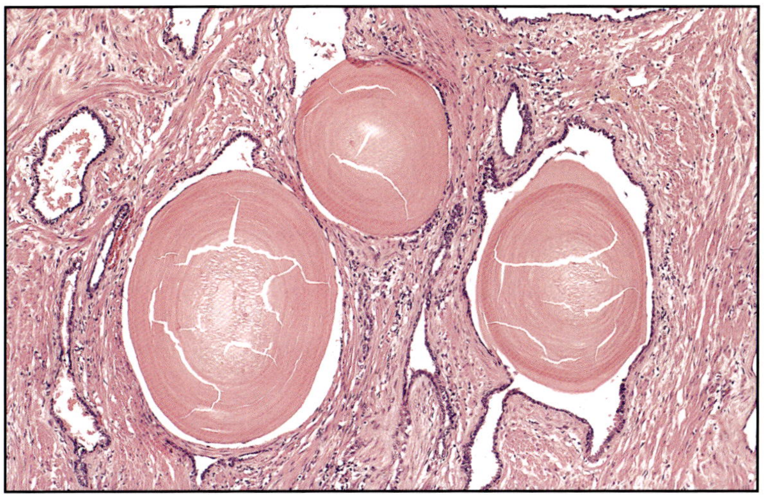

■ **i5.8** *Concentrically lamellated corpora amylacea filling and distending atrophic glands.*

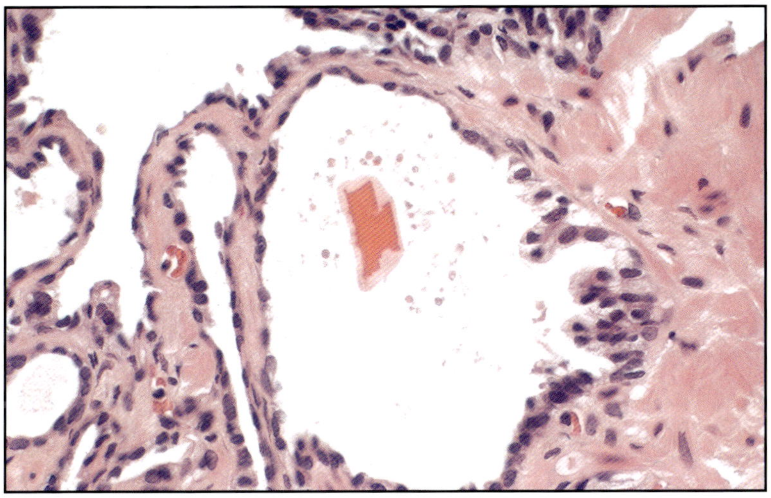

■ **i5.9** *Intraluminal crystalloid in an atrophic gland.*

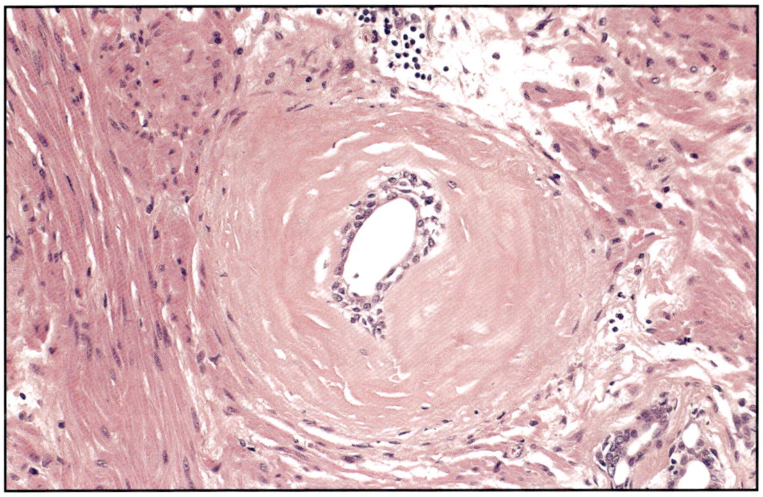

■ **i5.10** *Sclerotic thickening of ductal wall, with atrophic epithelial lining of the duct.*

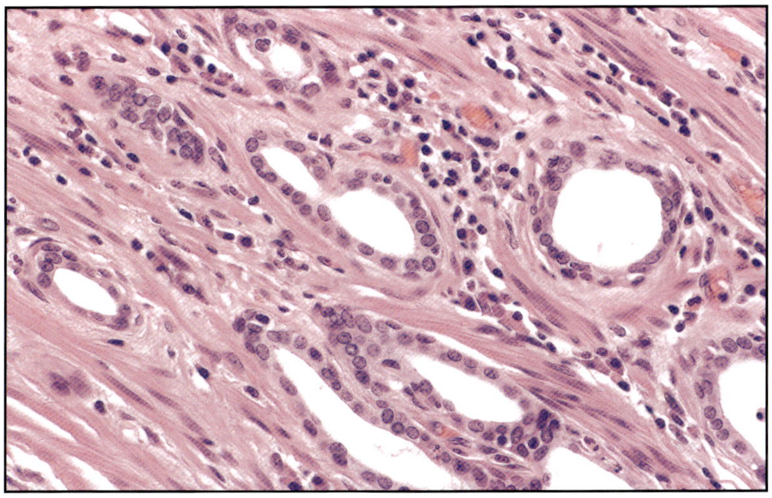

■ **i5.11** *Scattered lymphocytes in atrophy.*

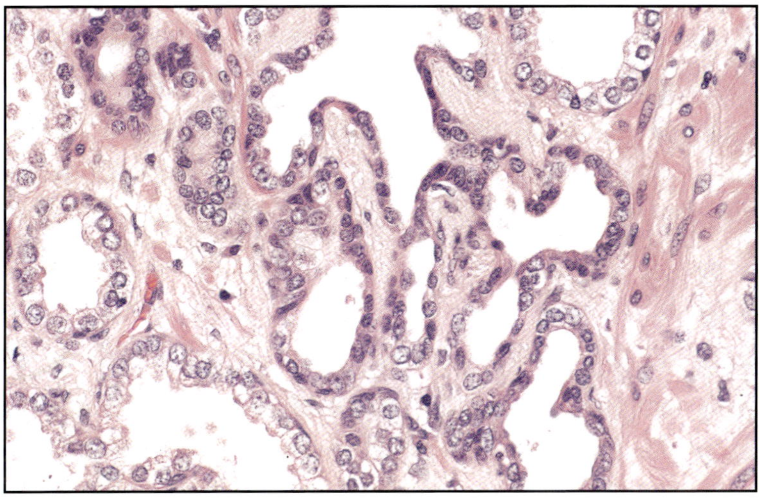

■ **i5.12** *Variable degree of cytoplasmic volume loss, with cuboidal to flattened cells.*

intraluminal wispy blue mucin are decidedly uncommon. The stroma in the lobule is often altered with pale fibrosis and sometimes with a thickening of periacinar collagen **i5.2** (Franks 1954). Sclerosis around ducts can be marked **i5.10**. Acute inflammation (of a moderate to severe grade) is observed in 15% of simple atrophy cases,whereas moderate to severe chronic inflammation is seen in 30% of cases **i5.11** (Ruska 1998). The luminal epithelial cells in the atrophic foci are cuboidal to flattened and have a high nuclear/cytoplasmic ratio **i5.12**. The nuclei

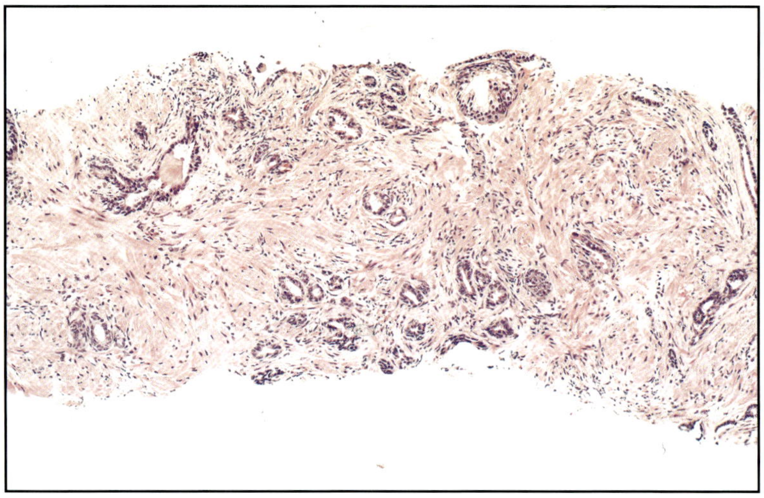

■ **i5.13** *Irregular arrangement of atrophic prostatic glands in needle biopsy tissue.*

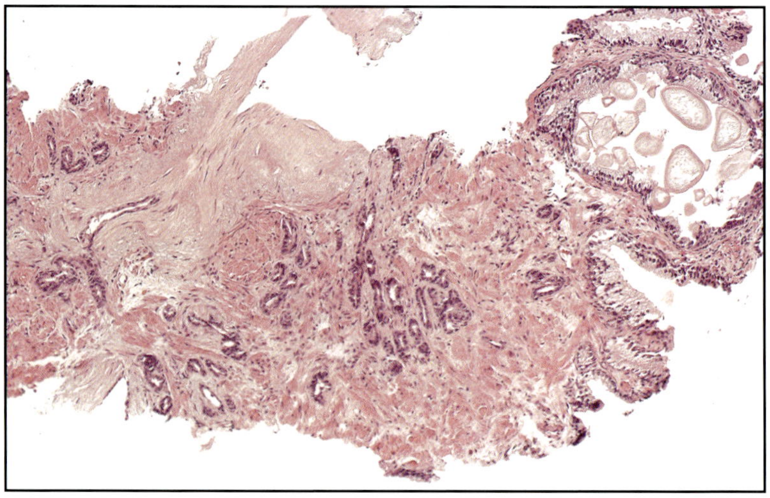

■ **i5.14** *Partial sampling of a lobule of atrophic glands by needle biopsy. On the left is the central duct within a band of stromal sclerosis.*

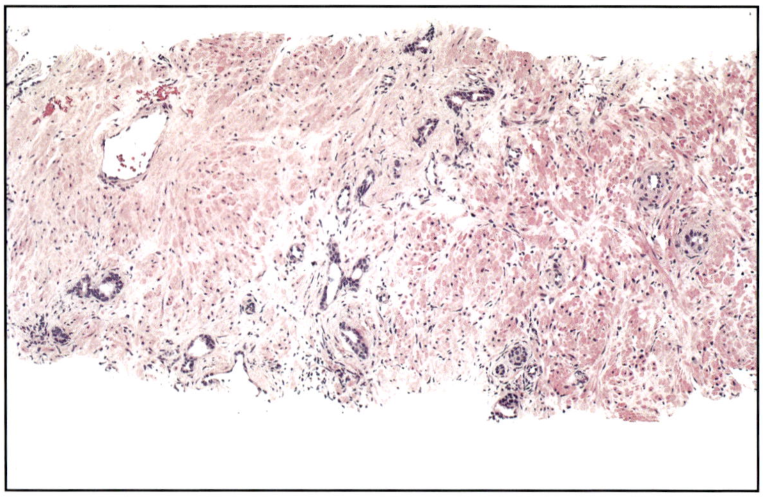

■ **i5.15** *Atrophic glands appear to grow as a column across the width of the needle core.*

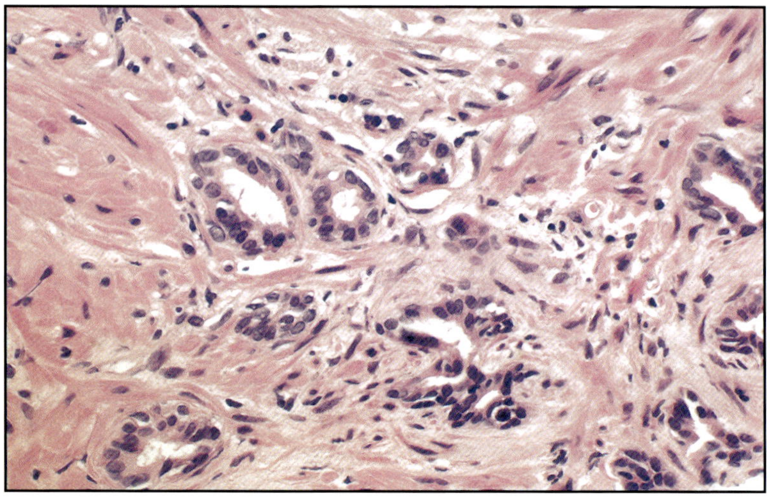

■ **i5.16** *Prostatic glandular atrophy: Round to oval to angulated, benign, atrophic glands.*

are typically not enlarged but are often deeply staining, with condensed chromatin (Franks 1954). However, in about 10% of cases with acute inflammation, nuclear enlargement occurs with prominent (>1 μm) nucleoli (Ruska 1998).

In needle biopsy, simple atrophy is eye-catching because it is often characterized by a haphazard distribution of small glands **i5.13, i5.14**. In some cases, there is a hint of a lobular grouping of the small dark acini **i5.14**. In other examples, the acini appear to stream across the width of the needle **i5.15**. At higher magnifications, the small acini are seen to have distorted and angulated outer contours **i5.16**. This appearance, along with the stromal fibrosis of the atrophic lobule, simulates an infiltrative process.

Cystic change in simple atrophy is a fairly common modification, with gland size varying from mild dilatation **i5.17** to the aforementioned 2cm cysts **t5.3;i 5.18**. The epithelium and nuclei in these glands are markedly flattened **i5.19, i5.20**. In the peripheral zone, a lobular arrangement of the cystically dilated, atrophic glands is sometimes evident **i5.21**, but with distortion the cystic, atrophic glands appear haphazardly arranged **i5.22**. Glands with cystic atrophy can masquerade as vessels **i5.23**. Simple cystic atrophy can also occur in areas of nodular hyperplasia in the transition zone **i5.24** (Franks 1954), where a flattened, atrophic-appearing epithelium can be found in continuity with usual epithelial hyperplasia.

Sclerotic atrophy is a frequently detected type of peripheral zone atrophy, having been found in 74% of cases of atrophy in the whole gland (Billis 1998). Like simple atrophy, it is usually admixed with other types of atrophy, and only 11% of atrophy cases were comprised of pure sclerotic atrophy (Billis 1998). This form of atrophy is remarkable for the lobular acinar disarray due to exuberant fibrosis. Accompanying chronic inflammation with often large collections of lymphocytes and histiocytes can be present **t5.4**. The acinar distortion and angulation in a background of stromal sclerosis can produce an infiltrative appearance **i5.25**,

■ **t5.4 Sclerotic Atrophy**

Small, distorted, dark acini
Scant epithelial cytoplasmic volume
Basal cells present but can be difficult to see
Fibrotic background
Inflammation common

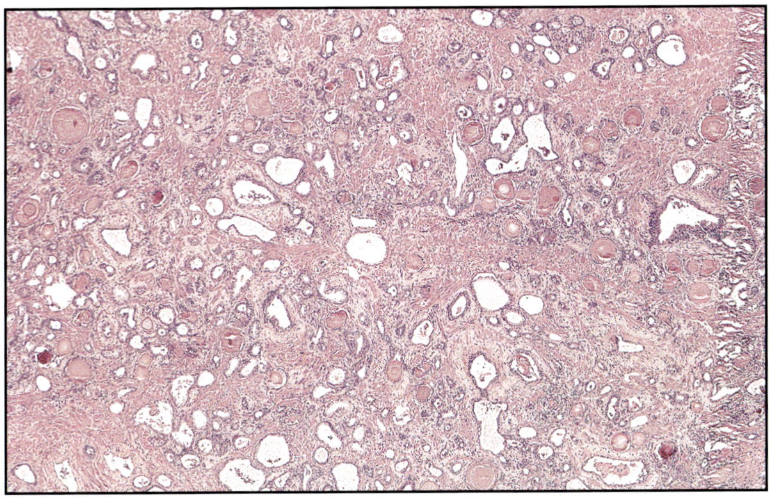

■ **i5.17** *Diffuse peripheral zone atrophy, with slight cystic change.*

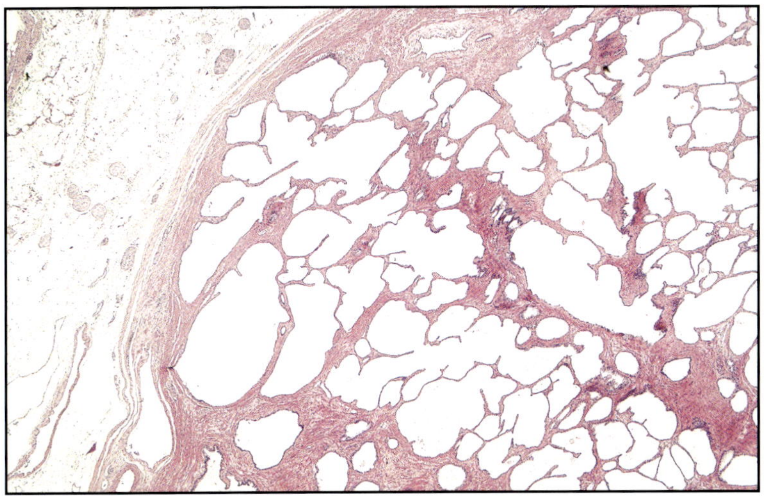

■ **i5.18** *Cystic atrophy in peripheral zone: Marked glandular dilatation.*

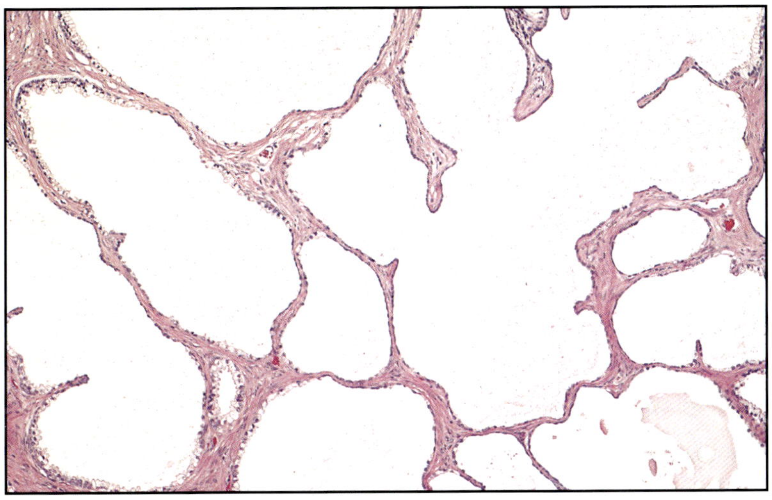

■ **i5.19** *Cystic atrophy with flattened epithelium.*

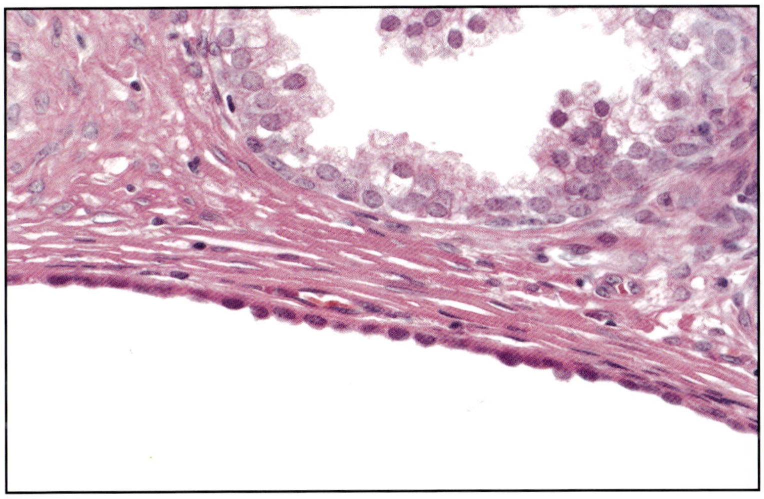

■ **i5.20** *Lining of cystic, atrophic gland (below), compared with that of benign gland with a normal amount of cytoplasm (above).*

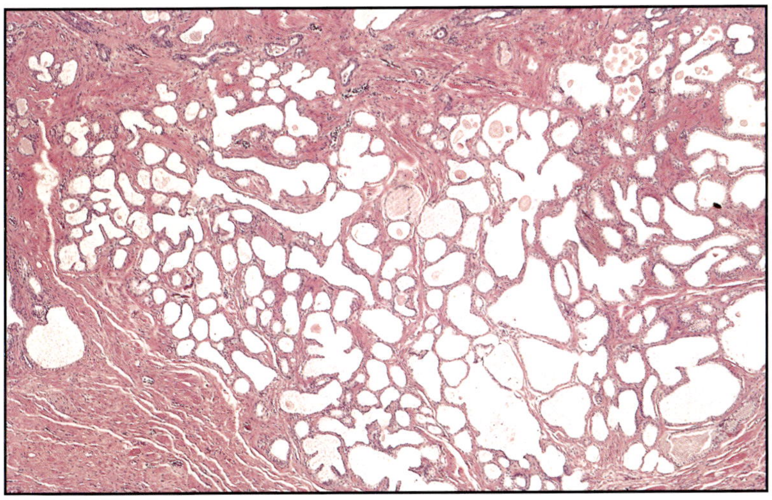

■ **i5.21** *Lobular arrangement of cystic and atrophic prostatic glands in peripheral zone.*

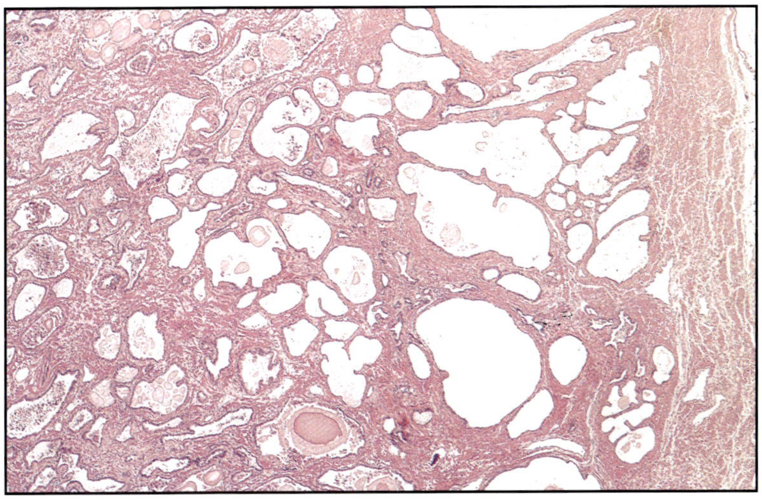

■ **i5.22** *Cystic atrophy with irregularly arranged glands.*

especially in needle biopsy. Such an image may be highly disturbing in needle biopsy, where lobular arrangements may be difficult or impossible to visualize **i5.25**. Yet, cytologically, the lining cells are small and bland; basal cells can be identified in some glands but not in all, owing to nuclear compression and crowding **i5.26**.

Partial atrophy is a variant of atrophy in which the atrophic glands have relatively scant cytoplasm, but the glands appear as a

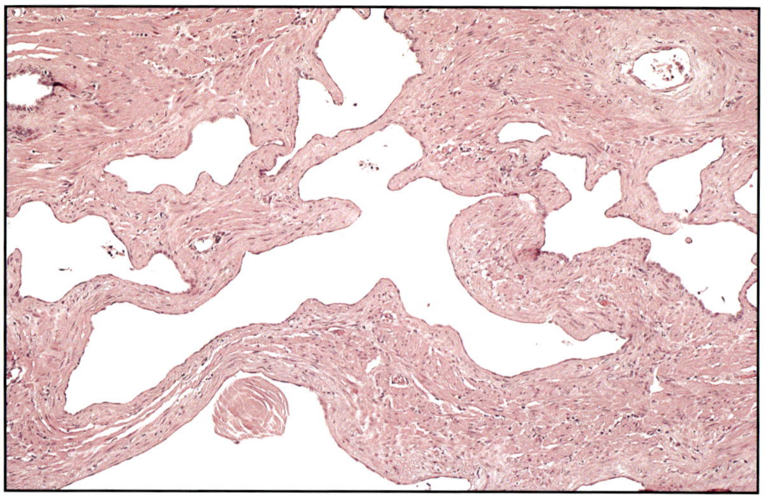

■ **i5.23** *Cystic atrophy with superficial resemblance to dilated vessels.*

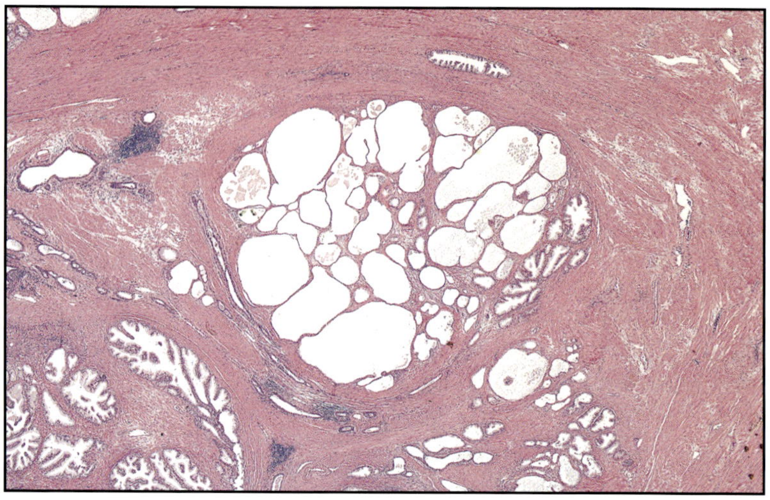

■ **i5.24** *BPH nodule with cystic atrophy.*

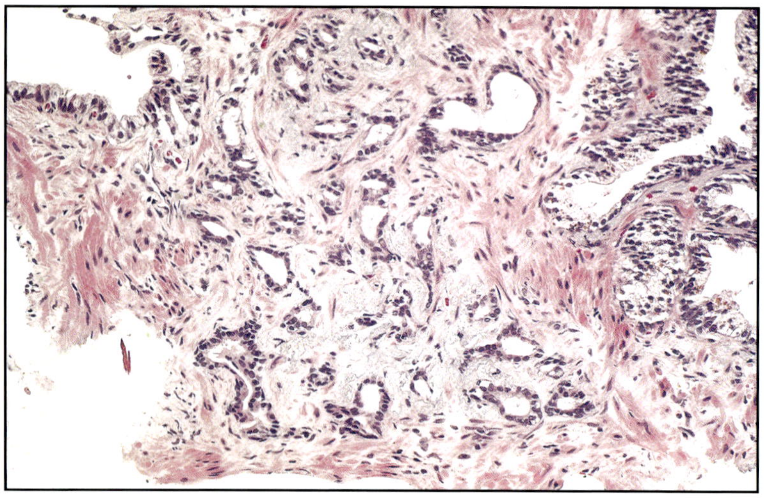

■ **i5.25** *Sclerotic atrophy in needle biopsy tissue. Small distorted, angular glands in a densely sclerotic background.*

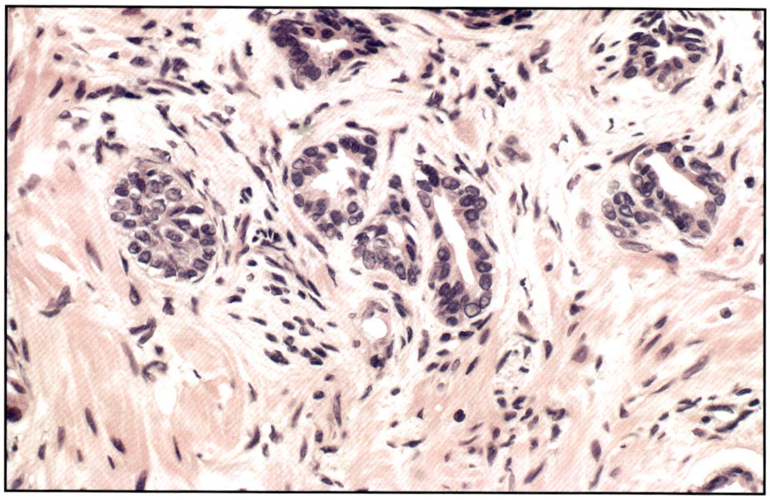

■ **i5.26** *Sclerotic atrophy: Basal cells can be seen in some glands, but are difficult to identify in others.*

crowded collection of pale glands rather than dark glands **t5.5; i5.27-i5.29**. In about one third of needle biopsies with partial atrophy, fully developed atrophy is also present (Oppenheimer 1998). The glandular outlines in partial atrophy vary from straight luminal borders to more undulating luminal surfaces and papillary projections **i5.27**, **i5.28**. A stellate shape is assumed by some glands **i5.30**. Intraluminal pale amorphous debris was observed in 33% of cases but intraluminal wispy blue mucin (blue-tinged mucinous secretions) and crystalloids, which are more often present in malignant than in benign glands, were not seen (Oppenheimer 1998). Nuclear/cytoplasmic ratios are 1:2 for most constituent epithelial cells, compared with 1:1 for fully developed atrophy **i5.29**. The nuclei of these cells are often abnormal, with an elongated, cylindrical shape and with visible nucleoli in one quarter of cases (Oppenheimer 1998).

■ **t5.5** **Partial Atrophy**
Crowded collection of pale glands
Variable gland profiles included undulating, papillary, stellate
Partial cytoplasmic volume loss
Nuclear/cytoplasmic ratios 1:2
Luminal epithelial cell nuclei, elongated and "crinkled"

Postatrophic hyperplasia (PAH) was originally felt to represent atrophic prostatic epithelium that underwent hyperplasia (Franks 1954). Accordingly, another term that has been used for postatrophic hyperplasia is hyperplastic atrophy (Billis 1998). (Of course, it is impossible to prove that this process is atrophy in hyperplastic acini or hyperplasia in atrophy.) Subtyping into categories of lobular hyperplasia and sclerotic atrophy with hyperplasia (postsclerotic hyperplasia) was proposed (Franks 1954) but has not been routinely applied. Postatrophic hyperplasia has an incidence of 2% to 4% in needle biopsy cases (Amin 1999) and of 13% to 78% in whole prostate glands (Billis 1998, Anton 1999, Cheville 1995, Amin 1999, Shah 2001). Most (about 90%) foci are identified in the peripheral zone (Anton 1999, Shah 2001), and this type of atrophy is always found admixed with other types of atrophy (simple and sclerotic) (Billis 1998). In addition, PAH is multicentric in 16% of needle biopsy cases (Amin 1999) and in 44% of whole glands (Cheville 1995).

Microscopically, postatrophic hyperplasia has a lobular outline, with a central duct surrounded by small, fairly regular, and closely packed acini **t5.6; i5.31, i5.32** (Franks 1954). The central "feeder" duct can show some slight cystic change and has a low, atrophic

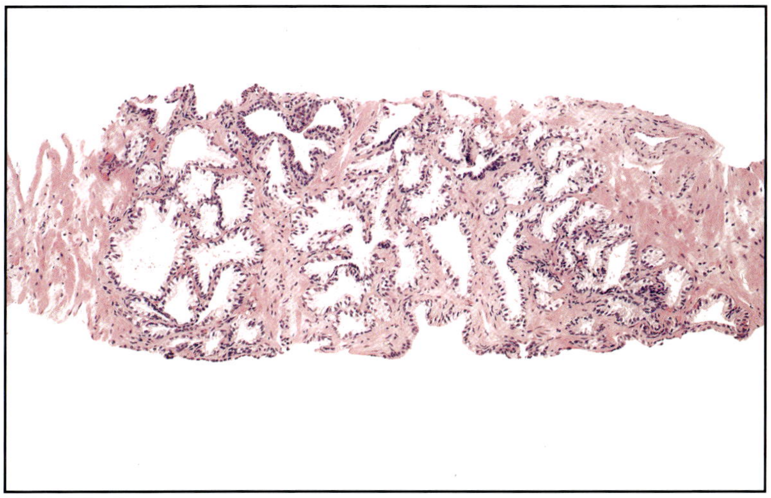

■ **i5.27** *Partial atrophy in needle biopsy tissue: Scanning magnification.*

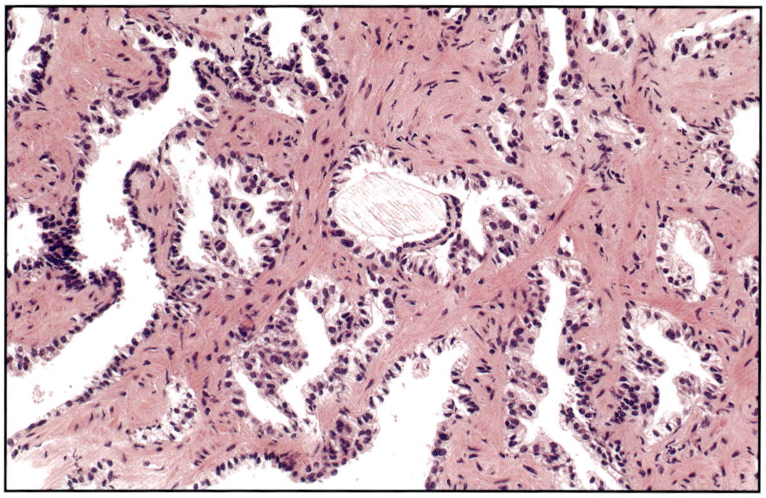

■ **i5.28** *Partial atrophy in needle biopsy tissue. Pale glands with partial cytoplasmic volume loss.*

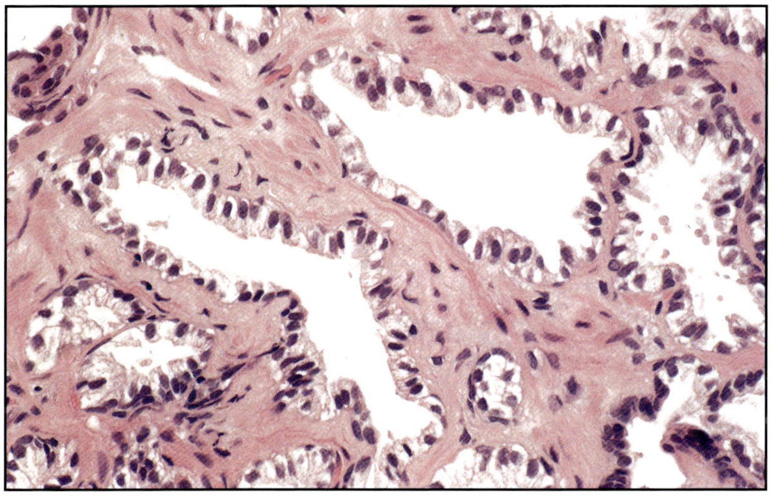

■ **i5.29** *Partial atrophy in needle biopsy tissue: Elongated luminal cell nuclei are oriented perpendicular to luminal surface.*

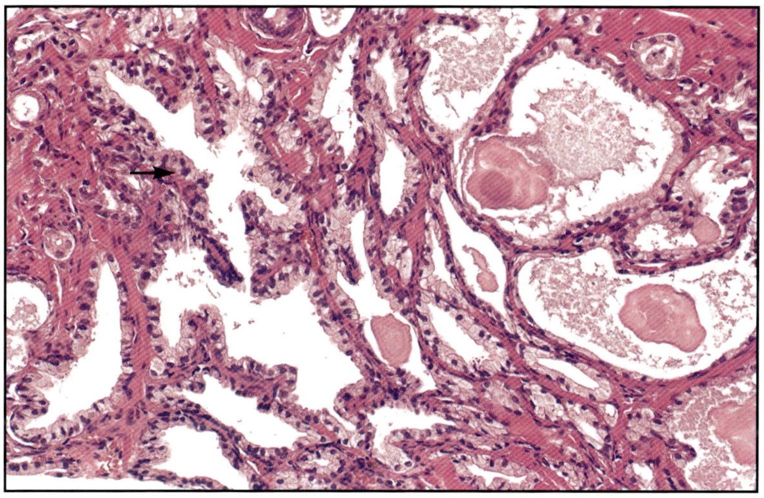

■ **i5.30** *Partial atrophy with crowded pale glands. One has a stellate luminal profile (arrow).*

epithelium. The surrounding, clustered acini number from about 10 to 20 (with a range of 5 to 88) and appear to bud from the central duct (Cheville 1995, Amin 1999). The acini are mainly small and oval to round, but there is variability in size and shape: a minority of acini show cystic change and round, oval, elongated, slit-like, and stellate glands may be observed (Amin 1999). The acinar epithelium is low cuboidal, and the luminal epithelial cell nuclei are mildly enlarged with fine, granular chromatin and small nucleoli (Franks 1954, Cheville 1995). Prominent (>1 μm) nucleoli can be noted in up to 26% of PAH cases, particularly when acute inflammation is present (Ruska 1998). The tinctoral character of the luminal cell cytoplasm is often condensed and basophilic but can be eosinophilic, finely granular to clear (Amin 1999). Basal cells can usually be seen in PAH using H&E stained sections **i5.32**, although, as for other forms of atrophy, their detection becomes difficult (or impossible) when epithelial flattening occurs. Basal cells are highlighted in all foci

■ **t5.6** **Postatrophic Hyperplasia**

Central feeder duct
Surrounding small, regular, closely packed acini
Low cuboidal acinar epithelium
Prominent nucleoli in 26%
Basal cells present
Stromal fibrosis and inflammation

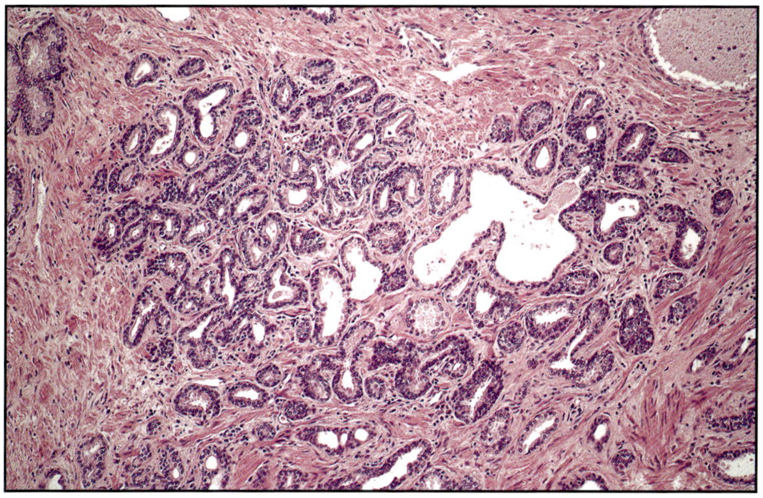

■ **i5.31** *Postatrophic hyperplasia (hyperplastic atrophy): High density collection of small acini with lobular arrangement and slightly dilated central duct.*

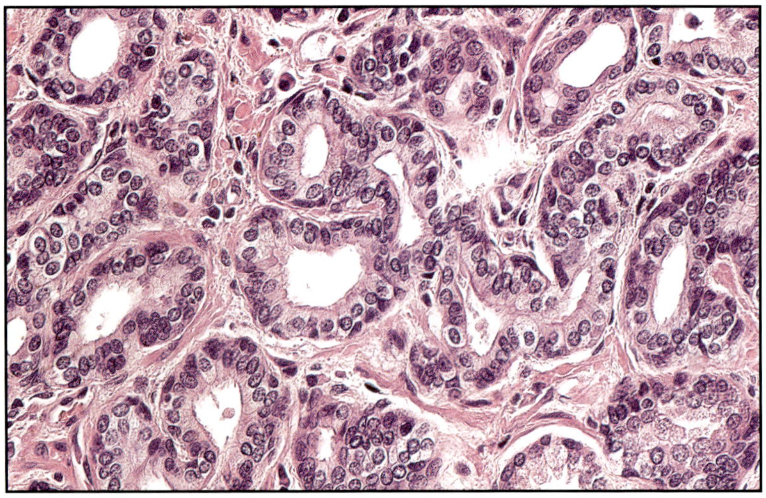

■ **i5.32** *Postatrophic hyperplasia : Round to oval small acini have cuboidal epithelium and two cell layers, with basal cells easily sighted.*

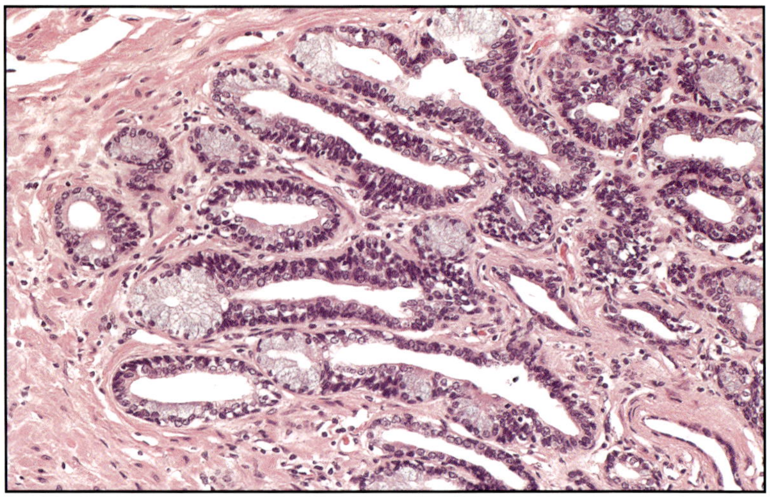

■ **i5.33** *Mucinous metaplasia in postatrophic hyperplasia .*

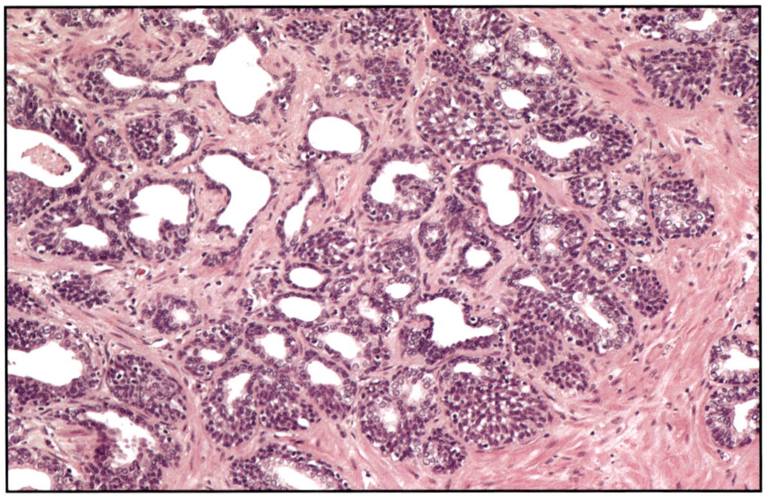

■ **i5.34** *Transitional cell metaplasia in postatrophic hyperplasia .*

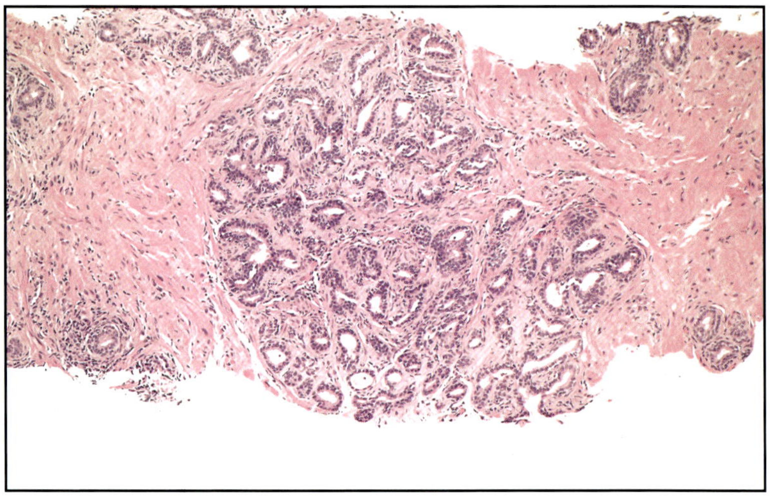

■ **i5.35** *Postatrophic hyperplasia in needle biopsy tissue. Here, there is nearly complete sampling of the lobule.*

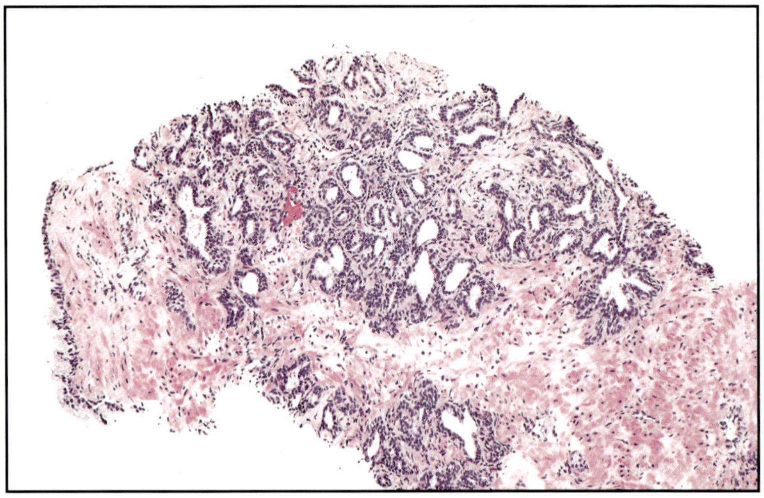

■ **i5.36** *Postatrophic hyperplasia in needle biopsy tissue. Partial sampling of several lobules.*

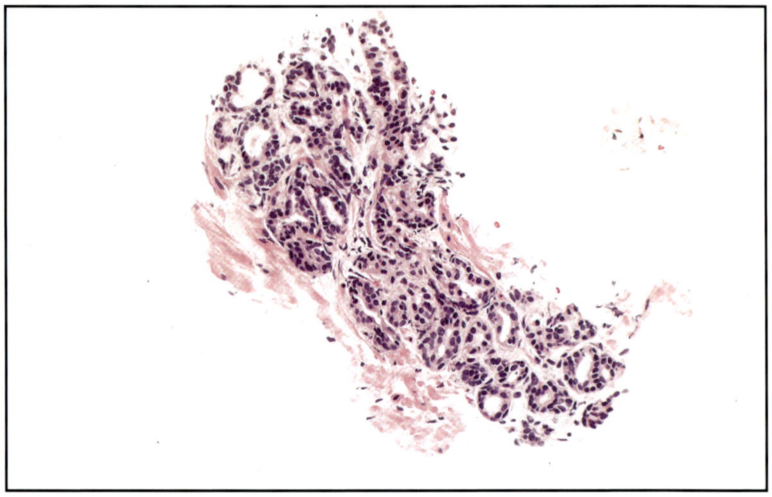

■ **i5.37** *Postatrophic hyperplasia in a small needle core fragment. This focus had been misdiagnosed as adenocarcinoma.*

with use of 34βE12 high-molecular-weight cytokeratin immunostains, although it is important to note that in about one quarter of cases, occasional glands will lack any staining at all (Amin 1999). Glandular lumina often contain corpora amylacea but lack crystalloids and intraluminal wispy blue mucin (Cheville 1995, Amin 1999). Intracytoplasmic blue mucin representing mucinous metaplasia can be found in PAH foci **i5.33**. Basal cell hyperplasia has also been seen in postatrophic hyperplasia (Cheville 1995), as has transitional cell metaplasia **i5.34**. Like all kinds of atrophy, stromal alterations occur commonly in the PAH and vary from smooth muscle atrophy to dense sclerosis (Cheville 1995) and elastosis (Billis 2000). In needle biopsy, lobules of postatrophic hyperplasia may be sampled nearly in toto **i5.35** or partially **i5.36, i5.37**. Complete loss of architectural context in a small biopsy fragment necessitates diagnostic reliance on densely packed small acini with cuboidal to flattened luminal cells, with basal cells identified. Postatrophic hyperplasia contains moderate to severe acute and chronic inflammatory cell infiltrates in 28% to 34% of needle biopsy cases (Ruska 1998). In the whole gland, PAH displays associated chronic inflammation in 43% to 88% of foci (Anton 1999, Shah 2001).

[5.3] Differential Diagnosis

The differential diagnosis of benign prostatic atrophy vs prostatic adenocarcinoma is one of the most important in diagnostic histopathology of the prostate. Other entities in the differential diagnosis with atrophy include basal cell hyperplasia and high-grade PIN. Atrophy is not a multilayered proliferation as is basal cell hyperplasia. Atrophy with prominent nucleoli, which is usually PAH, could be confused with the flat type of high-grade PIN, but flat PIN is usually a focal finding and does not involve entire lobules, as PAH does.

The differential distinction of prostatic atrophy and carcinoma should rely on a collection of light microscopic findings **t5.7, t5.8**. Clinical data, including age, serum prostate significant antigen (PSA) level, digital rectal examination findings, and transrectal ultrasound appearance, do not influence the light microscopic interpretation. The gross appearance in TURP chips and radical prostatectomy cut surfaces is similarly not often of utility, although grossly evident cystic change favors benignancy.

At scanning magnification, one should assess for the retention of a lobular architecture. In needle biopsies, such lobularity may be entirely sampled, partially sampled, or not evident at all. If, at low-power magnification, one detects small, dark acini in a lobular

■ t5.7 Differential Diagnosis: Prostatic Atrophy vs Prostatic Adenocarcinoma

Histologic Feature	Atrophy	Carcinoma
Architecture	Lobular	Infiltrative (except for circumscribed, well-differentiated, Gleason score 2-4 carcinomas)
Low-power image	Cluster of dark, small, acini	Low-grade[1]: aggregate of pale, small acini Intermediate-grade[2]: haphazardly arranged small glands
Luminal cell nuclei	Typically slightly enlarged with small nucleoli[3]	Nucleomegaly and nucleolomegaly
Luminal cell cytoplasm	Scanty to minimal, basophilic	Moderate amount, cleared to amphophilic
Basal cells		
H&E	Present, but may be inconspicuous	Absent
34βE12 IHC[4]	Usually continuous, occasionally fragmented, absent in rare glands	Absent
Luminal contents		
Corpora amylacea	Common	Uncommon
Crystalloids	Rare	May be present
Wispy blue mucin	Rare	May be present
Stromal response		
Sclerosis	Present	Variable
Inflammation	Common	Uncommon

[1]Low-grade carcinoma = well-differentiated, Gleason score 2-4
[2] Intermediate-grade carcinoma = moderately differentiated, Gleason score 5-6. Additional low-power patterns can be seen (Chapter 15)
[3]Prominent nucleoli can be seen in 26% of postatrophic hyperplasia cases (Ruska 1998)
[4]IHC = immunohistochemistry. Antibody 34βE12 binds to high-molecular cell cytokeratins in basal cells and not luminal epithelial cells

■ t5.8 Benign Atrophy vs Atrophic Carcinoma

Histologic Feature	Benign Atrophy	Atrophic Carcinoma*	χ^2	P
Macronucleoli	0/32 (0)	30/32 (94)	52.8	.0
Infiltrative growth	1/32 (3)	31/32 (97)	52.6	.0
Amphophilic cytoplasm	0/32 (0)	29/32 (91)	49.4	.0
Nuclear enlargement	3/32 (9)	27/32 (84)	33.2	.0
Intraluminal amorphous pink material	1/32 (3)	11/32 (34)	8.3	.004
Intraluminal wispy blue mucin	0/32 (0)	8/32 (25)	7	.0
Intraluminal crystalloids	0/32 (0)	6/32 (19)	4.6	.032
Perineural invasion	0/32 (0)	5/32 (16)	3.5	.062
Collagenous micronodules	0/32 (0)	4/32 (13)	2.4	.12
Mitotic figures	0/32 (0)	2/32 (6)	0.5	.47
Associated high-grade prostatic intraepithelial neoplasia	3/32 (9)	6/32 (19)	0.5	.47

*Data (Kaleem 1998) are given as number (percentage)

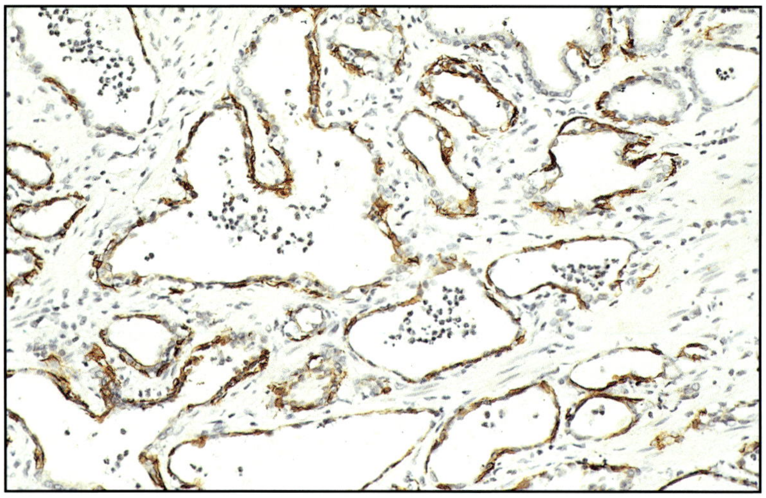

■ **i5.38** *Basal cells identified in inflamed atrophy with variable cystic changes: 34βE12 immunohistochemical stain.*

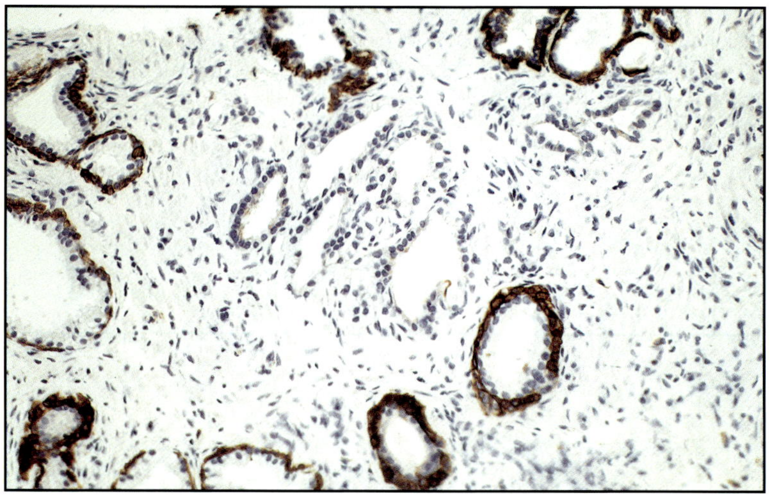

■ **i5.39** *Group of benign atrophic glands with absence of basal cells by 34βE12 immunostain.*

arrangement, this is strong presumptive evidence of atrophy. As prostate needle biopsies should be surveyed with both low- and high-power views, one may then confirm a benign diagnosis at high power, where the presence of basal cells and bland luminal cell nuclei in the setting of significant cytoplasmic volume loss is diagnostic of atrophy. Frequently, however, all architectural orientation is lost in needle biopsies, and the histopathologist is confronted with haphazardly disposed dark acini. The hyperchromasia of the small acini is actually a low-power clue that these might be atrophic glands, because most prostatic carcinomas have a moderate amount of cleared to amphophilic cytoplasm and will not appear as dark as the benign atrophic glands. The dark appearance of the benign atrophic glands is due to the high nuclear/cytoplasmic ratios and basophilic cytoplasm. The architecture can even appear infiltrative owing to small, distorted glands embedded in a fibrous background, as can be found in sclerotic atrophy. These benign glands assume the guise of a small-gland carcinoma that has elicited a fibrogenic response. Prostate cancers are not usually associated with such a stromal response and, in fact, may not manifest any evidence of a stromal sclerotic response. In a case initially misdiagnosed as carcinoma, the atrophic glands in a case of sclerotic atrophy seemed to stream across the width of the needle core **i5.25**. This pattern is most likely to be misdiagnosed as an intermediate-grade Gleason pattern 3 adenocarcinoma. High-power examination of this focus disclosed features of benignancy, ie, small, bland, luminal cell nuclei and basal cells.

A second pattern that can be recognized at low-magnification reconnaissance is that of partial atrophy. Here, instead of dark, small acini of fully developed atrophy, the glands appear pale, owing to only partial loss of cytoplasm. A clue that this represents a benign process is the lobular collection of pale glands, with luminal undulations and papillary infoldings. Secondly, a transition to usual, well-developed atrophy is reassurance that the partial atrophy glands are benign. High-power interrogation of these glands discloses basal cells and occasional, elongated nuclei. Visible nucleoli are allowable in this setting. The differential diagnosis for partial atrophy includes well-differentiated adenocarcinoma, which is, in contrast, a rounded small acinar proliferation without the glandular complexity of either partial atrophy or the recently described pseudohyperplastic prostatic adenocarcinoma (Humphrey 1998). This latter proliferation can have luminal undulations and papillary infoldings, yet totally lacks basal cells and has a high degree of nuclear atypia. In addition, instead of a transition to well-developed atrophy that partial atrophy shows, the transition for pseudohyperplastic prostatic adenocarcinoma is to a small acinar adenocarcinoma (Humphrey 1998).

Another pattern that usually does not cause concern during light microscopic examination at high altitudes is linear and compressed or obliquely sectioned strips of atrophic epithelium. These should not be confused with the cordlike growth of a high-grade prostatic carcinoma. Basal cell presence and bland cytology will confirm benignancy.

Diagnostic traps also await the histopathologist at high-power scrutiny of atrophic glands. First, it has become increasingly apparent that luminal cell nuclear atypia can be observed in atrophy. Although this atypia is usually of a mild degree, with slight nuclear enlargement and small, pinpoint nucleoli, prominent nucleoli, >1 μm in diameter, can be found in postatrophic hyperplasia (Ruska 1998). This is most often a reactive atypia secondary to acute inflammation (Ruska 1998). One should be cautious in diagnosing carcinoma in the setting of inflammation, since this reactive, inflammatory nuclear atypia can, on occasion, simulate the nuclear atypia of carcinoma. Secondly, because of cellular compression and nuclear flattening, basal cells in atrophy can be inconspicuous in H&E stained sections. Here, an immunohistochemical stain for basal cells can be supportive, in the appropriate context, of a diagnosis of atrophy. Most foci of atrophy have a continuous or fragmented basal cell layer by 34βE12 immunolabeling **i5.38**, but a potential diagnostic pitfall is that scattered atrophic glands can be negative for this stain in up to 11% to 23% of cases **i5.39, i5.40** (Amin 1999, Varma 1997, Hedrick 1989). A positive labeling is therefore useful in confirming a diagnostic impression of atrophy, but a negative result, especially in cases in which only a few glands fail to stain and atrophy on the H&E sections is suspected, is noncontributory.

Minor or "soft" diagnostic criteria that favor benign atrophy over carcinoma include the presence of corpora amylacea, stromal fibrosis, and inflammation, and the absence of intraluminal crystalloids and wispy blue mucin **t5.7**. However, these are not absolutely specific findings and should be incorporated into the consideration of all the findings.

Finally, prostatic adenocarcinoma with atrophic features is in the differential diagnosis with benign atrophy. Atrophic change, ie, loss of cytoplasmic volume, can occur in both treated (Reuter 1997) (see

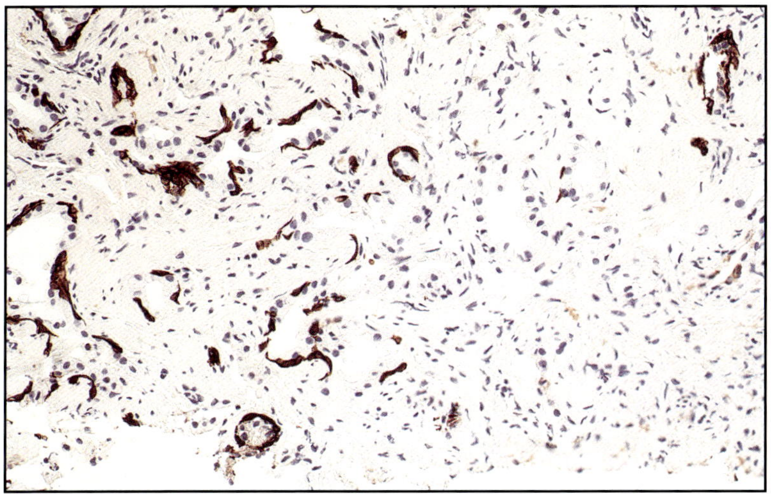

■ **i5.40** *Partial atrophy with failure of 34βE12 immunostain to detect basal cells in several benign atrophic glands (right).*

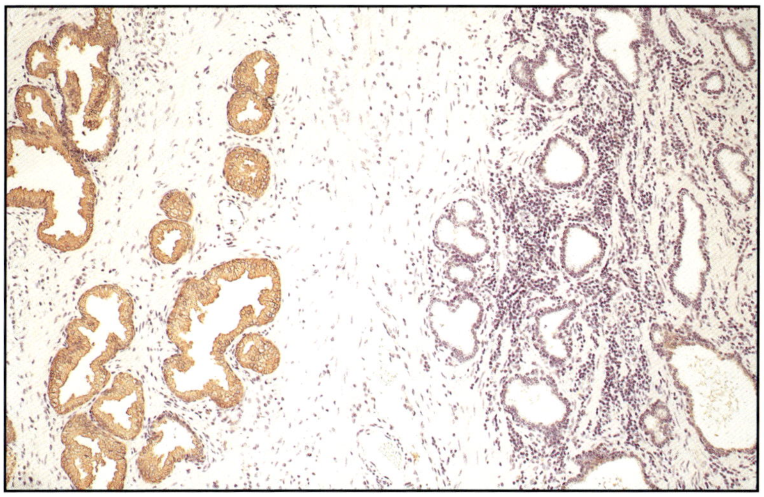

■ **i5.41** *PSA immunolabeling of benign prostatic glands (left), with minimal staining in inflamed, atrophic glands (right).*

chapter 19) and untreated (Cina 1997, Egan 1997, Kaleem 1998) prostatic adenocarcinoma. The features that we found most valuable in the differential separation of benign atrophy from atrophic pattern adenocarcinoma are given in **t5.8**. The absence of infiltrative growth, macronucleoli, and nucleomegaly, and the presence of basal cells were factors with the greatest discriminatory power; whereas the absence of intraluminal amorphous pink material, crystalloids, and wispy blue mucin also favored benign atrophy. Specific for benign atrophy but not of statistical significance due to low-event frequency were the lack of perineural invasion, collagenous micronodules, and mitotic figures **t5.8**.

Special studies other than 34βE12 immunohistochemical staining for basal cells are currently not indicated in addressing the differential diagnosis of benign atrophy vs adenocarcinoma.

[5.4] Biological Significance

Immunohistochemical marker studies have suggested that atrophy in epithelium in the prostate does not necessarily imply biological inactivity. Even though the atrophic epithelium has lost much secretory capacity, as reflected by markedly reduced or absent immunostaining for PSA **i5.41** and prostatic specific acid phosphate (PSAP) (McNeal 1988), the proliferation index of atrophic glands is 2.2 to 11 times that of nonatrophic benign glands (Ruska 1998, Shah 2001, De Marzo 1999, Feneley 1996), and neuroendocrine products are commonly detected (Speights 1994). Furthermore, atrophic glands in the prostate are not actively dying, because the apoptotic rate is low (Ruska 1998, De Marzo 1999, Kaleem 1998).

In the 1950s and 1960s it was speculated that postatrophic hyperplasia might be a precursor to carcinoma (Liavåg 1968, Franks 1954). Recently, proliferative inflammatory atrophy was advanced as a regenerative lesion that was a potential precursor to PIN and carcinoma (De Marzo 1999). The status of atrophy as a potential premalignant condition is currently unsettled (Anton 1999, Cheville 1995, Shah 2001, De Marzo 1999, Billis 2001). Postatrophic hyperplasia has a proliferation index that is intermediate between benign glands and high-grade PIN and demonstrates a gain of chromosome 8c (Shah 2001). Proliferative inflammatory atrophy, compared with normal-appearing nonatrophic epithelium, exhibits a 10.7 median fold increase in Ki-67 proliferation index, increased bcl-2 and GSTP1 staining, and reduced p27Kip1 (De Marzo 1999). These abnormalities are provocative but do not prove a precursor-product relationship. Such a relationship would require multiple lines of evidence including, but not limited to, direct physical continuity, evidence of increased incidence and increasing extent of PAH and PIA in prostate glands harboring carcinoma as opposed to glands that do not, animal models showing PAH and PIA preceding PIN and/or carcinoma, and an increased risk for subsequent detection of PIN and/or carcinoma for patients initially diagnosed with PAH or PIA. The idea that carcinogenesis (and possibly atrophy) in the prostate might be related to oxidative stress secondary to inflammatory cells in the prostate (De Marzo 1999) is, however, attractive. Further research is needed.

References

Amin MB, Tamboli P, Varma M, et al. Post-atrophic hyperplasia of the prostate gland: a detailed analysis of its morphology in needle biopsy specimens. *Am J Surg Pathol* 23:925-931, 1999.

Anton RC, Kattan MW, Chakraborty S, et al. Postatrophic hyperplasia of the prostate. *Am J Surg Pathol* 23:932-936, 1999.

Billis A. Prostatic atrophy: an autopsy study of a histologic mimic of adenocarcinoma. *Mod Pathol* 11:47-54, 1998.

Billis A, Magna LA. Prostate elastosis: a microscopic feature useful for the diagnosis of postatrophic hyperplasia. *Arch Pathol Lab Med* 124:1306-1309, 2000.

Billis A, Magna LA. Inflammatory atrophy of the prostate: prevalence and significance [abstract]. *Mod Pathol* 14:102A, 2001.

Cheville JC, Bostwick DG. Postatrophic hyperplasia of the prostate: a histologic mimic of prostatic adenocarcinoma. *Am J Surg Pathol* 19:1068-1076, 1995.

Cina SJ, Epstein JI. Adenocarcinoma of the prostate with atrophic features. *Am J Surg Pathol* 21:287-295, 1997.

De Marzo AM, Marchi VL, Epstein JI, et al. Proliferative inflammatory atrophy of the prostate: implications for prostatic carcinogenesis. *Am J Pathol* 155:1985-1992, 1999.

Egan AJM, Lopez-Beltran A, Bostwick DG. Prostatic adenocarcinoma with atrophic features: malignancy mimicking a benign process. *Am J Surg Pathol* 21:931-935, 1997.

Emmett JL, Braasch WF. Cysts of the prostate gland. *J Urol* 36:236-249, 1936.

Epstein JI, Walsh PC, Sanfilippo F. Clinical and cost impact of second-opinion pathology: review of prostate biopsies prior to radical prostatectomy. *Am J Surg Pathol* 20:851-857, 1996.

Feneley MR, Young MPA, Chinyama C, et al. Ki-67 expression in early prostate cancer and associated pathological lesions. *J Clin Pathol* 49:741-748, 1996.

Franks LM. Atrophy and hyperplasia in the prostate proper. *J Pathol Bacteriol* 68:617-621,1954.

Gardner WA Jr, Culberson DE. Atrophy and proliferation in the young adult prostate. *J Urol* 137:53-56, 1987.

Hedrick L, Epstein JI. Use of keratin 903 as an adjunct in the diagnosis of prostate carcinoma. *Am J Surg Pathol* 13:389-396, 1989.

Humphrey PA, Kaleem Z, Swanson PE, et al. Pseudohyperplastic prostatic adenocarcinoma. *Am J Surg Pathol* 22:1239-1246, 1998.

Jones EC, Young RH. The differential diagnosis of prostatic carcinoma: its distinction from premalignant and pseudocarcinomatous lesions of the prostate gland. *Am J Clin Pathol* 101:48-64, 1994.

Kaleem Z, Swanson PE, Vollmer RT, et al. Prostatic adenocarcinoma with atrophic features: a study of 202 consecutive, completely-embedded radical prostatectomy specimens. *Am J Clin Pathol* 109:695-703, 1998.

Liavåg I. Atrophy and regeneration in the pathogenesis of prostatic carcinoma. *Acta Pathol Microbiol Scand* 73:338-350, .

McNeal JE. Normal histology of the prostate. *Am J Surg Pathol* 12:619-633, 1988.

Moore RA. The evolution and involution of the prostate gland. *Am J Pathol* 12:599-624, 1936.

Oppenheimer JR, Wills ML, Epstein JI. Partial atrophy in prostate needle cores: another diagnostic pitfall for the surgical pathologist. *Am J Surg Pathol* 22:440-445, 1998.

Reuter VE. Pathological changes in benign and malignant tissue following androgen deprivation therapy. *Urology* 49(suppl 5):16-22, 1997.

Ruska KM, Sauvageot J, Epstein JI. Histology and cellular kinetics of prostatic atrophy. *Am J Surg Pathol* 22:1073-1077, 1998.

Shah R, Mucci NR, Amin A, et al. Postatrophic hyperplasia of the prostate gland: neoplastic precursor or innocent bystander? *Am J Pathol* 158:1767-1773, 2001.

Speights VO Jr, Cohen MK, Coffield KS, et al. Neuroendocrine staining in malignant, hyperplastic, and atrophic prostate tissue. *Appl Immunohistochem Mol Morphol* 2:212-217, 1994.

Thorson P, Swanson PE, Humphrey PA. Basal cell proliferations in needle biopsies of the peripheral zone of the prostate gland [abstract]. *Mod Pathol* 12:108A, 1999.

Varma M, Amin MB, Linden MD, et al. Discriminant staining patterns of small glandular and preneoplastic lesions of the prostate using high molecular weight cytokeratin (HMCK): a study of 301 consecutive needle biopsies [abstract]. *Mod Pathol* 10:93A, 1997.

Young RH. Pseudoneoplastic lesions of the urinary bladder, prostate gland, and urethra. In: Wick MR, Humphrey PA, Ritter JH, eds. *Pathology of Pseudoneoplastic Lesions*. New York: Lippincott-Raven; 223-224, 1997.

Metaplasia

[6.1] Squamous Cell Metaplasia **115**

[6.2] Transitional Cell Metaplasia **119**

[6.3] Mucinous Metaplasia **121**

[6.4] Paneth Cell–Like Metaplasia **122**

[6.5] Nephrogenic Metaplasia (Adenoma) and Stromal Metaplasia **123**

CHAPTER 6

M*etaplasia,* from the Greek *metaplasis,* means transformation (SMD 1976). This transformation is a change in cell type rather than neoplastic transformation. Although *metaplasia* has been used to describe divergent differentiation in malignancy, we use it here to refer to change in cell type in benign prostatic cells. In the prostate, it is epithelium that undergoes metaplastic change, and the metaplasia may involve prostatic glandular epithelium or epithelium of the prostatic urethra. Urothelial metaplasias are discussed in Chapter 23. Metaplastic change usually is secondary to inflammation, alteration in the hormonal milieu, or injury. Metaplasias can also occur as a result of therapy, such as hormonal therapy, radiation therapy, transurethral resection of the prostate (TURP), and cryosurgery. (See Chapter 19.) I have also seen squamous metaplastic epithelium adjacent to needle biopsy tracks. Four major categories of prostatic glandular cell metaplasia are presented: squamous cell metaplasia, transitional cell metaplasia, mucinous metaplasia, and Paneth cell–like metaplasia. The diagnostic significance of metaplasia resides in its pseudoneoplastic status. That is, it is possible to mistake some forms of metaplasia for neoplastic growth. These metaplastic proliferations are not precursors for prostatic carcinoma and do not constitute a risk factor for detection of carcinoma.

[6.1] Squamous Cell Metaplasia

The most common clinical settings for the occurrence of squamous cell metaplasia in the nontreated prostate are prostatitis and benign prostatic hyperplasia (BPH). Histologically, squamous cell metaplasia is most often an incidental finding associated with inflammation and infarction in BPH nodules. Inflammation and BPH, with or without infarction, can elevate serum prostate-specific antigen (PSA) levels (Brawn 1994, Humphrey 1998, Nadler 1995) and prompt needle biopsy, leading to detection of squamous cell metaplasia. The incidence of squamous cell metaplasia varies from 5% to 94%, depending on the type of tissue sample and the clinical and histologic context (Culp 1939, Golden 1953, Kasman 1933, Moore 1943, Mostofi 1951, Nanson 1950, Roth 1949, Spiro 1974) **t6.1**. The incidence in core needle biopsies was 5% (Helpap 1995), and the highest incidence was in the setting of BPH with infarction, where the incidence varied from 37% to 94%. The specimen type for this latter figure was not specified.

Treatment generally produces a higher incidence of squamous cell metaplasia than in nontreated glands, with the exception of infarcts **t6.1**. Surgical, medical, and radiation treatments can all induce squamous cell metaplasia (Andriole 1994, Bainborough 1952, Borkowski 1996, Bostwick 1982, Civantos 1995, Montironi 1996, Shabaik 1995, Sheaff 1997, Vaillancourt 1996). For patients who underwent repeat TURP for BPH, 52% had squamous cell metaplastic epithelium in the second set of TURP chips (Sutton 1943), and squamous cell metaplasia was noted in 21% to 23% of needle biopsies after cryosurgery (Borkowski 1996, Shabaik 1995). The incidence of squamous cell metaplasia after radiation therapy is quite high at about 60%, although it has been claimed that it is nonexistent after irradiation (Dhom 1982, Helpap 1995). Similarly, it has been written that squamous cell metaplasia is focal and rare in hormone-treated prostate glands (Armas 1994), but others report an incidence of around 30% to 50% (Civantos 1995, Vaillancourt 1996). These differences probably result from the definition of squamous cell metaplasia, where "mature" squamous cell metaplasia with overt keratinization may be uncommon after therapy but where "immature" squamous cell metaplasia, usually seen in association with basal cell prominence and hyperplasia, is common (Reuter 1997).

Squamous cell metaplastic epithelium in the prostate is not grossly evident (Sutton 1943). Microscopically, the presence of small, solid nests with admixed inflammation is one low-magnification clue to the presence of squamous cell metaplasia **i6.1, i6.2**. This is usually a focal finding unless the patient has been treated. Glands may be partially or completely involved by squamous cell metaplasia **i6.1-i6.5**. Sometimes only a small glandular lumen persists **i6.5**. The involved glands can be atrophic **i6.2, i6.3**. At higher-power scrutiny, intercellular bridges and an eosinophilic, squamoid cytoplasm are indicators of squamous cell metaplasia **i6.4, i6.5**. So-called immature squamous cell metaplasia has much less squamoid cytoplasm **i6.6**. Keratin pearls can be found but are unusual (Sutton 1943). The metaplastic epithelium can occasionally

t6.1 Incidence of Prostatic Squamous Metaplasia

Specimen type	Prior Treatment	Incidence	Reference(s)
Needle biopsy	None	5%	Helpap 1995
Needle biopsy with infarct	None	93%	Milford 2000
TURP[1] chips	None	16%	Sutton 1943
TURP chips with infarct	None	37%[2]	Sutton 1943
Radical prostatectomy	None	2-12%	Civantos 1995, Vaillancourt 1996
Cystoprostatectomy	None	8%	Sheaff 1997
Whole gland: autopsy	None	2%	Kahler 1939
TURP chips	TURP	52%	Sutton 1943
Needle biopsy	Cryosurgery	21-23%	Shabaik 1995, Borkowski 1996
Needle biopsy, cystoprostatectomy	Radiation	59-63%	Bostwick 1982, Sheaff 1997
Radical prostatectomy	Hormonal[3]	28-53%	Civantos 1995, Vaillancourt 1996

[1]TURP = transurethral resection of the prostate
[2]In one series (Mostofi 1951), up to 94% of infarcts had adjacent squamous metaplasia but specimen type was not given in this study
[3]Hormonal treatment = Neoadjuvant pre-operative androgen deprivation therapy using leuprolide, an LHRH agonist, and flutamide, an antiandrogen

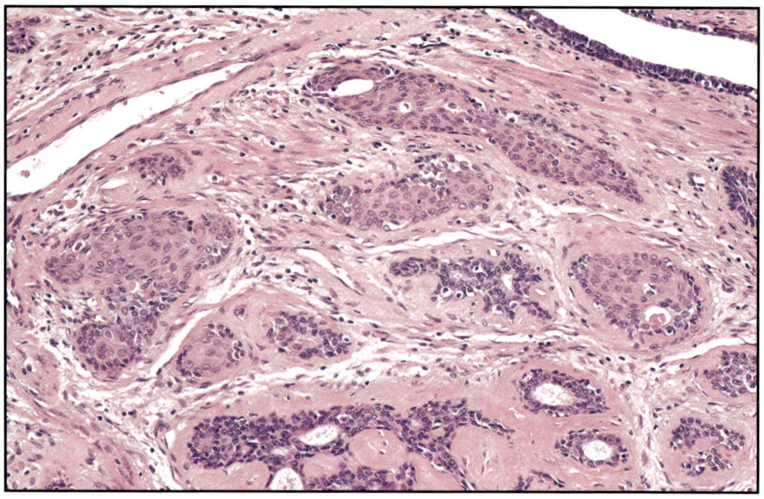

■ **i6.1** *Nests of squamous metaplasia in the prostate.*

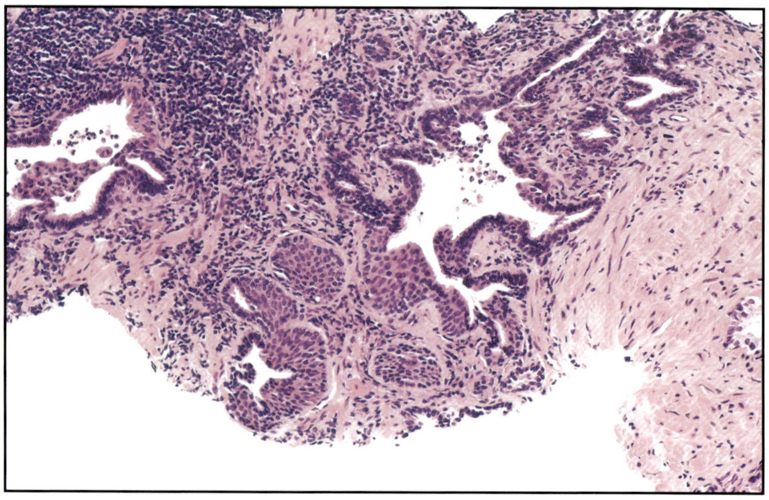

■ **i6.2** *Needle biopsy tissue with focal squamous metaplasia and chronic inflammation.*

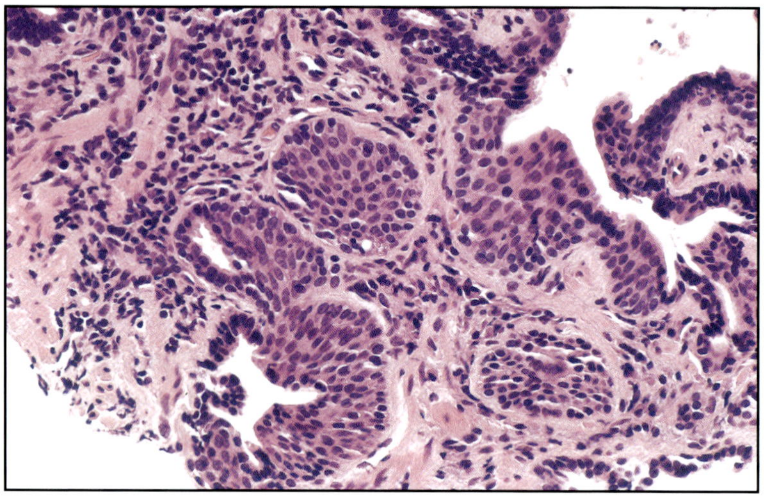

■ **i6.3** *Needle biopsy tissue with focal squamous metaplasia : Higher-power view of small, solid nests admixed with partial involvement of inflamed, atrophic glands.*

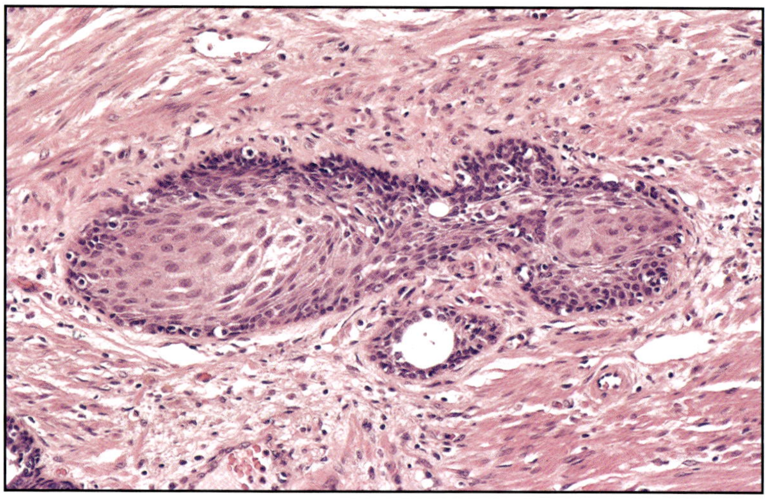

■ **i6.4** *Larger solid nest of squamous metaplasia.*

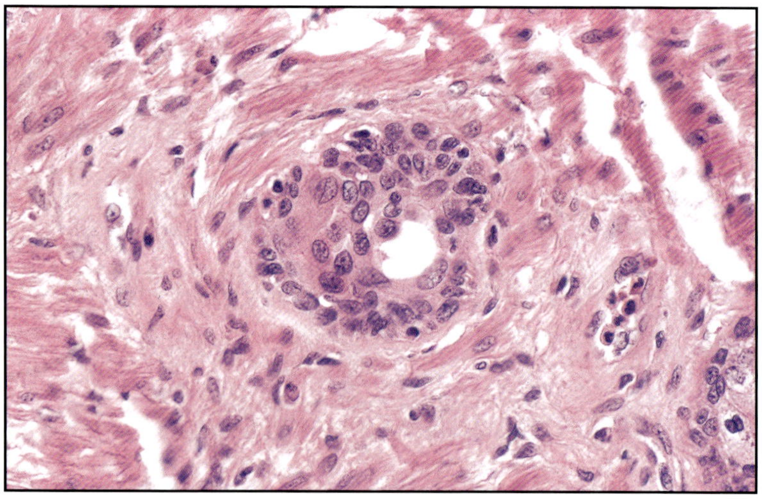

■ **i6.5** *Squamous metaplasia with near complete gland replacement. There is a variable amount of eosinophilic, squamoid cytoplasm.*

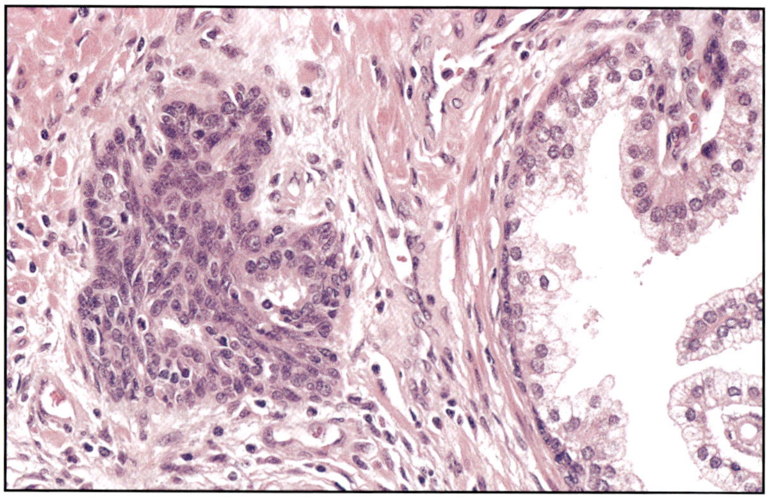

■ **i6.6** *Squamous metaplasia with little eosinophilic cytoplasm (left) versus normal-appearing gland (right).*

surround corpora amylacea (Sutton 1943). Squamous cell metaplasia can also be found lining large, central prostatic ducts containing stones and cellular debris **i6.7**. Finally, inflamed and disrupted glands can form slitlike spaces lined by a thinned squamous cell metaplastic epithelium **i6.8**, which could represent an attempt at reparative reepithelialization.

Squamous cell metaplasia associated with infarcts is first seen at about 4 days as a reactive rim immediately adjacent to infarcted,

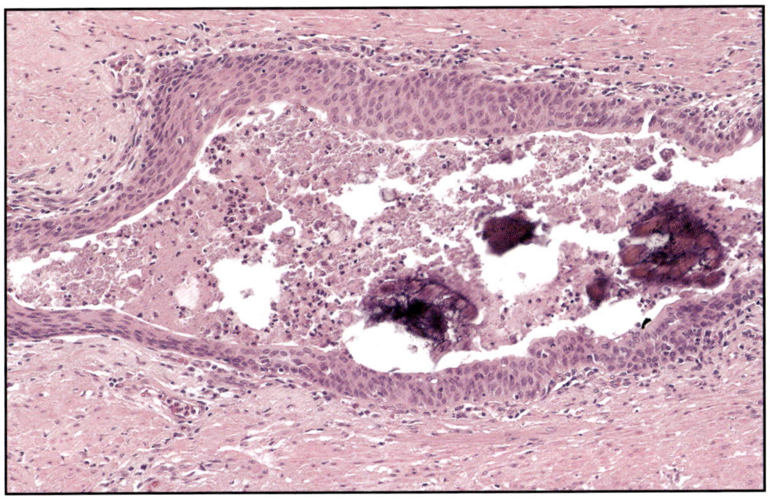

■ **i6.7** *Squamous metaplasia in large prostatic duct which has several calcified prostatic calculi.*

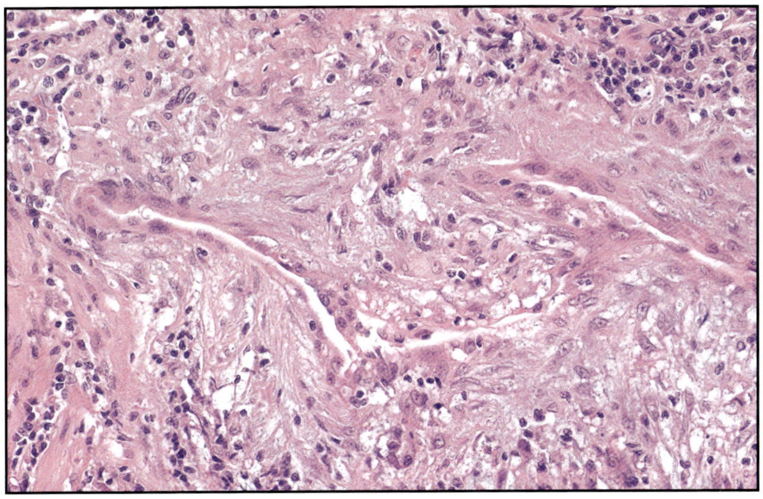

■ **i6.8** *Squamous metaplasia: A thinned metaplastic epithelium in inflamed, disrupted glands with slit-like luminal spaces and with periglandular fibrosis.*

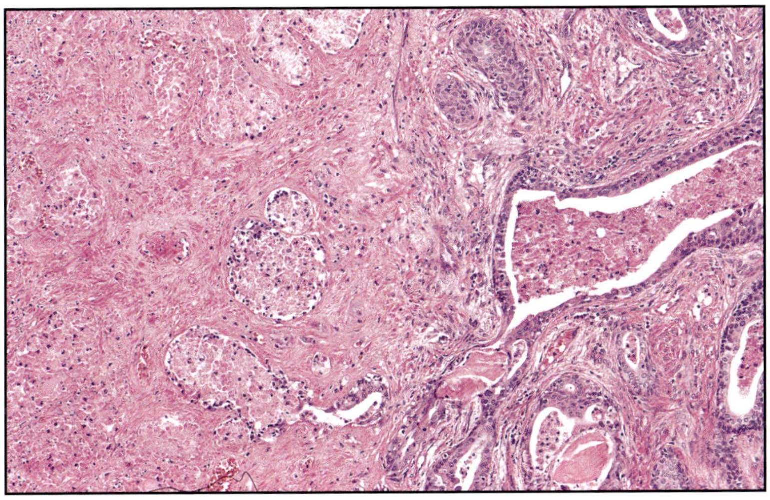

■ **i6.9** *Squamous metaplasia immediately adjacent to infarct (left).*

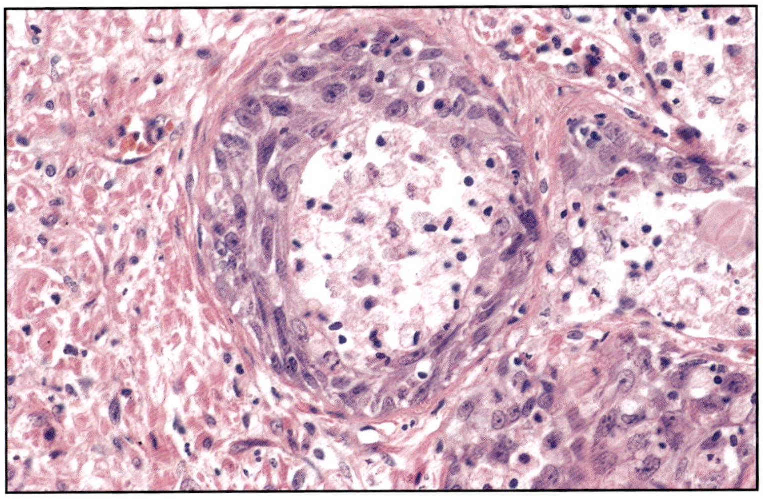

■ **i6.10** *Squamous metaplasia with central degenerated cells.*

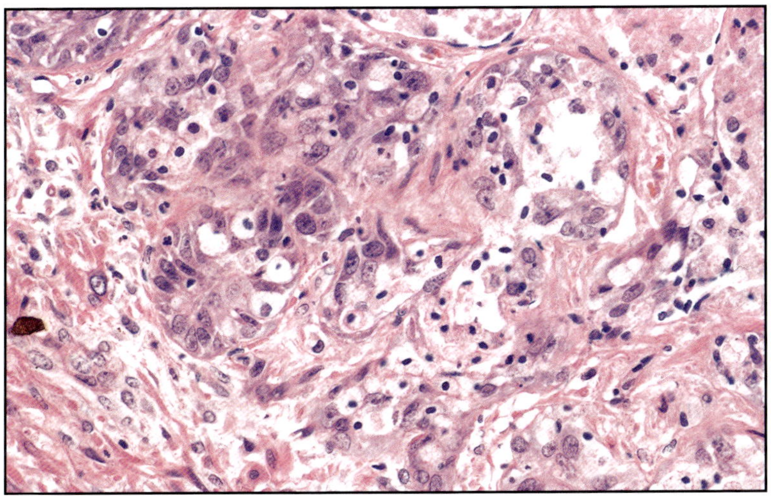

■ **i6.11** *Disrupted and distorted glands with squamous metaplasia should not be diagnosed as invasive carcinoma.*

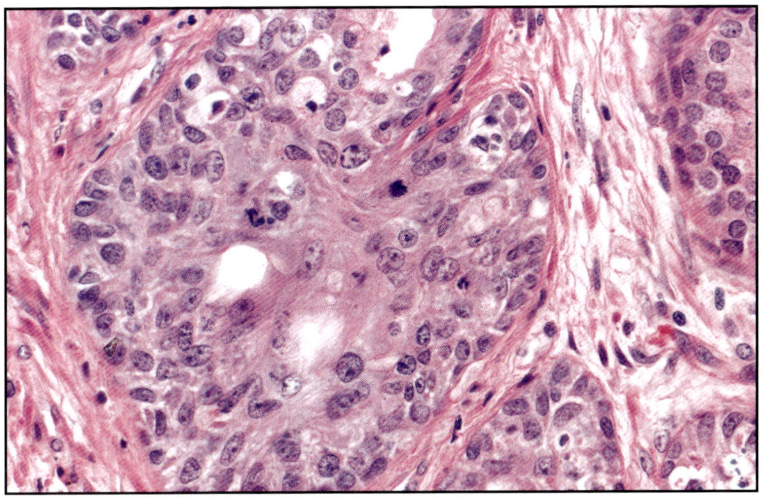

■ **i6.12** *Nuclear atypia with nucleoli in squamous metaplasia.*

hyperplastic tissue **i6.9**. Here the metaplastic epithelium is arranged as irregularly shaped, solid islands, partially involved glands, nests with central degenerated cells **i6.10**, and distorted groups **i6.11**. The cells are polygonal and often pavemented, with distinct intercellular borders. The cytoplasm is acidophilic or vacuolated, with large nuclei (Mostofi 1951). True macronucleoli can be seen **i6.12, i6.13**, along with squamous cell cytologic atypia and mitotic figures (Milford 2000). With healing, the necrotic tissue is replaced by fibrous tissue, which

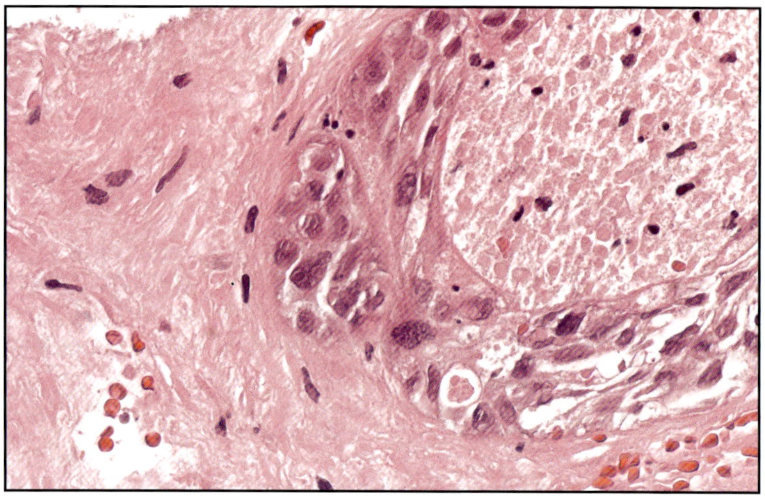

■ **i6.13** *Nest of squamous metaplasia adjacent to infarct seen in needle biopsy tissue. There is nuclear atypia. The central debris should not be mistaken for comedo necrosis of Gleason grade 5 comedocarcinoma.*

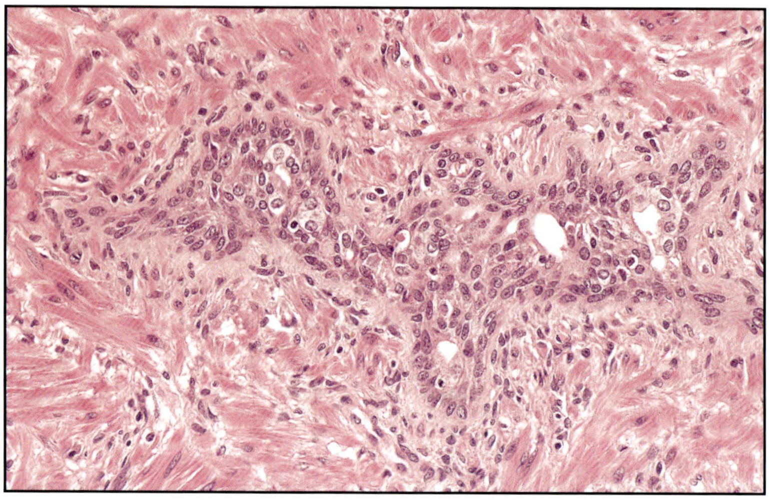

■ **i6.14** *Squamous metaplasia, immature type, posthormonal therapy.*

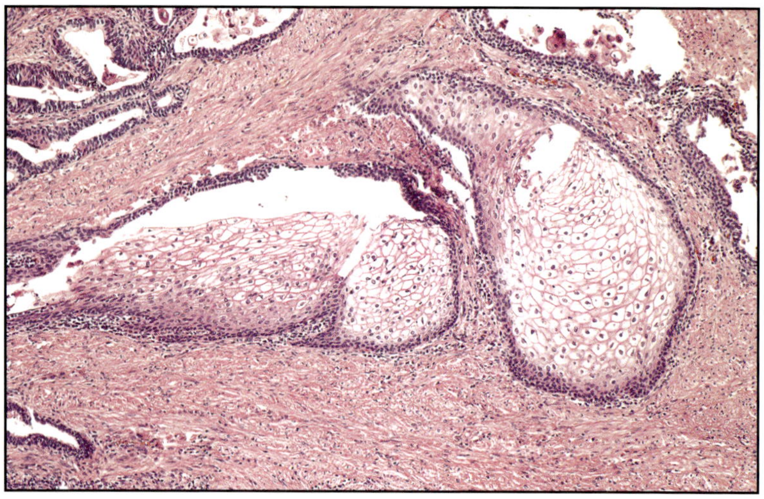

■ **i6.15** *Squamous metaplasia, mature glycogenated type, postestrogen therapy.*

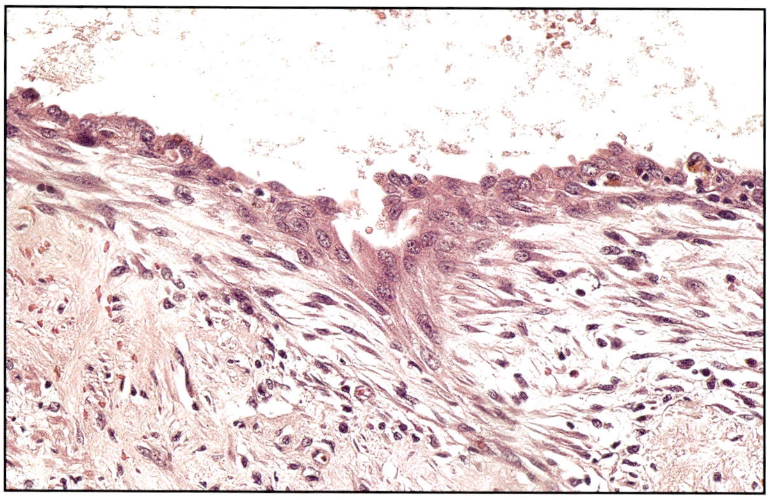

■ **i6.16** *Squamous metaplasia in gland adjacent to needle biopsy tract.*

can contain persistent solid or acinar nests of metaplastic cells (Mostofi 1951).

Squamous cell metaplasia induced by radiation and hormonal therapy often is of the immature type (Têtu 1991, Vaillancourt 1996), with less abundant, nonglycogenated cytoplasm, larger nuclei, and absence of keratinization **i6.14**. An exception to this is use of estrogen as hormonal therapy (a common form of prostate cancer therapy in the past), which can cause diffuse squamous cell metaplasia with glycogenated cytoplasm and small, shrunken nuclei (Bainborough 1952, Nanson 1950) **i6.15**. Prostatic urethral urothelium and prostatic ducts and acini can also be involved by such glycogenated mature squamous cell metaplasia (Bainborough 1952, Nanson 1950, Têtu 1991). Previous needle biopsy can induce a squamous cell metaplastic response in glands entrapped or immediately adjacent to the fibrous needle track **i6.16**.

The differential diagnosis of squamous cell metaplasia centers on carcinoma, and mainly squamous cell carcinoma **t6.2**. Squamous cell carcinoma does occur in the prostate, but it is rare (Randolph 1997) and should be diagnosed with caution (Culp 1939). In the first half of the last century, it was recognized that prostatic squamous cell metaplasia could easily be misdiagnosed as carcinoma (Culp 1939, Mostofi 1951). Indeed, in one series of 47 cases of metaplasia adjacent to an infarct, 10 (21%) had been diagnosed as carcinoma (Mostofi 1951). Diagnostic difficulties arise if reactive, metaplastic squamous epithelium is viewed out of context. Therefore, if inflammation or an adjacent infarct is ignored and reactive, metaplastic squamous epithelium is studied at high-power magnification, the reactive, nuclear atypia could be misinterpreted as evidence of malignancy. Architecturally, the nests of metaplastic squamous epithelium adjacent to infarcts may appear to be arranged in a disordered way, but infiltration into tissue surrounding the reactive rim does not occur (Mostofi 1951). Also, the individual metaplastic cells do not show anaplasia, hyperchromatism, or abnormal mitotic figures (Mostofi 1951). Prominent nucleoli in this situation should not be misconstrued

■ **t6.2 Squamous Metaplasia of Prostate**

Usual setting: Inflammation, infarcts, posttreatment

"Mature" form: Glycogenated cytoplasm and small, shrunken nuclei

"Immature" form: Less abundant, amphophilic cytoplasm, larger nuclei, and occasional macronucleoli

Differential diagnosis vs squamous cell carcinoma: No infiltration, no nuclear anaplasia or hyperchromasia, no atypical mitoses

■ **t6.3 Incidence of Prostatic Transitional Cell Metaplasia**

Specimen type	Prior Treatment	Incidence	Reference
Needle biopsy	None	6%	Helpap 1995
Needle biopsy	None	34%	Yantiss 1997
Radical prostatectomy	None	3%	Civantos 1995
Radical prostatectomy	Hormonal[1]	59%	Civantos 1995

[1]Hormonal therapy: Neoadjuvant pre-operative androgen deprivation therapy with an LHRH agonist (leuprolide) and flutamide, an antiandrogen

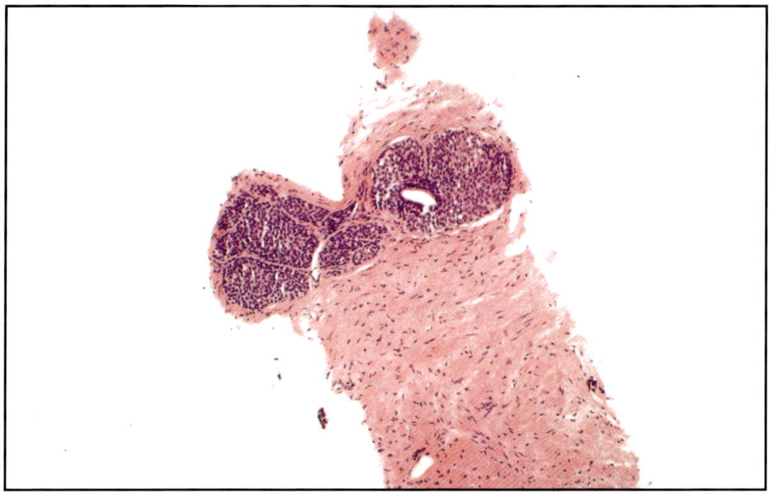

■ **i6.17** *Transitional cell metaplasia in needle biopsy: Solid nests, with of one glandular lumen.*

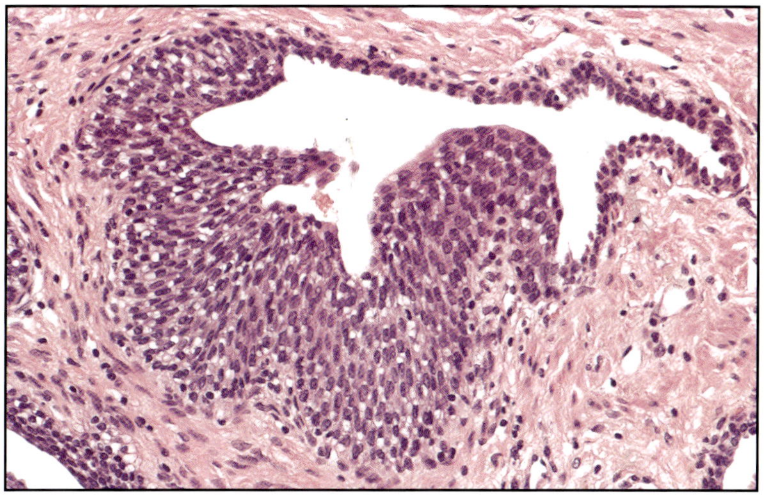

■ **i6.18** *Transitional cell metaplasia: Partial gland involvement.*

as evidence of malignancy. In the framework of treatment effect, there is even a greater diagnostic conundrum because glandular disarray, squamous epithelial cell cytologic atypia, and fibrosis can be found. For example, interpretation of prostate needle biopsies after radiation therapy can be difficult because almost every case with squamous cell metaplasia had cytologic atypia (Bostwick 1982). Immunohistochemical evaluation using antibody 34βE12 can be invaluable in difficult cases to confirm the presence of immature squamous cell metaplasia in these patients after radiation treatment (Brawer 1989, Shabaik 1995). Other special studies are not of diagnostic relevance but have proven loss of ability of the metaplastic squamous cells to synthesize PSA and PSAP (Lager 1988, Shabaik 1995). The proliferation index of squamous cell metaplasia is 4.3% (Helpap 1975), consistent with a weakly proliferative process and the observation of rare mitoses. By electron microscopy, prostatic squamous cell metaplastic cells have ultrastructural features of squamous differentiation, such as tonofibrils, broad desmosomes, and glycogen deposits (Kastendieck 1975).

[6.2] Transitional Cell Metaplasia

Transitional cells, that is, urothelial cells, normally line the prostatic urethra and extend for a variable distance into the main prostatic ducts (McNeal 1988) (Chapter 1). Because of this variability, there can be difficulty in determining whether a transitional cell proliferation represents a variation of normal anatomy or a metaplastic process. There is wide variation in the reported incidence of transitional cell metaplasia, from 3% to 34% (Civantos 1995, Helpap 1975, Yantiss 1997) **t6.3**. The development of transitional cell metaplasia may be related to damage or androgen deprivation because about one third of cases are associated with inflammation (Yantiss 1997), and transitional cell metaplasia has been detected adjacent to infarcts (Mostofi 1951), after cryosurgery (Borkowski 1996), and after androgen deprivation hormonal therapy (Civantos 1995). No clinical or radiologic findings are specific for transitional cell metaplasia. It is usually a focal, incidental histologic finding. It has a low proliferation index of 0.3% (Helpap 1975) and no premalignant potential.

Histologically, usually only a few glands are involved in a single focus **i6.17** (Yantiss 1997), but extent ranges from partial gland involvement **i6.18** to more florid gland involvement **i6.19, i6.20**. At low magnification the glands are eye-catching because they are hypercellular and therefore appear dark. Small, solid nests are commonly noted, but often there is preservation of a small central lumen **i6.21**. The glands exhibit proliferation of elongated cells beneath a bland-appearing luminal secretory cell layer **t6.4; i6.22**. The nuclei are elongated and are arranged perpendicularly to the basal membrane. Because of the elongation and stratification, the cells can appear to stream toward the luminal surface **i6.22**. At high power, the elongated nuclei have frequent nuclear grooves, and the faint eosinophilic cytoplasm exhibits frequent perinuclear clearing (Yantiss 1997) **i6.22, i6.23**. The nuclei are cytologically small and bland, with inconspicuous nucleoli and little to no mitotic activity.

The most important entity in the differential diagnosis is prostatic intraepithelial neoplasia (PIN). Transitional cell metaplasia can grow as PIN does, with tufted and micropapillary architectures. Yet high-grade PIN shows appreciable nuclear enlargement and usually nucleolomegaly. Also, the nuclei in high-grade

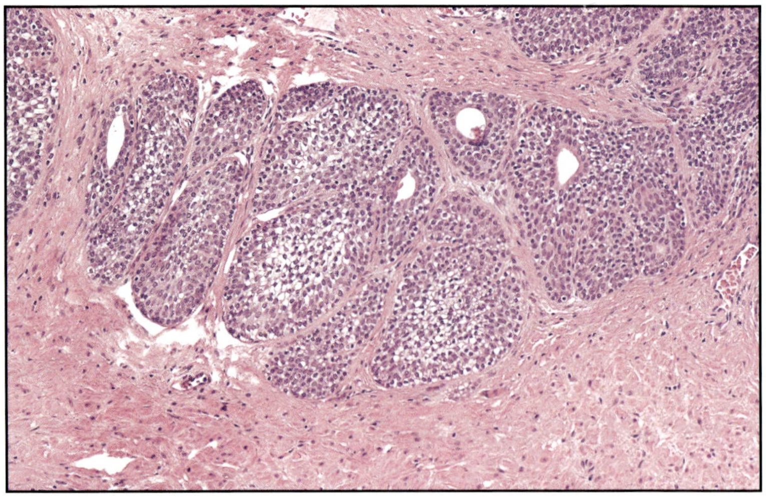

■ **i6.19** *Numerous glands involved by transitional cell metaplasia.*

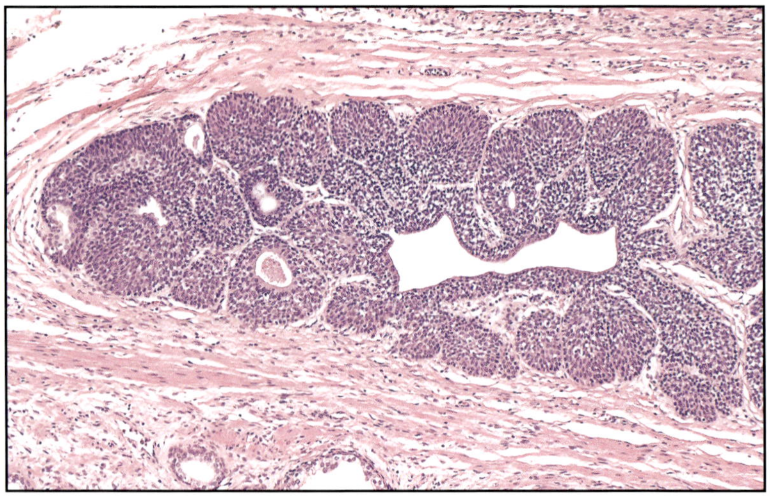

■ **i6.20** *Cloverleaf-like pattern of transitional cell metaplasia involvement of acini around a central duct.*

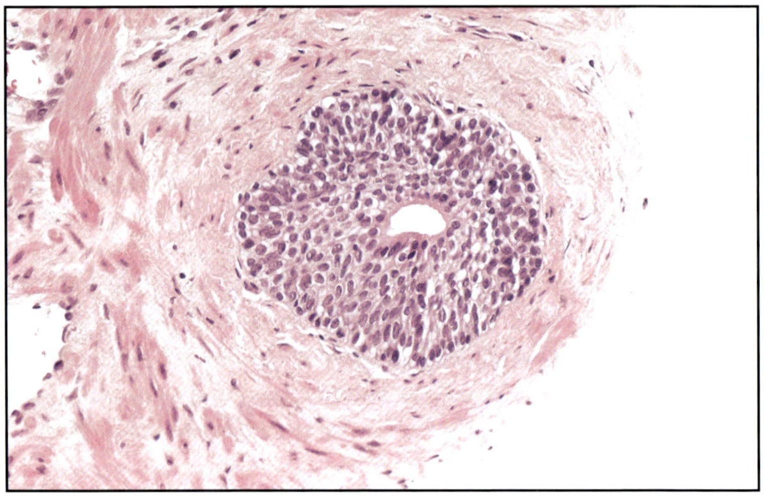

■ **i6.21** *Transitional cell metaplasia in needle biopsy: Multilayered, elongated transitional cells with preservation of a small, central lumen.*

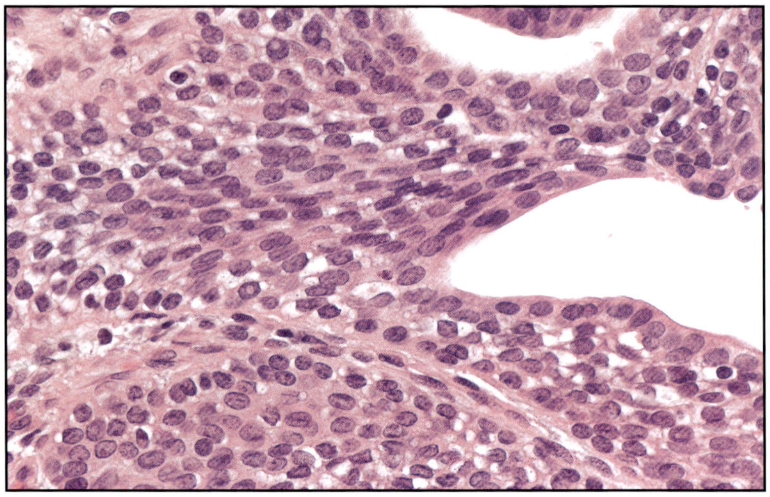

■ **i6.22** *Streaming of elongated transitional cells toward preserved luminal secretory cells in transitional cell metaplasia.*

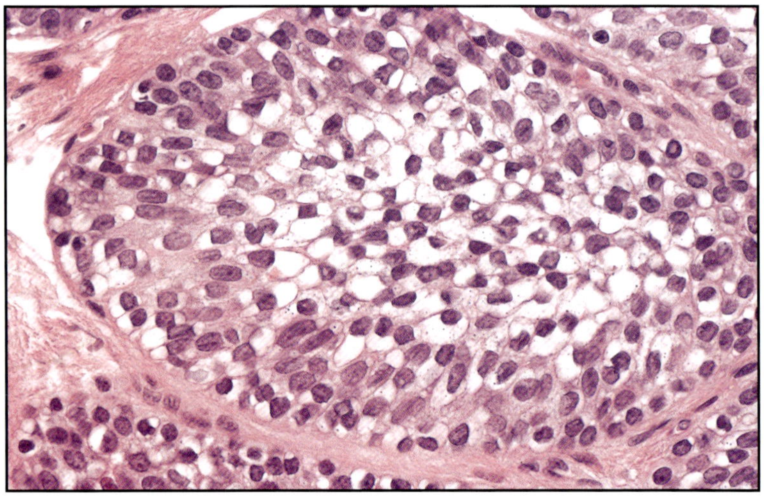

■ **i6.23** *Transitional cell metaplasia: Perinuclear clearing.*

PIN can be more hyperchromatic and rounded. The other neoplastic proliferation in the differential diagnosis is transitional cell carcinoma, but most transitional cell carcinomas that involve the prostate are cytologically high grade and are unlikely to be mistaken for transitional cell metaplasia. Basal cell hyperplasia and squamous cell metaplasia could also be confused with transitional cell metaplasia, but basal cell hyperplasia nuclei are typified by a rounded profile and lack nuclear grooves. The cells of squamous cell metaplasia can have distinct intercellular borders, as do the cells in transitional cell metaplasia, but in squamous cell metaplasia there are intercellular bridges, and the cells have a more densely eosinophilic cytoplasm without perinuclear clearing. On occasion, transitional cell metaplasia can merge with squamous cell metaplasia or basal cell hyperplasia. Special studies are not indicated in the evaluation of transitional cell metaplasia.

■ **t6.4 Transitional Cell Metaplasia of Prostate**

Associated with inflammation and androgen deprivation therapy
Proliferation of piled-up elongated cells underneath secretory layer
Elongated cells are perpendicular to basement membrane and "stream" toward lumen
Bland metaplastic cells with oblong nuclei with occasional nuclear grooves and perinuclear cytoplasmic clearing
Differential diagnosis: PIN, basal cell hyperplasia, and squamous metaplasia

■ **t6.5 Incidence of Prostatic Mucinous Metaplasia**

Specimen Type	Incidence	Stain	Reference
Needle biopsy	8%	H&E	Hu 1998
Mixture[1]	1%	H&E	Grignon 1993
Whole gland: autopsy	1%	H&E	Shiraishi 1993
Simple prostatectomy	30%	Mucin[2]	Gal 1996
Whole gland: autopsy	55%	Mucin[2]	Gal 1996

[1]Mixture of specimen types, including needle biopsies, TURP chips, and prostatectomies
[2]Mucin staining using PAS for neutral mucins and Alcian blue (pH 2.5) for acidic mucins

[6.3] Mucinous Metaplasia

Mucinous metaplasia, which has also been called mucous gland metaplasia, may be defined as the replacement of benign luminal epithelium by benign mucin-secreting cells (Gal 1996, Grignon 1993, Hu 1998, Shiraishi 1993). This alteration most often refers to cellular changes detected with hematoxylin and eosin (H&E)-stained sections (Grignon 1993, Hu 1998, Shiraishi 1993), but some have used histochemical staining for intracytoplasmic mucin to define mucinous metaplasia (Gal 1996). Mucin production by benign prostatic luminal epithelial cells is common when histochemical methods are used to detect it (Franks 1964, Hukill 1967). (This mucin is predominantly neutral and can be highlighted with a periodic acid-Schiff [PAS] stain, with prior diastase digestion.) However, mucinous metaplasia is uncommonly evident in benign glands by H&E staining, with an incidence of 1% to 8% (Grignon 1993, Hu 1998, Shiraishi 1993) **t6.5**.

No specific clinical or radiologic features are associated with mucinous metaplasia, which is an incidental histologic finding. Mucinous metaplasia has no known premalignant potential: we did not find mucinous metaplasia adjacent to examples of mucinous high-grade PIN (Reyes 1997), and mucinous carcinoma of the prostate (Randolph 1997) does not have a reported association with mucinous metaplasia. Finally, mucinous metaplasia occurred with equal frequency in needle biopsies with and without carcinoma (Hu 1998), and this also points to a lack of association with malignancy.

Mucinous metaplasia is a focal, incidental histologic finding **t6.6**. It can be located centrally or peripherally (Shiraishi 1993). Microscopically, the metaplastic cells are grouped in clusters of 5 to 10 **i6.24**, although occasionally individual, isolated glands **i6.25** or cells can be found **i6.26** (Grignon 1993). Rare foci are extensive **i6.27**, with only a few examples greater than 1 mm^2 (Shiraishi 1993). The constituent cells are tall and columnar, with a cytoplasm filled with bluish mucin **i6.28, i6.29**. A suggestion of goblet cell–like vacuolization may be seen in a few cells, but mostly the cytoplasm has a diffuse granular blue character. Rarely, this mucin is released into the glandular lumen. The nuclei of the metaplastic cells are small, dark, and basally situated; some nuclei can show slight enlargement and pinpoint nucleoli. Mucinous metaplasia is most often found against a background of atrophy, including both sclerotic and postatrophic hyperplasia types, transitional cell metaplasia, usual epithelial hyperplasia, and basal cell hyperplasia. Basal cells usually are seen easily **i6.29**, although difficulty may arise because of the basal distribution of the nuclei of the metaplastic cells.

Special stains usually are not needed to diagnose mucinous metaplasia. The mucin is of mixed neutral and acidic types, as indicated by positive PAS and Alcian blue (pH 2.5) stains, respectively.

■ **t6.6 Mucinous Metaplasia of Prostate**

Associated with atrophy, hyperplasia, transitional cell metaplasia
Usually clusters of 5-10 glands with tall columnar cells
Cytoplasm foamy and pink to goblet-like with bluish mucin
Bland, small basally-located nuclei
Differential diagnosis: Well-differentiated adenocarcinoma, mucinous high-grade PIN, Cowper's glands

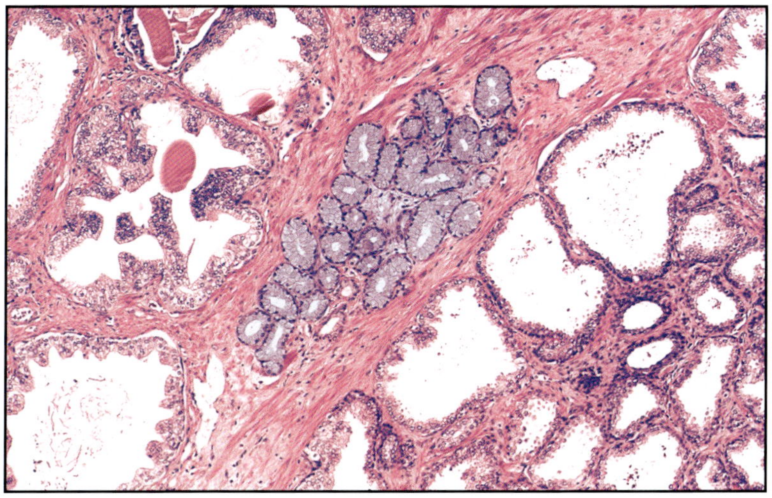

■ **i6.24** *Mucinous metaplasia: A small, well-circumscribed cluster of glands with pale-blue cytoplasm.*

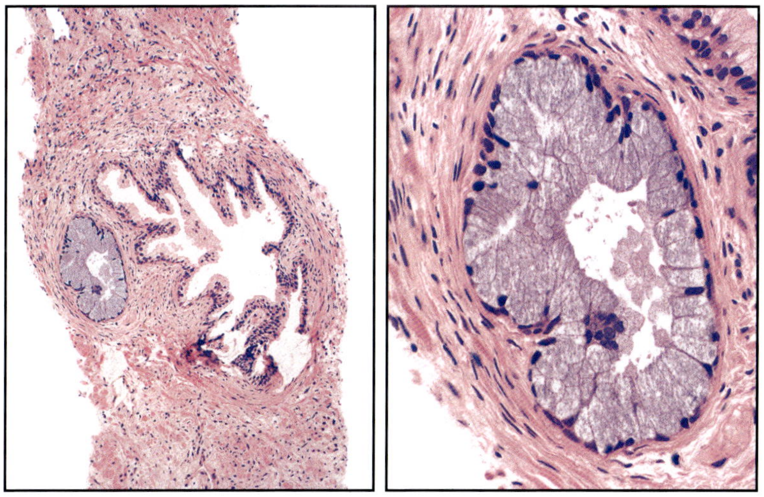

■ **i6.25** *Single gland of mucinous metaplasia in needle biopsy (high power view at right).*

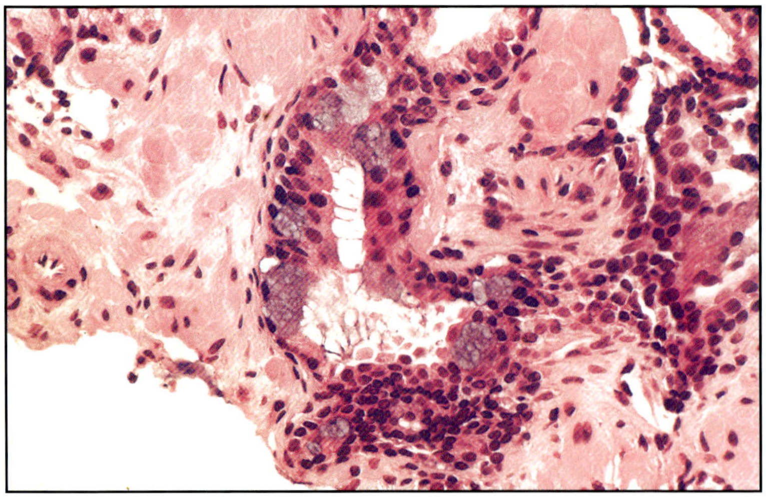

■ **i6.26** *Single gland with partial mucinous metaplasia of a few cells with subtle intracytoplasmic blue mucin.*

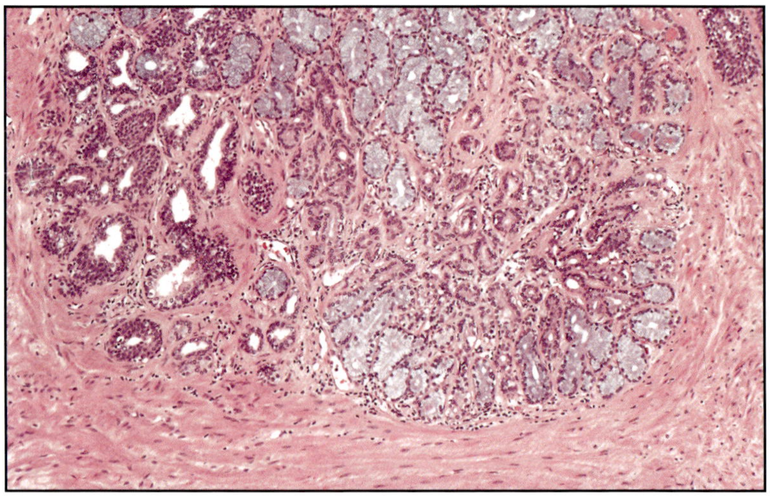

■ **i6.27** *Extensive mucinous metaplasia.*

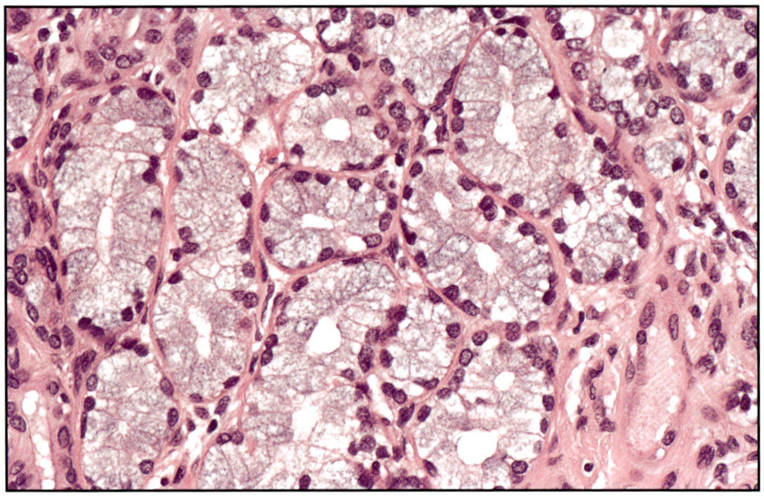

■ **i6.28** *Mucinous metaplasia with bland, basally-situated nuclei.*

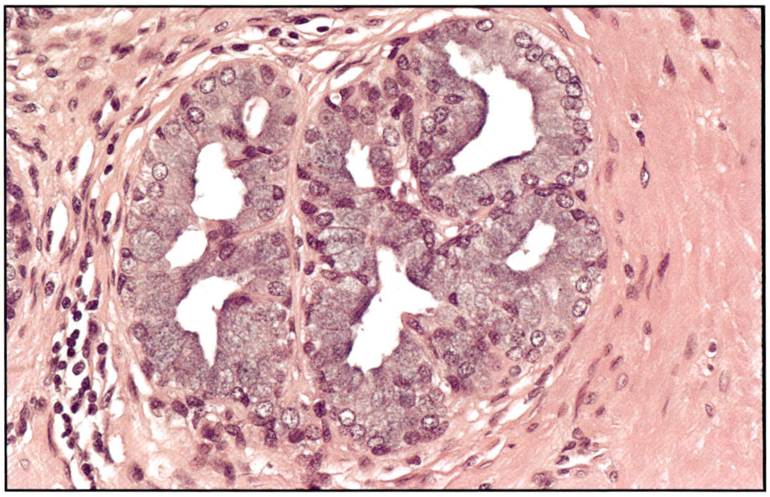

■ **i6.29** *Mucinous metaplasia with blue, granular cytoplasm.*

These mucinous cells are nonreactive, using antibodies directed against PSA and PSAP (Gal 1996, Grignon 1993, Shiraishi 1993). An intact basal cell layer can be confirmed by a 34βE12 immunostain.

The entity of greatest import in the differential diagnosis is a well-differentiated adenocarcinoma. Occasional carcinomas, including foamy gland carcinomas (Nelson 1996), can have small, basally situated nuclei and a fine, foamy cytoplasm. These carcinomas are not found in hyperplastic or atrophic prostatic glands or glands with transitional cell metaplasia, as mucinous metaplastic cells can be. Also, well-differentiated carcinomas lack basal cells, and these cells are detectable in mucinous metaplasia. Mucinous adenocarcinoma is not in the differential diagnosis because a substantial volume (at least 25%) of such tumors is made up of extracellular lakes of mucin with embedded tumor cells (Randolph 1997). Extracellular, stromal-based lakes of mucin are not seen in mucinous metaplasia. Mucinous high-grade PIN is not a prominent consideration because the mucin in these glands is intraluminal rather than intracytoplasmic (Reyes 1997) and because the high-grade PIN nuclei are atypical, with nucleomegaly and nucleolomegaly, unlike in mucinous metaplasia. Finally, the epithelium that mucinous metaplasia most resembles is that of Cowper's glands, which differ in being mucinous glands in a complete lobule, often with a central feeder duct and surrounding skeletal muscle. Cowper's glands are not seen against a background of hyperplasia, atrophy, or transitional cell metaplasia, as mucinous metaplasia can be. The lectin binding profile of mucinous metaplasia differs from that of Cowper's glands (Shiraishi 1993), but such lectin histochemical stains are not needed because this differential is best addressed with H&E-stained sections.

[6.4] Paneth Cell–Like Metaplasia

This cellular alteration is characterized by the presence of large, cytoplasmic, eosinophilic granules and therefore has been called Paneth cell–like metaplasia or change (Adlakha 1994, di Sant'Agnese 1994, Frydman 1992, Gaudin 1998, van de Voorde 1994, Weaver 1992A, 1992B). This terminology is misleading because this cytoplasmic granularity seems to result from several different processes. It has been proposed that the basis for this morphologic appearance may depend on the nature of epithelial proliferation. Thus, in benign epithelium it may be caused by exocrine differentiation with lysosomelike granules (Weaver 1992A, 1992B), neuroendocrine differentiation (Gaudin 1998), or even true Paneth cell differentiation (Cheng 1997), whereas in PIN and carcinoma the granules appear to reflect neuroendocrine differentiation (Adlakha 1994, di Sant'Agnese

1994). Accordingly, it has been suggested that the designation *Paneth cell–like metaplasia* be abandoned (Adlakha 1994, di Sant'Agnese 1994). For Paneth cell–like change in prostatic adenocarcinoma, the moniker *neuroendocrine cells with large eosinophilic granules* has been proposed (Adlakha 1994). A unifying terminology has not been proposed for benign epithelium with large eosinophilic granules.

The incidence of eosinophilic granules in benign prostatic epithelium is not well established, with reported ranges of 0% to 23% (Cheng 1997, Shabaik 1995). In one study (Cheng 1997), these large, supranuclear, eosinophilic granules were seen in benign epithelium in 16% of benign needle biopsies, 23% of needle biopsies with high-grade PIN, and 12% of needle biopsies with adenocarcinoma. Of radical prostatectomy specimens from untreated patients, 0% (Shabaik 1995) to 20% (Cheng 1997) had evidence of this change in benign epithelium. Only a few ($n = 4$) untreated cases have been reported in detail (Weaver 1992A, 1992B). Focal groups of cells (and in one case single cells) with eosinophilic granules were found in normal prostatic epithelium ($n = 1$) and usual epithelial hyperplasia ($n = 3$). There seems to be a preference for involvement of ductal over acinar epithelium (Cheng 1997). An association with inflammation has been noted (Cheng 1997). In all cases, bright eosinophilic granules filled the apical cytoplasm of luminal cells. Apical blebs also contained granules (Weaver 1992A). The granules are PAS-positive, diastase-resistant, and immunopositive for PSA, PSAP, lysozyme, and α-1-antichymotrypsin while failing to stain for chromogranin, serotonin, and neuron specific enolase by immunohistochemistry (Cheng 1997). Exocrine-like granules 400 to 690 nm in diameter have been observed by electron microscopy. It is intriguing that fixation conditions affect the detection of eosinophilic secretory granules in prostatic epithelium: if fixed in strong (>2.5%) glutaraldehyde, benign prostatic luminal cells are found to possess myriad intensely staining eosinophilic granules (Cohen 1998). After androgen deprivation therapy, Paneth cell–like change is uncommon (Civantos 1995), whereas these cells were found in 32% of postradiation biopsies and were always found in benign epithelium (Gaudin 1998, 1999). In the latter posttherapy setting, this cellular change indicates neuroendocrine differentiation rather than exocrine secretory granules because almost all were chromogranin positive and lysozyme negative in immunohistochemistry (Gaudin 1998). Further study is needed to better characterize eosinophilic granules in benign prostatic epithelium and to determine whether such granules in benign prostatic epithelium are exocrine secretory granules or indicative of neuroendocrine differentiation.

The differential diagnosis of eosinophilic granules in benign prostatic epithelium centers on the distinction between high-grade PIN and adenocarcinoma with neuroendocrine cells with large eosinophilic granules. These granules are seen in 15% of prostatic adenocarcinomas (Adlakha 1994). This intracytoplasmic pigment should also be distinguished from other prostatic cytoplasmic inclusions, such as lipofuscin pigment (Chapter 1) and viral inclusions (Weaver 1992A).

[6.5] Nephrogenic "Metaplasia" (Adenoma) and Stromal Metaplasia

This urothelial metaplasia is considered in Chapter 23. Metaplasia of benign mesenchymal cells in the prostate is vanishingly rare. There is a single case report of cartilaginous stromal metaplasia (Bedrosian 1983).

References

Adlakha H, Bostwick DG. Paneth cell–like change in prostatic adenocarcinoma represents neuroendocrine differentiation. Report of 30 cases. *Hum Pathol* 25:135-139, 1994.

Andriole GL, Hasson MU, Humphrey P. Finasteride induced changes in prostate histomorphology [abstract]. *J Urol* 151:507A, 1994.

Armas OA, Aprikian AG, Melamed J, et al. Clinical and pathobiological effects of neoadjuvant total androgen ablation therapy on clinically localized prostatic adenocarcinoma. *Am J Surg Pathol* 18:979-991, 1994.

Bainborough AR. Squamous metaplasia of prostate following estrogen therapy. *J Urol* 68:329-336, 1952.

Bedrosian SA, Goldman RL, Sung MA. Heterotopic cartilage in prostate. *Urology* 21:536-537, 1983.

Borkowski P, Robinson MJ, Poppiti RJ, et al. Histologic findings in postcryosurgical prostatic biopsies. *Mod Pathol* 9:807-811, 1996.

Bostwick DG, Egbert BM, Fajardo LF. Radiation injury of the normal and neoplastic prostate. *Am J Surg Pathol* 6:541-551, 1982.

Brawer MK, Nagle RB, Pitts W, et al. Keratin immunoreactivity as an aid to the diagnosis of persistent adenocarcinoma in irradiated human prostates. *Cancer* 63:454-460, 1989.

Brawn PN, Johnson EH, Foster DM, et al. Characteristics of prostatic infarcts and their effect on serum prostate-specific antigen and prostatic acid phosphatase. *Urology* 44:71-75, 1994.

Cheng L, MacLennan GT, Bostwick DG, et al. Paneth cell differentiation in the benign prostate [abstract]. *Mod Pathol* 10:71A, 1997.

Civantos F, Marcial MA, Banks ER, et al. Pathology of androgen deprivation therapy in prostate carcinoma. *Cancer* 75:1634-1641, 1995.

Cohen RJ, McNeal JE, Edgar SG, et al. Characterization of cytoplasmic secretory granules (PSG) in prostatic epithelium and their transformation-induced loss in dysplasia and adenocarcinoma. *Hum Pathol* 29:1488-1494, 1998.

Culp OS. Squamous metaplasia, simulating carcinoma, associated with prostatic infarction. *Bull Johns Hopkins Hosp* 65:239-252, 1939.

Dhom G, Degro S. Therapy of prostatic cancer and histopathologic follow-up. *Prostate* 3:531-542, 1982.

di Sant'Agnese PA. Neuroendocrine differentiation in prostatic adenocarcinoma does not represent true Paneth cell differentiation [editorial]. *Hum Pathol* 25:115-116, 1994.

Fergusson JD, Franks LM. The response of prostatic carcinoma to oestrogen treatment. *Br J Surg* 40:422-428, 1953.

Franks LM, O'Shea JD, Thomson AER. Mucin in the prostate: a histochemical study in normal glands, latent, clinical, and colloid cancers. *Cancer* 17:983-991, 1964.

Frydman CP, Bleiweiss IJ, Unger PD, et al. Paneth cell–like metaplasia of the prostate gland. *Arch Pathol Lab Med* 116:274-276, 1992.

Gal R, Koren R, Nofech-Mozes S, et al. Evaluation of mucinous metaplasia of the prostate gland by mucin histochemistry. *Br J Urol* 77:113-117, 1996.

Gaudin PB, Zelefsky MJ, Hutchinson B, et al. Paneth cell–like change in benign prostatic ducts and acini post-radiation therapy represents neuroendocrine differentiation [abstract]. *Mod Pathol* 11:83A, 1998.

Gaudin PB, Zelefsky MJ, Leibel SA, et al. Histopathologic effects of three-dimensional conformal external beam radiation therapy on benign and malignant prostate tissue. *Am J Surg Pathol* 23:1021-1031, 1999.

Golden MR, Abeshouse BS. A further clinical and pathological study of prostatic infarction. *J Urol* 70:930-936, 1953.

Grignon DJ, O'Malley FP. Mucinous metaplasia in the prostate gland. *Am J Surg Pathol* 17:287-290, 1993.

Helpap B, Stiens R. The cell proliferation of epithelial metaplasia in the prostate gland. An autoradiographic in vitro study. *Virchows Arch B Cell Pathol* 19:69-76, 1975.

Helpap B. Treated prostatic carcinoma. Histological, immunohistochemical and cell kinetic studies. *Appl Pathol* 3:230-241, 1995.

Hu JC, Palapattu GS, Kattan MW, et al. The association of selected pathological features with prostate cancer in a single-needle biopsy accession. *Hum Pathol* 29:1536-1538, 1998.

Hukill PB, Vidone RA. Histochemistry of mucus and other polysaccharides in tumors. II. Carcinoma of the prostate. *Lab Invest* 16:395-406, 1967.

Humphrey PA, Vollmer RT. Relationships between serum prostate-specific antigen and histopathologic appearances of prostate carcinoma. In: Foster CS, Bostwick DG, eds. *Pathology of the Prostate.* Philadelphia: WB Saunders; 253-281, 1998.

Kahler JE. Carcinoma of the prostate: a pathology study. *J Urol* 41:557-574, 1939.

Kasman LP, Gold J. Metaplastic changes in the prostate gland. *J Lab Clin Med* 19:301-308, 1933.

Kastendieck H, Altenahr E. Morphogenesis and significance of epithelial metaplasia in the human prostate gland. An electron-microscopic study [in German]. *Virchows Archiv A Pathol Anat Histol* 365:137-150, 1975.

Lager DJ, Goeken JA, Kemp JD, et al. Squamous metaplasia of the prostate. An immunohistochemical study. *Am J Clin Pathol* 90:597-601, 1988.

McNeal JE. Normal histology of the prostate. *Am J Surg Pathol* 12:619-633, 1988.

Milford RA, Kahane H, Epstein JI. Infarct of the prostate gland: experience on needle biopsy specimens. *Am J Surg Pathol* 24: 1378-1384, 2000.

Montironi R, Diamanti L. Morphologic changes in benign prostatic hyperplasia following chronic treatment with the 5-a-reductase inhibitor finasteride. Comparison with the effect of combination endocrine therapy. *J Urol Pathol* 4:123-135, 1996.

Moore RA. Benign hypertrophy of the prostate. A morphological study. *J Urol* 50:680-710, 1943.

Mostofi FK, Morse WH. Epithelial metaplasia in "prostatic infarction." *Arch Pathol* 51:340-345, 1951.

Nadler RB, Humphrey PA, Smith DS, et al. Effect of inflammation and benign prostatic hyperplasia on elevated serum prostate specific antigen levels. *J Urol* 154:407-413, 1995.

Nanson EM. Squamous metaplasia of the prostate gland. *J Urol* 22:394-403, 1950.

Nelson RS, Epstein JI. Prostatic carcinoma with abundant xanthomatous cytoplasm: foamy gland carcinoma. *Am J Surg Pathol* 20:419-426, 1996.

Randolph TL, Amin MB, Ro JY, et al. Histologic variants of adenocarcinoma and other carcinomas of the prostate: pathologic criteria and clinical significance. *Mod Pathol* 10:612-629, 1997.

Reuter VE. Pathological changes in benign and malignant prostatic tissue following androgen deprivation therapy. *Urology* 49(suppl 3A):16-22, 1997.

Reyes AO, Swanson PE, Carbone JM, et al. Unusual histologic types of high-grade prostatic intraepithelial neoplasia. *Am J Surg Pathol* 21:1215-1222, 1997.

Roth RB. Prostatic infarction. *J Urol* 62:474-479, 1949.

Shabaik A, Wilson S, Bidair M, et al. Pathologic changes in prostate biopsies following cryoablation therapy of prostate carcinoma. *J Urol Pathol* 3:183-193, 1995.

Sheaff MT, Baithun SI. Effects of radiation on the normal prostate gland. *Histopathology* 30:341-348, 1997.

Shiraishi T, Kusano I, Watanabe M, et al. Mucous gland metaplasia of the prostate. *Am J Surg Pathol* 17:618-622, 1993.

SMD (Stedman's Medical Dictionary). 23rd ed. Baltimore: Williams & Wilkins; 859, 1976.

Spiro LH, Labay G, Orkin LA. Prostatic infarction: role in acute urinary retention. *Urology* 3:345-347, 1974.

Sutton EB, McDonald JR. Metaplasia of the prostatic epithelium: a lesion sometimes mistaken for carcinoma. *Am J Clin Pathol* 13:607-615, 1943.

Têtu B, Srigley JR, Boivin JC, et al. Effect of combination endocrine therapy (LHRH agonist and flutamide) on normal prostate and prostatic adenocarcinoma. A histopathologic and immunohistochemical study. *Am J Surg Pathol* 15:111-120, 1991.

Vaillancourt L, Têtu B, Fradet Y, et al. Effect of neoadjuvant endocrine therapy (combined androgen blockade) on normal prostate and prostatic carcinoma. A randomized study. *Am J Surg Pathol* 20:86-93, 1996.

van de Voorde W, van Poppel H, Haustermans K, et al. Mucin-secreting adenocarcinoma of the prostate with neuroendocrine differentiation and Paneth-like cells. *Am J Surg Pathol* 18:200-207, 1994.

Weaver MG, Abdul-Karim FW, Srigley J, et al. Paneth cell–like change of the prostate gland. A histological, immunohistochemical, and electron microscopic study. *Am J Surg Pathol* 16:62-68, 1992A.

Weaver MG, Abdul-Karim FW, Srigley JR. Paneth cell–like change and small cell carcinoma of the prostate. Two divergent forms of prostatic neuroendocrine differentiation. *Am J Surg Pathol* 16:1013-1016, 1992B.

Yantiss RK, Young RK. Transitional cell "metaplasia" in the prostate gland. A survey of its frequency and features based on 104 consecutive prostatic biopsy specimens. *J Urol Pathol* 7:71-80, 1997.

CHAPTER 7

Hyperplasia

[7.1] Incidence **127**

[7.2] Etiology **127**

[7.3] Pathogenesis **127**

[7.4] Clinical Features **128**

[7.5] Usual Nodular Epithelial and Stromal Hyperplasia **129**

[7.6] Basal Cell Hyperplasia **140**

[7.7] Cribriform Hyperplasia **144**

[7.8] Mesonephric Remnant Hyperplasia **145**

[7.9] Verumontanum Mucosal Gland Hyperplasia **147**

Benign prostatic hyperplasia (BPH) is one of the most common diseases to affect men. Precisely how common depends on the definition used for BPH. One way to classify BPH is as microscopic BPH, macroscopic BPH, and clinical BPH (Isaacs 1989, Lepor 2002). In this conceptual framework, microscopic BPH is the histologic diagnosis of usual glandular or stromal hyperplasia. Macroscopic BPH describes an enlarged prostate, which can be detected by digital rectal examination (DRE) or by radiologic means, usually transrectal ultrasonography (TRUS) or, less commonly, magnetic resonance imaging. Clinical BPH is a diagnosis based on urinary tract symptoms and bladder dysfunction (Lepor 2002, Ziada 1999). In fact, the clinical diagnosis of BPH often is made by a combination of assessments for macroscopic and clinical BPH, which includes evaluation of prostate size, urinary symptoms, and reduced urinary flow rate (McConnell 1998). This definition of BPH has also been used as a basis to model the natural history of BPH, where microscopic BPH progresses in one half of cases to macroscopic BPH, of which in turn one half progress to clinical BPH. This is a useful conceptual model but it is probably imprecise because histologic presence of BPH and prostate gland size do not correlate well with clinical symptoms of BPH.

The diagnosis of BPH is a clinical one. A histologic diagnosis of BPH is not needed for treatment. Epithelial and stromal hyperplasia can be diagnosed in all types of prostatic tissue samples, but the main histologic significance of prostatic hyperplasia is not to mistake usual prostatic hyperplasia or one of its variants with carcinoma (Gaudin 1997, Young 1988, 1997A, 1997B) and, conversely, not to misdiagnose pseudohyperplastic prostatic carcinoma as prostate hyperplasia (Humphrey 1998).

[7.1] Incidence

Histologic evidence of BPH at autopsy is found in a majority of men over 60 years of age (Fang-Liu 1993, Moore 1943). This proliferative process is strongly related to age, with only a few percent of men under 40 having histologic BPH, whereas almost all men (88%) over 80 have histologic BPH (Berry 1984, Fang-Liu 1993, Moore 1943) **t7.1**. The prevalence of histologic BPH at autopsy is the same in different countries around the world (Fang-Liu 1993, Isaacs 1989).

BPH is a common clinical diagnosis, with the prevalence dependent on the clinical criteria used **t7.1**. Some studies have used only symptoms (Sagnier 1994) in its definition, whereas other studies have included prostate size or urinary flow rates. Also, different methods for measuring symptom scores and prostate size have been applied. BPH is a worldwide problem, with increasing severity of symptoms with age documented in several countries, including the United States (Chute 1993), France (Sagnier 1994), Japan (Tsukamoto 1995), New Zealand (Nacey 1995), and Spain (Chicharro-Molero 1998). It has been difficult to compare BPH prevalence in different countries because of different clinical definitions and the inherent difficulty in quantifying symptoms, but there does appear to be a lower prevalence in Japanese men (Tsukamoto 1995).

■ t7.1 Age-Related Incidence of Benign Prostatic Hyperplasia

Age	Histological Incidence[1]	Clinical Incidence[2]
1-10	0%	—
11-20	0%	—
21-30	0%	—
31-40	8%	—
41-50	23%	5%-27%
51-60	42%	8%-50%
61-70	71%	37%-69%
71-80	82%	40%-79%
81-90	88%	85%

[1]Incidence at autopsy. Data from Berry 1984
[2]Data from Guess 1990, Garaway 1991, Chute 1993, Chicharro-Molero 1998

■ t7.2 Risk Factors for Benign Prostatic Hyperplasia

Age
Intact androgen axis
Family history

[7.2] Etiology

Established etiologic risk factors for BPH are aging and an intact androgen axis (Foster 2000, Guess 1995, Lee 1995, Ziada 1999). Patients castrated before puberty do not develop BPH. The role of androgens in the development of BPH is felt to be permissive rather than directly causative. An emerging risk factor for BPH is a positive family history, indicative of an inheritable genetic basis, with an autosomal dominant mode of inheritance (Partin 1994, Roberts 1995, Sanda 1994, 1997) **t7.2**. As in general for inherited disease, hereditary BPH tends to strike younger patients: It is estimated that about 50% of men under 60 years of age who undergo surgery (prostatectomy) for BPH could have hereditary BPH, whereas only about 9% of men over 60 with BPH have the inherited form of the disease (Sanda 1994). Men with hereditary BPH have larger prostate glands, with a mean volume of 83 cm^3, compared with a mean volume of 56 cm^3 for men with sporadic BPH (Sanda 1997). The gene (or, more likely, genes) responsible for hereditary BPH have not been identified. Smoking, alcohol intake, vasectomy, and sexual activity have little or no association with BPH (Guess 1995). Histologically, hereditary BPH exhibits a higher stromal-epithelial ratio than sporadic BPH nodules (Sanda 1997).

[7.3] Pathogenesis

The molecular pathogenesis of BPH has not been elucidated, but epithelial-stromal cellular interactions and various growth-promoting molecules probably are involved, including androgens, estrogens, and polypeptide growth factors (Lawson 1997, Lee 1995, Roehrborn 2002, Steiner 1995). Because BPH is a benign increase in cell number, it fundamentally must represent an imbalance between cell proliferation and cell death. Therefore, it is probably a combination of growth promotion and impaired programmed cell death (apoptosis) that leads to BPH.

Androgens are the most potent growth promoters (mitogens) in BPH. For the prostate, the most important androgens are testosterone, which is mainly of testicular origin (with 10% contributed from the adrenals) and dihydrotestosterone (DHT), which is produced from testosterone by the enzyme 5α-reductase. DHT is the main active androgen in BPH and mediates its effects via a nuclear androgen receptor. The crucial nature of this pathway is underscored by several observations. First, BPH does not occur in patients with prepubertal surgical castration, with the resultant drop in circulating testosterone (Wilson 1980). Second, reduction in size of established BPH occurs with medical castration (Peters 1987). Third, in male pseudohermaphrodites with a genetic deficiency in 5α-reductase, BPH does not develop (Imperato-McGinley 1974). Fourth, drugs that block 5α-reductase can be used to treat BPH (Lepor 2002). Finally, abnormalities in the androgen receptor gene seem to influence the development of BPH. Specifically, shortened CAG repeats in exon 1 of the androgen receptor have been linked to a higher risk of BPH development (Giovannucci 1999). The role of other steroid hormones such as estrogen and progesterone has not been established, although BPH does express the estrogen receptor (Ehara 1995, Ekman 1983, Fenely 1995), and serum estrogen levels in men do increase with age. Polypeptide growth factors such as fibroblast growth factors, prolactin, insulinlike growth factors, transforming growth factors TGF-α and TGF-β, platelet-derived growth factor, and epidermal growth factor have also been implicated in BPH (Deshmukh 1997, Kyprianou 1996, Roehrborn 2002, Steiner 1995). Some of these growth factors and the extracellular matrix undoubtedly are involved in stromal-epithelial cell interactions that could affect BPH development. The apparent polarization of new gland branches in BPH toward BPH stroma suggests an inductive stromal influence, similar to embryonic development, and thus one proposal is that BPH represents a "reawakening" or reactivation of embryonic stromal inductive capacities (McConnell 1998).

The cell cycle, cell proliferation, and apoptosis are all intimately related to these steroid and polypeptide growth factors. Cell proliferation in BPH, though low, exceeds the cell death rate (Colombel 1998, Kyprianou 1996), which results in overall growth of BPH nodules. Apoptosis is inhibited, at least in part, by elevated levels of bcl-2 (an anti–cell death protein) in BPH (Colombel 1998, Kyprianou 1996). One of the molecular abnormalities related to the increased cell proliferation rate is loss of the negative cell cycle regulator $p27^{KIP1}$ (Cordon-Cardo 1998).

Mechanisms for BPH development have also been forwarded based on animal studies. Although it is often written in the literature that only dogs (Berry 1986) and humans develop BPH (McConnell 1998), nonhuman primates also can get BPH (Ferreira 1995, Lewis 1981). The inflammation that so commonly accompanies BPH in men may be involved in cellular proliferation via cytokine production; in rats, induced chronic inflammation was associated with hyperplasia (Kessler 1998). Transgenic mouse models have implicated specific polypeptide growth in BPH factor formation: Mice overexpressing a fibroblast growth factor (Tutrone 1993) or a prolactin transgene (Wennbo 1997) developed BPH. Mice with knockout of the aforementioned $p27^{KIP1}$ gene also developed BPH (Cordon-Cardo 1998).

[7.4] Clinical Features

Patients with BPH present with symptoms often called prostatism, which can be separated into obstructive and irritative symptoms **t7.3**. The obstructive symptoms may be caused by impaired bladder contractibility or outlet obstruction, whereas irritative symptoms probably are caused by bladder instability or decreased bladder compliance (Madsen 1995). Symptoms of prostatism are not specific for BPH, and other diseases must be ruled out in the workup for BPH. For example, urinary tract infections and bladder cancer may produce symptoms such as frequency and urgency that mimic BPH (Madsen 1995). Other diseases that can clinically simulate BPH include urethral stricture, bladder neck contracture, bladder calculus, and neurogenic bladder (Madsen 1995). Again, prostate size and histologic BPH presence correlate poorly with the degree of obstruction and these clinical symptoms (Madsen 1995, McConnell 1998).

t7.3 BPH "Prostatism" Symptoms

I. Obstructive symptoms
   - Hesitancy in initiating urination
   - Postvoid dribbling
   - Sensation of incomplete emptying of bladder
   - Urinary retention

II. Irritative symptoms
   - Frequency
   - Urgency
   - Nocturia
   - Urge incontinence
   - Dysuria

From Madsen 1995

The initial clinical evaluation for BPH includes a medical history, a physical examination including DRE, urinalysis (to exclude urinary tract infection and hematuria), serum creatinine measurement (to rule out renal insufficiency due to obstruction), serum prostate-specific antigen (PSA), and symptom assessment (Madsen 1995, McConnell 1998). On DRE, BPH often produces a "smooth, elastic enlargement of the prostate" (Madsen 1995). However, BPH can produce the classic "palpable prostatic nodule," which differs little from carcinoma in palpable abnormalities (Jewett 1956). Indeed, BPH and other benign nodules can simulate a malignant nodule by exhibiting stony indurations on palpation (Jewett 1956). The size of the prostate gland can be estimated by DRE, but prostate size alone is not a factor in determining whether active treatment is needed (McConnell 1998). Serum PSA is used in conjunction with DRE to assess for malignancy in the patient who presents with prostatism. An elevation in serum PSA (above 4 ng/mL) and an abnormal DRE are indications for transrectal ultrasound-guided sextant biopsy. Symptom assessment in the United States and worldwide is most often accomplished using the International Prostate Symptom Score (IPSS), which was initially developed and validated as the American Urological Association symptom index (Barry 2001).

It is essential to know that BPH alone can elevate the serum PSA, and indeed, BPH is the most common cause of an elevated serum PSA. Total serum PSA levels correlate directly with the total size of the prostate and seem to be most closely linked to volume of the transition zone, where BPH develops (Hammerer 1995, Lloyd 1994). Studies of patients with histologically confirmed BPH have shown that 21% to 86% have had an elevated serum PSA level (Armbruster 1993, Hudson 1989, Oesterling 1991, Stamey 1987). In our experience, high ultrasound-determined prostate volume (reflective of BPH) and inflammation, as identified on needle biopsy, were the most important factors contributing to an elevated serum PSA in men without clinically detectable prostate cancer (Nadler 1995). Most elevations are modest, in the 4 to 10 ng/mL range (Hudson 1989). Therefore, neither DRE nor serum PSA can discriminate between BPH and carcinoma, and histologic examination of needle biopsies is necessary to rule out (or rule in) malignancy.

Various permutations of serum PSA have been used in attempts to improve the distinction between BPH and prostatic carcinoma. These include PSA density (Seaman 1993), age-referenced serum PSA cutoffs (Oesterling 1993), PSA velocity (Carter 1993), and percentage of free (uncomplexed) PSA (Lilja 1993). PSA density attempts to correct for the contribution of BPH to serum PSA by dividing the serum PSA level by the volume of the prostate gland (as determined by ultrasound measurements). Age-referenced serum PSA cutoffs also attempt to control for BPH, which increases with age, by increasing PSA cutoff points with increasing age, where a level of 2.8 ng/mL is recommended for age 50 and 7.0 ng/mL for age 79 (Oesterling 1993). A major concern with these two approaches is the sacrifice of sensitivity at the expense of specificity in cancer detection (Catalona 1994). For PSA velocity, differences in doubling times of PSA elevation are used. Men with BPH have lower rates of change (increase) of PSA levels in serum over time than men with carcinoma, but there is overlap. Patients with BPH have linear doubling times of 2 to 17 years, whereas men with localized prostate cancer have linear and exponential phases with a mean doubling time of 2 years (Seaman 1993). A recommended cutoff for the decision to biopsy is a rate of PSA rise of 0.75 ng/mL/year (Smith 1994). Finally, percentage of free PSA has been used as an adjunct to total serum PSA to improve specificity (Catalona 1995). Patients with BPH tend to have a higher percentage of PSA that is unbound to carrier proteins in the serum, which is probably caused at least in part by failure of BPH nodules to synthesize one of these carrier proteins, α1-antichymotrypsin (Björk 1994). Patients with a free PSA above 25% are more likely to have BPH than carcinoma as the basis for an elevated total serum PSA (Björk 1994). In current clinical practice, almost all practicing urologists use total serum PSA in the workup of BPH (Gee 1998), and some use free PSA in addition to a total serum PSA.

Additional tests ordered in clinical evaluation of patients with BPH include postvoid residual measurement (71%), uroflow (48%), cystoscopy (29%), intravenous pyelography (9%) and urodynamics (5%) (Gee 1998). These are usually done when there is a concern that the patient's lower urinary tract symptoms may not be due to BPH. Radiologic evaluation of BPH can be performed by ultrasonography, intravenous urography, urethrography, computed tomography, and magnetic resonance imaging (Scheckowitz 1995) but is not routinely done in the initial evaluation of the patient with prostatism. Direct imaging of BPH probably is most often done with ultrasonography in the setting of ultrasound-guided biopsy. Here, a demarcation between the generally hypoechoic transition zone with BPH and more isoechoic peripheral zone can be seen (Scheckowitz 1995). With increasing size, the transition zone with BPH can be seen to compress the central and peripheral zones. Ultrasound findings of hypoechogenicity and transition zone location are not specific for BPH because carcinoma can also exhibit these attributes. Prostatic ultrasound is also useful in calculating the volume of the prostate (Scheckowitz 1995).

Clinical complications of BPH related to obstruction include urinary retention, urinary tract infections, hematuria, bladder decompensation, bladder stones, bladder diverticula, and rarely, renal failure (Girman 1998, McConnell 1998). The development of cancer is not associated with BPH; there is no evidence to suggest that usual (nonatypical) prostatic hyperplasia is a precursor to prostatic carcinoma. In one large study with long follow-up, the percentage of patients with and without BPH who developed prostate cancer was nearly identical (Greenwald 1974).

Treatment of BPH should be tailored to the individual patient and is often based on gland size and the bothersomeness of symptoms. When BPH clearly causes refractory urinary retention, recurrent or persistent gross hematuria, bladder stones, or renal insufficiency, surgery is indicated (McConnell 1998). Algorithms for evaluation and treatment of BPH have been developed (McConnell 1998, Roehrborn 2001). The management options include watchful waiting, medical therapy, minimally invasive therapies, and surgery (Fitzpatrick 2002, Lepor 2002). Medical (drug) treatments include α-blockade (α-adrenergic receptor blockage of prostate smooth muscle contractility) and androgen suppression (mainly 5α-reductase blockade by finasteride) (Debruyne 2000, Kaplan 2001, Lepor 1996, 2002, McConnell 1995). Minimally invasive therapies include high-intensity focused ultrasound, laser therapy, transurethral balloon dilation, hyperthermia and thermotherapy, transurethral electrovaporization, intraurethral stents, and transurethral needle ablation of the prostate (Blute 2001, Fitzpatrick 2002). The classic surgical treatment of BPH is transurethral prostatectomy, also known as TURP (Holtgrewe 1995, Fitzpatrick 2002). Since 1987, TURP rates have declined by roughly 50%, probably because of increasing availability of less invasive medical and surgical treatment alternatives, changes in reimbursement, and greater involvement of patients in decision making (Wasson 2000). Open or simple retropubic or suprapubic prostatectomy is another type of surgery performed in BPH patients with large (greater than 75g) prostates, a concomitant bladder condition that needs treatment such as a sizable diverticulum or large bladder stone, inguinal hernia, marked hip ankylosis or a urethral condition such as stricture (Han 2002).

[7.5] Usual Nodular Epithelial and Stromal Hyperplasia

This histopathologic diagnostic term is the appropriate designation for the most common morphologic presentation of BPH. The terms *benign prostatic hypertrophy* and *prostatic adenoma* are to be avoided. Even though BPH is sometimes called a neoplasm (adenoma), it is currently viewed as a true hyperplasia, that is, a nonneoplastic increase in cell number. Usual prostatic hyperplasia can be diagnosed in all types of prostatic tissue samples, but its recognition is most straightforward in tissue samples larger than the needle core biopsy. Hyperplasia is actually uncommon in prostatic needle biopsies because the zone of origin of BPH—the transition zone—usually is not biopsied and because hyperplasia is uncommon in the peripheral zone, which is targeted. Histopathologists routinely diagnose hyperplasia when benign, complex glands are appreciated in a needle biopsy **i7.1**, yet normal glands also have this appearance. Also, it is not possible to recognize in needle biopsy the nodularity of BPH glands. Finally, it is not necessary to diagnose usual prostatic hyperplasia in needle biopsy because treatment of BPH is driven by the clinical diagnosis. I use the term *benign prostatic tissue* for all

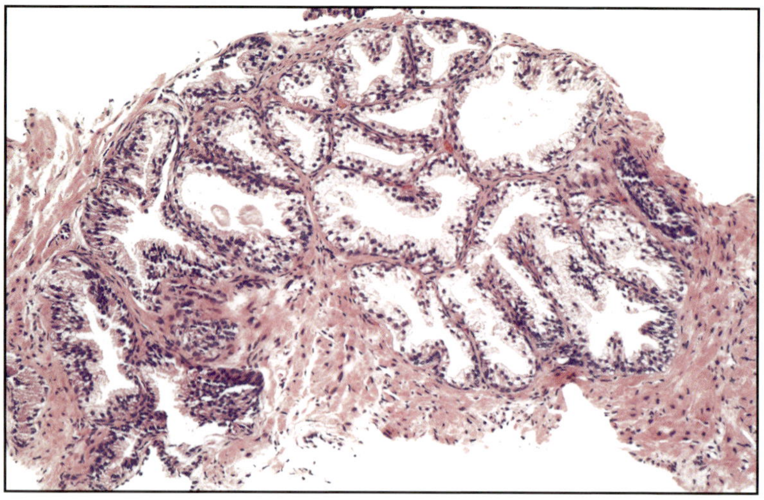

■ **i7.1** *Complex, benign glands should not be diagnosed as hyperplasia in needle biopsy tissue from the peripheral zone. Here the benign glands assume a nodular configuration (no typical hyperplastic stroma).*

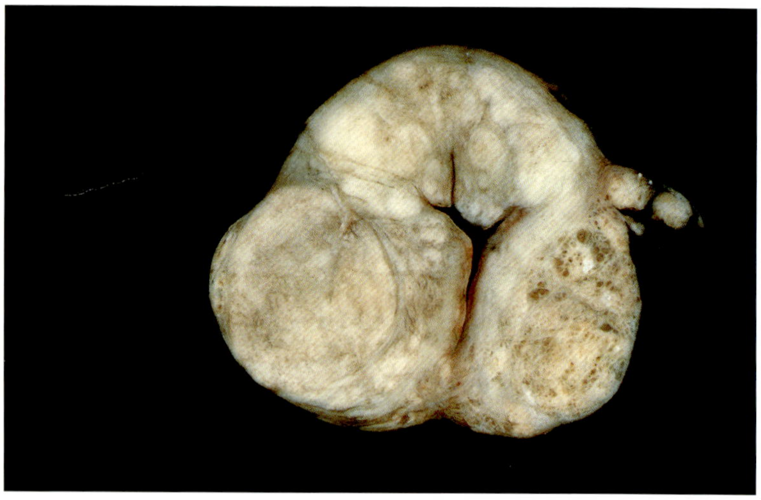

■ **i7.2** *BPH nodules surrounding central prostatic urethra in simple prostatectomy specimen.*

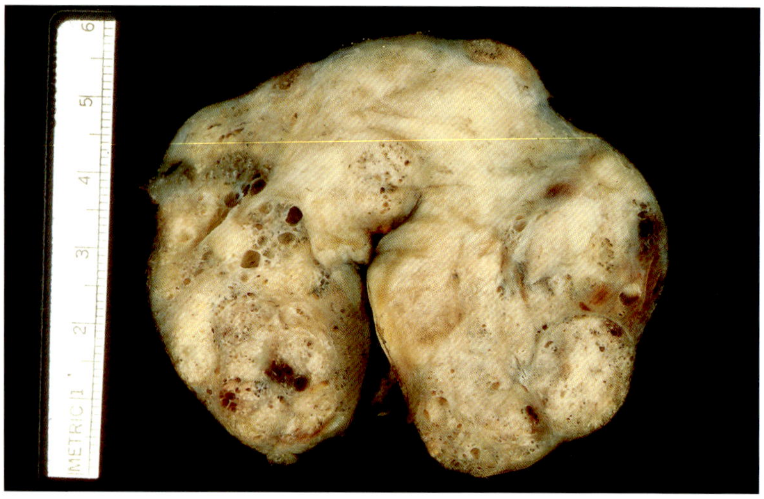

■ **i7.3** *BPH nodules with admixture of solid component and cystic change in simple prostatectomy specimen.*

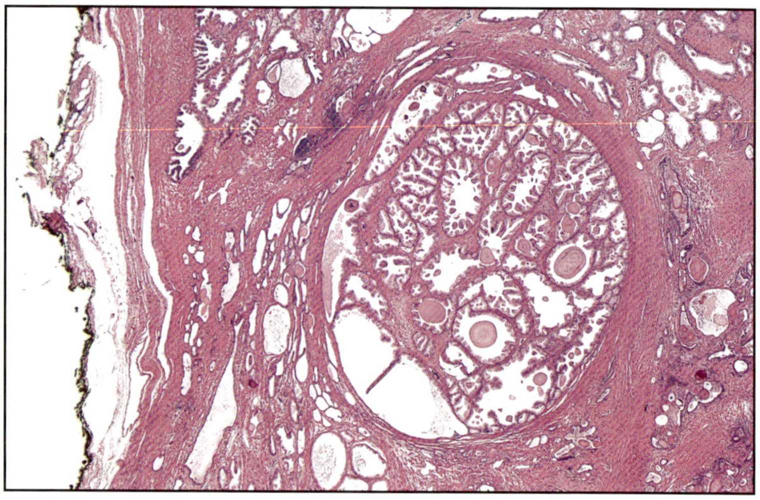

■ **i7.4** *Small peripheral zone BPH nodule.*

benign glands. I rarely diagnose usual prostatic hyperplasia in needle cores because this diagnosis usually is neither necessary nor possible in needle core biopsies.

Grossly, nodule formation is the hallmark of usual prostatic hyperplasia. Such nodularity can be seen in TURP chips, simple prostatectomy specimens, and whole glands (from radical prostatectomy, cystoprostatectomy, and autopsy specimens) but not needle biopsies. In TURP chips, most nodules (more than 80%) are less than 4 mm in diameter, whereas in simple prostatectomies (enucleations), most nodules are greater than 4 mm (Price 1990) **i7.2, i7.3**. In the whole gland, most nodules are found in the transition zone or periurethral areas (McNeal 1978), with peripheral zone hyperplastic nodules detected in 0.1% to 19% of prostates (Hamper 1991, Kerley 1997, Moore 1943, Ohori 1994, Oyen 1993, van de Voorde 1995) **t7.4; i7.4**. The periurethral and peripheral zone

■ **t7.4** **Hyperplastic Nodules: Anatomic Sites**

	Anatomic Site		
Characteristic	**Transition zone**	**Periurethral area**	**Peripheral zone**
Frequency	High	High	Low (0.1%-18%)
Number per gland	Multiple[1]	Several to multiple[2]	Usually solitary
Size	mm to cm	1-2 mm[3]	6 mm[4]
Histologic composition	Variable[5]	Usually stromal cells	Mixed glandular-stromal

[1]A mean of 11 nodules/whole gland in one series of intermediate involvement (McNeal 1978)
[2]A mean of 3 to 8 nodules/whole gland in two series of intermediate involvement (McNeal 1978, Bierhoff 1996)
[3]Mean nodule size before age of 70 years. After 70 the nodules can become large (McNeal 1978)
[4]Mean nodule size. Range = 1-13 mm
[5]Variable from pure stromal to mixed glandular-stromal to predominantly glandular

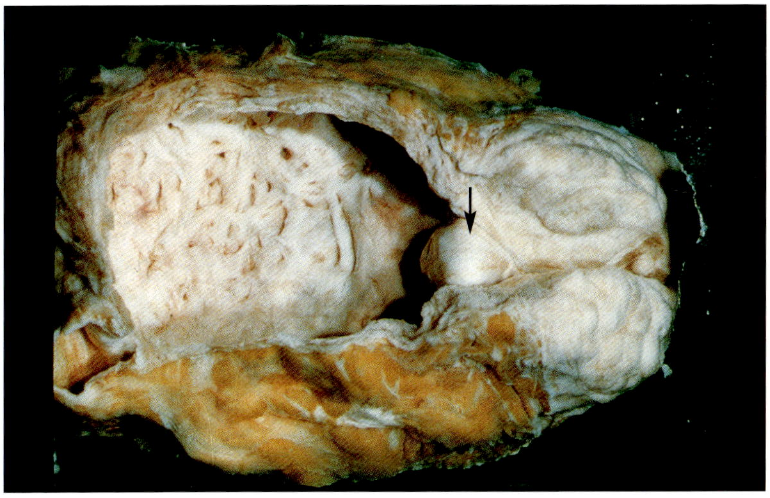

■ **i7.5** *BPH: Ball-like projection of median lobe (arrow) into bladder, which has a trabeculated appearance. (Reprinted from Royal College of Surgeons of England Slide Atlas of Pathology, 1985, slide 100.)*

hyperplastic nodules tend to be smaller than the transition zone nodules (Kerley 1997, Moore 1943, Ohori 1994). Transition zone and periurethral area nodules typically are multiple, whereas peripheral zone nodules usually are solitary (Bierhoff 1996, Kerley 1997, McNeal 1978). The number and size of hyperplastic nodules increases with age (Franks 1954A, McNeal 1978), with the greatest number of large nodules found in men over 60 years of age (Bierhoff 1996, McNeal 1978). This increase in BPH nodules correlates with the overall age-related increase in whole gland weight **t1.1**. The weight of BPH tissue resected by transurethral or open prostatectomy also increases with age and averages 21 g in the third decade, 43 g in the sixth decade, and 54 g in the ninth decade (Berry 1984). The weight range of surgically excised hyperplastic tissue is 5 g to several hundred grams (and even up to 800g). The transition zone nodules exhibit expansile growth, and larger ones in the transition zone can compress the urethra and peripheral zone. In the periurethral zone, the nodules are randomly scattered along the length of the proximal segment of the urethra, with extension to the bladder neck. When these proximal periurethral nodules become significantly enlarged, the mass can project into the bladder as an enlarged median or middle lobe (McNeal 1983) **i7.5**, which can obstruct the urethra in a ball-and-valve–like fashion. The peripheral zone nodules can produce a subcapsular bulge that can simulate carcinoma by DRE and TRUS. The gross appearance and texture of the nodules depend on the histologic cellular composition. Periurethral nodules made up of pure stromal cells are round, elliptical, dense, white nodules with a suggestion of a fibrillary or whorled cut surface (Moore 1943). The whorled look is reminiscent of a leiomyoma. Mixed glandular and stromal nodules may be hard or soft; the more epithelial ones can seem spongy with cystic change **i7.3**.

Microscopically, usual prostatic hyperplasia is a proliferation of either pure stromal cells or epithelial and stromal cells. Various classifications of usual prostatic hyperplasia have been forwarded (Franks 1954A, Price 1990) **t7.5**, and their main utility is diagnostic recognition.

Pure stromal cell hyperplasias may be either nodular or diffuse (Franks 1954A, Price 1990). The stromal cell nodules **t7.6**, which are thought to represent the first signs of BPH (Franks 1954A, McNeal 1983), are found predominantly in suburothelial tissues above the distal region of the verumontanum (Bierhoff 1996, Franks 1954A) but have also been reported in the central zone, and a few examples have been found in the peripheral zone (Bierhoff 1996). They are characterized by a well-circumscribed mass of spindled to star-shaped cells embedded in a myxoid **i7.6** or, more commonly, hyalinized **i7.7** matrix (Bierhoff 1996, Franks 1954A, Price 1990). The

■ **t7.5 Histologic Categories of Usual Hyperplasia**

I. Stromal nodules
   - Fibrous or fibrovascular nodule
   - Fibromuscular nodule
   - Muscular nodule ("leiomyoma")

II. Diffuse stromal hyperplasia

III. Glandular nodules[1]
   - Fibroadenomatous nodule
   - Fibromyoepithelial nodule

Modified from Price 1990, Franks 1954A

[1]Another way to classify glandular nodules is as high, medium, or low epithelial stromal nodules and cystic nodules (Price 1990)

■ **t7.6 Stromal Cell Hyperplastic Nodules**

Usually periurethral
Myxoid to hyalinized nodules
Composed of spindled, oval, or stellate cells
Hypocellular myxoid nodules
Hyalinized nodules with bundles and whorls
Matrix with prominent vascularity and scattered lymphocytes

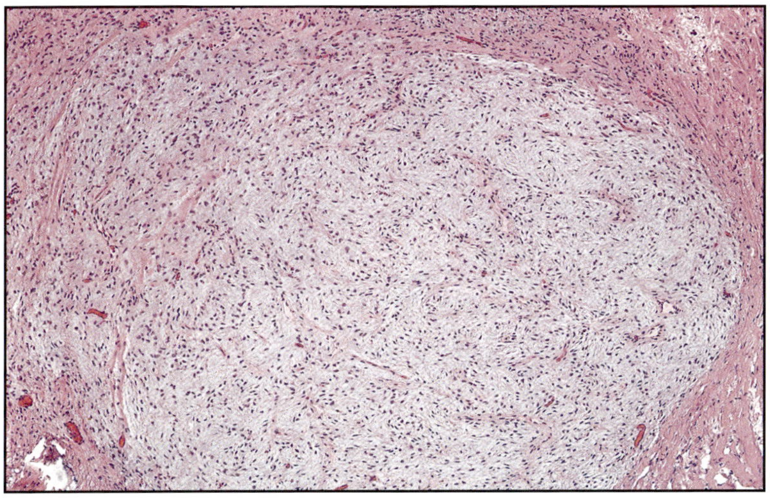

■ **i7.6** *Stromal hyperplasia (stromal nodule), with myxoid matrix.*

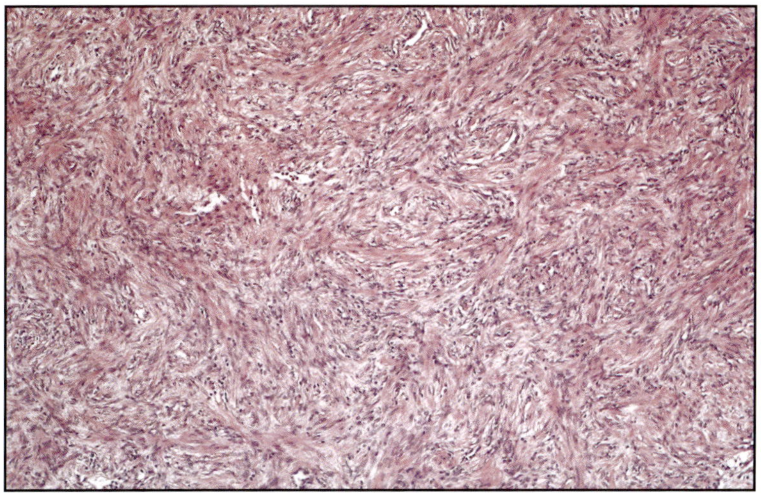

■ **i7.7** *Stromal hyperplasia (stromal nodule), with haphazardly-arranged, small bundles of fibromuscular spindle cells.*

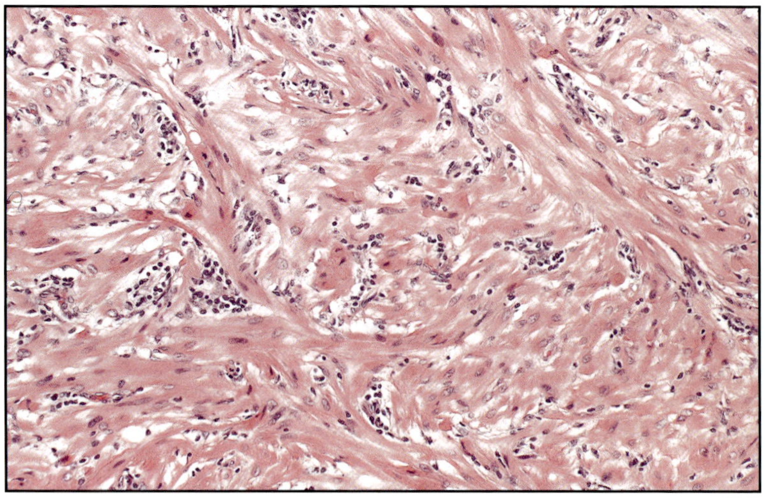

■ **i7.8** *Stromal hyperplasia with bundles and whorls of smooth muscle cells, the so-called "leiomyomatous variant."*

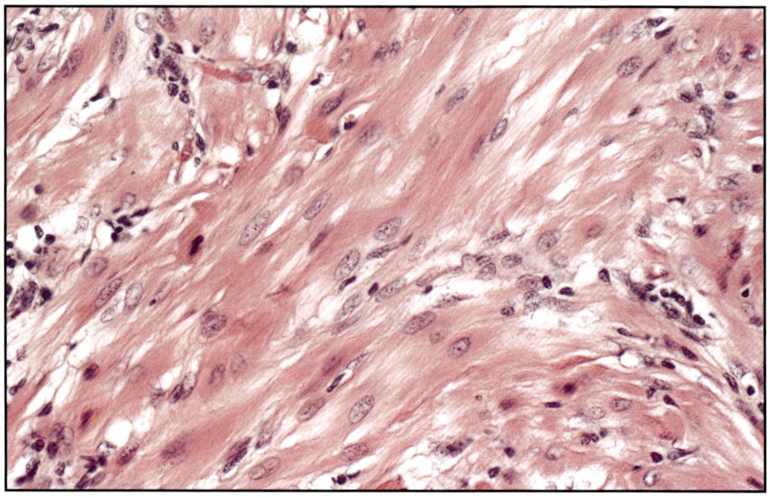

■ **i7.9** *Smooth muscle cells in stromal hyperplasia ("leiomyomatous variant").*

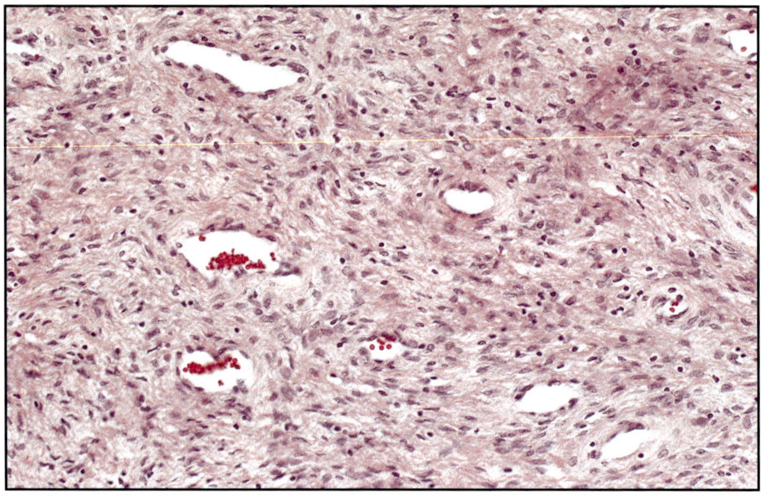

■ **i7.10** *Stromal hyperplasia with conspicuous vessels and scattered lymphocytes.*

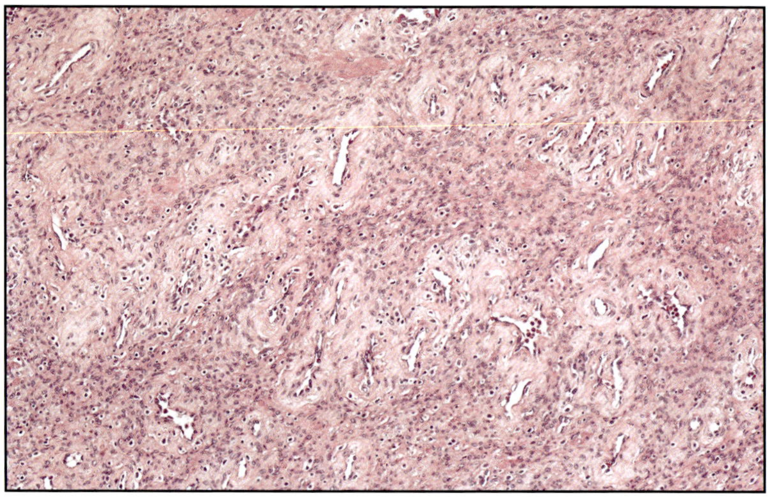

■ **i7.11** *Stromal hyperplasia with thick-walled blood vessels.*

spindled cells in the more hyalinized nodules can be arranged in bundles or whorls **i7.7, i7.8**. Some cells have a denser, more eosinophilic cytoplasm **i7.9**. There is a prominent vasculature **i7.10-i7.12**, which is made up of capillaries in the myxoid nodules and thick-walled vessels in the more hyalinized form **i7.11, i7.12**. Singly dispersed mature, small lymphocytes (which are mainly T-lymphocytes) are common in stromal nodules **i7.10** (Bierhoff 1996). Cytologic atypia and mitoses are lacking (Bierhoff 1996).

Stromal nodules have been classified as fibrous or fibrovascular, fibromuscular, and muscular (Franks 1954A) or as fibroblastic, fibromuscular, smooth muscular, and immature mesenchymal (Bierhoff 1996). This ordering is not diagnostically necessary but rather speaks to mesenchymal cell types that compose these nodules. These spindled cells mark by immunohistochemistry as immature mesenchymal cells (vimentin–, smooth muscle actin–, desmin–, myosin–), fibroblasts (vimentin+, smooth muscle actin–, desmin–, myosin–), smooth muscle cells (smooth muscle actin+, desmin+, myosin+), and myofibroblasts (vimentin+, smooth muscle actin+) (Bierhoff 1996). The most common immunophenotype is fibroblastic (62%), followed by fibromuscular (22%), immature mesenchymal (9%), and smooth muscular (4%). Diffuse stromal hyperplasia is less common than the nodular form and is distinguished from stromal nodules only by being larger and having a border that merges gradually with surrounding normal smooth muscle stroma (Price 1990). Stromal hyperplasia can be seen in needle biopsies **i7.13**, where it is not possible to determine whether it is nodular or diffuse.

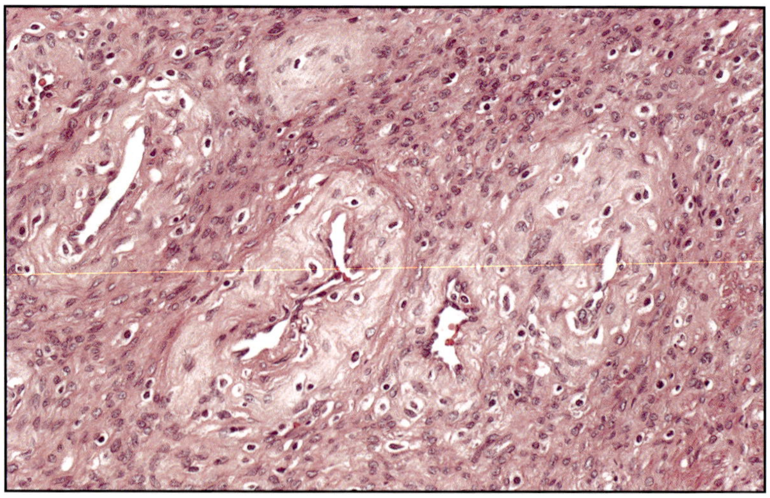

■ **i7.12** *Stromal hyperplasia with thick-walled blood vessels: Higher-power perspective showing hyalinization of vessel walls.*

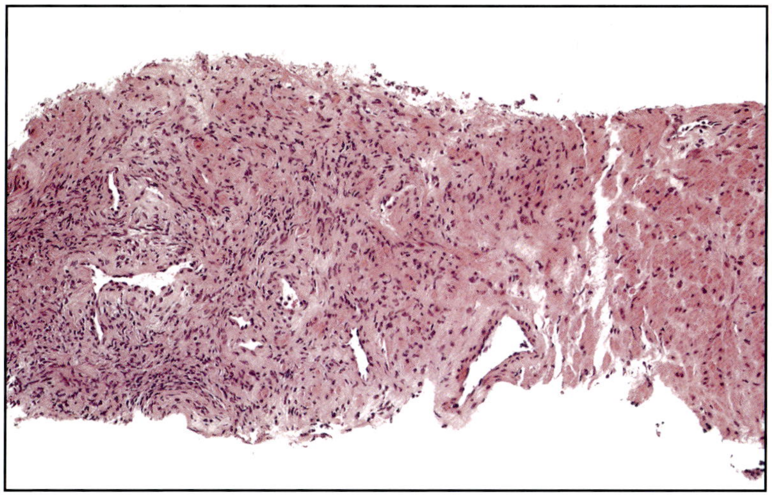

■ **i7.13** *Stromal hyperplasia in needle biopsy tissue (left) compared to normal prostatic stroma (right).*

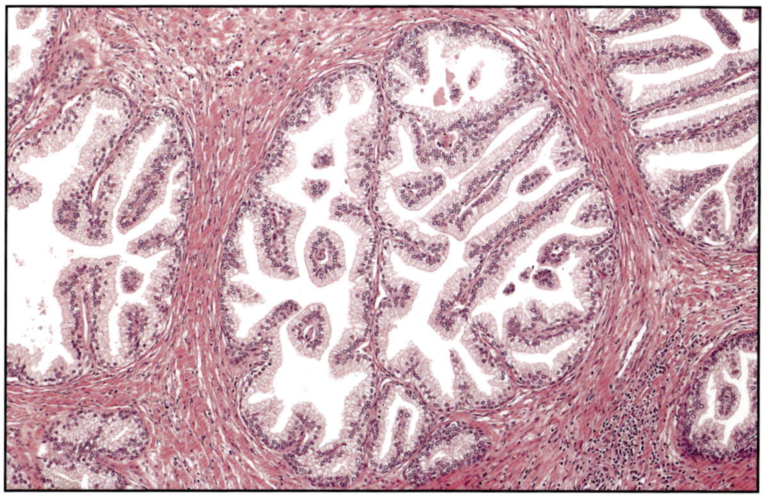

■ **i7.14** *Small hyperplastic nodule: A circumscribed collection of complex glands with a rounded border.*

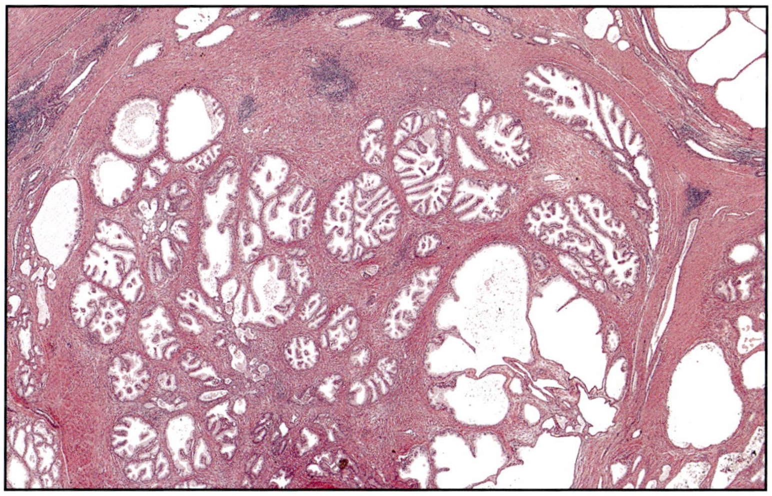

■ **i7.15** *BPH nodule with mixed glandular epithelial and stromal hyperplasia. The glands are complex with focal cystic change.*

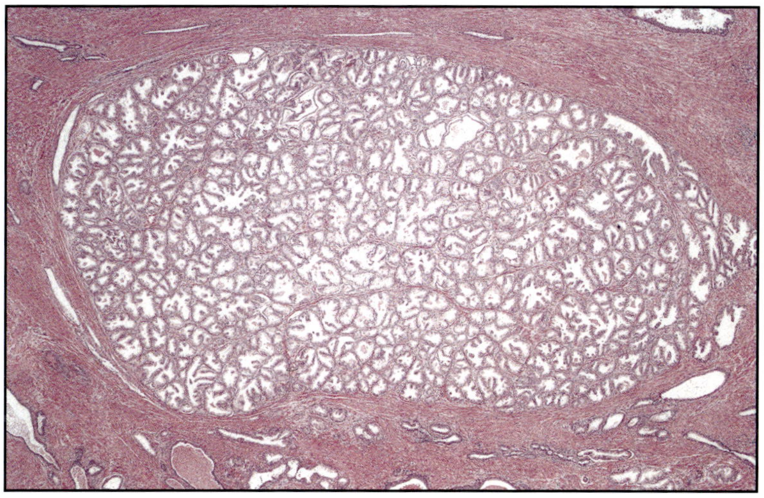

■ **i7.16** *Epithelial predominant BPH nodule.*

■ t7.7 **Glandular Hyperplastic Nodules**

Usually transition zone location
Expansile growth of hyperplastic epithelial and stromal cells
Variable epithelial:stromal ratio
Complex, branching glands with papillary projections and luminal undulations
Luminal cells: High-columnar with cleared/granular cytoplasm and small, bland, basally-situated nuclei without macronucleoli
Basal cells present and sometimes hyperplastic
Stromal cell component variable, from thin bands to dominant
Stromal cells: spindled to oval, bland

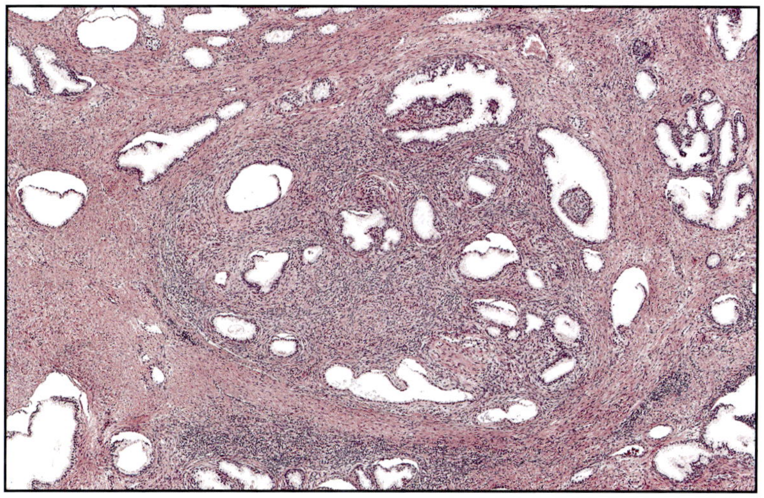

■ **i7.17** *Stromal predominant BPH nodule.*

Glandular nodules **t7.7**, which are a variable mixture of epithelial and stromal hyperplastic cells, usually are found in the transition zone but can also be seen in the periurethral area, central zone, and peripheral zone. In the transition zone, these hyperplastic nodules are thought to be glandular from their inception (McNeal 1983). The smallest or earliest growths can be difficult to identify because there is only an increased density of small glands with little in the way of an expansile border (Bierhoff 1996) **i7.14.**

Larger and better-developed glandular nodules are readily appreciated at scanning magnification **i7.15**. The variable amount of hyperplastic epithelium and stroma can also be noted at this level of examination. Epithelial predominant nodules **i7.16** have an epithelial-stromal ratio of about 2:1, whereas for stromal predominant nodules the ratio is reversed at 1:2 **i7.17** (Price 1990). The epithelial hyperplasia in

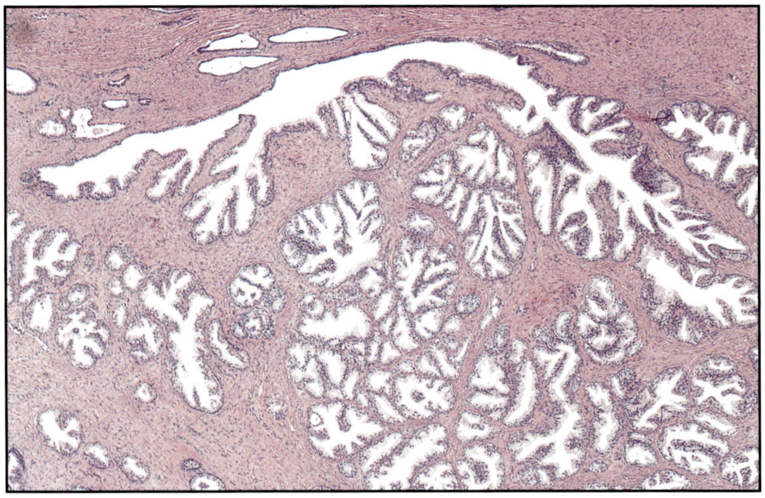

■ **i7.18** *BPH nodule with outer rimming gland demonstrating polarization of epithelial proliferation: There is ingrowth of new glands toward the nodule while the opposite luminal aspect is flattened.*

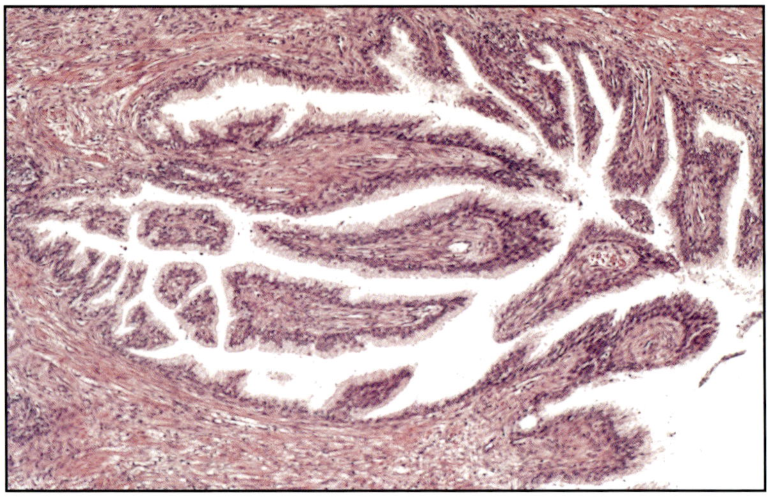

■ **i7.19** *Ingrowth of glands in BPH stroma from large outer duct (partially seen in lower right).*

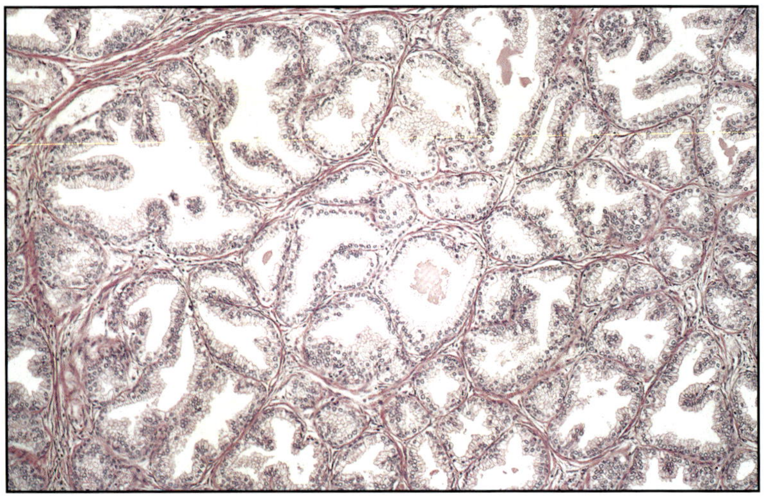

■ **i7.20** *BPH glands with variable size and shape.*

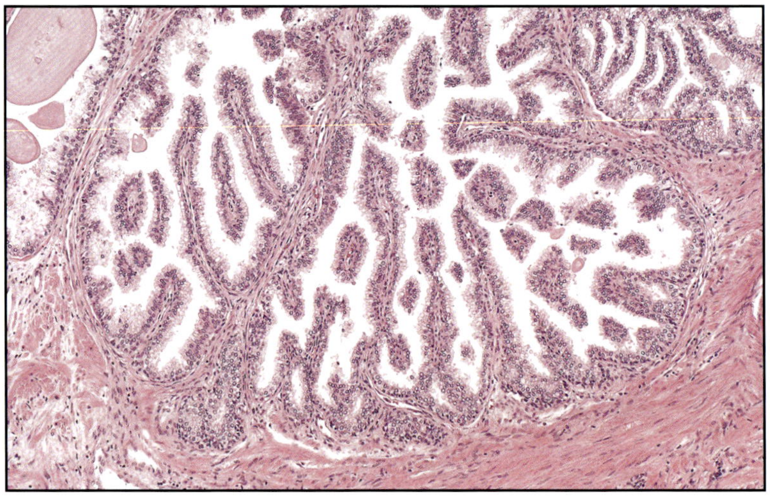

■ **i7.21** *BPH nodule with complex branching and papillary architecture.*

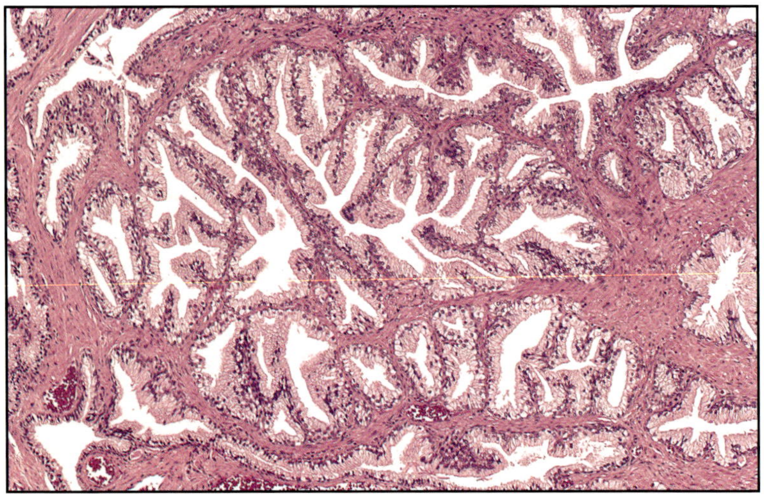

■ **i7.22** *Luminal papillary projections and undulations create a complex gland appearance.*

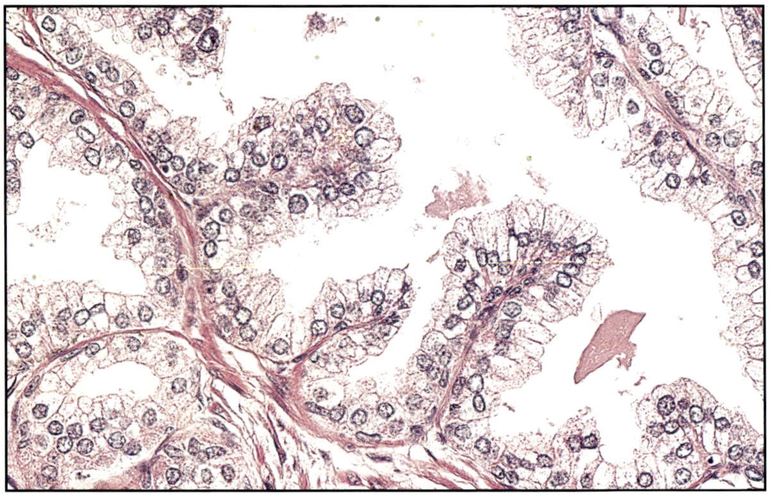

■ **i7.23** *Double layer epithelium in BPH. The luminal cells have a moderate amount of cleared, slightly granular cytoplasm. Basal cells are interspersed between luminal cells and surrounding stroma.*

glandular nodules is typified by a complex, branching arrangement of glands. In many nodules, it is possible to recognize the budding of new glands from preexisting ducts **i7.18, i7.19** (McNeal 1983). This distinctive pattern of growth often can be seen at the periphery of nodules, where ductal branches demonstrate inward ramifications, whereas the outer portion of the duct has a more flattened epithelial layer **i7.18**. Variable size and shape of glands, with complexity, true papillary projections, luminal undulations, and

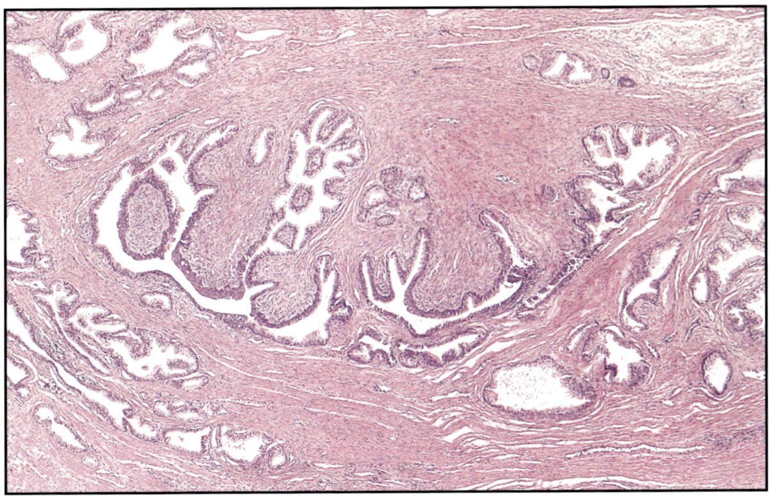

■ **i7.24** *Fibroadenomatoid BPH nodule.*

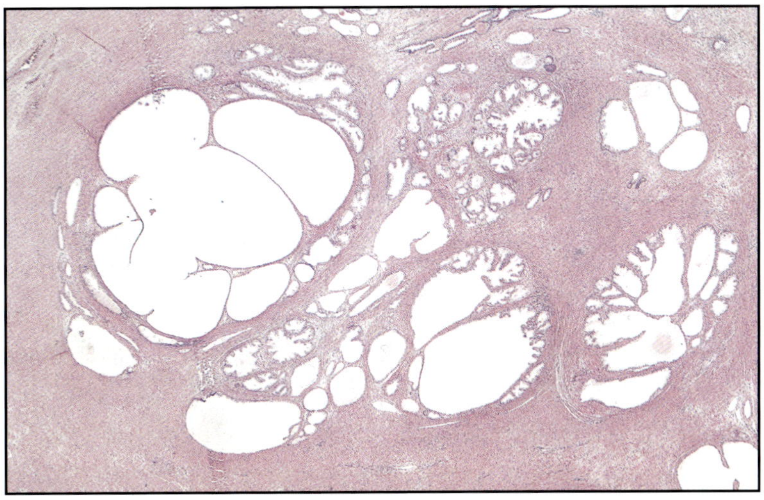

■ **i7.25** *Cyst formation in BPH nodules.*

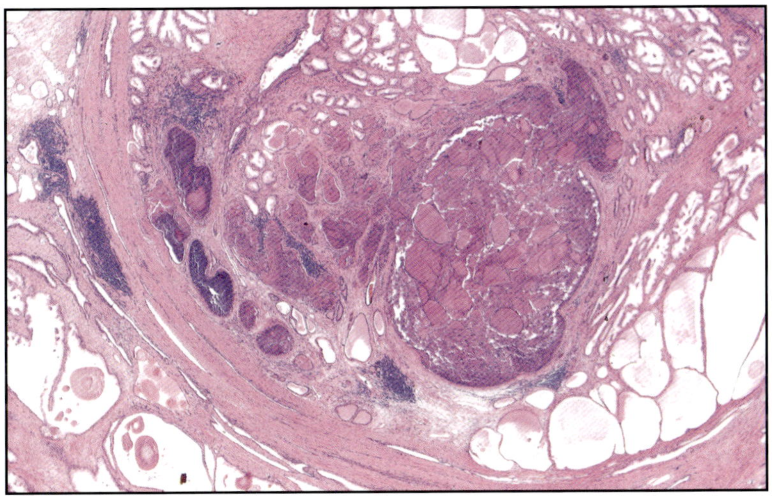

■ **i7.26** *Inflamed BPH nodule with duct-acinar expansion by inflammatory exudate.*

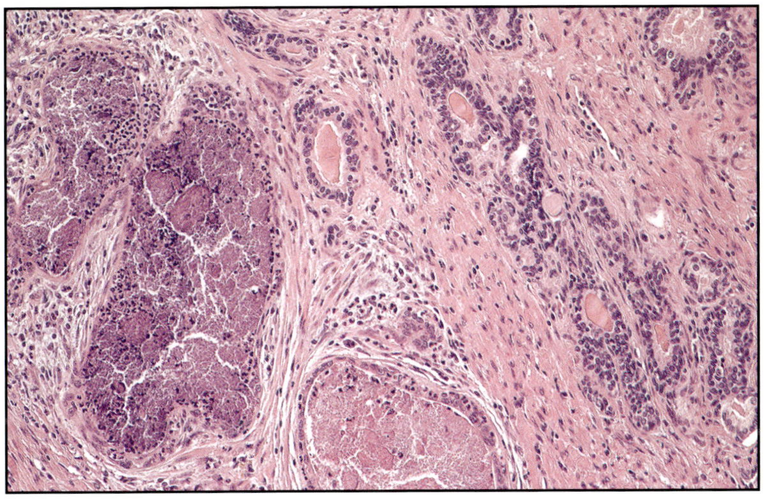

■ **i7.27** *BPH with intraglandular inflammatory exudate (left) and adjacent, reactive basal cell hyperplasia (right).*

branching, are all emblems of epithelial hyperplasia in the prostate **i7.20-i7.22**. The constituent epithelial cells of the glandular hyperplastic nodule include high columnar luminal cells and basal cells **i7.23**. The luminal cells have cleared to granular cytoplasm and basally situated, bland, regular nuclei without prominent nucleoli. In a minority of glands, the epithelium is low columnar to cuboidal, and in cystically dilated glands, the lining can be flattened and atrophic. Basal cells are readily detected in hyperplastic nodules, and not uncommonly this epithelial population also shows hyperplasia. (See section on basal cell hyperplasia later in this chapter.) Mitotic figures and apoptotic bodies in the hyperplastic luminal and basal cells are exceedingly rare. The luminal contents of hyperplastic glands include shed epithelial cells and corpora amylacea, while atypical intraluminal findings such as crystalloids and wispy blue mucin are rare. The appearance of stroma in glandular hyperplastic nodules varies from narrow smooth muscle bands between glands to broad bands to most of the nodule being composed of bland spindled cells similar to those in stromal nodules.

It is not necessary for diagnostic purposes to subtype the glandular hyperplastic nodules **t7.5**. One scheme (Franks 1954A) uses the terms *fibromyoepithelial nodule* and *fibroadenomatous nodule.* Foci resembling the mammary fibroadenoma do occur within the spectrum of nodular prostatic hyperplasia **i7.24**, but this is uncommon, with an incidence of 1% (Kafandaris 1983). A second scheme (Price 1990) uses the categories of high, medium, and low epithelial or stromal nodules and cystic nodules, but again, their main usefulness is in stimulating awareness of the range of morphologic presentation of glandular prostatic hyperplasia.

Secondary histologic alterations in hyperplastic nodules include cystic change, inflammation, duct or acinar rupture, squamous cell metaplasia, and infarction. Cystic glandular dilatation is common in BPH **i7.25**. The epithelial lining of the cysts often is flattened, with an atrophic appearance. Inflammation is also common in BPH, with 20% to 98% of BPH cases showing acute inflammation and 85% to 100% of cases harboring chronic inflammation **i7.26, i7.27** (Brawer 1989, Hasui 1994, Kohnen 1979). Duct or acinar expansion by inflammatory exudate can be associated with this inflammatory infiltrate **i7.26, i7.27**. Squamous cell metaplasia can be found in inflamed or infarcted BPH areas (Chapter 6).

Infarction is a reasonably common histologic finding in large BPH tissue samples (TURP chips, simple prostatectomy specimens, and whole glands from autopsy), with an overall incidence of 18% (451 of 2 563 cases), with a range of 3% to 85% (Baird 1950, Golden 1953,

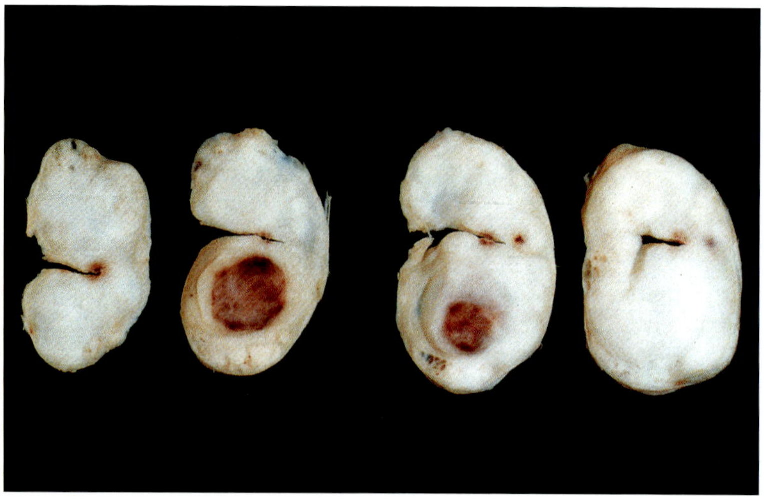

■ **i7.28** *Infarct in BPH: A rounded red-brown to tan nodule. (Reprinted from* Royal College of Surgeons of England Slide Atlas of Pathology, *1985, slide 99.)*

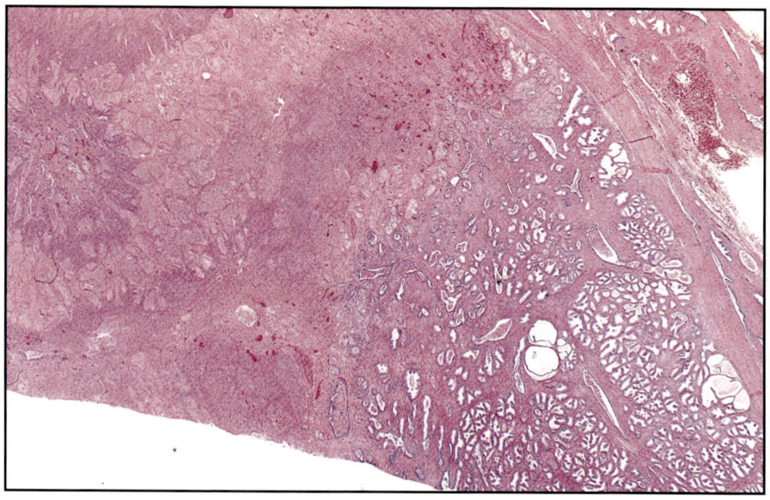

■ **i7.29** *Infarct of prostate: Large geographic zone of coagulative necrosis.*

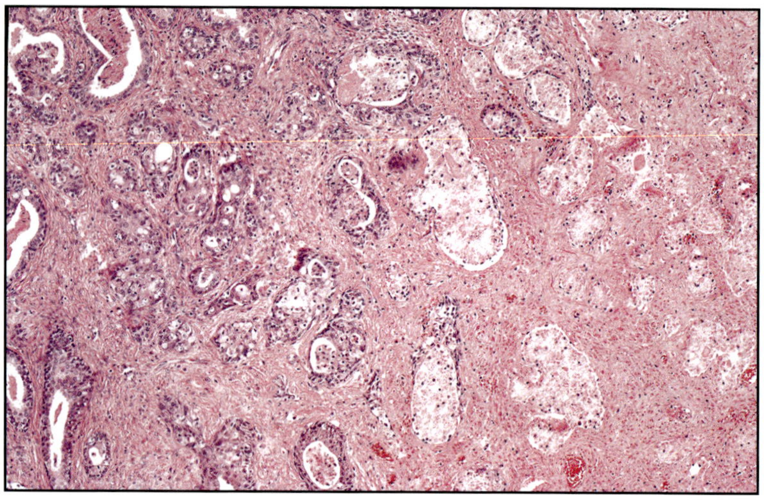

■ **i7.30** *Infarct with squamous metaplasia of glands in border region between infarct (right) and viable prostate.*

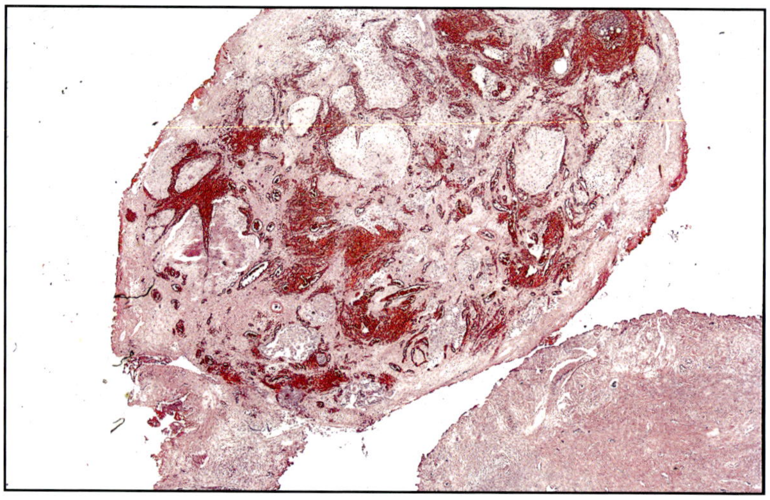

■ **i7.31** *Hemorrhagic infarct in TURP chip.*

Moore 1943, Roth 1949, Spiro 1974, Strachan 1993, Sutton 1943) **t7.8**. However, infarcts are rarely identified in needle biopsy tissue (Milford 2000), mainly because the transition zone, where BPH arises, typically is not targeted. The remarkably high incidence of 85% was found in patients who presented with acute urinary retention (Spiro 1974). Infarction has also been clinically associated with gross hematuria, advanced patient age, and large volume BPH (Baird 1950, Golden 1953). Clinically, infarcts can mimic prostate cancer because they can present (rarely) as a palpable nodule (Jewett 1956) or be associated with an elevated serum PSA (Brawn 1994, Garvin 1990), which can range from 6.9 ng/mL to 287 ng/mL, a level that is often associated with metastatic prostate carcinoma. Various possible causes have been proposed for prostatic infarct development, including urethral instrumentation and catheterization, infection, atherosclerosis, thromboembolism, smoking, compression of vascular supply by BPH mass effect, and hypotension (Baird 1950, Feero 1990, Golden 1953, Roth 1949, Spiro 1974, Strachan 1993, Taussig 1984). (Hypotension and urethral catheterization can also cause infarcts in the nonhyperplastic prostate [Jones 1986]). Grossly, prostatic infarcts in BPH appear bright and red to mottled, dull, reddish-brown or gray, and round to oval **i7.28**. They can be single or multiple and measure up to several centimeters in diameter (Golden 1953). Microscopically, the appearance depends on the age of the infarct (Spiro 1974). Coagulative necrosis, with a ghostlike outline of hyperplastic glands, is typical **i7.29-i7.33**. During the first 1 to 2 days, neutrophilic infiltrates are minimal. By day 4 neutrophilic infiltrates, stromal edema, and parenchymal necrosis are maximal (Spiro 1974). Hemorrhage and squamous cell metaplasia are common in the border zone between necrotic and viable tissue **i7.30**. Hemorrhagic infarcts can also be seen **i7.31, i7.32**. Significant nuclear atypia, including macronucleoli, and mitotic figures can be visualized in these foci of squamous metaplasia. Repair takes place during the third to sixth week, with the only residue being squamous cell metaplasia, lymphocytes, and fibrosis (Moore 1943, Spiro 1974).

There is no histologic evidence of a significant physical transition between usual epithelial hyperplasia and prostatic neoplasia. Both prostatic intraepithelial neoplasia (PIN) and carcinoma preferentially

■ **t7.8 Prostatic Infarcts**

18% of BPH cases have infarcts
Can elevate serum PSA
Grossly: Red to brown to gray, single or multiple, round to ovoid areas measuring up to several cm
Microscopically: Coagulative necrosis with hemorrhage, neutrophils, and squamous metaplasia

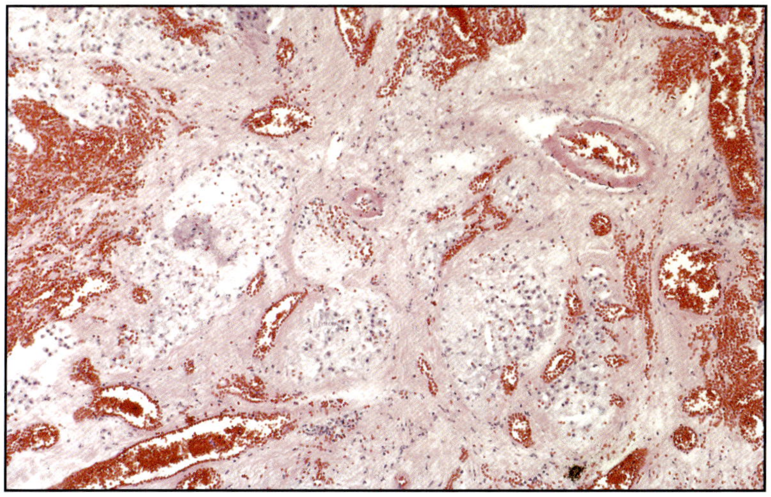

■ **i7.32** *Hemorrhagic infarct in TURP chip: Higher magnification of* **i7.31** *showing congested vessels, with stromal hemorrhage and early necrosis of glands.*

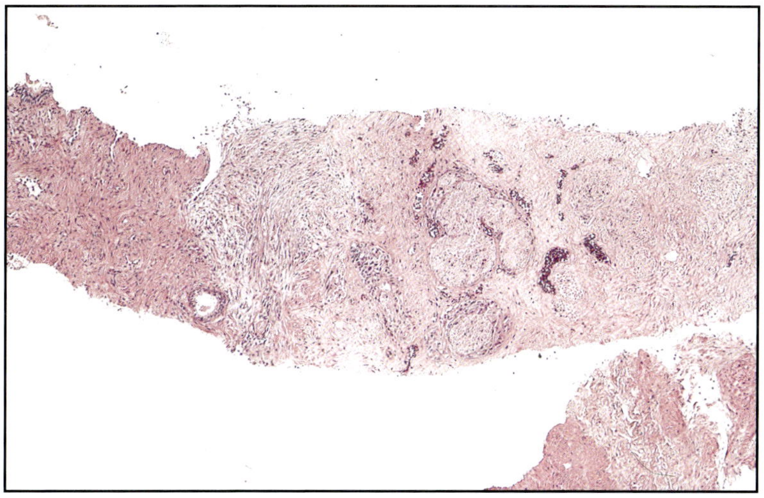

■ **i7.33** *Infarct in needle biopsy tissue: Infarct is swollen, pale tissue (right).*

involve the peripheral zone, whereas BPH most commonly occurs in the transition zone. Only 5% of cases of high-grade PIN involve BPH nodules (Bostwick 1993A), whereas about 20% of prostatic carcinomas are found within the transition zone (Greene 1991, Grignon 1994, McNeal 1988), where they can involve BPH nodules. Yet the incidence of usual hyperplasia is the same in glands with and without prostatic carcinoma (Kahler 1939). Also, the amount (volume) of nodular hyperplasia has no effect on the likelihood or size of associated carcinoma arising in the transition zone (Ewton 1998). For carcinomas that arise in the transition zone, there does not appear to be direct physical continuity with usual epithelial hyperplasia.

The differential diagnosis of usual prostatic hyperplasia can be divided into stromal-based and epithelial-based lists. For stromal hyperplasia of the prostate, the differential diagnosis includes normal prostatic stroma, prostatic reactive and reparative conditions, benign stromal neoplasms, and malignant stromal neoplasms **t7.9**. Compared with normal prostatic stroma, stromal hyperplasia is more hypercellular, is more vascular, and has a myxoid or hyalinized matrix. Reactive or reparative spindled granulation tissue, fibrosis, and postoperative spindle cell nodules could simulate prostatic stromal hyperplasia, but the former two usually are not nodular, and patients with postoperative spindle cell nodule have a previous history of surgery (usually TURP). A few stromal cell proliferations have enlarged, bizarre nuclei, with or without a phyllodes (leaflike) pattern of growth. These lesions have been designated as pseudosarcomatous (Young 1987), atypical stromal hyperplasia (Attah 1976, 1977, Leong 1988, Reese 1987, Wang 1997), and prostatic stromal proliferation of uncertain malignant potential (Gaudin 1998). It is not clear whether these rare cases represent a reactive or neoplastic proliferation (see Chapter 18). Usual prostatic stromal hyperplasia lacks the nuclear atypia of these proliferations and does not grow as broad fronds projecting into an epithelial line space, like phyllodes tumors. Cases diagnosed as "leiomyoma" of the prostate (Kaufmann 1951, Vassilakis 1978) probably represent the smooth muscular variant of nodular stromal hyperplasia. Myxoid neurofibroma could be confused with myxoid stromal hyperplasia, but there are only a few reported cases of prostatic neurofibroma (Chung 1996, McDonnell 1936). Prostatic stromal hyperplastic lesions can have fibrous histiocytomalike areas, but fibrous histiocytomas have not been reported in the prostate. Inflammatory myofibroblastic tumor, also known as pseudosarcomatous fibromyxoid tumor (Ro 1993, Sahin 1991), can involve the prostate and has more of an infiltrative appearance with cytologic pleomorphism than myxoid stromal hyperplasia. Lastly, prostatic sarcomas such as rhabdomyosarcoma, leiomyosarcoma, malignant phyllodes tumor (cystosarcoma phyllodes), and sarcomatoid carcinomas (carcinosarcomas) should be excluded (Cheville 1995, Dundore 1995, Gaudin 1998, Lauwers 1993, Lopez-Beltran 1990, Loughlin 1989, Shannon 1992, Wick 1984). In contrast to usual prostatic stromal hyperplasia, these malignancies demonstrate cytologic atypia, invasiveness or stromal overgrowth, necrosis, and mitotic activity. Sarcomatoid carcinomas can show an admixed adenocarcinoma and heterologous elements (with differentiation along the lines of bone, skeletal muscle, fat, or cartilage), which are not present in usual prostatic stromal hyperplasia.

The main differential diagnostic concerns for usual epithelial hyperplasia in the prostate are normal prostatic epithelium, PIN, atypical adenomatous hyperplasia (adenosis), well-differentiated adenocarcinoma, and pseudohyperplastic adenocarcinoma **t7.10**.

Normal prostatic epithelium often is misinterpreted as hyperplastic prostatic epithelium, particularly in needle biopsies. Yet most prostatic needle biopsies are directed to the peripheral zone, where

■ **t7.9 Prostatic Stromal Hyperplasia: Differential Diagnosis**

Normal prostatic stroma
Granulation tissue and fibrosis
Postoperative spindle cell nodule
Prostatic stromal proliferation of uncertain malignant potential (PSPUMP)
Benign mesenchymal neoplasms: leiomyoma, neurofibroma
Inflammatory myofibroblastic tumor (pseudosarcomatous fibromyxoid tumor)
Prostatic sarcoma
Sarcomatoid prostatic carcinoma (carcinosarcoma)

■ **t7.10 Prostatic Usual Epithelial Hyperplasia: Differential Diagnosis**

Normal prostatic epithelium
Prostatic intraepithelial neoplasia
Atypical adenomatous hyperplasia (adenosis)
Well-differentiated adenocarcinoma
Pseudohyperplastic prostatic adenocarcinoma

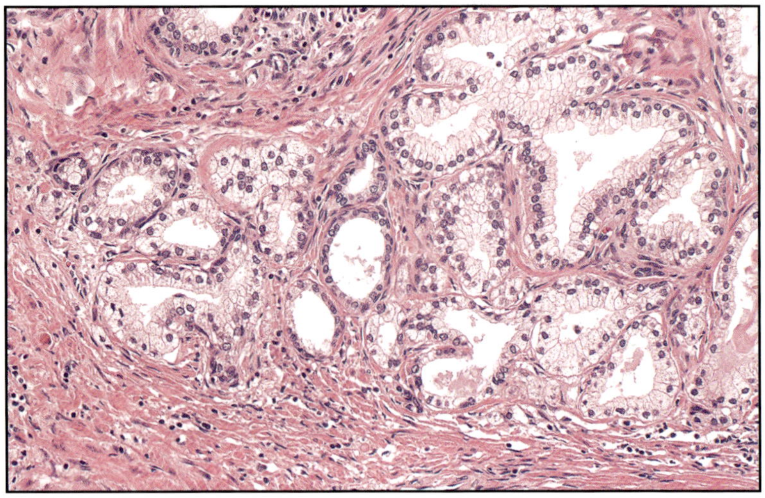

■ **i7.34** *BPH nodules can have a few small gland buds at the periphery.*

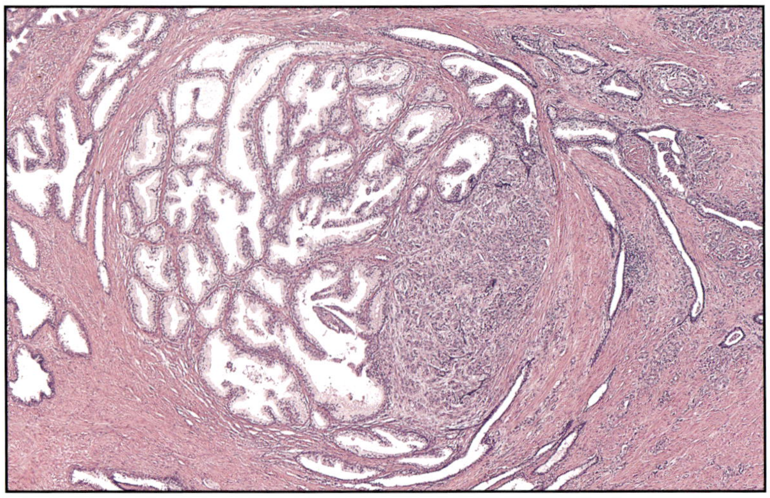

■ **i7.35** *BPH nodule secondarily involved by high-grade carcinoma (the solid nodule within the BPH nodule).*

prostatic carcinoma is most common and where BPH is decidedly uncommon. Both normal prostatic epithelium and hyperplastic epithelium share complex glandular configurations, with papillary infoldings, branching, and luminal undulations. Cytologically, the constituent basal cells and luminal cells are similar. One clue that the needle biopsy might have sampled a BPH nodule is if the background stroma also appears hyperplastic. Benign prostate needle biopsy cases should be signed out as "benign prostatic tissue" and not BPH (Viglione 2002).

Usual epithelial hyperplasia can be difficult to impossible to distinguish from low-grade PIN, whereas the distinction from high-grade PIN usually is easily made. Hyperplastic and PIN glands resemble each other in gland structure, but hyperplastic glands appear paler than PIN glands. Cytologically, the nuclear abnormalities of nucleomegaly and size variability are present in low-grade PIN (McNeal 1986) but not noninflamed usual epithelial hyperplasia. Any reactive changes in hyperplasia, oblique sectioning, poor preservation, or thick sections can create real problems in separating hyperplasia from low-grade PIN. This separation is not very reproducible (Epstein 1995B, Tsuchiya 1993) and also is not necessary because low-grade PIN is not a risk factor for detection of carcinoma. High-grade PIN is readily distinguished from hyperplasia based on the malignant-appearing nuclei in high-grade PIN.

Small acinar buds from usual glandular hyperplasia **i7.34** can be misinterpreted as atypical adenomatous hyperplasia (adenosis). Yet these small acini in usual hyperplastic nodules are scattered and few in number. In contrast, atypical adenomatous hyperplasia (adenosis) has a higher density of small, closely packed glands (Bostwick 1993B, Gaudin 1994, 1995A). Adenosis also more often has intraluminal crystalloids than usual hyperplasia, and the basal cell layer is fragmented rather than complete. Significant nuclear atypia (nuclear enlargement and macronucleoli) is not a trait of either usual epithelial hyperplasia or atypical adenomatous hyperplasia.

A historical diagnostic dilemma is distinguishing usual prostatic epithelial hyperplasia from well-differentiated adenocarcinoma (Ackerman 1964, Andrews 1949, Franks 1954A, Moore 1935, Muir 1934, Totten 1953, Willis 1948). Indeed, in 1934 Muir (Muir 1934) noted this diagnostic difficulty and stated, "The appearance (of well-differentiated carcinomas) may closely resemble benign hypertrophy and render diagnosis difficult." Actually, the typical small acinar prostatic carcinoma does not resemble the complex gland formations of usual epithelial hyperplasia. Rather, it is an uncommon variant, pseudohyperplastic prostatic adenocarcinoma, that can cause immense diagnostic difficulty. Both usual epithelial hyperplasia and pseudohyperplastic prostatic adenocarcinoma generate complex medium to large-sized gland formations with papillary infoldings, luminal undulations, branching, and cystic dilatation (Humphrey 1998, Levi 2000). It should be emphasized that these growth patterns are more typically associated with benign, usual epithelial hyperplasia but are not specific for hyperplasia. Compared with pseudohyperplastic prostatic adenocarcinoma, usual epithelial hyperplasia has basal cells and lacks luminal cell nuclear atypia. Small, pinpoint nucleoli can be found in a minority of nuclei, but prominent nucleoli larger than 1 μm in diameter should not be seen in noninflamed usual epithelial hyperplasia (Gleason 1985). Prominent nucleoli in hyperplastic epithelium can be seen in inflamed and reactive, metaplastic epithelium, especially at the edge of infarcts. Most nucleoli in hyperplastic cells are single and more centrally located than in neoplastic epithelium (Montironi 1992). Additionally, most cases of pseudohyperplastic variant of prostate adenocarcinoma exhibit a transition to, or admixture with, a typical small acinar adenocarcinomatous component (Humphrey 1998). However, it should be kept in mind that carcinoma can secondarily invade BPH nodules **i7.35** or even appear to arise within BPH nodules. In difficult cases, including needle biopsy sampling, immunohistochemical staining with antibody 34βE12 to identify basal cells can be a helpful confirmatory measure. The similarity in the low-power appearance of usual epithelial hyperplasia and pseudohyperplastic prostatic adenocarcinoma underscores the importance of examining prostatic tissues at both scanning and higher-power magnifications.

The special diagnostic technique most often applied in cases of usual epithelial hyperplasia is immunohistochemistry for basal cells using antibody 34βE12 (Brawer 1985, Okada 1992). Additional histochemical, immunohistochemical, and genetic studies have been performed in BPH tissues, but these are not currently being applied for diagnostic purposes. Histochemical studies have shown that silver staining for argyrophilic nucleolar organizer regions (AgNORs) yields AgNOR counts for usual epithelial hyperplasia that are less than those of PIN or carcinoma (Masai 1992, Mukherjee 1997, Sesterhenn 1991), but there is overlap in some cases (Cheville 1990, Mukherjee 1997, Sesterhenn 1991). Histochemical staining for mucins likewise does not definitely distinguish between hyperplastic and neoplastic

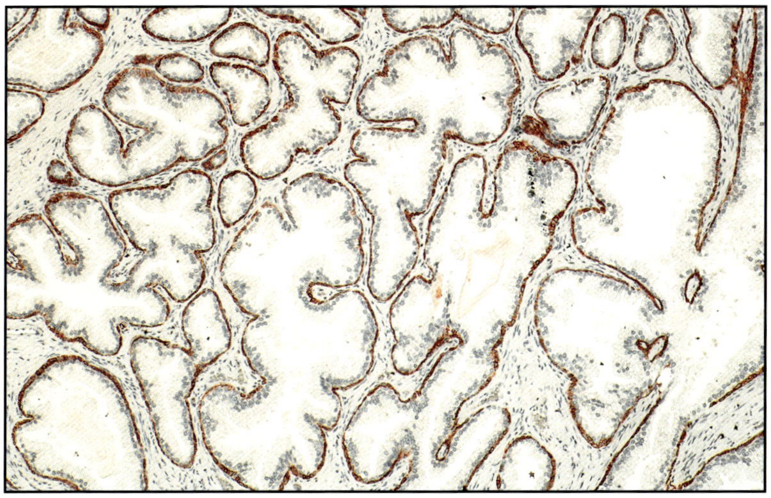

■ **i7.36** *Intact basal cell layer in BPH (34βE12 immunostain for high-molecular weight cytokeratins).*

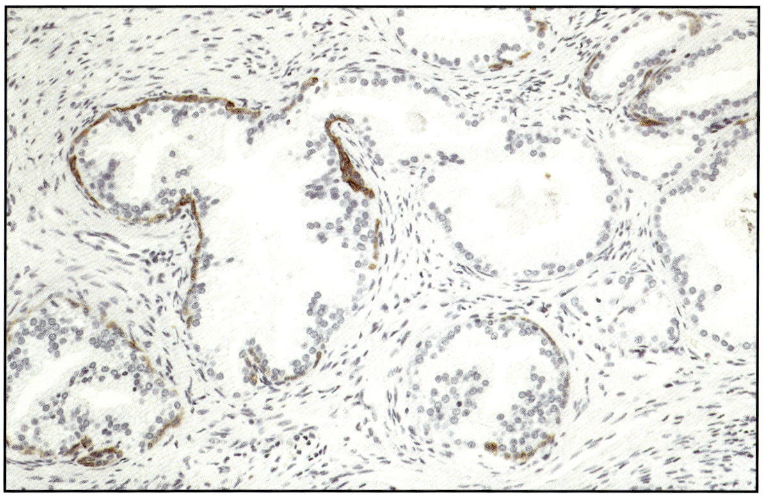

■ **i7.37** *Focal absence of basal cell staining should not be taken as evidence of malignancy (34βE12 immunostain of basal cell high-molecular weight cytokeratins).*

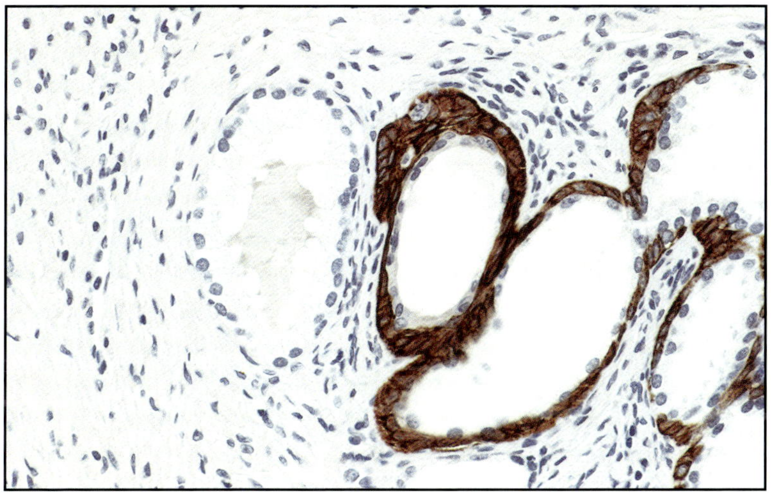

■ **i7.38** *Absence of basal cell staining in benign gland, using the 34βE12 antibody in immunohistochemistry.*

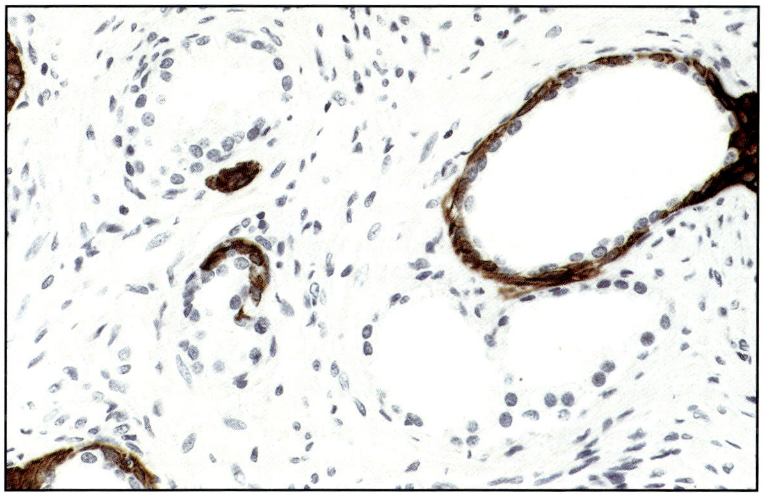

■ **i7.39** *Absence of basal cell staining in several benign glands, using the 34βE12 antibody in immunohistochemistry.*

prostatic epithelial proliferations, although acid mucin staining (with Alcian blue, pH 2.5) is commonly present in high-grade PIN (Humphrey 1991, Sentinelli 1993) and carcinoma (Allsbrook 1998) but is only occasionally seen in small acinar foci in BPH (Epstein 1992A).

The immunophenotype of usual epithelial hyperplasia is similar to that of normal prostatic glands (**t1.3, p7**). Of prime significance diagnostically, usual epithelial hyperplasia is similar to normal prostatic epithelium in that it has an intact basal cell layer that can be demonstrated by antibodies directed against basal cell–specific high-molecular-weight cytokeratins, such as 34βE12 (also called antibody 903), CK8.12, and 312C8-1 (Brawer 1985, Okada 1992) **i7.36**. Focal loss of staining can occur in BPH **i7.37-i7.39**, including in areas of inflammation, and should not be misconstrued as evidence of malignancy. In most cases of hyperplasia, this immunostain is not needed because basal cells can be easily seen on hematoxylin and eosin (H&E)-stained sections. Immunohistologic differences from normal prostatic epithelium include detection of antigens related to cell turnover, cell adhesion molecules, stromal cell proteoglycans, and microvessel density. Although the frequency of mitotic figures in BPH by H&E staining is only 0.001% (Giannulis 1993), the proliferation index of BPH, as judged by immunohistochemistry using antibodies against proliferating cell nuclear antigen or Ki-67 (including the MIB-1 antibody, which reacts with the Ki-67 antigen in formalin-fixed, paraffin-embedded tissue sections), is 0.6% to 4.0% (Bonkhoff 1994, Colombel 1998, Gallee 1989, Kyprianou 1996, McLoughin 1993, Montironi 1993B, Oomens 1991, Raymond 1988). This mean proliferation index is higher than normal epithelium at 0.1% to 0.9% (Colombel 1998, Kyprianou 1996) and in general less than means for PIN (at 6% to 14%) and carcinoma (at 3% to 16%), but overlap of ranges precludes diagnostic application for individual patients (Bostwick 1998, Gallee 1989, Kaleem 1998, McLoughin 1993, Montironi 1993B, Oomens 1991, Raymond 1988). Immunohistochemical staining for the cell cycle regulator $p27^{KIP1}$ is lost in BPH compared with normal epithelium (Cordon-Cardo 1998), which could be related to the somewhat increased proliferation rate. p53 Protein, which is also related to cell proliferation and death, has been found to focally accumulate in up to 36% of BPH cases, as detected by immunohistochemistry (Humphrey 1995, Kallakury 1994B, Wertz 1996). Bcl-2, an anti–cell death protein, is higher, by immunohistochemical assessment, in BPH than in normal prostatic epithelium (Colombel 1998, Kyprianou 1996). Other immunohistologic abnormalities in usual hyperplasia in comparison to normal epithelium include decreased staining for the epithelial cell adhesion protein C-CAM (Kleinerman 1995) and an increase in microvessel density (using an antibody against factor VIII–related antigen) (Deering 1995).

DNA and genetic abnormalities are ill-defined in BPH. p53 gene mutation, which is one of the most common alterations in human neoplasia (Humphrey 1994), has been found in 5% to 56% of BPH cases (Kallakury 1994A, Meyers 1993, Schlechte 1998, Wertz 1996). Although this finding has been suggested as a risk factor for carcinoma development (Schlechte 1998), this remains speculative. DNA fragmentation, detected by in situ terminal deoxynucleotidyl transferase (TdT)-mediated dUTP-biotin nick end labeling (TUNEL staining), indicative of apoptosis, was found in 0.5% to 1% of BPH epithelial cells, and this was somewhat lower than in normal prostatic epithelium (Kyprianou 1996). (Counting of apoptotic bodies on H&E-stained slides yields similar results for BPH at 0.3% to 1.4% [Kyprianou 1996, Montironi 1993A], and this former figure is significantly lower than that in PIN and carcinoma [Montironi 1993A].) A provocative finding is a high level of microsatellite instability in BPH (Werely 1996), where 38% of cases exhibited this abnormality (compared with 77% of prostatic carcinomas). The specific genes involved at these putative sites of somatic mutation and the specific gene abnormalities in germ-line DNA mutation in hereditary BPH are not known.

Finally, special tissue-based techniques do not currently allow prediction of response to BPH therapy, but proposals to develop such methods have been made. For example, because successful medical treatment of BPH may depend on the histologic composition of the BPH nodules, efforts have been made to quantitate, by morphometric analysis and immunohistochemistry, the amount of smooth muscle in BPH tissue (Robert 1995, Shapiro 1992). This approach remains experimental.

[7.6] Basal Cell Hyperplasia

Basal cell hyperplasia, also called fetalization or embryonal hyperplasia because of its resemblance to developing fetal glands, is positioned at one end of the spectrum of basaloid proliferations in the prostate (Bennett 1985, Bonkhoff 1994, Cleary 1983, Dermer 1978, Devaraj 1993, Epstein 1992B, Grignon 1988, Mittal 1989, Sarma 1982, Thorson 1999, van de Voorde 1994A) **t7.11**. Basal cell hyperplasia is uncommon, with an incidence of 3% to 15% (Bennett 1985, Devaraj 1993, Mittal 1989, Thorson 1999). Though often viewed as a transition zone proliferation found in the setting of usual epithelial hyperplasia, it can also be found in the peripheral zone, associated with inflammation (Thorson 2000). Finally, basal cell hyperplasia is a common reactive response to therapy effect on the prostate.

Basal cell hyperplasia usually is an incidental histologic finding in TURP chips (Cleary 1983, Devaraj 1993, Mittal 1989) or needle biopsies of the peripheral zone performed to rule out carcinoma (Thorson 1999). Patients typically are 60 to 80 years of age and present with prostatism symptoms that results in prostatectomy or with an abnormal DRE or serum PSA that results in needle biopsy.

■ t7.11 Prostatic Basal Cell Proliferations

Usual basal cell hyperplasia
Atypical basal cell hyperplasia (basal cell hyperplasia with prominent nucleoli)
Basal cell adenoma (nodular basal cell hyperplasia)
Adenoid basal cell tumor (adenoid cystic tumor; adenoid cystic-like tumor; adenoid cystic/basal cell carcinoma)

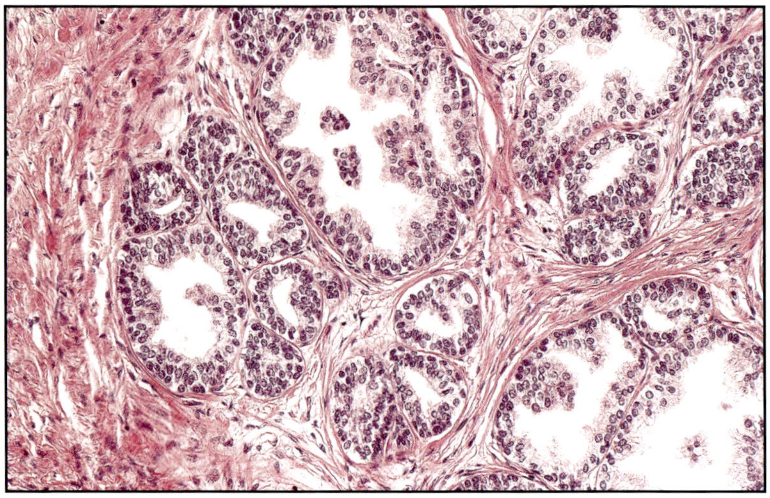

■ i7.40 *Basal cell hyperplasia in a few glands in a BPH nodule.*

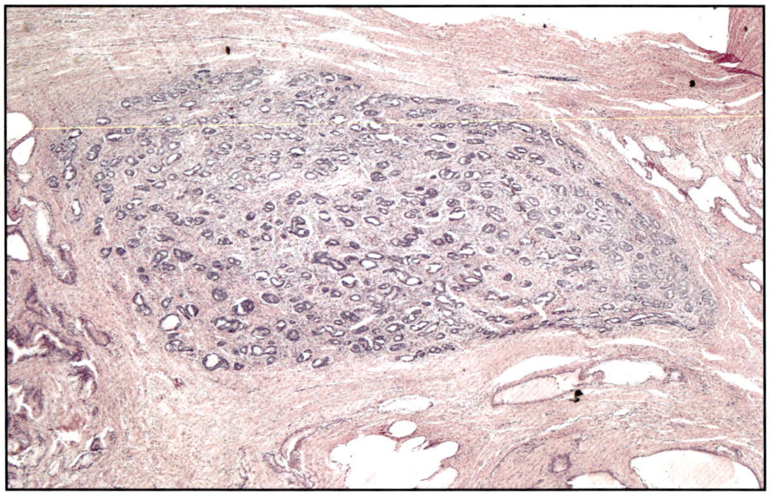

■ i7.41 *Nodular basal cell hyperplasia.*

Histologically, basal cell hyperplasia may be divided into usual (or ordinary) and atypical types (Devaraj 1993, Epstein 1992B). Currently, this is purely a morphologic distinction, and there is no known clinical meaning attached to a diagnosis of atypical basal cell hyperplasia. Usual basal cell hyperplasia often is multifocal (Cleary 1983, Epstein 1992B) and is characterized by two or more layers of basal cells with a range of growth features **t7.12**. These glands or nests often are focal **i7.40** but can form nodules (Oyen 1993) **i7.41**. In some cases the glands can appear to infiltrate between normal or hyperplastic glands **i7.42**. The glandular forms vary from tubular to cribriform to solid configurations **i7.43-i7.45**. The patterns vary from focal, eccentric, partial gland involvement **i7.46** to a symmetric, circumferential proliferation with central retention of secretory cell layer **i7.43**,

■ t7.12 Basal Cell Hyperplasia (BCH)

Two or more layers of basal cells
Acinar, cribriform and solid growth patterns
Usual BCH: Cytologically bland ovoid to elongated cells
Atypical BCH: BCH with prominent nucleoli

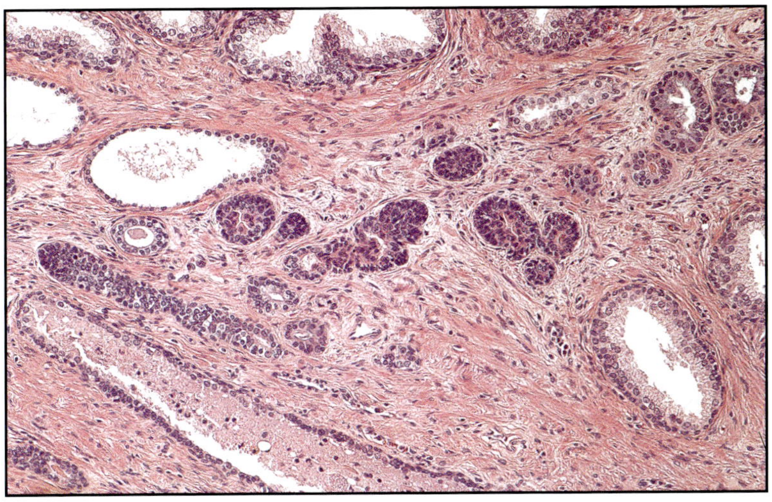

■ **i7.42** *Pseudoinfiltrative appearance of small, solid nests and tubules of basal cell hyperplasia.*

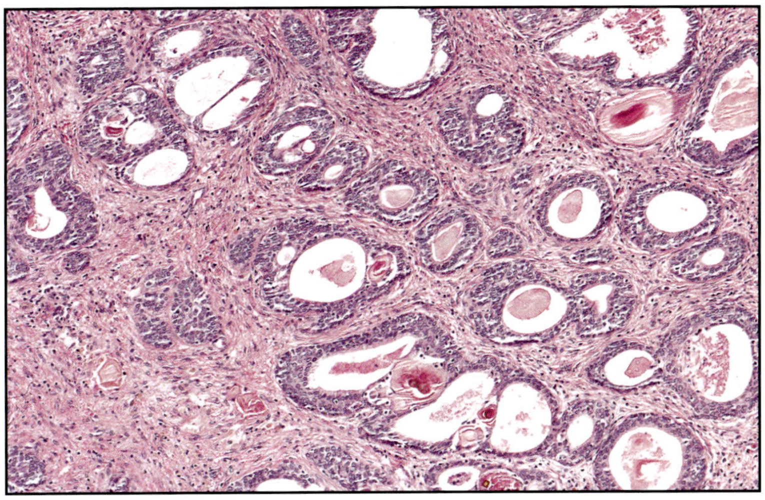

■ **i7.43** *Basal cell hyperplasia: Admixture of glands and focal solid forms.*

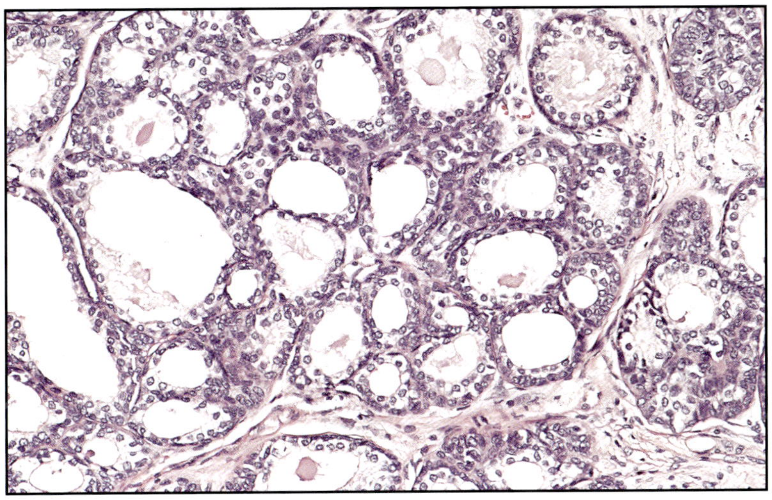

■ **i7.44** *Cribriform basal cell hyperplasia.*

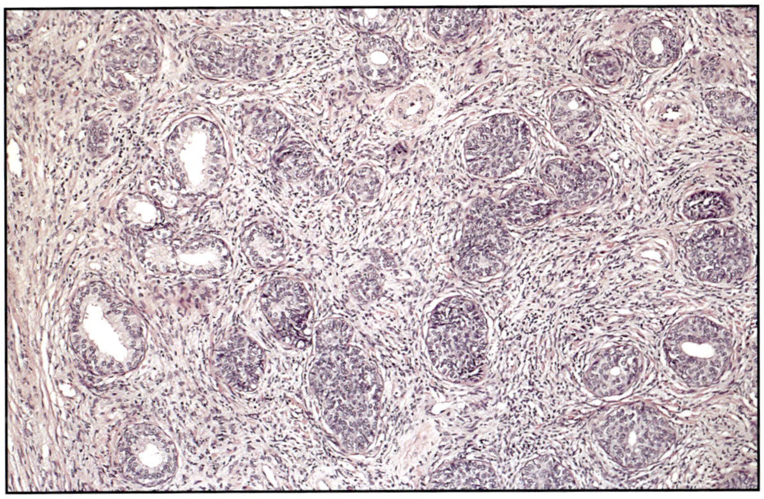

■ **i7.45** *Solid nests of basal cell hyperplasia within a hypercellular stroma.*

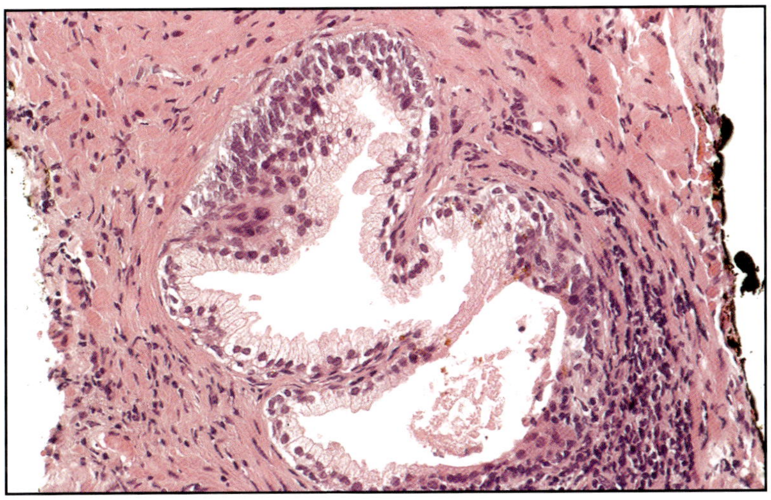

■ **i7.46** *Basal cell hyperplasia partially involving one gland in needle biopsy tissue.*

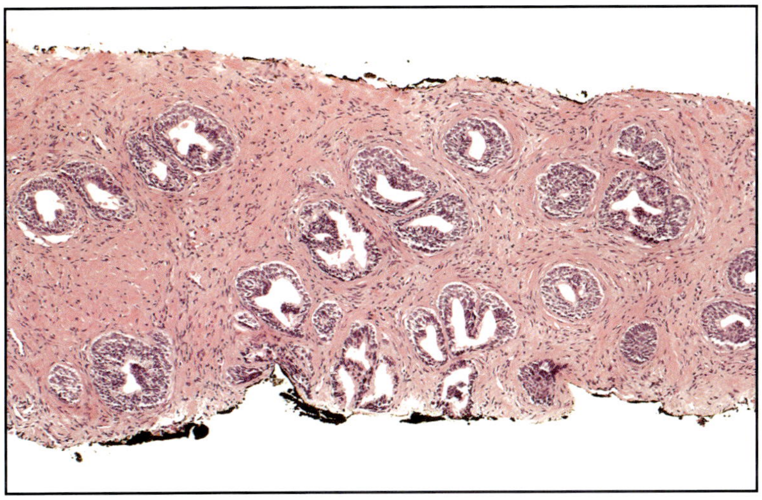

■ **i7.47** *Basal cell hyperplasia in needle biopsy tissue: PIN is in the differential diagnosis.*

i7.47, i7.48 to nearly complete luminal obliteration **i7.43, i7.47, i7.48** (Devaraj 1993). Solid, small nests are also common **i7.43, i7.45, i7.47, i7.48**, and these can occasionally demonstrate peripheral palisading (Grignon 1988). The cribriform (adenoid basal cell) pattern has been reported to be rare (Devaraj 1993, Rioux-Leclercq 2002) **i7.44**. Additional unusual morphologic patterns include basal hyperplasia with intracytoplasmic globules and squamous features (Rioux-Leclercq 2002). The surrounding stroma may be similar to adjacent uninvolved gland

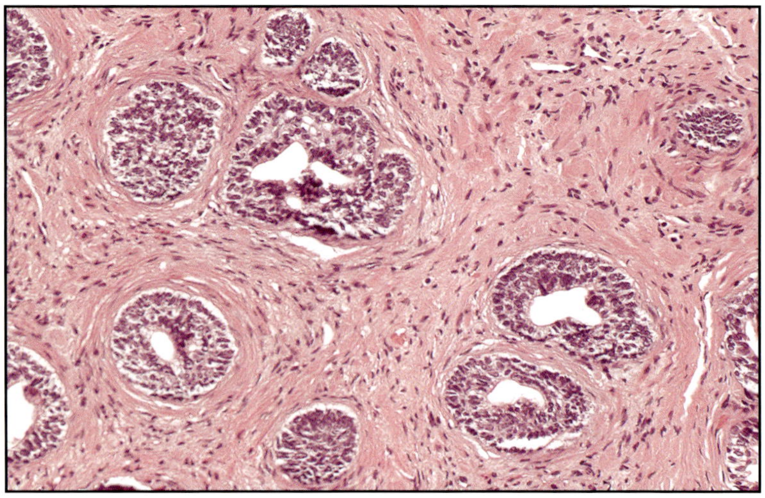

■ **i7.48** *Basal cell hyperplasia in needle biopsy tissue: Higher magnification view of* **i7.47** *showing circumferential gland involvement and solid nests.*

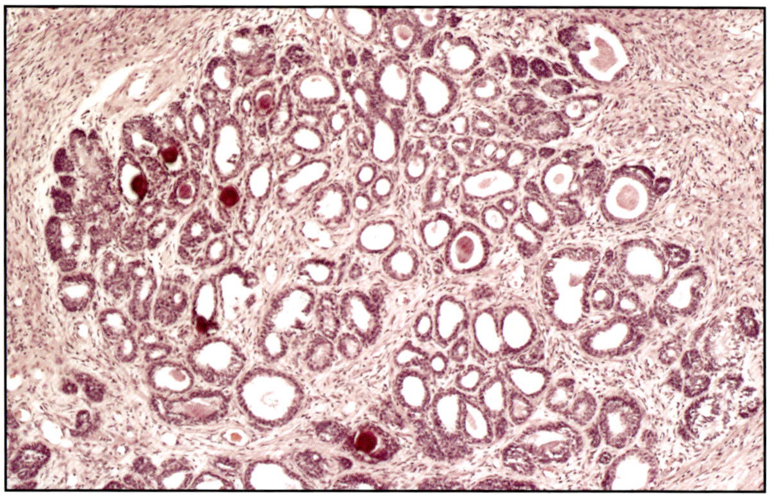

■ **i7.49** *Calcifications in basal cell hyperplasia.*

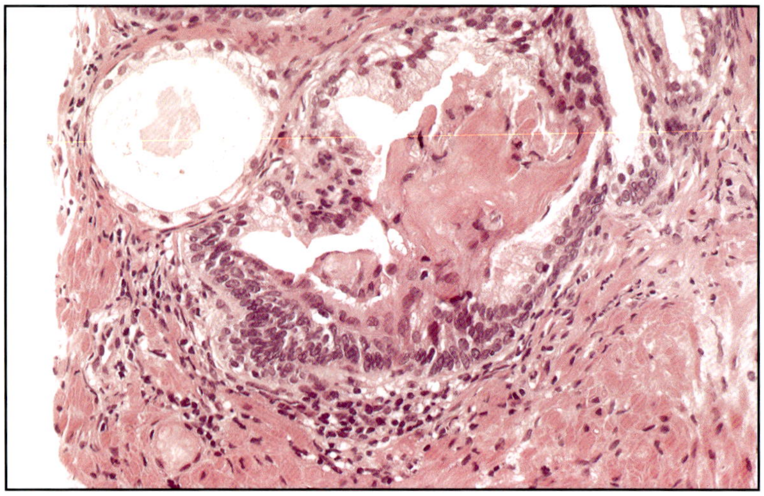

■ **i7.50** *Basal cell hyperplasia in association with a lymphocytic inflammatory cell infiltrate.*

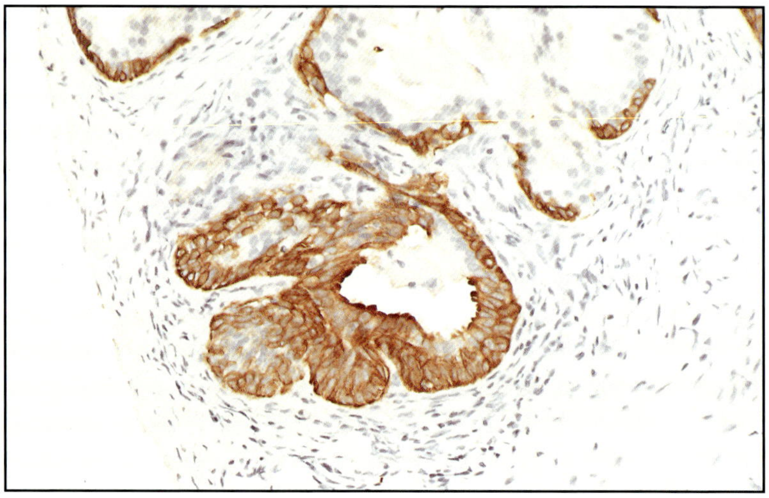

■ **i7.51** *Basal cell hyperplasia binds antibody 34βE12 in immunohistochemical reactions.*

(Bennett 1985), may reveal a few concentric layers of cellular or myxoid compressed stroma, or may show a hypercellular, hyperplastic stroma **i7.45**, which has been called sclerosing basal cell hyperplasia (Devaraj 1993). Microcalcifications are seen in nests in about one half of cases (Grignon 1988) **i7.49**. Cytologically, the basal cells are ovoid to occasionally elongated. Cytoplasmic volume is scanty and usually dense, but some cells can have cytoplasmic clearing. The nuclei are uniform, with finely dispersed chromatin without prominent (>1 μm) nucleoli or pleomorphism. The nuclei often are enlarged relative to those of normal basal cells, and few may exhibit hyperchromasia (Devaraj 1993, Epstein 1992B). Mitoses are rare (Epstein 1992B). Lymphocytes are commonly found in foci of basal cell hyperplasia (Devaraj 1993, Epstein 1992B, Thorson 1999) **i7.50**, suggesting that this may be a reactive proliferation. No physical transition between basal cell hyperplasia and neoplasia, including PIN and carcinoma, has been noted (Thorson 1999). In fact, in needle biopsy, basal cell hyperplasia in the peripheral zone is much more often found in benign biopsies rather than biopsies with carcinoma (Thorson 1999).

Special histochemical stains have shown acid and neutral mucin in basal cell hyperplasia (Grignon 1988), whereas immunohistochemical stains demonstrate an immunophenotype similar to normal basal cells **t1.3**. Of diagnostic importance, intense immunolabeling using antibody 34βE12 is found (Brawer 1985, Devaraj 1993, Epstein 1992B, Grignon 1988, Hedrik 1989) **i7.51**. Weak to absent PSA and prostate-specific acid phosphatase (PSAP) immunoreactivity in basal cells has been reported (Devaraj 1993, Grignon 1988), and preserved secretory cells are strongly positive for these two markers. Rare basal cells have stained for chromogranin, neuron-specific enolase, and smooth muscle actin (Devaraj 1993, Grignon 1988, van de Voorde 1994A). bcl-2 immunostains are negative to weakly positive, and weakly positive p53 immunoreactivity has been detected (Yang 1998). The mean proliferation index for usual basal cell hyperplasia (based on Ki-67 immunopositive cells) has been quantitated at 1.3% (Thorson 2000, Yang 1998). Compared with normal basal cells, basal cell hyperplasia exhibits a coordinate increase in proliferation index and a decrease in apoptotic index, which may account for the increased cell number in basal cell hyperplasia (Kyprianou 1996, Thorson 2000).

Atypical basal cell hyperplasia has been only recently described, and a limited number of cases have been studied (Devaraj 1993, Epstein 1992B, Rioux-Leclercq 2002, Thorson 1999, Yang 1998). Because its clinical significance as a risk factor for neoplasia is not established, the designation of "basal cell hyperplasia with prominent nucleoli" has also been used (Yang 1998). The incidence in peripheral zone needle biopsies is 2% (Thorson 1999); the incidence in other types of tissue specimens has

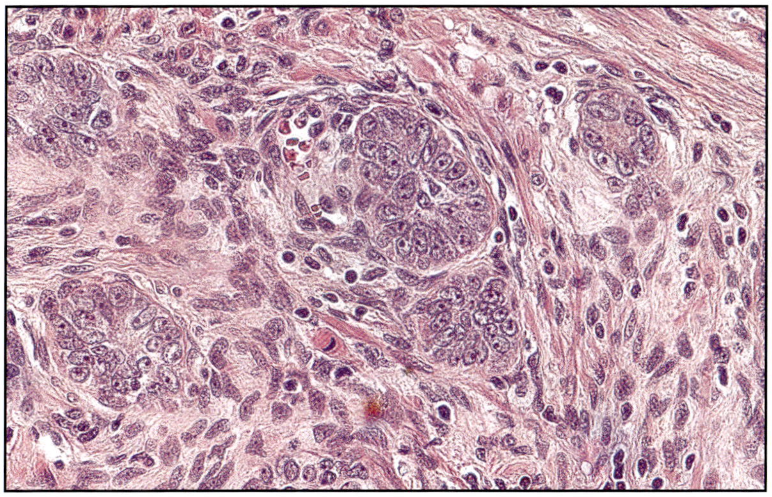

■ **i7.52** *Basal cell hyperplasia with prominent nucleoli.*

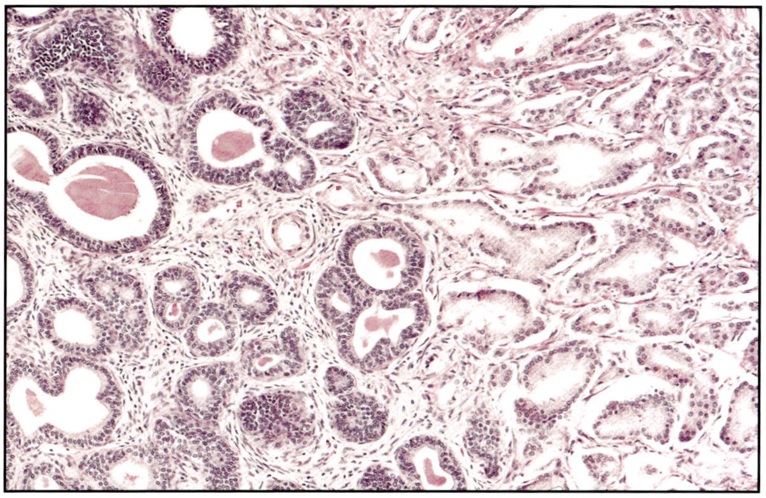

■ **i7.53** *Multilayered basal cell hyperplastic glands (left) juxtaposed to adenocarcinoma glands with single cell lining layer (right).*

■ **t7.13 Usual Basal Cell Hyperplasia: Differential Diagnosis**

Adenocarcinoma
Transitional cell carcinoma
High-grade PIN
Adenoid basal cell tumor
Basal cell adenoma
Basal cell prominence
Sclerosing adenosis
Benign seminal vesicle/ejaculatory duct epithelium
Squamous metaplasia
Transitional cell metaplasia

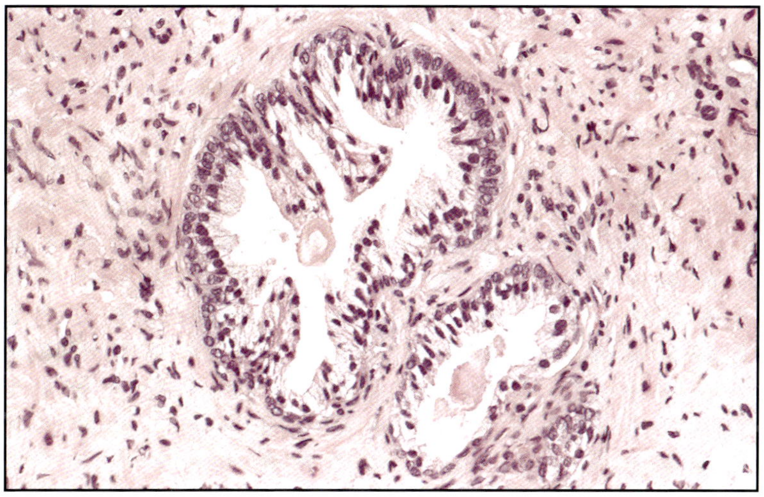

■ **i7.54** *Basal cell prominence, with single layer of crowded basal cells.*

not been defined. The sole histologic difference between usual and atypical basal cell hyperplasia is the presence of prominent nucleoli measuring more than 1.3 μm in atypical basal cell hyperplasia **i7.52** (Devaraj 1993). The percentage of these prominently nucleolated nuclei varied from 10% of basal cells to diffuse involvement (Devaraj 1993, Epstein 1992B). A few cases of atypical basal cell hyperplasia also had individually necrotic cells, necrotic intraluminal secretions, and intraluminal wispy blue mucin (Epstein 1992B), but these findings have been absent in our experience (Thorson 1999). The immunophenotype is the same as that of usual basal cell hyperplasia (Devaraj 1993, Yang 1998). These basal cells with prominent nucleoli have a mean proliferation index that is very close, at 3.4%, to that of usual basal cell hyperplasia. Inflammation is commonly observed in association with atypical basal cell hyperplasia (Devaraj 1993, Epstein 1992B, Thorson 1999), suggesting that the nucleolar prominence is reactive in nature. Another presentation of basal cell hyperplasia suggesting that it is a reactive response to injury is that it is common after various treatments. Therefore, basal cell hyperplasia has been seen in the prostate after hormonal (androgen deprivation) therapy, radiation therapy, and cryosurgery (Armas 1994, Grignon 1995, Montironi 1998, Reuter 1997, Sheaff 1997, Shuman 1997, Têtu 1991, Vaillancourt 1996, van de Voorde 1994A) (Chapter 19).

The differential diagnostic list for usual basal cell hyperplasia is lengthy **t7.13**. Of prime concern is the possibility that basal cell hyperplasia might be misdiagnosed as adenocarcinoma. For the acinar pattern the pitfall can be avoided if the multilayered nature of the basal cell proliferation is appreciated **i7.53**. The small, solid nests of basal cell hyperplasia should not be confused with the solid growth of invasive, neoplastic prostatic epithelial cells because this is usually high-grade (Gleason pattern 5) carcinoma that is sheetlike and solid. Also, high-grade carcinoma cells are cytologically much more atypical than the hyperplastic basal cells. Transitional cell carcinoma can exhibit solid growth as small, rounded aggregates when it extends as in situ disease in prostatic ducts and acini, but these malignant cells typically are quite pleomorphic. Cribriform basal cell hyperplasia could be initially be worrisome for PIN or carcinoma, but the bland basaloid cells do not appear neoplastic at high-power magnifications. Noncribriform basal cell hyperplasia is readily confused with PIN, particularly low-grade PIN, but in PIN the nuclear abnormalities are in the luminal cells, and the basal cells should appear unremarkable. Other prostatic basal cell proliferations that should be in one's mental checklist include basal cell adenoma, adenoid basal cell tumor (also known as adenoid cystic tumor), adenoid cystic–like tumor, adenoid cystic carcinoma, and basal cell carcinoma. Lesions called basal cell adenomas of the prostate probably represent nodular hyperplasia (Young 1997A), whereas the exceedingly rare basaloid carcinomas differ from usual basal cell hyperplasia by the extensive infiltration between normal prostatic glands, extraprostatic extension, perineural invasion, and necrosis (Epstein 1992B, Randolph 1997). Basal cell prominence is an apparent increase in number of basal cells, which are still in a single layer rather than forming multiple layers **i7.54**. Although this

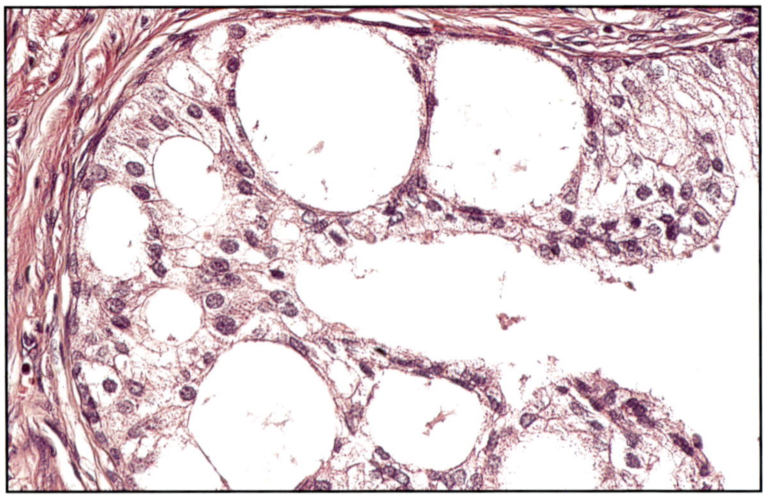

■ **i7.55** *Cribriform hyperplasia. (Cribriform is derived from the Latin* cribrum *or sieve and means pierced with small holes).*

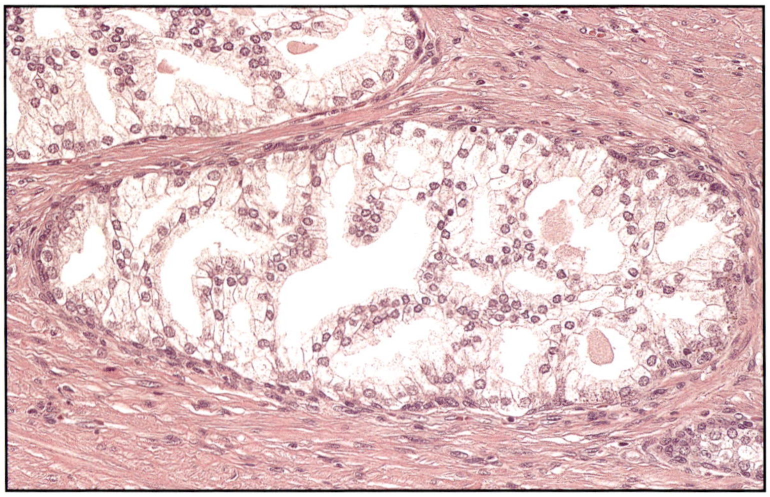

■ **i7.56** *Cribriform hyperplasia with partial gland involvement by rounded spaces.*

prominence also may represent basal cell hyperplasia, the current definition requires two or more layers of basal cells. Sclerosing adenosis is a small acinar proliferation without multilayering of basal cells in the acini. It contains S-100 and muscle-specific actin immunoreactive myoepithelial cells, which are not present in basal cell hyperplasia. In one case, sclerosing adenosis was found in association with basal cell hyperplasia (Ronnett 1989). Seminal vesicle and ejaculatory duct epithelium is also multilayered but usually contains monstrocellular smudge cells with hyperchromatic nuclei with smudged chromatin. Immature squamous cell metaplasia and transitional cell metaplasia can merge morphologically with basal cell hyperplasia, but one should specifically find intercellular bridges and elongated nuclei with grooves, respectively, in these two metaplasias.

Atypical basal cell hyperplasia is alarming because of its nucleolar enlargement, but compared with those of high-grade PIN, the cells with prominent nucleoli are basally situated, without atypia in the overlying luminal cell nuclei. In difficult cases, a 34βE12 immunostain marks atypical basal cells but not the atypical secretory high-grade PIN cells. The multilayering of the atypical basal cells helps distinguish atypical basal cell hyperplasia in acini from small acinar adenocarcinoma.

[7.7] Cribriform Hyperplasia

Cribriform hyperplasia is a variant of usual epithelial hyperplasia that is found in about 8% of untreated prostate glands (Civantos 1995). Cribriform hyperplasia can also be seen after androgen deprivation therapy (Civantos 1995, Montironi 1996); this therapy does not affect its incidence (Civantos 1995). Although they are called clear cell cribriform hyperplasia (Ayala 1986, Frauenhoffer 1991), not all such proliferations have cleared cells, so the term *cribriform hyperplasia* is preferable (Young 1997A). It was initially recognized in 1980 by the World Health Organization (Mostofi 1980) and has also been described as florid, benign papillary or cribriform hyperplasia (Gleason 1985). Despite early concerns (Brooks 1987, Vollmer 1987), these proliferations appear to be completely benign and do not constitute a risk factor for subsequent development of neoplasia.

Patients with cribriform hyperplasia are of a mean age of 64 to 72 years and usually present with a clinical diagnosis of BPH. Almost all of the initially reported cases of cribriform hyperplasia were TURP chip cases (Ayala 1986, Frauenhoffer 1991); cribriform hyperplasia can also be detected in needle biopsy (Frauenhoffer 1991), radical prostatectomy (Civantos 1995), and cystoprostatectomy (Frauenhoffer 1991).

Histologically, cribriform hyperplasia usually is seen in nodules of usual hyperplasia in the transition zone and is characterized by a sievelike glandular profile **i7.55, i7.56**, with or without admixed papillary proliferations **t7.14**. This can be a single focus or multiple foci (Ayala 1986). Partial gland involvement is possible. The constituent cells have bland nuclei with only rare, small, inconspicuous nucleoli and cleared cytoplasm. A peripheral basal cell layer is readily detected on H&E sections and by 34βE12 immunostains (Frauenhoffer 1991). On occasion this basal cell layer can be hyperplastic. No necrosis or mitotic figures should be evident. The DNA content of cribriform hyperplastic nuclei is diploid, whereas that of cribriform carcinoma often is aneuploid (Frauenhoffer 1991).

The differential diagnosis of cribriform hyperplasia centers on other cribriform proliferations in the prostate **t7.15**. One must be aware that central zone epithelium can normally form cribriform glands. Basal cell hyperplasia can be found admixed with cribriform hyperplasia, and pure cribriform basal cell hyperplasia does exist but is unusual. These basaloid cells have a much smaller volume of cytoplasm than clear cell cribriform hyperplasia. The rare adenoid

■ **t7.14 Cribriform Hyperplasia**

Seen in usual nodular hyperplasia
Admixed papillary-cribriform gland profiles
Cleared cytoplasm
Small bland nuclei without prominent nucleoli
Basal cells present

■ **t7.15 Cribriform Hyperplasia: Differential diagnosis**

Normal central zone epithelium
Cribriform basal cell hyperplasia
Cribriform adenoid basal cell tumor (adenoid cystic-like lesion)
Cribriform prostatic intraepithelial neoplasia
Cribriform, invasive Gleason pattern 3 or 4 carcinoma

■ **t7.16 Mesonephric Remnant Hyperplasia**

Case	Patient age	Specimen type	Location	Histologic features	Immunostains[1]	Reference
1	65	TURP[2]	Bladder neck	Small, single-layered tubules in muscle	PSA– PSAP– 34βE12+	Gikas 1993
2	64	Radical prostatectomy	Soft tissue around base of prostate	Tubules, some dilated, some atrophic, with intraluminal colloid-like material	PSA– PSAP– 34βE12+	Gikas 1993
3	63	TURP	Prostatic urethra	Irregular tubular structures	PSA– CK–	Andersen 1994
4	66	TURP	Predominantly bladder neck	Infiltrative single-layer tubules with intraluminal colloid-like material	PSA– PSAP– 34βE12– CEA– Chromogranin– Serotonin– Synaptophysin– NSE–	
5	85	TURP	Prostatic tissue	Small to medium-sized tubules with cuboidal epithelium and intraluminal colloid-like secretion	PSA– PSAP– 34βE12–	Jimenez 1998
6	50	Radical prostatectomy	Periprostatic soft tissue	Small tubules with some cystic change and bland cytology	PSA– PSAP– 34βE12±	Jimenez 1998
7	56	Needle biopsy	Prostatic tissue	Small, infiltrative bland tubules with cuboidal to flattened epithelium with colloid-like secretion	PSA– 34βE12–	i7.57, i7.58, i7.62, i7.63
8	64	Radical prostatectomy	Prostatic tissue	Lobular to infiltrative small acini	34βE12–	i7.59-i7.61, i7.64
9-16	75 mean	TURP	not given	Lobular or infiltrative acini with single layer of cuboidal cells and eosinophilic colloid-like secretions	PSA–	Pacelli 1997

[1]PSA = prostate specific antigen; PSAP = prostatic specific acid phosphatase; 34βE12 = high molecular weight cytokeratin antibody; CK = cytokeratin; CEA = carcinoembryonic antigen; NSE = neuron specific enolase
[2]TURP = transurethral resection of the prostate

basal cell tumor or adenoid-cystic tumorlike lesion can have cribriform areas, but the spaces contain basophilic secretions and basement membrane material (Grignon 1988). Unlike in high-grade PIN, the cells forming the round, regular glands in cribriform hyperplasia do not exhibit nuclear atypia. Also, although clear cell change can occur in PIN, the cytoplasm of PIN cells usually is amphophilic. Finally, in contrast to cribriform hyperplasia, cribriform carcinoma often grows as confluent masses, often is admixed with an adjacent small acinar adenocarcinomatous component, and lacks a basal cell layer (Amin 1994).

[7.8] Mesonephric Remnant Hyperplasia

Mesonephric remnant hyperplasia is well known in the female genital tract but is an uncommon proliferation in the prostate and periprostatic tissues, with 16 cases reported, including 8 in abstract form (Andersen 1994, Gikas 1993, Jimenez 1998, Pacelli 1997, Val-Bernal 1995) and 2 presented here **t7.16**. The incidence in TURP cases is estimated to be 0.6% (4/698) (Pacelli 1997). It is always an incidental histologic finding. The mean age of the patients was 70 (range 50 to 85), and most patients presented with prostatism and underwent transurethral resection of the prostate. A few patients had the proliferation detected in radical prostatectomy tissues, and one patient had these glands in needle biopsy performed to rule out prostate cancer. The clinical and pathological significance of this proliferation is that it can be confused microscopically with adenocarcinoma. Indeed, this happened in one case, and the patient underwent an unnecessary radical prostatectomy (Gikas 1993).

Histologically, mesonephric remnant hyperplasia is most often characterized by a vaguely lobular or infiltrative growth of small tubules with cuboidal epithelium and intraluminal, eosinophilic colloidlike secretions **i7.57-i7.62; t7.17**. These tubules can infiltrate prostatic tissue, in and around smooth muscle bundles of the bladder neck, and in periprostatic soft tissue. In three cases (Gikas 1993, Jimenez 1998) there was an association with nerve tissue. Sometimes the tubules form aggregates or can stream in columns. The tubules have a single-cell lining layer and usually are simple acini, but intraluminal micropapillary projections can be seen in some instances. The lining epithelium is most often cuboidal but can be flattened and

■ **t7.17 Mesonephric Remnant Hyperplasia: Diagnostic Features**

Vaguely lobular to infiltrative growth
Microacini with cuboidal to flattened single cell lining layer
Occasional acini with cystic dilation with flattened epithelium
Micropapillary tufts can be seen
Bland, regular nuclei and scant cytoplasm
Negative PSA, PSAP immunostains

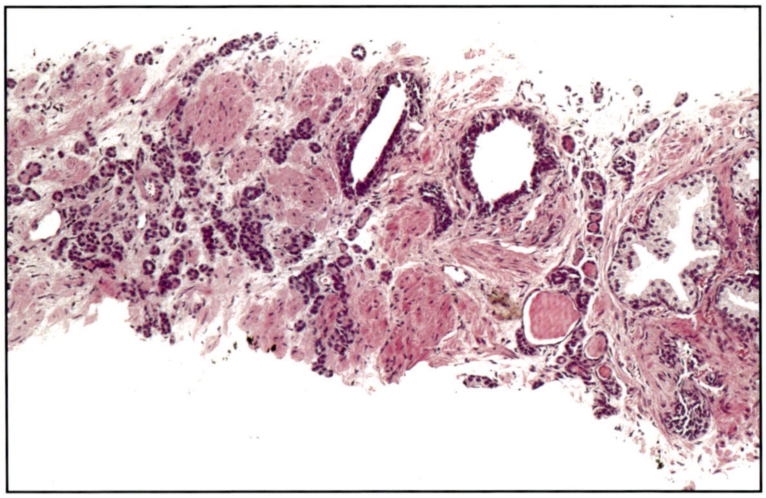

■ **i7.57** *Mesonephric remnant hyperplasia in needle biopsy tissue: Infiltrative-appearing small tubules.*

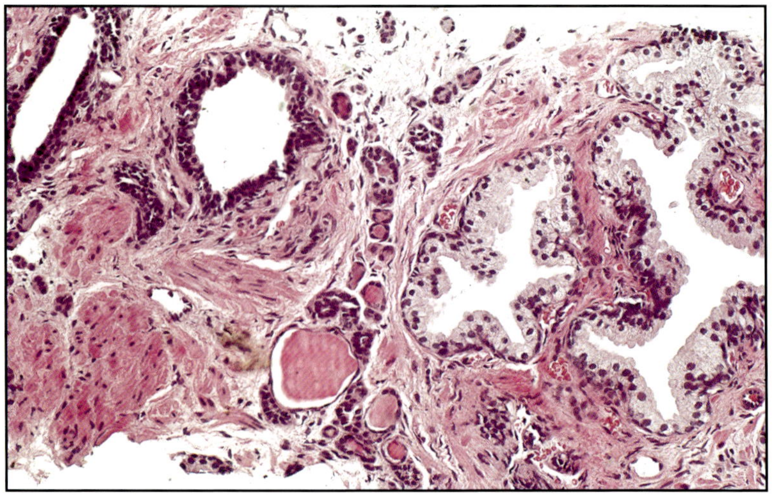

■ **i7.58** *Mesonephric remnant hyperplasia in needle biopsy tissue : Small tubules with bland nuclei and intraluminal colloid secretions.*

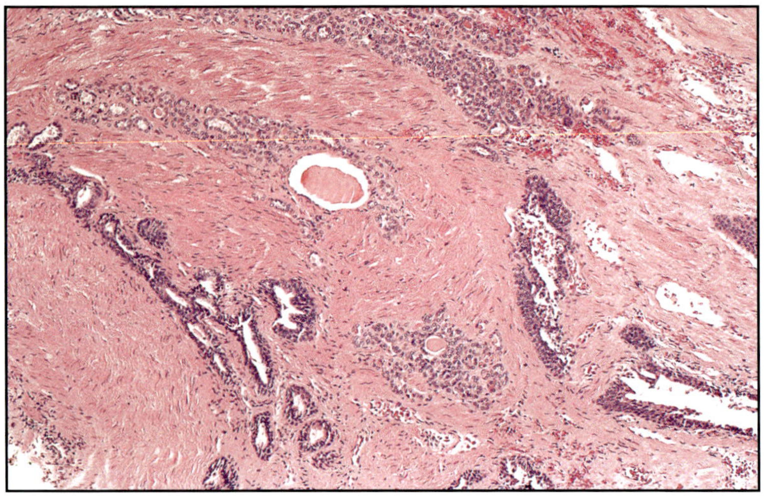

■ **i7.59** *Mesonephric remnant hyperplasia: Small acini arranged in lobular aggregates.*

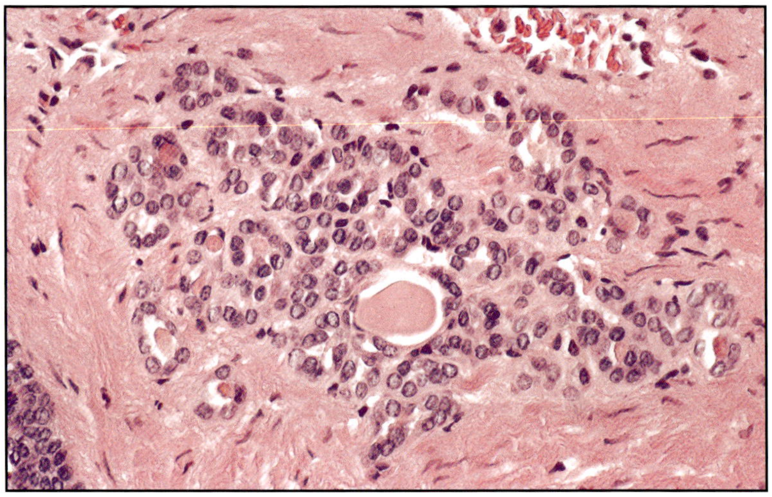

■ **i7.60** *Mesonephric remnant hyperplasia: Small acini admixed with solid nests.*

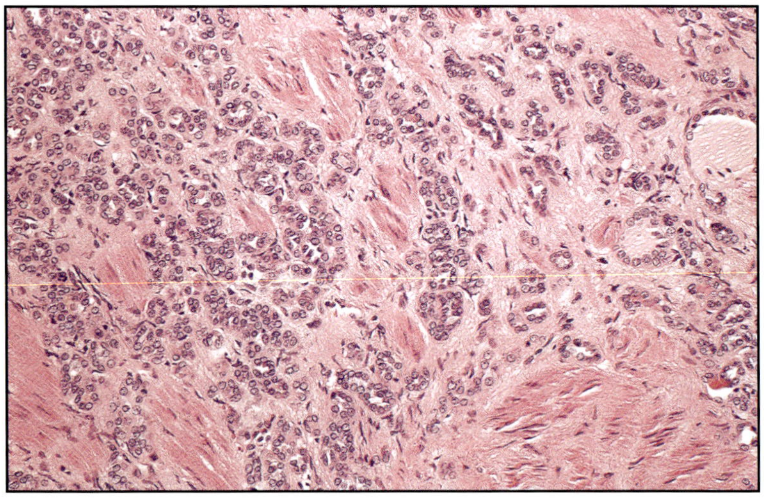

■ **i7.61** *Mesonephric remnant hyperplasia: The small tubules can assume an infiltrative appearance. The stromal sclerosis seen here is an unusual finding.*

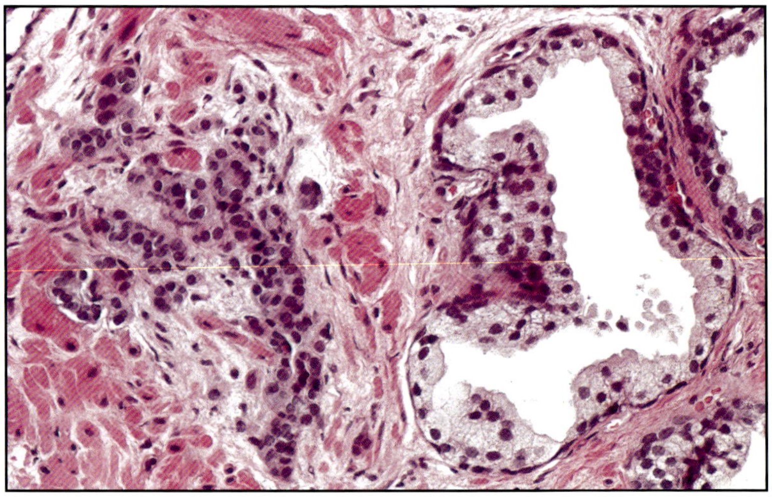

■ **i7.62** *Aggregate of hyperplastic mesonephric remnants (left) adjacent to benign gland (right).*

atrophic, especially in medium-sized tubules with cystic dilatation. Cytologically, the cells are bland, usually with no evidence of nuclear enlargement or prominent nucleoli **i7.60**. Occasionally, "punctate" (Pacelli 1997) or "conspicuous" (Gikas 1993, Val-Bernal 1995) nucleoli are visualized. There is generally not a stromal proliferation or response to the acini, although in one case a stromal, cellular, spindle cell proliferation that was negative for S-100 and muscle-specific actin was detected (Jimenez 1998). Histochemically,

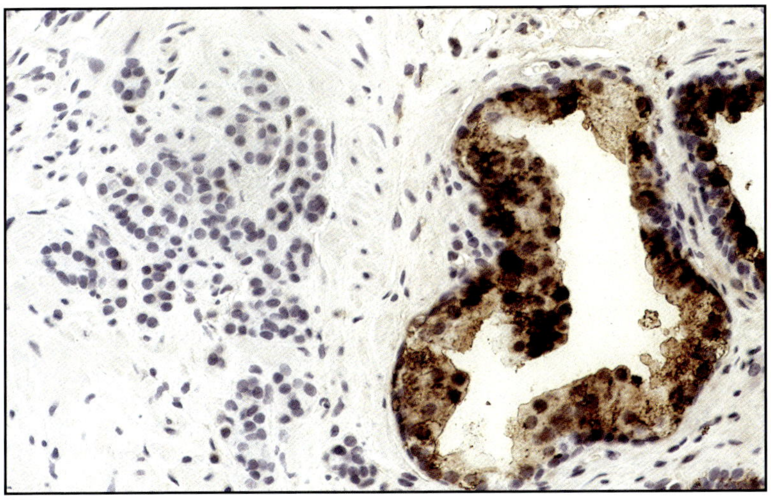

■ **i7.63** *PSA immunostain shows negativity in mesonephric remnants (left) and positivity in benign glands (right).*

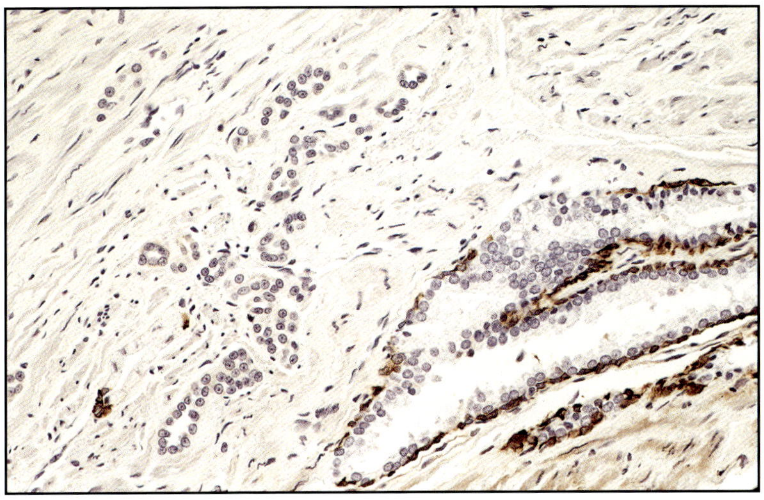

■ **i7.64** *A potential diagnostic pitfall: Small acini of mesonephric hyperplasia can be negative for high molecular weight cytokeratin. There is internal positive control staining of basal cells in adjacent benign glands (right).*

■ **t7.18 Mesonephric Remnant Hyperplasia: Differential Diagnosis**

Adenocarcinoma of prostate
Adenocarcinoma of bladder
Nephrogenic metaplasia (adenoma)
Atypical adenomatous hyperplasia (adenosis)
Sclerosing adenosis
Atrophy
Postatrophic hyperplasia

secretions in the acini are positive for periodic acid-Schiff (Andersen 1994, Jimenez 1998) and Alcian blue (Andersen 1994). Immunohistochemically, the critical finding is lack of staining for PSA **i7.63** and PSAP. Variable results have been obtained with the 34βE12 immunostain **t7.16**, but it can be negative in mesonephric hyperplasia **i7.64**.

The differential diagnostic checklist for mesonephric remnant hyperplasia is long **t7.18,** but obviously the most crucial entity to exclude is intermediate-grade, small acinar adenocarcinoma of the prostate. A number of findings could initially provoke concern for adenocarcinoma, including the presence of infiltrating small acini, a single-cell lining layer, conspicuous nucleoli, and involvement of bladder neck smooth muscle, periprostatic soft tissue, and nerves. The vague lobular aggregation of the acini is an important finding, but this architecture is lost in needle biopsy. The small acini of mesonephric remnant hyperplasia have a scant amount of cytoplasm and little to no nuclear atypia, whereas most prostatic adenocarcinomas have a moderate amount of cytoplasm and significant nucleomegaly and nucleolomegaly. Prostatic adenocarcinoma glands can uncommonly assume an atrophic or dilated profile (Kaleem 1998, Levi 2000), but the nuclei of the glandular lining cells are markedly atypical. The single-cell lining layer can also be disconcerting, especially when a 34βE12 immunostain is negative, but this one finding of lack of basal cells should not, by itself, be considered diagnostic of malignancy. The colloid-type secretions are characteristic of mesonephric remnant hyperplasia, but amphophilic to eosinophilic intraluminal secretions can also be seen in prostatic adenocarcinoma (Epstein 1995A, Thorson 1998), so this finding is helpful only in the correct histologic context. A critical procedure is immunostaining for PSA and PSAP. In all cases, mesonephric remnant hyperplastic glands are globally negative for these two markers, whereas intermediate-grade prostatic adenocarcinomas should be positive. Overall, the combination of aggregates of microacini with a single-cell lining layer, lining cells with regular, bland nuclei, intraluminal colloidlike material, and PSA and PSAP immunonegativity points toward a diagnosis of mesonephric remnant hyperplasia. Clear cell adenocarcinomas primary in the urethra or bladder should also be considered because they can form tubules, but sheets of cells, mitotic figures, and cytologic atypia are also present. Of less concern are the benign small acinar proliferations. Of these, nephrogenic metaplasia (adenoma) is the one that most closely resembles mesonephric remnant hyperplasia. This process can have small tubules but tends to be periurethral and associated with urothelial damage. Sclerosing adenosis, in contrast to mesonephric remnant hyperplasia, shows a hypercellular stroma that immunostains for S-100 and muscle-specific actin. Atypical adenomatous hyperplasia demonstrates a transition between crowded, small, pale acini and larger, more complex glands. The small acini in adenosis possess a (fragmented) basal cell layer. Atrophy, including postatrophic hyperplasia, has glands with basal cells and an altered periglandular stroma.

Although a few cases have been seen in the same gland as prostatic adenocarcinoma, it is not thought that mesonephric remnant hyperplasia is a risk factor for malignancy.

[7.9] Verumontanum Mucosal Gland Hyperplasia

This is a benign microacinar proliferation of the verumontanum and adjacent posterior urethra where the ejaculatory ducts and utricle empty into the urethra (Gagucas 1995). Its incidence in whole glands (from radical prostatectomies and cystoprostatectomies) is 14% (Gagucas 1995). Although it has been reported in needle biopsies (Gaudin 1995B), the incidence in this type of tissue specimen and in TURP chips has not been defined. Verumontanum mucosal gland hyperplasia is an incidental histologic finding in men 47 to 87 years of age (Gagucas 1995). Its clinical and pathologic significance is that it can potentially mimic small acinar prostatic adenocarcinoma.

■ t7.19 Verumontanum Mucosal Gland Hyperplasia: Diagnostic Features

Nodular growth
Back-to-back small acini
Bland cytology
Basal cells present
Urothelium nearby
Intraluminal orange-red concretions common
No intraluminal crystalloids

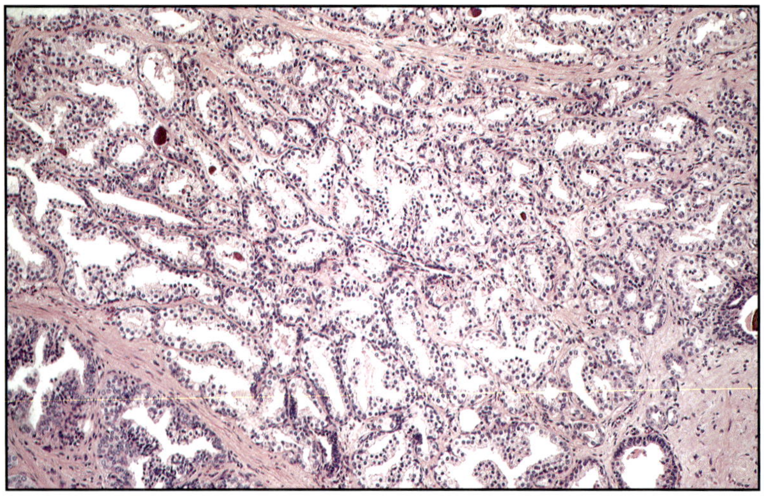

■ i7.65 *Verumontanum mucosal gland hyperplasia.*

Histologically, verumontanum mucosal gland hyperplasia **t7.19** is more often multifocal than solitary (Gagucas 1995). In needle biopsy the mean focus size was 2.9 mm, with involvement from 10% to 50% of needle cores (Gaudin 1995B). The majority of the foci in the whole gland are less than 1 mm and contain 6 to 25 glands (Gagucas 1995). The glands exhibit a nodular growth, regularly centered around ejaculatory or prostatic ducts. Urothelium is identified immediately adjacent to hyperplastic verumontanum mucosal gland nodules, in both needle biopsy and the whole gland. The small acini are positioned back-to-back with scanty, interspersed stroma **i7.65**. These acini are lined by cuboidal to columnar cells with small bland nuclei and rare, small nucleoli. The tinctorial character of the cytoplasm varies from eosinophilic to amphophilic to cleared. Basal cells are readily recognized. Numerous intraluminal, small, fragmented orange-red concretions and corpora amylacea are present, but crystalloids and wispy blue mucin are absent to rare, respectively (Gagucas 1995, Gaudin 1995B). Immunohistochemically, the luminal cells are strongly positive for PSA, and the basal cells mark with 34βE12. S-100 immunostains are negative (Gagucas 1995).

The main entity to exclude in the differential diagnosis is low-grade or well-differentiated adenocarcinoma of the prostate, which also is a well-circumscribed collection of back-to-back glands. Yet verumontanum mucosal gland hyperplasia lacks luminal cell nuclear atypia and intraluminal crystalloids and does possess basal cells and orange-red concentrations. Other small acinar proliferations in the differential diagnosis include atypical adenomatous hyperplasia (adenosis), sclerosing adenosis, nephrogenic metaplasia (adenoma), mesonephric remnant hyperplasia, basal cell hyperplasia , and postatrophic hyperplasia (Gagucas 1995, Gaudin 1995B). Of these, only atypical adenomatous hyperplasia (adenosis) can display nodular, crowded, back-to-back, small, pale acini. However, these small acini in adenosis are in continuity with larger, more complex usual-type hyperplastic glands, the basal cell layer in adenosis is fragmented, and intraluminal crystalloids are common in adenosis, whereas corpora are uncommon.

Verumontanum mucosal gland hyperplasia has been associated with the presence of atypical adenomatous hyperplasia (adenosis) (Muezzinoglu 2001), but it is not a risk factor for malignancy.

References

Ackerman LV. Male reproductive system. In: *Surgical Pathology.* St. Louis: CV Mosby; 651, 1964.

Allsbrook WC Jr, Pfeifer EA. Histochemistry of the prostate. In: Foster CS, Bostwick DG, eds. *Pathology of the Prostate.* Philadelphia: WB Saunders; 296-298, 1998.

Amin MB, Schultz DS, Zarbo RJ. Analysis of cribriform morphology in prostatic neoplasia using antibody to high-molecular-weight cytokeratins. *Arch Pathol Lab Med* 118:260-264, 1994.

Andersen CB, Horn T, Rasmussen F, et al. Mesonephric remnants involving renal pelvis and prostatic urethra: a diagnostic problem towards adenocarcinoma. *Scand J Urol Nephrol* 157(suppl):119-122, 1994.

Andrews GS. Latent carcinoma of the prostate. *J Clin Pathol* 2:197-208, 1949.

Armas OA, Aprikian AG, Melamed J, et al. Clinical and pathobiological effects of neoadjuvant total androgen ablation therapy on clinically localized prostatic adenocarcinoma. *Am J Surg Pathol* 18:979-991, 1994.

Armbruster DA. Prostate-specific antigen: biochemistry, analytical methods, and clinical application. *Clin Chem* 39:181-195, 1993.

Attah EB, Nkposong EO. Phyllodes type of atypical prostatic hyperplasia. *J Urol* 115:762-764, 1976.

Attah EB, Powell MEA. Atypical stromal hyperplasia of the prostate gland. *Am J Clin Pathol* 67:324-327, 1977.

Ayala AG, Srigley JR, Ro JY, et al. Clear cell cribriform hyperplasia of prostate. Report of 10 cases. *Am J Surg Pathol* 10:665-671, 1986.

Baird HH, McKay HW, Kimmelstiel P. Ischemic infarction of the prostate gland. *South Med J* 43:234-239, 1950.

Barry MJ. Evaluation of symptoms and quality of life in men with benign prostatic hyperplasia. *Urology* 58(suppl 6A):25-32, 2001.

Bennett BD, Gardner WA Jr. Embryonal hyperplasia of the prostate. *Prostate* 7:411-417, 1985.

Berry SJ, Coffey DS, Walsh PC, et al. The development of human benign prostatic hyperplasia with age. *J Urol* 132:474-479, 1984.

Berry SJ, Strandberg JD, Saunders WJ, et al. Development of canine benign prostatic hyperplasia with age. *Prostate* 9:363-373, 1986.

Bierhoff E, Vogel J, Benz M, et al. Stromal nodules in benign prostatic hyperplasia. *Eur Urol* 29:345-356, 1996.

Björk T, Hulkko S, Bjartell A, et al. Alpha$_1$-antichymotrypsin production in PSA-producing cells is common in prostate cancer but rare in benign prostatic hyperplasia. *Urology* 43:427-434, 1994.

Blute ML, Larson T. Minimally invasive therapies for benign prostatic hyperplasia. *Urology* 58(suppl 6A):33-41, 2001.

Bonkhoff H, Stein U, Remberger K. The proliferative function of basal cells in the normal and hyperplastic human prostate. *Prostate* 24:114-118, 1994.

Bostwick DG, Amin MB, Dundore P, et al. Architectural patterns of high-grade prostatic intraepithelial neoplasia. *Hum Pathol* 24:298-310, 1993A.

Bostwick DG, Srigley J, Grignon D, et al. Atypical adenomatous hyperplasia of the prostate: morphologic criteria for its distinction from well-differentiated carcinoma. *Hum Pathol* 24:819-832, 1993B.

Bostwick DG. Practical clinical application of predictive factors in prostate cancer. A review with an emphasis on quantitative methods in tissue specimens. *Anal Quant Cytol Histol* 20:323-342, 1998.

Brawer MK, Peehl DM, Stamey TA, et al. Keratin immunoreactivity in the benign and neoplastic human prostate. *Cancer Res* 45:3663-3667, 1985.

Brawer MK, Rennels MA, Nagle RB, et al. Serum prostate-specific antigen and prostate pathology in men having simple prostatectomy. *Am J Clin Pathol* 92:760-764, 1989.

Brawn PN, Foster DM, Kuhl D, et al. Characteristics of prostatic infarcts and their effect on serum prostate-specific antigen and prostatic acid phosphatase. *Urology* 44:71-75, 1994.

Brooks JJ, LiVolsi VA, Tomaszewski JE, et al. Cribriform hyperplasia of prostate [letter]. *Am J Surg Pathol* 11:488-489, 1987.

Carter HB, Morrell CH, Pearson JD, et al. Estimation of prostatic growth using serial prostate specific antigen measurement in men with and without prostate disease. *Cancer Res* 52:3323-3328, 1992.

Carter HB, Pearson JD. PSA velocity for the diagnosis of early prostate cancer. *Urol Clin North Am* 20:665-670, 1993.

Catalona WJ, Smith DS. Comparison of different serum prostate specific antigen measures for early prostate cancer detection. *Cancer* 74:1516-1518, 1994.

Catalona WJ, Smith DS, Wolfert RL, et al. Evaluation of percentage of free serum prostate-specific antigen to improve specificity of prostate cancer screening. *JAMA* 274:1214-1220, 1995.

Cheville J, Dundore PA, Nascimento AG, et al. Leiomyosarcoma of the prostate: report of 23 cases. *Cancer* 76:1422-1427, 1995.

Cheville JC, Clamon GH, Robinson RA. Silver-stained nucleolar organizer regions in the differentiation of prostatic hyperplasia, intraepithelial neoplasia, and adenocarcinoma. *Mod Pathol* 3:596-598, 1990.

Chicharro-Molero JA, Burgos-Rodriguez R, Sanchez-Cruz JJ, et al. Prevalence of benign prostatic hyperplasia in Spanish men 40 years old or older. *J Urol* 159:878-882, 1998.

Chung AK, Michels V, Poland GA, et al. Neurofibromatosis with involvement of the prostate gland. *Urology* 47:448-451, 1996.

Chute CG, Panser LA, Girman CJ, et al. The prevalence of prostatism: a population-based survey of urinary symptoms. *J Urol* 150:85-89, 1993.

Civantos F, Marcial MA, Banks ER, et al. Pathology of androgen deprivation therapy in prostate carcinoma. A comparative study of 173 patients. *Cancer* 75:1634-1641, 1995.

Cleary KR, Choi HY, Ayala AG. Basal cell hyperplasia of the prostate. *Am J Clin Pathol* 80:850-854, 1983.

Colombel M, Vacherot F, Gil Diez S, et al. Zonal variation of apoptosis and proliferation in the normal prostate and in benign prostatic hyperplasia. *Br J Urol* 82:380-385, 1998.

Cordon-Cardo C, Koff A, Drobnjak M, et al. Distinct altered patterns of $p27^{KIP1}$ gene expression in benign prostatic hyperplasia and prostatic carcinoma. *J Natl Cancer Inst* 90:1284-1291, 1998.

Debruyne FJM. Alpha blockers: are all created equal? *Urology* 56(suppl 5A):20-22, 2000.

Deering RE, Bigler SA, Brown M, et al. Microvascularity in benign prostatic hyperplasia. *Prostate* 26:111-115, 1995.

Dermer GB. Basal cell proliferation in benign prostatic hyperplasia. *Cancer* 41:1857-1862, 1978.

Deshmukh N, Scotson J, Dodson AR, et al. Differential expression of acidic and basic fibroblast growth factors in benign prostatic hyperplasia identified by immunohistochemistry. *Br J Urol* 80:869-874, 1997.

Devaraj LT, Bostwick DG. Atypical basal cell hyperplasia of the prostate. Immunophenotypic profile and proposed classification of basal cell proliferations. *Am J Surg Pathol* 17:645-659, 1993.

Dundore PA, Nascimento AG, Cheville JC, et al. Carcinosarcoma of the prostate. Report of 22 cases. *Cancer* 76:1035-1042, 1995.

Ehara H, Koji T, Deguchi T, et al. Expression of estrogen receptor in diseased human prostate assessed by non-radioactive in situ hybridization and immunohistochemistry. *Prostate* 27:304-313, 1995.

Ekman P, Barrack ER, Greene GL, et al. Estrogen receptors in human prostate: evidence for multiple binding sites. *J Clin Endocrinol Metab* 57:166-176, 1983.

Epstein JI, Fynheer J. Acidic mucin in the prostate: can it differentiate adenosis from adenocarcinoma? *Hum Pathol* 23:1321-1325, 1992A.

Epstein JI, Armas OA. Atypical basal cell hyperplasia of the prostate. *Am J Surg Pathol* 16:1205-1214, 1992B.

Epstein JI. Diagnostic criteria of limited adenocarcinoma of the prostate on needle biopsy. *Hum Pathol* 26:223-229, 1995A.

Epstein JI, Grignon DJ, Humphrey PA, et al. Interobserver reproducibility in the diagnosis of prostatic intraepithelial neoplasia. *Am J Surg Pathol* 19:873-886, 1995B.

Ewton AA, Kattan MW, Shimura S, et al. Clinical and pathological interrelationships between nodular hyperplasia and prostate cancer (abstract). *Mod Pathol* 11:82A, 1998.

Fang-Liu G. Incidence of benign prostatic hyperplasia and prostate cancer in China. *Chin J Surg* 31:323-326, 1993.

Feero P, Nickel JC, Brown P, et al. Prostatic infarction associated with aortic and iliac aneurysm repair. *J Urol* 143:367-368, 1990.

Feneley MR, Puddefoot JR, Xia S, et al. Zonal biochemical and morphological characteristics in BPH. *Br J Urol* 75:608-613, 1995.

Ferreira BR, Bechara GH, Pissinatti A, et al. Benign prostatic hyperplasia in the nonhuman primate *Leontopithecus. Folia Primatol* 65:48-53, 1995.

Fitzpatrick JM, Mebust WK. Minimally invasive and endoscopic management of benign prostatic hyperplasia. In: Walsh PC, Retik AB, Vaughan ED Jr, et al, eds. *Campbell's Urology*, 8th ed. Philadelphia. Saunders; 1379-1422, 2002.

Foster CS. Pathology of benign prostatic hyperplasia. *Prostate* (suppl) 9:4-14, 2000.

Franks LM. Benign nodular hyperplasia of the prostate: a review. *Ann R Coll Surg Engl* 14:92-106, 1954A.

Franks LM: Latent carcinoma of the prostate. *J Pathol Bacteriol* 68:603-616, 1954B.

Frauenhoffer EE, Ro JY, El-Naggar AK, et al. Clear cell cribriform hyperplasia of the prostate. Immunohistochemical and DNA flow cytometric study. *Am J Clin Pathol* 95:446-453, 1991.

Gagucas RJ, Brown RW, Wheeler TM. Verumontanum mucosal gland hyperplasia. *Am J Surg Pathol* 19:30-36, 1995.

Gallee MP, Visser de Jong E, Ten-Kate FJW, et al. Monoclonal antibody Ki-67 defined growth fraction in benign prostatic hyperplasia and prostatic cancer. *J Urol* 142:1242-1246, 1989.

Garraway WM, Collins GN, Lee RJ. High prevalence of benign prostatic hypertrophy in the community. *Lancet* 338:469-471, 1991.

Garvin TJ. Prostatic infarction associated with aortic and iliac aneurysm repair (letter). *J Urol* 144:1485, 1990.

Gaudin PB, Epstein JI. Adenosis of the prostate. Histologic features in transurethral resection specimens. *Am J Surg Pathol* 17:863-870, 1994.

Gaudin PB, Epstein JI. Adenosis of the prostate. Histologic features in needle biopsy specimens. *Am J Surg Pathol* 19:737-747, 1995A.

Gaudin PB, Wheeler TM, Epstein JI. Verumontanum mucosal gland hyperplasia in prostatic needle biopsy specimens. A mimic of low grade prostatic adenocarcinoma. *Am J Clin Pathol* 104:620-626, 1995B.

Gaudin P, Reuter VE. Benign mimics of prostatic adenocarcinoma on needle biopsy. In: Fechner RE, Rosen PP, eds. *Anatomic Pathology 1997.* Chicago: ASCP Press; 111-134, 1997.

Gaudin PB, Rosai J, Epstein JI. Sarcomas and related proliferative lesions of specialized prostatic stroma. A clinicopathologic study of 22 cases. *Am J Surg Pathol* 22:148-162, 1998.

Gee WF, Holtgrewe HL, Blute ML, et al. 1997 American Urological Association Gallup Survey: changes in diagnosis and management of prostate cancer and benign prostatic hyperplasia, and other practice trends from 1994 to 1997. *J Urol* 160:1804-1807, 1998.

Giannulis I, Montironi R, Magi Galluzzi C, et al. Frequency and location of mitoses in prostate intraepithelial neoplasia (PIN). *Anticancer Res* 13:2447-2452, 1993.

Gikas PW, Del Buono EA, Epstein JI. Florid hyperplasia of mesonephric remnants involving prostate and periprostatic tissue. Possible confusion with adenocarcinoma. *Am J Surg Pathol* 17:454-480, 1993.

Giovannucci E, Platz EA, Stampfer MJ, et al. The CAG repeat within the androgen receptor gene and benign prostatic hyperplasia. *Urology* 53:121-125, 1999.

Girman CJ. Population-based studies of the epidemiology of benign prostatic hyperplasia. *Br J Urol* 82:34-43, 1998.

Gleason DF. Atypical hyperplasia, benign hyperplasia, and well-differentiated adenocarcinoma of the prostate. *Am J Surg Pathol* 9(suppl):53-67, 1985.

Golden MR, Abeshouse BS. A further clinical and pathological study of prostate infarction. *J Urol* 70:930-936, 1953.

Greene DR, Wheeler TM, Egawa S, et al. A comparison of the morphological features of cancer arising in the transition zone and in the peripheral zone of the prostate. *J Urol* 146:1069-1076, 1991.

Greenwald P, Kirmiss V, Polan AK, et al. Cancer of the prostate among men with benign prostatic hyperplasia. *J Natl Cancer Inst* 53:335-340, 1974.

Grignon DJ, Ro JY, Ordóñez NG, et al. Basal cell hyperplasia, adenoid basal cell tumor, and adenoid cystic carcinoma of the prostate gland: an immunohistochemical study. *Hum Pathol* 19:1425-1433, 1988.

Grignon DJ, Sakr WA. Zonal origin of prostatic adenocarcinoma: are there biologic differences between transition zone and peripheral zone adenocarcinomas of the prostate gland? *J Cell Biochem* 19:267-269, 1994.

Grignon DJ, Sakr WA. Histologic effects of radiation therapy and total androgen blockage on prostate cancer. *Cancer* 75:1837-1841, 1995.

Guess HA, Arrighi HM, Metter EJ, et al. The cumulative prevalence of prostatism matches the autopsy prevalence of benign prostatic hyperplasia. *Prostate* 17:241-246, 1990.

Guess HA. Epidemiology and natural history of benign prostatic hyperplasia . *Urol Clin North Am* 22:247-261, 1995.

Hammerer PG, McNeal JE, Stamey TA. Correlation between serum prostate specific antigen levels and the volume of the individual glandular zones of the human prostate. *J Urol* 153:111-114, 1995.

Hamper U, Sheth S, Walsh P, et al. Stage B adenocarcinoma of the prostate: transrectal ultrasound and pathologic correlation of nonmalignant hypoechoic peripheral zone lesions. *Radiology* 180:101-104, 1991.

Han M, Alfert HJ, Partin AW. Retropubic and suprapubic open prostatectomy. In: Walsh PC, Retik AB, Vaughan ED Jr, et al, eds. *Campbell's Urology*, 8th ed. Philadelphia. Saunders; 1423-1434, 2002.

Hasui Y, Marutsuka K, Asada Y, et al. Relationship between serum prostate specific antigen and histological prostatitis in patients with benign prostatic hyperplasia. *Prostate* 25:91-96, 1994.

Hedrick L, Epstein JI. Use of keratin 903 as an adjunct in the diagnosis of prostate carcinoma. *Am J Surg Pathol* 13:389-396, 1989.

Holtgrewe HL: Transurethral prostatectomy. *Urol Clin North Am* 22:357-368, 1995.

Hudson MA, Bahnson RR, Catalona WJ. Clinical use of prostate specific antigen in patients with prostate cancer. *J Urol* 142:1011-1017, 1989.

Humphrey PA. Mucin in severe dysplasia in the prostate. *Surg Pathol* 4:137-143, 1991.

Humphrey PA. p53: mutations and immunohistochemical detection, with a focus on alterations in urologic malignancies. In: Weinstein RS, Graham AR, Anderson RE, et al, eds. *Advances in Pathology and Laboratory Medicine.* Vol 1. Chicago: Mosby; 579-606, 1994.

Humphrey PA, Swanson PE. Immunoreactive p53 protein in high-grade prostatic intraepithelial neoplasia. *Pathol Res Pract* 191:881-889, 1995.

Humphrey PA, Kaleem Z, Swanson PE, et al. Pseudohyperplastic prostatic adenocarcinoma. *Am J Surg Pathol* 22:1239-1246, 1998.

Imperato-McGinley J, Guerrero L, Gautier T, et al. Steroid 5-alpha-reductase deficiency in man: an inherited form of male pseudohermaphroditism. *Science* 186:1213-1215, 1974.

Isaacs JT, Coffey DS. Etiology and disease process of benign prostatic hyperplasia. *Prostate* 2(suppl 2):33-50, 1989.

Jewett HJ. Significance of the palpable prostatic nodule. *JAMA* 160:838-839, 1956.

Jimenez RE, Raval MFT, Spanto R, et al. Mesonephric remnants hyperplasia. Pitfall in the diagnosis of prostatic adenocarcinoma. *J Urol Pathol* 9:83-92, 1998.

Jones TJ, Howie AJ. Necropsy study of infarcts of prostate and prostatic urethra. *J Clin Pathol* 39:1221-1223, 1986.

Kafandaris PM, Polyzonis MB. Fibroadenoma-like foci in human prostatic nodular hyperplasia. *Prostate* 4:33-36, 1983.

Kahler JE. Carcinoma of the prostate: a pathologic study. *J Urol* 41:557-574, 1939.

Kaleem Z, Swanson PE, Vollmer RT, et al. Prostatic adenocarcinoma with atrophic features. A study of 202 consecutive completely embedded radical prostatectomy specimens. *Am J Clin Pathol* 109:695-703, 1998.

Kallakury BVS, Jennings TA, Ross JS, et al. Alteration of the p53 locus in benign hyperplastic epithelium associated with high-grade prostatic adenocarcinoma. *Diagn Mol Pathol* 3:227-232, 1994A.

Kallakury BV, Figge J, Ross JS, et al. Association of p53 immunoreactivity with high Gleason tumor grade in prostatic adenocarcinoma. *Hum Pathol* 25:92-97, 1994B.

Kaplan SA. 5-alpha-reductase inhibitors: what role should they play? *Urology* 58(suppl 6A):65-70, 2001.

Kaufmann JJ, Berneike RR. Leiomyoma of the prostate. *J Urol* 65:299-310, 1951.

Kerley SW, Corica FA, Qian J, et al. Peripheral zone involvement by prostatic hyperplasia. *J Urol Pathol* 6:87-94, 1997.

Kessler OJ, Keisari Y, Servadio C, et al. Role of chronic inflammation in the promotion of prostatic hyperplasia in rats. *J Urol* 159:1049-1053, 1998.

Kleinerman DI, Troncoso P, Lin SH, et al. Consistent expression of an epithelial cell adhesion molecule (C-CAM) during human prostate development and loss of expression in prostate cancer: implication as a tumor suppressor. *Cancer Res* 55:1215-1220, 1995.

Kohnen PW, Drach GW. Patterns of inflammation in prostatic hyperplasia: a histologic and bacteriologic study. *J Urol* 121:755-760, 1979.

Kyprianou N, Tu H, Jacobs SC. Apoptotic versus proliferative activities in human benign prostatic hyperplasia. *Hum Pathol* 27:668-675, 1996.

Lauwers GY, Schevchuk M, Armenakas N, et al. Carcinosarcoma of the prostate. *Am J Surg Pathol* 17:342-349, 1993.

Lawson RK. Role of growth factors in benign prostatic hyperplasia. *Eur Urol* 32(suppl 1):22-27, 1997.

Lee C, Kozlowski JM, Grayhack JT. Etiology of benign prostatic hyperplasia. *Urol Clin North Am* 22:237-246, 1995.

Leong SS, Vogt PJ, Yu GSM. Atypical stromal smooth muscle hyperplasia of prostate. *Urology* 31:163-167, 1988.

Lepor H, Williford WO, Barry MJ, et al, for the Veterans Affairs Cooperative Studies Benign Prostatic Hyperplasia Study Group. The efficiency of terazosin, finasteride, or both in benign prostate hyperplasia. *N Engl J Med* 335:533-539, 1996.

Lepor H, Lowe FC. Evaluation and nonsurgical management of benign prostatic hyperplasia. In: Walsh PC, Retik AB, Vaughan ED Jr, et al, eds. *Campbell's Urology.* 8th ed. Philadelphia: Saunders; 1337-1378, 2002.

Levi AW, Epstein JI. Pseudohyperplastic prostatic adenocarcinoma on needle biopsy and simple prostatectomy. *Am J Surg Pathol* 24:1039-1046, 2000.

Lewis RW, Kim JCS, Irani D, et al. The prostate of the nonhuman primate: normal anatomy and pathology. *Prostate* 2:51-70, 1981.

Lilja H. Significance of different molecular forms of serum PSA. The free, noncomplexed form of PSA versus that complexed to alpha-1-antichymotrypsin. *Urol Clin North Am* 20:681-686, 1993.

Lloyd SN, Collins GN, McKelvie GB, et al. Predicted and actual change in serum PSA following prostatectomy for BPH. *Urology* 43:472-479, 1994.

Lopez-Beltran A, Gaeta JF, Huben R, et al. Malignant phyllodes tumor of the prostate. *Urology* 35:164-167, 1990.

Loughlin KR, Retik AB, Weinstein HJ, et al. Genitourinary rhabdomyosarcoma in children. *Cancer* 63:1600-1606, 1989.

Madsen FA, Bruskewitz RC. Clinical manifestations of benign prostatic hyperplasia. *Urol Clin North Am* 22:291-298, 1995.

Masai M, Abe K, Akimoto S, et al. Argyrophilic nucleolar organizer regions in benign hyperplastic and cancerous human prostates. *Prostate* 20:1-13, 1992.

McConnell JD. Benign prostatic hyperplasia. Hormonal treatment. *Urol Clin North Am* 22:387-400, 1995.

McConnell JD. Epidemiology, etiology, pathophysiology, and diagnosis of benign prostatic hyperplasia. In: Walsh PC, Retik AB, Vaughan ED Jr, et al, eds. *Campbell's Urology.* 7th ed. Philadelphia: WB Saunders; 1429-1452, 1998.

McDonnell CH. Neurofibromatosis of bladder and prostate. *Am J Surg* 34:90-93, 1936.

McLoughlin J, Foster CS, Price P, et al. Evaluation of Ki-67 monoclonal antibody as prognostic indicator for prostatic carcinoma. *Br J Urol* 72:92-97, 1993.

McNeal JE. Origin and evolution of benign prostatic enlargement. *Invest Urol* 15:340-345, 1978.

McNeal JE. The prostate gland: morphology and pathobiology. *Monogr Urol* 4:3-33, 1983.

McNeal JE, Bostwick DG. Intraductal dysplasia: a premalignant lesion of the prostate. *Hum Pathol* 17:64-71, 1986.

McNeal JE, Redwine EA, Freiha FS, et al. Zonal distribution of prostatic adenocarcinoma. *Am J Surg Pathol* 12:897-906, 1988.

Meyers FJ, Chi SG, Fishman JR, et al. p53 Mutations in benign prostatic hyperplasia. *J Natl Cancer Inst* 85:1856-1858, 1993.

Milord RA, Kahane H, Epstein JI. Infarct of the prostate gland: experience on needle biopsy specimens. *Am J Surg Pathol* 24:1378-1384, 2000.

Mittal BV, Amin MB, Kinare SG. Spectrum of histological lesions in 185 consecutive prostatic specimens. *J Postgrad Med* 35:157-161, 1989.

Montironi R, Braccishi A, Matera G, et al. Quantitation of prostatic intra-epithelial neoplasia. Analysis of nucleolar size, number and location. *Pathol Res Pract* 187:307-314, 1992.

Montironi R, Magi Galluzzi C, Scarpelli M, et al. Occurrence of cell death (apoptosis) in prostatic intra-epithelial neoplasia. *Virchows Archiv A Pathol Anat* 423:351-357, 1993A.

Montironi R, Magi Galluzzi C, Diamanti L, et al. Prostatic intra-epithelial neoplasia: expression and location of proliferating cell nuclear antigen (PCNA) in epithelial, endothelial, and stromal nuclei. *Virchows Arch* 422:185-192, 1993B.

Montironi R, Diamanti L. Morphologic changes in benign prostatic hyperplasia following chronic treatment with the 5-α-reductase inhibitor finasteride. Comparison with the effect of combination endocrine therapy. *J Urol Pathol* 4:123-135, 1996.

Montironi R, Schulman CC. Pathological changes in prostate lesions after androgen manipulation. *J Clin Pathol* 51:5-12, 1998.

Moore RA. The morphology of small prostatic carcinoma. *J Urol* 33:224-234, 1935.

Moore RA. Benign hypertrophy of the prostate. A morphological study. *J Urol* 50:680-710, 1943.

Mostofi FK, Sesterhenn I, Sobin LH. *Histological Typing of Prostate Tumor.* Geneva: World Health Organization; 17-23, 1980.

Muezzinoglu B, Erdamar S, Chakraborty S. Verumontanum mucosal gland hyperplasia is associated with atypical adenomatous hyperplasia of the prostate. *Arch Pathol Lab Med* 125:358-360, 2001.

Muir EG. Carcinoma of the prostate. *Lancet* 1:667-672, 1934.

Mukherjee J, Misra V, Gupta SC, et al. Argyrophilic nucleolar organizer regions in atypical adenomatous hyperplasias, prostatic intraepithelial neoplasias and prostatic neoplasms. *Urol Int* 58:75-79, 1997.

Nacey JN, Morum P, Delahunt B. Analysis of the prevalence of voiding symptoms in Maori, Pacific Island and Caucasian New Zealand men. *Urology* 46:506-511, 1995.

Nadler RB, Humphrey PA, Smith DS, et al. Effect of inflammation and benign prostatic hyperplasia on elevated serum prostate specific antigen levels. *J Urol* 154:407-413, 1995.

Oesterling JE. Prostate specific antigen: a critical assessment of the most useful tumor marker for adenocarcinoma of the prostate. *J Urol* 145:907-923, 1991.

Oesterling JE, Cooner WH, Jacobsen SJ, et al. Influence of patient age on serum PSA concentration: an important clinical observation. *Urol Clin North Am* 20:671-680, 1993.

Ohori M, Egawa S, Wheeler TM: Nodules resembling nodular hyperplasia in the peripheral zone of the prostate gland. J Urol Pathol 2:223-233, 1994.

Okada H, Tsubura A, Okamura A, et al. Keratin profiles in normal/hyperplastic prostate and prostate carcinoma. *Virchows Archiv A Pathol Anat* 421:157-161, 1992.

Oomens EHGM, van Steenbrugge GJ, van der Kwast TK, et al. Application of the monoclonal antibody Ki-67 on prostate biopsies to assess the proliferative cell fraction of human prostatic carcinoma. *J Urol* 145:81-85, 1991.

Oyen R, Van de Voorde W, Van Poppel H, et al. Benign hyperplastic nodules that originate in the peripheral zone of the prostate gland. *Radiology* 189:707-711, 1993.

Pacelli A, Farrow GM, Bostwick DG. Mesonephric remnants of the prostate: incidence and clinical significance [abstract]. *Mod Pathol* 10:83A, 1997.

Partin AW, Page WF, Lee BR, et al. Concordance rates for benign prostatic disease among twins suggest hereditary influence. *Urology* 44:646-650, 1994.

Peters CA, Walsh PC. The effect of nafarelin acetate, a luteinizing-hormone-releasing–hormone agonist, on benign prostatic hyperplasia. *N Engl J Med* 317:599-604, 1987.

Price H, McNeal JE, Stamey TA. Evolving patterns of tissue composition in benign prostatic hyperplasia as a function of specimen size. *Hum Pathol* 21:578-585, 1990.

Randolph TL, Amin MB, Ro JY, et al. Histologic variants of adenocarcinoma and other carcinomas of prostate: pathologic criteria and clinical significance. *Mod Pathol* 10:612-629, 1997.

Raymond WA, Leong ASY, Bolt JW, et al. Growth fractions in human prostatic carcinoma determined by Ki-67 immunostaining. *J Pathol* 156:161-167, 1988.

Reese JH, Lombard CM, Krone K, et al. Phyllodes type of atypical prostatic hyperplasia: a report of 3 new cases. *J Urol* 138:623-626, 1987.

Reuter VE. Pathological changes in benign and malignant prostatic tissue following androgen deprivation therapy. *Urology* 49:16-22, 1997.

Rioux-Leclercq N, Epstein JI. Unusual morphologic patterns of basal cell hyperplasia of the prostate. *Am J Surg Pathol* 26:237-243, 2002.

Ro JY, El-Naggar A, Amin MB, et al. Pseudosarcomatous fibromyxoid tumor of the urinary bladder and prostate: immunohistochemical, ultrastructural, and DNA flow cytometric analysis of nine cases. *Hum Pathol* 24:1203-1210, 1993.

Robert M, Costa P, Bressolle F, et al. Percentage area density of epithelial and mesenchymal components in benign prostatic hyperplasia: comparison of results between single biopsy, multiple biopsies and multiple tissue specimens. *Br J Urol* 75:317-324, 1995.

Roberts RO, Rhodes T, Panser LA, et al. Association between family history of benign prostatic hyperplasia and urinary symptoms: results of a population-based study. *Am J Epidemiol* 142:965-973, 1995.

Roehrborn CG, Bartsch G, Kirby R, et al. Guidelines for the diagnosis and treatment of benign prostatic hyperplasia: a comparative, international overview. *Urology* 58:642-650, 2001.

Roehrborn CG, McConnell JD. Etiology, pathophysiology, epidemiology, and natural history of benign prostatic hyperplasia. In: Walsh PC, Retik AB, Vaughan ED Jr, et al, eds. *Campbell's Urology*, 8th ed. Philadelphia: Saunders; 1297-1336, 2002.

Ronnett BM, Epstein JI. A case showing sclerosing adenosis and an unusual form of basal cell hyperplasia of the prostate. *Am J Surg Pathol* 13:866-872, 1989.

Roth RB. Prostatic infarction . *J Urol* 57:474-479, 1949.

Sagnier PP, MacFarlane G, Richard F, et al. Results of an epidemiological survey using a modified American Urological Association symptom index for benign prostatic hyperplasia in France. *J Urol* 151:1266-1270, 1994.

Sahin AA, Ro JY, El-Naggar AK, et al. Pseudosarcomatous fibromyxoid tumor of prostate. *Am J Clin Pathol* 96:253-258, 1991.

Sanda MG, Beaty TH, Stutzman RE, et al. Genetic susceptibility of benign prostatic hyperplasia. *J Urol* 152:115-119, 1994.

Sanda MG, Doehring CB, Binkowitz B, et al. Clinical and biological characterization of familial benign prostatic hyperplasia. *J Urol* 157:876-879, 1997.

Sarma DP, Guileyardo JM. Basal cell hyperplasia of the prostate. *J La State Med Soc* 134:23-24, 1982.

Scheckowitz EM, Resnick MI. Imaging of the prostate. Benign prostatic hyperplasia. *Urol Clin North Am* 22:321-332, 1995.

Schlechte H, Lenk SV, Löning T, et al. p53 Tumour suppressor gene mutations in benign prostatic hyperplasia and prostate cancer. *Eur Urol* 34:433-440, 1998.

Seaman E, Whang M, Olsson CA, et al. PSA density (PSAD): role in patient evaluation and management. *Urol Clin North Am* 20:653-663, 1993.

Sentinelli S. Mucins in prostatic intra-epithelial neoplasia and prostatic carcinoma. *Histopathology* 22:271-274, 1993.

Sesterhenn IA, Becker RL, Avallone FA, et al. Image analysis of nucleoli and nucleolar organizer regions in prostatic hyperplasia, intraepithelial neoplasia, and prostatic carcinoma. *J Urogen Pathol* 1:61-74, 1991.

Shannon RL, Ro JY, Grignon DJ, et al. Sarcomatoid carcinoma of the prostate: a clinicopathologic study of 12 cases. *Cancer* 69:2676-2682, 1992.

Shapiro E, Hartanto V, Lepor H. The response to alpha blockade in benign prostatic hyperplasia is related to the percent area density of prostate smooth muscle. *Prostate* 21:297-307, 1992.

Sheaff MT, Baithun SI. Effects of radiation on the normal prostate gland. *Histopathology* 30:341-348, 1997.

Shuman BA, Cohen JK, Miller RJ Jr, et al. Histological presence of viable prostatic glands on routine biopsy following cryosurgical ablation of the prostate. *J Urol* 157:552-555, 1997.

SMD (*Stedman's Medical Dictionary*). 23rd ed. Baltimore: Williams & Wilkins; 673, 1976.

Smith DS, Catalona WJ. Rate of change in serum prostate specific antigen levels as a method for prostate cancer detection. *J Urol* 152:1163-1167, 1994.

Spiro LH, Labay G, Orkin LA. Prostatic infarction: Role in acute urinary retention. *Urology* 3:345-347, 1974.

Stamey TA, Yang N, Hay AR, et al. Prostate-specific antigen as a serum marker for adenocarcinoma of the prostate. *N Engl J Med* 317:909-916, 1987.

Steiner MS. Review of peptide growth factors in benign prostatic hyperplasia and urological malignancy. *J Urol* 153:1085-1096, 1995.

Strachan JR, Corbishley CM, Shearer RJ. Post-operative retention associated with acute prostatic infarction. *Br J Urol* 72:311-313, 1993.

Sutton EB, McDonald JR. Metaplasia of prostatic epithelium: a lesion sometimes mistaken for carcinoma. *Am J Clin Pathol* 13:607-624, 1943.

Taussig AS, Hurst JW, Ambrose SS, et al. Massive prostatic infarction following aortocoronary bypass surgery: a report of two cases. *Clin Cardiol* 7:113-116, 1984.

Têtu B, Srigley JR, Boivin JC, et al. Effect of combination endocrine therapy (LHRH agonist and flutamide) on normal prostate and prostatic adenocarcinoma. A histopathologic and immunohistochemical study. *Am J Surg Pathol* 15:111-120, 1991.

Thorson P, Vollmer RT, Arcangeli C, et al. Minimal carcinoma in prostate needle biopsy specimens: diagnostic features and radical prostatectomy follow-up. *Mod Pathol* 11:543-551, 1998.

Thorson P, Swanson PE, Humphrey PA. Basal cell proliferations of the peripheral zone of the prostate gland [abstract]. *Mod Pathol* 12:108A, 1999.

Thorson P, Swanson PE, Humphrey PA. Comparative incidence, proliferation index, and apoptotic index of peripheral zone versus transition zone basal cell hyperplasia of prostate [abstract]. *Mod Pathol* 13:116A, 2000.

Totten RS, Heinemann MW, Hudson PB, et al. Microscopic differential diagnosis of latent carcinoma of prostate. *Arch Pathol* 55:131-141, 1953.

Tsuchiya K, Lynch J, True L. Prostatic intraepithelial neoplasia: interobserver variability in grading [abstract]. *Mod Pathol* 6:71A, 1993.

Tsukamoto T, Kumamoto Y, Masumori N, et al. Prevalence of prostatism in Japanese men in a community-based study with comparison to a similar American study. *J Urol* 154:391-395, 1995.

Tutrone RF, Ball RA, Ornitz DM. Benign prostatic hyperplasia in a transgenic mouse: a new hormonally sensitive investigatory model. *J Urol* 149:633-639, 1993.

Vaillancourt L, Têtu B, Fradet Y, et al. Effect of neoadjuvant endocrine therapy (combined androgen blockade) on normal prostate and prostatic carcinoma. A randomized study. *Am J Surg Pathol* 20:86-93, 1996.

Val-Bernal JF, Gómez-Ortega JM. Hyperplasia of prostatic mesonephric remnants: a potential pitfall in the evaluation of prostate gland biopsy. *J Urol* 154:1138-1139, 1995.

van de Voorde W, Baldewijns M, Lauweryns J. Florid basal cell hyperplasia of the prostate. *Histopathology* 24:341-346, 1994A.

van de Voorde WM, Elgamal AA, Van Poppel HP, et al. Morphologic and immunohistochemical changes in prostate cancer after preoperative hormonal therapy. A comparative study of radical prostatectomies. *Cancer* 74:3164-3175, 1994B.

van de Voorde W, Oyen R, Van Poppel H, et al. Peripherally localized benign prostatic nodules of the prostate. *Mod Pathol* 8:46-60, 1995.

Vassilakis GB. Pure leiomyoma of prostate. *Urology* 11:93-94, 1978.

Viglione MP, Potter S, Partin AW, et al. Should the diagnosis of benign prostatic hyperplasia be made on prostate needle biopsy? *Hum Pathol* 33:796-800, 2002.

Vollmer RT. Letter to the editor. *Am J Surg Pathol* 11:489, 1987.

Wang X, Bostwick DG. Prostatic stromal hyperplasia with atypia: a study of 11 cases. *J Urol Pathol* 6:15-26, 1997.

Wasson JH, Bubolz TA, Lu-Yao GL, et al, Transurethral resection of the prostate among medicare beneficiaries: 1984 1997. For The Patient Outcomes Research Team for Prostatic Diseases. *J Urol* 164:1212-1215, 2000.

Wennbo H, Kindblom J, Isaksson OG, et al. Transgenic mice overexpressing the prolactin gene develop dramatic enlargement of the prostate gland. *Endocrinology* 138:4410-4415, 1997.

Werely CJ, Heyns CF, Van Velden DJJ, et al. DNA fingerprint detection of somatic mutations in benign prostatic hyperplasia and prostatic adenocarcinoma. *Genes Chromosomes Cancer* 17:31-36, 1996.

Wertz IE, Deitch AD, Gumerlock PH, et al. Correlation of genetic and immunodetection of TP53 mutations in malignant and benign prostate tissue. *Hum Pathol* 27:573-580, 1996.

Wick MR, Young RH, Malvesta R, et al. Prostatic carcinosarcoma: clinical, histologic, and immunohistochemical data on two cases, with a review of the literature. *Am J Clin Pathol* 92:131-139, 1984.

Willis RA. Carcinoma of the prostate. In: *Pathology of Tumors.* St Louis: CV Mosby; 587, 1948.

Wilson JD. The pathogenesis of benign prostatic hyperplasia. *Am J Med* 68:745-756, 1980.

Yang XJ, McEntee M, Epstein JI. Distinction of basaloid carcinoma of the prostate from benign basal cell lesions by using immunohistochemistry for bcl-2 and Ki-67. *Hum Pathol* 29:1447-1450, 1998.

Young RH, Scully RE. Pseudosarcomatous lesions of the urinary bladder, prostate gland, and urethra. *Arch Pathol Lab Med* 111:354-358, 1987.

Young RH. Pseudoneoplastic lesions of the prostate gland. *Pathol Annu* 23(1):105-128, 1988.

Young RH. Pseudoneoplastic lesions of the urinary bladder, prostate gland, and urethra. In: Wick MR, Humphrey PA, Ritter JR, eds. *Pathology of Pseudoneoplastic Lesions.* New York: Lippincott-Raven; 223-235, 1997A.

Young RH. Tumor-like lesions of the prostate gland. *Am J Clin Pathol* 104:607-610, 1997B.

Ziada A, Rosenblum M, Crawford ED. Benign prostatic hyperplasia: an overview. *Urology* 53:1-6, 1999.

Atypical Adenomatous Hyperplasia (Adenosis)

[8.1] Atypical Adenomatous Hyperplasia (Adenosis) **155**

[8.2] Sclerosing Adenosis **162**

CHAPTER 8

A*typical hyperplasia* and *adenosis* are terms that have been widely applied to diagnose prostatic cellular proliferations. *Atypical hyperplasia,* in particular, has been used to designate many different proliferations in the prostate (Andrews 1949, Baron 1941, Brawn 1989, Garnett 1989, Gleason 1985, Harbitz 1972, Helpap 1980, Kastendieck 1980, 1989, Kovi 1985, 1988, 1989, McNeal 1965, Moore 1943, Mostofi 1973, Tannenbaum 1977, Wernert 1984) **t8.1**. In the past there has been a lack of uniformity in use of these varying diagnostic terms for atypical epithelial hyperplasia. Indeed, *prostatic atypical hyperplasia* has been a broad diagnostic umbrella, covering a wide variety of cytologic and architectural atypia that has some but not all the features of malignancy. Therefore, a diagnosis of atypical hyperplasia has been rendered for a spectrum of epithelial atypias in the prostate, ranging from reactive atypia to intraepithelial neoplasia (or dysplasia) to small foci of adenocarcinoma. *Atypical hyperplasia of the prostate,* when so broadly defined and used, does not have a specific clinicopathologic meaning and should not be used as a diagnostic label.

Recently, there has been a movement to limit and focus the use of atypical epithelial hyperplasia terms to two categories: atypical adenomatous hyperplasia (AAH) and atypical basal cell hyperplasia. Even here, there is controversy regarding the most appropriate terminology because of a lack of understanding of the biologic potential of these two proliferations. Therefore, AAH is also known as adenosis, and atypical basal cell hyperplasia is also called basal cell hyperplasia with prominent nucleoli (Yang 1998).

Adenosis is most commonly used as a synonym for *atypical adenomatous hyperplasia.* Sclerosing adenosis is a second, distinctive type of adenosis in the prostate.

t8.1 Atypical Epithelial Hyperplasia: Diagnostic Terms

Previously Used Terminology
Atypical hyperplasia
Atypical epithelial hyperplasia
Atypical glandular hyperplasia
Atypical primary hyperplasia
Atypical postatrophic hyperplasia
Atypical small acinar hyperplasia
Atypical large acinar hyperplasia
Atypical adenomatous hyperplasia
Atypical cribriform hyperplasia
Atypical basal cell hyperplasia
Hyperplasia with cellular anaplasia
Atypical adenosis

Currently Used Terminology
Atypical adenomatous hyperplasia = adenosis
Atypical basal cell hyperplasia = basal cell hyperplasia with prominent nucleoli

t8.2 Incidence of Atypical Adenomatous Hyperplasia (Adenosis)

Specimen Type	Number (%)	Reference
Needle biopsy	1/795 (0.1)	Reyes 1998
Needle biopsy	3/1,009 (0.3)	Cheville 1997
Needle biopsy	6/719 (0.8)	Gaudin 1995
TURP	NA (1.6)	Gaudin 1994
TURP	24/752 (3.2)	Doll 1999
TURP	68/731 (9)	Skjorten 1997
TURP	152/975 (16)	Mai 2000
Simple prostatectomy	17/325 (5.2)	Skjorten 1997
Radical prostatectomy	50/217 (23)	Bostwick 1995
Radical prostatectomy	22/80 (27)	Troncoso 1995
Radical prostatectomy	40/120 (33)	Muezzinoglu 1997
Radical prostatectomy	43/72 (60)	Srigley 1986
Cystoprostatectomy	13/59 (22)	Muezzinoglu 1997

NA = not available

[8.1] Atypical Adenomatous Hyperplasia (Adenosis)

AAH, also known as adenosis, is a small glandular proliferation that has been defined as "a localized proliferation of small glands within the prostate that may be mistaken for carcinoma" (Bostwick 1993) or "a relatively well-circumscribed nodule of closely packed glands with a lobular growth pattern" (Gaudin 1994; reviews: Amin 1993, Bostwick 1996, Epstein 1995, Grignon 1996, Parkinson 1995, Sakr 1998). The term *atypical adenomatous hyperplasia* was used as early as 1941 (Baron 1941), but only recently have these definitions generated a more standardized approach to the diagnosis.

AAH is invariably an incidental histologic finding. There are no clinical findings that are specific for AAH. The mean age of patients diagnosed with AAH is 64 to 70 years, with a range of 45 to 83 (Bostwick 1995, Gaudin 1994, 1995). The volume of AAH and number of AAH foci increases with age (Bostwick 1995). It is not known whether AAH can elevate the serum prostate-specific antigen (PSA) or produce a mass palpable by digital rectal examination, but except for a few examples of larger-volume AAH cases, this seems unlikely because most AAH foci are microscopic in size.

The incidence of AAH depends on the type of tissue sample (Bostwick 1995, Cheville 1997, Doll 1999, Gaudin 1994, 1995, Mai 2000, Muezzinoglu 1997, Reyes 1998, Skjorten 1997, Srigley 1984, Troncoso 1995), with a wide range from less than 1% on needle biopsies (Cheville 1997, Gaudin 1995, Reyes 1998) to 22% to 60% in whole glands (Bostwick 1995, Muezzinoglu 1997, Srigley 1986, Troncoso 1995). In transurethral and simple prostatectomy specimens, there is an intermediate incidence of 2% to 16% (Doll 1999, Gaudin 1994, Mai 2000, Skjorten 1997) **t8.2**.

Grossly, AAH is not recognizable because it is usually a minute proliferation. The largest reported AAH nodule (at 21 cm^3) was not macroscopically distinguishable from other large hyperplastic nodules in the same 124-cm^3 prostate (Humphrey 1998A). Microscopically, most foci of AAH are extremely small, as the mean diameter in needle biopsy is 1.4 mm and in transurethral resection of the prostate (TURP) chips, 2.5 mm (Gaudin 1994, 1995). In radical prostatectomy tissues the average volume is 0.029 cm^3 (Bostwick 1995) **t8.3**. Multifocality is found in a majority of TURP chips but only in a minority of needle biopsy and radical prostatectomy tissues (Bostwick 1995, Gaudin 1994, 1995, Muezzinoglu 1997) **t8.3**. In needle biopsy, most multifocal AAH cases had 2 separate foci, and rare cases had 3 foci (Gaudin 1995). TURP chips had an average of 3.3 AAH foci per case (range, 1 to 16 foci), but this extent still usually made up less than 1%

■ **t8.3 Atypical Adenomatous Hyperplasia: Extent and Location[1]**

Specimen Type	Size	Multifocality	Location
Needle biopsy	Mean = 1.4 mm Range: 0.3-8 mm	16%	NA
TURP chips[2]	Mean = 2.5 mm Range: 0.5-0 mm	68%	NA
Radical prostatectomy	Mean = 0.029 cc Range: 0-1.29 cc	30%-46%	86%-100% transition zone

[1]Data from Gaudin 1994, Gaudin 1995, Bostwick 1995, Troncoso 1995, Muezzinoglu 1997
[2]TURP mainly samples transition zone
NA = Not available

■ **t8.4 Diagnostic Features of Atypical Adenomatous Hyperplasia (Adenosis)**

Typically a circumscribed nodule of small glands admixed with larger, complex glands
Densely packed arrangement of small glands
Fragmented basal cell layer
Luminal cell nuclei typically small and bland

of the tissue area (Gaudin 1994). Radical prostatectomies usually had only a single focus (range 1 to 10), and when they were multifocal, usually 2 or 3 foci were seen (Bostwick 1995). The reason for more frequent multifocal AAH in TURP chips than in radical prostatectomy specimens probably relates to the greater amount and multifocality of nodular hyperplasia in TURP chips than in radical prostatectomy tissues. Even in radical prostatectomy tissue, there is a strong correlation between amount of benign prostatic hyperplasia (BPH) tissue and the number of AAH foci (Bostwick 1995). Most AAH foci (86% to 100%) are discovered in the periurethral or transition zone region, with a minority in the peripheral and central zones or in both transition and nontransition zones (Bostwick 1995, Troncoso 1995).

Histologically, AAH typically is a well-circumscribed collection of densely packed small, pale, acini, which merge with larger, more complex glands **t8.4; i8.1, i8.2**. The periphery of the aggregate is characteristically rounded **i8.1, i8.3, i8.4**, but in a minority of cases, the small acini can extend into surrounding stroma in an infiltrative pattern **i8.5-i8.7; t8.5**. The small acini in AAH can be localized to the periphery of the nodule in ringlike or crescentic fashion **i8.6-i8.9**, or can be intermixed with the larger, complex glands **i8.1, i8.10**. The

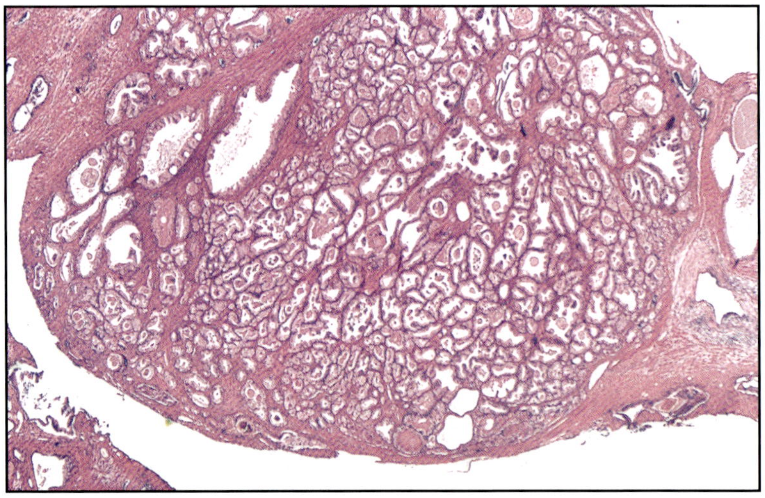

■ **i8.1** *Nodule of AAH (adenosis) in TURP chip*

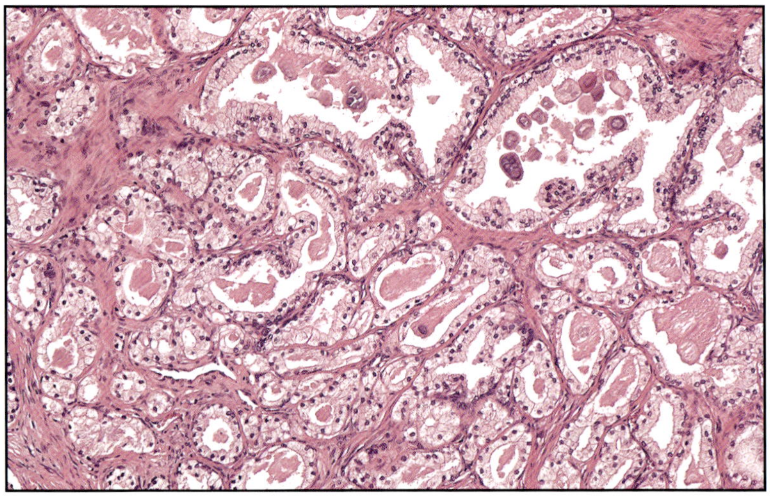

■ **i8.2** *Crowded, small acini merge with larger usual hyperplastic-like glands.*

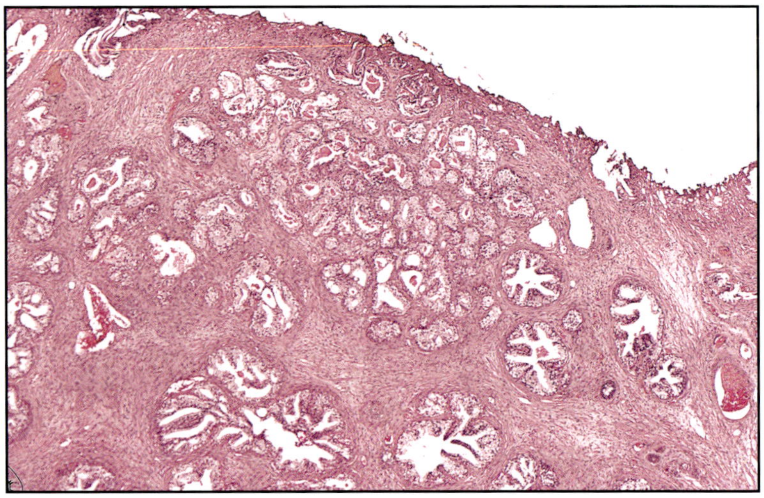

■ **i8.3** *Localized aggregate of small AAH glands in TURP chip.*

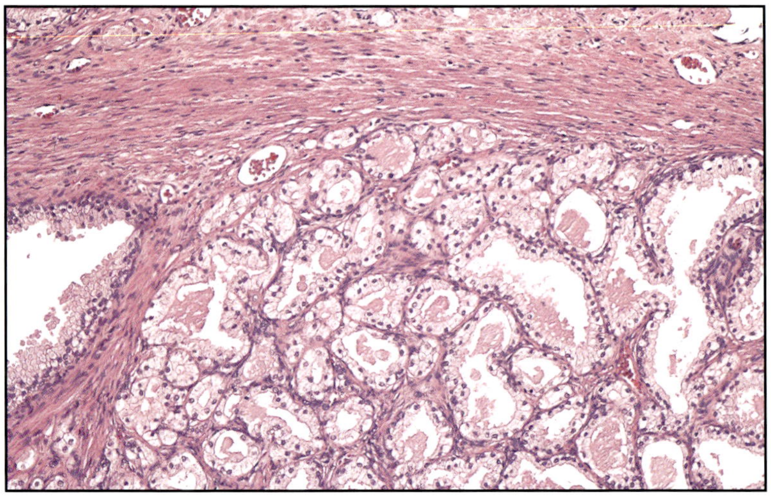

■ **i8.4** *AAH with rounded glandular-stromal interface.*

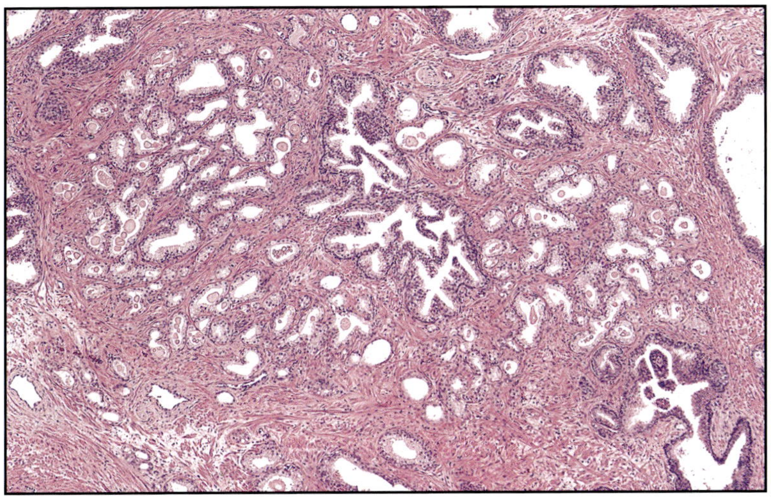

■ **i8.5** *Atypical adenomatous hyperplasia with extension of small acini between larger, more complex glands (right).*

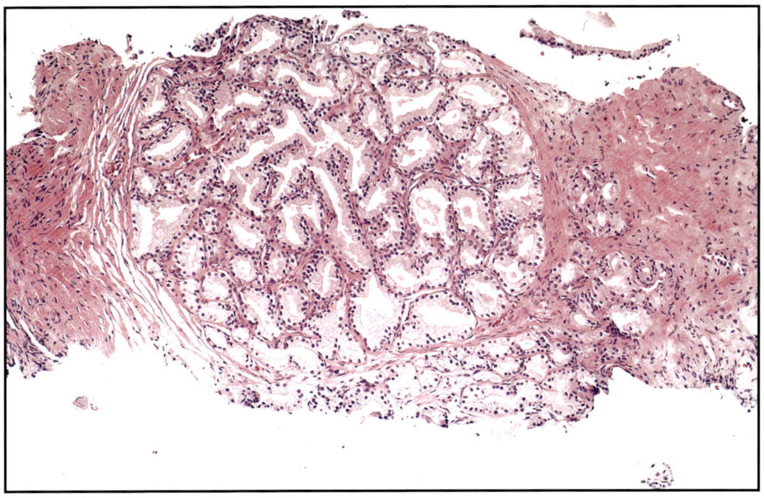

■ **i8.6** *Atypical adenomatous hyperplasia in needle biopsy tissue: Nodule surrounded by small acini.*

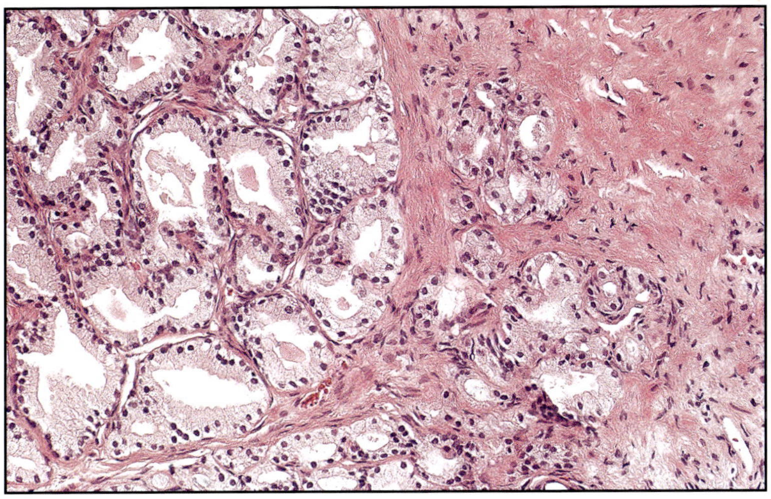

■ **i8.7** *Atypical adenomatous hyperplasia: The smaller, peripheral acini appear to be infiltrating the stroma.*

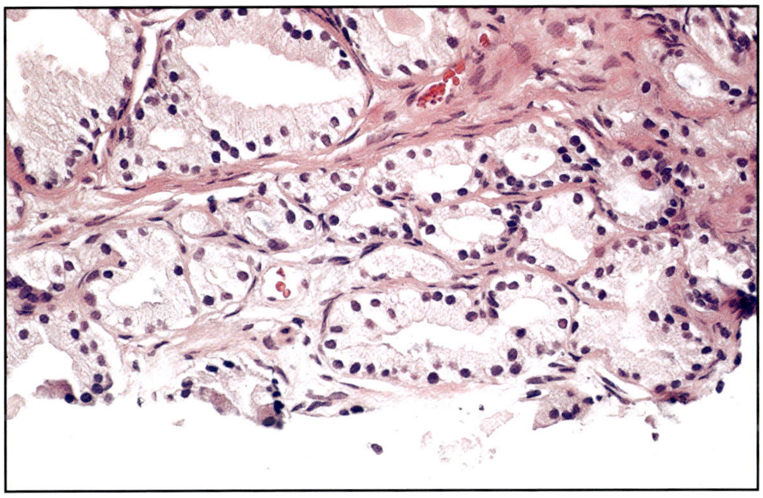

■ **i8.8** *Atypical adenomatous hyperplasia: Crowded small glands from peripheral band in* **i8.6** *extend to the edge of the needle core.*

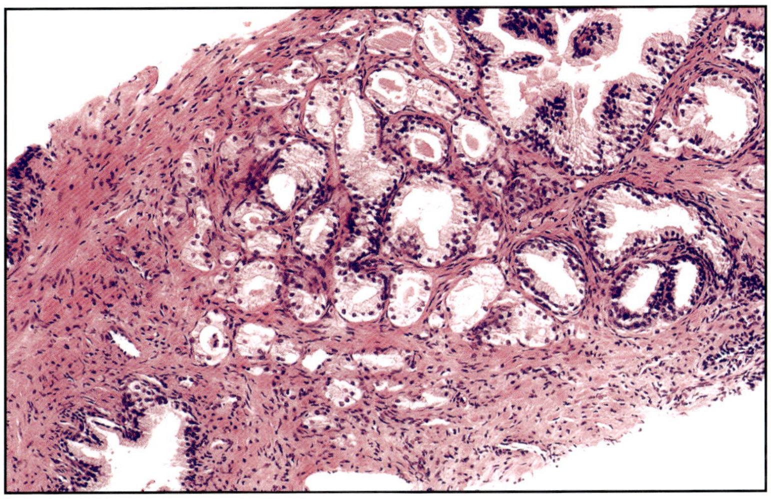

■ **i8.9** *AAH (adenosis) in needle biopsy tissue, with small glands at one pole of the glandular proliferation.*

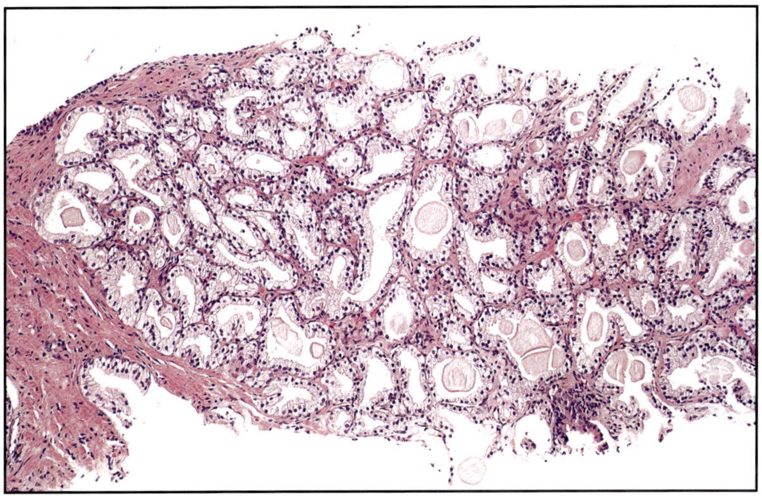

■ **i8.10** *AAH (adenosis) in needle biopsy with haphazardly arranged small acini, intermingled with larger acini.*

number of small acini is variable, and they can make up a minority **i8.11** or majority **i8.12**, of the glandular proliferation. Many of these small glands are round and regular **i8.13**, or elongated **i8.14**, with open lumens. There is usually little intervening stroma **i8.2, i8.4**, but this is not an absolute diagnostic requirement **i8.5**. A transition is present between the small AAH glands and larger, usual hyperplastic glands with luminal undulations, branching and papillary infoldings **i8.2**. These larger glands clearly possess basal cells and on occasion basal

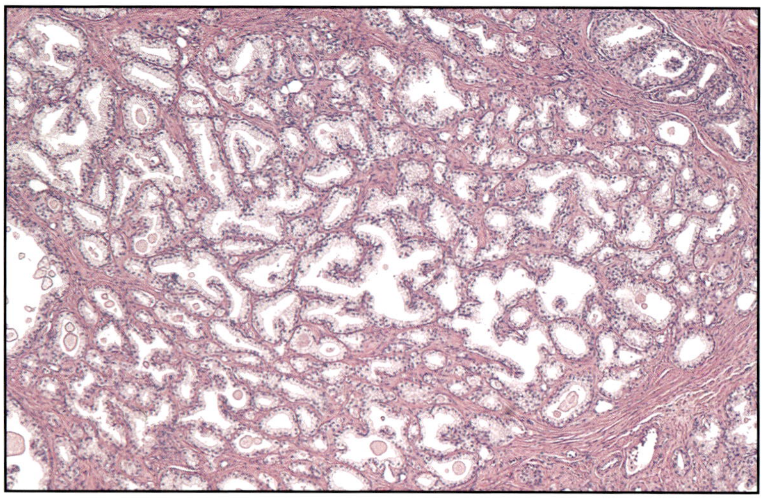

■ **i8.11** *AAH nodule with a minor small acinar population.*

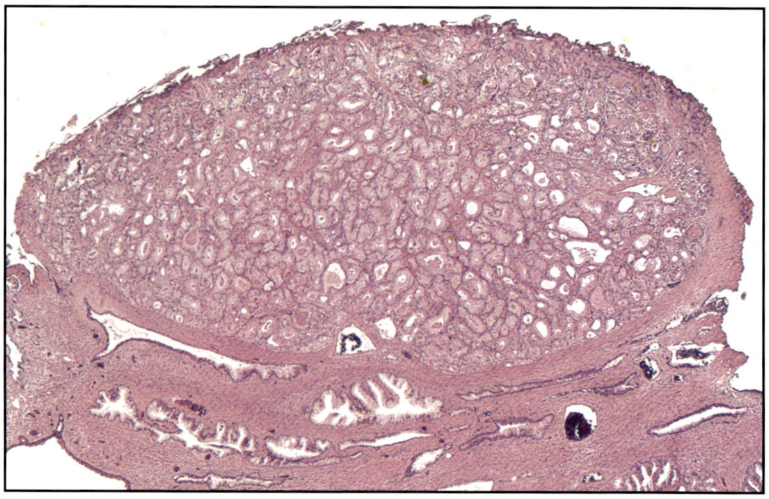

■ **i8.12** *AAH nodule in TURP chip with mainly closed packed small acini. Well-differentiated adenocarcinoma was excluded by the presence of basal cells and lack of nuclear atypia.*

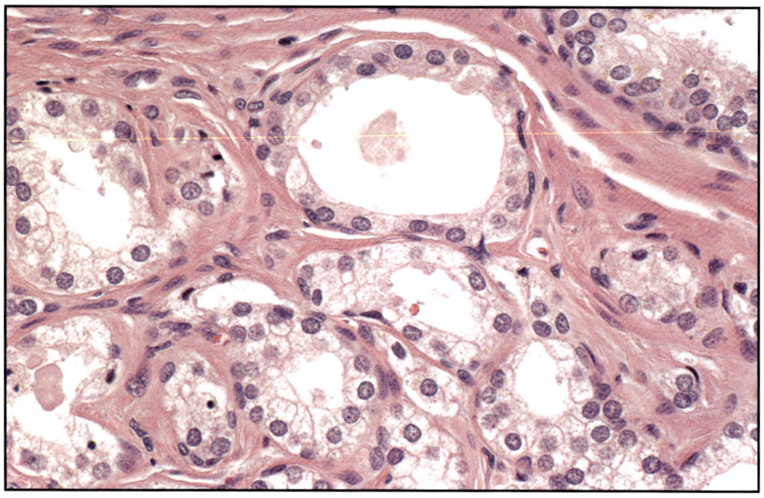

■ **i8.13** *Small, round acini of AAH (adenosis) with two cell layers and bland luminal cell nuclear features.*

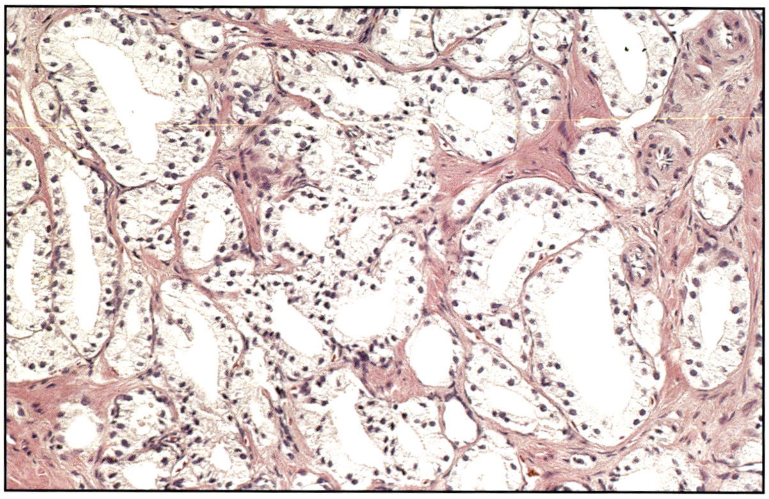

■ **i8.14** *AAH acini with more elongated forms.*

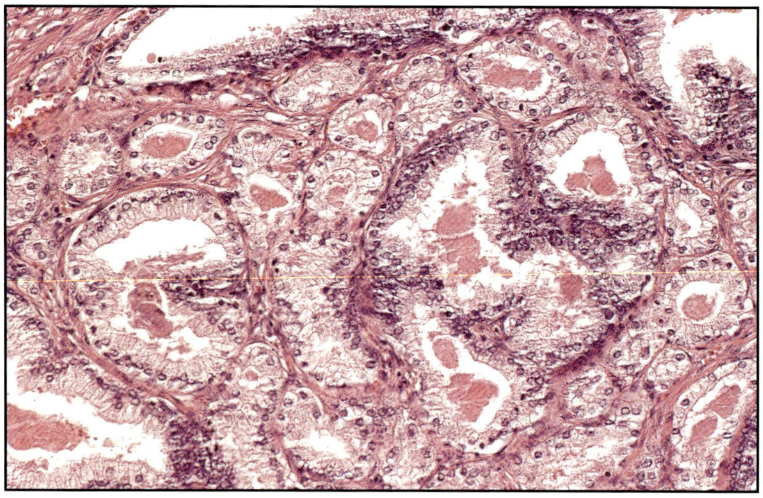

■ **i8.15** *Atypical adenomatous hyperplasia: Basal cell prominence in larger AAH glands.*

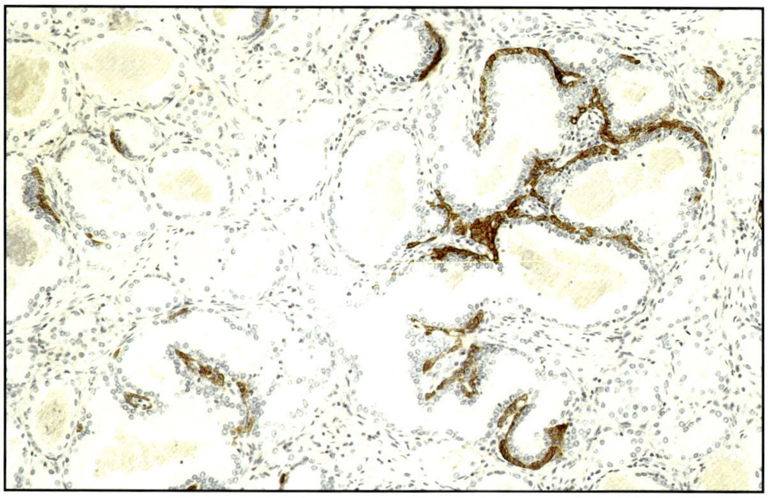

■ **i8.16** *Atypical adenomatous hyperplasia: Basal cell immunostain (34βE12 antibody) marks numerous basal cells in larger glands. Note some small acini do not have basal cells.*

cell prominence **i8.15, i8.16**, or cystic change **i8.17** can be noted. Of critical diagnostic importance, the small, tubular acini have a fragmented basal layer. Basal cells can be found in the majority of foci of adenosis (78% in one needle biopsy study [Gaudin 1995]) by careful scrutiny of hematoxylin and eosin (H&E)-stained sections **i8.13** but can be difficult to discern in some foci **i8.15**. Confirmation of a discontinuous basal cell layer can be accomplished by use of immunohistochemical staining with antibody 34βE12 **i8.16, i8.20**. On

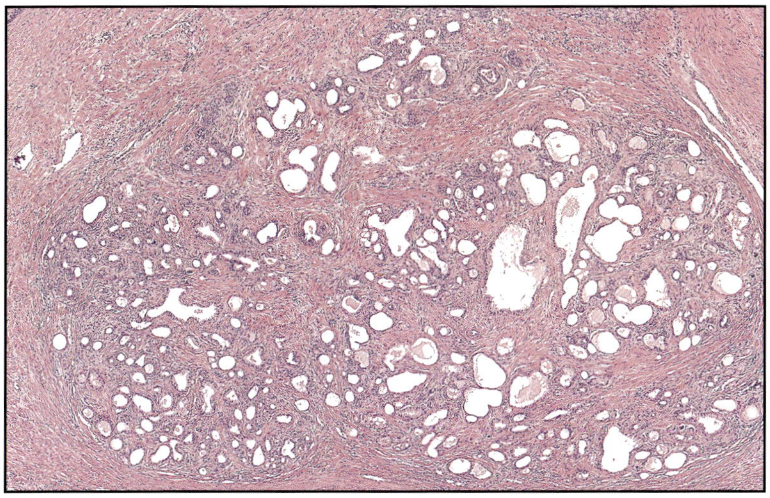

■ **i8.17** *AAH nodule with small acini admixed with cystically dilated glands. The AAH glands in this nodule exhibit atrophic features.*

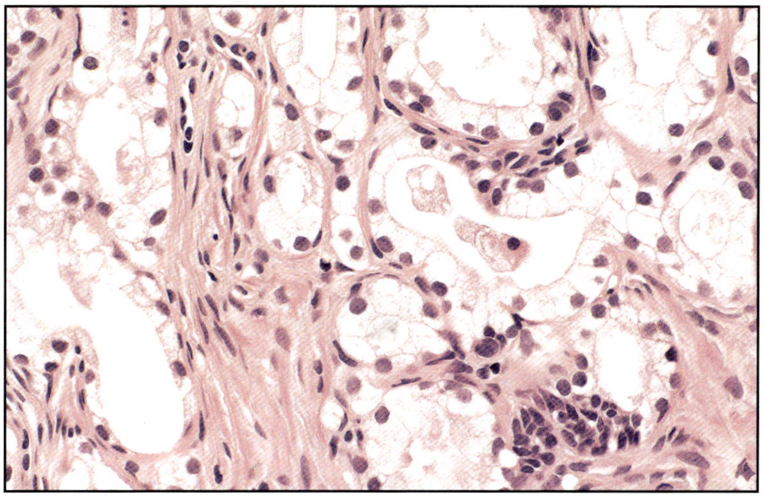

■ **i8.18** *AAH at high-power magnification. Only a few basal cells are present in this field.*

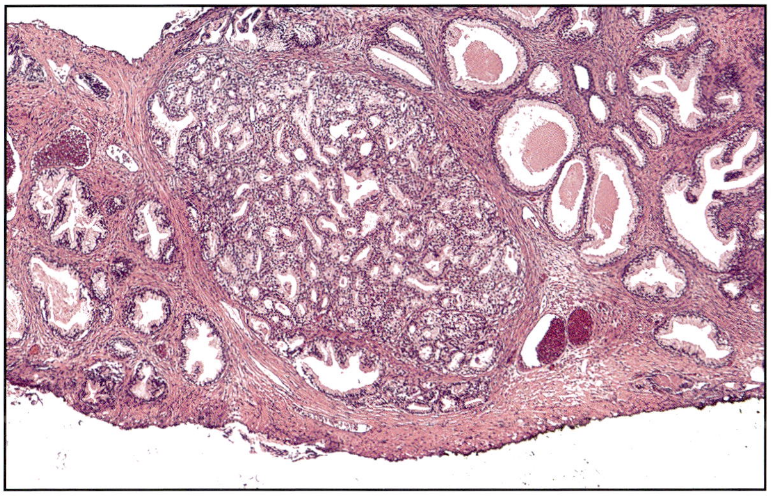

■ **i8.19** *Nodule of AAH.*

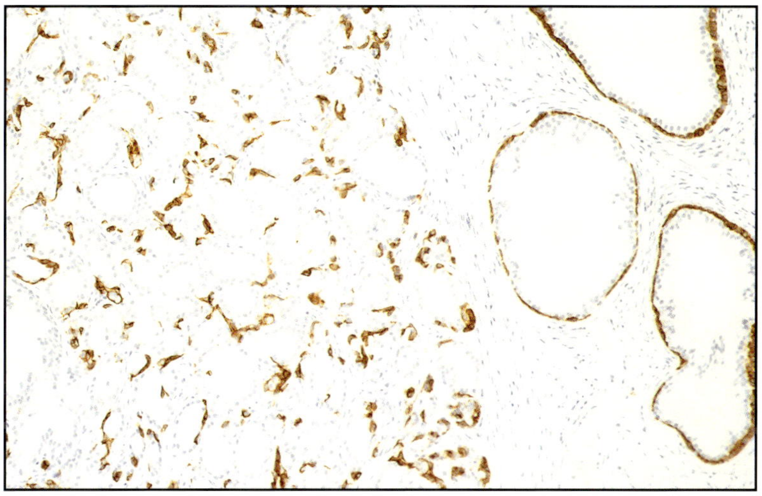

■ **i8.20** *Atypical adenomatous hyperplasia: Fragmented basal cell layer in AAH nodule in* **i8.19***, as revealed by 34βE12 immunostain for high molecular weight cytokeratins.*

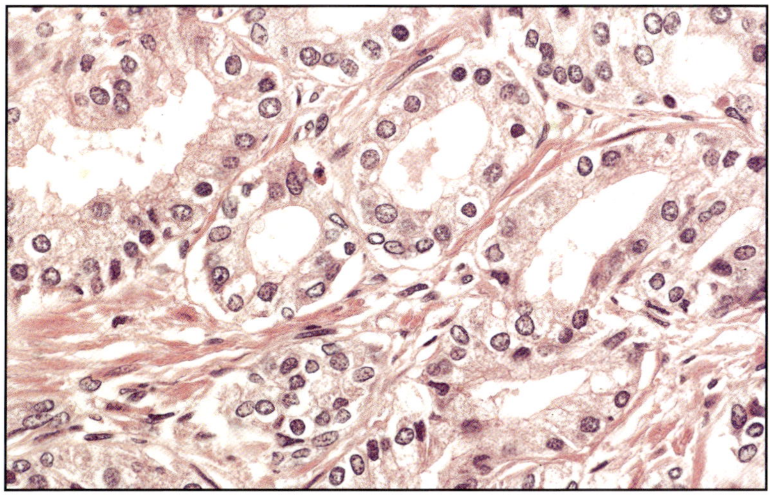

■ **i8.21** *Small acini of AAH (adenosis) with slight nuclear enlargement and infrequent nucleoli. Basal cells are present.*

average, more than one half of the glands in a particular focus are positive with this immunostain, but the range is 10% to 90% (Bostwick 1993, Gaudin 1995). Also of substantial importance, the nuclei of AAH should be bland **i8.13, i8.18**. That is, the nuclei should be small with little variation in size and shape, and any detectable nucleoli should be small. The nuclei in the small acini should appear similar to those of complex, benign-appearing glands both within the AAH focus and distant from the AAH focus. The chromatin in AAH luminal cell nuclei should be finely punctate and uniformly dispersed (Bostwick 1993, Gaudin 1995). However, a degree of nuclear atypia is allowable in AAH **i8.21**. The nucleoli in AAH usually are inconspicuous, but in 13% to 28% of cases, prominent nucleoli (greater than 1 μm in diameter) are present. These nucleoli typically are solitary and centrally located within the nuclei (Helpap 1995). Additional atypical features that can be found in a minority of AAH cases include intraluminal crystalloids, mitotic figures, and intraluminal wispy blue mucin **t8.5**. Attempts have been made to grade AAH based on the degree of the atypical findings. Therefore, schemes separating AAH into low and high grades (Helpap 1995) and classifying adenosis (AAH) into mild, moderate, and severe forms (Brawn 1982) have been published, but grading of AAH is not routine practice.

The differential diagnostic list for AAH (adenosis) is dominated by well-differentiated, Gleason score 2 to 4 adenocarcinoma **t8.6**. Both are circumscribed proliferations of small, pale glands, but AAH merges with hyperplastic-appearing glands, whereas most well-differentiated carcinomas consist of tubular glands with

■ **t8.5 Atypical Adenomatous Hyperplasia (Adenosis): Incidence of Histologic Features[1]**

	Specimen Type	
Histologic Feature	**Needle Biopsy**	**TURP**
Infiltrative growth	13%	5%-19%
Glands with basal cells	60% (range 10%-90%)	20%-50%
Prominent nucleoli[2]	13%	15%
Mitotic figures	2%	11%
Intraluminal material		
Corpora amylacea	43%	32%
Crystalloids	24%	18%-40%
Wispy blue mucin	3%	2%

[1]Data from Bostwick 1993, Gaudin 1994, Gaudin 1995
[2]Nucleoli larger than 1 μm in one study (Bostwick 1993) and greater than 1.6 μm in another (Kramer 1993)

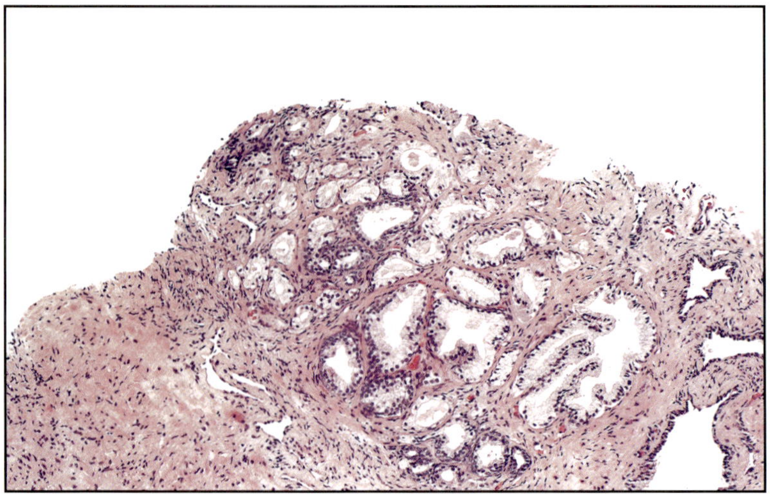

■ **i8.22** *AAH (adenosis) in needle biopsy with transection of small acinar proliferation.*

straight luminal borders. Also, the high-power identification of basal cells and bland luminal cell nuclei in AAH allows separation of these entities in most cases, based on examination of H&E-stained slides alone. Difficulty arises when atypical features such as infiltrative growth, prominent nucleoli, intraluminal crystalloids, and intraluminal wispy blue mucin are detected **t8.5**. In needle biopsy, the lobular character of AAH can be difficult to appreciate because in only 7% of foci is the entire lobular lesion sampled (Gaudin 1994) **i8.6, i8.8, i8.22**. In about one half of needle cases, AAH extends to both sides of the needle (Gaudin 1994), and this can cause concern for invasion. Furthermore, in some cases, basal cells can be a challenge to definitively identify on H&E-stained sections. In such cases, immunohistochemical staining for basal cells using antibody 34βE12 can help confirm basal cell presence. Overall, however, only a minority (15% to 20%) of adenosis cases warrants a 34βE12 immunostain (Wojno 1995), and the diagnosis usually can be established with H&E-stained slides. In a small minority of cases, particularly when only a few closely packed, small, pale glands with atypical features are present, a descriptive diagnosis of atypia, without commitment as to the precise nature of the proliferation, is a viable choice. One suggested designation for these cases is "atypical small acinar proliferation" with or without the qualifier of "of uncertain significance" (Bostwick 1993) (Chapter 12). Also in the differential diagnosis is the recently described pseudohyperplastic prostatic carcinoma (Humphrey 1998A, Levi 2000). Here, there can be an admixture of small, pale glands and complex hyperplastic-appearing glands. Yet these glands completely lack basal cells, and the nuclei exhibit substantial nucleomegaly with macronucleoli. Usual, moderately to poorly differentiated (Gleason score 5 to 10) adenocarcinomas are not likely to be confused with AAH because these carcinomas are clearly infiltrative, typically have amphophilic (rather than cleared) cytoplasm, lack basal cells, and usually have atypical nuclei.

A number of benign conditions must be differentiated from AAH **t8.6**. Usual epithelial hyperplasia has a predominance of larger, complex glands, but some recognize a small glandular variant of nodular hyperplasia, called adenomatous hyperplasia (Bostwick 1995). Compared with AAH, usual adenomatous hyperplasia has only small glands, with an intact basal cell layer. The other benign entities in **t8.6** are also made up of small glands, but only those with cleared cytoplasm merit mention. Basal cell hyperplasia can uncommonly have cells with cleared cytoplasm, but a crowded arrangement of back-to-back small glands with hyperplasia of basal cells with cleared cytoplasm is not expected. Verumontanum gland hyperplasia can mimic AAH but can be distinguished based on a continuous basal cell layer, intraluminal orange-red concretions, and the presence of nearby urothelium.

As noted earlier, the one special study that can be most helpful in diagnosis is immunohistochemical staining for basal cell cytokeratins using antibody 34βE12. Additional morphometric, histochemical, immunohistochemical, and genotypic studies have been performed to characterize AAH **t8.7**, but currently they are not of practical diagnostic applicability. Many of these investigations have been pursued to determine whether AAH more closely resembles usual hyperplasia or carcinoma. The preponderance of these data suggest a closer relationship between AAH and usual hyperplasia than AAH and carcinoma **t8.7**. Morphometrically, the nuclei of AAH are slightly but not significantly larger than those of usual hyperplasia (Lopez-Beltran 2000). Histochemically, AAH resembles BPH in failure to express D-galactose-β-[1→3]-*N*-acetyl-D-galactosamine (Shamsuddin 1994), and the number of silver-stained nucleolar organizing regions (AgNORs), which can be used as a marker of cell proliferation, is intermediate in AAH compared with BPH and low-grade carcinoma (Helpap 1995). The histochemical detection of acid mucin (by Alcian blue) is common in AAH (Epstein 1992A, Goldstein 1995, Luna-More 1997), and AAH resembles carcinoma more than BPH in this staining procedure. The

■ **t8.6 Differential Diagnosis of Atypical Adenomatous Hyperplasia (Adenosis)**

Well-differentiated adenocarcinoma (Gleason score 2-4)
Pseudohyperplastic prostatic adenocarcinoma
Atypical small acinar proliferation (of uncertain significance)
Usual epithelial hyperplasia
Basal cell hyperplasia
Postatrophic hyperplasia
Verumontanum gland hyperplasia
Mesonephric remnant hyperplasia
Nephrogenic metaplasia (adenoma)
Atrophy
Cowper's glands
Sclerosing adenosis

■ t8.7 Phenotype and Genotype of AAH (Adenosis)

Morphometric analysis
Nuclear volume for AAH = 237 μm^3 vs 209 μm^3 for usual hyperplasia vs. 436 μm^3 for well-differentiated carcinoma (Lopez-Beltran 2000)
Median nucleolar diameter for AAH = 0.7 μm vs 1.9 μm for well-differentiated carcinoma (Bostwick 1993)

Histochemical analysis
AgNORs per nucleus = 3.7 for AAH vs 2.6 for usual hyperplasia and 5.0 for low-grade carcinoma (Helpap 1995)
Neutral mucins (PAS positive) in 77% and acid mucins (Alcian blue positive) in 54%-63% of cases (Epstein 1992A, Goldstein 1995, Luna-More 1997)
Gal-GalNac: 0% adenosis foci vs 95% of adenocarcinomas and 0% normal and BPH (Shamsuddin 1994)
Peanut agglutinin receptor: 50% of adenosis cases vs 0% BPH cases and 100% of well-differentiated carcinomas (Chastonay 1986)

Immunophenotype
Proliferation index by Ki-67/MIB1 and PCNA immunolabeling = 1.2% to 4% (Helpap 1995, Haussler 1999)
PCNA immunolabeling: AAH = 0.07% vs 0.05% for BPH and 0.15% for carcinoma (Lopez-Beltran 1996)
ABH blood group isoantigens: 60% of adenosis cases vs 75% BPH cases and 25% of well-differentiated carcinomas (Chastonay 1986)
Androgen receptor: Negative to 1+ (on a scale of 3) (Harper 1998)
Epidermal growth factor receptor: Negative (Harper 1998)
c-erbB-2: Negative to low expression (Harper 1998, Haussler 1999)
c-erbB-3: Low (Haussler 1999)
E-Cadherin: 1+ to 2+ (on a scale of 3) (Harper 1998)
TGF-α: Negative (Harper 1998)
FGF-2: 1+ (on a scale of 3) (Harper 1998)
VEGF: Negative (Harper 1998)
bcl-2: Negative in luminal cells (Haussler 1999)
p53: Negative (Haussler 1999)
α-Methylacyl-CoA racemase (P504S): diffusely positive in 8% of cases (Yang 2002)

Genotype
Diploid DNA content (Humphrey 1998A, Lopez-Beltran 1996)
Loss of chromosome 7 and chromosome 8 foci by FISH uncommon (4% and 9%, respectively) (Qian 1995)
Allelic imbalance found in 12% of 25 cases without cancer (and only on chromosome 8p11-12) by PCR using microsatellite markers on 10 chromosomal arms (Doll 1999)
Allelic imbalance found in 47% of 15 cases in the presence of cancer by PCR using microsatellite polymorphic markers on 4 chromosome arms (Cheng 1998)
Frequency = 7q31-35: 9%, 18q12.2: 9%, 8q22.2: 15%, 8p12-21: 18%-60%

AgNOR = silver-stained nucleolar organizing regions; FGF-2 = fibroblast growth factor-2; FISH = fluorescence in-situ hybridization; PCNA = proliferating cell nuclear antigen; PCR = polymerase chain reaction; TGF-α = transforming growth factor-alpha; VEGF = vascular endothelial growth factor

immunophenotype of AAH indicates a paucity of growth factors and growth factor receptors, unlike carcinoma **t8.7**. The proliferation index of AAH is similar to that of BPH and lower than that of prostatic intraepithelial neoplasia (PIN) or carcinoma (Häussler 1999). ABH blood group antigen immunoreactivity resembles BPH more than well-differentiated carcinoma (Chastonay 1986), whereas peanut agglutinin receptors are at an intermediate level between BPH and carcinoma. AAH is negative for immunodetectable p53 and luminal cell bcl-2 (Häussler 1999). Genotypically, AAH nuclei have a diploid DNA content (Humphrey 1998A, Lopez-Beltran 1996), and some cases have loss of chromosomal DNA. In our experience, allelic loss in AAH in TURP chips without cancer was a low-frequency event at 6% to 12% **i8.23** (Doll 1999, Furman 1996), whereas in the presence of cancer AAH lesions had a 47% rate of allelic loss (Cheng 1998) **t8.7**. Tumor suppressor genes may reside at these foci of chromosomal loss, but to date specific genes have not been identified. Such genes could have diagnostic significance in the future.

Morphologic and clinical linkage of AAH to PIN or carcinoma is weak to absent. AAH, which is predominantly a transition zone proliferation, is rarely physically associated with high-grade PIN, which is usually a peripheral zone proliferation (Skjorten 1997), although the number of foci of AAH has been associated with volume of high-grade PIN (Bostwick 1995). There is evidence of a higher incidence of AAH in glands with carcinoma than in those without carcinoma (Helpap 1995, Srigley 1984, 1986). In one series, AAH overall was actually much more common in glands without carcinoma (82% of AAH cases) than in glands with carcinoma (18% of AAH cases), but so-called high-grade AAH was seen more often in glands with malignancy (Helpap 1995). In cystoprostatectomy specimens, AAH showed a slight but nonsignificant association (P = .073) with prostatic carcinoma presence (Muezzinoglu 1997). AAH is either slightly but nonsignificantly (P = .085) associated with transition zone carcinoma (Muezzinoglu 1997) or not associated with transition zone cancer (P = .5) (Troncoso 1995), which is a low-grade carcinoma that has been forwarded as the form of carcinoma most likely to evolve from AAH. Another lower-grade prostatic adenocarcinoma that did not

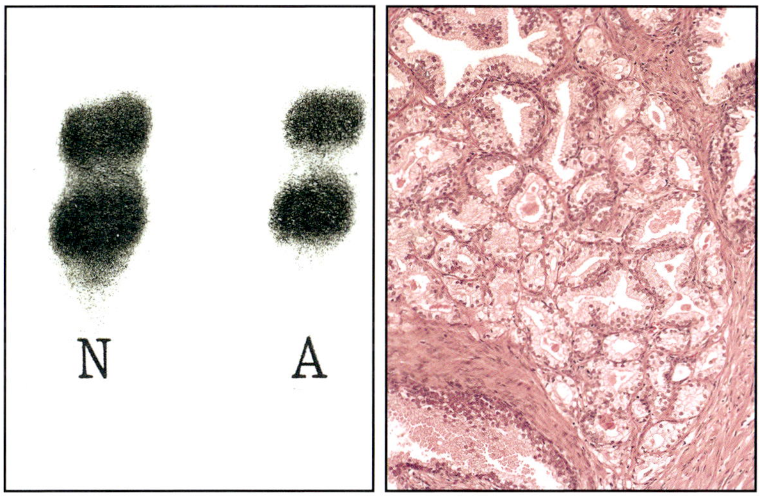

■ i8.23 *No evidence of allelic loss at chromosome 8p22 (left) in microdissected focus of AAH (right), using a polymorphic microsatellite marker and PCR. N= normal tissue DNA lane; A = AAH tissue DNA lane. Both alleles show equal band intensity in each lane.*

■ **t8.8 Sclerosing Adenosis of Prostate**

Study (year)	No. of Patients	Age (mean)	Tissue Type	Microscopic Findings
Chen 1983	1	62	TURP	7 mm nodule with irregular gland spaces and fibrous stroma
Young 1987	1	76	TURP	3 of 25 TUR chips with nodules of "irregular crowded acini, small nests, and single cells in a cellular stroma"
Hulman 1989	1	73	TURP	Well-circumscribed 5 mm nodule of small glands and slit-like spaces
Ronnnett 1989	1	78	TURP	Multiple foci of well-circumscribed nodules of closely packed small glands within a cellular stroma; merged with basal cell hyperplasia
Sakamoto 1991	5	72.3 (67-80)	3 TURP 1 simple prostatectomy 1 needle biopsy	4 mm nodule to multiple foci of closely packed small glands in a cellular stroma
Jones 1991	11	72.8 (62-84)	9 TURP 1 simple prostatectomy 1 needle biposy	Cellular nodule(s) of elongated, branched and compressed glands in a spindle cell stroma
Grignon 1992	15	71.5 (62-87)	10 TURP 3 cystoprostatectomy 2 simple prostatectomy	4.2 mm (range 1.5-11.1) nodules of small, round, and relatively uniform glands in a cellular stroma
Collina 1992	3	71.6 (65-78)	Simple prostatectomy	Single nodules of small packed glands in a cellular stroma
Barsky 1993	2	65,67	Biopsy, followed by simple prostatectomy	8-10 mm lesions of variably-sized, crowded acini
Redonodo Martinez 1997	4	73	TURP, simple prostatectomy	Incidental small gland proliferation in transition zone

have a physical association with AAH is pseudohyperplastic adenocarcinoma (Humphrey 1998A). AAH can be found within 2 mm of cancer in 34% of cases (Bostwick 1995), but a direct transition between the two seems to be uncommon to rare (Bostwick 1995, Helpap 1998, Jones 1994, Troncoso 1995).

Clinical follow-up of AAH is limited, and its natural history is unclear. Only a few patients with AAH (adenosis) have been followed, and based on 2 abstract reports (Renedo 1995, Srigley 1984), AAH does not seem to impart an increased risk for subsequent clinical detection of carcinoma. A third study (Brawn 1994) found that adenosis in TURP chips did not affect patient survival. However, these are preliminary data based on a low number of patients, and the risk of being diagnosed with malignancy after a diagnosis of AAH has not been established. Consequently, no established guidelines exist for follow-up of patients with AAH (adenosis) in needle biopsy or TURP chips.

[8.2] Sclerosing Adenosis

Sclerosing adenosis of the prostate, which also has been called "adenomatoid prostatic tumor" (Chen 1983), "pseudoadenomatoid tumor of prostate" (Hulman 1989), and "fibroepithelial nodule," is an uncommon, benign, small acinar proliferation embedded in a spindle cell background (Barsky 1993, Chen 1983, Collina 1992, Grignon 1992, Hulman 1989, Jones 1991, Meister 1996, Redonodo Martinez 1997, Ronnett 1989, Sakamoto 1991, Young 1987) **t8.8**. This proliferation usually is an incidental, microscopic finding in men in their 60s or 70s who present with BPH symptoms related to urinary tract obstruction. Serum PSA elevations have been reported (Barsky 1993, Sakamoto 1991), and this probably results from coexisting usual glandular and stromal hyperplasia. Most cases have been diagnosed in TURP chips, consistent with a transition zone predilection for sclerosing adenosis. Other specimen types with sclerosing adenosis include simple prostatectomy and radical cystoprostatectomy. The incidence of sclerosing adenosis in these tissue specimens is 2% (Grignon 1992, Sakamoto 1991). Sclerosing adenosis is rarely seen in needle core biopsies (Jones 1991).

■ **t8.9 Sclerosing Adenosis: Diagnostic Attributes**

- Well-circumscribed solitary or multiple nodules, 1-11 mm, in transition zone (usually in TURP chips)
- Crowded small acini in cellular spindle cell stroma
- Acini rounded to oval to compressed
- Epithelial cords, small nests, and single cells also seen
- Double cell layer present in some glands
- Myoepithelial cells present in basal cell and spindle cell populations (proof of this requires immunohistochemical staining)

Histologically, sclerosing adenosis is a circumscribed small nodule, usually about 4 mm in maximal dimension, with a size range of 1.5 to 11 mm (Grignon 1992). The nodules can be solitary or multifocal **t8.9**. At scanning magnification, there is a high density of small glands **i8.24, i8.25**. Closer inspection discloses an admixture of a small gland proliferation and cellular spindle cell growth **i8.26**. The small acini are crowded and irregular in shape with rounded, oval, and uniform to branching and compressed profiles seen. Compression of glandular lamina can lead to the appearance of cords, small clusters of epithelial cells, and single epithelial cells. In a minority of cases, cystically dilated glands can be found. A double cell layer made up of luminal and basal cells can be found in some of

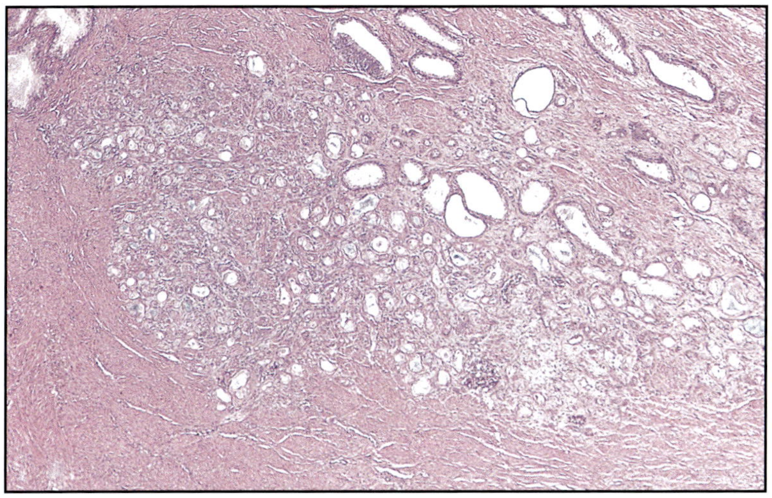

■ **i8.24** *Sclerosing adenosis with a well-delimited, compact arrangement of small acini, a few of which contain intraluminal wispy blue mucin.*

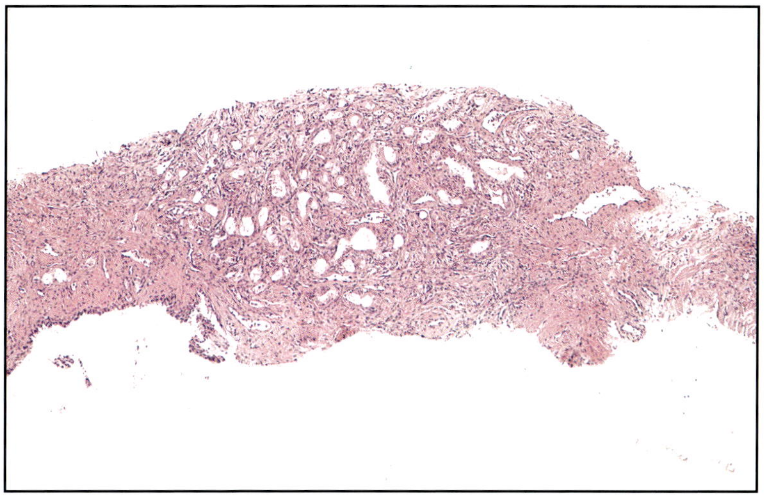

■ **i8.25** *Sclerosing adenosis in prostate needle biopsy tissue: Nodule of acini embedded within a spindle cell background.*

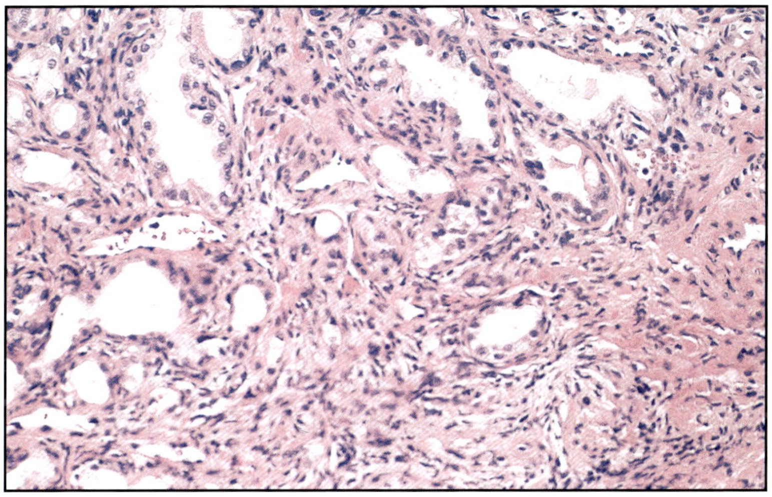

■ **i8.26** *Sclerosing adenosis in prostate needle biopsy tissue: Higher magnification of* **i8.25** *showing crowded small acini, with some being atrophic.*

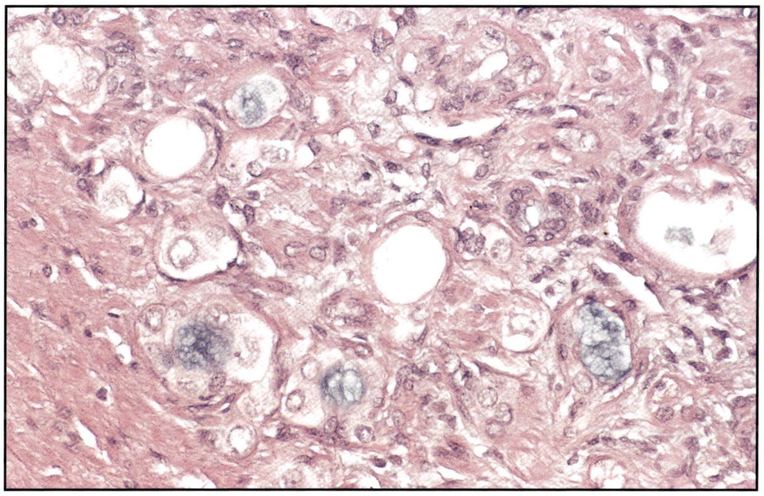

■ **i8.27** *Sclerosing adenosis with intraluminal blue mucin.*

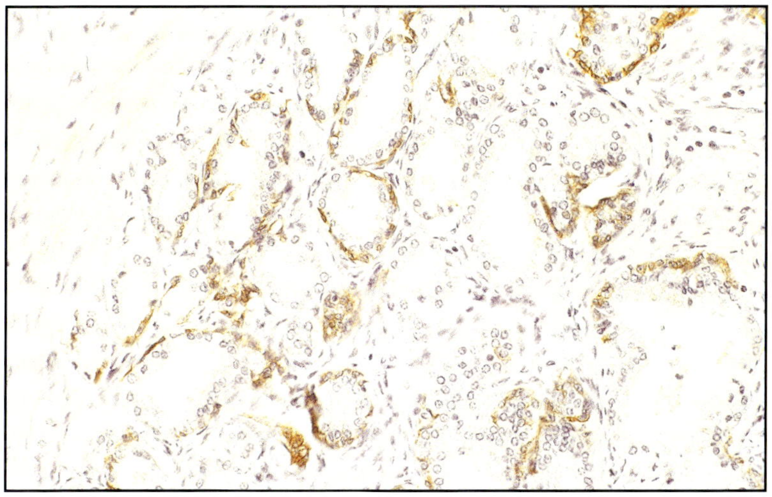

■ **i8.28** *Basal cells in sclerosing adenosis marked by a 34βE12 immunostain. These cells also bound antibodies reactive against smooth muscle actin.*

the acini, but in other glands the basal cell layer is not visualized (on H&E-stained sections) because of glandular distortion and flattening of luminal cells. The cytoplasm of the luminal cells is cuboidal to scanty and amphophilic to vacuolated. The vacuolated cytoplasm can occasionally impart a signet-ring cell image (Jones 1991). The luminal cell nuclei are round to oval and can exhibit a slight degree of atypia, but enlarged, prominent nucleoli can be detected only in a minority of cases (Jones 1991). Mitotic figures are rare to absent. The gland lumina often are empty but can contain eosinophilic or basophilic secretions; intraluminal wispy blue mucin can be present **i8.27**. Intraluminal crystalloids have been found in 16% of cases (Grignon 1992, Jones 1991) and intraluminal corpora amylacea are uncommon. The glands of sclerosing adenosis are surrounded by a thick eosinophilic membranous structure in a majority of cases (Grignon 1992). The adjacent stroma is highly cellular and is composed of spindled cells within a collagenous or myxoid, lightly basophilic matrix (Jones 1991). The spindled cells lack atypia and mitoses. Occasional lymphocytes and plasma cells can be noted within the stroma (Jones 1991).

Special studies play an important confirmatory role in establishing a definitive diagnosis of sclerosing adenosis. Specifically, an immunohistochemical marker panel is of great value in defining the presence of myoepithelial cells that mark with antibodies reactive with muscle-specific actin, S-100 protein, and high-molecular-weight cytokeratin (using antibody 34βE12) **i8.28; t8.10**. These myoepithelial cells, which are required for the diagnosis of prostatic sclerosing adenosis, are found within the basal cell lining layer of the glands and

t8.10 Sclerosing Adenosis: Immunophenotype

Basal and stromal cells:	MSA +
	S-100 +
	High molecular weight cytokeratin (34βE12) +
	Pan-cytokeratin (AE1/AE3) +
	Vimentin +
	PSA –
	PSAP –
Luminal Cells:	MSA –
	S-100 –
	34βE12 –
	AE1/AE3 +
	Vimentin +
	PSA +
	PSAP +
	CEA: focal +
	EMA: focal +

MSA = muscle-specific antigen; PSA = prostate-specific antigen; PSAP = prostatic specific acid phosphatase; CEA = carcinoembryonic antigen; EMA = epithelial membrane antigen

also in the spindle cell population of the stroma (Grignon 1992, Jones 1991). Some glandular basal cells do not show myoepithelial differentiation and mark only with the 34βE12 immunostain (Grignon 1992).

Additional special studies, including histochemical stains and ultrastructural examinations, are not required for the diagnosis but have provided additional information about the nature of sclerosing adenosis of the prostate. The glands of sclerosing adenosis are positive for intraluminal neutral mucin, using periodic acid-Schiff with diastase and mucicarmine, and for intraluminal acid mucin, using Alcian blue (Grignon 1992, Hulman 1989, Jones 1991, Sakamoto 1991, Young 1987). This acid mucin, which corresponds to the presence of wispy blue mucin, should not be taken as a sign of atypia. Masson histochemical stains have shown a lower amount of smooth muscle in sclerosing adenosis nodules than in adjacent prostatic stroma (Jones 1991). Electron microscopic characterization of basal cells in sclerosing adenosis shows abundant microfilaments with prominent dense bodies, which is in accord with myoepithelium (Grignon 1992).

The main differential diagnostic concern for sclerosing adenosis is adenocarcinoma. Mainly well-differentiated, Gleason score 2 to 4 adenocarcinomas of the prostate are under consideration because these are nodular growths. Yet these prostatic carcinoma glands are more uniformly rounded and do not reside in a densely cellular spindled stroma. Intermediate-grade carcinomas invading into stromal hyperplasia in BPH could also be confused with sclerosing adenosis if the infiltrative carcinoma surrounding the BPH or stromal nodule is not appreciated. Adenocarcinoma is readily excluded if one detects basal cells and myoepithelial cells in the lesional glands. Also, the nuclear atypia in sclerosing adenosis generally is mild compared with the significant nucleomegaly and nucleolomegaly seen in prostatic adenocarcinoma. Finally, the other form of adenosis in the prostate, usual adenosis or AAH, is also a differential diagnostic concern, but it lacks myoepithelial cells and the cellular spindled stroma of sclerosing adenosis.

Sclerosing adenosis of the prostate is currently viewed as a metaplastic proliferation arising from basal cells (Grignon 1992). It has no known malignant potential. No physical continuity between PIN or carcinoma and sclerosing adenosis has been demonstrated. Follow-up of patients with sclerosing adenosis has revealed a benign course.

References

Amin MB, Ro JY, Ayala AG. Putative precursor lesions of prostatic adenocarcinoma: fact or fiction. *Mod Pathol* 6:476-483, 1993.

Andrews GS. Latent carcinoma of the prostate. *J Clin Pathol* 2:197-208, 1949.

Baron E, Angrist A. Incidence of occult adenocarcinoma of the prostate after fifty years of age. *Arch Pathol* 32:787-793, 1941.

Barsky SH, Sassoon A. Sclerosing adenosis of the prostate as a cause of very high PSA levels. *J Urol Pathol* 1:313-331, 1993.

Bostwick DG, Srigley J, Grignon D, et al. Atypical adenomatous hyperplasia of the prostate: morphologic criteria for its distinction from well-differentiated carcinoma. *Hum Pathol* 24:819-832, 1993.

Bostwick DG, Qian J. Atypical adenomatous hyperplasia of the prostate. Relationship with carcinoma in 217 whole-mount radical prostatectomies. *Am J Surg Pathol* 19:506-518, 1995.

Bostwick DG. Prospective origins of prostate carcinoma. Prostatic intraepithelial neoplasia and atypical adenomatous hyperplasia. *Cancer* 78:330-336, 1996.

Brawn PN. Adenosis of the prostate: a dysplastic lesion that can be confused with prostate adenocarcinoma. *Cancer* 49:826-833, 1982.

Brawn PN, Speights VO, Contin JU, et al. Atypical hyperplasia in prostates of 20 to 40 year-old men. *J Clin Pathol* 42:383-386, 1989.

Brawn PN, Johnson EH, Speights VO, et al. Long-term survival of stage A carcinoma, atypical hyperplasia/adenosis and BPH. *Br J Cancer* 69:1098-1101, 1994.

Chastonay P, Hurlimannn J, Gardiol D. Biological tissue markers in benign and malignant disease of the human prostate. *Virchows Arch* A 410:221-229, 1986.

Chen KTK, Schiff JJ. Adenomatoid prostatic tumor. *Urology* 21:88-89, 1983.

Cheng L, Shan A, Cheville JC, et al. Atypical adenomatous hyperplasia of the prostate: a premalignant lesion? *Cancer Res* 58:389-391, 1998.

Cheville JC, Reznicek MJ, Bostwick DG. The focus of "atypical glands, suspicious for malignancy" in prostatic needle biopsy specimens. Incidence, histologic features, and clinical follow-up of cases diagnosed in a community practice. *Am J Clin Pathol* 108:633-640, 1997.

Collina G, Botticelli AR, Martinelli AM, et al. Sclerosing adenosis of the prostate. Report of three cases with electron microscopy and immunohistochemical study. *Histopathology* 20:505-510, 1992.

Devaraj LT, Bostwick DG. Atypical basal cell hyperplasia of the prostate. Immunophenotypic profile and proposed classification of basal cell proliferations. *Am J Surg Pathol* 17:645-659, 1993.

Doll JA, Zhu X, Furman J, et al. Genetic analysis of prostatic atypical adenomatous hyperplasia (adenosis). *Am J Pathol* 155:967-971,1999.

Epstein JI, Fynheer J. Acid mucin in the prostate: can it differentiate adenosis from adenocarcinoma? *Hum Pathol* 23:1321-1325, 1992A.

Epstein JI, Armas OA. Atypical basal cell hyperplasia of the prostate. *Am J Surg Pathol* 16:1205-1214, 1992B.

Epstein JI. Adenosis (atypical adenomatous hyperplasia): histopathology and relationship to carcinoma. *Pathol Res Pract* 191:888-898, 1995.

Furman J, Zhu X, Kaleem Z, et al. Chromosome 8p22 allelic loss in atypical adenomatous hyperplasia (adenosis) and carcinoma in the prostate [abstract]. *Mod Pathol* 9:73A, 1996.

Garnett JE, Oyasu R. Urologic evaluation of atypical prostatic hyperplasia. *Urology* 34(suppl):66-69, 1989.

Gaudin PB, Epstein JI. Adenosis of the prostate. Histologic features in transurethral resection specimens. *Am J Surg Pathol* 18:863-870, 1994.

Gaudin PB, Epstein JI. Adenosis of the prostate. Histologic features in needle biopsy specimens. *Am J Surg Pathol* 19:737-747, 1995.

Gleason DF. Atypical hyperplasia, benign hyperplasia, and well-differentiated adenocarcinoma of the prostate. *Am J Surg Pathol* 9(suppl):53-67, 1985.

Goldstein NS, Qian J, Bostwick DG. Mucin expression in atypical adenomatous hyperplasia of the prostate. *Hum Pathol* 26:887-891, 1995.

Grignon DJ, Ro JY, Srigley JR, et al. Sclerosing adenosis of the prostate. A lesion showing myoepithelial differentiation. *Am J Surg Pathol* 16:383-391, 1992.

Grignon DJ, Sakr WA. Atypical adenomatous hyperplasia of the prostate: a critical review. *Eur Urol* 30:206-211, 1996.

Harbitz TB, Haugen OA. Histology of the prostate in elderly men. A study in an autopsy series. *Acta Pathol Scand* A 80:756-768, 1972.

Harper ME, Glynne-Jones E, Goddard L, et al. Expression of androgen receptor and growth factors in premalignant lesions of the prostate. *J Pathol* 186:169-177, 1998.

Häussler O, Epstein JI, Amin MB, et al Cell proliferation, apoptosis, oncogene and tumor suppressor gene status in adenosis with comparison to benign prostatic hyperplasia, prostatic intraepithelial neoplasia, and cancer. *Hum Pathol* 30:1077-1086, 1999.

Helpap B. The biological significance of atypical hyperplasia of the prostate. *Virchows Arch* 387:307-317, 1980.

Helpap B, Riede C. Nucleolar and AgNOR-analysis of prostatic intraepithelial neoplasia (PIN), atypical adenomatous hyperplasia (AAH) and prostatic carcinoma. *Pathol Res Pract* 191:381-390, 1995.

Helpap B. Differential diagnosis of glandular proliferations in the prostate. A conventional and immunohistochemical approach. *Virchows Arch* 433:397-405, 1998.

Hulman G. "Pseudoadenomatoid" tumour of prostate. *Histopathology* 14:317-319, 1989.

Humphrey PA, Zhu X, Crouch EC, et al. Mass-formative atypical adenomatous hyperplasia of prostate. *J Urol Pathol* 9:73-81, 1998A.

Humphrey PA, Kaleem Z, Swanson PE, et al. Pseudohyperplastic prostatic adenocarcinoma. *Am J Surg Pathol* 22:1239-1246, 1998B.

Jones EC, Clement PB, Young RH. Sclerosing adenosis of the prostate gland. A clinicopathologic and immunohistochemical study of 11 cases. *Am J Surg Pathol* 15:1171-1180, 1991.

Jones EC, Young RH. The differential diagnosis of prostatic carcinoma. Its distinction from premalignant and pseudocarcinomatous lesions of the prostate gland. *Am J Clin Pathol* 101:48-64, 1994.

Kastendieck H. Correlations between atypical primary hyperplasia and carcinoma of the prostate. *Pathol Res Pract* 169:366-387, 1980.

Kastendieck H, Helpap B. Prostatic "dysplasia/atypical hyperplasia." Terminology, histopathology, pathobiology, and significance. *Urology* 34(suppl):28-42, 1989.

Kovi J. Microscopic differential diagnosis of small acinar adenocarcinoma of prostate. In: Sommers SC, Rosen PP, Fechner RE, eds. *Pathology Annual 20.* Part 1. Norwalk, CT: Appleton-Century-Crofts; 157-196, 1985.

Kovi J, Mostofi FK, Heshmat MY, et al. Large acinar atypical hyperplasia and carcinoma of the prostate. *Cancer* 61:555-561, 1988.

Kovi J, Mostofi FK. Atypical hyperplasia of prostate. *Urology* 34(suppl):23-27, 1989.

Kramer CE, Epstein JI. Nucleoli in low-grade prostate adenocarcinoma and adenosis. *Hum Pathol* 24:618-623, 1993.

Levi AW, Epstein JI. Pseudohyperplastic prostatic adenocarcinoma on needle biopsy and simple prostatectomy. *Am J Surg Pathol* 24:1039-1046, 2000.

Lopez-Beltran A, Pacelli A, Qian J, et al. Atypical adenomatous hyperplasia of the prostate: immunophenotype, genotype and DNA ploidy analysis [abstract]. *Mod Pathol* 9:77A, 1996.

Lopez-Beltran A, Artacho-Perula E, Luque-Barona RJ, et al. Nuclear volume estimates in prostatic atypical adenomatous hyperplasia. *Anal Quant Cytol Histol* 22:438-444, 2000.

Luna-More S, Florez P, Ayala A, et al. Neutral and acid mucins and eosinophil and argyrophil crystalloids in carcinoma and atypical adenomatous hyperplasia of the prostate. *Pathol Res Pract* 193:291-298, 1997.

Mai KT, Isotalo PA, Green J, et al. Incidental prostatic adenocarcinomas and putative premalignant lesions in TURP specimens collected before and after introduction of prostate specific antigen screening. *Arch Pathol Lab Med* 124:1454-1456, 2000.

McNeal JE. Morphogenesis of prostate carcinoma. *Cancer* 18:1659-1666, 1965.

Meister P. Sclerosing adenosis of the prostate. Carcinoma simulation [in German]. *Pathologe* 17:157-162, 1996.

Moore RA. Benign hypertrophy of the prostate. A morphological study. *J Urol* 50:680-710, 1943.

Mostofi FK, Price EB. Tumors of the male genital system. *Atlas of Tumor Pathology,* Fascicle 8. Washington, DC: Armed Forces Institute of Pathology, 1973.

Muezzinoglu B, Kattan M, Wheeler TM. Atypical adenomatous hyperplasia in radical prostatectomy and cystoprostatectomy specimens [abstract]. *Mod Pathol* 10:83A, 1997.

Parkinson MC. Pre-neoplastic lesions of the prostate. *Histopathology* 27:301-311, 1995.

Qian J, Jenkins RB, Bostwick DG. Chromosomal anomalies in atypical adenomatous hyperplasia and carcinoma of the prostate using fluorescence in situ hybridization. *Urology* 46:837-842, 1995.

Redonodo Martinez E, Lopez AR, de la Vega Perez M, et al. Sclerosing adenosis of the prostate [in Spanish]. *Arch Esp Urol* 50:935-940, 1997.

Renedo PE, Poy E, Wojno KJ. Clinical significance and distinction of adenosis of low grade adenocarcinoma of the prostate on TURP [abstract]. *Mod Pathol* 8:82A, 1995.

Reyes AO, Humphrey PA. Diagnostic effect of complete histologic sampling of prostate needle biopsy specimens. *Am J Clin Pathol* 109:416-422, 1998.

Ronnett BM, Epstein JI. A case showing sclerosing adenosis and an unusual form of basal cell hyperplasia of the prostate. *Am J Surg Pathol* 13:866-872, 1989.

Sakamoto N, Tsuneyoshi M, Enjoji M. Sclerosing adenosis of the prostate. Histopathologic and immunohistochemical analysis. *Am J Surg Pathol* 15:660-667, 1991.

Sakr WA, Grignon DJ. Prostatic intraepithelial neoplasia and atypical adenomatous hyperplasia. Relationship to pathologic parameters, volume and spatial distribution of carcinoma of the prostate. *Anal Quant Cytol Histol* 20:417-423, 1998.

Shamsuddin AM, Beasly WM. Expression of the tumor marker D-galactose-β-[1→3]-*N*-acetyl-D-galactosamine by premalignant and malignant prostate. *Arch Pathol Lab Med* 118:48-51, 1994.

Skjorten F, Berner A, Harvei S, et al. Prostatic intraepithelial neoplasia in surgical resections: relationship to coexistent adenocarcinoma and atypical adenomatous hyperplasia of the prostate. *Cancer* 79:1172-1179, 1997.

Srigley J, Toth P, Hartwick RWJ. Atypical histological patterns in cases of benign prostatic hyperplasia [abstract]. *Lab Invest* 60:90A, 1984.

Srigley J, King S, Van Nostrand AWP, Robinette M. The "preneoplastic" prostate: a giant section whole organ study of 72 radical prostatectomies [abstract]. *Lab Invest* 54:61A, 1986.

Tannenbaum M. Histopathology of the prostate gland. In: Tannenbaum M, ed. *Urologic Pathology: The Prostate.* Philadelphia: Lee & Febiger; 303-397, 1977.

Troncoso P, Ordonez NG, Ayala AG. Atypical adenomatous hyperplasia in radical prostatectomy and cystoprostatectomy specimens [abstract]. *Mod Pathol* 8:4A, 1995.

Wernert N, Dhom G. Morphologie und differential-diagnose der cribriformen prostatahyperplasie. *Pathologe* 5:27-32, 1984.

Wojno KJ, Epstein JI. The utility of basal cell-specific anti-cytokeratin antibody (34βE12) in the diagnosis of prostate. A review of 228 cases. *Am J Surg Pathol* 19:251-260, 1995.

Yang XJ, McEntee M, Epstein JI. Distinction of basaloid carcinoma of the prostate from benign basal cell lesions by using immunohistochemistry for bcl-2 and Ki-67. *Hum Pathol* 29:1447-1450, 1998.

Yang XJ, Wu CL, Woda BA, et al. Expression of α-methylacyl-CoA racemase (P504S) in atypical adenomatous hyperplasia of the prostate. *Am J Surg Pathol* 26:921-925, 2002.

Young RH, Clement PB. Sclerosing adenosis of the prostate. *Arch Pathol Lab Med* 111:363-366, 1987.

Unusual Benign Conditions

[9.1] Pigment Disorders: Melanosis, Blue Nevus, and Ochronosis **167**
[9.2] Amyloid in the Prostate **169**
[9.3] Collagenous Spherulosis **169**
[9.4] Postoperative Spindle Cell Nodule **170**
[9.5] Endometriosis **171**
[9.6] Extramedullary Hematopoiesis **171**
[9.7] Teratoma **171**
[9.8] Cowper's Glands **172**

CHAPTER 9

Assembled in this chapter is a potpourri of various unusual, benign conditions that affect the prostate gland. The types of maladies range from pigment disorders (melanosis, blue nevus, and ochronosis) to deposits of amyloid to a procedural-related, reactive, spindle cell proliferation (postoperative spindle cell nodule) to endometriosis, extramedullary hematopoiesis, and teratoma. Finally, a normal extraprostatic anatomic structure, Cowper's glands, is discussed because they can be misinterpreted as prostatic adenocarcinoma.

[9.1] Pigment Disorders: Melanosis, Blue Nevus, and Ochronosis

Melanin presence in prostatic stromal melanocytes has been called a blue nevus, and the apparent appearance of melanin in glandular epithelium with or without associated stromal melanocytes has been called melanosis (Block 1972, Botticelli 1989, Gardner 1971, Guillan 1970, Jao 1971, Kovi 1978, Rios 1976, Scarani 1972) **t9.1**. However, the existence of true melanosis with intraepithelial melanin has been questioned (Amin 1996, Brennick 1994), and it has been suggested that lipofuscin, which is common in prostatic epithelium (Brennick 1994, Goldman 1968, Leung 1995, Seman 1982), could be confused with melanin (Amin 1996, Azzopardi 1971, Brennick 1994). The source of this confusion in the past was the interpretation of a positive Lillie's ferrous iron (Azzopardi 1971) and Fontana-Masson stains as being indicative of melanin, yet these stains are not specific for melanin (Amin 1996, Azzopardi 1971, Brennick 1994, Mower 1994), and lipofuscin pigment is also positive for the Fontana-Masson stain (Amin 1996, Brennick 1994). Lipofuscin can be distinguished from melanin by using a Luxol fast blue histochemical stain, which stains lipofuscin blue but does not stain melanin, and melanocytic cellular differentiation in pigmented cells can be substantiated by a positive S-100 immunostain and by electron microscopic detection of premelanosomes and melanosomes. Also, lipofuscin stains positively with periodic acid-Schiff with diastase, Congo red, and oil red O and exhibits a yellow autofluorescence (Brennick 1994). (Schmorl's technique has been used to stain for lipofuscin [Ro 1988] but also stains melanin [Mower 1994]). A requirement for immunohistochemical or ultrastructural demonstration of melanocytic features in pigmented prostatic epithelium results in identification of only a few reported cases of prostatic melanosis in the literature **t9.2**. A single case of melanin pigmentation

■ t9.1 Melanin in the Prostate

Blue nevus:	Melanin in spindled stromal cells
Melanosis:	Defined in the past as melanin in epithelial cells with or without stromal cell melanin but melanin-like pigment in prostatic epithelium usually represents lipofuscin. True melanosis = Extremely rare cases (n=2) that have melanosomes in the pigmented epithelium.
Melanoma:	Rare

■ t9.2 Melanosis and Blue Nevus of the Prostate

Study	No. of Patients	Age	Tissue Specimen	Morphologic Findings	Diagnosis
Aguilar 1982	1	64	TURP	Gross: Black chips Micro: Dark brown-black pigment in spindled stromal cells, and benign and malignant epithelium. EM: Melanosomes	Melanosis
Ro 1988	1	75	TURP	Gross: Black chips Micro: Brown or black pigment in stromal and epithelial cells. EM: Melanosomes	Melanosis
Nigogosyan 1963	1	50	Autopsy	Gross: 2cm brown-black areas Micro: Ovoid or elongated pigmented cells.	Blue nevus
Simard 1964	1	70	Simple prostatectomy	Stromal pigmented cells	Blue nevus
Jao 1971	1	76	Simple prostatectomy	Gross: Dark brown streaks Micro: Single cells and clumps of pigmented stellate to spindle cells.	Blue nevus
Block 1972	3	66,69,70	Not available	Fusiform, dendritic, pigmented cells in BPH areas	Blue nevus
Langely 1974	6	Not available	TURP or simple prostatectomy	Stromal pigmented bipolar and ovoid cells	Blue nevus
Kovi 1977	1	65	TURP	Dendritic stromal melanocytes	Blue nevus
Ro 1988	2	68,76	TURP	Multiple chips with stromal pigmented, S-100+ cells	Blue nevus
Botticelli 1989	1	66	Simple prostatectomy	Gross: Irregular, brown streaks Micro: Pigmented spindle cells in concentric arrangements around glands and vessels	Blue nevus
Lew 1991	1	80	Simple prostatectomy	Gross: Black areas 0.1cm to 1cm Micro: Pigmented, S-100+ stromal cells	Blue nevus
Martinez 1992	2	69,81	Simple prostatectomy	Gross: Deep brown to black areas Micro: Pigmented, spindle cells with dendritic processes	Blue nevus
This book 2003	1	70	Needle biopsy	Pigmented stromal spindle cells	Blue nevus

■ **t9.3 Prostatic Blue Nevus: Essential Features**

Incidental finding in BPH nodules (usually)
Gross: Brown to black streaks or areas
Micro: Pigmented, stromal, spindle cells with elongated cytoplasmic processes

in urothelium of the prostatic urethra has also been published (Alroy 1986). About 22 cases of prostatic blue nevus have been reported **t9.3**.

Prostatic melanosis, with an ultrastructural finding of melanosomes, is extraordinarily rare, with 2 reported cases (Aguilar 1982, Ro 1988) **t9.2**. In both cases the prostatic chips, resected for benign prostatic hyperplasia (BPH) symptoms, were of a striking black color. Microscopically, finely granular brown to black pigment was present in the cytoplasm of stromal cells and in benign and malignant epithelial cells. The stromal cells were rounded, polygonal, or spindled, with dendritic cytoplasmic processes (Ro 1988). Extracellular stromal dispersion of the pigment was noted in 1 case (Ro 1988). The pigmented stromal cells but not pigmented epithelial cells marked with S-100 antibodies in an immunohistochemical reaction (Ro 1988). By electron microscopy, the stromal cells contained melanosomes of different maturation stages, whereas only mature stage IV melanosomes were seen in the pigmented epithelium (Aguilar 1982, Ro 1988). These immunohistochemical and ultrastructural findings have prompted the proposal that the melanin was transferred to the glandular epithelium from stromal melanocytes. The differential diagnosis of prostatic melanosis includes lipofuscin pigmentation of prostatic epithelium, blue nevus, and melanoma. When pigment is encountered in prostatic epithelium, it is far more likely to be lipofuscin than melanin. A Luxol fast blue stain is a straightforward method to distinguish them. Also, melanin in prostatic epithelium typically is seen adjacent to stromal cells with melanin. Blue nevus describes the presence of stromal melanocytes and can coexist with prostatic melanosis; some have used the terms interchangeably. The black macroscopic appearance of prostatic tissue with melanosis raises the possibility of malignant melanoma involving the prostate (Abeshouse 1958, Bamberger 1990, Berry 1953, Das Gupta 1965, Grignon 1989, Hubler 1980, Stein 1984, Wang 1995). Malignant melanoma of the prostate usually represents metastatic spread, and clinical history is helpful here.

Blue nevus of the prostate, which has also been called pigmented melanocytosis (Têtu 1988) and prostatic pigmentary nevohyperplasia (Simard 1964), is similar to the more common cutaneous blue nevus in being composed of spindled melanin-laden cells in stroma (Block 1972, Furusato 1989, Jao 1971, Kovi 1978, Langley 1974, Lew 1991, Martinez Marinez 1992, Nigogosyan 1963, Ro 1988, Scarani 1972, Simard 1964). Prostatic blue nevus is an incidental histologic finding, usually seen in patients who underwent transurethral or simple prostatectomy for BPH symptoms. The incidence is 0.03% (Ro 1988) to 4% (Langley 1974) of prostatic tissue samples. The average age at detection is 66 (with a range of 50 to 80 years) **t9.2**. Grossly, brown to black streaks or brown to black areas 0.1cm to 2cm in diameter can be appreciated in some cases. Microscopically, finely granular brown or black pigment can be found in stromal cells and sometimes in the extracellular matrix. In transurethral resection chips, the pigment often is noted in multiple chips and is detected in stromal hyperplasia in BPH nodules. We have seen blue nevus in needle biopsy of prostate **t9.2**. The stromal cells containing the pigment often are haphazardly dispersed **i9.1**, with single cells and clumps of cells; a pattern of concentric arrangement around glands and vessels has also been described (Têtu 1988). The pigment-laden cells are spindled, with bipolar, long, dendritic, cytoplasmic processes **i9.1**, but can also be round, ovoid, or polygonal. The cytoplasmic pigmentation can be so intense as to obscure nuclear detail **i9.2**.

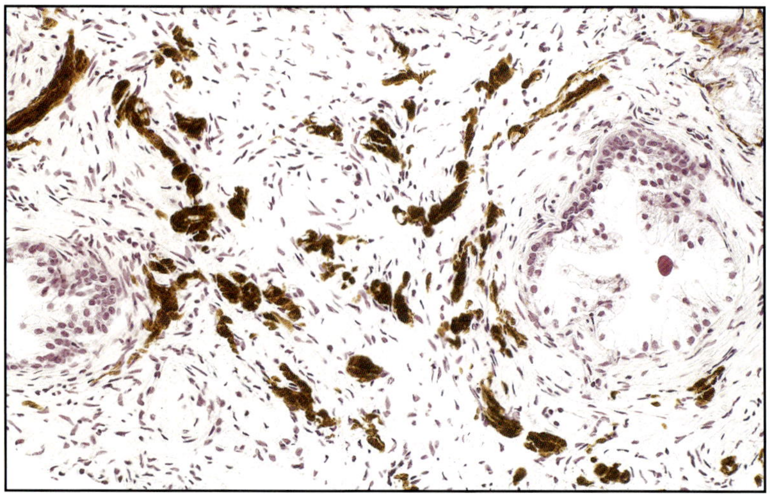

■ **i9.1** *Blue nevus of prostate is typified by scattered, heavily pigmented, single cells or clumps of cells in the stroma. Spindled shapes predominate.*

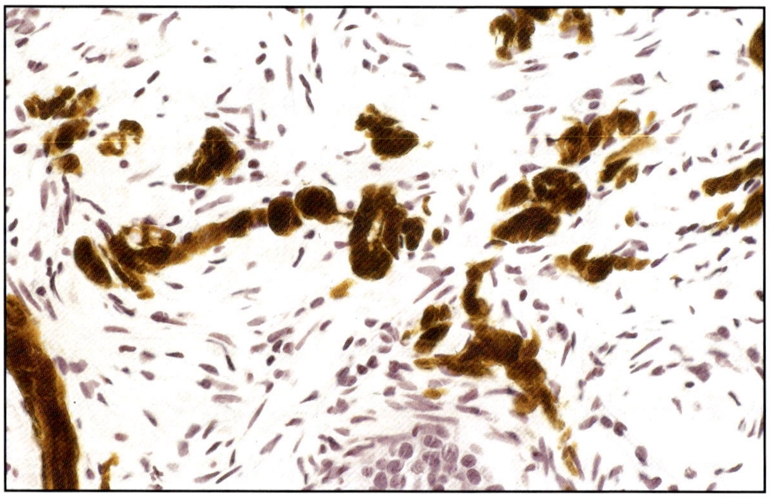

■ **i9.2** *Blue nevus: Nuclear features can be difficult to visualize due to the amount of brown, granular, cytoplasmic melanin.*

Special studies have documented melanin and melanocytic differentiation in prostatic blue nevus cells. Histochemically, the pigment stains black with Fontana-Masson and disappears after bleaching with potassium permanganate. Iron and lipofuscin (Luxol fast blue) stains are negative. Immunohistochemical staining of the pigmented cells can be accomplished using S-100, whereas prostate-specific antigen (PSA), prostate-specific acid phosphatase (PSAP), carcinoembryonic antigen (CEA), and lysozyme immunostains are negative (Lew 1991, Martinez Marinez 1992, Ro 1988, Têtu 1988). HMB-45 has also been negative in two cases (Martinez Marinez 1992). Ultrastructurally, melanosomes of variable maturation stages have been visualized in the pigmented cells in a number of cases (Jao 1971, Lew 1991, Martinez Marinez 1992, Ro 1988, Têtu 1988).

The main entities in the differential diagnosis with prostatic blue nevus include hemosiderin-laden stromal macrophages and malignant melanoma. Iron in the prostate in the form of

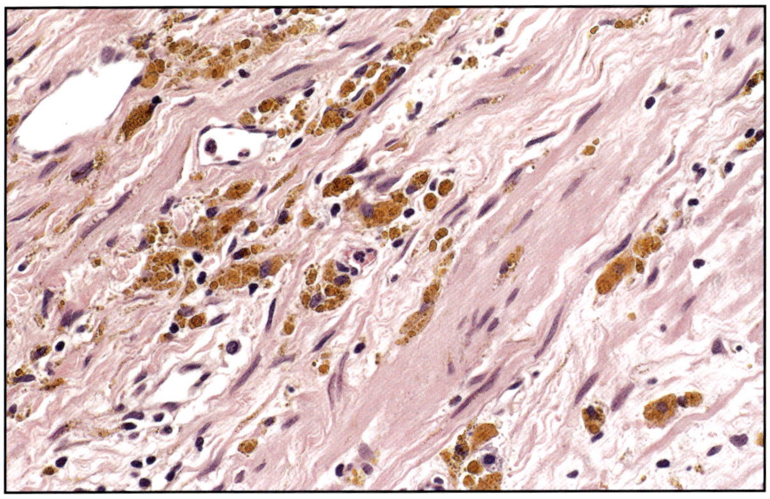

■ **i9.3** *Hemosiderin in the prostate after biopsy.*

hemosiderin results from hemorrhage and usually is related to a previous procedure, such as biopsy or transurethral resection. Iron overload as in hemochromatosis has not been reported. Hemosiderin is characterized by clumps of golden yellow pigment **i9.3**, whereas melanin is brown-black and more uniformly and finely granular. An iron stain will rule in hemosiderin. Malignant melanoma is rare in the prostate and exhibits nuclear atypia and mitotic figures, unlike prostatic blue nevus. Usually there is a clinical history of a cutaneous melanoma with widespread metastases.

The presence of melanocytes in the stroma of the adult prostate probably reflects migration of neural crest cells to the prostate at an early stage in embryogenesis (Aguilar 1982, Ro 1988). Prostatic blue nevus is not a known risk factor for the development of malignancy, including malignant melanoma.

There is a single case report of another pigmentary disorder, ochronosis, involving the prostate (Suarez 1983). Ochronosis is the clinical sequela of alkaptonuria, a rare hereditary metabolic disease (Suarez 1983). Clinically, the patient had a rock-hard prostate by digital rectal examination and needle biopsy revealed dark brown melanin-like pigment, representing homogentisic acid, in corpora amylacea and prostatic epithelium.

[9.2] Amyloid in the Prostate

Amyloid can be found in the prostate as an incidental finding in corpora amylacea, stroma, and blood vessels (Coyne 1993, Cross 1992, Dahlin 1949, Edit 1989, Lupovitch 1972, McDonald 1956, Tripathi 1969, Wilson 1973) **t9.4**. Most corpora amylacea in the prostate stain for amyloid because they are Congo red positive, with apple-green birefringence obtained by crossed polarizing filters (Cross 1992, Lupovitch 1972). The amyloid protein in prostatic corpora amylacea is β2 microglobulin, as shown by immunohistochemical staining (Cross 1992). In primary prostatic amyloidosis both stromal and blood vessel wall involvement have been documented (Dahlin 1949, Lupovitch 1972, McDonald 1956, Wilson 1973). The incidence in consecutive unselected cases has varied from 0.6% (1/167 cases) (McDonald 1956) to 10% (8/75) of patients (Wilson 1973). The reason for this wide range is not clear. In our experience, the incidence is closer to the former, lower figure.

■ **t9.4 Amyloid in the Prostate**

In corpora amylacea, stroma, small blood vessels
Most corpora Congo red-positive
1°: 1 to 10% of unselected patients have prostatic amyloid
2°: 38% of multiple myeloma patients have prostatic amyloid
Amount and location in stroma variable
Differentiate from collagen

We stained 50 radical prostatectomy specimens with Congo red and found amyloid in 1 case, in the wall of a sclerotic duct. The average age of patients with prostatic amyloidosis ranges from 66 (Wilson 1973) to 86 (Lupovitch 1972). Secondary, incidental prostatic amyloidosis has been reported in patients with multiple myeloma (Coyne 1993, Wilson 1973), with an incidence of 38% (Wilson 1973). No patient with secondary amyloidosis has been initially diagnosed with amyloidosis based on finding amyloid in the prostate. No gross abnormalities referable to prostatic amyloidosis have been communicated. Microscopically, prostatic stromal amyloid has been portrayed as stromal areas of irregular nodules of amorphous, highly eosinophilic material (McDonald 1956). The amount of amyloid deposition is variable (Dahlin 1949). The location within the stroma is also variable and can be periglandular (and adjacent to either normal or neoplastic glands) or distant from glandular epithelium (Lupovitch 1972, Wilson 1973). Congo red has been the most commonly used special technique in the characterization of prostatic amyloid; crystal violet has also been used. Little is known of the type of amyloid deposited in prostatic stromal and vascular amyloidosis because immunohistochemical characterization has not been performed (except in 1 case) (Coyne 1993). In contrast, seminal vesicle amyloidosis, which is present in about 10% to 15% of patients (Coyne 1993, Pitkänen 1983) has been much better characterized (Cornwell 1992, Coyne 1993, Pitkänen 1983, Unger 1997). It is not known whether prostatic amyloidosis is related to seminal vesicle amyloidosis. The pathogenetic basis for the primary accumulation of amyloid in the prostate is also unknown.

Prostatic amyloidosis should not be confused with prostatic stromal collagen, including collagenous micronodules in prostatic carcinoma (Bostwick 1995). When injected periurethrally to treat incontinence, collagen could also be sampled by prostate or prostatic fossa (Bejarano 1996) needle biopsy and is also in the differential of urethral (Stillwell 1989) and prostatic amyloidosis. (Note: This injected collagen can form a mass that can clinically simulate malignancy [Bejarano 1996].) Blood vessel hyalinization should not be mistaken for prostatic vascular amyloidosis. A Congo red stain will resolve any questions about the nature of amorphous deposits in prostatic stroma or vessels. It has not been established whether identification of amyloid in prostatic tissue should prompt a search for systemic amyloidosis.

[9.3] Collagenous Spherulosis

A single case of BPH with intraductal spherules resembling collagenous spherulosis of the breast has been illustrated (Melamed 1998). Small corpora amylacea and collagenous micronodules can simulate this appearance.

■ **t9.5 Prostatic Postoperative Spindle Cell Nodule**

Rare (n = 7)
Discovered 1-3 months after transurethral resection
Most cases initially misdiagnosed as leiomyosarcoma
Microscopically
 Infiltrative fascicles of bland spindle cells with edematous and vascular stroma
 Mitotic rate often 5-10 per 10 high-power fields
Beware keratin immunoreactivity in spindle cells; this does not equate with epithelial differentiation in this context

[9.4] Postoperative Spindle Cell Nodule

Postoperative spindle cell nodule is a rare, pseudoneoplastic and pseudosarcomatous, benign reactive proliferation in the prostate that occurs in response to transurethral resection **t9.5** (Huang 1990, Proppe 1984). Only a handful of cases ($n = 7$) have been described. These men averaged 65 years of age (range 45 to 79), and most had undergone transurethral resection of the prostate for BPH symptoms. Two patients had undergone several transurethral resections of bladder tumors (Huang 1990). After a mean interval of 2 months (range 1 to 3 months), the patients returned, usually because of recurrent symptoms such as obstruction and hematuria. Cystoscopically, 3 lesions were described as an "unusual-appearing mass or heaped-up tumor" (Proppe 1984). In 4 other cases, the proliferation was an incidental histologic finding in repeat tissue samples. The repeat tissue sampling included needle biopsy for a palpable prostatic nodule in 1 case, repeat transurethral resection of prostate, and in 1 case, cystoprostatectomy for transitional cell carcinoma (Huang 1990). An initial microscopic diagnosis of leiomyosarcoma was rendered in the repeat tissue samples in 5 of the 7 cases. However, those spindle cell proliferations were reclassified as postoperative spindle cell nodule based on the microscopic features, the close temporal relationship with recent surgical instrumentation, and benign outcome (Proppe 1984).

Grossly, the only descriptions of prostatic postoperative spindle cell nodule are the aforementioned cystoscopic depictions. Microscopically, the lesions measured 5mm to 9mm in 1 series (Huang 1990). The are poorly delimited and can infiltrate surrounding tissue, with replacement and destruction of stroma (Huang 1990, Proppe 1984). Intersecting fascicles are formed by spindle cells with tapered ends **i9.4**. The background stroma is edematous, with little hyalinization and few inflammatory cells. The spindle cells are uniform, with a moderate amount of eosinophilic to amphophilic cytoplasm and nuclei lacking in pleomorphism **i9.5**. The mitotic rate can be strikingly high, with up to 25 mitoses per 10 high-power fields. However, no atypical mitosis should be found. By immunohistochemistry, vimentin and desmin stains were positive (Huang 1990).

The differential diagnosis of postoperative spindle cell nodule converges on spindle cell malignancies, especially sarcomas. Although diagnoses such as spindle cell sarcoma, malignant fibrous histiocytoma, and Kaposi's sarcoma have been made in cases of postoperative spindle cell nodule (Proppe 1984), leiomyosarcoma is the major concern. Shared features of postoperative spindle cell nodule and leiomyosarcoma include interlacing fascicles, plump spindle cells, and mitotic activity. However, distinction from moderately to poorly differentiated leiomyosarcoma usually is not a problem because nuclear atypia is appreciable in these cases, unlike postoperative spindle cell nodule (Young 1997). Prominent vascularity favors postoperative spindle cell nodule (Young 1997). Well-differentiated leiomyosarcoma can be difficult or impossible to distinguish histologically from postoperative spindle cell nodule, and a clinical history of recent transurethral resection often is a key arbitrating factor (Huang 1990, Young 1997). Sarcomatoid (spindle cell) carcinoma is also in the differential diagnosis, but these are cytologically atypical spindle cell proliferations, with or without heterologous elements. A malignant epithelial component should be specifically sought, although it may not be sampled in a small biopsy. An important diagnostic pitfall is that cytokeratin immunoreactivity can be seen in postoperative spindle cell nodule (Wick 1988), and this finding should not immediately prompt a diagnosis of an epithelial proliferation. Inflammatory myofibroblastic tumor (also known as pseudosarcomatous fibromyxoid tumor, inflammatory pseudotumor, pseudosarcoma, and nodular fasciitis), which is a spindle cell proliferation with a myxoid or vascular, compact spindle cell or hypocellular fibrous patterns (Coffin 1998), can also be confused with postoperative spindle cell nodule (Ro 1993), but these lesions are not related to previous surgery. Finally, BPH stromal nodules, especially those with

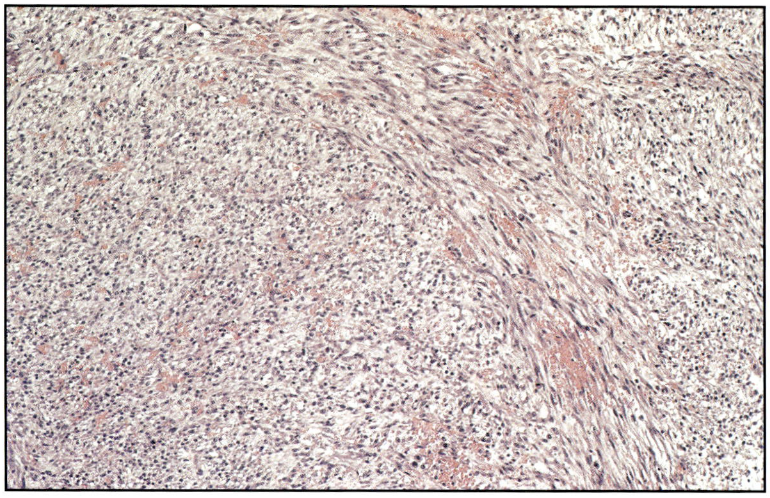

■ **i9.4** *Postoperative spindle cell nodule with fascicular growth of spindle cells.*

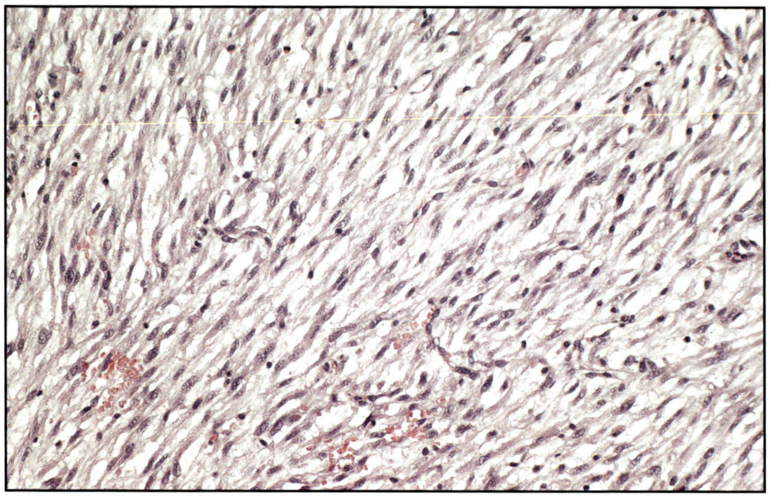

■ **i9.5** *Postoperative spindle cell nodule with bland spindle cells.*

myxoid stroma, are a possibility, but these stromal nodules lack infiltrative growth and the cellularity and mitotic activity of postoperative spindle cell nodules.

Postoperative spindle cell nodules appear to represent an exaggerated reparative response to surgical procedures. They are benign, although recurrences (which were cured by local reexcision) have been detected at other anatomic sites (Proppe 1984). Their clinicopathologic significance is in their mimicry of sarcoma, which led to unnecessary radical surgery (cystoprostatectomy) in several cases (Huang 1990, Proppe 1984).

[9.5] Endometriosis

There is a single case report of prostatic endometriosis that occurred in a 78-year-old man after prolonged estrogen therapy (Beckman 1985). After a clinical diagnosis of adenocarcinoma, the patient took the estrogen chlorotrianisene for almost 6 years and developed hematuria. A transurethral resection of a small, raised prostatic urethral nodule demonstrated multiple zones of endometriosis involving 25% of examined prostatic chips. Endometriotic gland stroma and hemosiderin were seen. Ductal adenocarcinoma of the prostate (called endometrioid carcinoma in the past) is in the differential diagnosis, but unlike endometriosis, ductal carcinomas of the prostate display cytologic atypia, are PSA immunoreactive, and lack endometriotic stroma.

[9.6] Extramedullary Hematopoiesis

We reported a single case of extramedullary hematopoiesis in the prostate (Humphrey 1991). This 75-year-old man had an 8-year history of myelofibrosis, massive hepatosplenomegaly, and a 5-year history of bladder outlet obstruction symptoms. Transurethrally resected prostate chips revealed a diffusely increased stromal hypercellularity **i9.6**. This hypercellularity was imparted by immature granulocytes, erythroid precursors, and atypical megakaryocytes **i9.7, i9.8**. The immature hematopoietic elements often were identified in perivascular **i9.7** and intravascular positions. The stromal megakaryocytes had irregularly shaped, hyperchromatic, large nuclei **i9.8**. A chloroacetate esterase (Leder's) stain was positive for numerous immature and mature cells of the granulocytic lineage. Upon initial review of the hematoxylin and eosin–stained slides (and uninformed of the myelofibrosis history), we were concerned about a stromal neoplasm, particularly after sighting of the atypical megakaryocytes. Identification of associated erythroid and myeloid precursors was crucial in ruling out a stromal neoplasm. The incidence of prostatic extramedullary hematopoiesis in bone marrow diseases resulting in high blood cell demand, such as myelofibrosis, is unknown.

[9.7] Teratoma

A single case of benign cystic teratoma (dermoid cyst) attached to the prostate has been reported in a 50-year-old man (Uthmann 1981). This attachment consisted of a solid cord. The teratoma itself was a 10cm × 6cm × 6cm cystic mass that contained brown paste and hair. No histologic images were published.

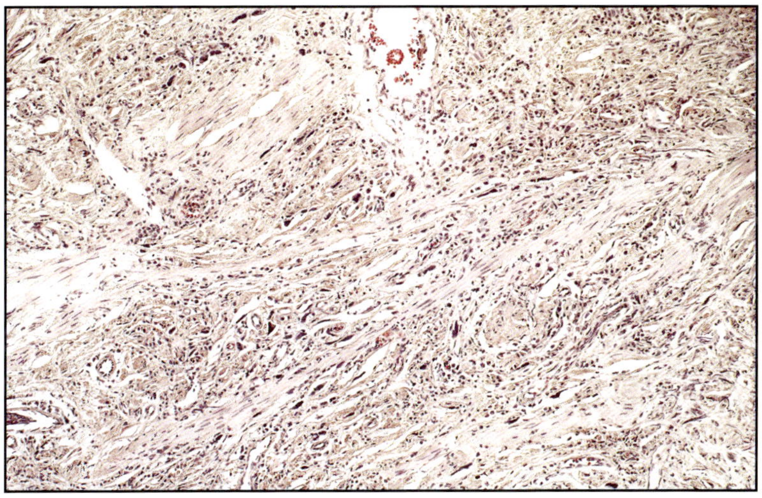

■ **i9.6** *Extramedullary hematopoiesis with stromal hypercellularity.*

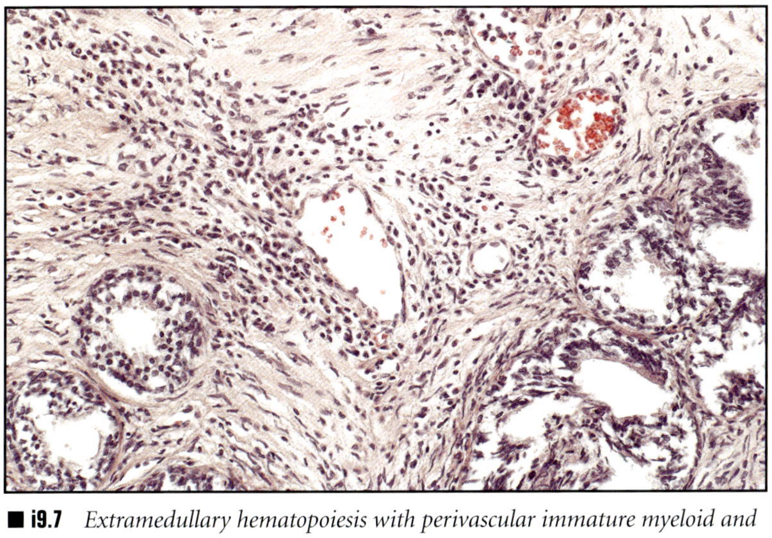

■ **i9.7** *Extramedullary hematopoiesis with perivascular immature myeloid and erythroid elements.*

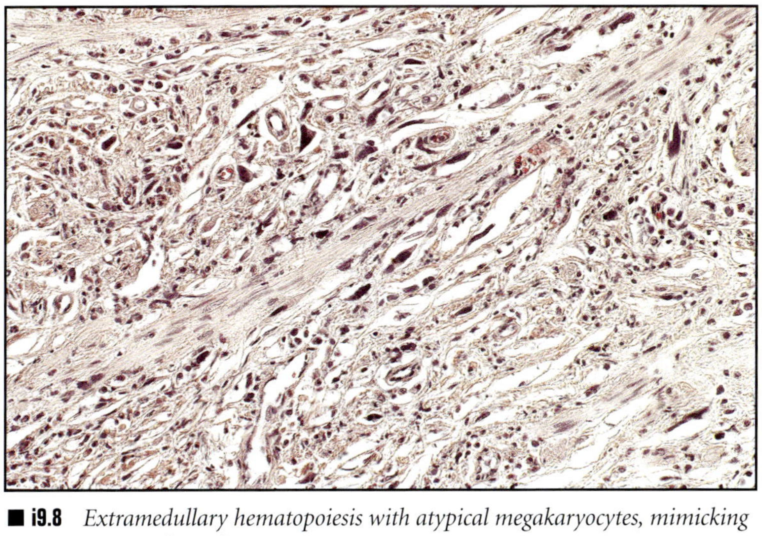

■ **i9.8** *Extramedullary hematopoiesis with atypical megakaryocytes, mimicking a stromal neoplasm.*

■ **t9.6 Normal Cowper's Glands**

Extraprostatic bulbourethral location, admixed with skeletal muscle
Rarely sampled by needle biopsy directed at prostate
Duct-acinar structure
Acini with mucinous cells with small, bland, basal nuclei
Differential diagnosis: mucinous metaplasia; low-grade adenocarcinoma

[9.8] Cowper's Glands

Cowper's bulbourethral glands are extrinsic to the prostate gland but are discussed here because they can be misdiagnosed as prostatic adenocarcinoma **t9.6** (Cina 1997, Saboorian 1997). In 1699 Cowper first described these paired glands (Cowper 1699). They are located in the urogenital diaphragm, just inferior to the prostate gland and lateral to the membranous urethra (**f1.1, p 4**). These small structures measure in average 10mm × 6mm × 5 mm in adult men (Sikorski 1982). Cowper's glands can be incidentally and inadvertently sampled by needle biopsy directed at the prostate gland (Cina 1997), by transurethral resection of the prostate (Melcher 1985), and by cystoprostatectomy (Elgamal 1994). The incidental sampling in needle biopsy is a rare event, with an incidence of 0.006% (Cina 1997). Microscopically, Cowper's glands are compound tubuloalveolar glands composed of lobules of acini, admixed with excretory ducts and ductules **i9.9**. Skeletal muscle fibers are seen associated with Cowper's gland in all needle biopsy cases **i9.10** (Cina 1997). The acinar lumens are small to occluded. Cuboidal to columnar pale-staining mucinous cells form the acini **i9.9-i9.11**, whereas more flattened hybrid mucinous-ductal cells line the ducts and ductules (Cina 1997). The mucinous cells are distended, with bluish, foamy cytoplasm, and possess small, bland, basally situated nuclei **i9.11**. An acinar basal cell layer often is not apparent on hematoxylin and eosin–stained sections **i9.11**. Histochemically, neutral and acid mucins have been detected by mucicarmine, periodic acid-Schiff with diastase, and Alcian blue stains (Cina 1997, Saboorian 1997, Sirigu 1993). Immunohistochemical studies have produced mixed findings. In particular, studies have found luminal cells in the acini to be PSA positive (Cina 1997, Elgamal 1994) or PSA-negative (Saboorian 1997) and PSAP positive (Elgamal 1994) or PSAP-negative (Cina 1997, Saboorian 1997). CEA and S-100 negativity has been reported in one series (Saboorian 1997). Similarly, whether the basal epithelial cells express high molecular weight cytokeratins recognized by antibody 34βE12 has not been determined (Cina 1997, Saboorian 1997). In most cases the basal cells are highlighted by antibodies to smooth muscle actin (SMA), which suggests myoepithelial differentiation, which has been confirmed by electron microscopy (Hellgren 1982, Riva 1988, Saboorian 1997).

The main differential diagnostic concern is low-grade prostatic adenocarcinoma. Both Cowper's glands and well-differentiated prostatic adenocarcinoma are well circumscribed, although discerning a lobular architecture can be troublesome in needle biopsy. Finding an excretory duct can direct one to the correct diagnosis for Cowper's gland, but in some cases the ducts are small and inconspicuous (Cina 1997). Immunohistochemical documentation of a basal cell and myoepithelial cell layer with 34βE12 and SMA immunostains can be helpful in difficult cases, but usually the hematoxylin and eosin–stained sections are diagnostic. The benign entity most likely to leave one flummoxed is mucinous metaplasia. However, unlike Cowper's glands, mucinous metaplasia is seen in prostatic glands, whereas Cowper's glands do not manifest such continuity. Finally, one should remember that Cowper's glands can be affected primarily by diseases such as retention cysts (Ansell 1976, Brock 1979, Colodny 1978, Maizels 1983) and carcinoma (Arduino 1969, Bourque 1970, Carpenter 1971, Keen 1970, Small 1992), but these are rare disorders.

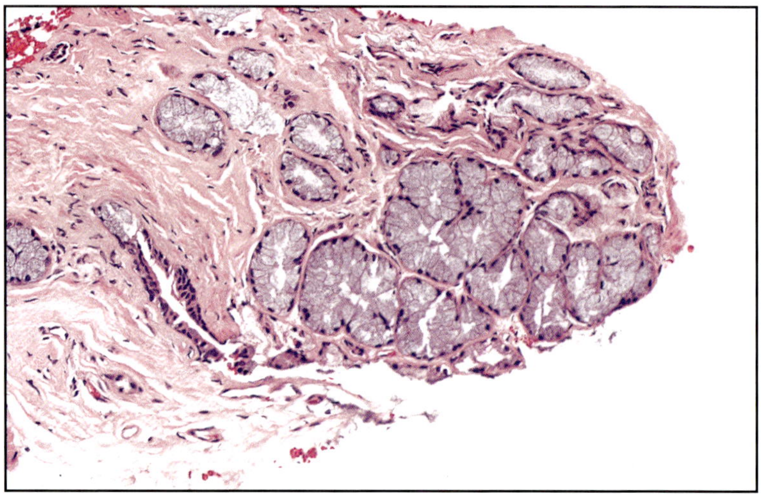

■ **i9.9** *Normal Cowper's glands sampled by needle biopsy. Note duct associated with acini of mucinous cells.*

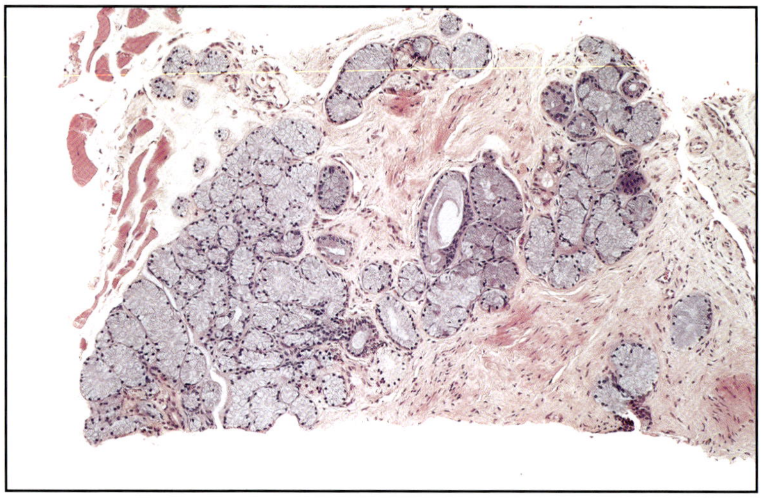

■ **i9.10** *Mucinous acini of Cowper's glands, with admixed skeletal muscle fibers (upper left), a helpful diagnostic clue.*

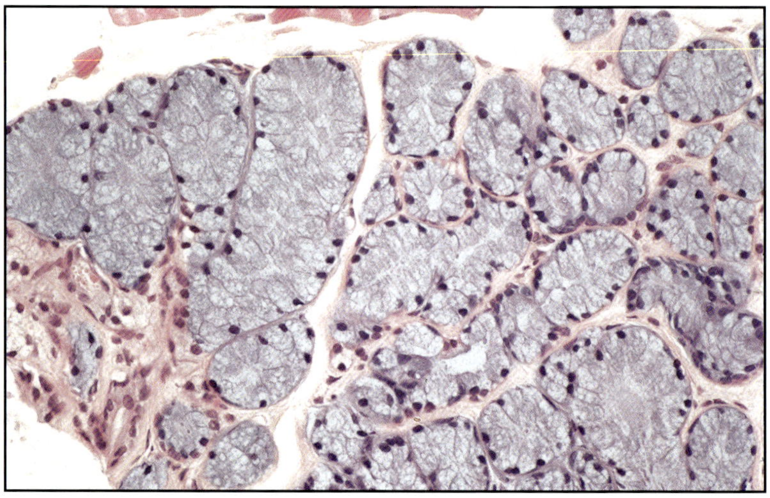

■ **i9.11** *Cowper's glands have acinar epithelium with bluish, foamy cytoplasm and small, basal nuclei.*

References

Abeshouse BS. Primary and secondary melanoma of the genitourinary tract. *South Med J* 51:994-1006, 1958.

Aguilar M, Gaffney EF, Finnerty DP. Prostatic melanosis with involvement of benign and malignant epithelium. *J Urol* 128:825-827, 1982.

Alroy J, Ucci AA, Heaney JA, et al. Multifocal pigmentation of prostatic and bladder urothelium. *J Urol* 136:96-97, 1986.

Amin MB, Bostwick DG. Pigment in prostatic epithelium and adenocarcinoma: a potential source of diagnostic confusion with seminal vesicular epithelium. *Mod Pathol* 9:791-795, 1996.

Ansell JS. Cysts of the ducts of Cowper's glands. *J Urol* 115:390-391, 1976.

Arduino LJ, Nuesse WE. Carcinoma of Cowper's gland: case report. *J Urol* 102:224-229, 1969.

Azzopardi JG, Evans DJ. Argentaffin cells in prostatic carcinoma: differentiation from lipofuscin and melanin in prostatic epithelium. *J Pathol* 104:247-250, 1971.

Bamberger MH, Romas NA. Clinically significant metastatic melanoma to the prostate. *Urology* 35:445-457, 1990.

Beckman EN, Pintado SO, Leonard GL, et al. Endometriosis of the prostate. *Am J Surg Pathol* 9:374-379, 1985.

Bejarano PA, Nestok B, Bracken RB. Collagen. A new cause for a mass in the prostatic fossa after radical prostatectomy. *J Urol Pathol* 4:99-105, 1996.

Berry NE, Reese L. Malignant melanoma which had its first presentation in the prostate gland. *J Urol* 69:286-290, 1953.

Block NL, Weber D, Schinella R. Blue nevi and other melanotic lesions of the prostate: report of 3 cases and review of the literature. *J Urol* 107:85-87, 1972.

Bostwick DG, Wollan P, Adlakha K. Collagenous micronodules in prostate cancer. A specific but infrequent diagnostic finding. *Arch Pathol Lab Med* 119:444-447, 1995.

Botticelli AR, Di Gregorio C, Losi L, et al. Melanosis (pigmented melanocytosis) of the prostate gland. *Eur Urol* 16:229-232, 1989.

Bourque JL, Charghi A, Gauthier GE, et al. Primary carcinoma of Cowper's gland. *J Urol* 103:758-761, 1970.

Brennick JB, O'Connell JX, Dickersin GR, et al. Lipofuscin pigmentation (so-called "melanosis") of the prostate. *Am J Surg Pathol* 18:446-454, 1994.

Brock WA, Kaplan GW. Lesions of Cowper's glands in children. *J Urol* 122:121-123, 1979.

Carpenter AA, Bernardo JR Jr. Adenoid cystic carcinoma of Cowper's gland: case report. *J Urol* 106:701-703, 1971.

Cina SJ, Silberman MA, Kahane H, et al. Diagnosis of Cowper's glands on prostate needle biopsy. *Am J Surg Pathol* 21:550-555, 1997.

Coffin CM, Humphrey PA, Dehner LP. Extrapulmonary inflammatory myofibroblastic tumor: a clinical and pathological survey. *Semin Diagn Pathol* 15:85-101, 1998.

Colodny AH, Lebowitz RL. Lesions of Cowper's ducts and glands in infants and children. *Urology* 11:321-325, 1978.

Cornwell GG III, Westermark GT, Pitkänen P, et al. Seminal vesicle amyloid: the first example of exocrine cell origin of an amyloid fibril precursor. *J Pathol* 167:297-303, 1992.

Cowper W. An account of two glands and their excretory ducts, in human bodies lately discovered. *Philos Trans R Soc London* 258:364, 1699.

Coyne JD, Kealy WF. Seminal vesicle amyloidosis: morphological, histochemical and immunohistochemical observations. *Histopathology* 22:173-176, 1993.

Cross PA, Bartley CJ, McClure J. Amyloid in prostatic corpora amylacea. *J Clin Pathol* 45:894-897, 1992.

Dahlin DC. Primary amyloidosis, with report of six cases. *Am J Pathol* 25:105-123, 1949.

Das Gupta T, Grabstald H. Melanoma of the genitourinary tract. *J Urol* 93:607-614, 1965.

Edit B, Ferenc S. A prostata amyloidosisa [in Hungarian]. *Orv Hetil* 130:2749-2750, 1989.

Elgamal AA, van de Voorde W, van Poppel H, et al. Immunohistochemical localization of prostate-specific markers within the accessory male sex glands of Cowper, Littre, and Morgagni. *Urology* 44:84-90, 1994.

Furusato M, Matsumoto I, Kato H, et al. Prostatic carcinoma with melanosis. *Prostate* 15:65-69, 1989.

Gardner WA Jr, Spitz WU. Melanosis of the prostate gland. *Am J Clin Pathol* 56:762-764, 1971.

Goldman RL. Melanogenic epithelium in the prostate gland. *Am J Clin Pathol* 49:75-78, 1968.

Grignon DJ, Ro JY, Ayala AG. Malignant melanoma with metastasis to adenocarcinoma of the prostate. *Cancer* 63:196-198, 1989.

Guillan RA, Zelman S. The incidence and possible origin of melanin in the prostate. *J Urol* 104:151-153, 1970.

Hellgren L, Mylius E, Vincent J. The ultrastructure of the human bulbourethral gland. *J Submicrosc Cytol* 14:683-689, 1982.

Huang WL, Ro JY, Grignon DJ, et al. Postoperative spindle cell nodule of the prostate and bladder. *J Urol* 143:824-826, 1990.

Hubler J, Pajor L, Kincses I. Primary malignant melanoma of the prostate [in German]. *Acta Chir Acad Sci Hung* 21:239-243, 1980.

Humphrey PA, Vollmer RT. Extramedullary hematopoiesis in the prostate. *Am J Surg Pathol* 15:486-490, 1991.

Jao W, Fretzin DF, Christ ML, et al. Blue nevus of the prostate gland. *Arch Pathol Lab Med* 91:187-191, 1971.

Keen MR, Golden RL, Richardson JF, et al. Carcinoma of Cowper's gland treated with chemotherapy. *J Urol* 104:854-859, 1970.

Kovi J, Jackson AG, Jackson MA. Blue nevus of the prostate: ultrastructural study. *Urology* 9:576-578, 1977.

Langley JW, Weitzner S. Blue nevus and melanosis of the prostate. *J Urol* 112:359-361, 1974.

Leung CS, Srigley JR. Distribution of lipochrome pigment in the prostate gland: biological and diagnostic implications. *Hum Pathol* 28:1302-1307, 1995.

Lew S, Richter S, Jelin N, et al. A blue naevus of the prostate: a light microscopic study including an investigation of S-100 protein positive cells in the normal and in the diseased gland. *Histopathology* 18:443-448, 1991.

Lupovitch A. The prostate and amyloidosis. *J Urol* 108:301-302, 1972.

Maizels M, Stephens FD, King LR, et al. Cowper's syringocele: a classification of dilatations of Cowper's gland duct based upon clinical characteristics of 8 boys. *J Urol* 129:111-114, 1983.

Martinez Marinez CJ, Garcia Gonzalez R, Castañeda Casanova AL. Blue nevus of the prostate: report of two new cases with immunohistochemical and electron-microscopic studies. *Eur Urol* 22:339-342, 1992.

McDonald JH, Heckel NJ. Primary amyloidosis of the lower genitourinary tract. *J Urol* 75:122-132, 1956.

Melamed MR. Letter to editor. *Am J Surg Pathol* 22:903-908, 1998.

Melcher MP. Bulbourethral glands of Cowper [letter]. *Arch Pathol Lab Med* 110:991, 1986.

Mower G. Pigments, minerals and other tissue deposits. In: Woods AE, Ellis RC, eds. *Laboratory Histopathology. A Complete Reference.* New York: Churchill Livingstone; 6.8, 1994.

Nigogosyan G, de la Pava S, Pickren JW, et al. Blue nevus of the prostate gland. *Cancer* 16:1097-1099, 1963.

Pitkänen P, Westermark P, Cornwell GG, et al. Amyloid of the seminal vesicles. A distinctive and common localized form of senile amyloidosis. *Am J Pathol* 110:64-69, 1983.

Proppe KH, Scully RE, Rosai J. Postoperative spindle cell nodules of genitourinary tract resembling sarcomas. A report of eight cases. *Am J Surg Pathol* 8:101-108, 1984.

Rios CN, Wright JR. Melanosis of the prostate gland: report of a case with neoplastic epithelium involvement. *J Urol* 115:616-617, 1976.

Riva A, Usai E, Cossu M, et al. The human bulbo-urethral glands. A transmission electron microscopy and scanning electron microscopy study. *J Androl* 9:133-141, 1988.

Ro JY, Grignon DJ, Ayala AG, et al. Blue nevus and melanosis of the prostate. Electron-microscopic and immunohistochemical studies. *Am J Clin Pathol* 90:530-535, 1988.

Ro JY, El-Naggar AK, Amin MB, et al. Pseudosarcomatous fibromyxoid tumor of the urinary bladder and prostate: immunohistochemical, ultrastructural, and DNA flow cytometric analyses of nine cases. *Hum Pathol* 24:1203-1210, 1993.

Saboorian MH, Huffman H, Ashfaq R, et al. Distinguishing Cowper's glands from neoplastic and pseudoneoplastic lesions of prostate. Immunohistochemical and ultrastructural studies. *Am J Surg Pathol* 21:1069-1074, 1997.

Scarani P, Lorenzini P. Nevo blu della prostata. *Pathologica* 71:563-568, 1979.

Seman G, Gallager HS, Johnson DE. Melanin-like pigment in the human prostate. *Prostate* 3:59-72, 1982.

Simard C, Rognon LM, Pilorce G. Le probleme du naevus bleu prostatique. *Ann Anat Pathol* 9:469-474, 1964.

Sirigu P, Turno F, Usai E, et al. Histochemical study of human bulbourethral (Cowper's glands). *Andrologia* 25:293-299, 1993.

Sikorski A. Human bulbourethral glands in the course of aging process in man. *Folia Morphol* 30:182-184, 1982.

Small JD, Albertsen PC, Graydon RJ, et al. Adenoid cystic carcinoma of Cowper's gland. *J Urol* 147:699-701, 1992.

Stein BS, Kendall AR. Malignant melanoma of the genitourinary tract. *J Urol* 132:859-868, 1984.

Stillwell TJ, Segura JW, Farrow GM. Amyloidosis of the urethra. *J Urol* 141:52-53, 1989.

Suarez GM, Roberts JA. Ochronosis of prostate presenting as advanced carcinoma. *Urology* 22:168-171, 1983.

Têtu B, Ro JY, Ayala AG, et al. Atypical spindle cell lesions of the prostate. *Semin Diagn Pathol* 5:284-293, 1988.

Tripathi VNP, Desautels RE. Primary amyloidosis of the urogenital system: a study of 16 cases and brief review. *J Urol* 102:96-101, 1969.

Unger PD, Wang Q, Gordon RE, et al. Localized amyloidosis of the seminal vesicle. Possible association with hormonally treated prostatic carcinoma. *Arch Pathol Lab Med* 121:1265-1268, 1997.

Uthmann U, Terhorst B. Dermoid cyst of the prostate with contralateral renal agenesis. *Br J Urol* 53:479, 1981.

Wang CJ, Chen YT, Shun CT, et al. Primary malignant melanoma of the prostate. *J Urol* 154:1865, 1995.

Wick MR, Brown BA, Young RH, et al. Spindle-cell proliferations of the urinary tract. An immunohistochemical study. *Am J Surg Pathol* 12:379-389, 1988.

Wilson SK, Buchanan RD, Stone WJ, et al. Amyloid deposition in the prostate. *J Urol* 110:322-323, 1973.

Young RH. Pseudoneoplastic lesions of the urinary bladder, prostate gland, and urethra. In: Wick MR, Humphrey PA, Ritter JH, eds. *Pathology of Pseudoneoplastic Lesions.* Philadelphia: Lippincott-Raven; 219-221, 235, 1997.

Pseudoneoplastic Lesions

[10.1] Pseudoneoplastic Lesions of Prostate **177**

[10.2] Pseudoneoplastic Lesions of Extraprostatic Tissues **177**

CHAPTER 10

One of the critical tasks in histopathologic differential diagnosis is to recognize benign conditions that may mimic a neoplasm, that is, pseudoneoplasms (Ackerman 1971, Wick 1997). In the previous chapters on normal tissues and benign diseases, a number of conditions have been discussed as pseudoneoplasms. Recent reviews have assembled and illustrated the conditions that can histologically simulate prostate cancer (Gaudin 1997, Young 1988, 1997A, 1997B). Provided in this chapter is a list of tumorlike lesions of the prostate. These specific prostatic lesions are not discussed here because they are covered in depth elsewhere in this book.

It is also important to note that extraprostatic benign tissues may masquerade as prostatic carcinoma. Benign seminal vesicle tissues, Cowper's glands, and lesions in lymph nodes excised at the time of radical prostatectomy can be misdiagnosed as prostate cancer. The misdiagnosis of normal seminal vesicle glands as prostate cancer is a classic pitfall in surgical pathology. Normal seminal vesicle and ejaculatory duct tissue are examined in Chapter 22, and Cowper's glands are reviewed in Chapter 9. Specific pseudocarcinomatous lesions in pelvic lymph nodes are discussed here.

[10.1] Pseudoneoplastic Lesions of Prostate

Listed in **t10.1** are benign entities in the prostate that may be mistaken for a neoplasm. Of these lesions, the first 3 are the ones most likely to be misdiagnosed as prostatic carcinoma. In a recent review of 535 consecutive needle biopsies, 7 (1.3%) were classified as false positives (Epstein 1996). These 7 cases consisted of 5 cases of adenosis (atypical adenomatous hyperplasia) and 2 cases of atrophy. In a study that focused on transurethral resection chips, findings misinterpreted as adenocarcinoma included atypical adenomatous hyperplasia (26% of the false-positive cases), basal cell hyperplasia (26%), atrophy (16%), sclerosing adenosis (10%), high-grade prostatic intraepithelial neoplasia (10%), xanthogranulomatous prostatitis (6%), florid cribriform hyperplasia (3%), and postatrophic hyperplasia (3%) (Bostwick 1999). Misinterpretation of benign conditions as cancer can have serious medical and medical-legal consequences (Troxel 1994).

t10.1 Pseudoneoplasms of the Prostate

Atypical adenomatous hyperplasia (adenosis)*
Atrophy*
Basal cell hyperplasia*
Sclerosing adenosis
Cribriform hyperplasia
Nephrogenic metaplasia (adenoma)
Verumontanum mucosal gland hyperplasia
Squamous metaplasia
Transitional cell metaplasia
Radiation atypia
Prostatitis (especially xanthogranulamotous prostatitis)
Malakoplakia
Endometriosis
Postoperative spindle cell nodule
Atypical stromal cells
Extramedullary hematopoiesis
Cowper's glands
Paraganglia in prostate
Benign glands adjacent to nerves and skeletal muscle
Signet ring change in benign lymphocytes and stromal cells secondary to cautery artifact
Signet ring change in stromal nodule (nodular stromal hyperplasia)
Florid cribriform hyperplasia

(Modified from Young 1988)
*Most likely to be misdiagnosed as carcinoma

[10.2] Pseudoneoplastic Lesions of Extraprostatic Tissues

Pelvic Lymph Nodes

In lymph nodes a large number of lymphoid hyperplasias, histiocytic and dendritic cell proliferations, and stromovascular proliferations can simulate neoplasms (Rosati 1997). In pelvic lymph nodes excised before or during radical prostatectomy, several benign conditions can specifically assume a carcinoma-like appearance. These conditions include benign glandular inclusions (Wilcox 1998), usual histiocytosis, foreign body histiocytosis (Bjornsson 1995, Peoch 1998), signet-ring histiocytosis, nodal nevi (Foitl 1992), and extramedullary hematopoiesis **t10.2**.

Benign glandular inclusions are a common incidental histologic finding in the pelvic and abdominal lymph nodes of women (Foitl 1992, Karp 1969) but are rare in the lymph nodes of men (Foitl 1992, Huntrakoon 1985, Karp 1969, Tazelaar 1986). Recently, 2 cases of benign glandular inclusions detected in pelvic lymph nodes removed during staging of prostate adenocarcinoma were reported (Wilcox 1998). Over a 15-year period I have seen a single case of such inclusions in a pelvic lymph node. This is an extremely rare finding, with an unknown incidence. A review of lymph nodes from 221 radical prostatectomy cases did not reveal a single case (Wilcox 1998). Histologically, the appearance has been described as that of tubular glands located beneath or within the lymph node capsule (Wilcox 1998). In our case, the glands were cystically dilated **i10.1-i10.3**. Intraluminal mucin and proteinaceous secretions can be identified. As in benign glandular inclusions at other anatomic sites, the lining cells are cuboidal to columnar **i10.2** (Wilcox 1998). Ciliated cells can be appreciated in some cases. Of critical importance, the glandular cells lack cytologic atypia and are devoid of mitotic figures. Immunostains for prostate-specific antigen (PSA) are

t10.2 Extraprostatic Tissues/Lesions That Can Mimic Prostatic Carcinoma

Seminal vesicles/ejaculatory duct
Cowper's glands
Pelvic lymph node lesions
- Benign glandular inclusions
- Histiocytosis, including usual, foreign body, and signet-ring histiocytosis
- Benign nodal nevi
- Extramedullary hematopoiesis

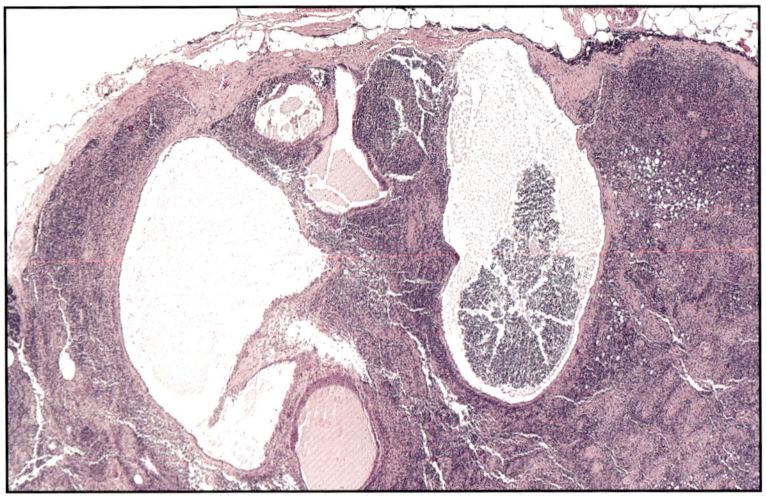

■ **i10.1** *Cystic benign glandular inclusion in pelvic lymph node removed at radical prostatectomy.*

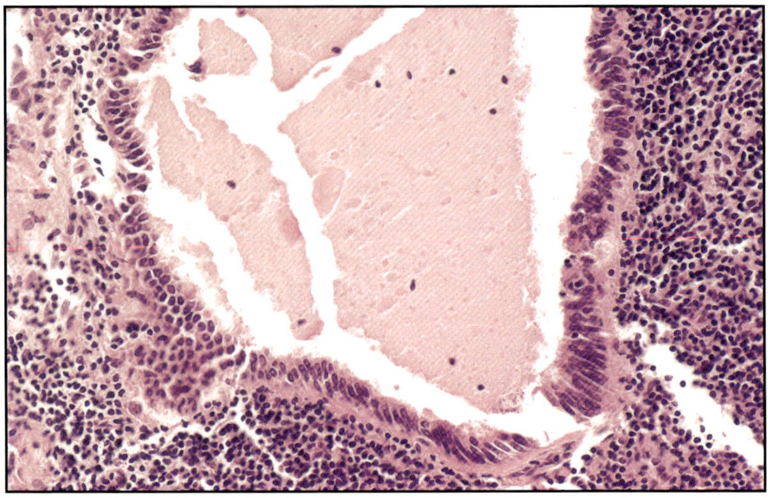

■ **i10.2** *Columnar cell lining and proteinaceous secretions of nodal benign glandular inclusion.*

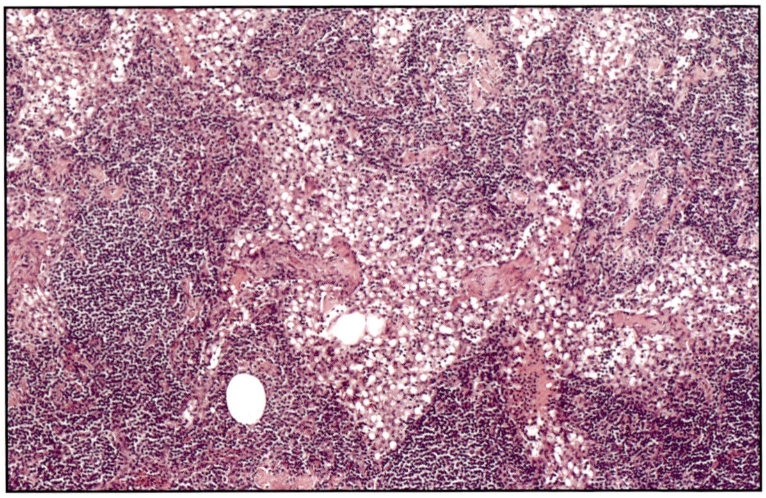

■ **i10.3** *Signet-ring histiocytosis of pelvic lymph node, with sinusoidal distribution pattern.*

negative. Leu-M-1 positivity has been reported in one case (Wilcox 1998), and in our case the immunophenotype was pan-cytokeratin positive, CA125 positive, EMA positive, B72.3 negative, LeuM1 negative, and PSA negative. Of course, the main differential diagnostic concern is metastatic adenocarcinoma. The tubular profiles of benign glandular inclusions could be mistaken for small acinar adenocarcinoma, and the dilated glands could be misinterpreted as cystic prostatic adenocarcinoma, which is a form of the uncommon pseudohyperplastic prostatic adenocarcinoma (Humphrey 1998). Comparison of the lymph node glands with morphologic features of the primary carcinoma in the prostate can be helpful, but the bland nuclear cytology and absence of PSA staining in the benign glandular inclusions are the most useful diagnostic characteristics. The histogenesis of these epithelial inclusions is thought to be related to a metaplastic proliferation of peritoneal mesothelium that becomes entrapped in lymph nodes during development (Foitl 1992, Karp 1969, Tazelaar 1986).

Histiocytosis of usual type, foreign body histiocytosis, and signet-ring histiocytosis are all benign macrophage proliferations that can masquerade as prostatic carcinoma. Usual histiocytosis can present as pale cells, sometimes with small nucleoli, that can mimic prostatic carcinoma metastatic to lymph nodes. The generation of spaces between the masses of histiocytes can specifically resemble glandlike spaces. Foamy gland prostatic carcinoma (Nelson 1996) and prostatic carcinoma with androgen deprivation treatment effect (Reuter 1997) are particularly high in the differential diagnosis. Valuable findings in favor of usual histiocytosis include a sinusoidal distribution pattern for the macrophages with preservation of nodal architecture, lack of nuclear pleomorphism, and maintenance of low nuclear-cytoplasmic ratios.

Foreign body histiocytosis and florid sinus histiocytosis have been reported for 12 patients with prostate cancer who underwent hip replacement (Bjornsson 1995, Peoch 1998) or lower limb joint prosthetic surgery (Winstanley 2002). Histologically, 30% to 80% of the pelvic node parenchyma was replaced by confluent, large histiocytes, with granular to foamy, eosinophilic to amphophilic cytoplasm (Bjornsson 1995). In nodes ipsilateral to the hip prosthesis, clear needle-shaped, polarizable particles were found (Bjornsson 1995). In many cases, admixed giant cells and histiocytes contained small, irregular, dark particles (Peoch 1998, Winstanley 2002). The needle-like foreign material was identified as polyethylene by histochemical staining (using a modified oil red 0 procedure [Bjornsson 1995]), and the small (1μm to 5μm) dark particles were metallic, with titanium, aluminum, chromium, cobalt, nickel, molybdenum, and tungsten identified by energy dispersive x-ray elemental analysis (Bjornsson 1995) and mass spectrometry (Peoch 1998). The polyethylene and metal particles were derived from the implanted synthetic prosthesis, and so this nodal reaction pattern has been called postprosthesis lymph node histiocytosis (Bjornsson 1995). The main diagnostic problem is misdiagnosis of the large numbers of histiocytes as metastatic prostatic adenocarcinoma, which occurred in one case and eventuated in inappropriate treatment (Bjornsson 1995). One should be aware that metastatic prostatic adenocarcinoma can be encountered in the same node as postprosthesis lymph node histiocytosis (Peoch 1998).

Signet-ring histiocytosis has been incidentally detected in about 1% (4/314) of pelvic lymph nodes extracted during radical prostatectomy operations (Guerrero-Medrano 1997). Microscopically, lymph node subcapsular and medullary sinuses are filled and distended by cytologically bland histiocytes with signet-ring vacuoles **i10.3, i10.4** (Guerrero-Medrano 1997). The signet-ring morphology is imparted by a single, large, cytoplasmic vacuole that displaces and compresses the nucleus, with indentation. The nuclei are small and dark and lack prominent nucleoli. No mitotic figures are present. Special studies demonstrate lack of mucin (negative periodic acid-Schiff, Alcian blue,

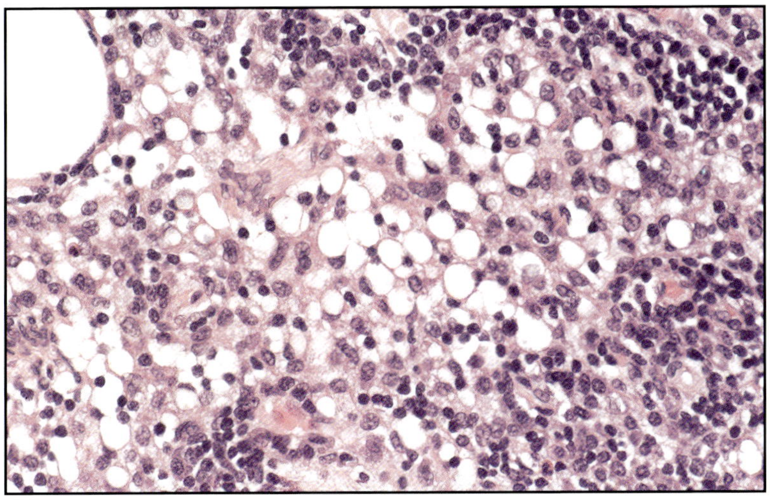

■ **i10.4** *Signet-ring histiocytosis—reactive proliferation of benign histiocytes mimicking signet-ring carcinoma.*

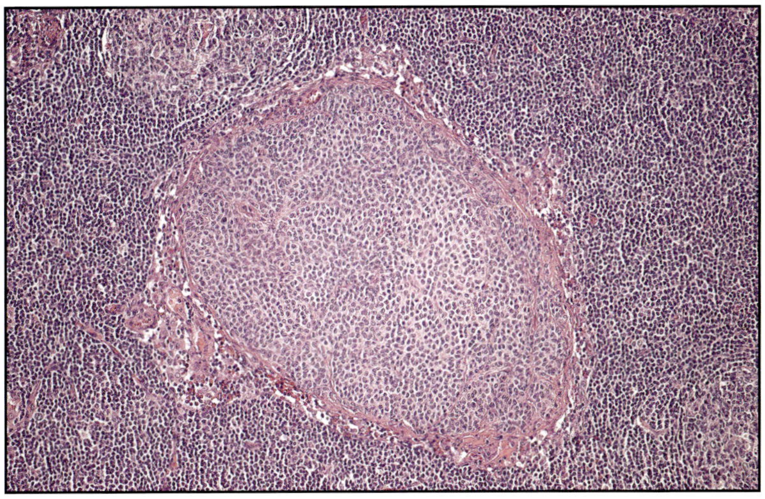

■ **i10.5** *Aggregate of benign nevus cells in pelvic lymph node.*

and mucicarmine stains) and reveal histiocytic differentiation in the signet-ring cells (positive CD68, HAM56, lysozyme, LN5, and cathepsin D immunostains), with negative pan-cytokeratin and PSA immunostains. The ultrastructural and etiologic basis for the formation of the vacuoles is not evident. It is necessary to exclude metastatic signet-ring prostatic adenocarcinoma in these cases, and a search for signet-ring cells in the carcinoma within the prostate gland is the first order of business. One should suspect that the correct diagnosis is signet-ring histiocytosis rather than metastatic signet-ring carcinoma based on confinement of the cells to sinuses (although small metastatic carcinoma deposits can also be sinus-confined) and, more importantly, the uniformly bland nuclei. In the few cases of signet-ring histiocytosis we have seen **i10.3, i10.4**, we have confirmed the histiocytic nature of the signet-ring cells by an immunostain panel of CD68, pan-cytokeratin, PSA, and prostate-specific acid phosphatase. Mucin stains are not very helpful because prostatic signet-ring adenocarcinoma usually are mucin-negative (Randolph 1997).

Nodal benign nevus cell aggregates are most commonly found in axillary lymph nodes (Foitl 1992) but can also be found in cervical, inguinal, and pelvic lymph nodes. We have seen a single case of a nevus cell aggregate in a pelvic lymph node taken out at radical prostatectomy **i10.5**. The incidence of this finding in nodes removed at radical prostatectomy is unknown. Nodal nevus is invariably an incidental histologic finding (Foitl 1992). Histologically, there is a concentration of the solid aggregates in capsular and pericapsular tissues, but ectopic nevus aggregates can be encountered in the substance of the node. In our case, we saw both capsular and parenchymal, small aggregates of uniformly bland cells without any mitotic activity. The aggregates were S-100 immunoreactive **i10.6** and pan-cytokeratin and PSA immunonegative. One should exclude metastatic melanoma, although this malignancy is vanishingly rare in the prostate. Minute nests of nodal nevus cells could masquerade as micrometastatic high-grade prostatic carcinoma, but the nevus cells lack cytologic atypia and often are embedded in the nodal capsule, whereas nodal prostate cancer metastases usually are first found in subcapsular sinuses. The aforementioned immunostains confirm the diagnosis. The presence of nevus cell aggregates in lymph nodes usually is hypothesized to result from benign metastasis of cutaneous nevi or arrested embryonic migration of neural crest cells (Foitl 1992).

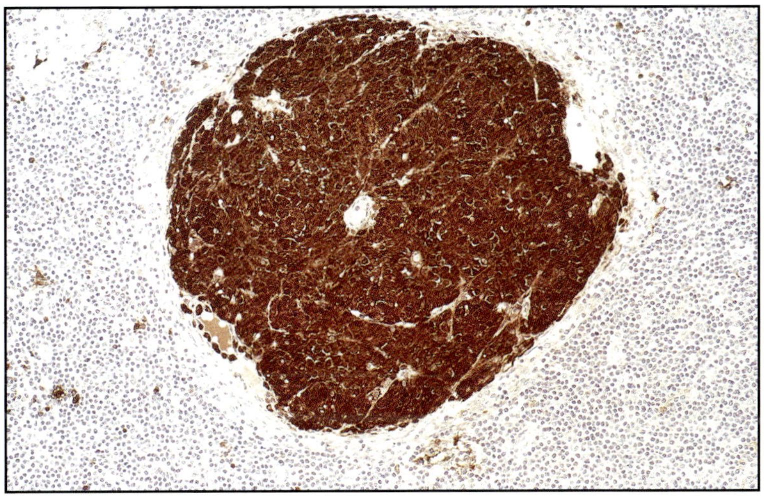

■ **i10.6** *S-100 positivity of benign nevus cell aggregate in* **i10.5**.

Finally, we have observed, as an incidental finding, a single case of pelvic lymph node extramedullary hematopoiesis in a patient who underwent radical prostatectomy. The immature myeloid cells and megakaryocytes could be confused with neoplastic cells. The incidence of extramedullary hematopoiesis in the pelvic lymph nodes of men with prostate cancer is unknown; the patients do need to be evaluated for a bone marrow disorder.

References

Ackerman LV, Rosai J. The pathology of tumors, part one. Introduction, precancerous lesions, benign lesions that resemble cancer. *CA Cancer J Clin* 21:163-173, 1971.

Bjornsson BL, Truong LD, Cartwright J, et al. Pelvic lymph node histiocytosis mimicking metastatic prostatic adenocarcinoma: association with hip prostheses. *J Urol* 154:470-473, 1995.

Bostwick DG, Cheng L. Overdiagnosis of prostatic adenocarcinoma. *Semin Urol Oncol* 17:199-205, 1999.

Epstein JI, Walsh PC, Sanfilippo F. Clinical and cost impact of second-opinion pathology. Review of prostate biopsies prior to radical prostatectomy. *Am J Surg Pathol* 20:851-857, 1996.

Foitl DR, Perzin KH, Knowles DM. Nonhematopoietic elements in lymph nodes. In: Knowles DM, ed. *Neoplastic Hematopathology.* Baltimore: Williams & Wilkins; 872-874, 1992.

Gaudin PB, Reuter VE. Benign mimics of prostatic adenocarcinoma on needle biopsy. In: Fechner RE, Rosen PP, eds. *Anatomic Pathology 1997.* Vol 2. Chicago: ASCP Press; 111-134, 1997.

Guerrero-Medrano J, Delgado R, Albores-Saavedra J. Signet-ring sinus histiocytosis. A reactive disorder that mimics metastatic adenocarcinoma. *Cancer* 80:277-285, 1997.

Humphrey PA, Kaleem Z, Swanson PE, et al. Pseudohyperplastic prostatic adenocarcinoma. *Am J Surg Pathol* 22:1239-1246, 1998.

Huntrakoon M. Benign glandular inclusions in the abdominal lymph nodes of a man. *Hum Pathol* 16:644-646, 1985.

Karp LA, Czernobilsky B. Glandular inclusions in pelvic and abdominal paraaortic lymph nodes. A study of autopsy and surgical material in males and females. *Am J Clin Pathol* 52:212-218, 1969.

Nelson RS, Epstein JI. Prostatic carcinoma with abundant xanthomatous cytoplasm: foamy gland carcinoma. *Am J Surg Pathol* 20:419-426, 1996.

Peoch M, Ducros V, Barnoud R, et al. Foreign body histiocytosis reaction after hip replacement with concomitant metastatic adenocarcinoma in the same lymph node. *Hum Pathol* 29:95-98, 1998.

Randolph TL, Amin MB, Ro JY, et al. Histologic variants of adenocarcinoma and other carcinomas of the prostate: pathologic criteria and clinical significance. *Mod Pathol* 10:612-629, 1997.

Reuter VE. Pathological changes in benign and malignant tissue following androgen deprivation therapy. *Urology* 49(suppl 3A):16-22, 1997.

Rosati S, Frizzera G. Pseudoneoplastic lesions of the hematolymphoid system. In: Wick MR, Humphrey PA, Ritter JR, eds. *Pathology of Pseudoneoplastic Lesions.* New York: Lippincott-Raven; 449-494, 1997.

Tazelaar HD, Vareska G. Benign glandular inclusions [letter]. *Hum Pathol* 17:100-101, 1986.

Troxel DB, Sabella JD. Problem areas in pathology practice. Uncovered by a review of malpractice claims. *Am J Surg Pathol* 18:821-831, 1994.

Wick MR, Humphrey PA, Ritter JH, eds. *Pathology of Pseudoneoplastic Lesions.* New York: Lippincott-Raven, 1997.

Wilcox GE, Conway EJ, Wheeler TM, et al. Benign glandular inclusions (BGI) detected in pelvic lymph nodes (PLN) during staging of prostate adenocarcinoma [abstract]. *Mod Pathol* 11:99A, 1998.

Winstanley AM, Sandison A, Bott SR, et al. Incidental findings in pelvic lymph nodes at radical prostatectomy. *J Clin Pathol* 55:623-626, 2002.

Young RH. Pseudoneoplastic lesions of the prostate gland. *Pathol Annu* 23(pt 1):105-128, 1988.

Young RH. Pseudoneoplastic lesions of the urinary bladder, prostate gland, and urethra. In: Wick MR, Humphrey PA, Ritter JR, eds. *Pathology of Pseudoneoplastic Lesions.* New York: Lippincott-Raven; 223-235, 1997A.

Young RH. Tumor-like lesions of the prostate gland. *Am J Clin Pathol* 104:607-610, 1997B.

CHAPTER 11

Prostatic Intraepithelial Neoplasia

[11.1] History of Diagnostic Terminology **183**

[11.2] Clinical Presentation **183**

[11.3] Incidence of PIN in Core Needle Biopsies **184**

[11.4] Incidence of High-Grade PIN in TURP Chips and Simple (Open) Prostatectomies **184**

[11.5] Incidence of High-Grade PIN in Whole Prostate Glands **185**

[11.6] Histologic Diagnosis of PIN **186**

[11.7] Low-Grade PIN **186**

[11.8] High-Grade PIN **188**

[11.9] Follow-up and Clinical Management of High-Grade PIN **203**

[11.10] PIN Reporting **205**

[11.11] PIN as Precursor **205**

[11.12] Summary **210**

Prostatic intraepithelial neoplasia (PIN) is the preferred diagnostic term for a putative premalignant proliferation of atypical epithelial cells within preexisting prostatic ducts and acini (reviews: Amin 1993B, 1994B, Bostwick 1995A, 1999, Epstein 1994B, Häggman 1997C, Jones 1994, Mostofi 1992, Parkinson 1995, Sakr 1998A, 1998B, 1999). PIN is still a putative premalignant lesion because the natural history of this lesion in humans remains ill-defined. Are human PIN cells even neoplastic? This has not been definitively proven because these cells have not been isolated and shown to exhibit autonomous in vitro growth in clonogenic assays in soft agar or in vivo in immunocompromised animals. Yet, as we will explore in this chapter, a wealth of compelling evidence links high-grade PIN with carcinoma. Although there is still debate regarding the appropriateness of PIN as a descriptive and diagnostic label (Drago 1989, Page 1991), the practical reality is that the PIN nomenclature is now well entrenched in urology and pathology literature and practice. It is vital that the diagnostic pathologist understand the diagnostic criteria for PIN, the difference between low-grade and high-grade PIN, the entities in the differential diagnosis of PIN, and the clinical implications of a diagnosis of PIN.

[11.1] History of Diagnostic Terminology

PIN probably was first described in 1926 by Ortel (Ortel 1926) as atypical (carcinoid) hyperplasia. Subsequently, in 1949 Andrews (Andrews 1949) reported "a characteristic type of hyperplasia" that he viewed as a precancerous condition of the prostate. Scrutiny of 2 of the illustrations in that article suggest depiction of micropapillary and cribriform patterns of PIN.

From midcentury until the 1980s, a plethora of diagnostic appellations have been applied to atypical but noninvasive epithelial proliferations in the prostate **t11.1**. Most of these were purely descriptive, and *atypical hyperplasia* was perhaps the most commonly used descriptor. Atypical hyperplasia has been linked to adenocarcinoma (Gleason 1985, Helpap 1980, Kastendieck 1980, 1989, Kovi 1989), but there have been difficulties with use of the term *atypical hyperplasia in the prostate.* Because of the many morphologic definitions, it has served for many as an umbrella diagnosis, encompassing any sort of atypia, architectural or cytologic, in prostatic tissue.

In 1965 McNeal (McNeal 1965) defined 2 potentially premalignant epithelial abnormalities in the prostate: adenomatous hyperplasia and intraductal dysplasia. This work has formed the foundation for current concepts on atypias in the prostate. Adenomatous hyperplasia is currently designated atypical adenomatous hyperplasia or adenosis, and intraductal dysplasia is now called PIN. The landmark article that rigorously defined grades of dysplasia and provided evidence of an association between dysplasia and invasive adenocarcinoma of the prostate was the 1986 article by McNeal and Bostwick (McNeal 1986). Here, the authors established the morphologic characteristics of 3 grades of dysplasia. These same basic criteria are the ones we use today in diagnosing PIN. In 1987, movement toward adoption of *PIN* and away from *dysplasia* was initiated by Bostwick and Brawer (Bostwick 1987), and *PIN* became widely accepted after a 1989 consensus conference (NPCDP 1989). At this same conference, compressed stratification of PIN into 2 grades, low-grade and high-grade PIN, rather than the previous 3 tiers of PIN 1, PIN 2, and PIN 3, was recommended (Drago 1989). As we shall see, this definition and separation of low-grade PIN and high-grade PIN has turned out to be critical from both histopathologic and clinical standpoints. Unfortunately, in the medical literature and in diagnostic practice, it is all too common to see the general diagnostic designation *PIN* rather than the more specific terms *low-grade PIN* and *high-grade PIN.* PIN always should be precisely defined as low-grade PIN or high-grade PIN. The evolutionary process in categorization from dysplasia to the 2 grades of PIN is displayed in **f11.1**.

■ **t11.1 Diagnostic Terms Previously Used for Atypical, Noninvasive, Epithelial Proliferations of the Prostate**

Atypical hyperplasia
Atypical epithelial hyperplasia
Atypical primary hyperplasia
Atypical postatrophic hyperplasia
Atypical cribriform hyperplasia
Atypical small acinar hyperplasia
Atypical large acinar hyperplasia
Atypical adenomatous hyperplasia
Adenosis
Hyperplasia with malignant change
Marked atypia
Atypism
Cellular atypia
Cytological atypia
Small alveolar proliferation
Dysplasia
Intraductal dysplasia
Duct-acinar dysplasia
Precancerous lesions
Preneoplasia
Carcinoma in situ

Modified from Table 1, Kastendieck 1989

[11.2] Clinical Presentation

Patients with isolated high-grade PIN in needle biopsy typically are 64 to 70 years old, although the age range is 46 to 87 (Aboseif 1995, Brawer 1991, Davidson 1995, Häggman 1997C, Keetch 1995, Langer 1996, Raviv 1996B) **t11.2**. These men usually present with an elevated serum prostate-specific antigen (PSA) of 5.6 to 11.2 ng/mL (where the normal cutoff is 4 ng/mL or less using the Hybritech assay). However, published

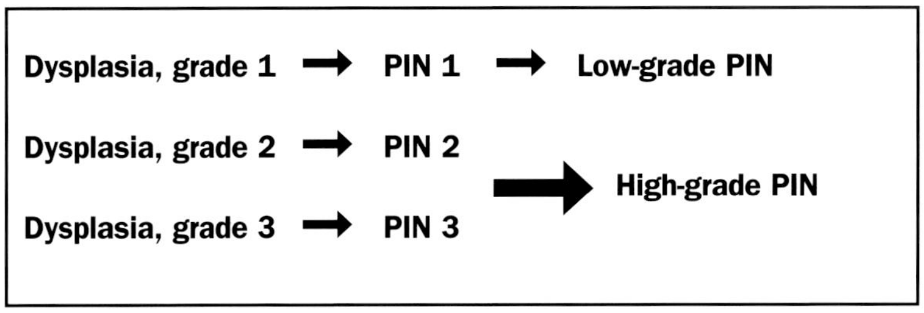

■ **f11.1** *PIN: Terminology evolution*

■ **t11.2 Clinical Presentation of Patients with High-grade PIN**

No clinical or radiological findings are specific for PIN
Most men are in their 60s
PIN does not raise serum PSA, but can be associated with modest elevations of total serum PSA
PIN does not form masses that are palpable by DRE
PIN does not exhibit specific sonographic findings

evidence suggests that PIN does not raise the serum PSA level (Alexander 1996, Ronnett 1993); it is probable that unsampled prostatic inflammation, hyperplasia, or carcinoma has caused the PSA elevation in these patients. There are conflicting data on whether high-grade PIN is associated with a low percentage of free PSA levels (Ramos 1999, Tarle 1997). Digital rectal examination (DRE) has been reported to be abnormal in 23% to 100% of patients with PIN (Aboseif 1995, Brawer 1991, Davidson 1995, Keetch 1995, Langer 1996, Raviv 1996B), but because PIN usually is not mass-formative, it is unlikely that this abnormality was caused by PIN. DRE is not considered to be a diagnostic modality for PIN detection. Similarly, although 49% to 100% of patients with PIN have an sonographic abnormality, and although PIN may be hypoechoic, similar to prostatic carcinoma (Tarle 1997), transrectal ultrasound (TRUS) also is not a diagnostic tool for PIN detection . It has been estimated that only 4% to 18% of hypoechoic foci harbor PIN (Brawer 1989A, Devonec 1990, Lee 1989).

There is no difference between low-grade PIN and high-grade PIN in patient age, DRE and TRUS findings, and serum PSA level **t11.3**.

In summary, patients with isolated PIN in needle biopsy do not present with clinical findings that are specific for this histopathologic diagnosis. However, these clinical findings may affect the relative risk of prostate cancer on repeat biopsy, as discussed in this chapter.

High-grade PIN may also be diagnosed in isolated form in transurethral resection of the prostate (TURP) chips and open (simple) prostatectomy tissues (Brawer 1989C, Gaudin 1997, Pacelli 1997, Samaratunga 1995, Skjorten 1997). The mean age for 85 patients with high-grade PIN in TURP resectates was 70 years (range 50 to 89), and for 13 of these patients a pre-TURP PSA level was available; the mean level was 15.1 ng/mL (range 1.0 to 100 ng/mL). No known clinical parameter allows presurgical identification of patients with high-grade PIN in TURP chips.

[11.3] Incidence of PIN in Core Needle Biopsies

The incidence of isolated high-grade PIN (without associated carcinoma) in needle biopsy has varied from 0.7% to 16.5%, with a literature mean of about 4% **t11.4, t11.5**. Most of these studies were retrospective; in our prospective series of 795 consecutive needle biopsies, the incidence was higher at 7.4% (Reyes 1998). An additional 4 studies (Brawer 1989B, Gohji 1995, Lee 1989, Richie 1994) report, in aggregate, a PIN detection rate of 60/677 (8.9%) in needle biopsy. In these 4 studies PIN grade was not supplied; as we shall see, it is vital that low-grade PIN be distinguished from high-grade PIN.

The basis for the wide range of reported incidence rates for high-grade PIN in needle biopsy probably is multifactorial. Different patient populations, differing degrees of prostate sampling (differing number of biopsies taken) (Rosser 1999), different fixatives (alcohol-based, Bouin's, or formalin), differing section thickness and quality, variable section staining, and varying thresholds for pathologists in the diagnosis of PIN, with variable application of criteria (Sakr 2001), are all probable factors. In 1 study (Kahn 1997), urologic pathologists were more likely to diagnose isolated high-grade PIN in needle biopsy (frequency = 7%) than general pathologists (frequency = 2%). The incidence figures in needle biopsy in **t11.4** should not be used as precise target figures for the frequency of high-grade PIN that should be diagnosed in any individual practice; rather, awareness of the reported incidence ranges may give the practitioner a general idea of how often high-grade PIN should be diagnosed in needle biopsy.

High-grade PIN is identified in 10% to 40% of needle biopsies that also harbor carcinoma (Epstein 1995A, Hu 1998, Mostofi 1995, Skjorten 1997, Thorson 1998).

■ **t11.3 Clinical Presentation of Patients with Isolated PIN on Needle Biopsy[1]**

	Low-grade PIN	High-grade PIN
Patients (number)	66	85
Age (mean)	67	70
Abnormal DRE (%)	32	36
Abnormal TRUS (%)	51	69
Serum PSA, mean	8.0	11.2
Serum PSA, median	5.2	5.7

[1]Compilation of data from Keetch 1995 and Raviv 1996B
DRE = digital rectal examination; TRUS = transrectal ultrasound

■ **t11.4 Incidence of High-grade PIN**

Tissue sample	Without carcinoma	With carcinoma
Needle biopsy	5%	10%-40%
TURP chips	2%-15%	3%-58%
Whole gland	35%	75%

[11.4] Incidence of High-Grade PIN in TURP Chips and Simple (Open) Prostatectomies

The incidence of high-grade PIN in TURP chips without carcinoma ranges from 2.3% to 15.2% (Gaudin 1997, Pacelli 1997, Samaratunga 1995, Skjorten 1997). In TURP chips with carcinoma, the incidence is reported at 3.2% to 58.1% (Epstein 1990B, Gaudin 1997, Pacelli 1997, Samaratunga 1995, Skjorten 1997). Most of the studies report incidence figures closer to the lower ones. The lower incidence percentages would make more biologic sense because high-grade PIN usually is a peripheral zone proliferation and TURP samples mainly the more centrally located transition zone.

In open or simple prostatectomy tissues (obtained by "enucleation" of benign prostatic hyperplasia [BPH] nodules) high-grade PIN has been identified in 67% and 66% of cases with and without carcinoma, respectively (Skjorten 1997). It is not clear why

■ **t11.5 Incidence of Isolated High-grade PIN in Core Needle Biopsy**

Study	Incidence	Comment
Bostwick 1995B	19/200 (9.5%) to 33/200 (16.5%)	9.5% incidence at private practice laboratory and 16.5% incidence at Mayo Clinic
Mostofi 1995	7/265 (2.6%)	Central review of patients in the American Cancer Society—National Prostate Cancer Detection Project
Langer 1996	48/1275 (3.8%)	Series of consecutive patients undergoing prostate needle biopsy at a university hospital from 1/1/91 to 8/30/93
Wills 1997	24/439 (5.5%)	Series of consecutive patients undergoing sextant biopsy from 1/1/92-7/1/94 at a university hospital
Skjorten 1997	12/79 (15.2%)	Core biopsies from a 1974-1975 at a Norwegian hospital. Includes PIN2 and PIN3 cases
Cheville 1997	15/1,009 (1.5%)	All prostate needle core biopsies at a community hospital from 11/1/93-8/1/95
Perachino 1997	21/148 (14.2%)	Series of Italian patients selected for re-biopsy
Renshaw 1998	98/2,219 (4.4%)	Prostate biopsies at a University hospital from 1989-1996
Kahn 1977	62/3309 (1.9%) to 53/752 (7%)	2% incidence for nonurologic pathologists vs 7% for urologic pathologists
Orozco 1998	2568/62,537 (4.1%)	Incidence from between 4/95 to 3/97 in a private laboratory
Weinstein 1998	81/5293 (1.5%)	Data on needle biopsies from 1/1/90 to 12/31/93 at three community hospitals, with average rates from 0%-2% at the three hospitals
Hu 1998	30/388 (7.7%)	Incidence in diagnosis by a urologic pathologist in community hospital needle biopsies.
Reyes 1998	59/795 (7.4%)	Data from a PSA-based screening program
Hoedemaeker 1999	12/1824 (0.7%)	Incidence in a prostate cancer screening program in the Netherlands
O'Dowd 2000	4,902/132,426 (3.7%)	Updated experience reported by Orozco 1998
Alsikafi 2001	21/485 (4.3%)	Consecutive series, with retrospective review by a single urologic pathologist
Vis 2001	33/4,057 (0.8%)	Expanded data from Hoedemaeker 1999
Fowler 2001	93/1,050 (8.9%)	Prevalence in African-American men significantly higher at 13.4% vs 5.9% for white men
Total	**5,611/154,389 (3.6%)**	

■ **t11.6 Incidence of High-grade PIN in Whole Prostate Glands**

Study	Without carcinoma (%)	With carcinoma (%)
McNeal 1986	26/43 (60.5%)	72/82 (88%)
Troncoso 1989	24/28 (86%)	57/61 (93%)
Sakr 1994B	6/174 (3%)	22/70 (31%)
Wiley 1997	19/26 (73%)	82/86 (95%)
Arakawa 1997	11/23 (48%)	38/49 (78%)
Abbas 1996	4/40 (10%)	15/40 (38%)
Silvestri 1995	91/260 (35%)	414/683 (61%)
Melhorn 1991	82/317 (26%)	105/133 (79%)
Billis 1996	108/135 (80%)	44/45 (98%)
Quinn 1990	—	40/40 (100%)
Humphrey 1992	—	71/81 (88%)
Qian 1997	—	169/195 (86%)
Greene 1991	—	85/96 (89%)
de la Torre 1993	—	46/54 (85%)
Yang 1999	11/31 (36%)	12/16 (75%)
Prange 2001	—	82/83 (99%)
Total	**382/1077 (35%)**	**1354/1814 (75%)**

these figures are so high in this single, large study. Examination of the transition zone corresponding to open prostatectomy tissues in whole glands has revealed a lower incidence of high-grade PIN.

[11.5] Incidence of High-Grade PIN in Whole Prostate Glands

High-grade PIN is extremely common in whole prostate glands removed by radical prostatectomy or cystoprostatectomy or at postmortem examination, with an aggregate incidence of 75% in glands with carcinoma and 35% of glands without carcinoma **t11.6**. This incidence increases dramatically with age, with an incidence of 5% to 10% in the fourth and fifth decades and >40% above age 50 **f11.2** (Sakr 1994B). Of note, despite the lower incidence of clinical prostate cancer in the Far East compared with the United States, the

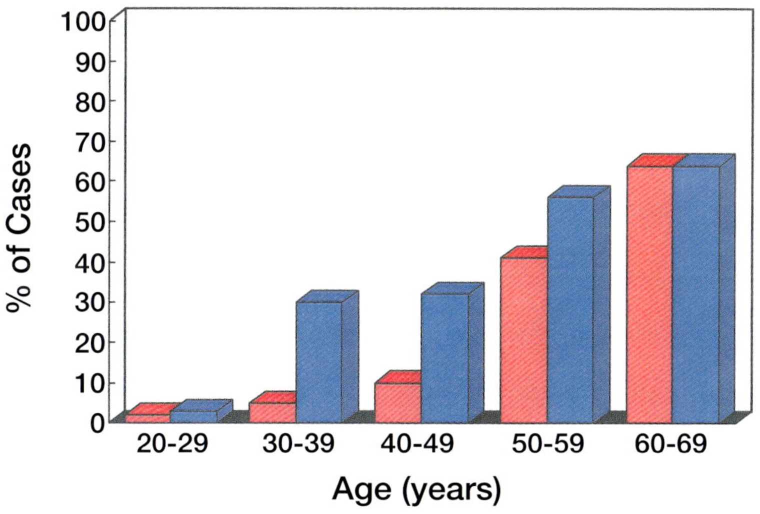

■ **f11.2** *Incidence of high-grade PIN (red bars) and invasive adenocarcinoma (blue bars) in whole prostate glands at autopsy, as related to age (Sakr 1994B).*

incidence of high-grade PIN in Japan and Taiwan appears to be similar to that of the United States (Fujita 1997, Yang 1999).

[11.6] Histologic Diagnosis of PIN

PIN may be diagnosed in all types of prostatic tissue samples, including core needle biopsies (14 or 18 gauge), transurethral resectates, and simple and radical prostatectomy tissues. The cytodiagnosis of PIN in fine needle aspirates of the prostate gland is difficult (see Chapter 3). The histologic diagnosis is based on both architectural and cytologic traits **t11.7**. The diagnosis is exclusively a microscopic one because PIN is not grossly visible.

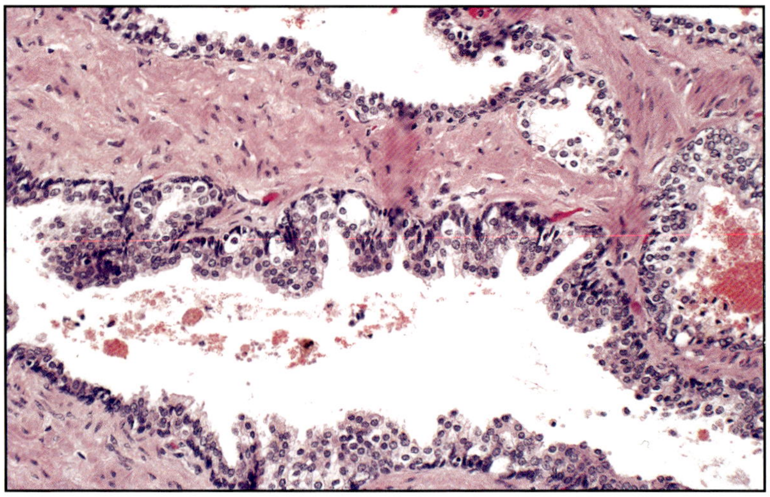

■ **i11.1** *Low-grade PIN with dark medium-sized glands with luminal undulations.*

[11.7] Low-Grade PIN

Low-grade PIN, previously known as mild dysplasia, grade I dysplasia (McNeal 1986), and PIN 1 (Bostwick 1987) **f11.1**, is an intraepithelial proliferation along preexisting ducts and acini that is recognizable at scanning magnification as darker, medium to large-sized, complex glands **i11.1**. The basis for this darker appearance is mainly the increase in density of nuclei per gland and often the increased staining of cytoplasm of the luminal cells in PIN, such that the cytoplasm is eosinophilic to amphophilic compared with the normal or hyperplastic luminal cell cytoplasm, which is slightly granular to cleared. Low-grade PIN usually is a focal finding in needle biopsy. In our experience (Keetch 1995), the mean size of low-grade PIN in needle biopsy was 0.9mm.

The architectural arrangement of cells in low-grade PIN is not as well defined as for high-grade PIN **t11.7**. The original description of low-grade PIN (grade 1 dysplasia) (McNeal 1986) emphasizes mainly the multilayering of cells and depicts a tufted pattern of growth. It seems that low-grade PIN can present with the same intraglandular structures as high-grade PIN, including the tufted, micropapillary, cribriform. and flat patterns (Bostwick 1993).

Basal cells are present in normal numbers in low-grade PIN, and identification of these cells confirms the intraepithelial nature of the process. These basal cells are morphologically identical to those in normal glands. That is, these cells have scanty cytoplasm and dark nuclei that abut the basement membrane. The nuclei often assume oblong and cigar shapes but may be triangular or rounded.

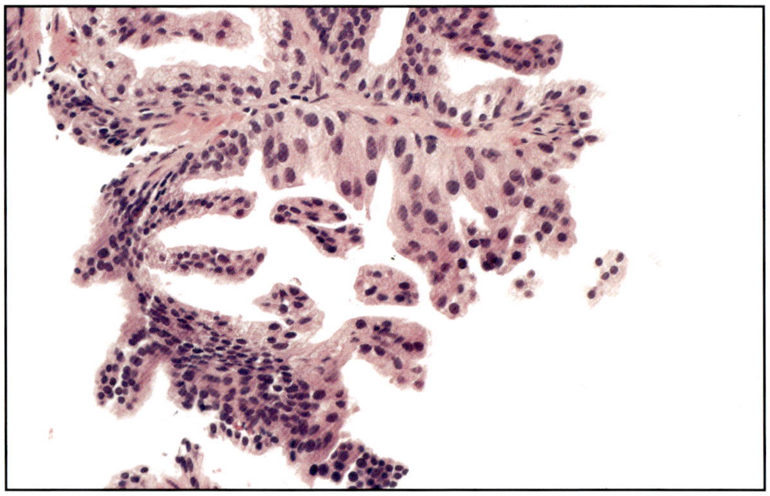

■ **i11.2** *Low-grade PIN in needle biopsy: Nuclear enlargement and nuclear size variability.*

Nuclear aberrations of low-grade PIN separate it from usual epithelial hyperplasia and from high-grade PIN **t11.7**. The most characteristic cytologic changes in low-grade PIN are a marked increase in nuclear size (nucleomegaly) **i11.2, i11.3** and markedly increased variability in nuclear size (anisokaryosis) (McNeal 1986) **i11.2**. Nucleoli are allowable in low-grade PIN, but they should be infrequent and small. Hyperchromasia of the nuclei should not be evident.

■ **t11.7 PIN Diagnostic Criteria**

Feature	Low-grade PIN	High-grade PIN
Architecture	Luminal cell crowding, irregular spacing, and multilayering	Similar to low-grade PIN but more pronounced. Patterns: Cribriform, tufting, micropapillary, and flat
Basal cell layer	Intact	May show decrease in basal cell number
Luminal cell cytology: (at 400×)		
Nuclei	Enlarged; marked size variation	Enlarged; size and shape variation
Chromatin	Normal	Increased density and clumping
Nucleoli	Rarely prominent	Large and prominent, sometimes multiple, similar to invasive carcinoma
Cytoplasm	Amphophilic	Amphophilic

Bostwick 1995A and McNeal 1986

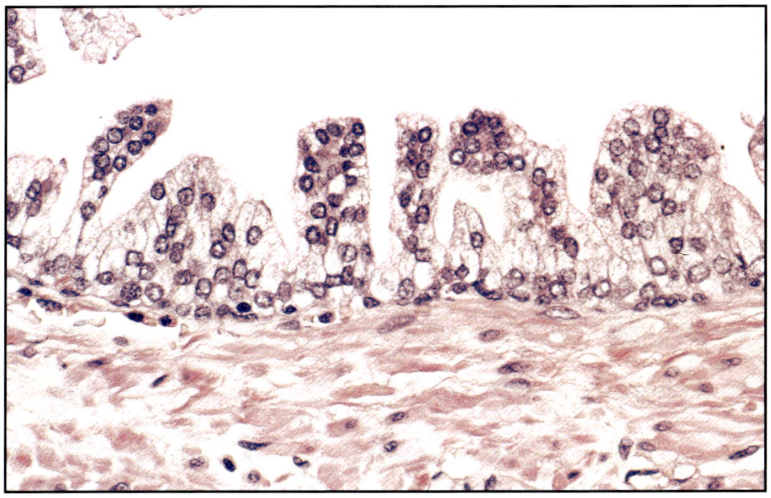

■ **i11.3** *Low-grade PIN with a mixed tufted and micropapillary growth pattern.*

Mitotic figures and apoptotic figures are difficult to detect in low-grade PIN, with frequencies of 0.05% and 0.7%, respectively (Giannulis 1993, Montironi 1993A). These levels are intermediate between usual hyperplasia and high-grade PIN.

The differential diagnosis of low-grade PIN encompasses many entities but centers on usual epithelial hyperplasia and high-grade PIN. Usual epithelial hyperplasia may be mistaken for low-grade PIN when oblique sectioning results in pseudostratification of nuclei or when there is nuclear enlargement. The distinction between benign hyperplastic glands and low-grade PIN is not very reproducible (Epstein 1995B, Tsuchiya 1993). In 1 interobserver study (Epstein 1995B), in no case was there uniform agreement between urologic pathologists on a diagnosis of low-grade PIN, and in a second study (Tsuchiya 1993) the lowest consensus occurred when the differential diagnosis was normal versus low-grade PIN. Thus, the mild nuclear changes of low-grade PIN may not constitute a viable diagnostic category. In this regard, the prostate is similar to other anatomic sites, where it can be difficult or impossible to distinguish mild dysplasia from reactive or hyperplastic change.

Adjunctive techniques that have been forwarded to aid in distinguishing usual hyperplasia from low-grade PIN include mitotic counting (Giannulis 1993) and nuclear volume estimates (Montironi 1991). The extremely low frequency of mitotic figures in low-grade PIN and the labor-intensive nature of both techniques do not support their routine use in daily practice. Additional reactive and hyperplastic conditions in the prostate that are difficult to distinguish from low-grade PIN include inflammatory atypia and basal cell hyperplasia. These differential distinctions are not discussed in detail in this chapter because at present low-grade PIN does not constitute a distinct clinicopathologic entity.

In addition to difficulty in pathologic recognition, a compelling reason to not diagnose low-grade PIN is that there is no proven association with invasive carcinoma. This was first suggested by a study of whole glands with and without carcinoma (McNeal 1986). Whereas high-grade PIN was more often found in glands with cancer than in those without cancer, low-grade PIN was actually found more often in benign glands. That it is not necessary to diagnose low-grade PIN in needle biopsy is supported by clinical follow-up data, which have demonstrated a uniformly low rate (mean of 8 series = 18%) of detection of carcinoma on rebiopsy **t11.8**. This rate is actually lower than the rate of subsequent carcinoma diagnosis when a benign diagnosis is given for the initial biopsy **t11.8**. Similarly, although the data are scanty ($n = 27$ patients), low-grade PIN in TURP chips and simple (open) prostatectomies does not constitute a risk factor for subsequent detection of carcinoma (Samaratunga 1995). This stance of not reporting low-grade PIN in needle biopsy or transurethral resectates has been advocated by a number of urologic pathologists (Epstein 1995B). The concern is that these patients might be subjected to unnecessary biopsies and that undue physician and patient concern might be elicited by noting the word *neoplasia* in a diagnosis of low-grade PIN. Therefore, our current practice is to report any changes thought to represent low-grade PIN as "benign prostatic tissue" in the diagnostic line. For these patients, persistent clinical abnormalities such as an elevated serum PSA or abnormal DRE should drive rebiopsy considerations (Raviv 1996B).

■ **t11.8 Incidence of Carcinoma in Follow-up Biopsy**

	Initial Core Biopsy Diagnosis		
Study	**Benign**	**Low-grade PIN**	**High-grade PIN**
Brawer 1991	—	2/11 18.2%)	10/10 (100%)
Weinstein 1993	—	—	10/33 (30%)
Keetch 1995	82/427 (19.2%)	4/21 (19.0%)	19/37 (51.3%)
Davidson 1995	15/112 (13.4%)	—	35/100 (35%)
Aboseif 1995	—	2/12 (16.7%)	19/24 (79.2%)
Ellis 1995	10/69 (14.5%)	0/9 (0%)	5/5 (100%)
Raviv 1996B	—	6/45 (13.3%)	23/48 (47.9%)
Langer 1996	—	2/5 (40%)	13/48 (27.1%)
Perachino 1997	41/107 (38.3%)	4/20 (20%)	15/21 (71.4%)
Fleshner 1997	39/103 (37.9%)	3/6 (50%)	9/16 (56.3%)
O'Dowd 2000	702/3,544 (19.8%)	—	295/1,306 (22.6%)
Alsikafi 2001	—	—	3/21 (14%)
Kamoi 2000	—	—	10/45 (22%)
Vis 2001	51/462 (11.0%)	—	3/30 (10%)
Kronz 2001B	—	—	79/245 (32.2%)
Park 2001	—	—	21/43 (48.8%)
Borboroglu 2001	—	—	20/45 (44%)
Total	**940/4,824 (20%)**	**23/129 (18%)**	**589/2,077 (28%)**

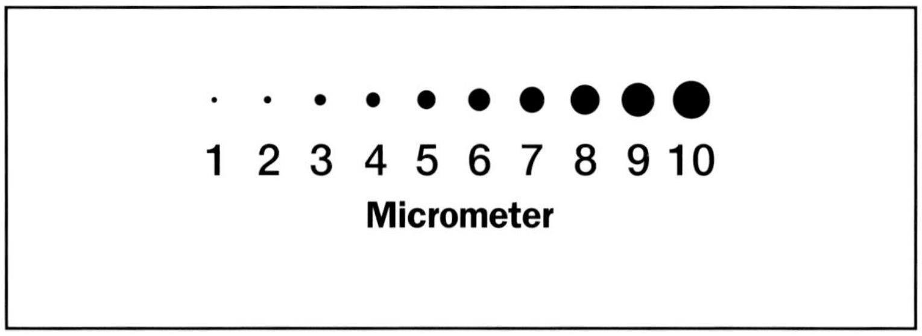

■ **f11.3** *Size of 1 to 10 micron diameter circles as they would appear under the light microscope at 400×.*

As discussed later in this chapter, high-grade PIN in needle biopsy and TURP chips is a significant risk factor for subsequent detection of adenocarcinoma, and rebiopsy is recommended, so distinguishing low-grade from high-grade PIN is most critical. It has been show that "good distinction" between them can be achieved (Tsuchiya 1993). Here, the best discriminator is prominent nucleoli, which should be 1μm to 3μm in diameter to diagnose high-grade PIN. Difficulty in excluding low-grade PIN arises when the nucleoli are not small and pinpoint but are more prominent, when only rare nuclei contain a large nucleolus, or when the nuclei are hyperchromatic but there is insufficient chromatin clearing to allow appreciation of intranuclear detail. First, short of morphometric measurements of nucleoli, which are not practical, it should be acknowledged that morphologic definition of a prominent nucleolus is imprecise in some cases. The 400× appearance of circles ranging from 1μm to 10μm in diameter is presented in **f11.3**. This figure shows how difficult it can be to distinguish between a nucleolus that is 1μm in diameter and one that is 2μm in diameter. If the nuclear atypia seems borderline between low- and high-grade PIN, sharing the case with colleagues or obtaining additional sections (levels) is advisable. A second common PIN grading question is how many nuclei with prominent nucleoli should one visualize in excluding low-grade PIN and diagnosing high-grade PIN. No data addressing this issue exist, but it has been our practice to exclude low-grade PIN if even a few cells are identified with profound nucleomegaly and with macronucleoli. Enlarged, hyperchromatic nuclei with clumped chromatin do rule out low-grade PIN. Finally, eccentrically positioned nucleoli and multiple nucleoli do not distinguish low-grade from high-grade PIN (Montironi 1991).

As in all grading schemes, there will always be an element of subjectivity in grading PIN. In the future, biomarkers or algorithmic methods (Montironi 1995B) may allow a more objective separation of low-grade and high grade PIN. A number of morphologic, histochemical, immunophenotypic, and genetic markers demonstrate differences between low-grade PIN and high-grade PIN, such as nuclear volume (Lopez-Beltran 2000), mucin (Sentinelli 1993), peanut agglutinin lectin binding (Janssen 1996), immunoreactive epidermal growth factor receptor (Turkeri 1994), immunoreactive androgen receptor (Magi-Galluzzi 1997), immunoreactive A-80 antigen (Gould 1996), and DNA content (Baretton 1994, Crissman 1993). However, at present these remain experimental markers, and the diagnostic distinction between low-grade and high-grade PIN is purely histomorphologic and based on interpretation of hematoxylin and eosin (H&E)-stained sections.

In summary, at this time low-grade PIN does not warrant recognition for routine diagnostic purposes.

[11.8] High-Grade PIN

High-grade PIN is a histologically well-defined entity, with distinctive architectural and cytologic abnormalities. There are 4 major structural patterns of high-grade PIN growth **f11.4** and several minor variations (Bostwick 1993) **t11.9**. The dominant patterns are the tufting **i11.4**, micropapillary **i11.5**, cribriform **i11.6**, and flat **i11.7** motifs. These patterns are important for diagnostic recognition but are not related to presence or absence of adjacent carcinoma and are not related to histologic grade of the invasive carcinoma (Bostwick 1993). Uncommon to rare variants include the solid pattern (at 5%) **i11.8** (Bostwick 1993), signet-ring high-grade PIN **i11.8, i11.9** (Reyes 1997B),

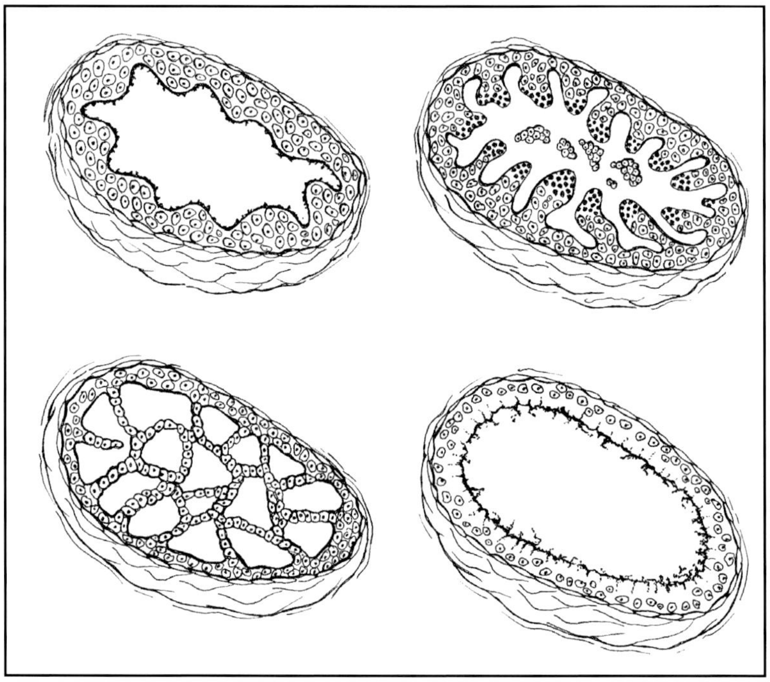

■ **f11.4** *Architectural patterns of high-grade PIN, as defined by Bostwick 1993. (Schematic illustration adapted from Bostwick 1993, with permission).*

■ **t11.9 Types of High-grade PIN**

Most common patterns: tufting, micropapillary, cribriform, flat
Uncommon variants: Solid pattern, signet ring type, small cell neuroendocrine type, mucinous type, foamy gland type, inverted pattern

■ **t11.10 Most Common High-Grade PIN Patterns**

Pattern	Needle Biopsy[1]	TURP Chips[2]	Radical Prostatectomy[3]
Tufting	56%	10%	97%
Micropapillary	29%	41%	66%
Flat	15%	3%	21%
Cribriform	0-5%	0%	19%

[1]Predominant pattern in cases without carcinoma (Davidson 1995, Reyes 1997A)
[2]Pure pattern in cases both with and without carcinoma. In additional cases micropapillary pattern was mixed with tufting or flat pattern (28%), and flat pattern was mixed with tufting pattern (17%) (Pacelli 1997)
[3]Expressed as percentage of PIN cases. From a series of 195 radical prostatectomy specimens with carcinoma (Qian 1997B)

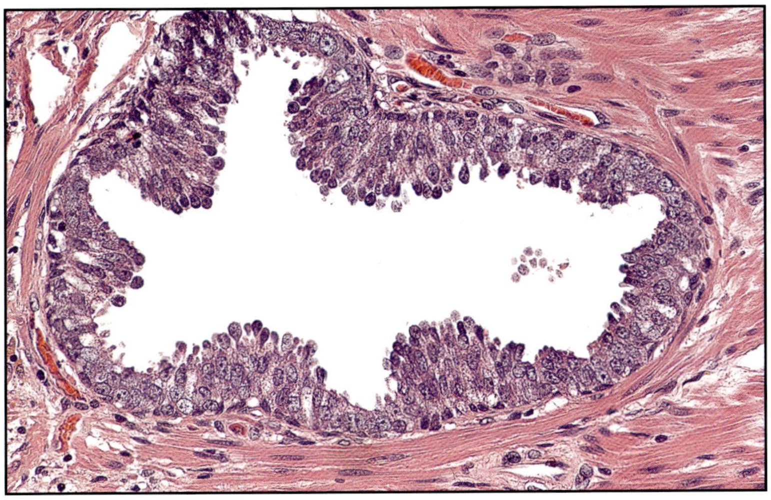

■ **i11.4** *Tufting or mound-like intraluminal projections in high-grade PIN.*

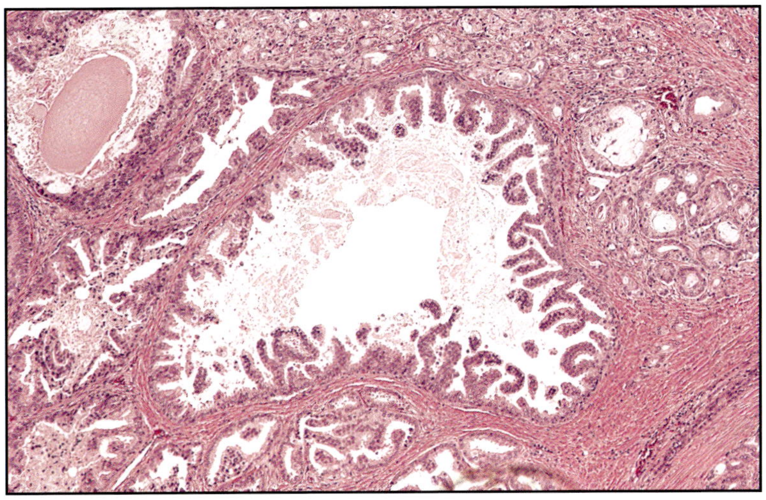

■ **i11.5** *Micropapillary high-grade PIN with adjacent invasive small acinar adenocarcinoma.*

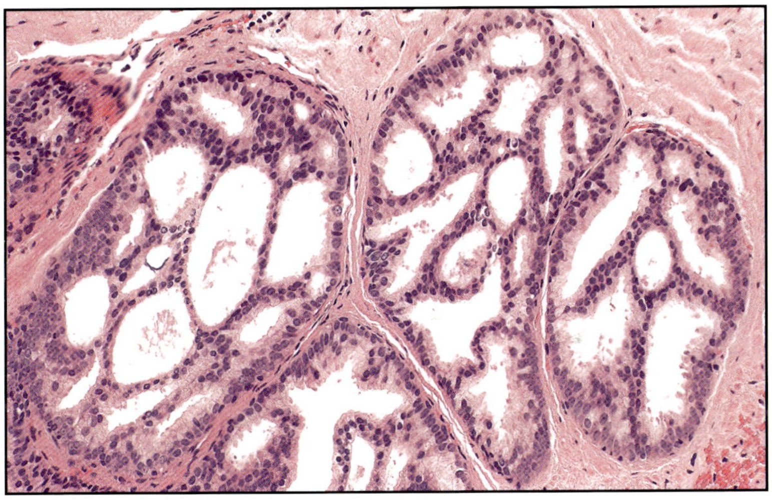

■ **i11.6** *Cribriform pattern of high-grade PIN.*

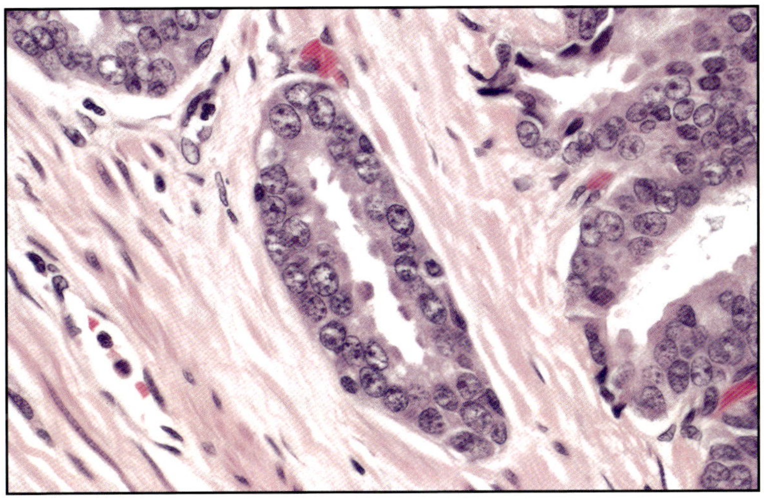

■ **i11.7** *Flat high-grade PIN. There are only a few cell layers and the luminal border is also flat. Without basal cells, this gland would be considered an example of usual invasive small acinar adenocarcinoma.*

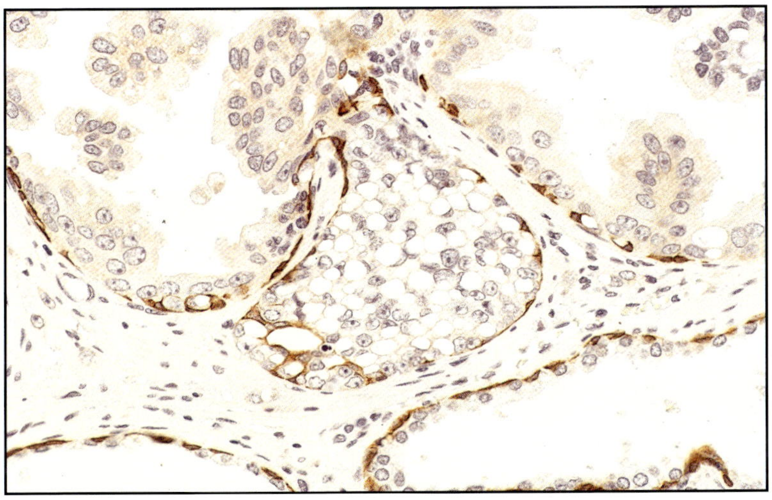

■ **i11.8** *Solid signet ring growth of high-grade PIN cells. The intraepithelial nature is substantiated by this 34βE12 immunohistochemical stain for basal cells.*

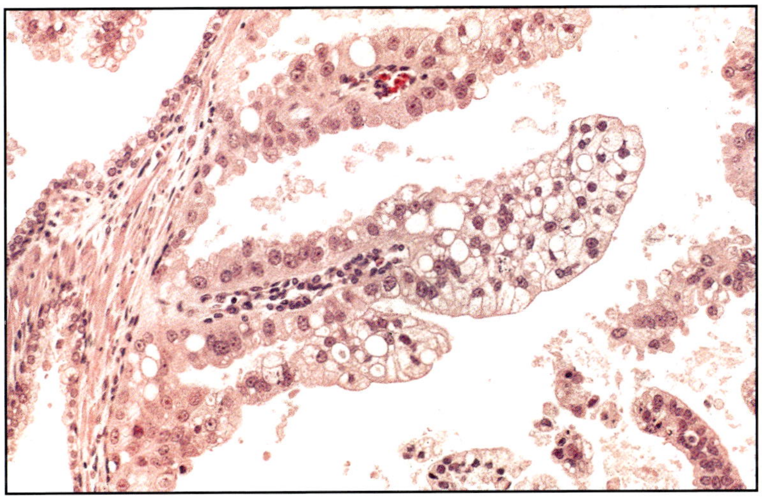

■ **i11.9** *Signet ring high-grade PIN: A rare variant.*

small cell neuroendocrine high-grade PIN **i11.10, i11.11** (Reyes 1997B), mucinous high-grade PIN **i11.12** (Reyes 1997B), foamy gland high-grade PIN **i11.13** (Berman 2000), "inverted" high-grade PIN **i11.14** (Argani 2001), and growth of high-grade PIN cells along fibrovascular stalks **i11.15**. Additional variations include arches **i11.16**, "Roman" bridges, and trabeculae (little beams) **i11.17** (Bostwick 1993).

The flat and cribriform patterns are less common, especially in pure form. The most frequently detected high-grade PIN structures

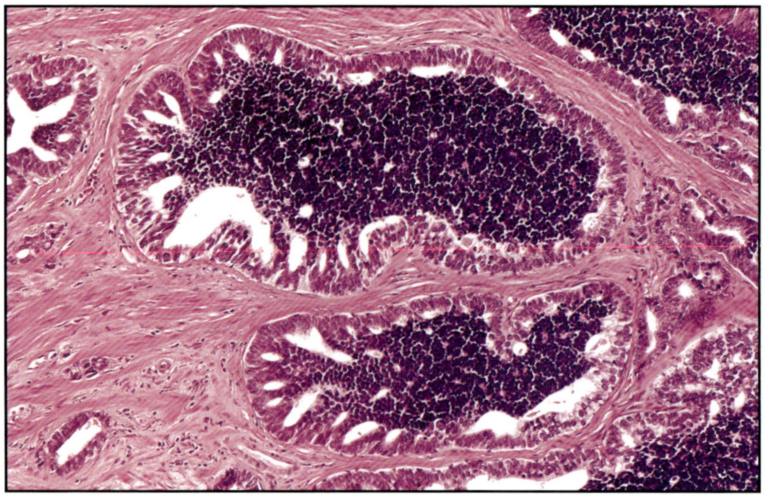

■ **i11.10** *Small cell neuroendocrine high-grade PIN with central neuroendocrine cells with rosette-like formations.*

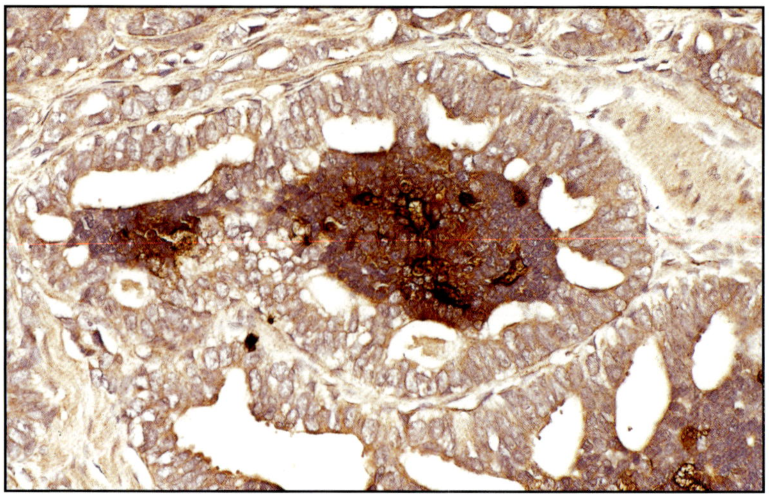

■ **i11.11** *Small cell neuroendocrine high-grade PIN: A chromogranin immunostain confirms neuroendocrine differentiation in the small cells.*

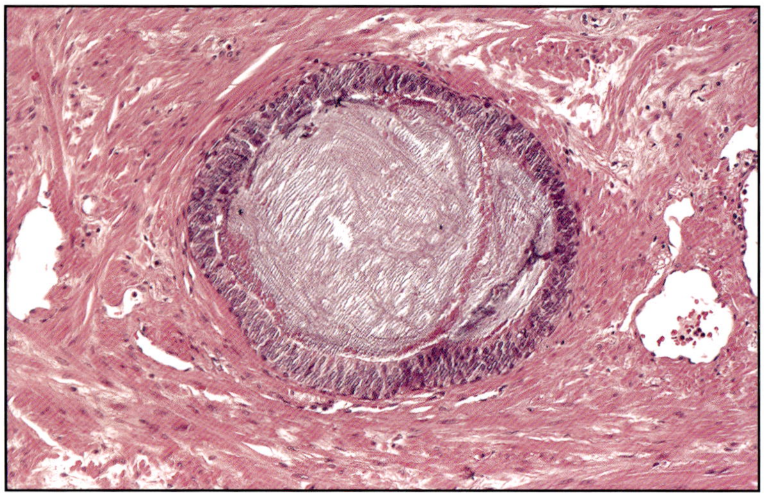

■ **i11.12** *Mucinous high-grade PIN. Blue mucin fills this flat high-grade PIN gland.*

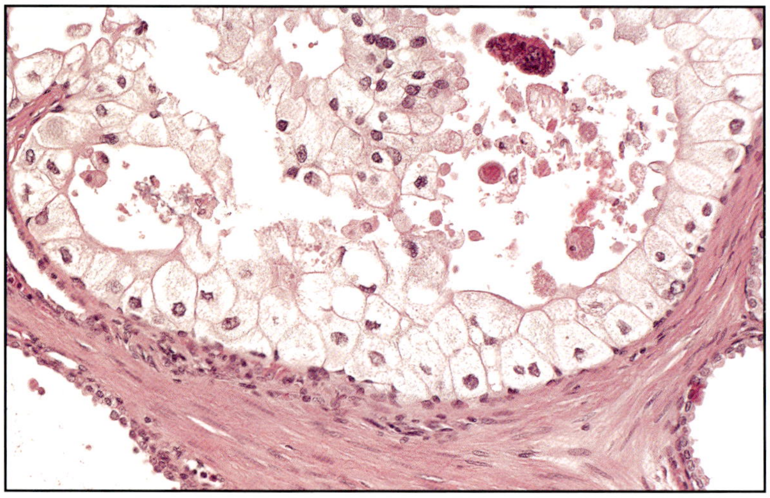

■ **i11.13** *Foamy gland high-grade PIN with xanthomatous cytoplasm.*

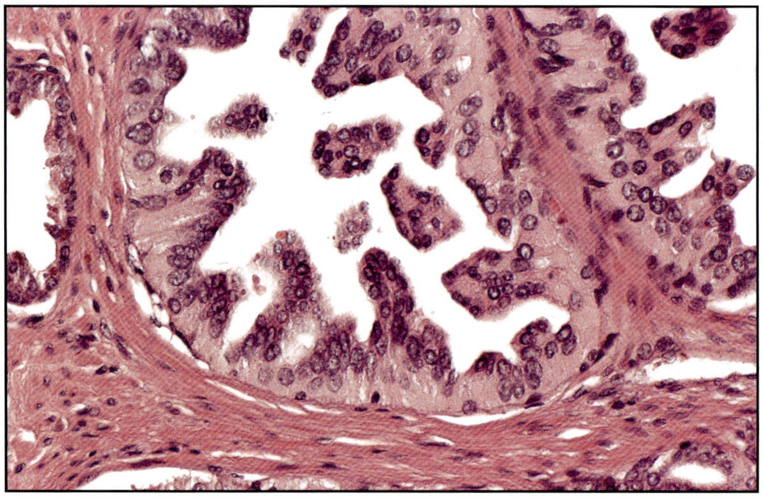

■ **i11.14** *"Inverted" pattern high-grade PIN with nuclei aligned along luminal border.*

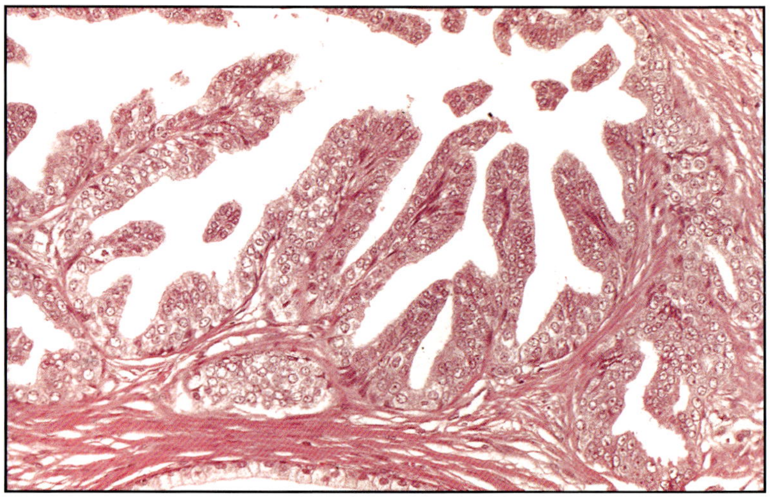

■ **i11.15** *Growth along fibrovascular stalks is uncommon in high-grade PIN.*

are the tufting and micropapillary ones **t11.10**. The tufting and micropapillary patterns are also the most voluminous (Qian 1997B).

The patterns often are found admixed in the same gland and in adjacent glands. In particular, partial gland involvement is also very common **i11.18** and is associated with the tufting and micropapillary patterns (Bostwick 1993). The tufting, or moundlike, pattern often is admixed with the micropapillary pattern **i11.19**. We found this mixed pattern in 58% of 156 cases of isolated

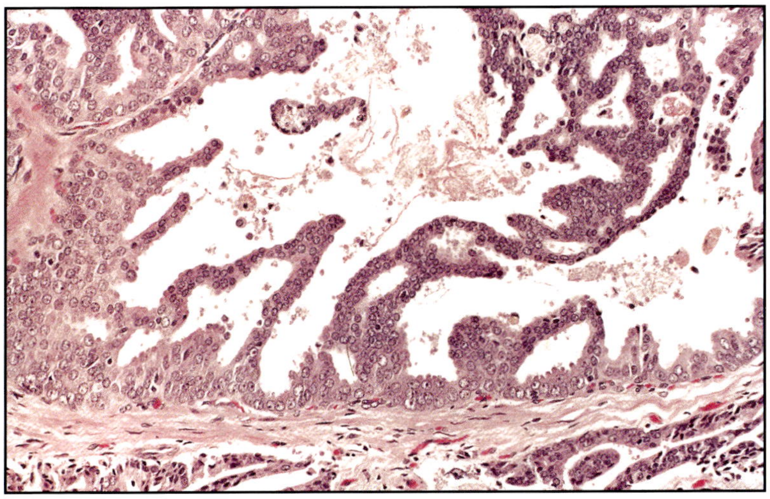

■ **i11.16** *Arch formation in high-grade PIN.*

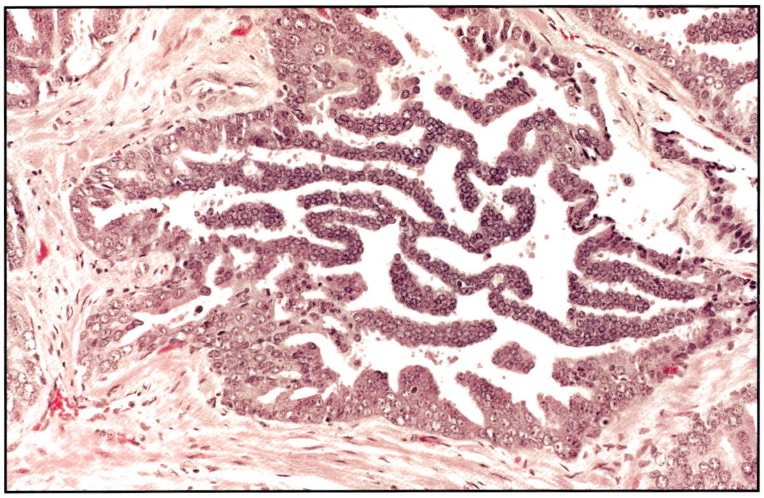

■ **i11.17** *Bars or small beams known as trabeculae span this high-grade PIN gland.*

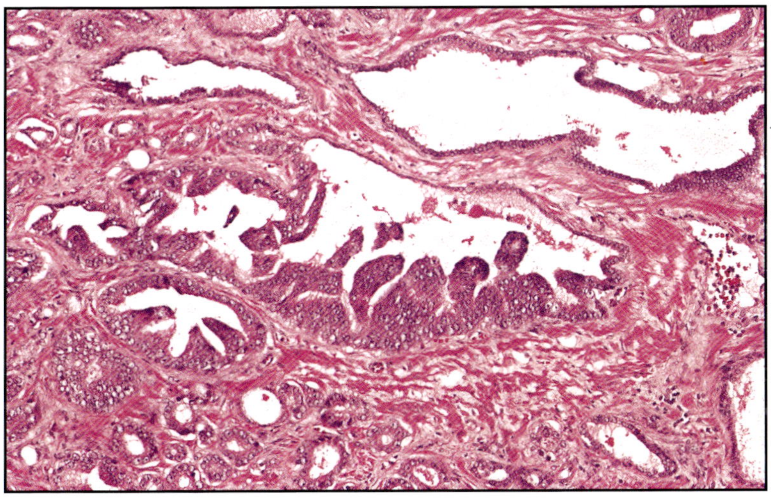

■ **i11.18** *Partial gland involvement in high-grade PIN with polarization along one side. There is an associated invasive small acinar adenocarcinoma.*

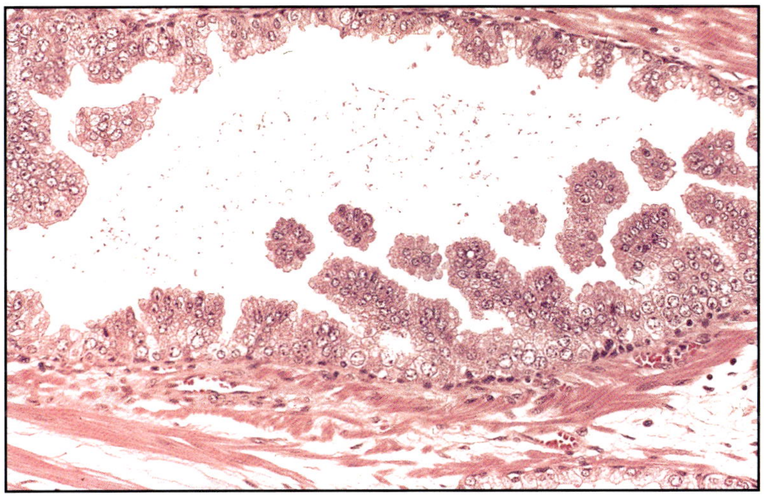

■ **i11.19** *Mixed tufting and micropapillary patterns in the same high-grade PIN gland.*

high-grade PIN in needle biopsy. Another 22% were mixed tufting and flat **i11.20** (Reyes 1997A).

Like low-grade PIN, high-grade PIN usually is recognizable at low magnifications. Accordingly, one should first survey all prostatic tissue at scanning magnification. In general, high-grade PIN glands will stand out as a cluster of darker, complex glands **i11.21**. The size and complexity of high-grade PIN resemble those of typical hyperplastic glands, yet high-grade PIN glands are darker because of their greater number of nuclei, stratification and crowding of nuclei, higher DNA content in the individual nuclei, and amphophilia of cytoplasm. High-grade PIN can present as large, complex, and branching glands **i11.21–i11.23** or as smaller glands closer in size to small acinar adenocarcinoma **i11.24**. Usually the high-grade PIN glands are regularly arranged, without any particular architectural order; uncommonly a lobular arrangement may be appreciated **i11.25**.

The extent of high-grade PIN in needle biopsy and TURP chips usually is focal **t11.11,** so a careful and thorough high-power search of all sampled tissue is necessary. In needle biopsy, isolated high-grade PIN usually is a single focus of <1mm in greatest dimension, with a mean of 0.68mm (Keetch 1995) **i11.26**. In most cases of high-grade PIN in TURP chips, the amount of high-grade PIN is focal, involving 1

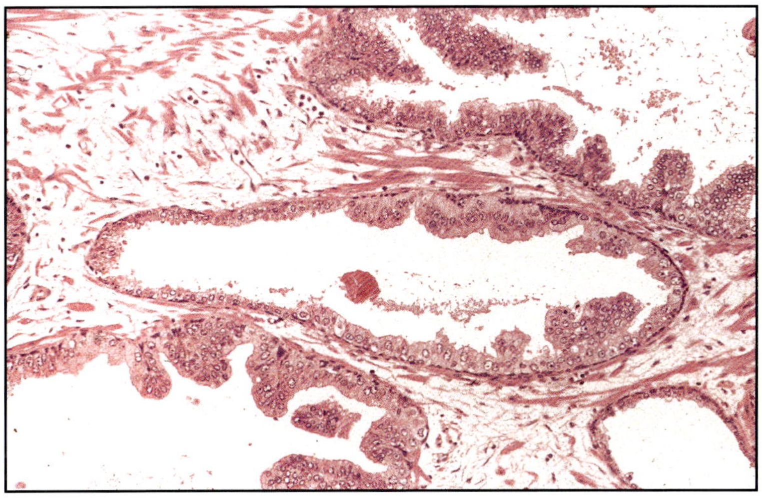

■ **i11.20** *Mixed tufting and flat patterns in the same high-grade PIN gland.*

prostatic chip (Pacelli 1997) and <1 low-power (4×) field in greatest diameter (Gaudin 1997) **i11.27**.

In the whole prostate gland (postmortem examination, cystoprostatectomy specimens, radical prostatectomy specimens),

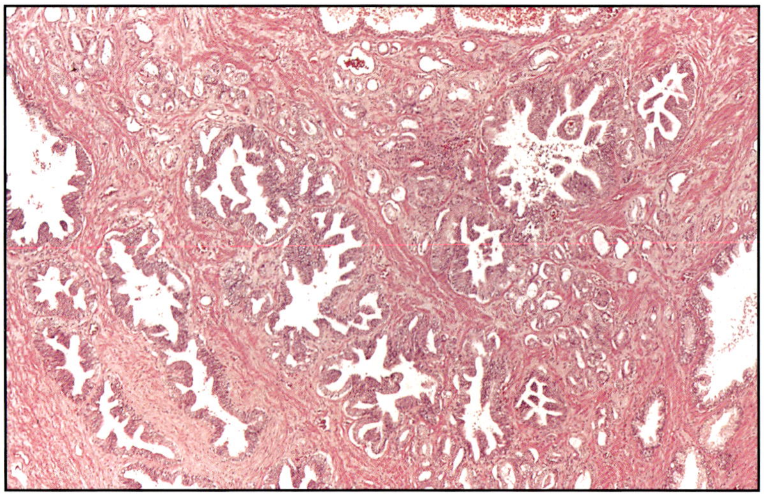

■ **i11.21** *At low magnification high-grade PIN glands are conspicuous by their medium size, complexity, and dark appearance. In this field, the haphazardly distributed small glands represent admixed invasive adenocarcinoma.*

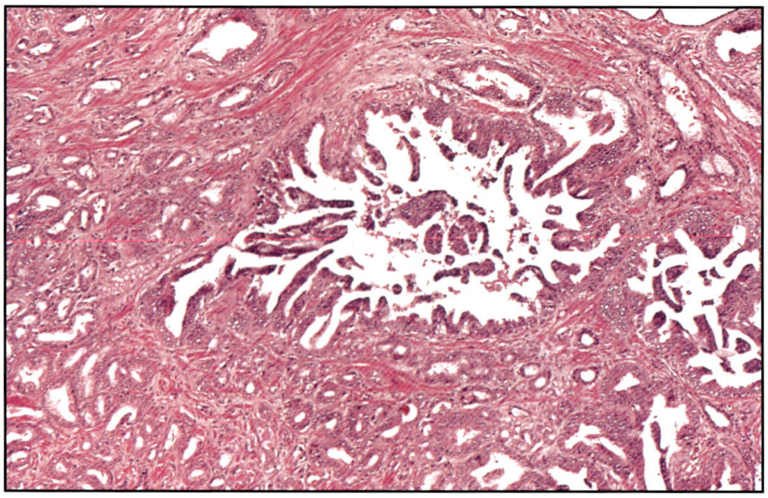

■ **i11.22** *Irregular, fairly large high-grade PIN gland with irregular outer contour and outpouchings. Invasive adenocarcinoma surrounds the high-grade PIN.*

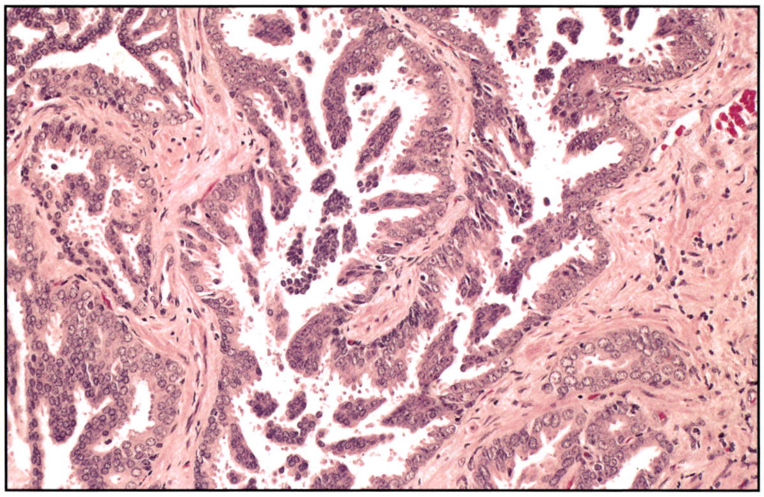

■ **i11.23** *Branching of high-grade PIN gland.*

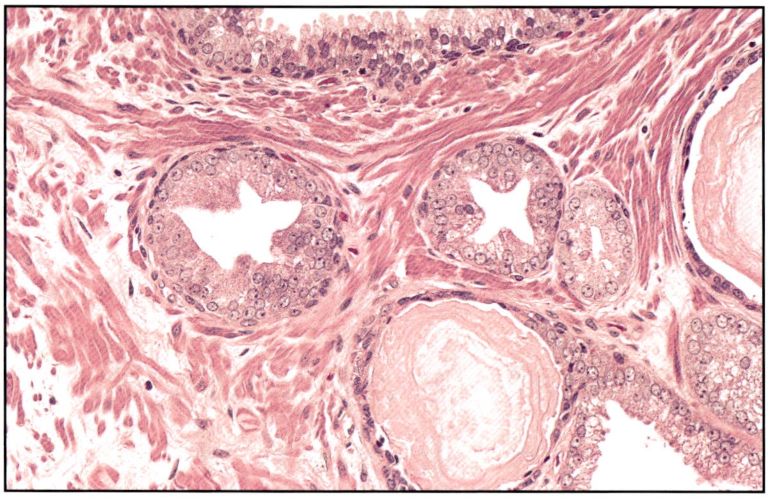

■ **i11.24** *Smaller gland profiles of high-grade PIN. These could be due to sectioning across outpouches of high-grade PIN.*

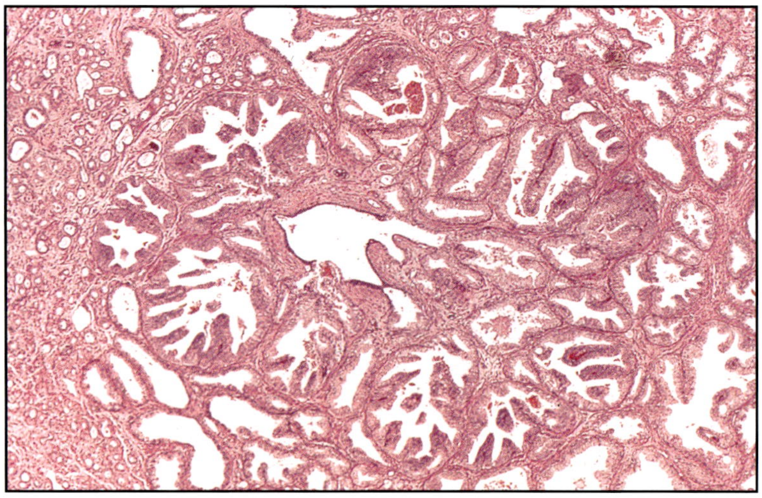

■ **i11.25** *Unusual lobular configuration of high-grade PIN glands surrounding an atrophic duct.*

■ t11.11 **Extent of High-grade PIN**

Needle biopsy tissue:	Usually a single focus less than 1mm
TURP chip tissue:	Involves a single chip and less than one 4× field
Radical prostatectomy tissues*:	Mean number of foci = 17 (range 1-62)
	5% of gland involved
	Mean volume 1.3cc-2.1cc (range 0cc-8.1cc)

*In the setting of admixed carcinoma

high-grade PIN usually is readily visualized. Here, high-grade PIN is most often a peripheral zone and multifocal process **i11.28**. High-grade PIN may exist as a pure, isolated proliferation without carcinoma or at a distance from carcinoma **i11.28**. It may also be found immediately adjacent to **i11.29** and admixed with invasive adenocarcinoma **i11.21**. Peripheral zone localization is found in the majority of whole glands, and the transition zone may be involved in 18% to 49% of cases (de la Torre 1993, Qian 1997A, Silvestri 1995). Transition zone involvement by itself is rare without concomitant peripheral zone involvement (Qian 1997B). Quite uncommon (at 5% [Bostwick 1993]) is the finding of high-grade PIN within nodular hyperplasia (BPH) in the transition zone **i11.27**. A single case of high-grade PIN involving the prostatic utricle has been reported (Erdamar 1998).

Although high-grade PIN is variable in extent in whole glands from different patients, overall it is easier to detect in whole glands removed for clinical stage T2 prostate cancer than in needle

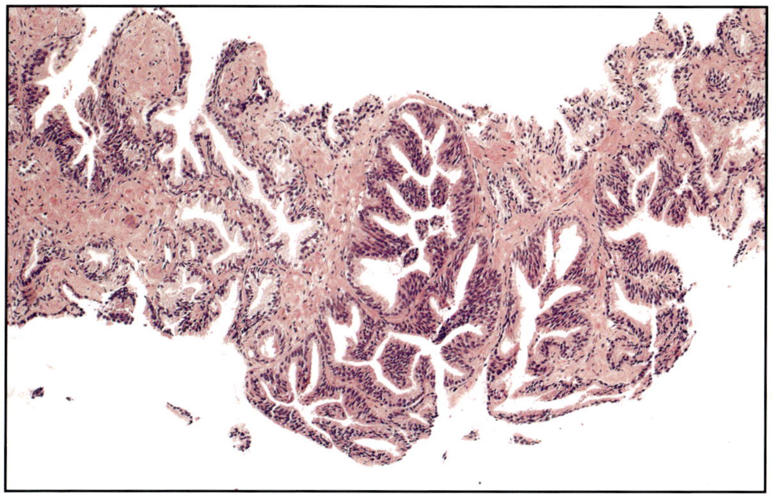

■ **i11.26** *Typical extent of high-grade PIN in needle biopsy tissue. Note darker appearance compared to adjacent paler benign glands.*

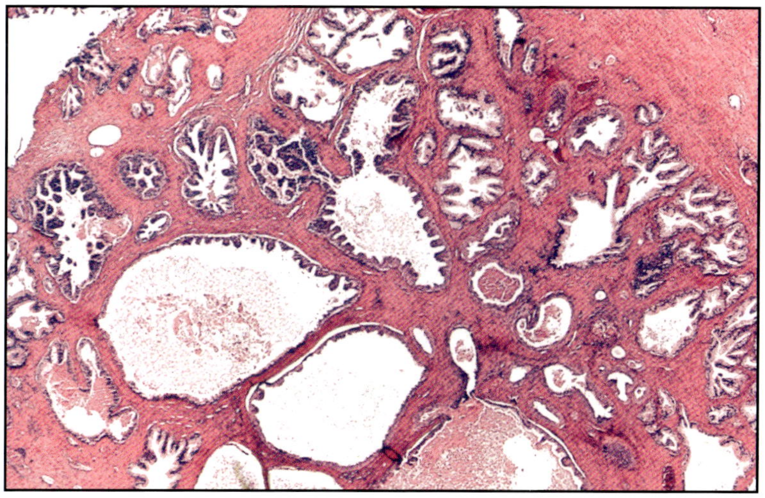

■ **i11.27** *Typical amount of high-grade PIN in TURP chips: A single nodule in a single chip is involved.*

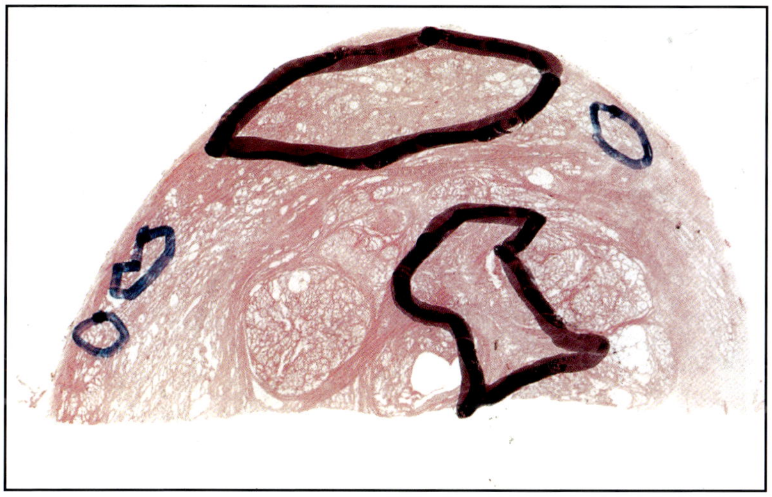

■ **i11.28** *Three small peripheral zone foci of high-grade PIN (blue) physically separate from a peripheral zone and a transition zone carcinoma (black).*

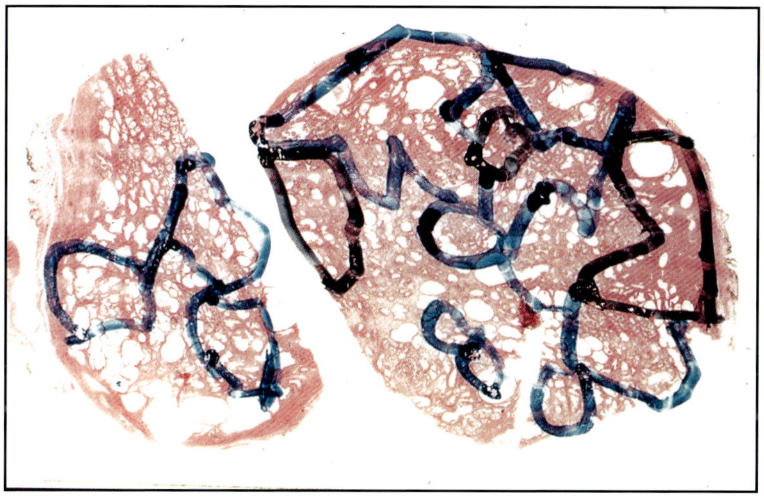

■ **i11.29** *Complex spatial relationship between high-grade PIN (blue) and carcinoma (black).*

biopsies. This is so because this high-grade PIN in this setting of carcinoma in the whole gland usually is intermediate (55% of cases) to extensive (35% of cases) in amount (Quinn 1990). Only 10% of cases were judged minimal (<1.8mm in diameter) (Quinn 1990) **i11.30**. The mean number of fields of high-grade PIN per gland is 17, with a range of 1 to 62 fields (Bostwick 1993). In glands removed for carcinoma, on average, 4.5% of the gland is involved by high-grade PIN (Humphrey 1992); mean volumes of 1.3cm^3 (range 0cm^3 to 8.1cm^3) and 2.1cm^3(range 0.04cm^3 to 6.9cm^3) have been reported (Häggman 1997B, Qian 1997B).

High-grade PIN may be more difficult to identify in glands removed for incidental T1a–T1b carcinoma (detected initially in TURP chips) and in whole glands without carcinoma. In 44% of T1a–T1b cases high-grade PIN was minimal in amount, with 44% being intermediate and 12% extensive (Quinn 1990). In whole glands without carcinoma, a mean of 0.7 foci were seen in 1 study, compared with 1.6 to 2.7 foci in glands with carcinoma (Silvestri 1995). Low-power recognition of high-grade PIN in whole glands may help pinpoint small foci of associated invasive carcinoma, but otherwise, as discussed later in this chapter, diagnosis of high-grade PIN in whole glands is not nearly as critical as its diagnosis in needle biopsy, TURP chips, and simple prostatectomy specimens.

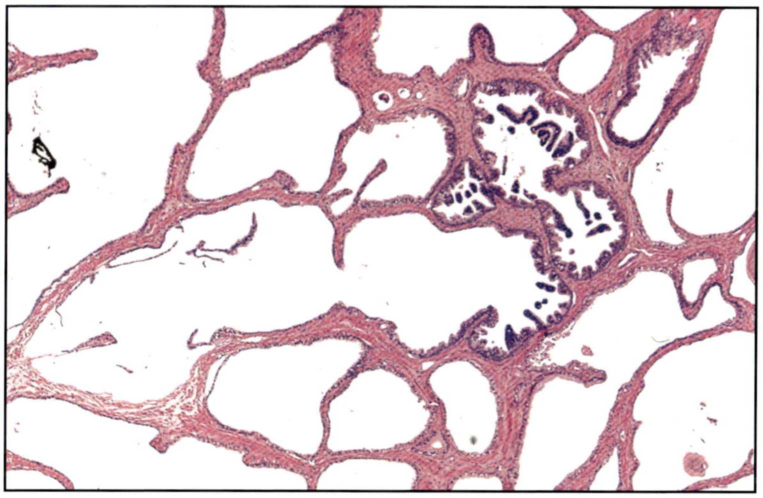

■ **i11.30** *Focal, isolated high-grade PIN found in a background of cystic atrophy.*

Most foci of PIN are recognizable as dark, complex glands at low power, with the notable exceptions of flat high-grade PIN (Reyes 1997A), PIN involvement of large, cystically dilated glands (Bostwick 1993), and high-grade PIN with cleared cytoplasm (Bostwick 1993). Flat

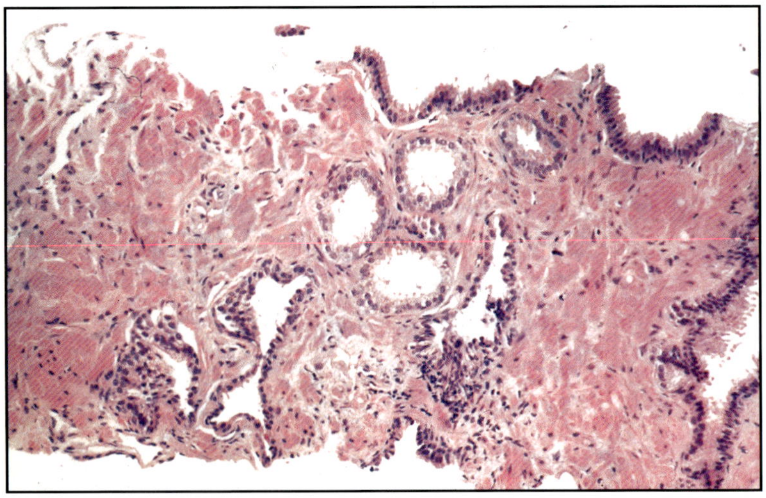

■ **i11.31** *Four pale glands of flat high-grade PIN in needle biopsy. Distinction from invasive carcinoma and benign glands is difficult (actually impossible) at this magnification.*

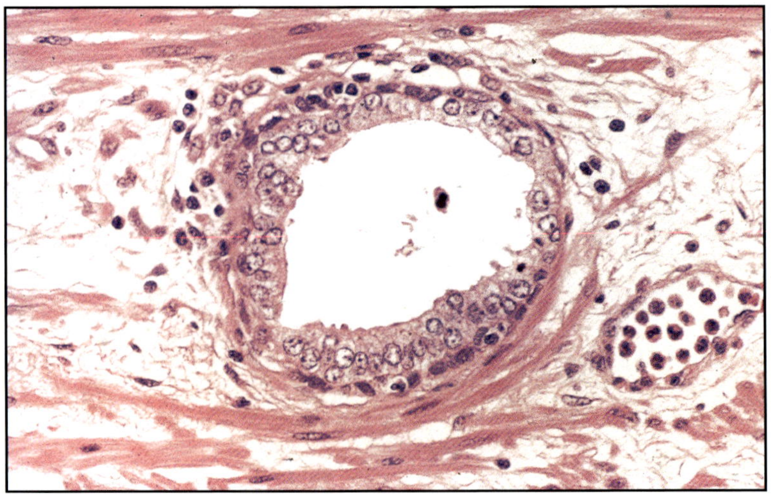

■ **i11.32** *A flat pattern high-grade PIN gland.*

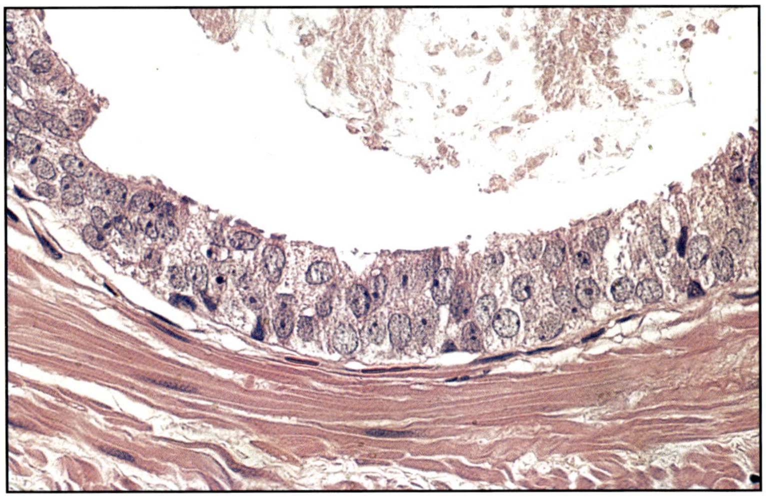

■ **i11.33** *Flat high-grade PIN: A flattened lining layer and flattened luminal surface.*

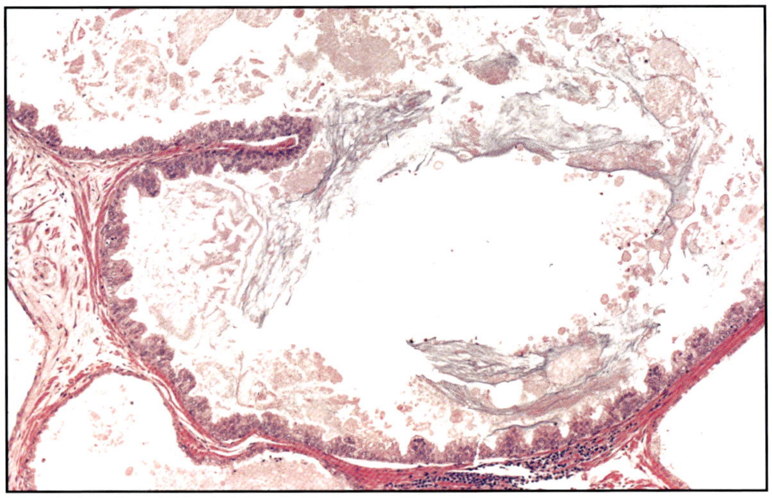

■ **i11.34** *High-grade PIN in a large, dilated gland. Note tufting pattern and intraluminal wispy blue mucin.*

high-grade PIN may be difficult to appreciate from a low-power perspective because these glands appear pale **i11.31** and less complex, and in needle biopsy the foci are of smaller mean size (mean = 0.37mm, range 0.07mm to 0.9mm) than that of the more common tufting and micropapillary pattern (mean = 0.67mm, range 0.1mm to 2mm) (Reyes 1997A). The pale nature of flat high-grade PIN glands results from the lack of significant multilayering of nuclei **i11.32, i11.33**. The flat pattern typically has only 1 or 2 layers of luminal cells (Bostwick 1993). It is easier to detect flat high-grade PIN when it is associated with production of intraluminal mucinous masses (Reyes 1997B). The glands in this unusual mucinous type of high-grade PIN are filled and distended with intraluminal blue mucin **i11.12**. High-grade PIN involvement of cystically dilated glands may also be missed by low-power examination **i11.34**. Such cystification of high-grade PIN glands has been noted in 10% of radical prostatectomy specimens (Bostwick 1993). Finally, high-grade PIN with cleared or foamy cytoplasm **i11.13** may confound attempts to identify high-grade PIN from "high altitudes."

At high-power magnifications, high-grade PIN displays basal cells and atypical luminal cells. Basal cell presence is a key criterion in the diagnosis of PIN, yet they may be difficult to find because increasing grades of PIN are associated with basal cell loss and disruption of the basal cell layer (Bostwick 1987). This is not a uniform finding, however, and the number of basal cells may be normal **i11.35** or even elevated **i11.36, i11.37**. A scattered distribution of a low number of basal cells is most common **i11.38**. Difficulties in basal cell recognition arise when there is a marked diminution in basal cell number, when oblique sectioning or thick sections render interpretation of number of cell layers difficult **i11.39**, and when distortion or poor preservation make the distinction between basal cells and luminal cells difficult. Indeed, elongated, hyperchromatic, and distorted luminal cell nuclei in invasive carcinoma are easily mistaken for basal cells. These difficulties are compounded by small size of high-grade PIN foci, such as that evident in needle biopsy.

Nuclear abnormalities in luminal cells that resemble those of invasive carcinoma are hallmarks of high-grade PIN **i11.40; t11.7**. In particular, the most characteristic nuclear aberrations in high-grade PIN glands are markedly increased nuclear size, increased chromatin clumping and content, and occasional to numerous, prominent nucleoli (Bostwick 1995A, McNeal 1986). Nuclear shape in high-grade PIN typically is rounded to somewhat oblong **i11.40** but can be quite elongated **i11.41**. Within the individual nuclei, the nucleoli may be single or multiple and centrally or eccentrically

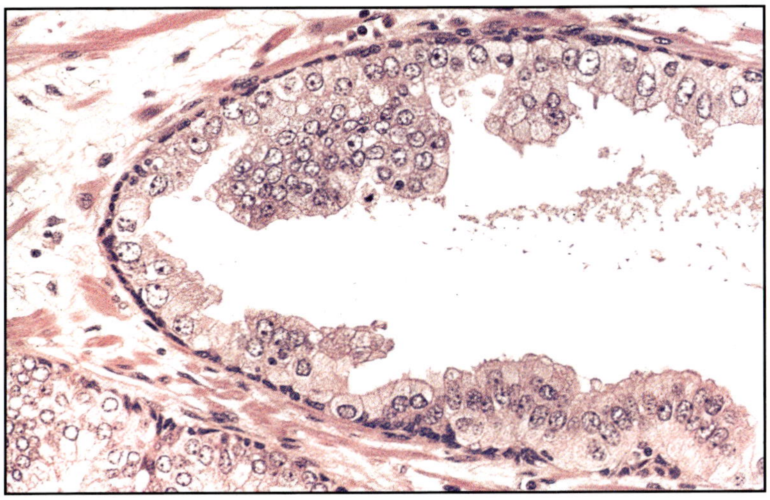

■ **i11.35** *Uniform, circumferential basal cell layer in high-grade PIN, here visualized as a thin rim at the rounded, outer contour of the gland.*

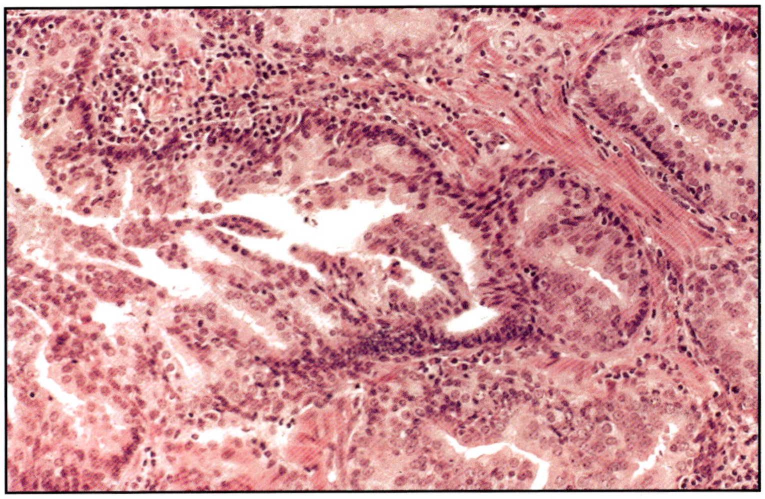

■ **i11.36** *Increased number of basal cells in high-grade PIN. This is an uncommon finding and is most likely a response to another uncommon feature, the presence of a chronic inflammatory cell infiltrate in this high-grade PIN focus.*

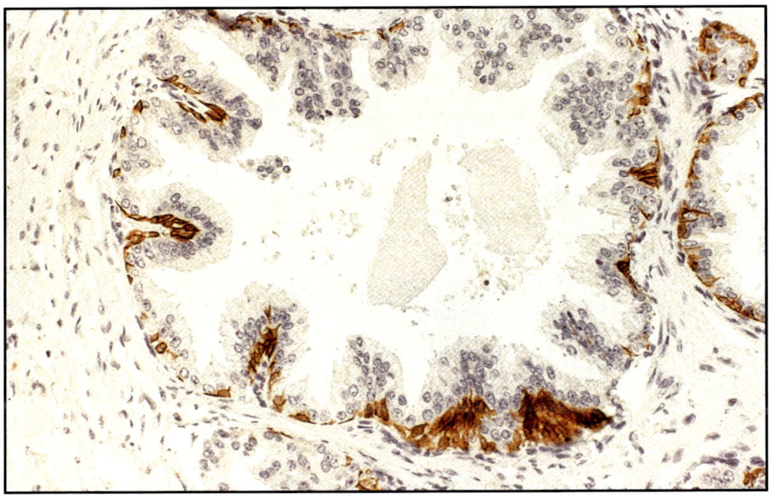

■ **i11.37** *High-grade PIN with focal increase in basal cells highlighted by this 34βE12 immunohistochemical stain.*

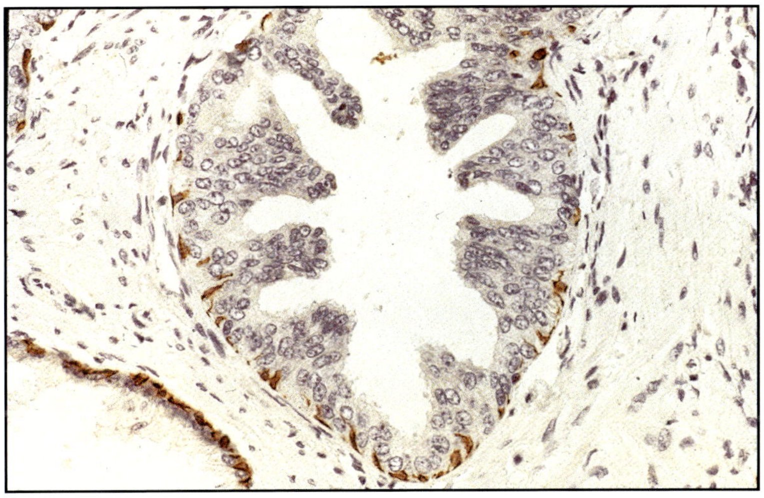

■ **i11.38** *Scattered basal cells in a high-grade PIN gland (34βE12 immunostain).*

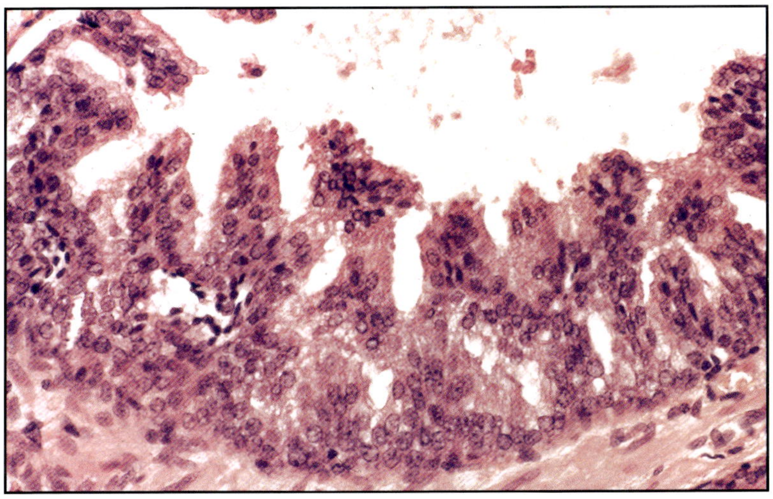

■ **i11.39** *A thick 10μm section of high-grade PIN. Recognition of basal cells is difficult, as is appreciation of nuclear detail.*

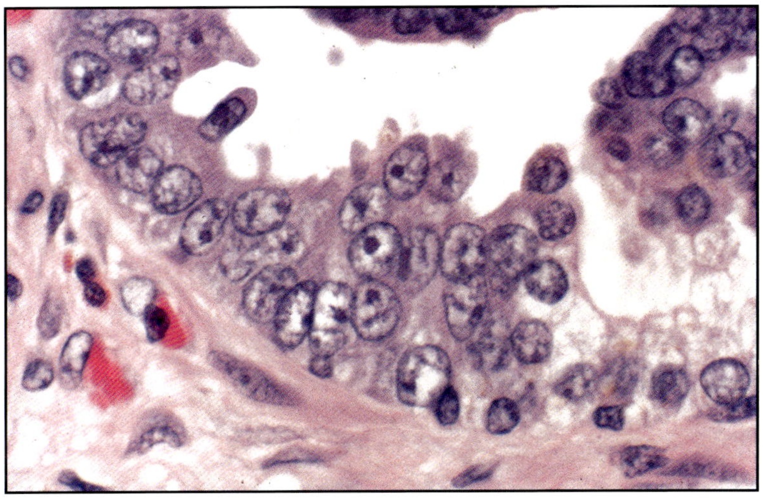

■ **i11.40** *Classical nuclear atypia in high-grade PIN. Note small, rounded, darker basal cell nuclei along the base of the gland.*

positioned. The frequency of mitotic figures and apoptotic bodies in high-grade PIN is exceedingly low but similar to that of carcinoma (Giannulis 1993, Montironi 1993A). Cells in the basal portion of the epithelial lining layer of high-grade PIN exhibit the highest turnover. Even in this location, the mitotic count was only 0.2% (Giannulis 1993), and the apoptotic body count was 1% (Montironi 1993A).

The most diagnostically straightforward high-grade PIN cases are those with classic architecture, easily visualized basal cells, and

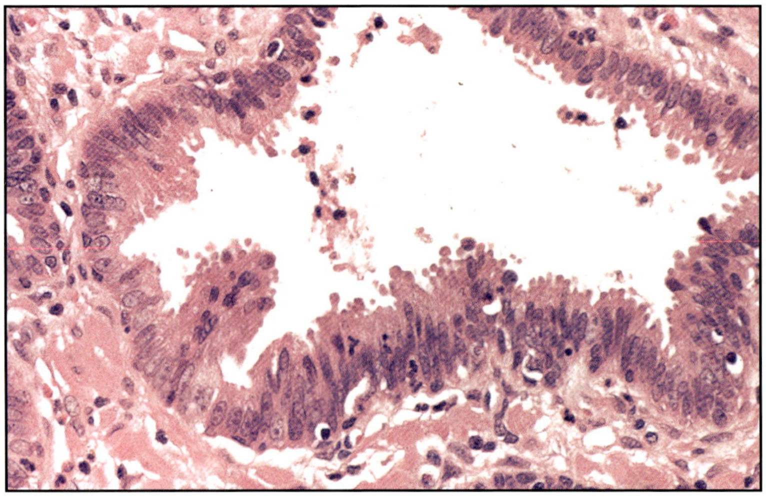

■ **i11.41** *Elongated nuclei in high-grade PIN.*

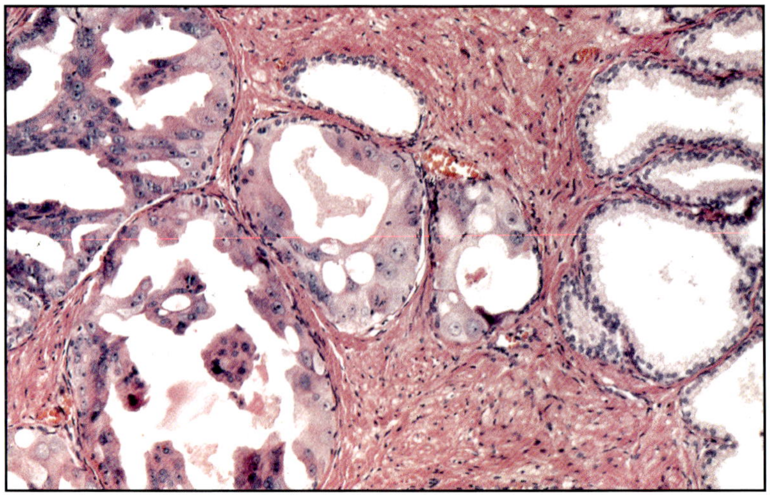

■ **i11.42** *High-grade PIN with architectural abnormalities. Compare with benign glands on right side.*

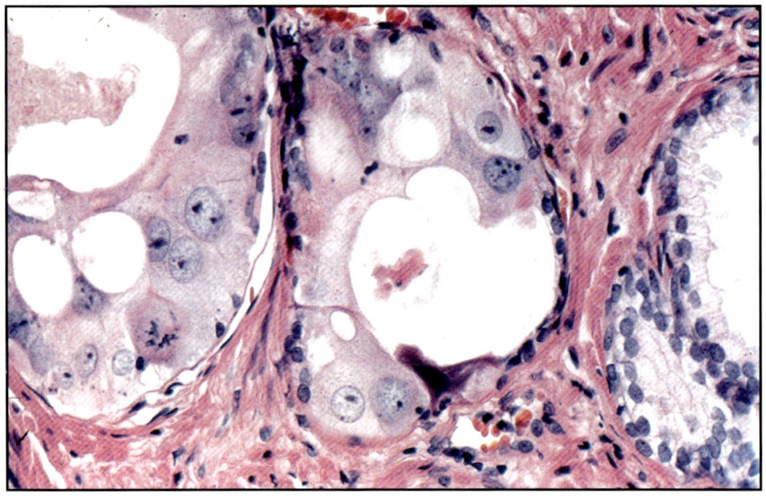

■ **i11.43** *High-grade PIN with cytologic abnormalities. Compare with benign glands on right side.*

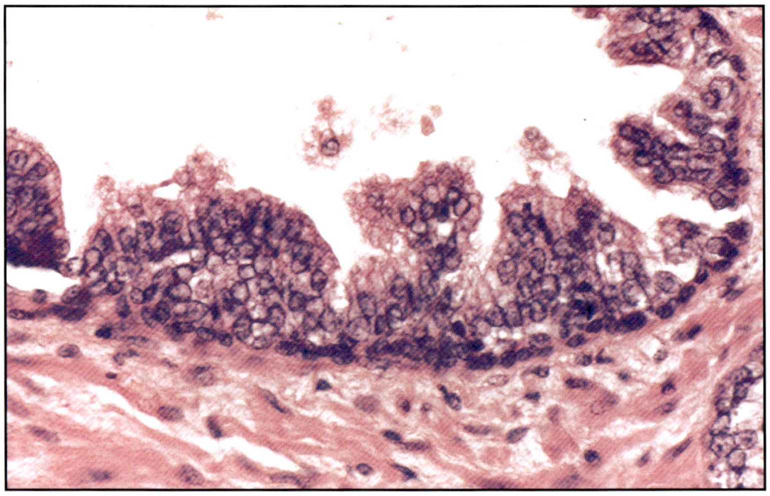

■ **i11.44** *Thick 10μm section of high-grade PIN creates problems in definition of nuclear detail due to nuclear overlap.*

luminal cell nuclear enlargement with numerous large (>3μm) macronucleoli that are easily seen because of chromatin clearing **i11.43**. The diagnosis becomes more difficult when the macronucleoli are present in only a few cells, when nucleoli are numerous but exhibit borderline enlargement, when the nucleoli are difficult to visualize (because of section thickness **i11.44**, overstaining, or intrinsic biologic lack of chromatin clearing), and when nucleoli are not evident at all but where there is massive nucleomegaly and striking, dense nuclear hyperchromasia **i11.45, i11.46**. In regard to the first circumstance, there is no minimum number of cells with macronucleoli needed to diagnose high-grade PIN. Also, nucleolar prominence is not quantitatively defined in the diagnosis of high-grade PIN, but nucleoli 1μm to 3μm in diameter would be sufficient. Even at 400× magnification, visually setting the lower limit of this threshold is a challenge **i11.3**. Morphometric measurements of nucleolar diameter are not indicated in the establishment of a high-grade PIN diagnosis. The diagnosis of high-grade PIN originally was not meant to be applied in the absence of prominent nucleoli, yet a number of pathologists, including this writer, have agreed to render a diagnosis of high-grade PIN in the unusual setting of significant nucleomegaly and hyperchromasia of such a degree that visualization of intranuclear detail is not possible (Allam 1996, Epstein 1995B).

It is important to study high-grade PIN nuclei that are more basally situated because in micropapillary and cribriform high-grade PIN, the centrally disposed nuclei appear smaller and more hyperchromatic **i11.47**. This difference in nuclear appearance based on intraglandular location is similar to that of mammary ductal carcinoma in situ (CIS) of micropapillary and cribriform types and is thought to be a degenerative, atrophic, or ischemic process. Such "maturation" does not always occur in micropapillary and cribriform high-grade PIN; in some cases highly atypical nuclei extend all the way to the luminal surface **i11.48**. It is a common misconception that nuclear atypia always must be of full thickness to diagnose high-grade PIN; this is definitely not the case. A peculiar pattern of nuclear distribution is an apical nuclear alignment along the luminal aspect of the gland, the so-called inverted pattern **i11.14** (Argani 2001).

Cytoplasmic features of high-grade PIN are not specific **t11.12**, and usually there is a moderate amount of amphophilic cytoplasm **i11.43**, similar to invasive moderately to poorly differentiated carcinoma. In the extremely rare cases of neuroendocrine small cell high-grade PIN **i11.10** (Reyes 1997B), the cytoplasm is scanty. Another variant with a diminished volume of cytoplasm is atrophic pattern high-grade PIN **i11.49** (de la Torre 1993); this pattern

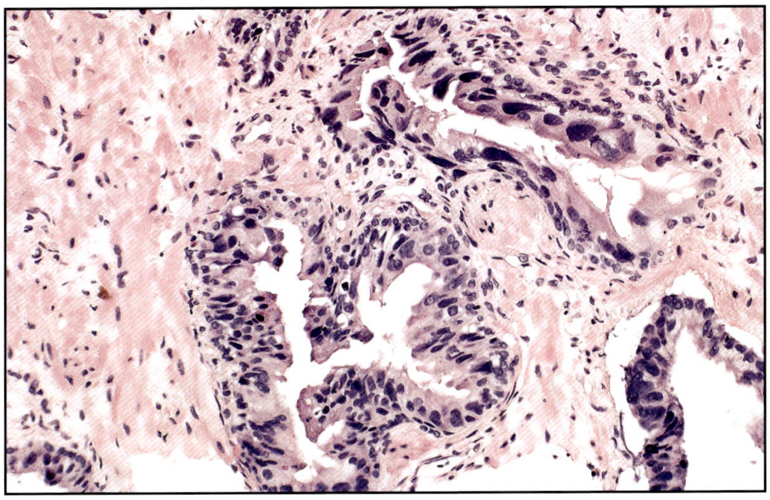

■ **i11.45** *Pleomorphic high-grade PIN with nuclear enlargement and hyperchromasia as the dominant manifestations of cytologic atypia.*

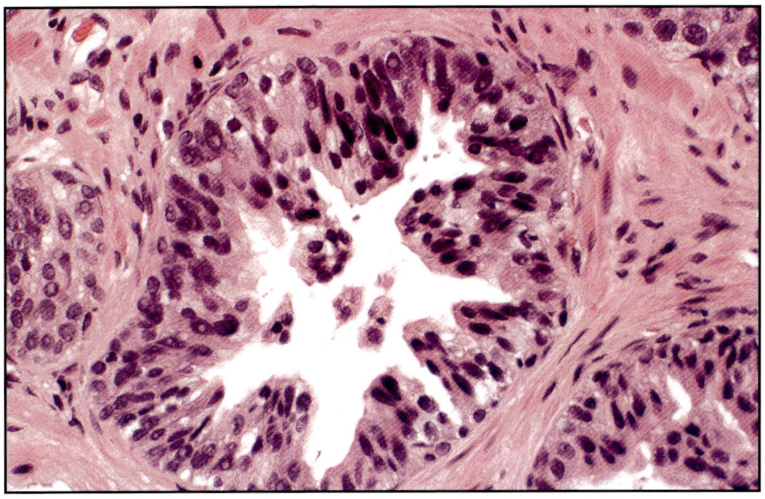

■ **i11.46** *High-grade PIN with nuclear enlargement and hyperchromasia as the dominant manifestations of cytologic atypia.*

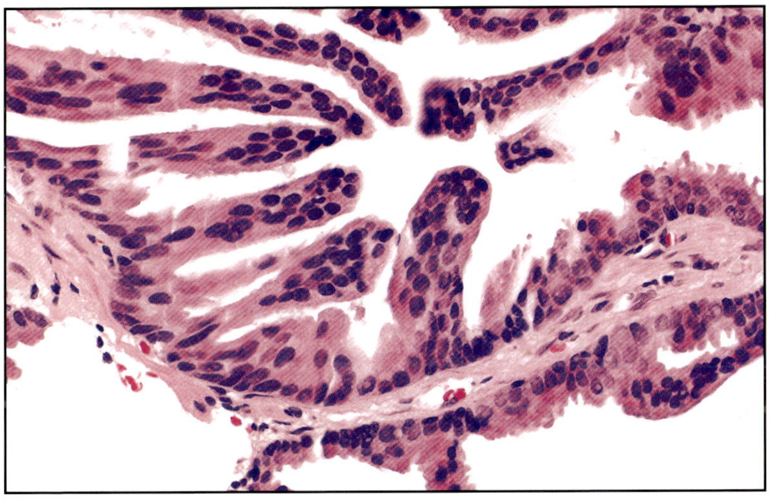

■ **i11.47** *Nuclei are smaller and more hyperchromatic at the tips of micropapillae of high-grade PIN.*

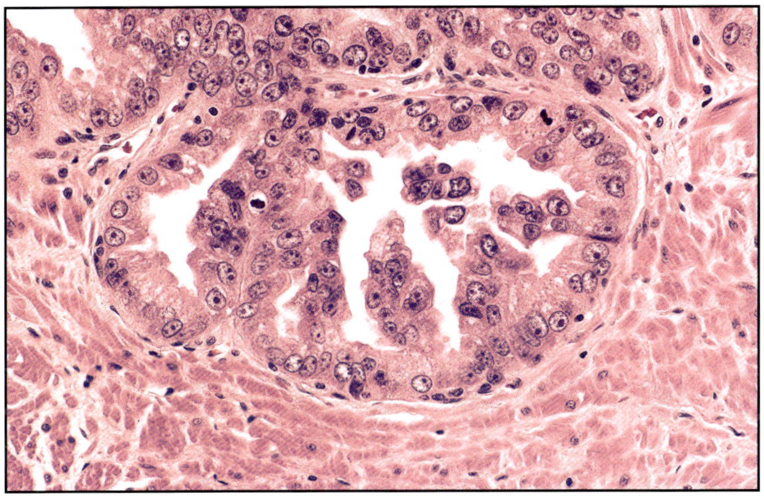

■ **i11.48** *Highly atypical nuclei from luminal aspect to base of high-grade PIN gland.*

■ t11.12 **Cytoplasm of High-grade PIN**

Usually amphophilic, moderate in amount	
Common:	Luminal blebs and pigment
Uncommon:	Clearing, goblet cell formalin, Paneth cell–like change, signet ring change, foamy cell change

has not been well characterized. Common cytoplasmic features include apical cytoplasmic luminal blebs (100% of radical prostatectomy cases) **i11.50** and pigment (30% to 78% of cases) that ranges from golden-yellow to purple to black **i11.51** (Amin 1996, Bostwick 1993). Uncommon cytoplasmic alterations include clearing (15% of cases), microcalcifications (8% of cases), goblet cell change (mucinous metaplasia) (5% of cases), Paneth cell–like change (2% of cases), signet-ring change (rare) (Bostwick 1993, Reyes 1997B) **i11.8, i11.9**, and foamy cell change (rare) **i11.13** (Berman 2000).

Luminal contents of high-grade PIN glands also are not specific for PIN **t11.13**. Corpora amylacea, which are more often present in benign than malignant glands, have been reported in 55% of high-grade PIN cases at radical prostatectomy **i11.52** (Bostwick 1993). Crystalloids, on the other hand, are more common in malignant

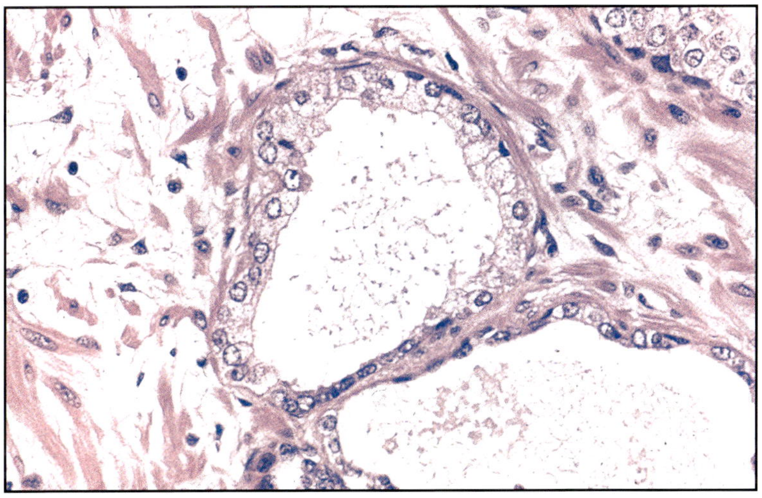

■ **i11.49** *Atrophic changes in high-grade PIN, with markedly decreased cytoplasmic volume. The flat high-grade PIN gland at center is partially atrophic; in the adjacent gland all cells have substantially reduced cytoplasmic volume.*

than benign glands; these structures were seen in 3% of high-grade PIN cases **i11.53** (Bostwick 1993). Amphophilic pink material (proteinaceous eosinophilic secretions) and wispy blue mucin have also been

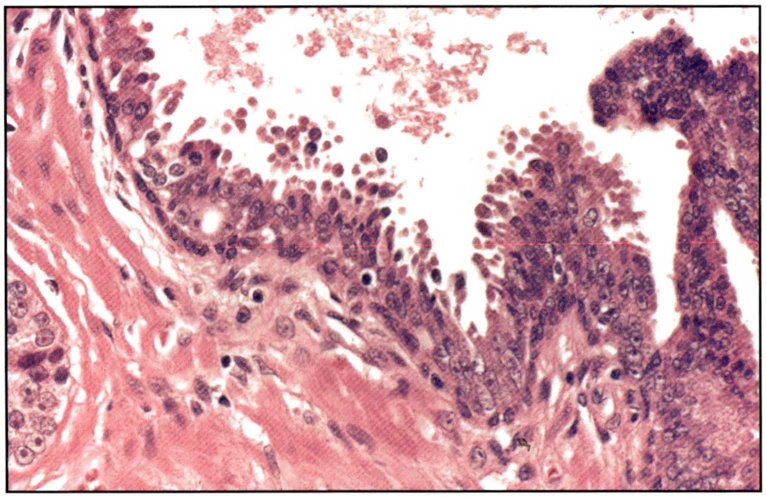

■ **i11.50** *Apocrine-like apical bleb formation in high-grade PIN.*

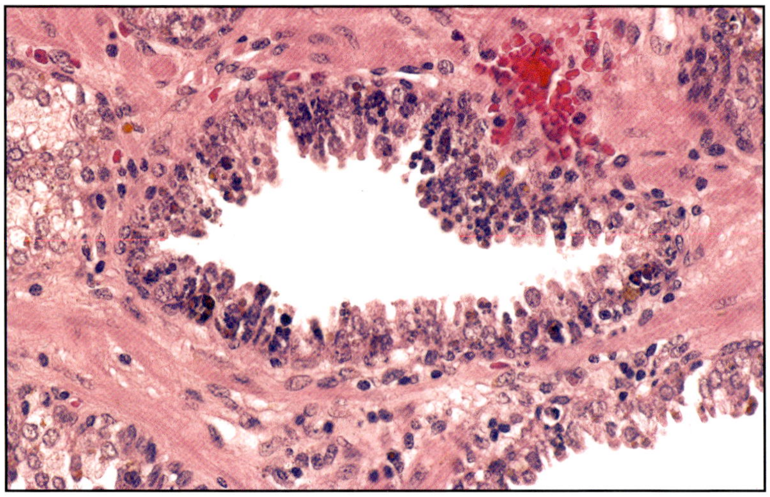

■ **i11.51** *Cytoplasmic pigment in high-grade PIN cells varies from finely granular to more voluminous and yellow-brown to purple to black. The darker pigment, shown here, can obscure nuclear detail.*

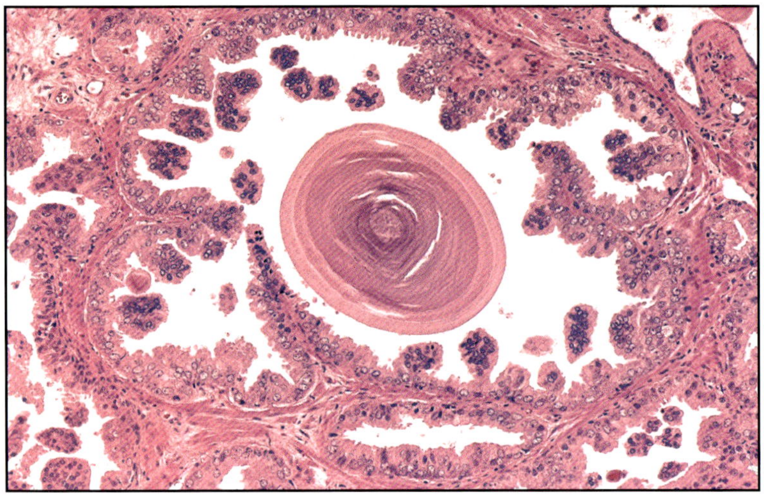

■ **i11.52** *Corpus amylaceum in lumen of high-grade PIN gland.*

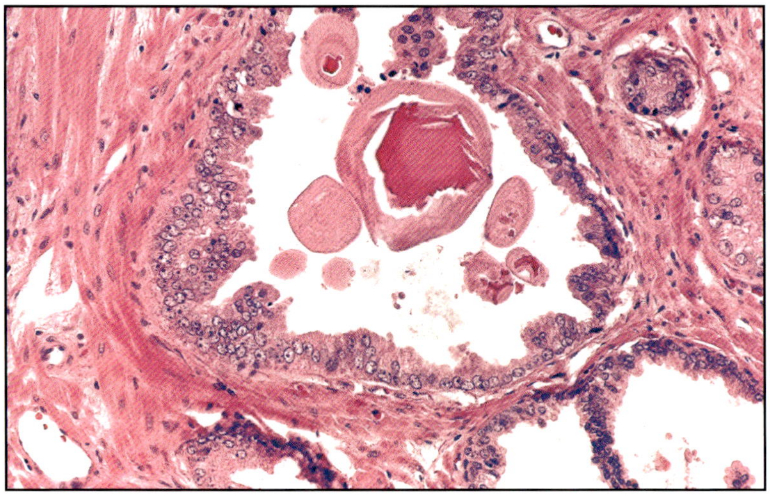

■ **i11.53** *Small to large brightly eosinophilic crystalloids with sharply-defined edges. Here, they are found in corpora amylacea in this high-grade PIN gland.*

seen more often in malignant than benign glands. The former secretions were observed in 62% of high-grade PIN cases (Bostwick 1993), whereas the incidence of wispy blue mucin in high-grade PIN **i11.34** is unknown. As noted earlier, in rare cases this mucin fills and distends high-grade PIN glands **i11.12** (Reyes 1997B). Intraluminal contents that do not segregate between benign and malignant proliferations include exfoliated cells (42% of cases) and hemorrhage (2% of cases) (Gaudin 1997). Intraluminal comedo necrosis has not been recognized in high-grade PIN (Gaudin 1997). Although none of these intraluminal materials is specific for high-grade PIN, intraluminal crystalloids and wispy blue mucin should be viewed as atypical findings and, when recognized in a low-power survey, should prompt further high-power study of the glands in question. This maneuver may be of benefit in detecting high-grade PIN glands that may not be readily seen at low-power, such as those with cleared or foamy cytoplasm and the flat type of high-grade PIN.

■ **t11.13 Luminal Contents in High-grade PIN**

Common:	Corpora amylacea, amphophilic pink proteinaceous secretions, exfoliated cells
Uncommon:	Hemorrhage, crystalloids
Not allowed:	Necrosis

Finally, hormonal (androgen deprivation) therapy and radiation therapy may complicate diagnostic recognition of high-grade PIN. Androgen deprivation therapy reduces the incidence and extent of high-grade PIN (Balaji 1999, Bostwick 2001, Civantos 1995, 1996, Ferguson 1994, Häggman 1993, Montironi 1995A, Reuter 1997, Shin 2000, Têtu 1991, Vaillancourt 1996, Wheeler 1996). Treated high-grade PIN glands demonstrate flattened intraluminal growth (van der Kwast 1999) **i11.54**, basal cell hyperplasia, and cytologic alterations in the luminal cells similar to that observed in invasive neoplastic cells, including the classic cytoplasmic vacuolization and nuclear pyknosis (see Chapter 19). These modifications can produce difficulty in low-power recognition of PIN because the glands appear less dark because of diminished cell crowding secondary to cytoplasmic clearing and expansion by coalescence of vacuoles (Häggman 1993). The nuclear pyknosis induced by androgen deprivation therapy can blur the boundary between low- and high-grade PIN, such that PIN grading may not be feasible (Montironi 1995A). Apoptotic bodies are increased (but still uncommon at 1.74% of PIN cells) in hormonally treated PIN, and it appears that this activation of cell death in combination with suppression of cell

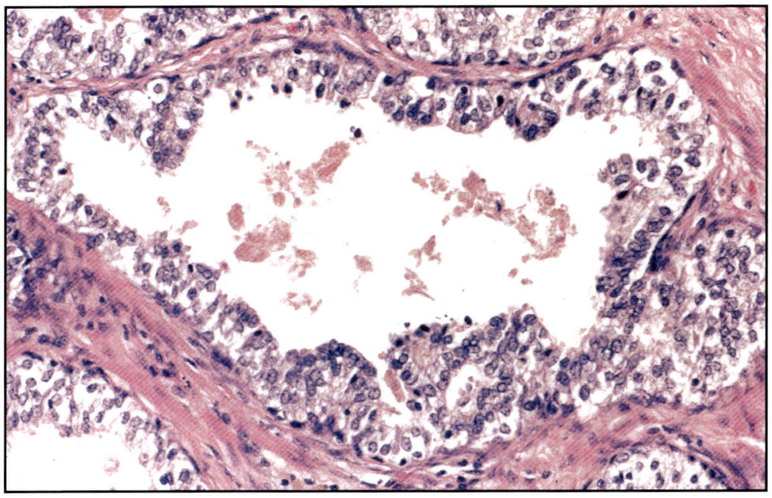

■ **i11.54** *Androgen-deprivation hormonal therapy effect on high-grade PIN: Cytoplasmic vacuolization and nuclear pyknosis are evident.*

■ **t11.14 Differential Diagnosis of High-Grade PIN**

Benign	
Fragments of ejaculatory duct/seminal vesicle	
Normal central zone epithelium	
Atrophy	
Transitional cell metaplasia	
Inflammation-induced atypia	
Infarction-induced atypia	
Radiation-induced atypia	
Usual hyperplasia	
Basal cell hyperplasia	
Basal cell hyperplasia with prominent nucleoli	
Low-grade PIN	
Malignant	
High-grade PIN with invasive adenocarcinoma	
Prostatic duct adenocarcinoma	
Invasive cribriform prostatic adenocarcinoma	
Transitional cell carcinoma	

proliferation may account for the reduction in PIN extent (Montironi 1994A, 1995A). Similar but less pronounced effects on high-grade PIN were noticed after treatment with finasteride (a drug used to treat BPH and baldness that inhibits the conversion of testosterone to dihydrotestosterone by blocking the enzyme 5α-reductase) (Civantos 1996, 1997).

Radiation therapy also reduces prevalence and extent of high-grade PIN (Arakawa 1995, Cheng 1999, Wheeler 1996) but does not appear to affect its architecture. There is some debate as to whether it is possible to diagnose high-grade PIN after radiation therapy; some pathologists do not believe that it is possible to distinguish high-grade PIN from postirradiation atypia induced in benign glands (Häggman 1997C).

The effect of emerging new therapies for BPH and prostate cancer on the morphology of high-grade PIN is unknown. Included among these BPH therapies are nonhormonal medical therapy, such as a-adrenergic receptor blockade and the delivery of energy to the prostate, including electromagnetic, radiofrequency, ultrasound, microwave, electrocautery, and laser energies. Although these therapies do not result in tissue removal for microscopic examination, these patients could undergo biopsy and prostatectomy (transurethral, open, or radical) in the future. Similarly, the morphologic impact of new modalities for treating prostate cancer, including cryosurgery (freezing of the prostate) and brachytherapy (interstitial radioactive seed implantation), on high-grade PIN is obscure. Again, tissue is not removed during these therapies, but follow-up tissue samples could be procured in the future.

The differential diagnosis for high-grade PIN is broad **t11.14** and often centers on its separation from low-grade PIN, basal cell hyperplasia, and PIN with associated atypical small acini or invasive carcinoma. The distinction between high- and low-grade PIN is discussed earlier in this chapter, and that between high-grade PIN and PIN adjacent to atypical acini or invasive carcinoma is discussed later. Basal cell hyperplasia may be readily mistaken for high-grade PIN because this proliferation is typified by a darker gland appearance at scanning magnification, with multilayering of cells that may cause concern for high-grade PIN. Yet basal cell hyperplasia does not resemble high-grade PIN in architectural configurations: basal cell hyperplasia often presents as a multilayered, concentric thickening, with eccentric thickening and solid nests also being common (Devaraj 1993). These cells do not form tufts and micropapillary projections, as do those of high-grade PIN. Nucleoli <1μm are common in usual basal cell hyperplasia, but large, prominent nucleoli (with a mean diameter of 2μm) may be seen in atypical basal cell hyperplasia (Devaraj 1993, Srigley 1998), also known as basal cell hyperplasia with prominent nuclei (Yang 1998). This nucleomegaly may represent a reactive change, as chronic inflammation was noted in association with most atypical basal cell hyperplasia cases (Devaraj 1993), whereas abundant chronic inflammation is rarely seen in high-grade PIN foci **i11.55, i11.56** (Bostwick 1993).

A number of additional benign and malignant conditions may be misdiagnosed as high-grade PIN **t11.14**. Normal anatomic structures such as fragments of ejaculatory duct or seminal vesicle and normal central zone epithelium may be confused with high-grade PIN (McNeal 1988C). Normal central zone epithelium may generate complex glandular images with intraluminal trabeculae and bridges with nuclear stratification that could be confused with high-grade PIN (Srodon 2002), but the normal central zone epithelium lacks the profound nuclear atypia of high-grade PIN. Central zone epithelium may further mirror high-grade PIN in a dark appearance of the glands resulting from a darker, more granular cytoplasm and nuclear crowding (McNeal 1988D). Although occasional ejaculatory duct and seminal vesicle structures may simulate high-grade PIN at intermediate magnification, these epithelia are mainly in the differential diagnosis of small glandular patterns (McNeal 1988C) rather than the typical medium to large acini and ducts involved by PIN. Although it has been written that PIN rarely, if ever, involves small acini (Montironi 1996C), we have found high-grade PIN involvement of small acini in some cases of flat high-grade PIN. Unlike flat high-grade PIN, ejaculatory duct and seminal vesicle epithelium exhibits irregularly dispersed large, monstrous cells. As noted earlier, golden lipofuscin pigment can be found in both PIN and seminal vesicle and ejaculatory duct epithelium. Atrophy is also distinguishable from flat high-grade PIN by the nuclear atypia of high-grade PIN. This is also true for inflammatory-induced atypia and infarction-induced atypia in epithelium at the edge of the infarct. In general, although nuclear enlargement and nucleoli may be seen in these atypias, the magnitude of the increased nuclear and nucleolar size usually is not at the level of high-grade PIN. Exceptions include the macronucleoli in basal cell hyperplasia with prominent nucleoli and the large nucleoli that can be seen in immature squamous metaplasia adjacent to infarcts. Huge nuclei and nucleoli that are induced in normal

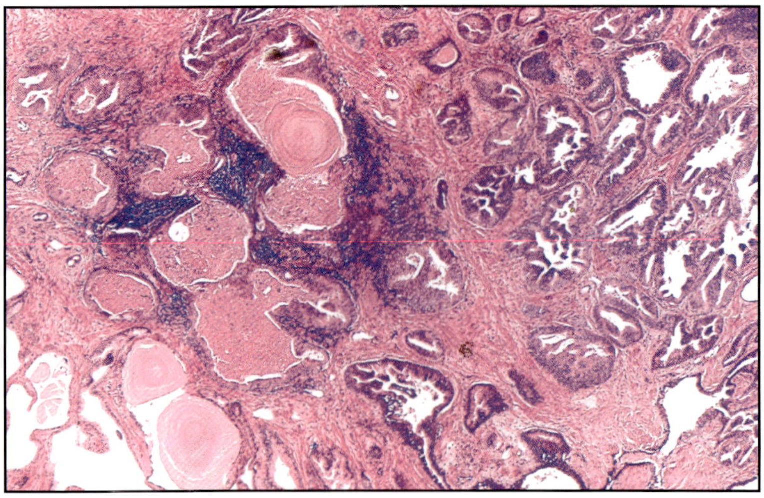

■ **i11.55** *Chronic inflammation with cystic dilatation of high-grade PIN glands.*

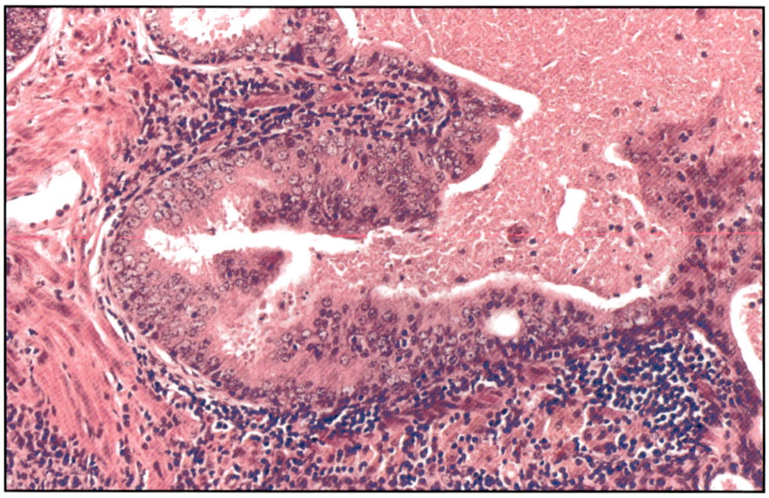

■ **i11.56** *High-grade PIN with inflammation: Most of the lymphocytes are in peri-glandular stroma, with a few intraepithelial lymphocytes.*

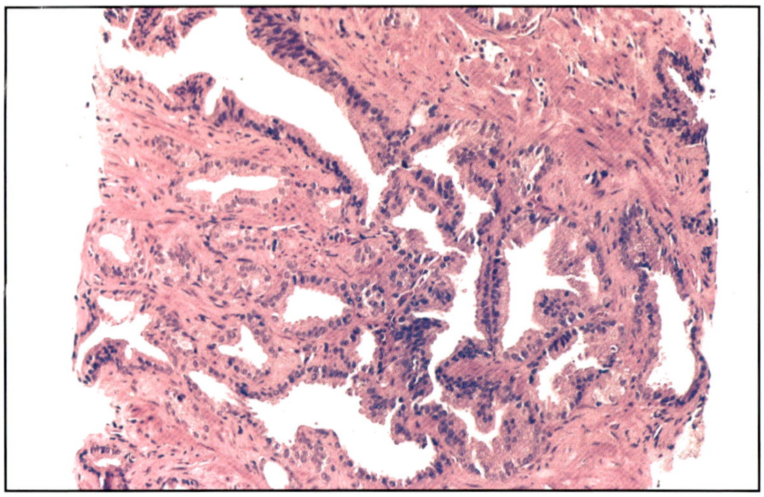

■ **i11.57** *High-grade PIN admixed with a few atypical small acini in needle biopsy.*

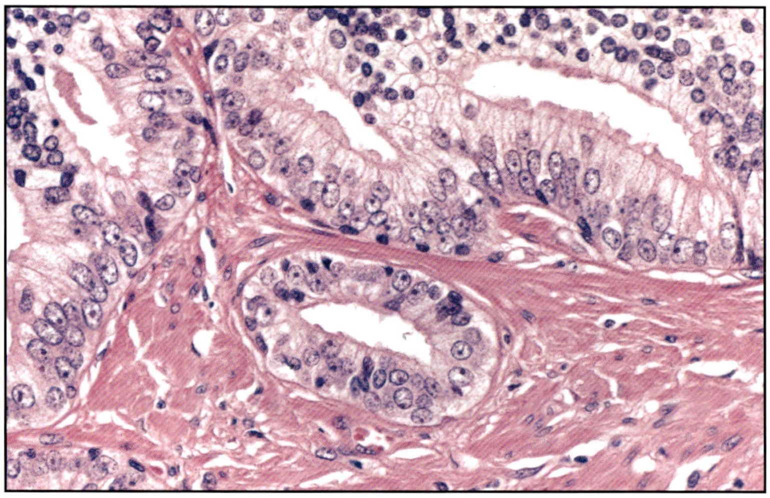

■ **i11.58** *Single atypical small gland adjacent to high-grade PIN. Basal cell presence indicates that this is an outpouching rather than "microinvasion."*

epithelium secondary to radiation therapy can also be confused with high-grade PIN, although nuclear variability typically is greater in radiation effect. In all these circumstances, the overall context in which these changes occur will help guide one toward the correct diagnosis. Finally, in the benign realm, transitional cell metaplasia and usual hyperplasia enter into the differential diagnosis of high-grade PIN. Transitional cell metaplasia might prompt consideration of solid high-grade PIN, but the constituent cells are typical benign transitional cells with some cleared cytoplasm and oblong nuclei containing occasional grooves. Usual hyperplasia, with its absence of multilayering, most often is contemplated in the differential diagnosis with flat high-grade PIN. The key discriminator here is the profound luminal cell nuclear atypia in high-grade PIN.

A difficult diagnostic problem arises when there are a few small acini or nests of cells immediately adjacent to high-grade PIN **i11.57–i11.60**. The differential diagnosis here is high-grade PIN with outpouching versus high-grade PIN with focal, invasive adenocarcinoma. Outpouching is the favored diagnosis when solid nests are visualized immediately adjacent to high-grade PIN; this usually represents oblique sectioning across the base of high-grade PIN **i11.59**. If only rare, atypical, small acini **i11.57, i11.58** or a few distorted, obliquely sectioned or poorly preserved small acini are found immediately adjacent to high-grade PIN, then caution is advised on the diagnosis of invasion. In such cases a descriptive diagnosis of high-grade PIN with adjacent small atypical glands may be rendered (Kronz 2001A). In the literature this has been abbreviated as PINATYP (Kronz 2001A) and also designated as small acinar glands suspicious for cancer with high-grade PIN (O'Dowd 2000) or high-grade PIN with adjacent atypical glands (Alsikafi 2001). The mean incidence of PINATYP is 0.3%, with a range of 0.1% to 2.5% of all prostate needle biopsies (Alsikafi 2001, Borboroglu 2001, O'Dowd 2000, Reyes 1998, Vis 2001). In one study on PINATYP the average number of small atypical glands was 5.3, and the average distance from the PIN glands was 0.12mm (Kronz 2001A). Though not a discrete pathologic entity, this descriptive diagnosis of small glandular atypia with PIN is a useful diagnostic category for cases indeterminate for invasion.

The first morphologic evidence of invasion from high-grade PIN has been called early invasive adenocarcinoma (Bostwick 1996B), transitive gland change (McNeal 1991), and microinvasive adenocarcinoma (Bostwick 1995A). However, no rigorous morphologic criteria exist for establishing a diagnosis of microinvasive prostatic carcinoma originating from high-grade PIN. Loss of basal cells clearly occurs as glands invade stroma **i11.61, i11.62**, but basal cell antibodies such as 34βE12 do not constitute definitive markers for invasion because

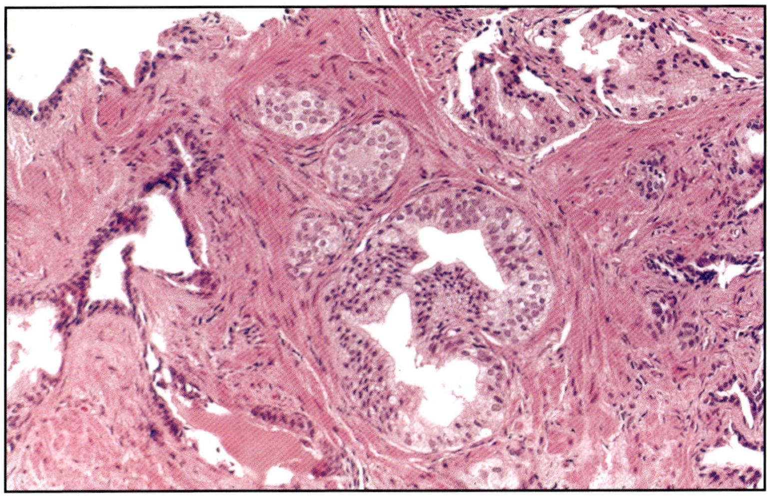

■ **i11.59** *Isolated high-grade PIN with adjacent solid nests with basal cells. This represents oblique sectioning across the base of high-grade PIN.*

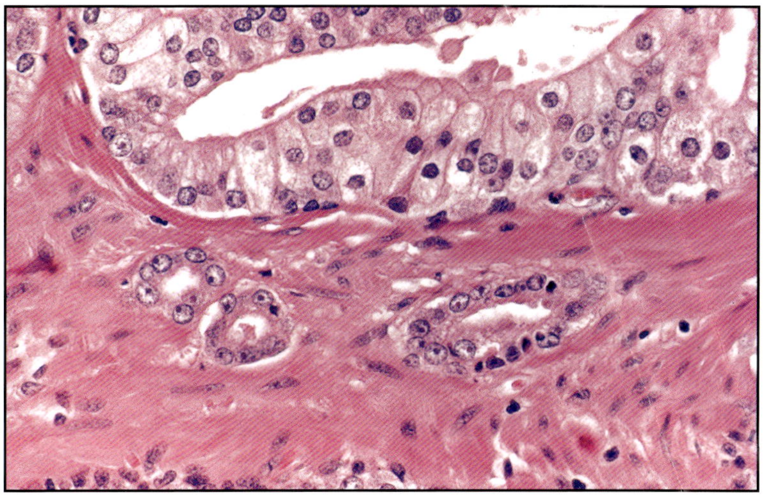

■ **i11.60** *Focal invasive adenocarcinoma adjacent to high-grade PIN.*

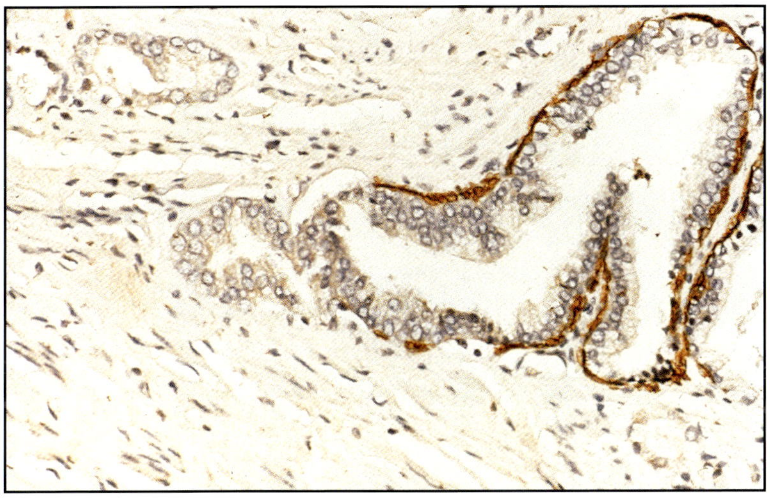

■ **i11.61** *Probable focal invasion from high-grade PIN: A budding gland with loss of basal cell layer, as highlighted by 34βE12 immunohistochemical stain. While this likely represents the earliest phase of invasion, it is not diagnostic of invasion and adenocarcinoma.*

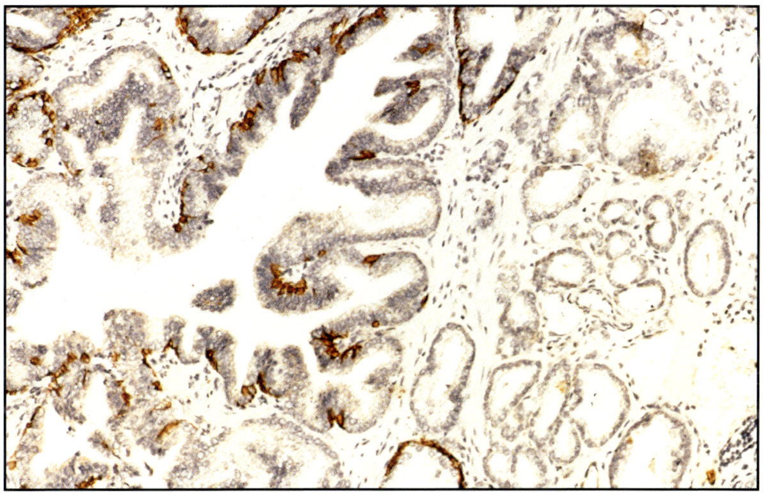

■ **i11.62** *Small acinar adenocarcinoma without basal cells adjacent to high-grade PIN with fragmented basal cell layer (34βE12 immunohistochemical stain).*

PIN glands can exhibit discontinuity of the basal cell layer. Accordingly, loss of basal cells in a few atypical glands next to PIN does not necessarily represent invasive adenocarcinoma (Kronz 2001A). Part of the difficulty in identifying microinvasive carcinoma emanating from high-grade PIN is that, unlike in many microinvasive carcinomas at other anatomic sites, there is little or no stromal response to invasive prostatic carcinoma; typically lacking are a fibrogenic and inflammatory response. Additionally, basement membrane immunohistochemical staining for laminin, type IV collagen, and heparan sulfate proteoglycan is not of value because many prostatic adenocarcinomas maintain a basement membrane (Bonkhoff 1991, 1992, Bostwick 1995C, Fuchs 1989, Sinha 1989, 1991).

High-grade PIN with invasive adenocarcinoma can be diagnosed when the immediately adjacent small atypical glands are too numerous and too crowded (Epstein 1995B) **i11.63**, but there are no quantitative thresholds for how many is too numerous and how crowded is too crowded. Different thresholds clearly exist for different pathologists for diagnosing carcinoma adjacent to high-grade PIN (Epstein 1995B). If the pattern of growth is infiltrative, with glands wrapping around a high-grade PIN gland or a fair number of atypical acini without basal cells and with requisite nuclear atypia, with some stromal separation, then high-grade PIN with invasive carcinoma can be diagnosed. Usually the focally invasive carcinoma adjacent to high-grade PIN is small acinar Gleason pattern 3 adenocarcinoma **i11.63**, but high-grade Gleason pattern 4 may also be seen **i11.64**.

Specific patterns of high-grade PIN generate particular difficulties in differentiating isolated high-grade PIN from invasive carcinoma. Isolated cribriform high-grade PIN can be difficult to distinguish from invasive cribriform carcinoma, especially when just a few cribriform glands are encountered in needle biopsy. Another problem is that in radical prostatectomy tissues, cribriform high-grade PIN and cribriform invasive carcinoma often coexist (Qian 1997B). One potential clue is that cribriform high-grade PIN more often exhibits irregular oblong to slitlike spaces, whereas cribriform carcinoma usually assumes a more classic sievelike pattern, with open, round spaces (Amin 1994A), although there is overlap here. The essential primary discriminating feature is the presence (in high-grade PIN) or absence (in carcinoma) of basal cells. Because there may be only a few of these basal cells in cribriform high-grade PIN glands, confirmation of basal cells by immunohistochemistry for basal cell–specific cytokeratins, as detected by monoclonal antibody 34βE12, can be helpful (Amin 1994A). A negative staining result in this context has less value, particularly if there is only a single atypical cribriform gland (Amin 1994A). Again, this is because there is a lack of uniform staining with this antibody even

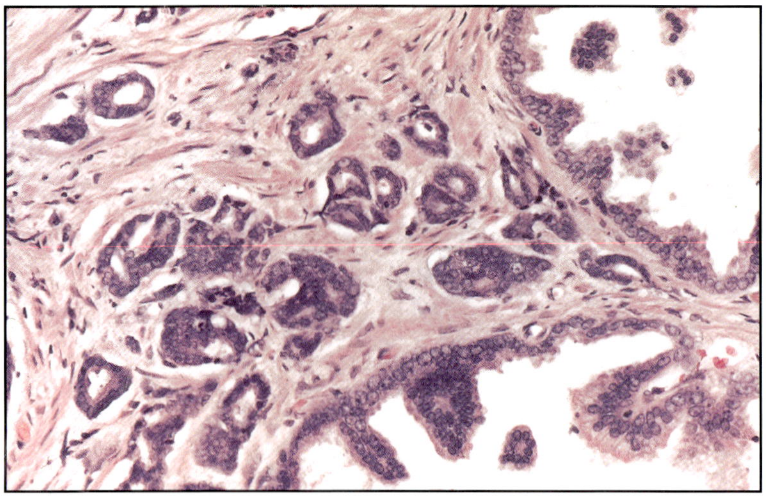

■ **i11.63** *Invasive adenocarcinoma adjacent to high-grade PIN: More than a few small acini, with stromal separation, are useful findings in diagnosing invasion.*

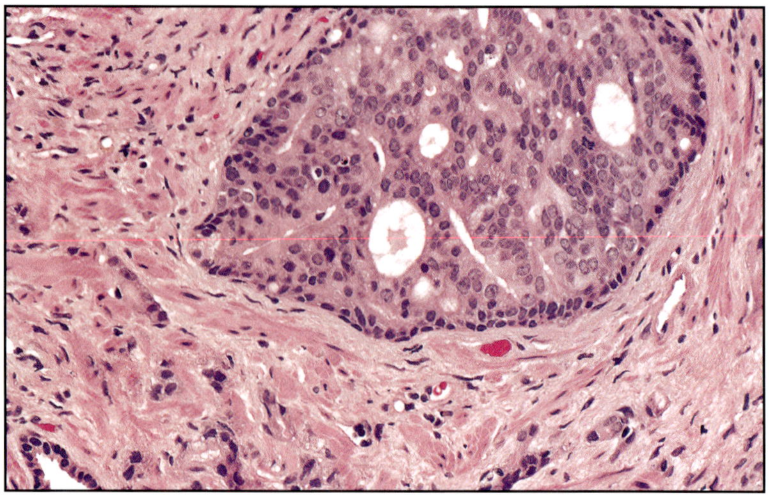

■ **i11.64** *Focal high-grade Gleason pattern 4 carcinoma, with cord-like growth, adjacent to high-grade PIN in needle biopsy.*

in benign glands (Amin 1994A, Hedrick 1989, Shah 1991, Wojno 1995). If the atypical cribriform proliferation is extensive or confluent or harbors necrosis, the index of suspicion for carcinoma should be increased (Amin 1994B, Jones 1991). No data exist as to the quantity of glands that qualifies as extensive. For some pathologists, the presence of necrosis excludes a diagnosis of high-grade PIN. Fortunately, the isolated cribriform pattern of high-grade PIN is quite uncommon to rare in pure form (Davidson 1995, Pacelli 1997, Reyes 1997A) **t11.10**. Invasive cribriform carcinoma is also highly unusual as a pure pattern; usually it is associated with an invasive small acinar component. The flat pattern of high-grade PIN is another uncommon pattern that when found in pure form may be hard to distinguish from invasive carcinoma. Pure flat pattern high-grade PIN may present as a few small pale glands that are suspicious for a minimal invasive adenocarcinoma at low power **i11.31**. Only at high power are basal cells evident **i11.7, i11.33**. If one does not have full confidence in basal cell identity on H&E-stained sections, confirmatory 34βE12 immunohistochemistry may be performed.

Prostatic duct carcinoma also figures prominently in the differential diagnosis of high-grade PIN. Ductal carcinomas of the prostate may closely resemble high-grade PIN at low-power examination because of a prominent intraductal component that demonstrates cribriform, comedo, solid, and papillary patterns. Prominent comedo necrosis in a high-grade intraepithelial neoplasm or papillary structures with creation of slitlike lumina favor ductal carcinoma over high-grade PIN. At higher-magnification scrutiny, these in situ ductal carcinomas display columnar cells with marked nuclear pleomorphism and striking mitotic activity that may exceed 10 mitotic figures per 10 high-power fields (Amin 1994B, Dube 1972, Kovi 1985, Ro 1988). In contrast, high-grade PIN cells are cuboidal to columnar, demonstrate nuclear monotony, and have an exceedingly low mitotic count (of only 0.2%). One should not confuse cellular or hemorrhagic debris in high-grade PIN **i11.65** with comedo necrosis.

Transitional cell carcinoma from primaries in the prostatic urethra, urinary bladder, or, rarely, the major prostatic ducts may involve prostatic ducts or acini by in situ spread and should be contemplated in the differential diagnosis with high-grade PIN. The patterns of this spread, which are not characteristic of high-grade PIN, include solid, comedo, undermining, and pagetoid. At low power there is an impression of expansion of ducts and acini. Another hint that this is not high-grade PIN is a chronic inflammatory cell infiltrate, which may be prominent in transitional cell carcinoma but

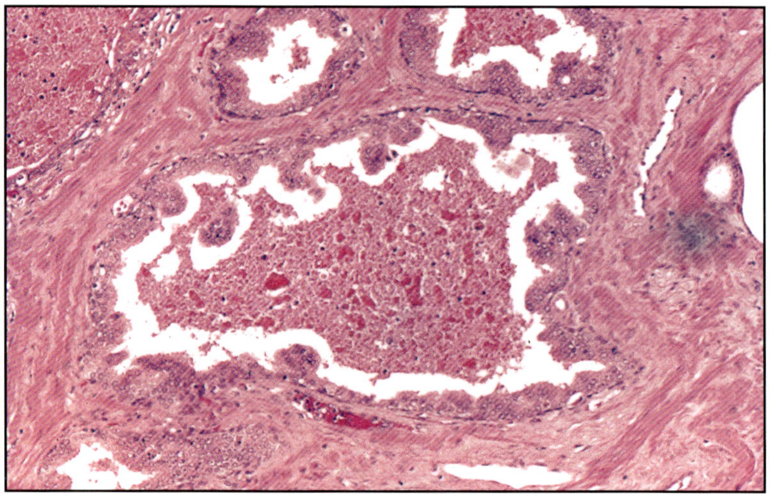

■ **i11.65** *Hemorrhagic and cellular debris, not comedo necrosis, in a high-grade PIN gland.*

is uncommon (at 2% [Bostwick 1993]) in high-grade PIN. The diagnosis of in situ spread of transitional cell carcinoma is easily substantiated at high magnification because transitional cell carcinoma nuclei are pleomorphic, and the cytoplasm of these cells often has a squamoid appearance. Solid and comedo patterns often are evident. A history of previous urothelial carcinoma is relevant, but uncommonly, previously undiagnosed transitional cell carcinoma may present in needle biopsy or TURP chip tissue. Although usually not necessary, immunostaining for PSA confirms the H&E impression; high-grade PIN is positive and transitional cell carcinoma negative.

A final entity that is in the differential diagnosis with high grade PIN but is not listed in **t11.14** is prostatic CIS, including in situ spread of prostatic acinar adenocarcinoma, representing "cancerization" of prostatic ducts and acini by an adjacent invasive carcinoma. Prostatic CIS, also known as intraductal carcinoma, is not in **t11.14** because this is currently not an established pathologic diagnosis with known clinical meaning and outcome. Does CIS of the prostate exist? Biologically, it must, and undoubtedly some examples of high-grade PIN must represent CIS. CIS of the ductal type of prostatic carcinoma also exists. Morphologic definitions for prostatic CIS and in situ spread of prostatic acinar adenocarcinoma have been forwarded (McNeal 1996, Rubin 1998, Wilcox 1998). Cribriform and solid patterns of high-grade PIN and comedo necrosis within intraductal neoplastic proliferations have been conceptualized as prostatic CIS (Cohen 2000, McNeal 1996, Rubin 1998, Stamey 2000, Wilcox 1998). However, no consensus exists on these definitions, and, more importantly, the clinical significance of isolated CIS in needle biopsy or TURP chips is unknown. In comparison, the clinical significance and clinical management of patients with isolated high-grade PIN is well established. A real concern is that if a diagnosis of prostatic CIS is rendered in biopsy or TURP tissue, therapy may be pursued when there is no evidence to support such a clinical approach. For these reasons, at present isolated CIS and intraductal adenocarcinoma of the prostate are not tenable diagnoses in the absence of associated invasive carcinoma. In the presence of carcinoma, these patterns of high-grade PIN or intraductal carcinoma, when identified in radical prostatectomy specimens, appear to indicate a more aggressive cancer (Cohen 2000, McNeal 1996, Rubin 1998, Stamey 2000, Wilcox 1998).

The differential diagnosis of high-grade PIN and the above-cited benign and malignant conditions is best addressed with standard H&E-stained tissue sections. Only a few studies have specifically asked how many sections are needed to detect high-grade PIN (Renshaw 1997, Reyes 1998). In one study of needle biopsies, all high-grade PIN lesions were detected on the first slide of 3 prepared H&E slides (Renshaw 1997). However, we have seen cases in which the high-grade PIN focus was present only in sections on the second or third slide. One must serially section through the entire block to detect all high-grade PIN lesions (Reyes 1998), but this is not practical because it requires 30 slides per block. Therefore, it is reasonable to follow the recommendations (Renshaw 1997, Reyes 1998) that 3 slides with several sections on each slide be examined as routine practice for prostate needle biopsy microscopic interpretation.

The optimum number of slides to prepare to detect high-grade PIN in other tissue samples, including TURP chips and open and radical prostatectomy specimens, is unknown.

Additional sections (levels) may be helpful in resolving some of the aforementioned differential diagnostic problems. This is particularly the case if the initial sections are too thick, folded, or overstained. If the sections are too thick or if there is hematoxylin overstaining, benign glands may appear dark at low power, mimicking high-grade PIN. In a high-power examination of a thick section it is difficult to assess for number of cell layers, multilayering, and nuclear morphology because of overlapping cells. A thin section at 3μm is optimal for demonstrating that glands of usual hyperplasia possess 2 cell layers, no nuclear stratification, and cells with bland cytology. Similarly, for high-grade PIN glands, well-fixed, well-sectioned, well-stained sections are invaluable in establishing a definitive diagnosis. Although additional sections may enhance the differential diagnostic approach, the evidence to date suggests that additional sections after a diagnosis of high-grade PIN in the initial 3 slides do not increase the detection rate of invasive adenocarcinoma (Reyes 1998).

The only special study that is of value in the differential diagnosis of high-grade PIN, is immunohistochemistry for basal cell–specific cytokeratins. In almost all cases, the diagnosis of high-grade PIN may be established based solely on H&E-stained sections. Indeed, in one study on the use of basal cell–specific anticytokeratin antibody 34βE12, this immunostain was used in <2% of all PIN cases and was mainly a confirmatory tool (Wojno 1995). The most common indications for use of this immunostain in the differential diagnosis of high-grade PIN are to distinguish pure cribriform high-grade PIN from invasive cribriform carcinoma (Wojno 1995) and flat high-grade PIN from invasive adenocarcinoma adjacent to high-grade PIN. It must be emphasized that, like all immunostains, this immunostain must be interpreted in the overall morphologic context. This is paramount here because one is relying on a negative result to diagnosis malignancy, and absence of proof is not proof of absence. Extreme caution is advised in use and interpretation of this immunostain, especially in the evaluation of a focal lesion, because its labeling of basal cells is not uniform, and entirely benign glands may be entirely negative with this immunostain (Amin 1994A, Hedrick 1989, Shah 1991, Wojno 1995).

[11.9] Follow-up and Clinical Management of High-Grade PIN

It is critical to recognize and diagnose isolated high-grade PIN in needle biopsy, TURP chips, and open (simple) prostatectomy specimens. This is so because high-grade PIN is a risk factor for the subsequent detection of carcinoma **t11.8; t11.15**. In needle biopsy, the mean incidence of carcinoma detection on rebiopsy is about 30% (range 10% to 100%) **t11.8**. Of these studies, only 3 were of 100 or more high-grade PIN patients (Davidson 1995, Kronz 2001B, O'Dowd 2000), and only 2 of these 3 had control patent populations with benign prostatic tissue on initial biopsy (Davidson 1995, O'Dowd 2000). The cancer detection rate of 23% on rebiopsy in the largest published series (O'Dowd 2000) is low compared with those of other studies, based on a single rebiopsy, with follow-up of only 1 year (Park 2001). The importance of follow-up beyond a first rebiopsy, if this tissue is negative for carcinoma, is underscored by 1 study that showed a 25% cancer detection rate in a single rebiopsy for high-grade PIN, with an increase to 32% for men with at least 1 follow-up rebiopsy (Kronz 2001B). Most (80% to 90%) cases of carcinoma detected on rebiopsy after an initial diagnosis of high-grade PIN are found in the first rebiopsy (Kronz 2001B, Park 2001). Rebiopsy may detect persistent high-grade PIN in anywhere from 5%

t11.15 Summary of High-Grade PIN Follow-up

	Incidence of Subsequent Carcinoma Detection				
	Core Needle biopsy			TURP Chips	
Initial Diagnosis	BPT	High-grade PIN	PINATYP	BPT	High-grade PIN
Patients with carcinoma	20%	28%	53%	3.7%	22%

BPT = benign prostatic tissue; PINATYP = high-grade PIN with adjacent small atypical glands

(Cheville 1997) to 26% (Kronz 2001B) to 43% of cases (Davidson 1995) and also benign prostatic tissue. In these cases the possibility of a third biopsy session should be discussed with the patient (Häggman 1997C). Atypia has been detected in up to 50% of patients rebiopsied for high-grade PIN (Kronz 2001B). A third set of biopsies should be procured in this group of patients because atypia is a high-risk category (see Chapter 12).

High-grade PIN with adjacent atypical glands seems to confer a higher risk for subsequent diagnosis of carcinoma than does high-grade PIN alone (Alsikafi 2001, Kronz 2001A, O'Dowd 2000). In 4 studies this risk ranged from 46% to 75%, with a summed risk for all 3 of 53% **t11.15**. In 1 series, younger age and predominantly flat high-grade PIN predicted a lower risk of cancer on repeat biopsy (Kronz 2001A). Because of the magnitude of the risk, all men with PINATYP should undergo rebiopsy (Kronz 2001A).

It is not settled whether serum PSA and DRE findings provide further information on risk for subsequent detection of carcinoma (Häggman 1997C, Kamoi 2000, Kronz 2001B, Park 2001). The data are mixed as to whether histologic findings relate to risk of subsequent diagnosis of carcinoma on rebiopsy (Davidson 1995, Keetch 1995, Kronz 2001B). Two studies did not find amount of high-grade PIN in needle biopsy to predict risk (Davidson 1995, Keetch 1995), whereas a third study found that the number of cores with high-grade PIN was an independent predictor of a cancer diagnosis (Kronz 2001B). Architectural pattern of PIN growth was not linked to cancer detection in 1 study (Davidson 1995), whereas in another investigation, for men with >1 follow-up biopsy, features including the presence of mitoses, the number of positive cores, predominant micropapillary and cribriform high-grade PIN patterns, and very large prominent nucleoli were associated with higher risk of carcinoma detection (Kronz 2001B). Mitotic count in high-grade PIN as a stratification feature is of little use because of the rarity of mitotic figures, and assessment of nucleolar size is subjective. Further studies are needed to validate whether amount and histologic characteristics of high-grade PIN are predictive measures. Serum PSA density (Raviv 1996A) and TRUS results do not appear to enhance the predictive capacity of high-grade PIN.

Patients with isolated high-grade PIN should be considered candidates for rebiopsy in 3 to 4 months, irrespective of the serum PSA level and DRE findings. The rebiopsy technique should entail at least systematic sextant rebiopsy of the entire gland (Kamoi 2000, Langer 1996, Perachino 1997, Shepherd 1996) because high-grade PIN is a general risk factor for carcinoma throughout the gland. To highlight this point, consider that if only the ipsilateral side of the prostate had been rebiopsied in 1 series, fully 36% of carcinomas would have been missed because they were on the other side of the prostate gland (Shepherd 1996).

More long-term follow-up and stratification research is needed to determine the risk of detecting carcinoma in patients with isolated high-grade PIN on initial biopsy and a nonmalignant diagnosis on subsequent biopsies. The future research on risk stratification of these patients with isolated initial or persistent high-grade PIN in needle biopsy should encompass clinical parameters such as serum PSA and its permutations, DRE, histologic features of PIN, and emerging avenues of research, such as genetic abnormalities in high-grade PIN.

What is the nature of prostate cancers that are being detected after an initial diagnosis of isolated high-grade PIN in needle biopsy? All 23 men in 1 series had clinically localized prostate cancer (as determined by bone scan, computed tomography of abdomen and pelvis, chest radiography, and serum enzymatic prostatic acid phosphatase) (Keetch 1995). Pathologically, the carcinomas in the whole gland were similar to other prostate cancers detected in our PSA-based screening program (Humphrey 1996B, 1997, Keetch 1995) in that 71% were organ confined and the mean Gleason score was 6.1 (range 5 to 7). The tumor volume was slightly smaller at a mean of $0.7cm^3$ (range $0.02cm^3$ to $3.4cm^3$), compared with a mean of $0.9cm^3$ for typical screen-detected carcinomas (Humphrey 1997). Most (65%) of these carcinomas were deemed pathologically significant, and 35% were insignificant using the Johns Hopkins definition of insignificant tumor ($<0.2cm^3$, organ-confined, no Gleason grade pattern 4 or 5) (Epstein 1994A). The patients in this series who had high-grade PIN only on initial needle biopsy had about twice the volume of high-grade PIN (at $0.7cm^3$) in the whole gland as patients with benign prostatic tissue on the initial biopsy (at $0.3cm^3$) (Humphrey 1997).

Patients with isolated high-grade PIN in TURP chips also appear to be at higher risk of subsequent detection of carcinoma (Gaudin 1997, Pacelli 1997, Samaratunga 1995), although the risk is not quite as high as for a diagnosis of isolated high-grade PIN in needle biopsy **t11.15**, and in 1 larger study high-grade PIN in TURP chips and enucleation specimens was not a risk factor for subsequent cancer detection (Harvei 1998). At a mean follow-up of 5 to 6 years, 21.4% to 22% (Gaudin 1997, Pacelli 1997) of patients with high-grade PIN in TURP chips were diagnosed with adenocarcinoma, compared with 0% of patients with BPH only in TURP chips (Pacelli 1997). Other studies (Greenwald 1974, Hammarsten 1994, Kearse 1993) have reported that a mean of 3.7% (48/1295; range 1.6% to 7.8%) of men with BPH in TURP chips were subsequently diagnosed with carcinoma after long-term follow-up. Serum PSA may help distinguish patients with high-grade PIN who are at higher risk of subsequent diagnosis of prostate cancer (Gaudin 1997, Pacelli 1997), although statistical analysis has not yet been applied to this question. After diagnosis of isolated high-grade PIN in TURP chips, it is probably prudent to submit all TURP chips for histologic examination, although no data exist on the effect of TURP chip sampling on high-grade PIN detection. The clinical management of high-grade PIN in TURP chips may be somewhat different from that of high-grade PIN in needle biopsy because the former patient population is somewhat older, and efforts to detect carcinoma by needle biopsy sampling of the peripheral zone may be less aggressive (Gaudin 1997, Häggman 1997C). If the patient is younger and fit for radical treatment, then systematic core needle biopsy of the peripheral zone should be contemplated (Häggman 1997C).

The meaning of discovering high-grade PIN in open (single) prostatectomy tissues where BPH nodules are enucleated is unknown (Samaratunga 1995) but probably is similar to that in TURP chips. However, 1 study found that high-grade PIN in 281 transvesical prostatic enucleations was not predictive, after 11 years of follow-up, of prostate cancer development (Harvei 1998).

Finally, the presence and extent of high-grade PIN in radical prostatectomy and cystoprostatectomy tissues does not appear to directly influence clinical outcome after this extirpative surgery. As noted earlier, although high-grade PIN presence and extent usually are related to the likelihood of carcinoma presence, small-volume, unifocal cancers may not be associated with high-grade PIN (Arakawa 1997, Häggman 1997B, Sakr 1994B), and mixed, conflicting data exist on the relationship between high-grade PIN extent and cancer grade (Qian 1997B, Sakr 1994B), cancer volume (de la Torre 1993, Häggman 1997B, Qian 1997A, Skjorten 1997, Wiley 1997), and cancer pathologic stage (Humphrey 1992, Qian 1997B). The extent of high-grade PIN is not correlated with biochemical failure after radical prostatectomy, as judged by an increased postoperative serum PSA (Humphrey 1993). Furthermore, the presence of high-grade PIN after radiation and radical prostatectomy did not have an effect on survival (Arakawa 1995). Therefore, high-grade PIN presence or extent in the whole gland does not affect clinical management of patients after surgical removal of the entire gland.

Treatment is not indicated after a diagnosis of high-grade PIN. A few ($n = 15$) patients have been treated by radical prostatectomy after a needle biopsy diagnosis of high-grade PIN (DiGiuseppe 1997, Häggman 1997C, Woderich 2001). The findings in the radical prostatectomy specimen were variable, from no cancer detected to minimal to significant amounts of cancer. In the future, patients with isolated high-grade PIN in needle biopsy may be a target population for chemoprevention therapy, especially with androgen deprivation (Aquilina 1997, Montironi 1996D, Nelson 1996, Sakr 1999). The problem here, of course, is that at least one third of these patients already have prostate cancer that has not been sampled by needle biopsy. The ideal candidates for chemoprevention would be patients with high-grade PIN only in the whole gland. It is not possible to identify these patients by needle biopsy alone.

[11.10] PIN Reporting

In needle biopsy tissue, one should report high-grade PIN and PIN with adjacent atypical small glands when detected in the absence of invasive carcinoma (Amin 1996B, Srigley 2000) **t11.16**. Reporting high-grade PIN in the presence of adenocarcinoma has been recommended (Srigley 2000), and preliminary data suggest that presence and amount of high-grade PIN in prostate needle biopsy tissue with carcinoma are associated with multifocal and bilateral carcinoma in the whole gland (Bock 1999, Trònscoso 1997). However, in another study the presence and amount of high-grade PIN in prostate needle biopsy tissue with adenocarcinoma were not predictive of Gleason grade, tumor volume, pathologic stage, or margin status in the whole gland (Bock 1999). Reporting the extent of high-grade PIN, architectural pattern of high-grade PIN, and other histologic features of PIN (such as mitoses and nucleolar prominence) should be viewed as optional because the data on the predictive value of these findings are conflicting or not validated (Davidson 1995, Keetch 1995, Kronz 2001B). One should not report low-grade PIN.

In TURP chips and open (enucleation) prostatectomy tissue, isolated high-grade PIN should be reported, but no data exist to suggest that features such as extent or pattern need be recorded. Low-grade PIN should not be reported.

Reporting high-grade PIN in radical prostatectomy and cystoprostatectomy is optimal but recommended.

■ t11.16 Reporting of PIN

Do not report low-grade PIN
Report presence of high-grade PIN in needle biopsy tissue, TURP chips and open prostatectomy tissues, with and without carcinoma
Reporting of presence of high-grade PIN in radical prostatectomies is optional (but recommended)
Reporting of extent and architectural pattern of high-grade PIN is optional

Recommendations for clinical follow-up to the treating physician are optional. Some pathologists may want to add "Rebiopsy is suggested" in a comment that explains the risk of subsequent detection of carcinoma after a diagnosis of isolated high-grade PIN or high-grade PIN with adjacent atypical small glands **t11.15**.

[11.11] PIN as Precursor

High-grade PIN is the most likely precursor proliferation for many moderately to poorly differentiated (Gleason score 5 to 10) carcinomas that arise in the peripheral zone. A wealth of morphologic, histochemical, immunophenotypic, molecular, genetic, and animal model data supports this concept **t11.17**. However, the prevailing notion is that high-grade PIN is not the universal precursor for prostate cancer. In particular, well-differentiated transition zone cancers have not been closely linked to high-grade PIN (Arakawa 1997, Epstein 1990B, Greene 1991), and recent data indicate that small, unifocal prostate cancers detected in whole glands at autopsy (Sakr 1994B), in cystoprostatectomy specimens (Arakawa 1997), and in radical prostatectomy tissues (Häggman 1997B) tend not to have physically associated, adjacent high-grade PIN. Based on these data, the role of high-grade PIN as even the main precursor lesion of all carcinomas of the prostate has been questioned (Arakawa 1997, Sakr 1994B), and additional epithelial abnormalities, including atypical adenomatous hyperplasia, postatrophic hyperplasia (Shah 2001), and proliferative inflammatory atrophy (De Marzo 1999), have been forwarded as candidate precursor proliferations. The possibility that high-grade PIN might be an epiphenomenon, a field effect, or "cancerization" of preexisting ducts and acini by adjacent invasive carcinoma has been raised. However, from a practical diagnostic and prognostic perspective, this debate does not change the diagnostic significance of high-grade PIN as a valid and important factor of risk for detecting invasive adenocarcinoma.

Elucidating the natural history of high-grade PIN has been extraordinarily difficult, and the natural course of this proliferation may only be inferred from age-based incidence studies. If high-grade PIN were a premalignant precursor lesion, given the low proliferation index of high-grade PIN, it should precede the development of invasive carcinoma by years, if not decades. The evidence supporting this idea is scanty. In fact, in an autopsy survey of the incidence of whole gland high-grade PIN and adenocarcinoma by decade, high-grade PIN incidence did not precede adenocarcinoma (Sakr 1994B) **f11.2**. In contrast, in a second autopsy study (Billis 1996), the frequency of high-grade PIN was higher than carcinoma at younger ages (40 to 64 years). For an age-related malignancy such as prostate cancer, one would expect a precursor lesion to increase in incidence and extent with age. Again, the results have been mixed. Although no correlation between age and frequency of all PIN grades was observed in the original McNeal and Bostwick article (McNeal 1986), the broadest age survey (Sakr 1994B) clearly shows an increase in incidence with age **f11.2**. A weak correlation of high-grade PIN volume with age was found in 1 study (Qian 1997B) but not 2 others (Humphrey 1992, Sakr 1995). Of interest, more extensive and more frequent high-grade PIN has been reported to arise earlier in African American (Sakr 1995, 1998A) and African Brazilian (Billis 1996) men than white men. These findings may contribute to an understanding of the higher incidence of prostate cancer in African

■ t11.17 High-grade PIN: Evidence in Support of Precursor Role

I. Clinical
- Incidence increases with age
- Occurs earlier and is more extensive in populations at risk (African Americans and Brazilian Americans)

II. Morphologic
- More often found in glands with vs without prostate cancer
- Physical association with clinical (but not incidental autopsy) cancers, including direct continuity
- Peripheral zone and multicentric
- Reduced number of basal cells, with basal cell loss at sites of invasion
- Nucleomegaly, nucleolomegaly and clumped chromatin
- Loss of secretory vacuoles (by electron microscopy)

III. Morphometric
- Increased nuclear and nucleolar size

IV. Histochemical
- Increased silver-stained NORs
- Aberrant lectin binding
- Aberrant mucin expression

V. Immunophenotypic
- Aberrant blood group antigen expression
- Dowregulation of neuroendocrine markers
- Aberrant enzyme expression, including decreased antioxidant enzyme expression
- Increased nuclear matrix protein expression
- Aberrant intermediate filament expression
- Increased cell proliferation index
- Abnormal expression of cell cycle regulators
- Increased polypeptide growth factor and growth factor receptors
- Increased bcl-2 protein (cell death antidote)
- Decreased expression of cell adhesive proteins
- Increased metalloproteinase expression
- Increased stromal angiogenesis

VI. Genetic
- Increased DNA content
- Increased DNA fragmentation (apoptosis)
- Gene amplification: *c-myc*
- Chromosomal gains: 7,8,10,12,17,X,Y
- Chromosomal losses: 7,8,10,Y
- Allelic loss: 7q,8p,8q,10q,16q,18q
- Mutator (RER+) phenotype
- p53 gene point mutation (14%)
- Methylation of GSTP1 gene

VII. Animal Models
- Spontaneous in Lobund-Wistar rats
- Spontaneous in dogs
- *N*-nitrosomethylurea and testosterone-induced in Loband-Wistar rats
- DES-induced in the Han:NMRI mice
- Testosterone/estradiol-induced in Noble rats
- Rat steroid binding protein C3 (1)-SV40 large T antigen transgenic mice
- Short probasin—SV40 early region transgenic mice
- Large probasin—SV40 large T antigen mice
- Fetal globin promoter-SV40 large T antigen transgenic mice
- C3 (1)-polyoma virus middle T transgenic mice
- Probasin-SV40 T antigen transgenic rats
- Probasin-EcoRI transgenic mice
- Probasin-FGF8 transgenic mice
- Probasin-androgen receptor transgenic mice
- BK5 promoter-insulin like growth factor-1 transgenic mice
- 2C (3)1-c-myc transgenic mice
- Cryptdin-2-SV40 early region transgenic mice
- PTEN +/– knockout mice
- Nkx3.1 knockout mice
- Conditional disruption of mouse retinoid x receptor alpha allele

[1]Note: Only some PIN animal models are proven precursors, with progression to invasive carcinoma

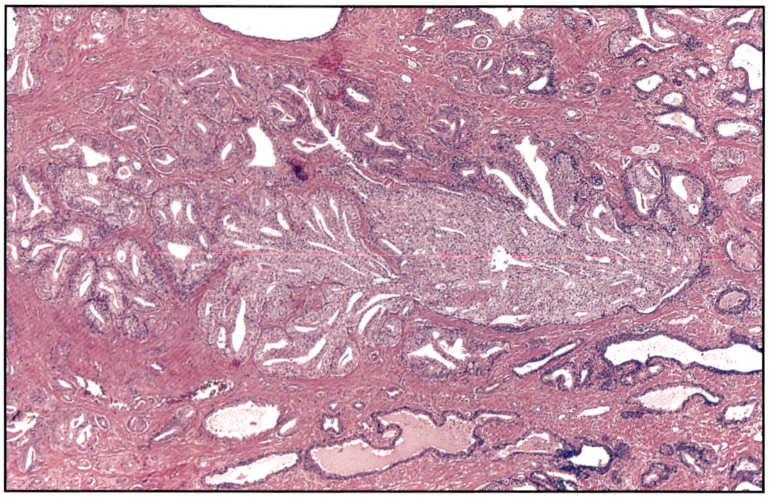

■ i11.66 *Expansile intraductal high-grade PIN, with branching into invasive carcinoma.*

Americans and African Brazilians. Although European men have a higher incidence of clinical prostatic cancer than Asian men, the frequency and volume of high-grade PIN do not differ between them (Anton 1998). Currently, there are many unanswered questions about the natural history of high-grade PIN:

- Does low-grade PIN progress to high-grade PIN, and if so, how often, and what is the time course?
- If high-grade PIN does progress to invasive carcinoma, how often does this occur, and what is the time course?
- Does PIN ever undergo regression (not induced by exogenous agents)?
- What are the cellular and molecular determinants of progression at each step?

The morphologic evidence linking high-grade PIN to clinical invasive carcinoma by examination of H&E slides is substantial. High-grade PIN often is physically associated with clinical (as opposed to incidental autopsy) invasive carcinoma, and both are multicentric and arise predominantly in the peripheral zone. It is often possible to visualize "buds" of high-grade PIN glands into adjacent stroma, which probably represents microinvasion **i11.61; i11.66, i11.67**. Cytologically, the luminal cells of high-grade PIN more closely resemble invasive carcinoma cells than benign luminal cells.

Electron microscopic study of high-grade PIN cells has demonstrated many shared ultrastructural characteristics with adenocarcinoma (Bostwick 1997). High-grade PIN cells were typified by dark and light cytoplasm, corresponding to amphophilic and cleared cytoplasm by H&E staining, respectively. Dark cytoplasm, which was found more often in carcinoma, contains a small number of secretory vacuoles and numerous mitochondria, lysosomes, microtubules, and free ribosomes. The light cells have an abundance of secretory vacuoles. Nuclei are large and rounded, with clumped chromatin and enlarged nucleoli **i11.68**.

Morphometric cell image analysis of high-grade PIN has supported the light and electron microscopic studies. Nuclear size calculations for high-grade PIN, quantified as nuclear area, nuclear perimeter, nuclear diameter, and nuclear volume, are closer to invasive carcinoma than benign epithelium (Lopez-Beltran 2000, Montironi 1990, 1991).

Histochemical staining reactions have highlighted aberrant high-grade PIN silver-stained nucleolar organizer regions

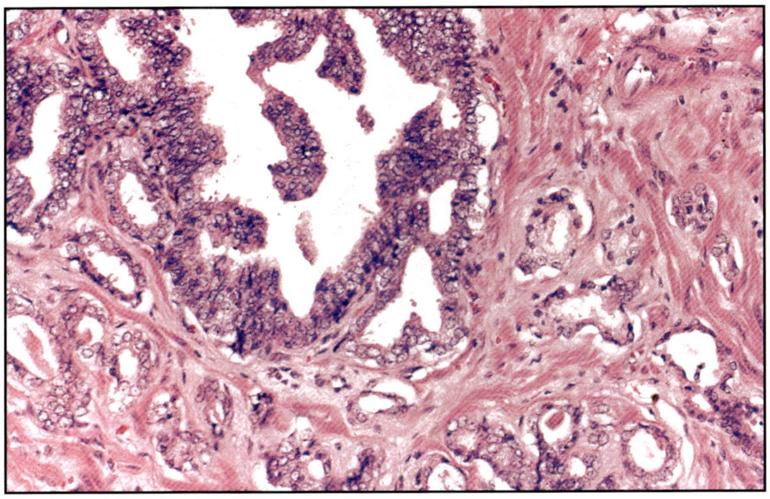

■ **i11.67** *"Budding" of invasive carcinoma from a high-grade PIN gland.*

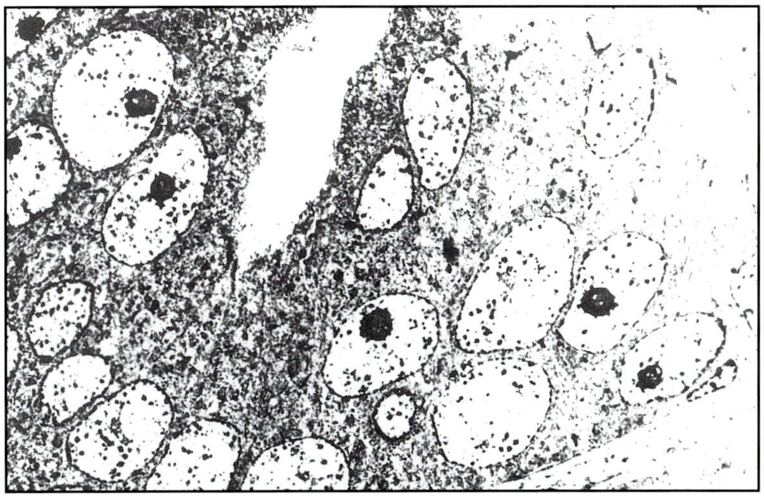

■ **i11.68** *Ultrastructural appearance of high-grade PIN cells.*

(AgNORs), lectin binding, and mucin synthesis. AgNORs are loops of chromosomal DNA that encode for ribosomal RNA, and AgNOR counts have been used as indicators of cell proliferation activity. Most investigators have found AgNOR levels in high-grade PIN to be elevated and close to those of invasive adenocarcinoma (Cheville 1990, Helpap 1995, Mukherjee 1997, Sakr 1993, Sentinelli 1990, Sesterhenn 1994). In ungraded PIN, anomalous binding by a number of lectins has been reported (McNeal 1988A). Aberrant glycoprotein expression, as reflected by lectin binding, has been recognized in high-grade PIN (Drachenberg 1995, Janssen 1996, Nagle 1991). High-grade PIN luminal cells synthesize both periodic acid-Schiff–positive neutral and Alcian blue–positive acid mucins (Humphrey 1991, Sentinelli 1993), which is typical of carcinoma as opposed to benign epithelial cells, which secrete mainly neutral mucins. In our experience acid mucin expression in high-grade PIN is exemplified by a thin mucin rimming of the luminal border **i11.69** (Humphrey 1991). Uncommonly, this mucin fills and distends high-grade glands, yielding the mucinous variant **i11.12** (Reyes 1997B). Only rarely do high-grade PIN cells harbor intracytoplasmic mucin.

The immunophenotype of high-grade PIN luminal cells is more concordant with invasive carcinoma than benign epithelium. Basal cells in PIN, which may be lower in number, have the same immunophenotype as basal cells in normal and hyperplastic glands. Abnormal expression of a large number of diverse molecules intimately involved in cell growth and differentiation has been shown in luminal cells of high-grade PIN (Bostwick 1996A, Häggman 1997C, Maygarden 1994A, Myers 1996A). That an impaired state of differentiation is present in high-grade PIN cells is buttressed by immunohistochemical detection of aberrant expression of blood group antigens (Perlman 1990), markers of neuroendocrine differentiation (with downregulation of serotonin, neuron-specific enolase, chromogranin, and human chorionic gonadotropin) (Bostwick 1994, di Sant'Agnese 1996), and enzymes such as pepsinogen II (Bostwick 1996C), human glandular kallikrein 2 (Darson 1997), glutathione S-transferase-pi (Cookson 1997, Moskaluk 1997), acid phosphatase (Darson 1997, McNeal 1988B, Monger 1994), 5'-nucleotidase (Monger 1994), hexosaminidase (Monger 1994), the antioxidant enzymes superoxidase dismutase and catalase (Bostwick 2000A), and PSA (Darson 1997, McNeal 1988B). PSA and prostatic acid phosphatase immunoreactivity in high-grade PIN is intermediate between a uniform, strong positivity in benign glands and diminished, heterogeneous expression in invasive carcinoma.

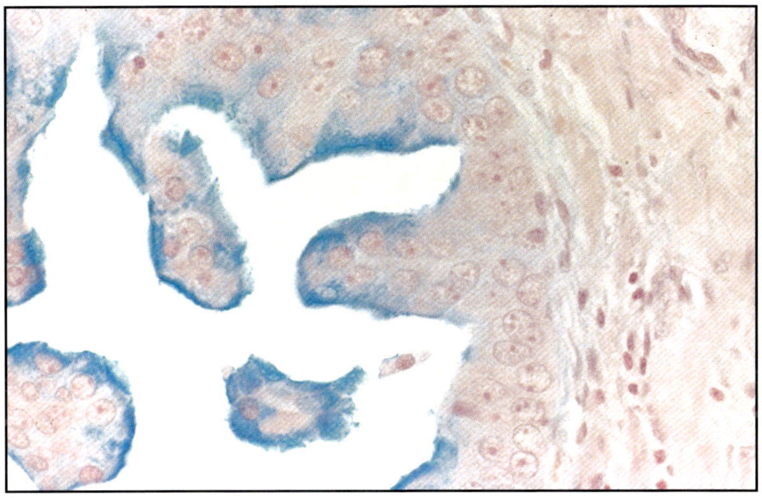

■ **i11.69** *Acidic mucin along luminal aspect of high-grade PIN gland (Alcian blue stain)*

Further evidence of perturbation of differentiation of high-grade PIN luminal cells in provided by aberrant intermediate filament expression where high-grade luminal cells exhibit loss of vimentin and expression of cytokeratins 15, 16, and 19, as in carcinoma (Nagle 1991, 1996, Yang 1997). Proliferation indices of high-grade PIN, as measured by immunohistochemical staining for the Ki-67 antigen (by monoclonal antibody MIB-1) and proliferating cell nuclear antigen, indicate that high-grade PIN has a proliferative activity intermediate between those of benign epithelium and invasive carcinoma (Berges 1995, Feneley 1996, Häussler 1999, Johnson 1998, Koch 2000, Montironi 1994B, Tamboli 1996). Also, there is a shift in the proliferative cell compartment from basal cells in benign epithelium to the luminal cells in high-grade PIN (Berges 1995, Montironi 1994B). Overall, the proliferative index exceeds that of the apoptotic index such that for isolated high-grade PIN there should be a slow but inexorable growth, with a doubling time estimated at 154 days (Berges 1995). The increased growth of high-grade PIN could be related to an increase in expression of growth factors such as parathormone-related protein (Iwamura 1995), platelet-derived growth factor (Fudge 1996), vascular endothelial growth factor (Kollermann 2001, Nassar 2001), fibroblast growth factors 6 (Ropiquet 2000) and 8 (Valve 2001), and growth factor receptors, including vascular endothelial growth factor receptor (Kollermann 2001), fibroblast growth factor receptors 1 and 2 (Valve 2001), Her-2/neu/c-erbB-2 (Haussler 1999, Ibrahim 1992, Myers 1994B), c-erbB-3 (Häussler 1999, Myers 1994B), insulin-like growth factor binding protein-2 (Tennant 1996), and the hepatocyte growth factor/scatter factor receptor (c-met proto-oncogene product) (Humphrey 1995A, Pisters 1995). Immunoreactive androgen receptor, which probably is also related to high-grade PIN cell proliferation, is present in high-grade PIN luminal cells but not basal cells (Harper 1998, Leav 1996A, Magi-Galluzzi 1997, Sweat 1999, van der Kwast 1996). Concomitant with increased cell proliferation of high-grade PIN luminal cells, there is enhanced immunoreactivity of the anti–cell death proteins bcl-2, bcl-X, and mcl-1 (Colombel 1993, Johnson 1998, Krajewska 1996, Stattin 1996) and also aberrant expression of the cell cycle regulator proteins p16INK4A (Henshall 2001), p21/WAF1 (Adsay 1997), and p27/Kipl (Fernández 1999, Nassar 2001). Proto-oncogene and tumor suppressor gene products in high-grade PIN have been characterized by immunohistochemistry. The aforementioned erb-B and c-met, as well as RET (Dawson 1998), proto-oncogene products are elevated in high-grade PIN. Downstream effectors of oncogenic signals such as mitogen-activated protein kinase phosphatase (MKP-1) are elevated in PIN (Magi-Galluzzi 1996). One of the most important tumor suppressor gene products, the p53 protein, exhibits abnormal accumulation in a minority of high-grade PIN cases in most series (Al-Maghrabi 2001, Häussler 1999, Hughes 1995, Humphrey 1995B, Lee 1994, Salem 1997, Tamboli 1998, Thomas 1993, Van Veldhuizen 1993) **i11.70**. Accumulation of the p53 protein, as judged by immunohistochemistry, is associated with mutations in the p53 gene (Humphrey 1996A), which is one of the most commonly mutated tumor suppressor genes in all human cancer. In high-grade PIN, p53 mutations have been detected in 14% to 22% of cases, with most mutations being missense point mutations (Takayama 2000, Yasunaga 1998). In several cases there was heterogeneity of p53 mutation, with silent or nonsense point mutations also discovered (Yasunaga 1998). There is also diminished expression of adhesive-related molecules, such as C-CAM (Kleinerman 1995), and β4 integrin (Allen 1998). A possible connection with stromal invasion from high-grade PIN is the presence of metalloproteinases, including type IV collagenase, in high-grade PIN cells (Boag 1993, 1994, Montironi 1996B, Upadhyay 1999). By laminin, collagen type VII, and heparan sulfate proteoglycan immunohistochemistry, an intact basement membrane is maintained in high-grade PIN (Bostwick 1995C, Nagle 1995), but there is a stromal response to high-grade PIN, exemplified by new blood vessel formation (angiogenesis) (Brawer 1994, Montironi 1993B, 1996A, Sinha 1995). Such increased microvessel density can be highlighted using antibodies to CD31, CD34, or factor VIII–related antigen. In addition to a higher number of microvessels around high-grade PIN glands than around benign glands, there is a remodeling of the capillary architecture, with a higher proportion of short, nontouching capillaries, which have an undulated external contour, an open lumen, and a higher number of endothelial cell nuclei (Montironi 1996A). Additional markers that are aberrantly expressed in high-grade PIN, as determined by immunohistochemistry, include cathepsin D (Maygarden 1994B), nm23-Hl (Jensen 1996, Myers 1996B), TAG-72 (Brenner 1995, Myers 1995A), glycoprotein A-80 (Gould 1997), estrogen-inducible pS2 protein (Bonkhoff 1995), Lewis Y antigen (Myers 1995B), OA-519 (fatty acid synthetase) (Epstein 1995C), nuclear matrix proteins (Mucci 1998), prostate inhibin peptide (Nangia 1998), Ep-CAM (Poczatek 1999), inducible nitric oxide synthase (Baltaci 2001), the DNA excision repair and redox enzyme Ape 1/ref-1 (Kelley 2001), and 15-lipoxygenase-2 (Jack 2000).

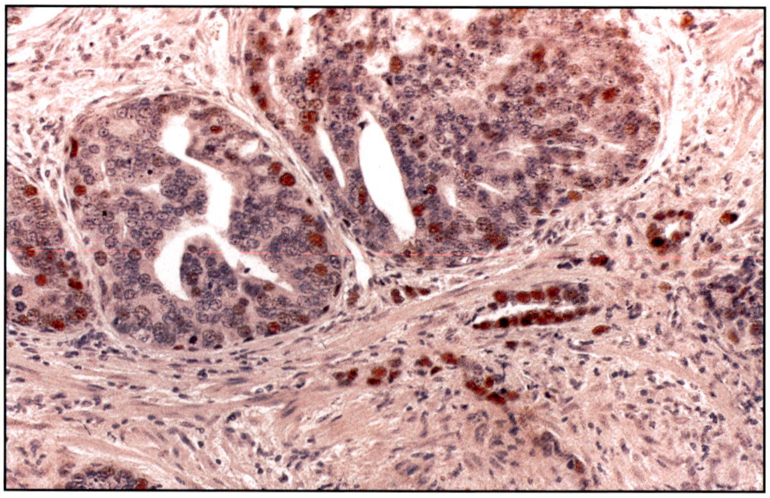

■ **i11.70** *p53 protein accumulation in cribriform high-grade PIN and adjacent invasive small acinar adenocarcinoma.*

DNA and genetic abnormalities in high-grade PIN also suggest a close relationship between high-grade PIN and invasive carcinoma **t11.17**. PIN luminal cell nuclei are aneuploid in 0% to 76% of cases, depending on the study and methodologic method (image analysis, flow cytometry, or in situ hybridization) (Alers 1995, Amin 1993B, Baretton 1994, Crissman 1993, de la Torre 1993, Petein 1991, Sakr 1995, Weinberg 1993). Data on concordance of ploidy status in high-grade PIN and invasive carcinoma in the same case are mixed (Amin 1993B, Baretton 1994, Crissman 1993). Whereas aneuploid high-grade PIN is highly associated with aneuploid invasive carcinoma in 70% to 87% of cases, diploid high-grade PIN is found with aneuploid invasive carcinoma in 32% to 57% of cases. These results suggest that not all high-grade PIN foci progress to invasive carcinoma. This might be particularly true for the diploid high-grade PIN foci. Alternatively, it is conceivable that for some cases genetic abnormalities as reflected by DNA content may accumulate not at the preinvasive high-grade PIN phase but later in the progression sequence. In addition to accumulation, DNA fragmentation that occurs in apoptosis is higher in high-grade PIN than in benign glands (Berges 1995, Drachenberg 1997). Apoptosis can be detected reliably by H&E staining of apoptotic bodies or by Tdt-mediated dUTP-biotin nick end labeling (Drachenberg 1997). To reiterate, cell proliferation rate in high-grade PIN exceeds the apoptotic cell death rate, so that overall the balance is shifted toward high-grade PIN growth (Berges 1995).

Chromosomal abnormalities are common in high-grade PIN (Al-Maghrabi 2002, Alcaraz 2001, Brooks 1998, Bull 2001, Doll 1997, Erbersdobler 1996, Häggman 1997A, Issacs 1998, Jenkins 1997, Miet 1999, Pihan 2000, Qian 1996, Sandberg 1998) **t11.17; f11.5** and are characterized by numerical gains and losses of specific chromosomes and loss of specific DNA sequences in specific chromosomal regions. Numerical chromosomal abnormalities have been detected in up to 67% of high-grade PIN foci, compared with 68% and 98% of locally invasive carcinoma and metastatic carcinoma foci, respectively (Jenkins 1997). The most common chromosomal anomaly for both high-grade PIN and carcinoma is a gain of chromosome 8. In general, carcinoma exhibits a more complex genotypic array of chromosomal gains and losses than high-grade PIN, but there is tremendous heterogeneity of genetic lesions even within the same gland. Therefore, some high-grade PIN foci do not exhibit any chromosomal abnormalities at all

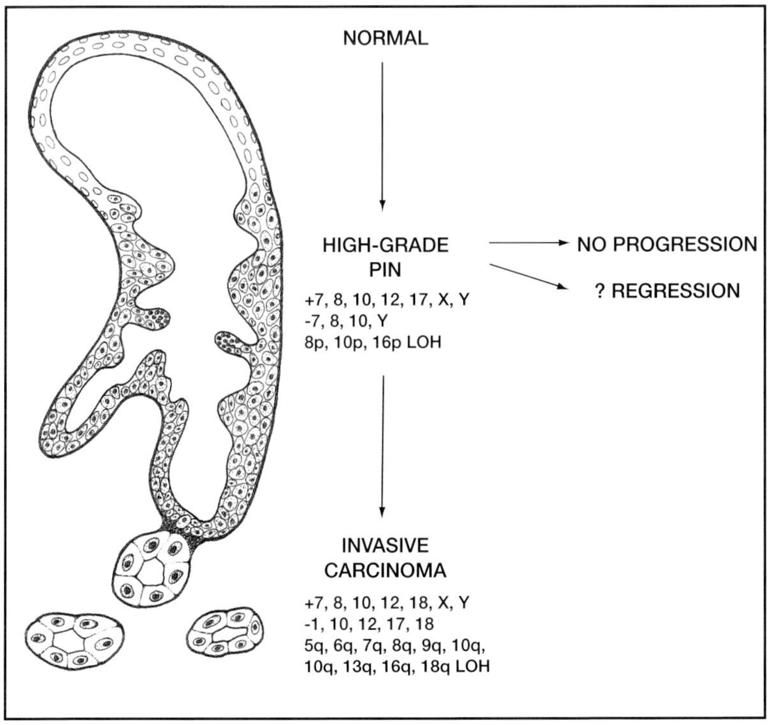

■ **f11.5** *Morphological and genetic progression of high-grade PIN.*

(at least using the current fluorescence in situ hybridization [FISH] probes), and some foci actually contain more genetic FISH anomalies than the coexisting carcinoma in the same case. The cribriform pattern of high-grade PIN more often has a gain in chromosomes 7, 12, and Y than the tufting pattern but not the micropapillary pattern. Of note, this genetic profile does not seem to impart a high risk for subsequent detection of adenocarcinoma in patients with isolated cribriform high-grade PIN in needle biopsy (Qian 1997A). Fractional loss of DNA at specific chromosomal loci (allelic loss) has been documented in high-grade PIN on chromosomes 7q, 8p, 8q, 10q, 16q, and 18q (Bostwick 1998, Emmert-Buck 1995, Häggman 1997A, Jenkins 1997, Macoska 1994, Sakr 1994A). Loss of DNA sequences and as yet unidentified tumor suppressor genes at 8p12–22 is likely to be particularly important in high-grade PIN initiation and progression. Of interest, there was loss of the same allele at 8p21 for high-grade PIN adjacent to invasive carcinoma, whereas distant high-grade PIN had different allele loss (Häggman 1997A). Also, there is concordance of *c-myc* gene amplification in high-grade PIN and invasive carcinoma (Jenkins 1997). Overall, although there is often a similar pattern of allelic loss in matched high-grade PIN and carcinoma foci from the same gland, the frequency of allelic loss is lower in PIN than in carcinoma. Both PIN and carcinoma exhibited significant genetic heterogeneity (Bostwick 1998, Saric 1999, Zitzelsberger 1998). Additional genetic alterations in high-grade PIN include abnormal centrosomes (which may contribute to aneuploidy) (Pihan 2000), a mutator (RER^+) phenotype in a minority of cases (Miet 1999), and, as in carcinoma, CG island methylation in the 5′-regulatory region of the GSTP1 gene is a majority of cases (Brooks 1998).

All of these genetic data implicate high-grade PIN as a precursor, but much remains to be learned, such as which specific genes are involved in the progression of high-grade PIN. Already, cDNA libraries have been constructed from microdissected PIN; such a library could be used in subtractive hybridizations and cDNA microarray technology to identify specific genes whose expression is altered in the course of prostate cancer initiation and progression (Krizman 1996). Preliminary gene expression profiling of PIN using cDNA microarrays has been accomplished, with identification of several novel overexpressed genes (Bull 2001). Genetic models of prostate cancer progression through high-grade PIN have been forwarded (Sandberg 1998), but these linear models are somewhat simplistic because multiple pathways through a wide variety of accumulated genetic aberrancies probably underlie high-grade PIN progression to invasive disease. Currently, genetic alterations in high-grade PIN detected by FISH on tissue sections or polymerase chain reaction using RNA or DNA extracted from PIN harbor potential as diagnostic or prognostic tools, yet such tests are still experimental.

A more temporally dynamic way to study the natural history of high-grade PIN is through the use of animal models (Abdulkadir 2001, Asamoto 2001, Bostwick 2000B, DiGiovanni 2000, Garabedian 1998, Greenberg 1995, Masumori 2001, Navone 1999, Podsypania 1999, Shappell 2002, Voelkel-Johnson 2000, Zhang 2000) **t11.17**, although these models are not perfect because animal prostate glands are not morphologically identical to human prostates. High-grade PIN may arise spontaneously in rats or dogs and may be induced in rats and mice by hormonal treatment or in rats with a combination of a carcinogen and testosterone. High-grade PIN has also been observed in transgenic mice by use of viral oncogenes, the androgen receptor (Stanbrough 2002), *Eco*R1, c-myc, the growth factor FGF8 (Song 2002), and IGF-1 genes in the transgene **t11.17**. Deletion (knockout) of the tumor suppressor gene *PTEN* (Podsypania 1999) or the homeodomain-containing transcription factor Nkx3.1 (Abdulkadir 2002), a putative tumor suppressor, can lead to high-grade PIN. Finally, delay of prostatic carcinogenesis at the PIN stage has been achieved by crossing SV40 early region transgenic mice with mice deficient in the transcription factor Egrl (Abdulkadir 2001). In some of these models low-grade and high-grade PIN precede the development of invasive carcinoma. Increase in extent of PIN with time has been noted, and architectural patterns of growth similar to those of human disease have been described (Garabedian 1998, Shibata 1996). These animal models will be useful in dissecting molecular events involved in prostate cancer progression and in testing treatments to prevent the development of high-grade PIN and thereby presumably prostate cancer. Cell lines derived from animal model PIN cells may be informative (Soares 2002). From a diagnostic standpoint, it will be of interest to study the earliest foci of microinvasion from high-grade PIN in these animal models. Knowledge gained from such study may translate into improvements in diagnosis of human high-grade PIN with and without focal invasion.

Determining the origin of high-grade PIN will require understanding of the genesis of prostate cancer itself. Clearly, age, androgens, and race all play a role. Heredity probably does as well, and it is probable that men with familial and hereditary prostate cancer also inherit a susceptibility for high-grade PIN development. It may be hypothesized that, as for other inherited epithelial malignancies, men with hereditary prostate cancer will develop multifocal, extensive precursor proliferations, such as high-grade PIN, at a young age. This remains to be proven, and the extent of high-grade PIN in the presence of carcinoma was not different between sporadic and inherited forms of prostate cancer (Bastacky 1995). Stem cells within the basal cell compartment of the normal prostate probably are the targets for neoplastic transformation (Bonkhoff 1996A, 1996B) and high-grade PIN development. Differentiation arrest, or perturbation of differentiation (as might occur in transformation) of prostatic stem cells is a process that may depend on bidirectional stromal cell–basal cell communication (Liu 1997), which could influence the formation of high-grade PIN.

[11.12] Summary

It is critical to recognize and diagnose isolated high-grade PIN in prostatic tissue samples, particularly core prostate needle biopsy, transurethral resectates, and open (simple) prostatectomy tissues. The differential diagnosis of high-grade PIN is extensive and includes low-grade PIN, which, according to current concepts should be not reported. Patients with isolated high-grade PIN are at risk for subsequent detection of carcinoma and are candidates for rebiopsy in 3 to 4 months. Currently, no biomarkers or genotypic abnormalities are useful in the diagnosis or prediction of prognosis for patients with high-grade PIN, but this remains an area of intensive investigation for the future.

References

Abbas F, Hochberg D, Civantos F, et al. Incidental prostatic adenocarcinoma in patients undergoing radical cystoprostatectomy for bladder cancer. *Urology* 30:322-326, 1996.

Abdulkadir SA, Magee JA, Peters TJ, et al. Conditional loss of Nkx3.1 in adult mice induces prostatic intraepithelial neoplasia. *Mol Cell Biol* 22:1495-1503, 2002.

Abdulkadir SA, Qu Z, Garabedian E, et al. Impaired prostate tumorigenesis in Eg1-deficient mice. *Nat Med* 7:101-107, 2001.

Aboseif S, Shinohara K, Weidner N, et al. The significance of prostatic intraepithelial neoplasia. *Br J Urol* 76:355-359, 1995.

Adsay V, Sakr W, Grignon D, et al. Distribution of WAFI (p21) in normal and neoplastic prostate tissue [abstract]. *Mod Pathol* 10:68A, 1997.

Al-Maghrabi J, Vorobyova L, Chapman W, et al. p53 Alteration of chromosomal instability in prostatic high-grade intraepithelial neoplasia and concurrent carcinoma: analysis by immunohistochemistry, interphase in situ hybridization, and sequencing of laser-captured microdissected specimens. *Mod Pathol* 14:1252-1262, 2001.

Al-Maghrabi J, Vorobyova L, Toi A, et al. Identification of numerical chromosomal changes detected by interphase fluorescence in situ hybridization in high-grade prostate intraepithelial neoplasia as a predictor of carcinoma. *Arch Pathol Lab Med* 126:165-169, 2002.

Alcaraz A, Barranco MA, Corral JM, et al. High-grade prostatic intraepithelial neoplasia shares cytogenetic alterations with invasive prostate cancer. *Prostate* 47:29-35, 2001.

Alers JC, Krijtenburg PJ, Vissers KJ, et al. Interphase cytogenetics of prostatic adenocarcinoma and precursor lesions: analysis of radical prostatectomies and 17 adjacent prostatic intraepithelial neoplasias. *Genes Chromosom Cancer* 12:241-250, 1995.

Alexander EE, Qian J, Wollan PC, et al. Prostatic intraepithelial neoplasia does not appear to raise serum prostate-specific antigen concentration. *Urology* 47:693-698, 1996.

Algaba F. Evolution of isolated high-grade prostatic intraepithelial neoplasia in a Mediterranean patient population. *Eur Urol* 35:496-497, 1999.

Allam CK, Bostwick DG, Hayes JA, et al. Interobserver variability in the diagnosis of high-grade prostatic intraepithelial neoplasia and adenocarcinoma. *Mod Pathol* 9:742-751, 1996.

Allen MV, Smith GJ, Juliano R, et al. Downregulation of ?B4 integrin subunit in prostatic carcinoma and prostatic intraepithelial neoplasia. *Hum Pathol* 29:311-318, 1998.

Alsikafi NF, Brendler CB, Gerber GS, et al. High-grade prostatic intraepithelial neoplasia with adjacent atypia is associated with a higher incidence of cancer on subsequent needle biopsy than high-grade prostatic intraepithelial neoplasia alone. *Urology* 57:296-300, 2001.

Amin MB, Schultz DS, Zarbo RJ, et al. Computerized static DNA ploidy analysis of prostatic intraepithelial neoplasia. *Arch Pathol Lab Med* 117:794-798, 1993A.

Amin MB, Ro JY, Ayala AG. Putative precursor lesions of prostatic adenocarcinoma: fact or fiction? *Mod Pathol* 6:476-483, 1993B.

Amin MB, Schultz DS, Zarbo RJ. Analysis of cribriform morphology in prostatic neoplasia using antibody to high-molecular-weight cytokeratins. *Arch Pathol Lab Med* 118:260-264, 1994A.

Amin MB, Ro JY, Ayala AG. Prostatic intraepithelial neoplasia: relationship to adenocarcinoma of prostate. *Pathol Ann* 29:1-30, 1994B.

Amin MB, Bostwick DG. Pigment in prostatic epithelium and adenocarcinoma: a potential source of diagnostic confusion with seminal vesicular epithelium. *Mod Pathol* 9:791-795, 1996.

Amin MB, Grignon D, Bostwick D, et al. Recommendations for the reporting of resected prostate carcinomas. ADASP (Association of Directors of Anatomic and Surgical Pathology). *Am J Clin Pathol* 105:667-670, 1996B.

Andrews GS. Latent carcinoma of the prostate. *J Clin Pathol* 2:197-208, 1949.

Anton RC, Wilcox GE, Maru N, et al. The incidence and extent of high-grade prostatic intraepithelial neoplasia (HGPIN) and prostate cancer (PCa) at autopsy in Central Asia. *Mod Pathol* 11:76A, 1998.

Aquilina JW, Lipsky JJ, Bostwick DG. Androgen deprivation as a strategy for prostate cancer chemoprevention. *J Natl Cancer Inst* 89:689-676, 1997.

Aquilina JW, McKinney L, Pacelli A, et al. High grade prostatic intraepithelial neoplasia in military working dogs with and without prostate cancer. *Prostate* 36:189-193, 1998.

Arakawa A, Song S, Scardino PT, et al. High-grade prostatic intraepithelial neoplasia in prostates removed following irradiation. Failure in the treatment of prostatic adenocarcinoma. *Pathol Res Pract* 191:868-872, 1995.

Arakawa A, Soh S, Wheeler TM. High-grade prostatic intraepithelial neoplasia in cystoprostatectomy specimens. *J Urol Pathol* 7:1-8, 1997.

Argani P, Epstein JI. Inverted (hobnail) high-grade prostatic intraepithelial neoplasia (PIN). Report of 15 cases of a previously undescribed pattern of high-grade PIN. *Am J Surg Pathol* 25:1534-1538, 2001.

Asamoto M, Hokaiwado N, Cho YM, et al. Prostate carcinomas developing in transgenic rats with SV40 T antigen expression under probasin promoter control are strictly androgen dependent. *Cancer Res* 61:4693-4700, 2001.

Balaji KC, Rabbani F, Tsai H, et al. Effect of neoadjuvant hormonal therapy on prostatic intraepithelial neoplasia and its prognostic significance. *J Urol* 162:753-757, 1999.

Baltaci S, Orhan D, Gogus C, et al. Inducible nitric oxide synthase expression in benign prostatic hyperplasia, low and high-grade prostatic intraepithelial neoplasia and prostatic carcinoma. *BJU Int* 88:100-103, 2001.

Baretton G, Vogt T, Valina C, et al. Prostate cancers and potential precancerous conditions: DNA cytometric investigations and interphase cytogenetics. *Verh Dtsch Ges Pathol* 77:86-92, 1993.

Baretton GB, Vogt T, Blasenbreu S, et al. Comparison of DNA ploidy in prostatic intraepithelial neoplasia and invasive carcinoma of the prostate. *Hum Pathol* 25:506-513, 1994.

Bastacky SI, Wojno KJ, Walsh PC, et al. Pathological features of hereditary prostate cancer. *J Urol* 153:987-992, 1995.

Berges RR, Vukanovic J, Epstein JI, et al. Implication of cell kinetic changes during progression of human prostate cancer. *Clin Cancer Res* 1:472-480, 1995.

Berman DM, Yang J, Epstein JI. Foamy gland high-grade prostatic intraepithelial neoplasia. *Am J Surg Pathol* 24:140-144, 2000.

Berner A, Danielsen HE, Pettersen EO, et al. DNA distribution in the prostate. Normal gland, benign and premalignant lesions and subsequent adenocarcinomas. *Anal Quant Cytol Histol* 15:247-252, 1993.

Bhatia-Gaur R, Donjacour AA, Sciavolino PJ, et al. Roles for Nkx3.1 in prostate development and cancer. *Genes Dev* 13:966-977, 1999.

Billis A. Age and race distribution of high-grade prostatic intraepithelial neoplasia. An autopsy study in Brazil (South America). *J Urol Pathol* 5:1-7, 1996.

Boag AH, Young ID. Immunohistochemical analysis of type IV collagenase expression in prostatic hyperplasia and adenocarcinoma. *Mod Pathol* 6:65-68, 1993.

Boag AH, Young ID. Increased expression of the 72-kd type IV collagenase in prostatic adenocarcinoma. Demonstration by immunohistochemistry and in situ hybridization. *Am J Pathol* 144:585-591, 1994.

Bock BJ, Sebo TJ, Cheville JC. High grade prostatic intraepithelial neoplasia associated with adenocarcinoma is predictive of tumor multifocality but not stage, margin status, or tumor volume at prostatectomy [abstract]. *Mod Pathol* 12:90A, 1999.

Bonkhoff H, Wernert N, Dhom G, et al. Basement membranes in fetal, adult normal, hyperplastic and neoplastic human prostate. *Virchows Arch-A, Pathol Anat Histopathol* 418:375-381, 1991.

Bonkhoff H, Wernert N, Dhom G, et al. Distribution of basement membranes in primary and metastatic carcinomas of the prostate. *Hum Pathol* 23:934-939, 1992.

Bonkhoff H, Stein U, Welter C, et al. Differential expression of the pS2 protein in the human prostate and prostate cancer: association with premalignant changes and neuroendocrine differentiation. *Hum Pathol* 26:824-828, 1995.

Bonkhoff H, Remberger K. Differentiation pathways and histogenetic aspects of normal and abnormal prostatic growth: a stem cell model. *Prostate* 28:98-106, 1996A.

Bonkhoff H. Role of the basal cells in premalignant changes of the human prostate: a stem cell concept for the development of prostatic cancer. *Eur Urol* 30:201-205, 1996B.

Borboroglu PG, Sur RL, Roberts JL, et al. Repeat biopsy strategy in patients with atypical small acinar proliferation or high grade prostatic intraepithelial neoplasia on initial prostate needle biopsy. *J Urol* 166:866-870, 2001.

Bostwick DG, Brawer MK. Prostatic intraepithelial neoplasia and early invasion in prostate cancer. *Cancer* 59:788-754, 1987.

Bostwick DG. Premalignant lesions of the prostate. *Semin Diagn Pathol* 5:240-253, 1988.

Bostwick DG, Amin MB, Dundore P, et al. Architectural patterns of high-grade prostatic intraepithelial neoplasia. *Hum Pathol* 24:298-310, 1993.

Bostwick DF, Dousa MK, Crawford BG, et al. Neuroendocrine differentiation in prostatic intraepithelial neoplasia and adenocarcinoma. *Am J Surg Pathol* 18:1240-1246, 1994.

Bostwick DG. High-grade prostatic intraepithelial neoplasia. The most likely precursor of prostate cancer. *Cancer* 75:1822-1836, 1995A.

Bostwick DG, Qian WJ, Frankel K. The incidence of high grade prostatic intraepithelial neoplasia in needle biopsies. *J Urol* 154:1791-1794, 1995B.

Bostwick DG, Leske DA, Qian J, et al. Prostatic intraepithelial neoplasia and well-differentiated adenocarcinoma maintain an intact basement membrane. *Pathol Res Pract* 191:850-855, 1995C.

Bostwick DG, Pacelli A, Lopez-Beltran A. Molecular biology of prostatic intraepithelial neoplasia. *Prostate* 29:117-134, 1996A.

Bostwick DG. Progression of prostatic intraepithelial neoplasia to early invasive adenocarcinoma. *Eur Urol* 30:145-152, 1996B.

Bostwick DG, Pacelli A, Lopez-Beltran A. Ultrastructure of prostatic intraepithelial neoplasia. *Prostate* 33:32-37, 1997.

Bostwick DG, Shan A, Qian JQ, et al. Independent origin of multiple foci of prostatic intraepithelial neoplasia-comparison with matched foci of prostate carcinoma. *Cancer* 83:1995-2002, 1998.

Bostwick DG. Prostatic intraepithelial neoplasia is a risk factor for cancer. *Semin Urol Oncol* 17:187-198, 1999.

Bostwick DG, Alexander EE, Singh R, et al. Antioxidant enzyme expression and reactive oxygen species damage in prostatic intraepithelial neoplasia and cancer. *Cancer* 89:123-134, 2000A.

Bostwick DG, Ramnani D, Qian J. Prostatic intraepithelial neoplasia: animal models 2000. *Prostate* 43:286-294, 2000B.

Bostwick DG, Qian J. Effect of androgen deprivation therapy on prostatic intraepithelial neoplasia. *Urology* 58:91-93, 2001.

Brawer MK, Rennels MA, Nagle RB, et al. Prostatic intraepithelial neoplasia: a lesion that may be confused with cancer on prostatic ultrasound. *J Urol* 142:1510-1512, 1989A.

Brawer MK. Prostatic intraepithelial neoplasia and prostate-specific antigen. *Urology* 346(suppl):62-65, 1989B.

Brawer MK, Rennels MA, Nagle RB, et al. Serum prostate-specific antigen and prostate pathology in men having simple prostatectomy. *Am J Clin Pathol* 92:760-764, 1989C.

Brawer MK, Bigler SA, Sohlberg OE, et al. Significance of prostatic intraepithelial neoplasia on prostate needle biopsy. *Urology* 38:103-107, 1991.

Brawer MK, Deering RE, Brown M, et al. Predictors of pathologic stage of prostatic carcinoma. The role of neovascularity. *Cancer* 73:678-687, 1994.

Breitkreuz T, Romanakis K, Lutz S, et al. Genotypic characterization of prostatic carcinomas: a combined cytogenetic, flow cytometry, and in situ hybridization study. *Cancer Res* 53:4035-4040, 1993.

Brenner PC, Rettig WJ, Sanz-Moncasi MP, et al. TAG-72 expression in primary, metastatic and hormonally treated prostate cancer as defined by monoclonal antibody CC49. *J Urol* 153:1575-1579, 1995.

Brooks JD, Weinstein M, Lin X, et al. CG island methylation changes near the GSTP1 gene in prostatic intraepithelial neoplasia. *Cancer Epidemiol Biomarkers Prev* 7:531-536, 1998.

Bull JH, Ellison G, Patel A, et al. Identification of potential diagnostic markers of prostate cancer and prostatic intraepithelial neoplasia using cDNA microarray. *Br J Cancer* 84:1512-1519, 2001.

Cheng L, Cheville JC, Pisansky TM, et al. Prevalence and distribution of prostatic intraepithelial neoplasia in salvage radical prostatectomy specimens after radiation therapy. *Am J Surg Pathol* 23:803-808, 1999.

Cheville JC, Clamon GH, Robinson RA. Silver-stained nucleolar organizer regions in the differentiation of prostatic hyperplasia, intraepithelial neoplasia, and adenocarcinoma. *Mod Pathol* 3:596-598, 1990.

Cheville JC, Reznicek MJ, Bostwick DG. Thc focus of "atypical glands, suspicious for malignancy" in prostatic needle biopsy specimens. Incidence, histologic features, and clinical follow-up of cases diagnosed in a community practice. *Am J Clin Pathol* 108:633-640, 1997.

Civantos F, Marcial MA, Banks ER, et al. Pathology of androgen deprivation therapy in prostate carcinoma. A comparative study of 173 patients. *Cancer* 75:1634-1641, 1995.

Civantos F, Soloway MS, Pinto JE. Histopathological effects of androgen deprivation in prostatic cancer. *Semin Urol Oncol* 14(2 suppl 2):22-31, 1996.

Civantos F, Watson RB, Pinto JE, et al. Finasteride effect on prostatic hyperplasia and prostate cancer. A comparative clinicopathologic study of radical prostatectomies. *J Urol Pathol* 6:1-13, 1997.

Cohen RJ, McNeal JE, Baillie T. Patterns of differentiation and proliferation in intraductal carcinoma of the prostate: significance for cancer progression. *Prostate* 43:11-19, 2000.

Colombel M, Symmans F, Gil S, et al. Detection of the apoptosis-suppressing oncoprotein bcl-2 in hormone-refractory human prostate cancers. *Am J Pathol* 143:390-400, 1993.

Cookson MS, Reuter VE, Linkov I, et al. Glutathione s-transferase PI (GST-pi) class expression by immunohistochemistry in benign and malignant prostate tissue. *J Urol* 157:673-676, 1997.

Crissman JD, Sakr WA, Hussein ME, et al. DNA quantitation of intraepithelial neoplasia and invasive carcinoma of the prostate. *Prostate* 22:155-162, 1993.

Darson MF, Pacelli A, Roche P, et al. Human glandular kallikrein (hK2) expression in prostatic intraepithelial neoplasia and adenocarcinoma : a novel prostate cancer marker. *Urology* 49:857-862, 1997.

Davidson D, Bostwick DG, Qian J, et al. Prostatic intraepithelial neoplasia is a risk factor for adenocarcinoma: predictive accuracy in needle biopsies. *J Urol* 154:1295-1299, 1995.

Dawson DM, Lawrence EG, MacLennan GT, et al. Altered expression of RET proto-oncogene product in prostatic intraepithelial neoplasia and prostate cancer. *J Natl Cancer Inst* 90:519-523, 1998.

de la Torre M, Häggman M, Brändtstedt S, et al. Prostatic intraepithelial neoplasia and invasive carcinoma in total prostatectomy specimens: distribution, volumes, and DNA ploidy. *Br J Urol* 72:207-213, 1993.

De Marzo AM, Marchi VL, Epstein JI, et al. Proliferative inflammatory atrophy of the prostate. *Am J Pathol* 155:1985-1992, 1999.

Devaraj LT, Bostwick DG. Atypical basal cell hyperplasia of the prostate. Immunophenotypic profile and proposed classification of basal cell proliferations. *Am J Surg Pathol* 17:645-659, 1993.

Devonec M, Fendler JP, Monsallier M, et al. The significance of the prostatic hypoechoic area: results in 226 ultrasonically guided prostatic biopsies. *J Urol* 143:316-319, 1990.

di Sant'Agnese PA. Neuroendocrine differentiation in the precursors of prostate cancer. *Eur Urol* 30:185-190, 1996.

DiGiovanni J, Kiguchi K, Frijhoff A, et al. Deregulated expression of insulin-like growth factor 1 in prostate epithelium leads to neoplasia in transgenic mice. *Proc Natl Acad Sci U S A* 97:3455-3460, 2000.

DiGiuseppe JA, Sauvageot J, Epstein JI. Increasing incidence of minimal residual cancer in radical prostatectomy specimens. *Am J Surg Pathol* 21:174-178, 1997.

Doll J, Sanjuro F, Helms C, et al. Chromosome 8p loss of heterozygosity in prostate tumors [abstract]. *Proc Am Assoc Cancer Res* 38:22, 1997.

Drachenberg CB, Papadimitriou JC. Aberrant pattern of lectin binding in low and high grade prostatic intraepithelial neoplasia. *Cancer* 75:2539-2544, 1995.

Drachenberg CB, Ioffe OB, Papadimitriou JC. Progressive increase of apoptosis in a prostatic intraepithelial neoplasia and carcinoma: comparison between in situ end-labeling of fragmented DNA and detection by routine hematoxylin-eosin staining. *Arch Pathol Lab Med* 121:54-58, 1997.

Drago JR, Mostofi FK, Lee F. Introductory remarks and workshop summary: workshop on prostatic intraepithelial neoplasia, significance and correlation with prostate-specific antigen and transrectal ultrasound. *Urology* 34(suppl):2-3, 1989.

Dube VE, Joyce GT, Kennedy E. Papillary primary duct adenocarcinoma of the prostate. *J Urol* 107:825-826, 1972.

Ellis WJ, Brawer MK. Repeat prostate needle biopsy: who needs it? *J Urol* 153:1496-1498, 1995.

Emmert-Buck MR, Vocke CD, Pozzatti RO, et al. Allelic loss on chromosome 8p12-21 in microdissected prostatic intraepithelial neoplasia. *Cancer Res* 55:2959-2962, 1995.

Epstein JI. Relationship of dysplasia to prostate carcinoma. *Semin Urol* 8:2-8, 1990A.

Epstein JI, Cho KR, Quinn BD. Relationship of severe dysplasia to stage A (incidental) adenocarcinoma of the prostate. *Cancer* 65:2321-2327, 1990B.

Epstein JI, Armas O. Atypical basal cell hyperplasia of the prostate. *Am J Surg Pathol* 16:1205-1214, 1992.

Epstein JI, Walsh PC, Carmichael M, et al. Pathologic and clinical findings to predict tumor extent of nonpalpable (stage T1c) prostate cancer. *JAMA* 271:368-374, 1994A.

Epstein JI. Prostatic intraepithelial neoplasia. *Adv Anat Pathol* 1:123-140, 1994B.

Epstein JI. Diagnostic criteria of limited adenocarcinoma of the prostate on needle biopsy. *Hum Pathol* 26:223-229, 1995A.

Epstein JI, Grignon DJ, Humphrey PA, et al. Interobserver reproducibility in the diagnosis of prostatic intraepithelial neoplasia. *Am J Surg Pathol* 19:873-886, 1995B.

Epstein JI, Carmichael M, Partin AW. OA-519 (fatty acid synthase) as an independent predictor of pathologic stage in adenocarcinoma of the prostate. *Urology* 45:81-86, 1995C.

Erbersdobler A, Gürses N, Henke RP. Numerical chromosomal changes in high-grade prostatic intraepithelial neoplasia (PIN) and concomitant invasive carcinoma. *Pathol Res Pract* 192:418-427, 1996.

Erdamar S, Slawin KM, Wheeler TM. High grade prostatic intraepithelial neoplasia involving the prostatic utricle. A case report. *J Urol Pathol* 8:167-10, 1998.

Feneley MR, Young MP, Chinyama C, et al. Ki-67 expression in early prostate cancer and associated pathological lesions. *J Clin Pathol* 49:741-748, 1996.

Feneley MB, Green JSA, Young MPA, et al. Prevalence of prostatic intraepithelial neoplasia (PIN) in biopsies from hospital practice and pilot screening-clinical implications. *Prostate Cancer Prostatic Dis* 1:79-83, 1997.

Ferguson J, Zincke H, Ellison E, et al. Decrease in prostatic intraepithelial neoplasia following androgen deprivation therapy in patients with stage T3 carcinoma treated by radical prostatectomy. *Urology* 44:91-95, 1994.

Fernández PL, Arce Y, Farré X, et al. Expression of p27/Kip 1 is down-regulated in prostate carcinoma progression. *J Pathol* 187:563-566, 1999.

Fleshner NE, O'Sullivan M, Fair WR. Prevalence and predictors of a positive repeat transrectal ultrasound guided needle biopsy of the prostate. *J Urol* 158:505-509, 1997.

Fowler JE Jr, Bigler SA, Lynch C, et al. Prospective study of correlations between biopsy detected high grade prostatic intraepithelial neoplasia, serum prostate specific antigen concentration and race. *Cancer* 91:1291-1296, 2001.

Fuchs ME, Brawer MK, Rennels MA, et al. The relationship of basement membrane to histologic grade of human prostatic tissue. *Mod Pathol* 2:105-111, 1989.

Fudge K, Bostwick DG, Stearns ME. Platelet-derived growth factor A and B chains and the alpha and beta receptor in prostatic intraepithelial neoplasia. *Prostate* 29:282-286, 1996.

Fujita MQ, Shin M, Yasunaga Y, et al. Incidence of prostatic intraepithelial neoplasia in Osaka, Japan. *Int J Cancer* 73:808-811, 1997.

Garabedian EM, Humphrey PA, Gordon JI. A transgenic mouse model of metastatic prostate cancer originating from neuroendocrine cells. *Proc Natl Acad Sci U S A* 95:15382-15387, 1998.

Gaudin PB, Sesterhenn IA, Wojno KJ, et al. Incidence and clinical significance of high-grade prostatic intraepithelial neoplasia in TURP specimens. *Urology* 49: 558-563, 1997.

Giannulis I, Montironi R, Galluzzi CM, et al. Frequency and location of mitoses in prostatic intraepithelial neoplasia (PIN). *Anticancer Res* 13:2447-2451, 1993.

Gingrich JR, Barrios RJ, Kattan MW, et al. Androgen-independent prostate cancer progression in the TRAMP model. *Cancer Res* 57:4687-4691, 1997.

Gleason DF. Atypical hyperplasia, benign hyperplasia and well-differentiated adenocarcinoma of the prostate. *Am J Surg Pathol* 9(suppl):53-67, 1985.

Gohji K, Okamoto M, Morisue K, et al. Usefulness of digital rectal examination, serum prostate-specific antigen, transrectal ultrasonography and systematic prostate biopsy for the detection of organ-confined prostate cancer. *Int J Urol* 2:116-120, 1995.

Gould VE, Doljanskaia V, Gooch G, et al. Immunolocalization of glycoprotein A-80 in prostatic carcinoma and prostatic intraepithelial neoplasia. *Hum Pathol* 27:547-552, 1996.

Gould VE, Doljanskaia V, Gooch GT, et al. Stability of glycoprotein A-80 in prostatic carcinoma subsequent to androgen deprivation therapy. *Am J Surg Pathol* 21:319-326, 1997.

Greenberg NM, DeMayo F, Finegold MJ, et al. Prostate cancer in a transgenic mouse. *Proc Natl Acad Sci U S A* 92:3439-3443, 1995.

Greene DR, Wheeler TM, Egawa S, et al. A comparison of the morphological features of cancer arising in the transition zone and in the peripheral zone of the prostate. *J Urol* 146:1069-1076, 1991.

Greenwald P, Kirmss V, Polan AK, et al. Cancer of the prostate among men with benign prostatic hyperplasia. *J Natl Cancer Inst* 53:335-340, 1974.

Häggman M, Hellström M, Aus G, et al. Neoadjuvant GnRH-agonist treatment (triptofelin and cyproterone acetate for flare protection) and total prostatectomy. *Eur Urol* 24:451-460, 1993.

Häggman MJ, Wojno KJ, Pearsall CP, et al. Allelic loss of 8p sequences in prostatic intraepithelial neoplasia and carcinoma. *Urology* 50:643-647, 1997A.

Häggman M, Nordin B, Mattson S, et al. Morphometric studies of intra-prostatic volume relationships in localized prostatic carcinoma. *Br J Urol* 80:612-617, 1997B.

Häggman MJ, Macoska JA, Wojno KJ, et al. The relationship between prostatic intraepithelial neoplasia and prostate cancer: critical issues. *J Urol* 158:12-22, 1997C.

Hammarsten J, Andersson S, Holmen A, et al. Does transurethral resection of a clinically benign gland increase the risk of developing clinical prostate cancer? A 10-year follow-up study. *Cancer* 74:2347-2351, 1994.

Harper ME, Glynne-Jones E, Goddard L, et al. Expression of androgen receptor and growth factors in premalignant lesions of the prostate. *J Pathol* 186:169-177, 1998.

Harvei S, Skjorten FJ, Robsahm TE, et al. Is prostatic intraepithelial neoplasia in the transition/central zone a true precursor of cancer? A long-term retrospective study in Norway. *Br J Cancer* 78:46-49, 1998.

Häussler O, Epstein JI, Amin MB, et al. Cell proliferation, apoptosis, oncogene, and tumor suppressor gene status in adenosis with comparison to benign prostatic hyperplasia, prostatic intraepithelial neoplasia, and cancer. *Hum Pathol* 30:1077-1086, 1999.

Hedrick L, Epstein JI. Use of keratin 903 as an adjuvant in the diagnosis of prostate carcinoma. *Am J Surg Pathol* 13:389-396, 1989.

Heidger PM Jr, Lubaroff DM, Cohen MB. Fine structural studies of induced tumors arising within the prostatic complex of Lobund-Wistar rats. *Prostate* 32:173-178, 1997.

Helpap B. The biological significance of atypical hyperplasia of the prostate. *Virchows Arch A Pathol Anat and Histol* 387:309-317, 1980.

Helpap B, Riede C. Nucleolar and AgNOR-analysis of prostatic intraepithelial neoplasia (PIN), atypical adenomatous hyperplasia (AAH) and prostatic carcinoma. *Pathol Res Pract* 191:381-390, 1995.

Henshall SM, Quinn DI, Lee CS, et al. Overexpression of the cell cycle inhibitor p16INK4A in high-grade prostatic intraepithelial neoplasia predicts early relapse in prostate cancer patients. *Clin Cancer Res* 7:544-550, 2001.

Hoedemaeker RF, Kranse R, Rietbergen JBW, et al. Evaluation of prostate needle biopsies in a population-based screening study. *Cancer* 85:145-152, 1999.

Hu JC, Palapattu GS, Kattan MW, et al. The association of selected pathological features with prostate cancer in a single-needle biopsy accession. *Hum Pathol* 29:1536-1538, 1998.

Huang J, Powell WC, Khodavirdi AC, et al. Prostatic intraepithelial neoplasia in mice with conditional disruption of the retinoid X receptor alpha allele in the prostate epithelium. *Cancer Res* 62: 4812-4819, 2002.

Hughes JH, Cohen MB, Robinson RA. p53 immunoreactivity in primary and metastatic prostatic adenocarcinoma. *Mod Pathol* 8:462-466, 1995.

Humphrey PA. Mucin in severe dysplasia in the prostate. *Surg Pathol* 4:137-143, 1991.

Humphrey PA, Frazier HA, Bollmer RT, et al. Stratification of pathologic features in radical prostatectomy specimens that are predictive of elevated initial postoperative serum prostate specific antigen levels. *Cancer* 71:1821-1827, 1993.

Humphrey PA, Frazier HA, Paulson DF, et al. Extent of severe dysplasia in the prostate is inversely related to pathologic stage (abstract). *Mod Pathol* 5:54A, 1992.

Humphrey PA, Zhu X, Zarnegar R, et al. Hepatocyte growth factor and its receptor in prostatic carcinoma. *Am J Pathol* 147:386-396, 1995A.

Humphrey PA, Swanson PE. Immunoreactive p53 protein n high-grade prostatic intraepithelial neoplasia. *Pathol Res Pract* 191:881-887, 1995B.

Humphrey PA. p53: Mutations and immunohistochemical detection, with a focus on alterations in urologic malignancies. In: Weinstein RS, Graham AR, Anderson RE, et al, eds. *Advances in Pathology and Laboratory Medicine.* Vol 7. Chicago: Mosby; 579-606, 1996A.

Humphrey PA, Keetch DW, Smith DS, et al. Prospective characterization of pathologic features of prostatic carcinomas detected via serum prostate specific-antigen-based screening. *J Urol* 155:816-820, 1996B.

Humphrey PA, Keetch DW. Morphometric analysis of prostate cancers detected because of rebiopsy for high-grade prostatic intraepithelial neoplasia (PIN) [abstract]. *J Urol* 157:229A, 1997.

Ibrahim GK, MacDonald JA, Kerns BJ, et al. Differential immunoreactivity of her-2/neu oncoprotein in prostatic tissues. *Surg Oncol* 1:151-155, 1992.

Issacs WB, Bosa GS. Prostate cancer. In: Vogelstein B, Kinzler KW, eds. *The Genetic Basis of Human Cancer.* New York: McGraw-Hill; 653-660, 1998.

Iwamura M, Gershagen S, Lapets O, et al. Immunohistochemical localization of parathyroid hormone-related protein in prostatic intraepithelial neoplasia. *Hum Pathol* 261:797-801, 1995.

Jack GS, Brash AR, Olson SJ, et al. Reduced 15-lipoxygenase-2 immunostaining in prostate adenocarcinoma: correlation with grade and expression in high-grade prostatic intraepithelial neoplasia. *Hum Pathol* 31:1146-1154, 2000.

Janssen T, Petein M, Van Velthoven R, et al. Differential histochemical peanut agglutinin stain in benign and malignant human prostate tumors: relationship with prostatic specific antigen immunostain and nuclear DNA content. *Hum Pathol* 27:1341-1347, 1996.

Jenkins RB, Qian J, Lieber MM, et al. Detection of c-myc oncogene amplification and chromosomal anomalies in metastatic prostatic carcinoma by fluorescence in situ hybridization. *Cancer Res* 57:524-531, 1997.

Jensen SL, Wood DP Jr, Banks ER, et al. Increased levels of nm23H1/nucleoside diphosphate kinase A mRNA associated with adenocarcinoma of the prostate. *World J Urol* 14(suppl 1):S21-S25, 1996.

Johnson MI, Robinson MC, Marsh C, et al. Expression of bcl-2, bax, and p53 in high-grade prostatic intraepithelial neoplasia and localized prostate cancer. Relationship with apoptosis and proliferation. *Prostate* 37:223-229, 1998.

Jones EC, Young RH. The differential diagnosis of prostatic carcinoma. Its distinctions from premalignant and pseudocarcinomatous lesions of the prostate gland. *Am J Clin Pathol* 101:48-64, 1994.

Kahn W, Sakr WA, Grignon DJ, et al. Analysis of 3300 consecutive prostate biopsies (Pbx): a 4 year institutional experience with the frequency of carcinoma (Pca), isolated high grade prostatic intraepithelial neoplasia (HGPIN) and "atypical" [abstract]. *Mod Pathol* 10:79A, 1997.

Kamoi K, Troncoso P, Babaian RJ. Strategy for repeat biopsy in patients with high grade prostatic intraepithelial neoplasia. J Urol 163:819-823, 2000.

Kasper S, Sheppard PC, Yan Y, et al. Development, progression and androgen-dependence of prostate tumors in transgenic mice: a model for prostate cancer. *Lab Invest* 78:319-333, 1998.

Kastendieck H. Correlations between atypical primary hyperplasia and carcinoma of the prostate. A histological study of 180 total prostatectomies. *Pathol Res Pract* 169:366-387, 1980.

Kastendieck H, Helpap B. Prostatic "dysplasia/atypical hyperplasia." Urology 34(6 suppl):28-42, 1989.

Kearse WS Jr., Seay TM, Thompson IM. The long-term risk of development of prostate cancer in patients with benign prostatic hyperplasia: correlation with stage A1 disease. *J Urol* 150:1746-1748, 1993.

Keetch DW, Humphrey P, Stahl D, et al. Morphometric analysis and clinical follow-up of isolated prostatic intraepithelial neoplasia in needle biopsy of the prostate. *J Urol* 154:347-351, 1995.

Kelley MR, Cheng L, Foster R, et al. Elevated and altered expression of the multifunctional DNA base excision repair and redox enzyme Ape 1/ref-1 in prostate cancer. *Clin Cancer Res* 7:824-830, 2001.

Kleinerman DI, Troncoso P, Lin SH, et al. Consistent expression of an epithelial cell adhesion molecule (C-CAM) during human prostate development and loss of expression in prostate cancer: implication as a tissue suppressor. *Cancer Res* 55:1215-1220, 1995.

Koch M, de Miguel M, Höfler H, et al. Kinetic profiles of intraepithelial and invasive prostatic neoplasias: the key role of down-regulated apoptosis in tumor progression. *Virchows Arch* 436:413-420, 2000.

Kollermann J, Helpap B. Expression of vascular endothelial growth factor (VEGF) and VEGF receptor Flk-1 in benign, premalignant, and malignant prostate tissue. *Am J Clin Pathol* 116:115-121, 2001.

Kovi J, Jackson MA, Heshmat MY. Ductal spread in prostatic carcinoma. *Cancer* 56:1566-1573, 1985.

Kovi J, Mostofi FK. Atypical hyperplasia of prostate. *Urology* 34(6 suppl):23-27, 1989.

Krajewska M, Krajewski S, Epstein JI, et al. Immunohistochemical analysis of bcl-2, bax, bcl-X, and mcl-1 expression in prostate cancers. *Am J Pathol* 148:1567-1596, 1996.

Krizman DB, Chuaqui RF, Meltzer DS, et al. Construction of a representative cDNA library from prostatic intraepithelial neoplasia. *Cancer Res* 56:5380-5383, 1996.

Kronz JD, Shaikh AA, Epstein JI. High-grade prostatic intraepithelial neoplasia with adjacent small atypical glands on prostate biopsy. *Hum Pathol* 32:389-395, 2001A.

Kronz JD, Allan CH, Shaikh AA, et al. Predicting cancer following a diagnosis of high-grade prostatic intraepithelial neoplasia on needle biopsy : data on men with more than one follow-up biopsy. *Am J Surg Pathol* 25:1079-1085, 2001B.

Langer JE, Rovner ES, Coleman BG, et al. Strategy for repeat biopsy of patients with prostatic intraepithelial neoplasia detected by prostate needle biopsy. *J Urol* 155:228-231, 1996.

Leav I, McNeal JE, Kwan PWL, et al. Androgen receptor expression in prostatic dysplasia (prostatic intraepithelial neoplasia) in the human prostate: an immunohistochemical and in situ hybridization study. *Prostate* 29:137-145, 1996A.

Leav I, Galluzzi CM, Ziar J, et al. Mitogen-activated protein kinase and mitogen-activated kinase phosphatase-1 expression in the Noble rat model of sex hormone-induced prostatic dysplasia and carcinoma. *Lab Invest* 75:361-370, 1996B.

Lee F, Torp-Pedersen ST, Carroll JT, et al. Use of transrectal ultrasound and prostate-specific antigen in diagnosis of prostatic intraepithelial neoplasia. Urology 34(6 suppl):4-8, 1989.

Lee S, Ro J, Park K, et al. Expression of p53 in the benign prostatic hyperplasia and prostate adenocarcinoma: an immunohistochemical study with PCNA expression [abstract]. *Mod Pathol* 7:78A, 1994.

Liu AY, True LD, LaTray L, et al. Cell-cell interaction in prostate gene regulation and cytodifferentiation. *Proc Natl Acad Sci U S A* 96:10705-10710, 1997.

Lopez-Beltran A, Artacho-Perula E, Roldan-Villalobos R, et al. Nuclear volume estimates in prostatic intraepithelial neoplasia. *Analyt Quant Cytol Histol* 22:37-44, 2000.

Macoska JA, Micale MA, Sakr WA, et al. Extensive genetic alterations in prostate cancer revealed by dual PCR and FISH analysis. *Genes Chromosomes Cancer* 8:88-97, 1993.

Macoska JA, Trybus TM, Sakr WA, et al. Fluorescence in situ hybridization analysis of 8p allelic loss and chromosome 8 instability in human prostate cancer. *Cancer Res* 54:3824-3830, 1994.

Magi-Galluzzi C, Loda M. Molecular events in the early phases of prostate carcinogenesis. *Eur Urol* 30:167-176, 1996.

Magi-Galluzzi C, Xu X, Hlatky L, et al. Heterogeneity of androgen receptor content in advanced prostate cancer. *Mod Pathol* 10:839-845, 1997.

Magi-Galluzzi C, Montironi R, Giulia Cangi M, et al. Mitogen-activated protein kinases and apoptosis in PIN. *Virchows Arch* 432:407-413, 1998.

Masumori N, Thomas TZ, Chaurand P, et al. A probasin-large T antigen transgenic mouse line develops prostate adenocarcinoma and neuroendocrine carcinoma with metastatic potential. *Cancer Res* 61:2239-2249, 2001.

Maygarden SJ. Applications of immunohistochemistry to the diagnosis and prognostication of prostate carcinoma and prostatic intraepithelial neoplasia. *Pathol Ann* 29:303-320, 1994A.

Maygarden SJ, Novotny DB, Moul JW, et al. Evaluation of cathepsin D and epidermal growth factor receptor in prostate carcinoma. *Mod Pathol* 7:930-936, 1994B.

McNeal JE. Morphogenesis of prostatic carcinoma. *Cancer* 18: 1659-1665, 1965.

McNeal JE, Bostwick DG. Intraductal dysplasia: a premalignant lesion of the prostate. *Hum Pathol* 17:64-71, 1986.

McNeal JE, Leav I, Alroy J, et al. Differential lectin staining of central and peripheral zones of the prostate and alterations in dysplasia. *Am J Clin Pathol* 89:41-48, 1988A.

McNeal JE, Alroy J, Leav J, et al. Immunohistochemical evidence for impaired cell differentiation in the premalignant phase of prostate carcinogenesis. *Am J Clin Pathol* 90:23-32, 1988B.

McNeal JE. Normal histology of the prostate. *Am J Surg Pathol* 12:619-633, 1988C.

McNeal JE, Villers A, Redwine EA, et al. Microcarcinoma in the prostate: its association with duct-acinar dysplasia. *Hum Pathol* 22:644-652, 1991.

McNeal JE, Yemoto EM. Spread of adenocarcinoma within prostatic ducts and acini. *Am J Surg Pathol* 20:802-814, 1996.

Melhorn J. The diagnostic value of "dysplastic" changes in the prostate. *Zentralbl Pathol* 137:395-401, 1991.

Miet SMD, Neyra M, Jaques R, et al. RER^+ phenotype in prostate intra-epithelial neoplasia associated with human prostate-carcinoma development. *Int J Cancer* 82:635-639, 1999.

Monger LE Jr, Nagabhushan M, Pretlow TG, et al. A novel approach to the characterization of whole prostate pathology in glycol methacrylate. *Am J Pathol* 145:54-60, 1994.

Montironi R, Scarpelli M, Sisti S, et al. Quantitative analysis of prostatic intraepithelial neoplasia on tissue sections. *Anal Quant Cytol Histol* 12:366-372, 1990.

Montironi R, Braccischi D, Matera G, et al. Quantitation of the prostatic intra-epithelial neoplasia. Analysis of nucleolar size, number, and location. *Pathol Res Pract* 187:307-314, 1991.

Montironi R, Magi-Galluzzi C, Scarpelli M, et al. Occurrence of cell death (apoptosis) in prostatic intraepithelial neoplasia. *Virchows Archiv Anat Histopathol* 423:351-357, 1993A.

Montironi R, Galluzzi CM, Diamanti L, et al. Prostatic intraepithelial neoplasia. Qualitative and quantitative analysis of the blood capillary architecture on thin tissue sections. *Pathol Res Pract* 189:542-548, 1993B.

Montironi R, Magi-Galluzzi C, Muzzonigro G, et al. Effects of combination endocrine treatment on normal prostate, prostatic intraepithelial neoplasia, and prostatic adenocarcinoma. *J Clin Pathol* 47:906-913, 1994A.

Montironi R, Magi-Galluzzi CM, Marina S, et al. Quantitative characterization of the frequency and location of cell proliferation and death in prostate pathology. *J Cell Biochem* 19(suppl):238-245, 1994B.

Montironi R, Magi-Galluzzi C, Fabris G. Apoptotic bodies in prostatic intraepithelial neoplasia and prostatic adenocarcinoma following total androgen ablation. *Pathol Res Pract* 191:873-880, 1995A.

Montironi R, Bartels PH, Thompson D, et al. Prostatic intraepithelial neoplasia (PIN). Performance of Bayesian belief network for diagnosis and grading. *J Pathol* 177:153-162, 1995B.

Montironi R, Diamanti L, Thompson D, et al. Analysis of the capillary architecture in the precursors of prostate cancer: recent findings and new concepts. *Eur Urol* 30:191-200, 1996A.

Montironi R, Lucarini G, Castaldini C, et al. Immunohistochemical evaluation of type IV collagenase (72-kd metalloproteinase) in prostatic intraepithelial neoplasia. *Anticancer Res* 16(4A):2057-2062, 1996B.

Montironi R, Bostwick DG, Bonkhoff H, et al. Origins of prostate cancer. Workgroup I. *Cancer* 78:362-365, 1996C.

Montironi R, Schulman CC. Precursors of prostatic cancer: progression, regression and chemoprevention. *Eur Urol* 30:133-137, 1996D.

Moskaluk CA, Duray PK, Cowan KH, et al. Immunohistochemical expression of pi-class glutathione s-transferase is down-regulated in adenocarcinoma of the prostate. *Cancer* 79:1595-1599, 1997.

Mostofi FK, Sesterhenn IA, Davis CJ Jr. Prostatic intraepithelial neoplasia (PIN): morphological clinical significance. *Prostate* 4(suppl):71-77, 1992.

Mostofi FK, Murphy GP, Mettlin C, et al. Pathology review in an early prostate cancer detection program: results from the American Cancer Society-National Prostate Cancer Detection Project. *Prostate* 27:7-12, 1995.

Mucci NR, Wojno K. Nuclear matrix proteins in human prostate cancer as detected by Pro:4-216 and Pro:8-133 [abstract]. *Mod Pathol* 11:90A, 1998.

Mukherjee J, Misra V, Gupta SC, et al. Argyrophilic nucleolar organizer regions in atypical adenomatous hyperplasias, prostatic intraepithelial neoplasias and prostatic neoplasms. *Urol Int* 58:75-79, 1997.

Myers RB, Oelschlager D, Srivastava S, et al. Accumulation of the p53 protein occurs more frequently in metastatic than in localized prostatic adenocarcinoma. *Prostate* 25:243-248, 1994A.

Myers RB, Srivastava S, Oelschlager DK, et al. Expression of p160^{erbB-3} and p185^{erbB-2} in prostatic intraepithelial neoplasia and prostatic adenocarcinoma. *J Natl Cancer Inst* 86:1140-1145, 1994B.

Myers RB, Schlom J, Srivastava S, et al. Expression of tumor-associated glycoprotein 72 in prostatic intraepithelial neoplasia and prostatic adenocarcinoma. *Mod Pathol* 8:260-265, 1995A.

Myers RB, Srivastava S, Grizzle WE. Lewis Y antigen as detected by monoclonal antibody BR96 as expressed strongly in prostatic adenocarcinoma. *J Urol* 153:1572-1574, 1995B.

Myers RB, Grizzle WE. Biomarker expression in prostatic intraepithelial neoplasia. *Eur Urol* 30:153-166, 1996A.

Myers RB, Srivastava S, Oelschlager DK, et al. Expression of nm23-Hl in prostatic intraepithelial neoplasia and adenocarcinoma. *Hum Pathol* 27:1021-1024, 1996B.

Nagle RB, Brawer MK, Kittelson J, et al. Phenotypic relationships of prostatic intraepithelial neoplasia to invasive carcinoma. *Am J Pathol* 138:119-128, 1991.

Nagle RB, Hao J, Knox JD, et al. Expression of hemidesmosomal and extracellular matrix proteins by normal and malignant human prostate tissue. *Am J Pathol* 146:1498-1507, 1995.

Nagle RB. Intermediate filament expression in prostate cancer. *Ca Metastasis Rev* 15:473-482, 1996.

Nangia R, Zhang PJ. Decreased immunoexpression of prostate inhibin peptide in prostatic carcinoma (PCA): a study with monoclonal antibody (MoAB) [abstract]. *Mod Pathol* 11:91A, 1998.

Nassar H, Butler C, Pansare V, et al. Low and high grade prostatic intraepithelial neoplasia (PIN), a biologic spectrum? Evaluation of cell cycle regulators and neovascularization [abstract]. *Mod Pathol* 114:118A, 2001.

Navone NM, Logothetis CJ, von Eschenbach AC, et al. Model systems of prostate cancer: uses and limitations. *Cancer Metastasis Rev* 17:361-371, 1999.

Nelson PS, Gleason TP, Brawer MK. Chemoprevention for prostatic intraepithelial neoplasia. *Eur Urol* 30:269-278, 1996.

NPCDP (National Prostate Cancer Detection Project). Prostatic intraepithelial neoplasia: significance and correlation with prostate-specific antigen and transrectal ultrasound. *Urology* 34(suppl):1-69, 1989.

O'Dowd GJ, Miller MC, Orozco R, et al. Analysis of repeated biopsy results within 1 year after a noncancer diagnosis. *Urology* 55:553-559, 2000.

Orozco R, O'Dowd G, Kunnel B, et al. Observations on pathology trends in 62,537 prostate biopsies obtained from urology private practices in the United States. *Urology* 51:186-195, 1998.

Ortel H. Involutionary changes on the prostate and female beast cancer in relation to cancer development. *Can Med Assoc J* 16:237-241, 1926.

Pacelli A, Bostwick DG. The clinical significance of high-grade prostatic intraepithelial neoplasia in transurethral resection specimens. *Urology* 50:355-359, 1997.

Page DL. Atypical hyperplasia, narrowly and broadly defined. *Hum Pathol* 22:631-632, 1991.

Park S, Shinohara K, Grossfeld GD, et al. Prostate cancer detection in men with prior high grade prostatic intraepithelial neoplasia or atypical prostate biopsy. *J Urol* 165:1409-1414, 2001.

Parkinson MC. Pre-neoplastic lesions of the prostate. *Histopathology* 27:301-311, 1995.

Perachino M, di Ciolo L, Barbetti V, et al. Results of rebiopsy for suspected prostate cancer in symptomatic men with elevated PSA levels. *Eur Urol* 32:155-159, 1997.

Perez-Stable C, Altman NH, Mehta PP, et al. Prostate cancer progression, metastasis, and gene expression in transgenic mice. *Cancer Res* 57:900-906, 1997.

Perlman EJ, Epstein JI. Blood group antigen expression in dysplasia and adenocarcinoma of the prostate. *Am J Surg Pathol* 14:810-818, 1990.

Petein M, Michel P, van Velthoven R, et al. Morphonuclear relationship between prostatic intraepithelial neoplasia and cancers as assessed by digital cell image analysis. *Am J Clin Pathol* 96:628-634, 1991.

Pihan G, Malhotra R, Xa XF, et al. Abnormal centrosomes in a fraction of high grade prostatic intraepithelial neoplasia (PIN) [abstract]. *Mod Pathol* 13:111A, 2000.

Pisters LL, Troncoso P, Zhau HE, et al. C-met proto-oncogene expression in benign and malignant human prostate tissues. *J Urol* 154:293-298, 1995.

Poczatek RB, Myers RB, Manne U, et al. Ep-CAM levels in prostatic adenocarcinoma and prostatic intraepithelial neoplasia. *J Urol* 162:1462-1466, 1999.

Podsypania K, Ellenson LH, Nemes A, et al. Mutations of Pten/Mmacl in mice causes neoplasia in multiple organ systems. *Proc Natl Acad Sci U S A* 96:1563-1568, 1999.

Prange W, Erbersdobler A, Hammerer P, et al. Significance of high-grade prostatic intraepithelial neoplasia in needle biopsy specimens. *Urology* 57:486-490, 2001.

Pylkkanen L, Makela S, Santti R. Animal models for the preneoplastic lesions of the prostate. *Eur Urol* 30:243-248, 1996.

Qian J, Bostwick DG, Takahashi S, et al. Chromosomal anomalies in prostatic intraepithelial neoplasia and carcinoma detected by fluorescence in situ hybridization. *Cancer Res* 55:5408-5414, 1995.

Qian J, Jenkins RB, Bostwick DG. Potential markers of aggressiveness in prostatic intraepithelial neoplasia detected by fluorescence in situ hybridization. *Eur Urol* 30:177-184, 1996.

Qian J, Jenkins RB, Bostwick DG. Detection of chromosomal anomalies and c-myc gene amplification in the cribriform pattern of prostate intraepithelial neoplasia and carcinoma by fluorescence in-situ hybridization. *Mod Pathol* 10:1113-1119, 1997A.

Qian J, Wollan P, Bostwick DG. The extent and multicentricity of high-grade prostatic intraepithelial neoplasia in clinically localized prostatic adenocarcinoma. *Hum Pathol* 28:143-148, 1997B.

Qian J, Jenkins RB, Bostwick DG. Determination of gene and chromosome dosage in prostatic intraepithelial neoplasia and carcinoma. *Analyt Quant Cytol Histol* 20:373-380, 1998.

Quinn BD, Cho KR, Epstein JI. Relationship of severe dysplasia to stage B adenocarcinoma of the prostate. *Cancer* 65:2328-2337, 1990.

Ramos CG, Carvalhal GF, Mager DE, et al. The effect of high-grade prostatic intraepithelial neoplasia on serum total and percentage of free prostate specific antigen levels. *J Urol* 162:1587-1590, 1999.

Raviv G, Zlotta AR, Janssen TH, et al. Does prostate-specific antigen and prostate-specific antigen density enhance the detection of prostate cancer in patients initially diagnosed to have prostatic intraepithelial neoplasia? *Cancer* 77:2103-2108, 1996A.

Raviv G, Janssen T, Zlotta AR, et al. Prostatic intraepithelial neoplasia: influence of clinical and pathological data on the detection of prostate cancer. *J Urol* 156:1050-1055, 1996B.

Renshaw AA. Adequate tissue sampling of prostate core needle biopsies. *Am J Clin Pathol* 107:26-29, 1997.

Renshaw AA, Santis WF, Richie JP. Clinicopathological characteristics of prostatic adenocarcinoma in men with atypical prostate needle biopsies. *J Urol* 159:2018-2022, 1998.

Reuter VE. Pathological changes in benign and malignant prostatic tissue following androgen deprivation therapy. *Urology* 49(3A suppl):16-22, 1997.

Reyes AO, Humphrey PA. Flat high-grade prostatic intraepithelial neoplasia (HGPIN) in needle biopsy [abstract]. *Mod Pathol* 10:86A, 1997A.

Reyes AO, Swanson PE, Carbone JM, et al. Unusual histologic types of high-grade prostatic intraepithelial neoplasia. *Am J Surg Pathol* 21:1215-1222, 1997B.

Reyes AO, Humphrey PA. Diagnostic effect of complete histologic sampling of prostate needle biopsies. *Am J Clin Pathol* 109:416-422, 1998.

Richie JP, Kavoussi LR, Ho GT, et al. Prostate cancer screening: role of the digital rectal examination and prostate-specific antigen. *Ann Surg Oncol* 1:117-120, 1994.

Ro JY, Ayala AG, Wishnow KI, et al. Prostatic duct adenocarcinoma with endometrioid features: immunohistochemical and electron microscopic study. *Semin Diagn Pathol* 5:301-311, 1988.

Ronnett BM, Carmichael MJ, Carter HB, et al. Does high-grade prostatic intraepithelial neoplasia result in elevated serum prostate specific antigen levels? *J Urol* 150:386-389, 1993.

Ropiquet F, Giri D, Kwabi-Addo B, et al. Increased expression of fibroblast growth factor 6 in human prostatic intraepithelial neoplasia and prostate cancer. *Cancer Res* 60:4245-4250, 2000.

Rosser CJ, Broberg J, Case D, et al. Detection of high-grade prostatic intra-epithelial neoplasia with the five-region biopsy technique. *Urology* 54:853-856, 1999.

Rubin MA, de la Taille A, Bagiella E, et al. Cribriform carcinoma of the prostate and cribriform prostatic intraepithelial neoplasia. *Am J Surg Pathol* 22:840-848, 1998.

Sakr WA, Sarkar FH, Sreepathi P, et al. Measurement of cellular proliferation in human prostate by AgNOR, PCNA, and SPF. *Prostate* 22:147-154, 1993.

Sakr WA, Macoska JA, Benson P, et al. Allelic loss in locally metastatic, multi-sampled prostate cancer. *Cancer Res* 54:3273-3277, 1994A.

Sakr WA, Grignon DJ, Crissman JD, et al. High grade prostatic intraepithelial neoplasia (HGPIN) and prostatic adenocarcinoma between the ages of 20-69: an autopsy study of 249 cases. *In Vivo* 8:439-444, 1994B.

Sakr WA, Grignon DJ, Haas GP, et al. Epidemiology of high grade prostatic intraepithelial neoplasia. *Pathol Res Pract* 191:838-841, 1995.

Sakr WA, Grignon DJ, Haas GP. Pathology of premalignant lesions and carcinoma of the prostate in African-American men. *Semin Urol Oncol* 16:214-220, 1998A.

Sakr WA, Grignon DJ. Prostatic intraepithelial neoplasia and atypical adenomatous hyperplasia. Relationship to pathologic parameters, volume and spatial distribution of carcinoma of the prostate. *Analyt Quant Cytol Histol* 20:417-423, 1998B.

Sakr WA. Prostatic intraepithelial neoplasia: a marker for high-risk groups and a potential target for chemoprevention. *Eur Urol* 35:474-478, 1999.

Sakr WA, Srigley JR, Dey J, et al. What features do urologic pathologists emphasize in diagnosing prostate lesions with equivocal changes of prostatic intraepithelial neoplasia (PIN)? A study of morphologic criteria and reproducibility [abstract]. *Mod Pathol* 14:122A, 2001.

Salem CE, Tomasic NA, Elmajian DA, et al. p53 protein and gene alterations in pathological stage C prostate carcinoma. *J Urol* 158:520-524, 1997.

Samaratunga H, Searle J. Significance of prostatic intraepithelial in transurethral resection and simple open resections of prostate [abstract]. *Int J Surg Pathol* 2(suppl):545, 1995.

Samaratunga H, Singh M. Distribution pattern of basal cells detected by cytokeratin 34 Beta E12 in primary prostatic duct adenocarcinoma. *Am J Surg Pathol* 21:435-440, 1997.

Sandberg AA. Chromosomal abnormalities in human prostate cancer: their detection and pathologic significance. In: Foster CS, Bostwick DG. *Pathology of the Prostate.* Philadelphia: WB Saunders; 400-427, 1998.

Saric T, Brkanac Z, Troyer DA, et al. Genetic pattern of prostate cancer progression. *Int J Cancer* 81:219-224, 1999.

Sentinelli S, Rondanelli E. Nucleolus organizer regions in prostatic intraepithelial neoplasm. *Pathologica* 82:405-412, 1990.

Sentinelli S. Mucins in prostatic intra-epithelial neoplasia and prostatic carcinoma. *Histopathology* 22:271-274, 1993.

Sesterhenn IA, Becker RL, Avallone FK, et al. Image analysis of nucleoli and nucleolar organizer regions in prostatic hyperplasia, intraepithelial neoplasia, and prostatic carcinoma. *J Urogen Pathol* 1:61-74, 1994.

Shah IA, Schlageter MO, Stinnett P, et al. Cytokeratin immunohistochemistry as a diagnostic tool for distinguishing malignant from benign epithelial lesions of the prostate. *Mod Pathol* 4:220-224, 1991.

Shah R, Mucci NR, Amin A, et al. Postatrophic hyperplasia of the prostate gland: neoplastic precursor or innocent bystander? *Am J Pathol* 158:1767-1773, 2001.

Shappell SB, Masumori N, Thomas T, et al. Transgenic mouse models of prostate carcinoma: anatomic, histopathologic, and molecular considerations. In: Lalani EW, Abel PD, eds. *Prostate Cancer: Scientific and Clinical Aspects: Bridging the Gap.* London: Imperial College Press; 2002.

Shepherd D, Keetch DW, Humphrey PA, et al. Repeat biopsy strategy in men with isolated prostatic intraepithelial neoplasia on prostate needle biopsy. *J Urol* 156:460-462, 1996.

Shibata MA, Ward JM, Devor DE, et al. Progression of prostatic intra-epithelial neoplasia to invasive carcinoma in C3(1) SV40 large T antigen transgenic mice: histopathological and molecular biological alterations. *Cancer Res* 56:4894-4903, 1996.

Shin M, Takayama H, Nonomura N, et al. Extent and zonal distribution of prostatic intraepithelial neoplasia in patients with prostatic intraepithelial neoplasia in patients with prostatic carcinoma in Japan: analysis of whole-mounted prostatectomy specimens. *Prostate* 42:81-87, 2000.

Silvestri F, Bussani R, Pavletic N, et al. Neoplastic and borderline lesions of the prostate: autopsy study and epidemiological data. *Pathol Res Pract* 191:908-916, 1995.

Sinha AA, Gleason DF, Wilson MJ, et al. Immunohistochemical localization of laminin in the basement membranes of normal, hyperplastic, and neoplastic human prostate. *Prostate* 15:299-313, 1989.

Sinha AA, Gleason DF, DeLeon OF, et al. Localization of type IV collagen in the basement membranes of human prostate and lymph nodes by immunoperoxidase and immunoalkaline phosphatase. *Prostate* 18:93-104, 1991.

Sinha AA, Gleason DF, Staley NA, et al. Cathepsin B in angiogenesis of human prostate: an immunohistochemical and immunoelectron microscopic analysis. *Anat Rec* 241:353-362, 1995.

Skjorten FJ, Berner A, Harvei S, et al. Prostatic intraepithelial neoplasia in surgical resections: relationship to coexistent adenocarcinoma and atypical adenomatous hyperplasia of the prostate. *Cancer* 79:1172-1179, 1997.

Soares CR, Shibata MA, Green JE, et al. Development of PIN and prostate adenocarcinoma cell lines: a model system for multistage progression. *Neoplasia* 4:112-120, 2002.

Song Z, Wu X, Powell WC, et al. Fibroblast growth factor 8 isoform B overexpression in prostate epithelium: a new mouse model for prostatic intraepithelial neoplasia. *Cancer Res* 62:5096-5105, 2002.

Srigley JR, Bullock M, Amin M. small glandular patterns in the prostate: differential diagnosis of small acinar carcinoma. In: Foster CS, Bostwick DG, eds. *Pathology of the Prostate.* Philadelphia: WB Saunders; 126-155, 1998.

Srigley JR, Amin MB, Bostwick DG, et al. Updated protocol for the examination of specimens from patients with carcinomas of the prostate gland. A basis for checklists. *Arch Pathol Lab Med* 124:1034-1039, 2000.

Srodon M, Epstein JI. Central zone histology of the prostate: a mimicker of high-grade prostatic intraepithelial neoplasia. *Hum Pathol* 33:518-523, 2002.

Stamey TA, Yemoto CM, McNeal JE, et al. Prostate cancer is highly predictable: a prognostic equation based on all morphological variables in radical prostatectomy specimens. *J Urol* 163:1155-1160, 2000.

Stanbrough MM, Lear I, Kwan PWL, et al. Prostatic intraepithelial neoplasia in mice expressing an androgen receptor transgene in prostate epithelium. PNAS 98: 10823-10828, 2001.

Stattin P, Damber JE, Karlberg L, et al. Bcl-2 immunoreactivity in prostate tumorigenesis in relation to prostatic intraepithelial neoplasia, grade, hormonal status, metastatic growth, and survival. *Urol Res* 24:259-264, 1996.

Sweat SD, Pacelli A, Bergstralh EJ, et al. Androgen receptor expression in prostatic intraepithelial neoplasia and cancer. *J Urol* 161:1229-1232, 1999.

Takahashi S, Qian J, Brown JA, et al. Potential markers of prostate cancer aggressiveness detected by fluorescence in situ hybridization in needle biopsies. *Cancer Res* 54:3574-3579, 1994.

Takayama H, Shin M, Nonomura N, et al. p53 mutations in prostatic intraepithelial neoplasia and concurrent carcinoma: analysis of laser capture microdissected specimens form non-transition and transition zones. *Jpn J Cancer Res* 91:941-947, 2000.

Tamano S, Rehm S, Waalkes MP, et al. High incidence and histogenesis of seminal vesicle adenocarcinoma and lower incidence of prostate carcinomas in the Lobund-Wister prostate cancer rat model using N-nitrosomethylurean and testosterone. *Vet Pathol* 33:557-567, 1996.

Tamboli P, Amin MB, Schultz DS, et al. Comparative analysis of the nuclear proliferative index (Ki-67) in benign prostate, prostatic intraepithelial neoplasia, and prostatic carcinoma. *Mod Pathol* 9:1015-1019, 1996.

Tamboli P, Amin MB, Xu HJ, et al. Immunohistochemical expression of retinoblastoma and p53 tumor suppressor genes in prostatic intraepithelial neoplasia. Comparison with prostatic adenocarcinoma and benign prostate. *Mod Pathol* 11:247-252, 1998.

Tarle M, Kraljic I. Free and total serum PSA values in patients with prostatic intraepithelial neoplasia (PIN), prostate cancer and BPH. Is F/T PSA a potential probe for dormant and manifest cancer? *Anticancer Res* 17:1531-1534, 1997.

Tehranian A, Morris DW, Min BH, et al. Neoplastic transformation of prostatic and urogenital epithelium by the polyoma virus middle T-gene. *Am J Pathol* 149:1177-1191, 1996.

Tennant MK, Thrasher JB, Twomey PA, et al. Insulin-like growth factor-binding protein-2 and -3 expression in benign human prostate epithelium, prostate intraepithelial neoplasia and adenocarcinoma of the prostate. *J Clin Endocrinol Metab* 81:411-420, 1996.

Têtu B, Srigley JR, Boivin JC, et al. Effect of combination endocrine therapy (LHRH agonist and Flutamide) on normal prostate and prostatic adenocarcinoma. *Am J Surg Pathol* 15:111-120, 1991.

Thomas DJ, Robinson M, King P, et al. p53 expression and clinical outcome in prostate cancer. *Br J Urol* 72:778-781, 1993.

Thorson P, Vollmer RT, Arcangeli C, et al. Minimal carcinoma in prostate needle biopsy specimens: diagnostic features and radical prostatectomy follow-up. *Mod Pathol* 11:543-551, 1998.

Tronscoso P, Babaian RJ, Ro JY, et al. Prostatic intraepithelial neoplasia and invasive prostatic adenocarcinoma in cystoprostatectomy specimens. Urology 34(suppl):52-56, 1989.

Tronscoso P, Reyes A, von Eschenbach A. High-grade prostatic intraepithelial neoplasia in sextant biopsies with CA [abstract]. *Mod Pathol* 10:92A, 1997.

Tsuchiya K, Lynch J, True L. Prostatic intraepithelial neoplasia: interobserver variability in grading [abstract]. *Mod Pathol* 6:71A, 1993.

Turkeri LN, Sakr WA, Wykes SM, et al. Comparative analysis of epidermal growth factor receptor gene expression and protein product in benign, premalignant, and malignant prostate tissue. *Prostate* 25:199-205, 1994.

Upadhyay J, Shekarriz B, Nemeth JA, et al. Membrane type 1–matrix metalloproteinase (MT1-MMP) and MMP-2 immunolocalization in human prostate: change in cellular localization associated with high-grade prostatic intraepithelial neoplasia. *Clin Cancer Res* 5:4105-4110, 1999.

Vaillancourt L, Têtu B, Fradet Y, et al. Effect of neoadjuvant endocrine therapy (combined androgen blockade) on normal prostate and prostatic carcinoma. A randomized study. *Am J Surg Pathol* 20:86-93, 1996.

Valve EM, Nevalainen MT, Nurmi MJ, et al. Increased expression of FGF-8 isoforms and FGF receptors in human premalignant prostatic intraepithelial neoplasia lesions and prostate cancer. *Lab Invest* 81:815-826, 2001.

van der Kwast TH, Têtu B. Androgen receptors in untreated and treated prostatic intraepithelial neoplasia. *Eur Urol* 30:265-268, 1996.

van der Kwast TH, Labrie F, Têtu B. Persistence of high-grade prostatic intraepithelial neoplasia under combined androgen blockade therapy. *Hum Pathol* 30:1503-1507, 1999.

Van Veldhuizen PJ, Sadasivan R, Cherian R, et al. p53 Expression in incidental prostatic cancer. *Am J Med Sci* 305:275-279, 1993.

Vis AN, Hoedemaeker RF, Roobol M, et al. The predictive value for prostate cancer of lesions that raise suspicion of concomitant carcinoma. An evaluation from a randomized, population-based study of screening for prostate cancer. *Cancer* 92:524-534, 2001.

Voelkel-Johnson C, Voeks DJ, Greenberg NM, et al. Genomic instability-based transgenic models of prostate cancer. *Carcinogenesis* 21:1623-1627, 2000.

Waters DJ, Hayden DW, Bell FW, et al. Prostatic intraepithelial neoplasia in dogs with spontaneous prostate cancer. *Prostate* 30:92-97, 1997A.

Waters DJ, Bostwick DG. Prostatic intraepithelial neoplasia occurs spontaneously in the canine prostate. *J Urol* 157:713-716, 1997B.

Weinberg DS, Weidner N. Concordance of DNA content between prostatic intraepithelial neoplasia and concomitant invasive carcinoma. Evidence that prostatic intraepithelial neoplasia is a precursor of invasive prostatic carcinoma. *Arch Pathol Lab Med* 117:1132-1137, 1993.

Weinstein MH, Epstein JI. Significance of high-grade prostatic intraepithelial neoplasia on needle biopsy. *Hum Pathol* 24:624-629, 1993.

Weinstein MH, Greenspan DL, Epstein JI. Diagnoses rendered on prostate needle biopsy in community hospitals. *Prostate* 35:50-55, 1998.

Wheeler TM. Influence of irradiation and androgen ablation on prostatic intraepithelial neoplasia. *Eur Urol* 30:261-264, 1996.

Wilcox G, Soh S, Chakraborty S, et al. Patterns of high-grade prostatic intraepithelial neoplasia associated with clinically aggressive prostate cancer. *Hum Pathol* 29:1119-1123, 1998.

Wiley EL, Davidson P, McIntire DD, et al. Risk of concurrent prostate cancer in cystoprostatectomy specimens is related to volume of high-grade prostatic intraepithelial neoplasia. *Urology* 49:692-696, 1997.

Wills ML, Hamper UM, Partin AW, et al. Incidence of high-grade prostatic intraepithelial neoplasia in sextant needle biopsy specimens. *Urology* 49:367-373, 1997.

Woderich R, McLoughlin J, Deen S. Radical prostatectomy for high grade prostatic intraepithelial neoplasia. *Int Urol Nephrol* 33:649-650, 2001.

Wojno KJ, Epstein JI. The utility of basal cell-specific anti-cytokeratin antibody (34 beta E12) in the diagnosis of prostate cancer. *Am J Surg Pathol* 19:251-260, 1995.

Yang Y, Hao J, Liu X, et al. Differential expression of cytokeratin mRNA and protein in normal prostate, prostatic intraepithelial neoplasia, and invasive carcinoma. *Am J Pathol* 150:693-704, 1997.

Yang XJ, McEntee M, Epstein JI. Distinction of basaloid carcinoma of the prostate from benign basal cell lesions by using immunohistochemistry for bcl-2 and Ki-67. *Hum Pathol* 29:1447-1450, 1998.

Yang CR, Ou YC, Ho CH, et al. Unsuspected prostate carcinoma and prostatic intraepithelial neoplasm in Taiwanese patients undergoing cystoprostatectomy. *Mol Urol* 3:33-39, 1999.

Yasunaga Y, Shin M, Fujita MQ, et al. Different patterns of p53 mutations in prostatic intraepithelial neoplasia and concurrent carcinoma: analysis of microdissected specimens. *Lab Invest* 78:1275-1279, 1998.

Zhang X, Lee C, Ng PY, et al. Prostatic neoplasia in transgenic mice with prostate-directed overexpression of the c-myc oncoprotein. *Prostate* 43:278-285, 2000.

Zitzelsberger H, Kulka U, Lehmann L, et al. Genetic heterogeneity in a prostatic carcinoma and associated prostatic intraepithelial neoplasia as demonstrated by combined use of laser-microdissection, degenerate oligonucleotide primed PCR and comparative genomic hybridization. *Virchows Arch* 433:297-304, 1998.

Focal Glandular Atypia

[12.1] FGA in Needle Biopsy 219

[12.2] FGA in TURP Chips and Simple Prostatectomy Specimens 224

CHAPTER 12

Focal glandular atypia (FGA) is a descriptive name for a gland or groups of glands with architectural or cytologic atypia that does not allow for a definitive diagnosis of reactive atypia, atypical adenomatous hyperplasia, prostatic intraepithelial neoplasia (PIN), or carcinoma (Reyes 1998). A number of synonymous monikers have been used, including atypia, atypical hyperplasia, atypical suspicious for carcinoma, borderline lesions, uncertain, and atypical small acinar proliferation (ASAP) (Amin 1998, Bostwick 1995, Chan 1999, Cheville 1997, Dundore 1998, Epstein 2001, Gleason 1985, Iczkowski 1998, Mostofi 1995, O'Dowd 2000, Reyes 1998, Weinstein 1998) **t12.1**. Most definitions in the literature state that the atypical glands harbor some but not all of the architectural and cytologic attributes of carcinoma. There is no uniformity as to precisely which features and how many of these features must be present to constitute atypia. This category undoubtedly is a broad diagnostic umbrella and encompasses benign and reactive but atypical epithelium to undersampled, small foci of carcinoma that harbor some but not all of the features needed for a definitive diagnosis of malignancy. A diagnosis of FGA, or ASAP, without further classification, is a valid diagnosis that is applied mainly to a small percentage of needle biopsies, where only limited sampling of the atypical epithelium has occurred.

[12.1] FGA in Needle Biopsy

The incidence of FGA in needle biopsies varies from 1% to 9% **t12.2**, with a mean aggregate in the literature of about 3%. No clinical features are contributory to or predictive of a diagnosis of atypia. The mean patient age is in the 60s, with a range of 40 to 95 **t12.3**. The men

■ t12.1 Focal Glandular Atypia: Diagnostic Terms

Focal glandular atypia
Borderline lesions
Uncertain
Atypia or atypical
Atypical hyperplasia
Atypical small acinar proliferation
Atypical suspicious for carcinoma/malignancy

■ t12.2 Incidence of Atypia in Prostate Needle Biopsy

Study	Diagnosis	Incidence
Bostwick 1995	1) Suspicious for carcinoma (Atypical small acinar proliferation = ASAP)	4/400 (1%)
	2) High-grade PIN and suspicious for cancer	4/400 (1%)
Mostofi 1995	Atypical glands or atypical hyperplasia	13/265 (4.9%)
Cheville 1997	Atypical focus suspicious for malignancy	48/1,009 (4.8%)
Khan 1997	Atypical	139/3,309 (4%)
Wills 1997	1) Atypical foci suspicious	18/439 (4.1 %)
	2) High-grade PIN and atypical suspicious	2/439 (0.5%)
Orozco 1998	Suspicious	1,814/62,537 (2.9%)
Reyes 1998	Focal glandular atypia	58/795 (7.3%)
Weinstein 1998	Atypical	75/5,240 (1.4%)
Renshaw 1998	Atypical	204/2,219 (9%)
Hoedemaker 1999	Borderline	43/1,824 (2.4%)
O'Dowd 2000	Suspicious	3,269/132,426 (2.5%)
	Suspicious and high-grade PIN	440/132,426 (0.3%)
Vis 2001	Suspicious	106/4,057 (2.6%)
	Suspicious and high-grade PIN	2/4,057 (0.1%)
Borboroglu 2001	ASAP	53/1,391 (3.8%)
	ASAP and high-grade PIN	8/1,391 (0.6%)
Alsikafi 2001	High-grade PIN with adjacent atypical glands	12/285 (4.2%)
Total		**4495/153,659 (2.9%)**

■ t12.3 Clinical Data: Patients with Atypia on Needle Biopsy

Study	Patient Number	Patient Age[1]	Serum PSA[2]	Abnormal DRE	TRUS
Bostwick 1995	3	66.9 (45-90)	5.9 (1-14)	75%	88%
Iczkowski 1997	33	61.6 (45-72)	7.3 (1-20)	22%	NA
Cheville 1997	41	69 (55-85)	7.3 (1-51)	50%	NA
Iczkowski 1998	295	68 (40-89)	NA	31%	NA
Renshaw 1998	64	65.8	7.5	23%	NA
Chan 1999	200	66 (41-95)	10.7 (0-200)	NA	NA
Park 2001	45	66 (50-81)	9.7 (1.6-33)	51%	NA

[1]Mean age (range)
[2]Median serum prostate specific antigen concentration in ng/mL (range), except for Chan 1999, where mean is provided
DRE =Digital rectal examination; TRUS = transrectal ultrasound; NA = not available

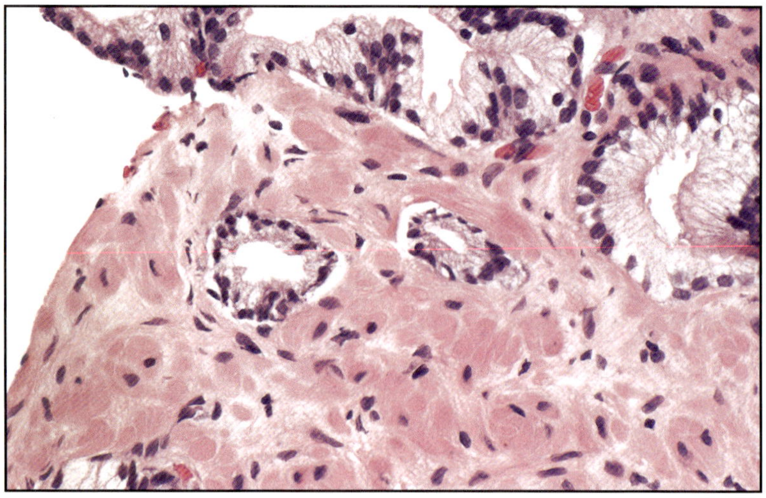

■ **i12.1** *Two small atypical acini adjacent to benign-appearing glands.*

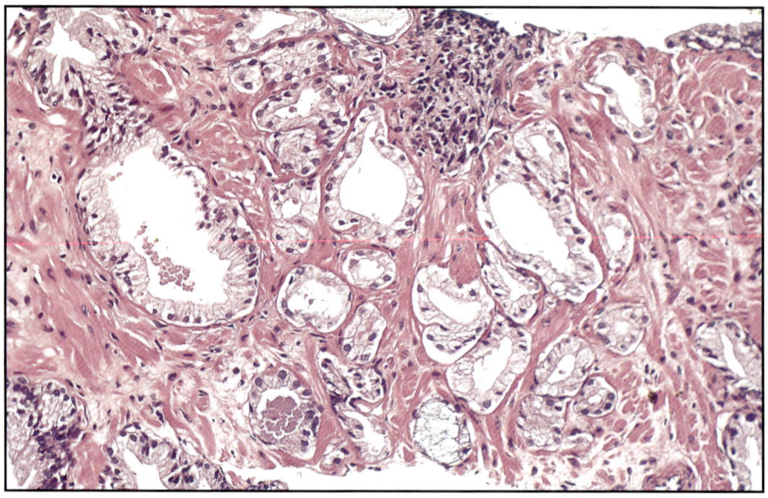

■ **i12.2** *Infiltrative appearance of small acini, coursing across the width of the needle core. Basal cells were present in several of the glands and there was minimal nuclear atypia at high power.*

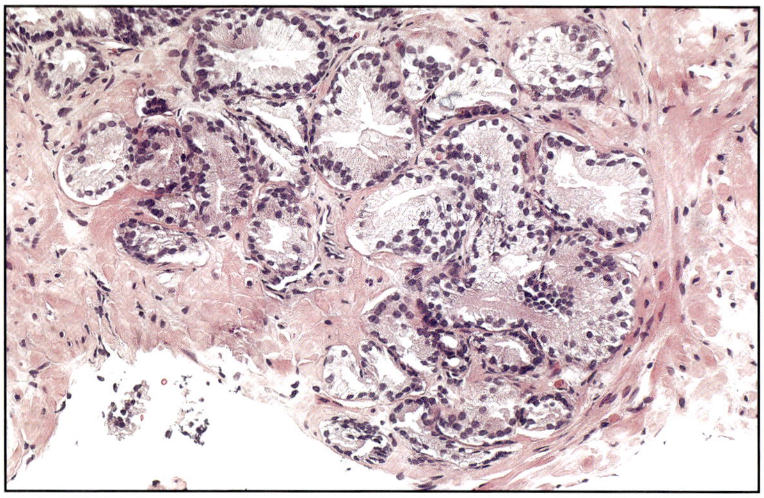

■ **i12.3** *Focal glandular atypia with crowded, small acini in a lobular cluster.*

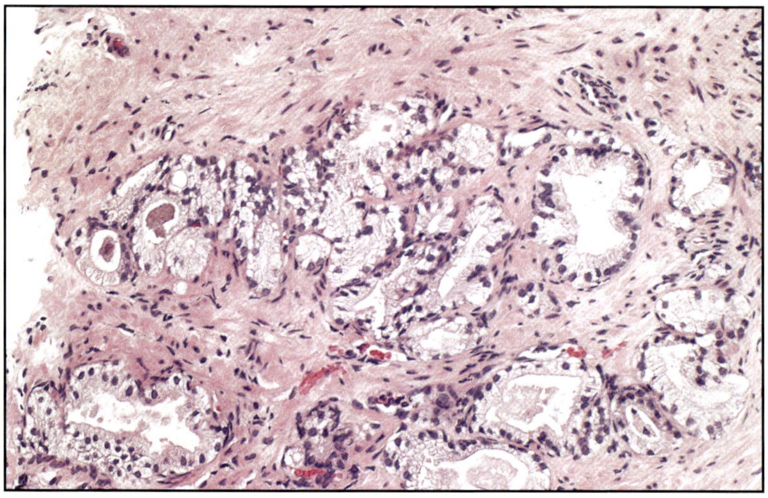

■ **i12.4** *Crowded, small acini of focal glandular atypia. Interpretation is compromised by tangential plane of sectioning.*

typically are biopsied to rule out prostate cancer, with the clinical indication being an elevated serum prostate-specific antigen (PSA) or abnormal digital rectal examination (DRE). The median PSA elevation usually is modest, ranging from 6 to 8 ng/mL, but very high PSA levels (>50 ng/mL) have been seen (Chan 1999, Cheville 1997). Only few transrectal ultrasound results have been reported (Bostwick 1995).

Histologically, FGA is an epithelial abnormality involving only a few glands **i12.1; t12.4**. Most often there is only 1 atypical focus, but in about 30% of cases there are 2 foci. In uncommon cases (7%), one can find FGA in different needle biopsies from both sides of the prostate (Cheville 1997). The number of glands per atypical focus has varied from a mean of 3.7 to 21, with a range of 1 to 67 (Cheville 1997, Iczkowski 1997, Wills 1997). The size of the atypical focus is small, generally <0.5mm to <1mm in linear dimension, with a range of 0.1mm to 1.4mm (Cheville 1997).

■ **t12.4 Histologic Features of Atypia in Needle Biopsy**

Architectural and/or cytologic atypia
Limited number of glands
Architectural: Haphazard arrangement of small acini that lack nuclear atypia
Cytologic atypia in rare glands: Nucleomegaly and nucleolomegaly
Intraluminal wispy blue mucin, crystalloids and/or pink proteinaceous secretions can be seen

An infiltrative growth pattern can be recognized in many cases of FGA **i12.2** and was present in 68% of cases in 1 series (Cheville 1997). In these cases a few acini are haphazardly distributed, but the cells lining the acini lack appreciable nuclear atypia such as nuclear enlargement and prominent nucleoli. In other cases, a lobular, clustered arrangement of small acini is the atypical finding (Cheville 1997) **i12.3, i12.4**. Another major histologic presentation of FGA is the presence of rare small acini that are worrisome for malignancy because they exhibit most of the cytologic features of carcinoma, but interpretation is comprised by the small number of acini (Iczkowski 1998) **i12.5–i12.8**. The nuclear abnormalities in these cases are not well developed, with mild to moderate nucleomegaly and nucleolomegaly in most examples (Cheville 1997, Iczkowski 1997). Amphophilic cytoplasm is an atypical cytologic finding in one third of cases (Cheville 1997).

Additional histologic findings in FGA (atypical small acinar proliferations suspicious for malignancy) include intraluminal wispy blue mucin in 39% to 42% of cases, intraluminal pink amorphous secretions in 74% of cases, intraluminal crystalloids in

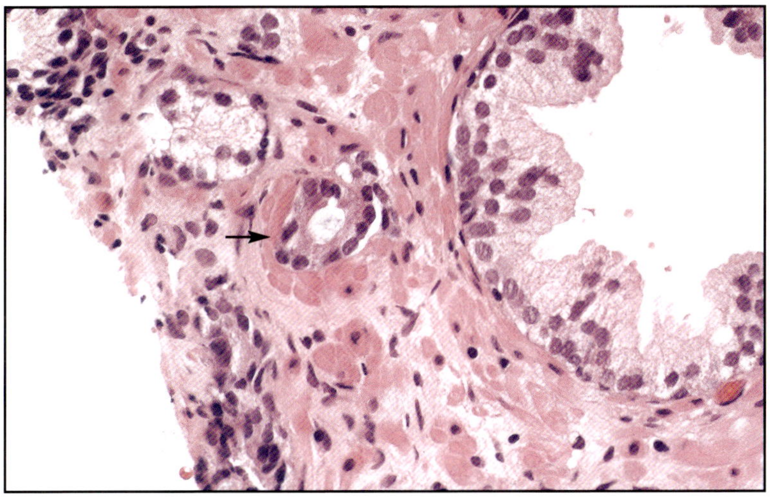

■ **i12.5** *Single small atypical acinus (arrow), adjacent to benign gland.*

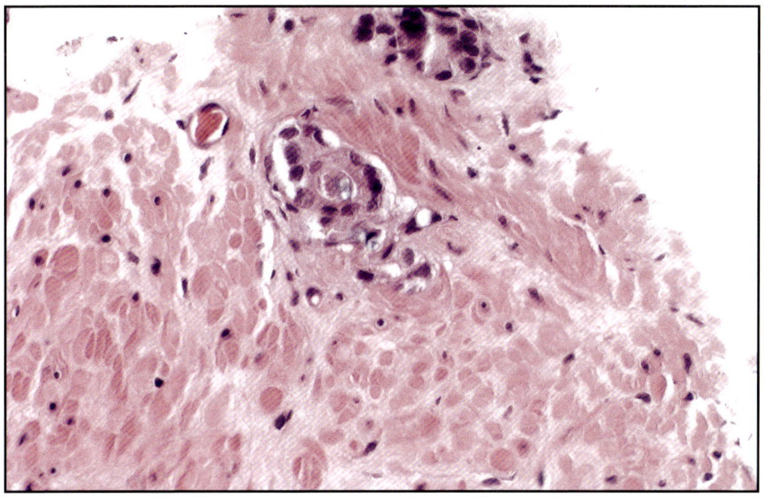

■ **i12.6** *Focal glandular atypia, suspicious for carcinoma.*

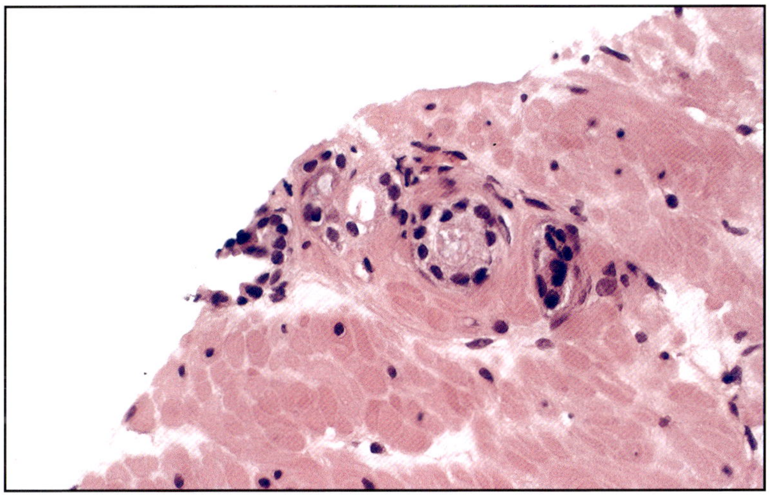

■ **i12.7** *Focal glandular atypia, also known as atypical small acinar proliferation (ASAP), suspicious for carcinoma.*

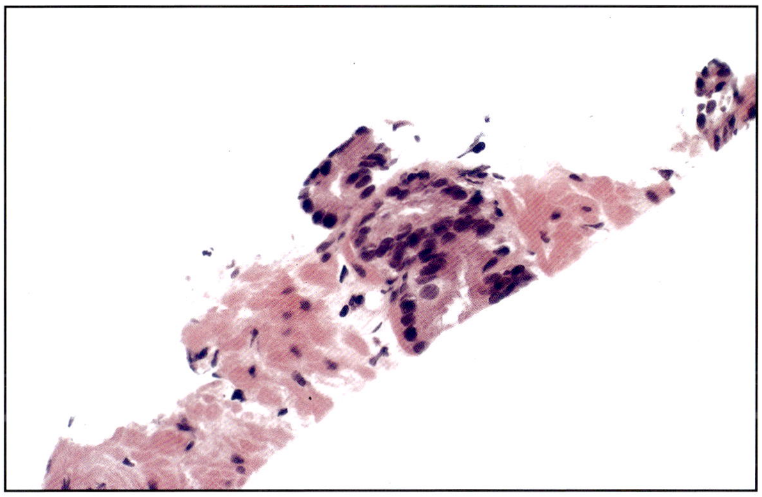

■ **i12.8** *Three small, atypical acini.*

22% of cases, focal chronic inflammation in 64% of cases, and adjacent high-grade PIN in 31% to 42% of cases (Cheville 1997, Iczkowski 1997).

The differential diagnosis of FGA is lengthy and includes benign and malignant epithelial conditions **t12.5**. Pseudoneoplasms of the prostate **t10.1** should be considered before a diagnosis of FGA is rendered. That benign entities account for a percentage of cases of FGA is underscored by reports that upon review, 4% (Iczkowski 1998) to 8% (Renshaw 1998) of prostate needle biopsies initially diagnosed as atypical were classified as benign prostatic tissue. In my experience, inflammatory atypia, particularly inflammation-related nuclear atypia in atrophy and basal cell hyperplasia, are the benign disorders most often diagnosed as FGA.

■ t12.5 **Focal Glandular Atypia: Differential Diagnosis**

Atrophy
Basal cell hyperplasia
Inflammatory atypia
Seminal vesicle/ejaculatory duct epithelium
Atypical adenomatous hyperplasia (adenosis)
Prostatic intraepithelial neoplasia
Radiation-induced atypia
Minimal adenocarcinoma

It is abundantly clear that some cases diagnosed as FGA or ASAP, suspicious for carcinoma, actually represent poorly sampled adenocarcinoma. Review of cases initially diagnosed as atypical has resulted in 18% (Iczkowski 1998) to 20% (Renshaw 1998) being reclassified as adenocarcinoma. A definitive diagnosis of minimal or limited adenocarcinoma in prostate should be based on a constellation of major and minor diagnostic criteria (Algaba 1996, Epstein 1995, Grignon 1998, Thorson 1998, 2000, Totten 1953). The major criteria are an infiltrative growth pattern, a single cell layer (absence of basal cells), and nuclear atypia in the form of nuclear and nucleolar enlargement (Algaba 1996, Totten 1953). FGA does not exhibit all of these criteria, but minimal carcinoma does not necessarily display all 3 attributes either (Epstein 1995, Thorson 1998). FGA and minimal carcinoma can both fulfill minor diagnostic criteria (Algaba 1996) for a diagnosis of malignancy, including intraluminal wispy blue mucin (blue-tinged mucinous secretions), pink amorphous secretions, mitotic figures, intraluminal crystalloids, adjacent high-grade PIN, amphophilic cytoplasm, and nuclear hyperchromasia.

The major confounding factors that prompt a diagnosis of FGA rather than adenocarcinoma are small lesion size, lack of an invasive

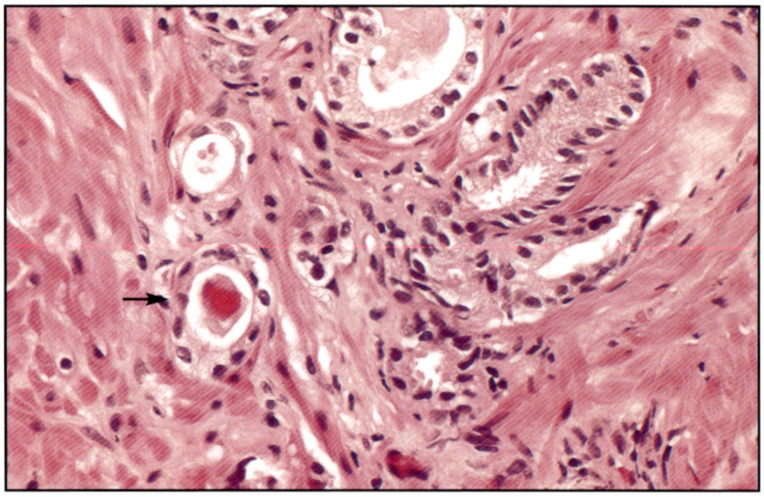

■ **i12.9** *Tangential sectioning of a focal, atypical glandular proliferation. One gland contains a crystalloid (arrow).*

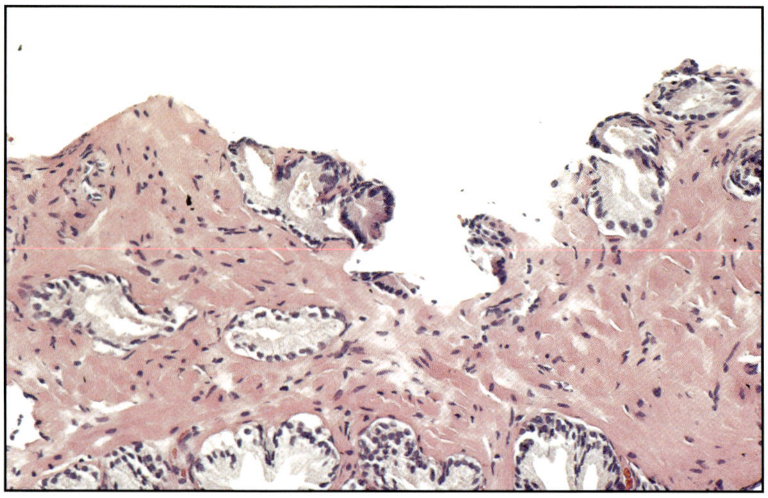

■ **i12.10** *Atypical, pale, small acinar proliferation, with several distorted glands at the edge of the needle core.*

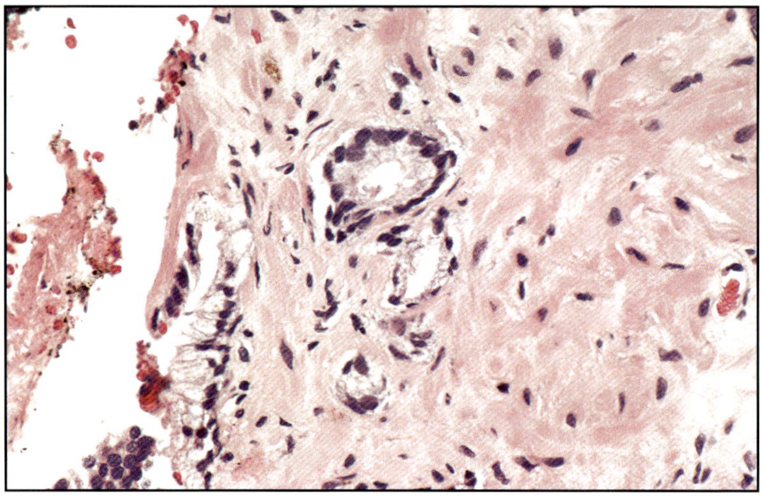

■ **i12.11** *Several atypical small glands with distorted nuclei.*

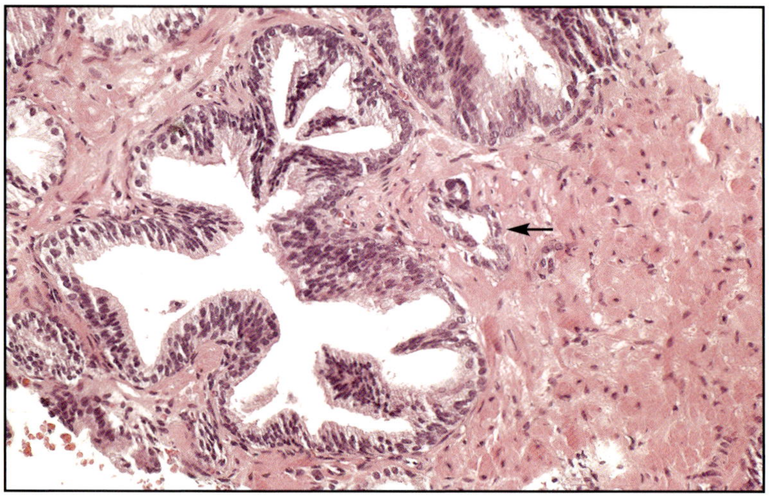

■ **i12.12** *High-grade prostatic intraepithelial neoplasia with adjacent atypical small acinar proliferation. This small gland (arrow) could represent protrusion from the PIN or focal invasion.*

growth pattern, and lack of cytologic abnormalities such as diffuse nucleolar enlargement (Cheville 1997, Iczkowski 1997). Moreover, the few acini may be difficult to assess because of tangential sectioning **i12.4, i12.9**, crush or distortion artifact **i12.10, i12.11**, section thickness, poor tissue fixation, or overstaining. These confounding factors can make evaluating nuclear atypia and cell layer number difficult. In particular, checking for basal cell presence or absence can be a problematic exercise where only a few distorted acini are present. Additional sources of difficulty in the diagnosis of focal atypical glands include unusual gland architectures and adjacent high-grade PIN. Most foci of glandular atypia have small acini (Cheville 1997). When the focal atypical glands possess hyperplastic-like features such as cystic change, branching, and papillary structures, a definitive diagnosis can be difficult to establish. Here the differential diagnosis is with minimal pseudohyperplastic prostatic adenocarcinoma (Humphrey 1998). Atrophic features in a small atypical focus can also create a diagnostic quagmire, where atrophic pattern prostatic adenocarcinoma (Cina 1997, Egan 1997, Kaleem 1998) lurks. Lastly, in a substantial percentage (10% to 50%) of FGA cases, high-grade PIN is observed adjacent to a focal ASAP **i12.12** (Bostwick 1995, Cheville 1997, Iczkowski 1997, Wills 1997). The differential diagnosis in this instance is outpouching of high-grade PIN versus high-grade PIN with focal invasive adenocarcinoma (see Chapter 11). The challenge of the differential diagnosis of atypia is underscored by the only fair to good interobserver agreement (Amin 1998, Renshaw 1998), with overall concordance rates of 62% to 78% (Iczkowski 1998, Renshaw 1998).

Additional studies can be of diagnostic value in distinguishing FGA from minimal adenocarcinoma. Clinical information such as serum PSA levels and DRE findings are not useful in addressing this purely morphologic diagnosis. Morphologic-based special studies can be of value, particularly additional sampling of the block and 34βE12 immunohistochemistry. We found that generating additional hematoxylin and eosin (H&E)-stained levels from the block resulted in a definitive diagnosis of adenocarcinoma in 10% of FGA cases (Reyes 1998). After a diagnosis of FGA was made in a set of initial 3 slides, the next additional H&E slide with several sections was diagnostic of malignancy in 4 of 40 cases. In these cases, the basis for the ability to render a definitive diagnosis of cancer was an increase in size of the atypical glandular focus.

Another valuable approach to these focal atypical epithelial proliferations is application of the 34βE12 (also incorrectly called CK903) immunostain for basal cells. This immunostain can be an important confirmatory tool to assess for basal cells, but it should not be used as a screening test for basal cells in all cases of atypical glands. Rather, its use should be specifically applied in selected cases with selection and the differential diagnosis driven by the H&E histologic appearance. As with all other ancillary reactions in surgical pathology, one should ask what one will do with the information. Here, absence of 34βE12 immunopositivity in a few atypical glands does not always mean that this is a focal carcinoma. Basal cell absence is an important criterion for the histologic diagnosis of prostatic carcinoma, but it is only one of several of the major criteria. Also, as Stout (Totten 1953) noted 50 years ago, based on examination of H&E-stained sections, not all benign glands have basal cells. This has been substantiated by the 34βE12 immunostain, as a minority of benign glands can have a discontinuous or absent basal cell layer. Indeed, one of the benign entities most often misdiagnosed as carcinoma—atrophy—can reveal scattered negative glands in up to 11% of cases (Hedrick 1989, Varma 1997). Up to 12% of basal cell hyperplasia glands fail to stain (Hedrick 1989), and 10% to 90% (average = 39%) of glands in atypical adenomatous hyperplasia do not stain (Hedrick 1989). Finally, this immunohistochemical stain is based on a negative result to render a positive diagnosis of malignancy. Many factors can cause failure of immunohistochemical staining (Iczkowski 1999, Ramnani 1999, Varma 1994), and absence of proof is not proof of absence. So, for a few atypical prostatic glands, the greatest meaning is a positive reaction indicating basal cell presence, thereby excluding invasive carcinoma. In one large series (Wojno 1995), this immunostain was ordered to assess a focus of 4 to 30 atypical glands, but the range was 1 to 200. Overall the immunostain was felt to be confirmatory in 46% of cases, was equivocal in 27% of cases, established the diagnosis in 14% of cases, and was of no used in 9% of cases (Wojno 1995). In needle biopsy cases stained with 34βE12, there was a tendency for cases with fewer glands to be diagnosed as equivocal rather than minimal cancer, but there was extensive overlap in number of glands on which a diagnosis was based, which again speaks to use of this immunostain as an supplementary tool. In another series of needle biopsies, it was concluded that the 34βE12 immunostain substantially reduced the percentage of prostate needle biopsy cases diagnosed as atypical (Kahane 1995).

Currently, our approach for FGA is to obtain additional H&E-stained sections (levels) (Reyes 1998) and a 34βE12 immunostain in selected cases. We rely on the H&E-stained sections to classify a focal atypical proliferation as FGA or minimal adenocarcinoma.

Clinical follow-up of a diagnosis of atypia in prostate needle biopsies indicates that this diagnosis places the patient at high risk for subsequent detection of adenocarcinoma on rebiopsy **t12.6**. After a diagnosis of atypia, the aggregate risk based on summation of the data in **t12.7** is 43% that the patient will be diagnosed with carcinoma on rebiopsy. This figure is higher than isolated high-grade PIN (at 28%) and should be compared with a risk of 20% for a subsequent diagnosis of carcinoma after a benign diagnosis **t12.7**. Atypical glands adjacent to high-grade PIN seem to impart an even higher risk of subsequent detection of carcinoma (at 53%), compared with atypia alone **t12.7**.

It is not currently possible to stratify for risk of detection of carcinoma after a diagnosis of atypia, based on clinical or pathologic features. Most (Chan 1999, Ellis 1995, Iczkowski 1997, 1998, Khan 1997, Renshaw 1998) but not all (Cheville 1997, O'Dowd 2000) studies have indicated that clinical features such as serum PSA level, DRE findings, and age do not add to the predictive information imparted by a diagnosis of atypia. At the histopathologic level, attempts have been made to place atypia into 3 tiers, such as favor benign, uncertain (or equivocal), and favor carcinoma (highly suspicious) (Chan 1999, Iczkowski 1997, 1998). However, this stratification is not significantly related to the risk of subsequent detection of carcinoma on rebiopsy (Chan 1999, Iczkowski 1997, 1998, Zhang 2000). Even when a benign diagnosis is favored for an atypical prostatic needle biopsy, up to 44% of patients (Iczkowski 1998) ([range 20% to 44%] [Chan 1999, Iczkowski 1997, 1998]) are diagnosed with carcinoma on rebiopsy. Finally this 3-tiered stratification is not very reproducible (Iczkowski 1998, Keane 1990), with 63% interobserver agreement in 1 study.

Rebiopsy probably should be performed in 3 to 4 months after an initial diagnosis of atypia. Most carcinomas on rebiopsy after an initial diagnosis of atypia were found within 6 months of that initial diagnosis (Chan 1999, Iczkowski 1998), but the reported timing of rebiopsy in the literature was quite variable with wide ranges, from 2 weeks to 3.5 years (Chan 1999, Iczkowski 1997, 1998, Renshaw 1998). To optimize cancer detection, the re-biopsy procedure should entail systematic rebiopsy of the entire gland (Borboroglu 2001, Chan 1999, Iczkowski 1998), not just the previous site of atypia. On rebiopsy only 23% to 48% of the cancers were in the same as the atypia, and 15% to 27% of carcinomas were in the other side of the prostate (Allen 1998, Iczkowski 1998). There is reported clinical variability in rebiopsy strategy and even whether rebiopsy is performed at all. In 2 series (Allen 1998, Renshaw 1998), 36% to 63% of patients with an atypical prostate needle biopsy had not undergone rebiopsy.

t12.6 Follow-up of Patients Diagnosed With Atypia on Prostate Needle Biopsy

Study		Patients with carcinoma on re-biopsy
Ellis 1995		5/17 (29%)
Iczkowski 1997		15/33 (45%)
Cheville 1997		15/25 (60%)
Iczkowski 1998		125/295 (42%)
Khan 1997		21/36 (58%)
Renshaw 1998		22/59 (37%)
Allen 1998		56/124 (45%)
Chan 1999		45/92 (49%)
O'Dowd 2000		639/1,525 (42%)
Zhang 2000		75/156 (48%)
Hoedemaker 1999		15/39 (38.5%)
O'Dowd 2000	Suspicious	529/1,321 (40%)
	Suspicious + HGPIN	111/209 (53%)
Vis 2001		36/93 (39%)
Borboroglu 2001	Suspicious	23/48 (48%)
	Suspicious + HGPIN	4/7 (57%)
Kronz 2001	Suspicious + HGPIN	28/56 (50%)
Alsikafi 2001	Suspicious + HGPIN	9/12 (75%)
Total		**1773/4147 (43%)**

HGPIN = high-grade prostatic intraepithelial neoplasia

t12.7 Risk of Detection of Carcinoma on Needle Core Rebiopsy Due to Atypia

Initial diagnosis	Patients with cancer on rebiopsy
Benign prostatic tissue	20%
High-grade PIN	28%
Atypia	43%
High-grade PIN + atypia	53%

Data from **t11.8** and **t12.6**

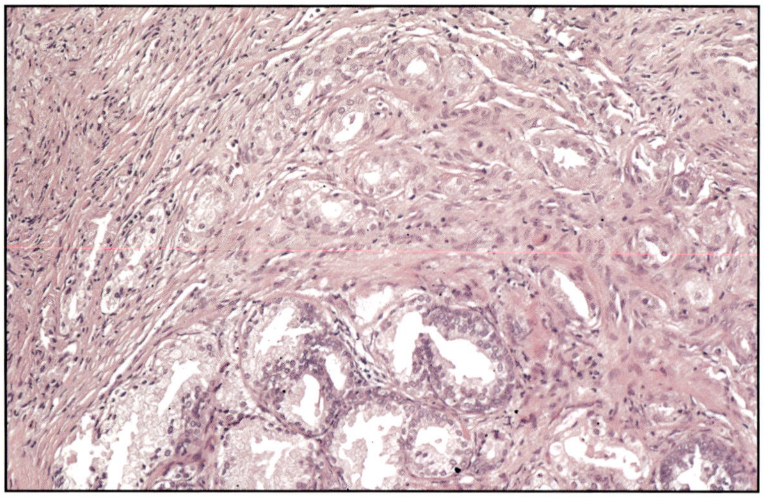

■ **i12.13** *Focal atypical small acinar proliferation at one pole of a BPH nodule.*

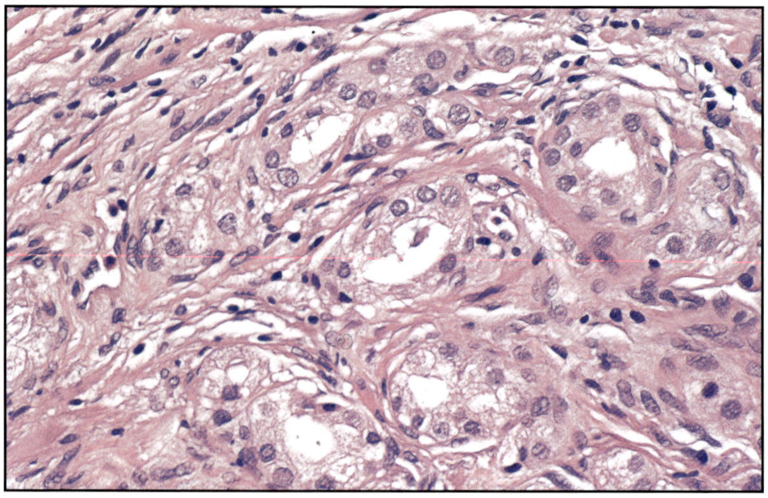

■ **i12.14** *Higher-power scrutiny of atypical small acini depicted in* **i12.13**.

■ t12.8 **Gleason Histologic Grade of Carcinomas Detected on Rebiopsy Due to Initial Diagnosis of Atypia**

Gleason Score	% of Patients
2-4	4%-12%
5,6	67%-68%
7	10%-24%
8-10	5%-10%

Data from Iczkowski 1998, Chan 1999

Repeat biopsy results in a second diagnosis of atypia in about 6% of cases (Chan 1999, Ellis 1995, Iczkowski 1997, 1998, Renshaw 1998). These patients probably should undergo a second rebiopsy. Consideration for additional rebiopsy sessions probably should be based on clinical findings (serum PSA and DRE results) and judgment.

The carcinomas detected on rebiopsy for a diagnosis of atypia are mainly of intermediate grade, with Gleason scores of 5 and 6 (Allen 1998, Iczkowski 1997, 1998, Renshaw 1998), but 30% are high grade, of Gleason scores 7 to 10 (Allen 1998, Iczkowski 1998) **t12.8**. Little is known of the characteristics of the tumors in the whole gland because only a few patients have been reported to undergo radical prostatectomy (Cheville 1997, Iczkowski 1997, Renshaw 1998).

[12.2] FGA in TURP Chips and Simple Prostatectomy Specimens

A diagnosis of FGA can also be given to tissue samples larger than needle cores, particularly transurethral resection of the prostate (TURP) chips or simple prostatectomy specimens (Bostwick 1993, Keane 1990). Synonymous terms applied to these specimens include "suspicious of malignancy" (Keane 1990) and "atypical small acinar proliferation of uncertain significance" (Bostwick 1993). The histologic criteria for this diagnosis in TURP chips are not established, but nuclear abnormalities, including number of enlarged nucleoli and nucleolar size, are intermediate between those of atypical adenomatous hyperplasia (adenosis) and well-differentiated adenocarcinoma (Bostwick 1993) **i12.13, i12.14**. What is clear is that there is substantial interobserver variability in rendering an atypical suspicious diagnosis in TURP chips (Bostwick 1993, Keane 1990). Concordance in one study was 41% (Bostwick 1993), and in 20% to 25% of cases, carcinoma was diagnosed by other observers (Bostwick 1993, Keane 1990). Only a few patients with atypia in TURP chips have been studied, and the clinical significance is unknown. If a diagnosis of atypia is contemplated for a TURP chip or open prostatectomy case, additional sampling (gross or histologic) should be pursued, and use of the 34βE12 immunostain and consultation should also be considered. If a diagnosis of atypia is proffered after these maneuvers, clinical follow-up probably should be recommended, including serum PSA draw and DRE.

References

Algaba F, Epstein JI, Aldape HC, et al. Assessment of prostate carcinoma in core needle biopsy-definition of minimal criteria for the diagnosis of cancer in biopsy material. *Cancer* 78:376-381, 1996.

Allen EA, Kahane H, Epstein JI. Repeat biopsy strategies for men with atypical diagnoses on initial prostate needle biopsy. *Urology* 52:803-807, 1998.

Alsikafi NF, Brendler CB, Gerber GS, et al. High-grade prostatic intraepithelial neoplasia with adjacent atypia is associated with a higher incidence of cancer on subsequent needle biopsy than high-grade prostatic intraepithelial neoplasia alone. *Urology* 57:296-300, 2001.

Amin MB, Bostwick DG, Epstein JI, et al. Interobserver reproducibility in the diagnosis of small foci of prostatic adenocarcinoma in needle biopsies [abstract]. *Mod Pathol* 11:76A, 1998.

Borboroglu PG, Sur RL, Roberts JL, et al. Repeat biopsy strategy in patients with atypical small acinar proliferation or high grade prostatic intraepithelial neoplasia in initial prostate needle biopsy. *J Urol* 166:866-870, 2001.

Bostwick DG, Srigley J, Grignon D, et al. Atypical adenomatous hyperplasia: morphologic criteria for its distinction from well-differentiated carcinoma. *Hum Pathol* 24:819-832, 1993.

Bostwick DG, Qian J, Frankel K. The incidence of high-grade prostatic intraepithelial neoplasia in needle biopsies. *J Urol* 154:1791-1794, 1995.

Chan TY, Epstein JI. Follow-up of atypical prostate needle biopsies suspicious for cancer. *Urology* 53:351-355, 1999.

Cheville JC, Reznicek MJ, Bostwick DG. The focus of atypical glands suspicious for malignancy in prostatic needle biopsy specimens. Incidence, histologic features, and clinical follow-up of cases diagnosed in a community practice. *Am J Clin Pathol* 108:633-640, 1997.

Cina SJ, Epstein JI. Adenocarcinoma of the prostate with atrophic features. *Am J Surg Pathol* 21:287-295, 1997.

Dundore PA. Atypical small acinar proliferations (ASAP) suspicious for malignancy in prostate needle biopsies. *J Urol Pathol* 8:21-29, 1998.

Egan AJ, Lopez-Beltran A, Bostwick DG. Prostatic adenocarcinoma with atrophic features: malignancy mimicking a benign process. *Am J Surg Pathol* 21:931-935, 1997.

Ellis WJ, Brawer MK. Repeat prostate needle biopsy: who needs it? *J Urol* 153:1496-1498, 1995.

Epstein JI. Diagnostic criteria of limited adenocarcinoma of the prostate on needle biopsy. *Hum Pathol* 26:223-229, 1995.

Epstein JI, Potter SR. The pathological interpretation and significance of prostate needle biopsy findings: implications and current controversies. *J Urol* 166:402-410, 2001.

Gleason DF. Atypical hyperplasia, benign hyperplasia, and well-differentiated adenocarcinoma of the prostate. *Am J Surg Pathol* 9(suppl):53-67, 1985.

Grignon DJ. Minimal diagnostic criteria for adenocarcinoma of the prostate. *J Urol Pathol* 8:31-43, 1998.

Hedrick L, Epstein JI. Use of keratin 903 as an adjunct in the diagnosis of prostate carcinoma. *Am J Surg Pathol* 13:389-396, 1989.

Hoedemaeker RF, Kranse R, Rietbergen JBW, et al. Evaluation of prostate needle biopsies in a population-based screening study. *Cancer* 85:145-152, 1999.

Humphrey PA, Kaleem Z, Swanson PE, et al. Pseudohyperplastic prostatic adenocarcinoma. *Am J Surg Pathol* 22:1239-1296, 1998.

Iczkowski KA, MacLennan GT, Bostwick DG. Atypical small acinar proliferation suspicious for malignancy in prostate needle biopsies. *Am J Surg Pathol* 21:1489-1495, 1997.

Iczkowski KA, Bassler TJ, Schwob VS, et al. Diagnosis of "suspicious for malignancy" in prostate biopsies: predictive value for cancer. *Urology* 51:749-758, 1998.

Iczkowski KA, Cheng L, Crawford BA, et al. Steam heat with an EDTA buffer and protease digestion optimizes immunohistochemical expression of basal cell–specific antikeratin 34βE12 to discriminate cancer in prostatic epithelium. *Mod Pathol* 12:1-4, 1999.

Kahane H, Sharp JW, Shuman GB, et al. Utilization of high molecular weight cytokeratin on prostate needle biopsies in an independent laboratory. *Urology* 45:981-986, 1995.

Kaleem Z, Swanson PE, Vollmer RT, et al. Prostatic adenocarcinoma with atrophic features: a study of 202 consecutive, completely-embedded radical prostatectomy specimens. *Am J Clin Pathol* 109:695-703, 1998.

Kambham N, Taylor JA, Troxel A, et al. Atypical small acinar proliferation in prostate needle biopsies. *J Urol Pathol* 10:177-187, 1999.

Keane PF, Ilesley IC, O'Donoghue EPN, et al. Pathological classification and follow-up of prostatic lesions initially diagnosed as "suspicious of malignancy." *Br J Urol* 66:306-311, 1990.

Khan W, Sakr WA, Grignon DJ, et al. Analysis of 3300 consecutive prostate biopsies (PBx): a 4 year institutional experience with the frequency of carcinoma (PCa), isolated high grade prostatic intraepithelial neoplasia (HGPIN) and "atypical" [abstract]. *Mod Pathol* 10:79A, 1997.

Kronz JD, Shaikh AA, Epstein JJ. High-grade prostatic intraepithelial neoplasia with adjacent small atypical glands on prostate biopsy. *Hum Pathol* 32:389-395, 2001.

Lessells AM, Burnett RA, Howatson SR, et al. Observer variability in the histopathological reporting of needle biopsy specimens of the prostate. *Hum Pathol* 28:646-649, 1997.

Mostofi F, Murphy GP, Mettlin C, et al. Pathology review in an early prostate cancer detection program: results from the American Cancer Society–National Prostate Cancer Detection Project. *Prostate* 27:7-12, 1995.

Novis DA, Zarbo RJ, Valenstein PA. Diagnostic uncertainty expressed in prostate needle biopsies. A College of American Pathologists Q-Probes study of 15,753 prostate needle biopsies in 332 institutions. *Arch Pathol Lab Med* 123:687-692, 1999.

O'Dowd GJ, Miller MC, Orozco R, et al. Analysis of repeated biopsy results within 1 year after a noncancer diagnosis. *Urology* 55:553-559, 2000.

Orozco R, O'Dowd G, Kunnel B, et al. Observations on pathology trends in 62, 537 prostate biopsies obtained from urology private practices in the United States. *Urology* 51:186-195, 1998.

Park S, Shinohara K, Grossfeld GD, et al. Prostate cancer detection in men with prior high grade prostatic intraepithelial neoplasia or atypical prostate biopsy. *J Urol* 165:1409-1414, 2001.

Ramnani DM, Bostwick DG. Basal cell-specific anti-keratin antibody 34βE12: optimizing its use in distinguishing benign prostate and cancer [editorial]. *Mod Pathol* 12:443-444, 1999.

Renshaw AA, Santis WF, Richie JP. Clinicopathological characteristics of prostatic adenocarcinoma in men with atypical prostate needle biopsies. *J Urol* 159:2018-2022, 1998.

Reyes AO, Humphrey PA. Diagnostic effect of complete histologic sampling of prostate needle biopsy specimens. *Am J Clin Pathol* 109:416-422, 1998.

Thorson P, Arcangeli C, Keetch DW, et al. Diagnostic features and follow-up of minimal carcinoma in prostate needle biopsies. *Mod Pathol* 11:543-551, 1998.

Thorson P, Humphrey PA. Minimal adenocarcinoma in prostate needle biopsy tissue. *Am J Clin Pathol* 114:896-909, 2000.

Totten RS, Heinemann MW, Hudson PB, et al. Microscopic differential diagnosis of latent carcinoma of the prostate. *Arch Pathol* 55:131-141, 1953.

Varma M, Linden MD, Amin MB. Effect of formalin fixation and epitope retrieval techniques on antibody 34βE12 immunostaining of prostatic tissues. *Mod Pathol* 12:472-478, 1994.

Varma M, Amin MB, Linden MD, et al. Discriminant staining patterns of small glandular and preneoplastic lesions of the prostate using high molecular weight cytokeratin (HMCK): a study of 301 consecutive needle biopsies [abstract]. *Mod Pathol* 10:93A, 1997.

Vis AN, Hoedemaeker RF, Roobol M, et al. The predictive value for prostate cancer of lesions that raise suspicion of concomitant carcinoma. An evaluation from a randomized, population-based study of screening for prostate cancer. *Cancer* 92:524-534, 2001.

Weinstein MH, Greenspan DL, Epstein JI. Diagnoses rendered on prostate needle biopsies in community hospitals. *Prostate* 35:50-55, 1998.

Wills ML, Hamper UM, Partin AW, et al. Incidence of high grade prostatic intraepithelial neoplasia in sextant needle biopsy specimens. *Urology* 49:367-373, 1997.

Wojno KJ, Epstein JI. The utility of basal cell-specific anti-cytokeratin antibody (34βE12) in the diagnosis of prostate cancer. A review of 228 cases. *Am J Surg Pathol* 19:251-260, 1995.

Zhang PL, Shuffler SH, Bihrle W III, et al. Subclassification of small atypical glands in prostate biopsies provides a clearer indication for re-biopsies [abstract]. *Mod Pathol* 13:105A, 2000.

Clinical Aspects of Prostatic Carcinoma, With Histopathologic Correlations

[13.1] Etiology **231**
[13.2] Clinical Presentation **234**
[13.3] Natural History and Mortality **241**
[13.4] Treatment **245**

CHAPTER 13

Prostatic carcinoma is the most common noncutaneous malignancy clinically diagnosed in men in the United States (Jemal 2002) **t13.1**. In 2002, it is estimated that 189,000 new cases of prostate cancer will be diagnosed in the United States (Jemal 2002). This incidence corresponds to about 30% of all new cancers diagnosed in men **f13.1**. The lifetime risk of developing prostate cancer for men in the United States is estimated to be 9.5% (Seidman 1985).

The clinical incidence of prostate cancer has changed remarkably over the last 2 centuries and particularly over the last 15 years. In the 19th century, prostate cancer was thought to be a rare disease (Bodie 1842, Bush 1977, Thompson 1883). Indeed, in a survey of cancer deaths in Paris from 1830 to 1840, only 5 of 1904 (0.3%) were reported to be due to a prostatic primary (Tanchou 1844, Thompson 1883). In the first half of the 20th century, there was an increase in longevity from 47 years in 1911 to 67 years in 1947 and a corresponding increase in incidence in clinically detected prostate cancer (Huggins 1947). This is not surprising because prostate cancer affects mainly men 60 years of age and older. Also contributing to this increase in incidence were clinical use of the digital rectal examination (DRE) to detect prostate cancer (Jewett 1956, Young 1926) and the use of the light microscope to diagnose malignancy in biopsy tissue sections (Jewett 1956, Rosai 1997, Rosen 1977) and in sections of prostatic tissue removed as treatment for benign prostatic hyperplasia (BPH) (transurethral resection of the prostate [TURP] chips and open prostatectomy tissues). In the latter part of the twentieth century, there has been a vast expansion in the number of patients diagnosed with prostate cancer in the United States **f13.2**. In particular, between 1987 and 1992, the incidence rate of prostate cancer increased 85%, followed by a decline of 28% between 1992 and 1995 (Ries 1998) **f13.2**. Most of this remarkable increase has been attributed to use of prostate-specific antigen (PSA) screening (Gann 1997, Wingo 1997). The increased incidence probably reflects earlier detection of lower-stage cancer, with the fall resulting from depletion of the prevalent cases found by screening. It is not known whether future incidence rates will stabilize at or above the pre-PSA testing level (Gann 1997).

Globally, clinically detected prostate cancer is the third most common male cancer, after malignancies of the lung and stomach (Parkin 1999, Pisani 2002). The incidence of prostate cancer is increasing around the world, in part because of the aging of the populations, but the age-adjusted incidence is also increasing (Boyle 1995, Brasso 1998). There are extraordinary differences between world regions and countries in clinically detected prostate cancer incidence (Boyle 1995, Parkin 1999) **f13.3**.

The age-adjusted incidence rates are highest in North America, Australia and New Zealand, Europe, and the Caribbean, where Jamaican men have the highest incidence in the world (Glover 1998B). In contrast, rates are far lower in Asia, and the difference between North America and China is >80-fold. Both genetic and environmental influences have been implicated in this dissimilarity. There

t13.1 Incidence of Clinically-detected Prostatic Carcinoma

Most common noncutaneous cancer in American men
189,000 estimated new cases in American men in 2002
Third most common cancer in men worldwide
Frequency varies greatly worldwide: with highest incidence in the West and much lower incidence in the Far East

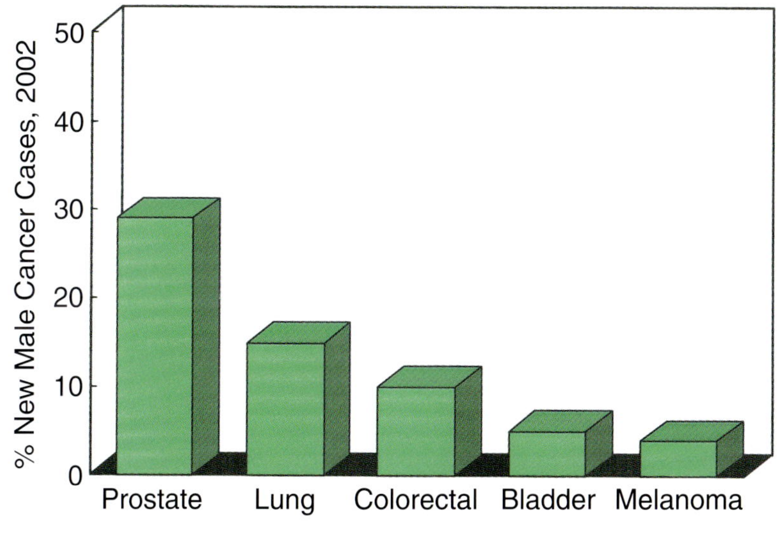

f13.1 *Prostate cancer is the most common non-cutaneous malignancy in American men, representing almost 30% of all new cancer cases.*

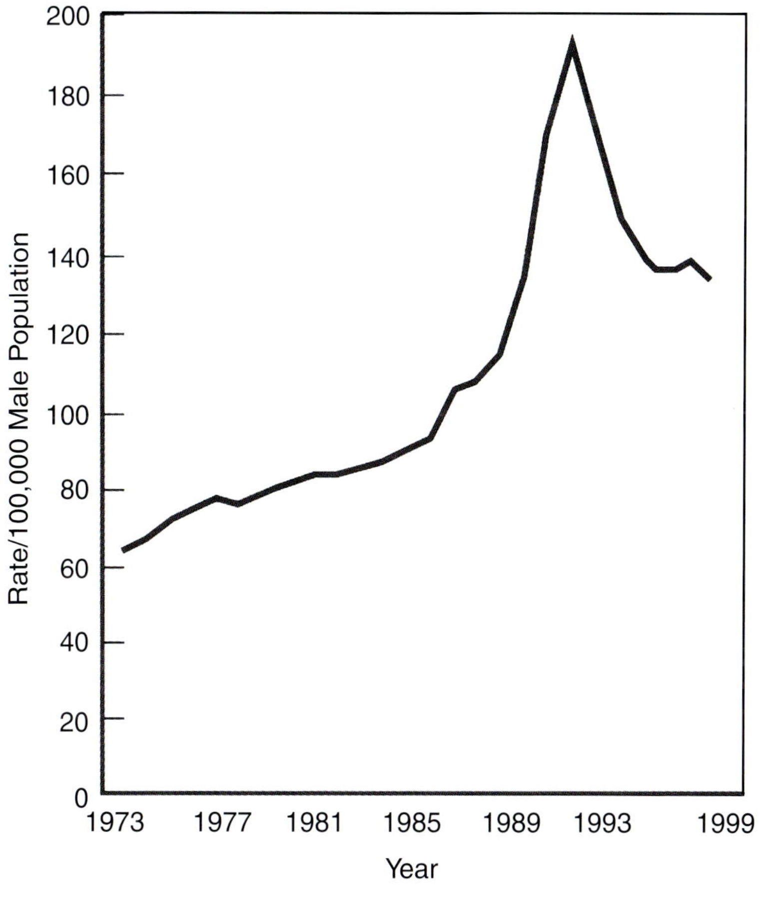

f13.2 *Prostate cancer incidence change with time. The peak is due to widespread use of PSA screening.*

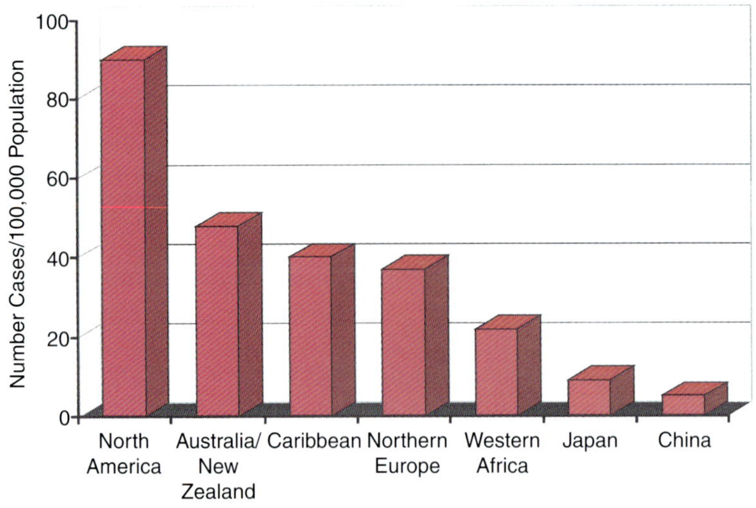

■ **f13.3** *Variation of prostate cancer incidence by geographic region around the world.*

is felt to be a major environmental component because the movement of low-risk Asian men to a high-risk geographic areas (the United States) results in a marked increase in prostate cancer, but the annual incidence for all generations of Asian Americans is still only roughly half that of white men born in the United States (Cook 1999).

Autopsy-Detected Prostatic Carcinoma

The prevalence of prostate cancer discovered at autopsy is extremely high, with an estimated range of 9% to 46% **t13.2, t13.3**. (Prevalence is the number of people at a particular time—here, at death—with a given disease [Parkin 1999]). These carcinomas discovered at autopsy, without a prior clinical diagnosis, have been called unsuspected carcinoma, early carcinoma, beginning carcinoma, histologic carcinoma, localized carcinoma, and latent

■ **t13.2 Prevalence of "Latent" Prostatic Carcinoma at Autopsy**

Study	Country	Sampling	Number (%)
Moore 1935	Germany	Completely-embedded	51/304 (17%)
Rich 1935	US	1 slide	27/292 (9%)
Gaynor 1938	Austria	Completely embedded	185/940 (20%)
Kahler 1939	US	2-3 slides	54/490 (11%)
Baron 1941	US	1-2 random sections	54/364 (15%)
		Completely embedded	23/50 (46%)
Andrews 1949	England	Completely embedded	17/142 (12%)
Edwards 1953	Canada	Completely embedded	41/254 (16%)
Franks 1954	England	Completely embedded	69/178 (39%)
Butler 1959	US	1 complete cross-section	71/220 (32%)
Karube 1961	Japan	Completely embedded	25/229 (11%)
Oota 1961	Japan	Completely embedded	47/259 (18%)
McNeal 1968	US	Completely embedded	36/94 (38%)
Liavåg 1968	Norway	3 slides	87/340 (26%)
Harbitz 1972	Norway	3-6 slides	66/202 (33%)
Akazaki 1973	US: Hawaii[1]	Completely embedded	46/158 (29%)
	Japan	Completely embedded	47/239 (20%)
Breslow 1977	Israel	Completely embedded	32/143 (22%)
	Hong Kong	Completely embedded	26/173 (15%)
	Uganda	Completely embedded	36/150 (24%)
	Jamaica	Completely embedded	55/168 (33%)
	Sweden	Completely embedded	123/306 (40%)
	Germany	Completely embedded	43/145 (30%)
	Singapore	Completely embedded	35/242 (14%)
Guileyardo 1980	US African-Americans	Completely embedded	65/207 (31%)
	US Whites	Completely embedded	85/293 (29%)
Høland 1980	Denmark	2 or more slides	50/223 (22%)
Yatani 1982	Columbia	Completely embedded	57/182 (31%)
	US: Hawaii	Completely embedded	107/417 (26%)
	Japan	Completely embedded	118/576 (21%)
	US Whites	Completely embedded	88/253 (35%)
	US African-Americans	Completely embedded	66/178 (37%)
Yatani 1988	Japan 1965-1979	Completely embedded	130/576 (23%)
	Japan 1982-1986	Completely embedded	228/660 (35%)
Sakr 1993	US Whites	Completely embedded	14/54 (26%)
	US African-Americans	Completely embedded	19/98 (19%)
Sakr 1994	US Whites	Completely embedded	34/96 (35%)
	US African-Americans	Completely embedded	36/159 (23%)
Brawn 1995	US	Completely embedded	79/209 (38%)
Silvestri 1995	Italy	Completely embedded	32/130 (25%)
Billis 2000	Brazil	Completely embedded	55/150 (37%)
Total			**2,559/10,447 (25%)**

[1]Japanese migrants to Hawaii

■ **t13.3 Autopsy-Detected Prostatic Carcinoma: Prevalence**

Extremely common worldwide, with a prevalence, based on complete gland sampling, of 15-20% in the Orient to 30-40% in the West
Prevalence depends on extent of gross prostate gland sampling
Prevalence is highly age-dependent

■ **t13.4 Lifetime Risk of Developing Prostate Cancer for a 50-Year-Old Man**

Lifetime risk of developing "autopsy" cancer = 42%
Lifetime risk of developing "clinical" cancer = 9.5%

From Scardino 1992

carcinoma (Karube 1961). Currently, *latent* (meaning a disease in which the usual symptoms are not manifest [Brown 1993]) *carcinoma* is the preferred designation. The detection rate of latent prostate cancers at autopsy varies with extent of gland sampling, age of the patient population, country, and criteria for a malignant diagnosis **t13.2**. If only 1 slide is generated per prostate gland, the prevalence can be as low as 9% for men 50 years or older (Rich 1935). In one study the prevalence was 15% for 1 or 2 random sections and 46% for complete embedding of all prostatic tissue (Baron 1941). The prevalence is exquisitely age-dependent, with rare cases discovered in the third decade (Sakr 1993) and an 83% prevalence in patients 90 years and older (Hirst 1954) **f13.4**. A recent surprising finding was a frequency of 29% in the fourth decade and 32% in the fifth decade (Sakr 1993). Prior studies of completely embedded glands had indicated that 5% of men under 50 had latent prostatic carcinoma at postmortem examination (Sakr 1993). There is also variation of the frequency of latent prostate cancer diagnosed at autopsy based on world region **t13.2**. Although this autopsy-based prevalence shows much less variation than that of clinical prostate cancer, the ethnicity-specific ranks are similar. Thus, latent prostate cancer incidence is lower in Singapore, Hong Kong, and Japan than in Western countries (Breslow 1977, Yatani 1982), but recent data suggest an increase in latent prostate cancer in Japan to Western levels (Yatani 1988) **t13.2**. It is of etiologic interest that the prevalence of latent carcinoma for Japanese Hawaiians (Japanese migrants to Hawaii) is intermediate between that of native Japanese and native Americans (Akazaki 1973, Yatani 1982) **t13.2**. This suggests an effect of environmental influences, such as diet, on the development of latent prostate cancer. In the United States, African Americans have a similar (Guileyardo 1980, Yatani 1982) or

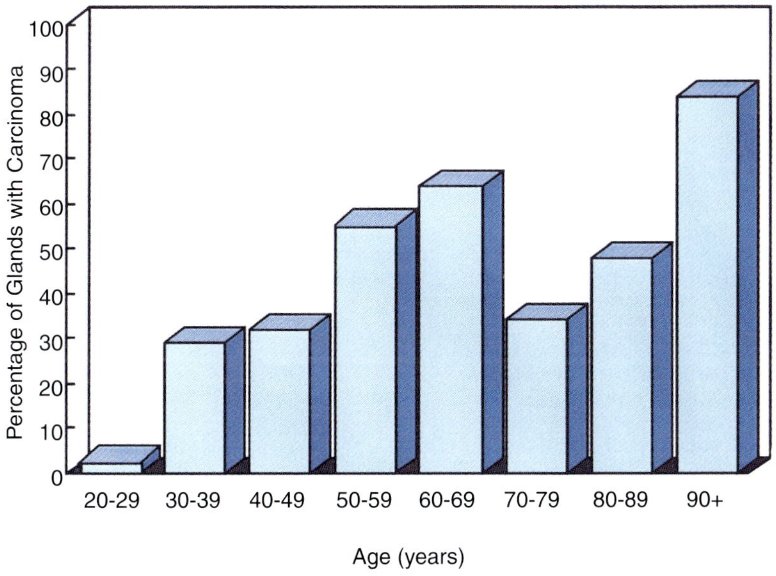

■ **f13.4** *Age-dependent prevalence of prostatic carcinoma detected at autopsy. Data for individuals 20-69 from Sakr 1994 and for 70-90+ from Hirst 1954. Both series were of completely-embedded glands.*

lower (Sakr 1993, 1994) prevalence of latent autopsy cancers than whites but a higher clinical incidence. Finally, given that most latent prostatic carcinomas are quite small, interobserver variability in diagnosis of malignancy will exist, but these differences in interpretation are small in effect compared with the effects of geographic region and age (Breslow 1977).

The lifetime risk of developing prostate cancer detected at autopsy for a 50-year-old man is, at 42%, 4.4 times greater than the lifetime risk of clinical detection of prostate cancer (Scardino 1992) **t13.4**. The basis for this difference has not been elucidated, but it may be that latent prostate cancers have acquired some but not all of the genotypic abnormalities necessary for progression to a histologic grade, stage, and size that would allow clinical detection (Watanabe 1996). It has been specifically postulated that low-grade carcinomas with a doubling time of >4 years are likely to remain latent, whereas the more proliferative tumors with a doubling time of <3 years may emerge as clinically detectable (Hirano 1998).

Prevalence of Prostatic Carcinoma in Radical Cystoprostatectomy Specimens

The incidental histologic discovery of prostatic adenocarcinoma in prostate glands from radical cystoprostatectomy specimens (typically removed for bladder cancer), like autopsy-detected prostate cancer, is exceptionally common **t13.5**, with a range of 27% to 70% for completely embedded glands. Just as for prostate cancers detected at postmortem examination, the frequency of identification is related to the degree of prostate gland sampling and patient age (Pritchett 1988). It is not known whether there is any worldwide geographic variation because almost all series are from the United States.

Pathologic Features of Latent Autopsy Cancers

Clinically unsuspected prostatic carcinomas diagnosed at postmortem examination are of lower grade, stage, and size than clinically detected cancers, although pathologic features associated with clinical carcinomas are found in a minority of cases **t13.6**. Grossly, prostatic carcinoma in glands from autopsy are difficult or impossible to identify (Baron 1941, Butler 1959, Franks 1954, Kahler 1939, Karube 1961, Moore 1935). In most series 0% to 23% of cancers could be seen macroscopically on cut surfaces. When recognized, descriptions of yellow to white to gray-white masses of increased consistency were given (Kahler 1939). Yet solid BPH nodules can also be yellow to firm and solid-white masses, such that the distinction can be guesswork (Baron 1941). Microscopically, most autopsy-detected prostatic cancer is small acinar adenocarcinoma **i13.1**. Most carcinomas are present in the peripheral zone, and multifocality is common. Of interest, there is little physical association of these carcinomatous foci with high-grade prostatic intraepithelial neoplasia (PIN) (Sakr 1993, 1994). There is

■ **t13.5 Incidence of "Latent" Prostatic Carcinoma at Cystoprostatectomy**

Study	Country	Sampling	Number (%)
Mahadevia 1986	US	Completely embedded	14/20 (70%)
Winfield 1987	US	NA	22/80 (28%)
Pritchett 1988	US	"Wide sampling"	45/165 (27%)
Baron 1989	France	NA	26/100 (26%)
Montie 1989	US	Completely embedded	39/84 (46%)
Kabalin 1989	US	Completely embedded	25/66 (38%)
Troncoso 1989	US	Completely embedded	61/100 (61%)
Abbas 1996	US	Completely embedded	18/40 (45%)
Wiley 1997	US	"Representative"	22/48 (46%)
Montzouris 1999	Greece	Completely embedded	16/59 (27%)

■ **13.6 Pathologic Features of Autopsy-Detected Prostatic Carcinoma**

Location:	Most in peripheral zone
Size:	Mean diameter: 2.3 mm (range 0.8 to 6 mm)[1]
	Median cc: 0.24 cc (range 0.01 to 10 cc)[2]
Grade:	Most well-differentiated Gleason score 2-4
Stage:	Usually organ-confined (T2), with up to 16% extraprostatic extension[2] and 8% seminal vesicle invasion (T3)[3]. Metastasis rare.

[1]Sakr 1993
[2]Brawn 1995
[3]Moore 1935

a wide size range from diameters of 0.1cm to 5cm **i13.2** (Franks 1954, Kahler 1939, Sakr 1993). A mean diameter of 0.2cm was obtained in one series (Sakr 1993). Volumes of $0.01cm^3$ to $12cm^3$ have been reported, with average volume estimates of $0.07cm^3$ to $1.1cm^3$ (Andrews 1949, Brawn 1995, Hirano 1998, Sakr 1993, Wada 1992), depending on the series. Most autopsy-detected carcinomas are well-differentiated Gleason score 2 to 4 carcinomas. It is curious that these well-differentiated carcinomas are localized to the peripheral zone, whereas for clinically detected carcinomas, most well-differentiated cancers reside in the transition zone. Intermediate-grade (Gleason score 5 and 6) **i13.3** and high-grade (Gleason score 7 or greater) **i13.4** carcinomas make up a minority of cases. In one large series (n = 814), Gleason score 7 or greater latent carcinoma was found in 1% of men under 60 and in 16% of men over 60 (Sakr 2000). Perineural invasion can be noticed in

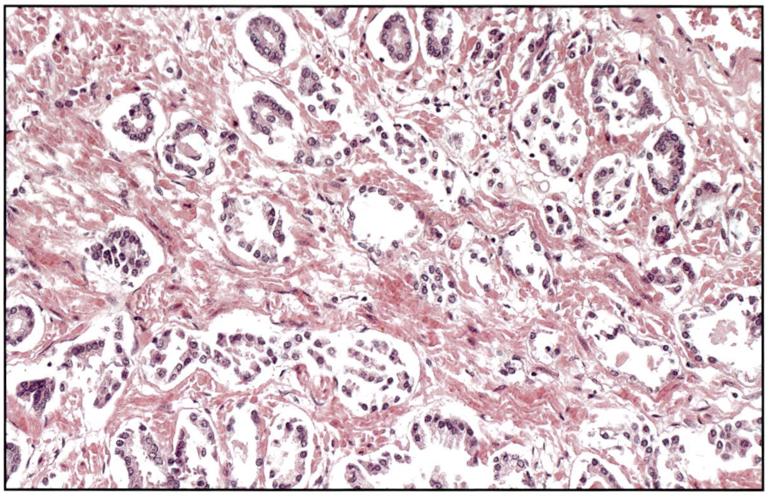

■ **i13.1** *Adenocarcinoma of the prostate detected at autopsy. Note artifactual separation of malignant glands from stroma due to autolysis and poor preservation, which can be a problem in sections from prostate glands at postmortem examination.*

one third to nearly all cases **i13.5** (Andrews 1949, Franks 1954, Moore 1935). Latent cancers that exhibit extraprostatic extension are of higher Gleason grade (Gleason score 5 to 8) and tumor volume ($3.3cm^3$) than organ-confined latent carcinoma (all Gleason score 2 to 4 and mean tumor volume $0.2cm^3$) (Moutzouris 1999). Extension into seminal vesicle wall is even less common **i13.6**, being reported in up to 6% of cases (Franks 1954, Moore 1935, Oota 1961). Metastases to regional lymph nodes and distant sites are absent or rare.

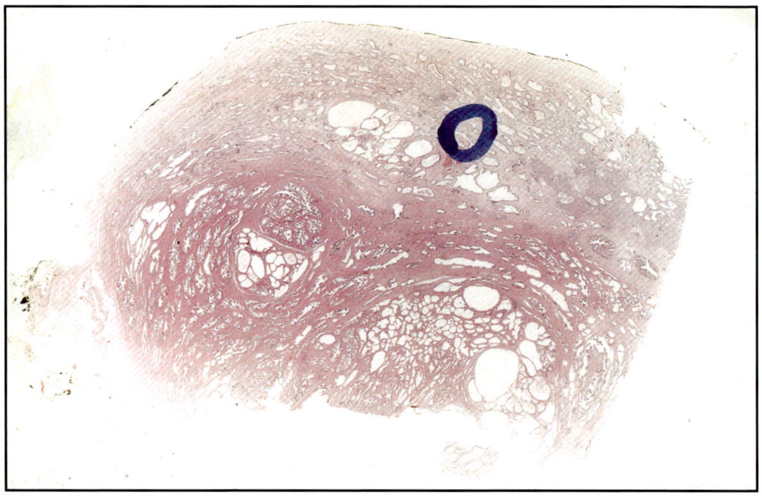

■ **i13.2** *Size of typical latent prostatic adenocarcinoma discovered at autopsy. In this quadrant section of prostate, the circled focus has a diameter of 2mm.*

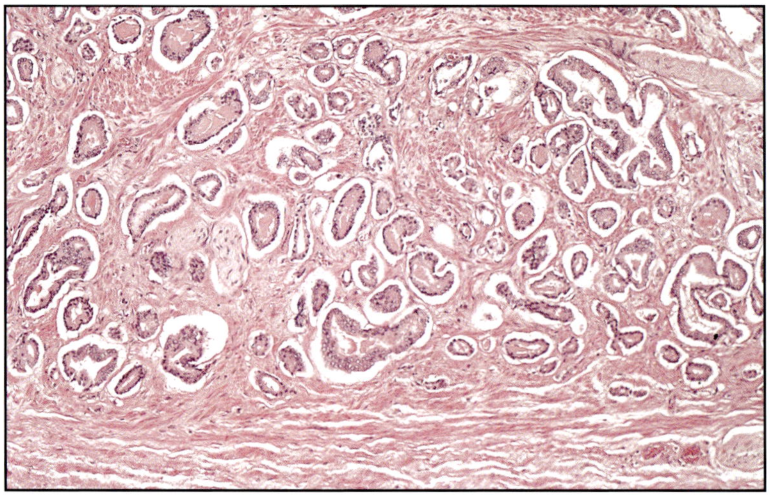

■ **i13.3** *Moderately differentiated adenocarcinoma of Gleason 3+3=score of 6, discovered at autopsy.*

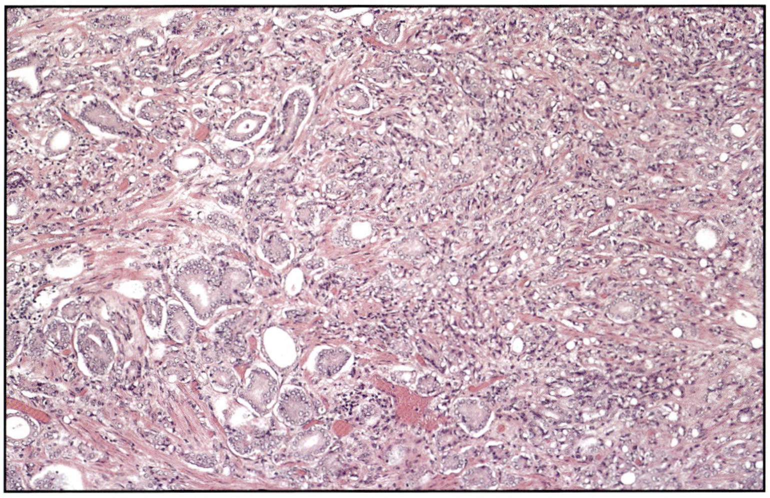

■ **i13.4** *Adenocarcinoma at autopsy, with high-grade component. Gleason grade is 4+3=score of 7.*

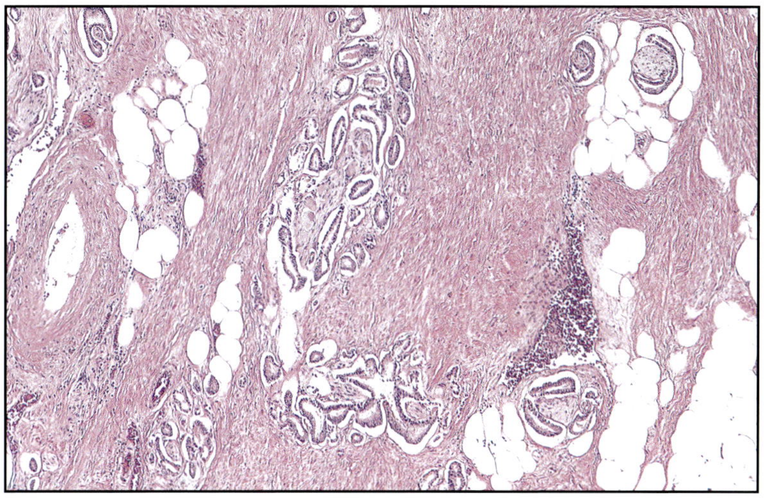

■ **i13.5** *Perineural invasion by a latent prostatic adenocarcinoma, with extraprostatic extension into periprostatic adipose tissue.*

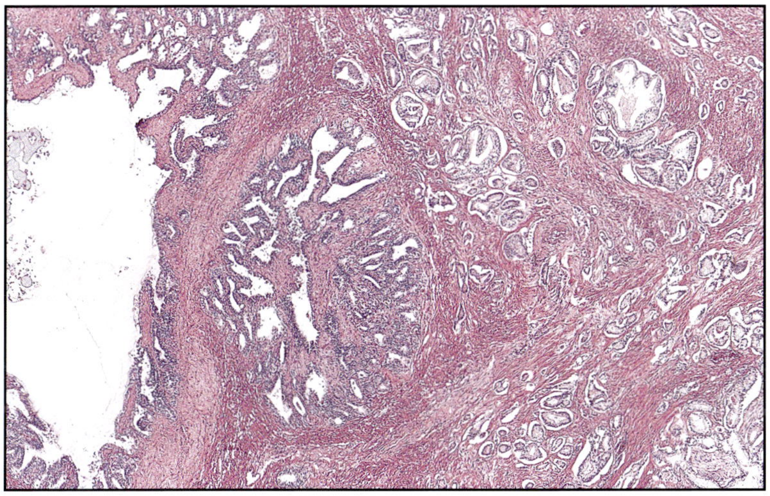

■ **i13.6** *Seminal vesicle wall invasion by a latent prostatic adenocarcinoma. This is an uncommon event.*

■ **t13.7 Risk Factors for Prostatic Carcinoma**

Definite	Probable	Potential
Age	Dietary fat	Cadmium
Family history	Androgens	Low vitamin D
Race		Low vitamin E
		Low selenium
		Herbicides
		Sedentary lifestyle

■ **t13.8 Age Distribution for Clinical Prostate Cancer Detection**

Age (years)	All Prostate Cancer Cases
25-49	0.5%
50-59	6.4%
60-79	31.7%
70-79	42.5%
≥80	18.9%

Ries 1994

The histopathologic features of incidentally detected prostatic carcinoma in radical cystoprostatectomy specimens removed for bladder cancer are similar to autopsy-detected cancers (Abbas 1996A, Baron 1989, Hirano 1998, Kabalin 1989, Mahadevia 1986, Montie 1989, Pritchett 1988, Troncoso 1989, Wiley 1997, Winfield 1987). Notable aspects of these series are that lymph node metastasis was found in a total of 3 patients (Mahadevia 1986, Winfield 1987), and the percentage of intermediate- to high-grade (Gleason score 5 to 7) prostate carcinoma cases was 44% in one series (Kabalin 1989). Still, most were well-differentiated, small (with mean and median volumes of 0.11 cm^3 [Montie 1989] and 0.04 cm^3 [Ohori 1994A], respectively), and organ-confined.

[13.1] Etiology

Ultimately it is the accumulation of genetic damage to prostate DNA that causes adenocarcinoma of the prostate. Alteration of specific chromosomes and genes has been associated with prostatic carcinoma (Isaacs 1998) (see Chapter 21). However, the precise initiating and promoting events that cause and result in the progression of prostate cancer are ill defined. Definite risk factors for the development of prostate cancer include age, family history, and race (Chan 1998B, Reiter 2002, Zlotta 1998) **t13.7**.

Age is strongly related to the detection of both clinical and autopsy prostate cancer. Clinically, carcinoma of the prostate is most often detected in men over 60 years of age (Ries 1994) **t13.8**. In 1985, the mean age at detection was 72 years, with a decrease in age to the current mean age of 68, because of PSA screening (Farkas 1998, Ries 1994). The hazard of detection is nearly 40 times greater for men over 65 than for men under 65 (Pienta 1998). Still, 18% of all prostate cancers detected by screening are found in men 50 to 59 years of age (Richie 1993). Carcinoma of the prostate is distinctly uncommon in men under 50, accounting for 1% of all patients with clinically detected prostate cancer (Aprikian 1994, Benson 1987, Byar 1969, Chow 1986, Cochran 1981, Culkin 1986, Ellner 1965, Heidenberg 1994, Immergut 1966, Jadeja 1994, Ruska 1999, Sandhu 1992, Shimada 1980, Weitzner 1980, Yamamoto 1990) and is exceedingly rare in children and adolescents, with only a few reported cases (Chow 1986, Ellner 1965, Immergut 1966, Sandhu 1992, Shimada 1980).

■ **t13.9 Family History and Risk of Prostate Cancer**

	Risk Ratio[1]	
Age at Diagnosis	**No Additional Relatives**	**Additional Relatives**
40	3	11
50	2	7
60	1.4	5
70	1	4

Cannon 1982, Steinberg 1990
[1]Fold-higher risk for having a first-degree relative (father or brother) with prostate cancer

■ **t13.10 Clinical and Pathologic Features of Hereditary Prostatic Carcinoma**

Accounts for 9% of all prostate cancers and 43% of cases diagnosed before age 55.
Clinically defined: 3 or more affected men in a nuclear family, or 2 relatives diagnosed before age 55 or prostate cancer in 3 successive generations.
Pathologically, no significant differences for localized cancer tumor size, stage and grade compared to sporadic cases, but HPC1-linked cancers tend to be higher grade and stage.
Clinically, there is no difference compared to sporadic prostate cancer in response to surgical treatment or survival.

Carcinoma of the prostate in the first 2 decades of life generally is high grade and high stage, with a correspondingly poor prognosis. For men 20 to 40, it has also been claimed that patients have poorly differentiated and aggressive tumors (Sandhu 1992, Weitzner 1980), but if small, palpable nodules are biopsied (Cochran 1981) or the serum PSA is <10 ng/mL (Ruska 1999), then chances for survival are favorable. For men under 50, there is greater multifocality of small tumors (DeGuia 2001); for these patients stage and histologic grade are the independent predictors of survival (Aprikian 1994). For all men with prostatic carcinoma, there is a suggestion of associated higher grade (Alexander 1989, Borek 1990, Stamey 1999), higher stage (Borek 1990, Gilliland 1999), and worse outcome (Carter 1999, Herold 1998, Partin 1992) with increasing age. However, the data are conflicting on this issue; other studies have not found age to be related to outcome (Bauer 1998, Catalona 1998, Stamey 1999) or found a younger age to be associated with a better response to therapy (surgery) (Smith 2000).

A family history of prostatic carcinoma places a man at higher risk than those without such a history (Cannon 1982, B Carter 1992, 1993, Glover 1998A, Keetch 1995, Page 1997, Schaid 1998, Spitz 1991, Steinberg 1990, Walsh 1997). About 25% of men with prostatic carcinoma have a known positive family history (Walsh 1997). The degree of risk is related to the age of the relatives at diagnosis and the number of relatives affected (Carter 1993) **t13.9**. The greatest risk (with a 11-fold increase) is for the father or brother of a man diagnosed at age 40 with prostate cancer, where an additional first-degree relative has prostate cancer (Carter 1993). Because of this heightened chance, it is recommended that screening for prostate cancer before age 50 be offered to men with a family history of prostate cancer (Walsh 1997). Men with a positive family history for prostatic carcinoma may be divided into two groups: familial and hereditary (Carter 1993). Familial prostate carcinoma is the simple clustering of disease, whereas hereditary prostate carcinoma is a subtype of familial carcinoma with a distribution pattern consistent with a Mendelian inheritance (Carter 1993, Walsh 1997). The clinical definition of hereditary prostate carcinoma is a clustering of 3 or more affected relatives in a nuclear family or 2 relatives with early disease onset (<55 years) or the occurrence of prostatic carcinoma in 3 generations (Carter 1993). Inherited prostate cancer probably is caused by autosomal dominant transmission of rare high-risk alleles leading to early onset (B Carter 1992). Overall, hereditary prostate cancer accounts for 9% of all cases of carcinoma of the prostate but 43% of cases diagnosed before age 55 **t13.10** (B Carter 1992). Recently, several susceptibility loci have been identified. The first discovered susceptibility locus is on chromosome 1q24-25 (HPC1) (Cooney 1997, Dunsmuir 1998, Grönberg 1997A, 1997B, Smith 1996) and is most strongly linked to large families with 5 or more affected men and with early age at diagnosis (Grönberg 1997A, Schaid 1998). This one locus accounts for a minority of familial clusters of prostate cancer. Additional susceptibility loci on chromosomes 1q42.2-43 (Berthon 1998), 1p36 (Gibbs 1999), Xq27-28 (Xu 1998), and others (Chapter 21, **t21.3**) have been reported, underscoring the likelihood that prostate cancer may be inherited by mutation of one of several genes.

The pathologic features of biopsy histologic Gleason grade and radical prostatectomy tumor size, Gleason grade, and pathologic stage do not appear to be substantially different for patients with or without a family history of prostate cancer (sporadic prostate cancer) **i13.7** (Bastacky 1995, Bauer 1998, Bova 1998, Grönberg 1998, Hanus 1999, Keetch 1996, Kupelian 1997B), except for a slightly lower Gleason grade in hereditary prostatic carcinoma (Bastacky 1995, Grönberg 1998, Keetch 1996) and more small multifocal cancers associated with PIN in the sporadic group (Bastacky 1995). No significant differences were discerned in prostate cancer p53, bcl-2, proliferation index, and microvessel density in patients with and without a positive family history (Bauer 1998). In two studies looking specifically at the comparative pathologic features of HPC1-linked and unlinked prostate cancers, this subgroup of hereditary prostate cancers was of higher grade and higher stage (Grönberg 1997A, Goode 2001). Key studies in the future should assess the pathologic features of prostate cancers found in patients with specific alterations in cloned and sequenced hereditary prostate cancer genes.

Patients with hereditary prostatic carcinoma do not differ from men with sporadic disease in their response to radical prostatectomy (Bova 1998) or survival (Grönberg 1998), but outcome data are mixed on analyses of familial prostate cancers (as opposed to the hereditary subset) (Hanus 1999, Kupelian 1997A, 1997B).

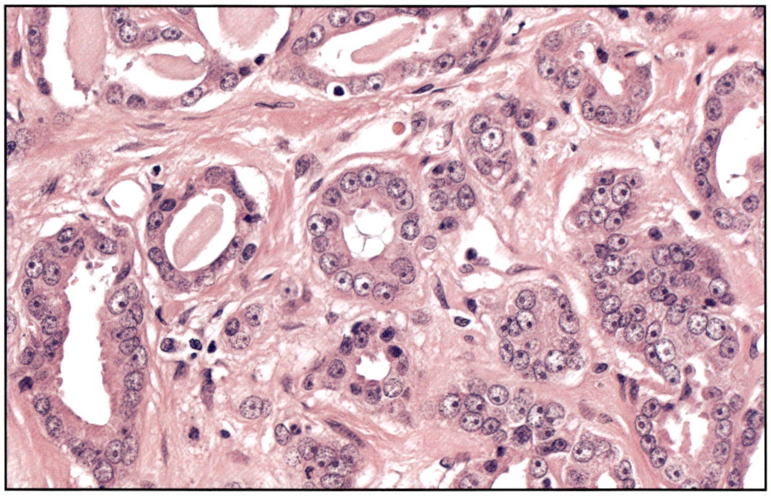

■ **i13.7** *Hereditary prostatic carcinoma: Most are intermediate-grade acinar adenocarcinomas.*

t13.11 Prostatic Carcinoma Incidence by Race in United States

Racial Group	Incidence/100,000
African-American	224.3
White	150.3
Hispanic	104.4
Asian/Pacific Islander	82.2
Native American	46.4

Jemal 2002

Family members of patients with hereditary prostatic carcinoma are at a small but statistically significant higher risk for development of central nervous system tumors but not breast, ovarian, or endometrial carcinomas (Walsh 1997). Conversely, men in families with a positive history of breast cancer are at increased risk of having prostate cancer (Goldgar 1994, Tulinius 1992) and of having fatal prostate cancer (Rodriguez 1998). For BRCA1 and BRCA2 mutant gene (breast and ovarian hereditary gene) carriers, the risk of prostate cancer is 3 to 4 times higher (Ford 1994, Linder 1998). There is no established risk of prostate cancer with other family cancer syndromes (Linder 1998).

Race is a definite risk factor for prostatic cancer incidence and detection. There are the remarkable worldwide differences discussed earlier, but there are also racial differences within countries. In the United States, African Americans have the highest incidence and Native Americans the lowest (Jemal 2002, Merrill 1997) **t13.11**. For African American men <65 years of age the comparative incidence is highest, with 79% more prostate cancer than in white men (Brawley 1998). African American men have a greater chance of a positive biopsy than white men when the serum PSA is elevated (D Smith 1997B, 1998). When the PSA is >4 ng/mL (the standard cutoff), 48% of black men have a positive biopsy, compared with 34% of white men (D Smith 1997B). African American men present with higher-stage disease and have a higher age-adjusted mortality rate (Austin 1993, Kim 1995, Moul 1996, Pienta 1995, Thompson 2001), even after controlling for stage and grade (Austin 1993, Moul 1996), than U.S. whites (Jemal 2002).

Racial differences in the histologic and molecular biologic features of prostatic carcinoma have been reported. Histologically, African American men, in comparison to white American men, more often have high-grade (Gleason score 7 to 10) and multifocal carcinoma, larger tumor size, and more frequent anterior and transition zone cancer localization (DeVere White 1998, Fowler 2000, Freeman 1997, Iselin 1998, Lee 1999, Pettaway 1998, Sakr 1993, 1998, Tiguert 1998). Prostate cancers from black and white American men exhibit a similar pattern and frequency of chromosomal alterations (Cher 1998, Zhau 1999) and do not differ in p53, p16, or bcl-2 expression (Bauer 1995, 1996, Gaddipati 1997). Molecular genetic differences include fewer CAG repeats in the androgen receptor gene in black men, polymorphic variation in a vitamin D binding protein gene, and polymorphic variation in the type 2 5α-reductase gene (Aronson 2000). U.S. Hispanic men have more tumor in sextant biopsies than white men but otherwise do not differ significantly in positive biopsy rate or Gleason grade (Orozco 1997). The basis of racial differences in clinical incidence and histologic features is not known but could relate to a number of factors including genetics, metabolism (in particular, testosterone levels and metabolism), health care accessibility, environment, lifestyle, and diet (Aronson 2000, Montie 1999). Histologic and molecular biologic differences may exist between prostate cancers in the United States and those in China and Japan (Konishi 1997, Shiraishi 1998, Watanabe 1994, Zhau 1997). Prostatic carcinoma detected in Chinese men tends more often to be poorly differentiated, with correspondingly higher levels of tumor microvessel density, serotonin, bombesin, and p53 protein accumulation (Zhau 1997). Ras gene mutations are rare in prostatic carcinoma in the United States but are more common in Japan (Konishi 1997, Shiraishi 1998, Wantanabe 1994).

Probable risk factors for development of prostate cancer include diet and steroid hormones (Chan 1998B, Pienta 1998, Schulman 2001). The strongest dietary link to prostate cancer development is high fat intake (Bairati 1998, Giles 1997, Giovannucci 1993, Kolonel 1988, 1999, Mettlin 1989, Snowdon 1984, West 1991), particularly in the form of red meat. It is not clear which fat components are responsible (Kolonel 1999), although α-linolenic fatty acid has been implicated (Gann 1994, Giovannucci 1993). Dietary fat could increase prostate cancer risk via one or more mechanisms, such as lipid peroxidation leading to DNA-damaging free radicals and alteration of serum sex hormone levels (Chan 1998B, Gann 1994, Pienta 1998). Conversely, dietary consumption of fruits and vegetables, especially tomatoes, appears to lower the risk of prostate cancer (Giovannucci 2002, Mills 1989). Lycopene, a carotenoid antioxidant, is an agent in tomatoes that has been associated with this diminished risk (Gann 1999, Giovannucci 2002). Lycopene levels in serum are also inversely related to aggressive prostate cancer, defined as malignancy of high histologic grade (Gleason score 7) or high stage (Giovannucci 2002). Vitamin E, another antioxidant, in the serum may also protect against prostate cancer (Heinonen 1998). Preliminary work suggests that dietary selenium may also guard against prostatic carcinoma development (Clark 1996, Yoshizawa 1998).

The steroid hormones that are likely to be involved in prostate cancer risk include vitamin D (1,25 $(OH)_2D_3$) and the sex hormones, especially testosterone. Men with high levels of serum vitamin D are at lower risk for prostate cancer, particularly poorly differentiated and higher-stage tumors (Corder 1993, Gann 1996). Interestingly, there is a greater risk of prostate cancer at higher latitudes, which could be related to decreased synthesis of vitamin D because of less ultraviolet light exposure (Hanchette 1992). Testosterone and its derivative, dihydrotestosterone, are important in prostate cancer growth, and prostate cancer is rare in men castrated before puberty. However, serum levels of these androgens have not been consistently associated with prostate cancer risk (Pienta 1998, Vatten 1997). Prostate carcinoma can be detected in men with low total and free testosterone levels. When the vitamin D and androgen receptor genes exhibit specific polymorphisms, there is a higher prostate cancer susceptibility (Hardy 1996, Ingles 1997, Stanford 1997, Taylor 1996). Short CAG trinucleotide microsatellites in exon 1 of the androgen receptor are related to a 2-fold greater risk (Hardy 1996, Ingles 1997, Stanford 1997), and polymorphisms in the vitamin D receptor may be associated with 3- to 5-fold greater risk (Ingles 1997). Polymorphisms in the genes involved in testosterone metabolism, such as cytochrome P459C17α and CYP3A4, may also confer increased prostate cancer risk (Reiter 2002).

Potential risk factors for prostate cancer include elevated plasma insulin-like growth factor I levels (Chan 1998A, Stattin 2000), a sedentary lifestyle (Chan 1998B), and occupational exposure in farming to herbicide spraying (Chan 1998B) and cadmium in welders (Brawley 1996).

Factors that have not been definitively linked to prostate cancer risk include BPH, smoking (Adami 1996, Chan 1998B, Lumey 1997, Rohan 1997), alcohol consumption (Breslow 1998), infection, including human papillomavirus (HPV) infection (Latil 1998), immunosuppression in the setting of organ transplantation (Konety 1998, Penn 1994), vasectomy (Cox 2002, Lesko 1999, Zhu 1996), sexual activity, and socioeconomic status (Brawley 1996). Most studies have not established a relationship between smoking and prostate cancer incidence, but smoking has been positively related to poorly differentiated carcinoma, higher stage, and a worse prognosis (Chan 1998B). The data on the role of HPV infection in prostatic carcinoma causation are controversial, and it is not possible to exclude HPV involvement in a small subset (20%) of cases (Serth 1999). Similarly, the evidence for risk imparted by vasectomy is inconsistent (Chan 1998B), but the risk probably is small to nonexistent (Cox 2002). Prostatic carcinoma arising in immunosuppressed renal transplant patients is uncommon at 2% (Penn 1994). These patients usually had low- to intermediate-grade, clinically localized disease (Konety 1998).

Prevention of prostate cancer could be pursued based on knowledge of these risk factors, and there is much interest in lycopenes, selenium, and vitamin E as potential chemoprevention agents. Green tea, vitamin D, and soy have also been forwarded as potential chemopreventives (Moyad 1999). Several agents, including finasteride, a 5α-reductase inhibitor that blocks the conversion of testosterone to dihydrotestosterone (Thompson 1996), and selenium and vitamin E (Klein 2001), are being tested in clinical trials for chemoprevention of prostate cancer.

[13.2] Clinical Presentation

Clinical Symptoms

Prostatic carcinoma generally does not cause symptoms until late in the course of the disease (Carter 2002, Kim 1996). Local symptoms mimic BPH, with an increase in frequency and difficulty in urination (Young 1909). This is because of growth of the carcinoma into the bladder neck or urethra. Acute urinary retention and hematuria are uncommon in patients with prostate cancer and are also nonspecific (Kim 1996). Hematospermia is rare and is caused by destruction of the ejaculatory ducts (Carter 2002, Kim 1996). Impotence can result from posterolateral extraprostatic extension of peripheral zone carcinoma into the adjacent neurovascular bundles. Rectal invasion, priapism, and uremia (due to renal failure secondary to ureteral obstruction) are rare, late manifestations of highly advanced local disease (Kim 1996).

The first symptoms of prostate cancer can be caused by metastasis. Regional pelvic lymph nodes and bones are the anatomic sites most commonly involved by metastatic spread, but only bone involvement consistently produces significant symptoms (Kim 1996). Thus, patients can present with pain in the lower back, chest and upper back, hip, leg, and shoulder caused by carcinoma in the spine, ribs, pelvis, femur, and shoulder bones, respectively. Infrequently, pathologic fractures due to metastatic spread to bones occur (Kim 1996). Neurologic symptoms, related to epidural cord compression, intracranial metastasis, cranial nerve palsy, and temporal bone involvement, are a common complaint in patients with metastatic disease but are not usually presenting symptoms. Rarely, spread to other sites can cause symptoms, and this usually occurs in the setting of known, widely disseminated disease. For example, lung involvement can cause cough, dyspnea, and hemoptysis, and spread into the liver can cause jaundice (Kim 1996). Metastasis to the adrenal, gastrointestinal tract, testis, skin, and head and neck have also been reported to generate symptoms (Kim 1996). Paraneoplastic syndromes such as Cushing's syndrome, syndrome of antidiuretic hormone secretion, limbic encephalitis, cerebellar degeneration, Eaton-Lambert syndrome, and hypercalcemia and hypocalcemia have been reported in a few patients (Kim 1996, Stern 1999). Neuroendocrine or small cell prostatic carcinoma is the histologic type most often associated with Cushing's syndrome and neurologic disorders in patients with prostate cancer, whereas the other syndromes have not been related to a specific histologic type of cancer. Hematologic abnormalities associated with metastatic prostatic carcinoma include anemia and disseminated intravascular coagulopathy (Kim 1996). These paraneoplastic syndromes and hematologic manifestations are uncommon.

Currently, prostate cancer in most cases in the United States is clinically detected by DRE and serum PSA abnormalities, not by clinical symptoms. This was not always the case. In the first half of the 20th century up to 95% of men with prostatic carcinoma presented with metastatic disease (Gleaves 1935, cited in Hudson 1954). Indeed, in 1947 Nobel Laureate Huggins, in a review on prostate cancer (Huggins 1947), wrote that the typical presentation in a case of prostate cancer was a man over 50 years of age who complained of a several-month history of dysfunctional voiding, weight loss, and lower back pain, the latter being indicative of bony metastasis.

Digital Rectal Examination

Digital palpation of the prostate via the rectum has long been an important clinical maneuver in detecting prostatic carcinoma (Muir 1934, Young 1926). Before the advent of serum PSA testing in 1980s, DRE was the primary method of detecting prostate cancer. Although PSA has a higher positive predictive value for prostate cancer detection at 31% for serum PSA and 21% for DRE (Catalona 1994B), current recommendations for early detection of prostate cancer are for combined use of DRE and PSA (ACS 2001, AUA 1999). This is so because PSA detects a number of cancers that are missed by DRE, and DRE detects some cancers that are diagnosed without serum PSA elevation (above 4 ng/mL). In one large screening series of 6630 men, an elevated serum PSA resulted in diagnosis of 82% of cancers, whereas DRE detected only 55% (Catalona 1994B). Moreover, another problem with the DRE is that it is subjective, with high interobserver variability (Philips 1991, Smith 1995).

A DRE suspicious for malignancy is not particularly sensitive, nor is it specific, for a diagnosis of carcinoma. The DRE is suspicious for malignancy in about 15% of all screened men. When these men underwent needle biopsy, a histopathologic diagnosis of malignancy was rendered in 21% of the biopsied men **t13.12**. Therefore, a pure DRE screening detects prostate cancer in about 3% of men over 50 (Catalona 1994B). In other series, higher positive predictive values of 27%

t13.12 Digital Rectal Examination (DRE) vs Serum Prostate Specific Antigen in Detection of Prostatic Carcinoma

Total number of men over 50 screened	6,630
Percentage with suspicious DRE	15%
Percentage with suspicious DRE and positive biopsy	3.2%
Percentage with elevated serum PSA	15%
Percentage with elevated PSA and positive biopsy	4.6%
Percentage with suspicious DRE and/or elevated PSA and positive biopsy	5.8%

Catalona 1994

t13.13 Positive Predictive Value of Suspicious DRE is Related to Serum PSA Level

Serum PSA Level (ng/mL)	Suspicious DRE Positive Predictive Value[1,2]
0-1	5%
1.1-2.5	14%
2.6-4.0	30%
4-9.9	41%
10 and above	69%

[1]Positive predictive value = The probability that cancer is present with an abnormal DRE
[2]Data from Catalona 1994, Schröder 1998

to 53% were obtained for an abnormal DRE (Brawer 1993, Cooner 1990, Ellis 1994A, Grayhack 1981, Jewett 1956, Schröeder 1998, Sika 1963, Smith 1995, Stone 1994). The 50% figure was reported for indurated, palpable nodules (Jewett 1956). The positive predictive value of the DRE is directly related to the serum PSA level (Carvalhal 1999, Catalona 1994B, Schröeder 1998) **t13.13**, which probably reflects the predilection of the DRE to detect larger-volume carcinomas that are associated with higher PSA levels.

The pathologic basis for an abnormal DRE in the absence of cancer usually is BPH or inflammation (Jewett 1956). Calculi, infarction, normal prostate, and postsurgical or postbiopsy changes can also be reasons for an abnormal DRE (Cooner 1990, Jewett 1956, Kim 1996).

Prostatic carcinomas detected by DRE usually are advanced, with extraprostatic extension (Epstein 1994, Thompson 1987). Clinically localized cancer is found in about 65% of patients with an abnormal DRE, but histopathologic study of radical prostatectomy specimens from these men reveals extraprostatic extension in up to 66% (Epstein 1994). That is, by the time a prostate cancer is palpable, it is more likely than not to have already spread beyond the confines of prostate gland. Histopathologic analysis of DRE-detected, palpable prostate cancers indicates that they are larger and of higher pathologic stage than PSA-detected prostatic carcinoma. In needle biopsy, DRE-detected prostatic carcinomas occupy twice as much of the needle core tissue at a mean of 39%, compared with PSA-detected carcinoma at 21% (Humphrey 1998). In radical prostatectomy tissue, DRE-detected carcinomas are, on average, twice the size of PSA-detected carcinomas and are more likely to exhibit extraprostatic extension, seminal vesicle invasion, and positive surgical margins (Epstein 1994) **t13.14**. In one series, only 34% of DRE-detected cancers were pathologically confined to the prostate, the mean Gleason score was a moderately differentiated 6, and the mean tumor size was 4cm^3 (Epstein 1994). The lowest size limit for DRE detection of prostatic carcinoma has been reported to be 0.3cm^3 to 1.3cm^3 (Stamey 1988), but DRE typically underestimates tumor size (Spigelman 1986), and many larger PSA-detected (T1c) prostate cancers are not palpable. Possible explanations for failure of DRE to detect T1c carcinomas include smaller size of some of the PSA-detected carcinomas because 30% are <0.5cm^3 (Epstein 1994, Humphrey 1996), anterior or central location, masking of palpability by BPH, and tumor-associated desmoplasia (Epstein 1994).

t13.14 Histopathologic Features of DRE-Detected vs PSA-Detected Carcinomas in Radical Prostatectomy Specimens

Pathologic Feature	PSA-Detected[1]	DRE-Detected[2]
Extraprostatic extension	43%	66%
Positive margins	34%	43%
Seminal vesicle invasion	6%	14%
Lymph node invasion	2%	7%
Tumor volume, mean	1.9 cc	4 cc
Gleason grade, mean	6	6

[1]Clinical stage Tlc. Pooled data, except tumor volume and grade from Humphrey 1998 review. Tumor volume and grade from Epstein 1994, Humphrey 1996.
[2]Clinical stage T2. Data from Epstein 1994.

In addition to detection of prostatic carcinoma, DRE is also used for clinical staging (Chapter 16). Therefore, DRE is used to determine whether prostatic carcinoma is clinically confined to the prostate (T2) or not (T3 to T4). However, DRE is not accurate in defining true stage, as determined by histologic examination of radical prostatectomy tissues. That is, clinical stage as ascertained by DRE often is incorrect when compared with pathologic stage. Both understaging and overstaging occur. When the DRE indicates clinically organ-confined disease, 48% of patients, on average, have microscopical evidence of spread beyond the prostatic capsule in radical prostatectomy slides (O'Dowd 1997). The 1997 TNM clinical substages of T2a (tumor confined to one lobe) and T2b (tumor involves both lobes) (Fleming 1997) also do not correlate well with pathologic substage. Clinical T2a disease is, in the majority (73%) of cases, pathologic T2b disease or greater (Öbek 1999). Clinical T2b tumors do tend to have more adverse pathologic findings (extraprostatic extension, positive margins, seminal vesicle invasion, lymph node metastasis, higher grade) in radical prostatectomy specimens than clinical T2a tumors (Ramos 1999). DRE is somewhat more accurate in the diagnosis of extraprostatic carcinoma, but 7% to 30% of cases deemed by DRE to represent tumor outside the gland (clinical stage T3) are in fact organ confined (pathologic stage T2) (O'Dowd 1997, Ohori 1994B, Partin 1993, Schröeder 1975).

Despite these flaws, DRE is still a valuable component of clinical staging models that use several pretreatment factors (usually DRE, serum PSA, and biopsy Gleason score) to predict pathologic stage (Carter 2002, Humphrey 1998, Kleer 1993, Partin 1993, 1997, Perrotti 1999) and outcome (D'Amico 2000, Kattan 1998, 2001).

It has not been established that screening for prostatic carcinoma with DRE will reduce mortality. Indeed, in one study many men who died of prostate cancer had a normal DRE at the time of histologic diagnosis (Thompson 1991). Recent radical prostatectomy series have demonstrated that 28% to 73% of patients experience biochemical failure (an elevated serum PSA level) after surgery for DRE-detected prostate cancer (Amling 1998, Ramos 1999, Stamey 1998B). Large, randomized clinical trials that are in progress (Prorok 2000) may provide information on whether DRE screening for prostate cancer reduces mortality due to prostate cancer.

In summary, DRE is a clinically important part of the physical examination that is useful in prostatic carcinoma detection and staging, but DRE suffers from only fair reproducibility, it misses a substantial proportion of cancers, and it detects cancers that are at a more advanced pathologic stage, when the chance for cure is diminished (Carter 2002).

Prostate-Specific Antigen

Serum PSA, as the most important tumor marker for adenocarcinoma of the prostate, has a vital role in detection, staging, and posttherapy monitoring of prostate cancer (Humphrey 1998, Polascik 1999). It has largely supplanted prostatic acid phosphatase as a serum prostatic tumor marker (Heller 1987, Lowe 1993, Romas 1993). Serum prostatic acid phosphatase level is related to extraprostatic spread of cancer, but it is insensitive and rarely provides additional staging in formation beyond that provided by serum PSA, DRE, and needle biopsy Gleason score (Burnett 1992, Carter 2002). The PSA protein was initially identified and characterized from 1966 to 1978 (Armbruster 1993), but it was not until the late 1980s that measurement of PSA protein levels in serum was widely used in clinical medicine.

PSA protein is a 33-kDa glycoprotein product of the 6-kb PSA gene that is located on chromosome 19 (Lundwall 1987, Riegman 1989). It is an enzyme that belongs to the kallikrein family of serum proteases and is also (less commonly) known as human kallikrein 3 (McCormack 1995). Its biological function is to liquefy seminal coagulum by breakdown of semenogelin, with resultant enhancement of sperm motility (Armbruster 1993). PSA is normally secreted by prostatic luminal cells into seminal fluid, where concentrations, at around 1 to 5 mg/mL, are up to 1 million times greater than serum levels, where normal is usually deemed 4 ng/mL or less. PSA can also be found in the urine (Breul 1994, Irani 1997, Iwakiri 1993, Pannek 1997, Takayama 1994), but this assay is not of established diagnostic value (Pannek 1997).

PSA expression is not, as the name *PSA* indicates, specific for the prostate gland **t13.15**. PSA expression is characteristic of benign and malignant prostatic luminal epithelial cells, but it has also been detected in male and female periurethral glands (Elgamal 1994, Frazier 1992, Kamoshida 1990, Pollen 1984, Tepper 1984) **i13.8**, urachal remnants (Golz 1989), cystitis cystica and glandularis (Nowels 1988), Cowper's glands (Elgamal 1994), male anal glands (Kamoshida 1990), endometrium (Clements 1994), normal salivary gland (Elgamal 1996, Tazawa 1999, Van Krieken 1993), normal breast tissue (Howarth 1997), and normal pancreatic tissue (Elgamal 1996). Nonprostatic tumors with detectable PSA include periurethral gland carcinomas (reviewed in Epstein 1993), rare bladder adenocarcinomas (Epstein 1993), salivary gland neoplasms (Elgamal 1996, Tazawa 1999, Van Krieken 1993), breast carcinoma (Howarth 1997, Monne 1994, Yu 1994), adrenal neoplasms, renal cell carcinomas (Levesque 1995), colon carcinoma (Levesque 1995), liver carcinoma (Levesque 1995), lung tumors (Zarghami 1997), ovarian carcinoma (Yu 1995), and neuroblastoma (Mannello 1999). Many nonprostatic carcinomas appear to express low levels of PSA such that the threshold for immunohistochemical detection of PSA protein in tissue and detection of PSA protein in serum may not be reached. PSA has also been detected in nipple fluid, milk, and amniotic fluid (Diamandis 1997, Melegos 1996). This lack of absolute cellular and tissue specificity does not detract from the practical diagnostic utility of immunohistochemical stains for PSA

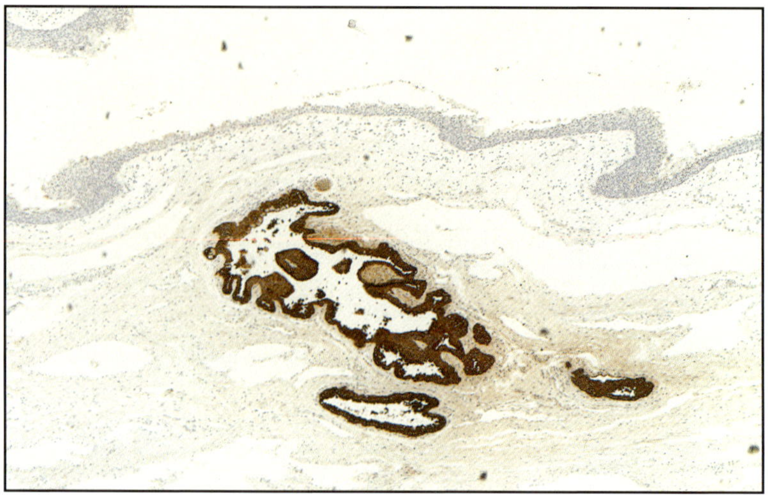

■ **i13.8** *Immunohistochemical detection of prostate-specific antigen in extraprostatic periurethral glands.*

■ **t13.15 Extraprostatic PSA Expression**

Tissue/cell Type	Detection Method	Comment	Reference
Benign:			
Periurethral glands	IHC	Female & male glands stain	Frazier 1992, Kamoshida 1990, Pollen 1984, Tepper 1984, Elgamal 1994
Urachal remnants	IHC		Golz 1989
Cystitis cystica and glandularis	IHC	PAP also present	Nowels 1988
Cowper's glands	IHC		Elgamal 1994
Male anal glands	IHC	PAP also present	Kamoshida 1996
Normal salivary gland ducts	IHC		Elgamal 1996, Tazawa 1999
Normal pancreatic ducts	IHC		Elgamal 1996
Normal endometrium	RT-PCR		Clements 1994
Benign breast tissue	IA,IHC	Normal and hyperplasia positive	Howarth 1997
Malignant:			
Ovarian carcinoma	IA, RT-PCR, IHC	Two cases	Levesque 1995, Yu 1995
Neuroblastoma	RT-PCR, Western blot	Cell lines	Mannello 1999
Salivary gland neoplasms	IHC, IA	Several tumor types positive[1]	Van Krieken 1993, Elgamal 1996, Levesque 1995, Tazawa 1999
Colon carcinoma	IA	Low levels	Levesque 1995
Liver carcinoma	IA	Low levels	Levesque 1995
Periurethral gland carcinoma	IHC	Two cases positive	Epstein 1993
Bladder adenocarcinoma	IHC	Rare cases positive	Epstein 1993
Breast carcinoma	IA,RT-PCR, IHC	May indicate favorable prognosis	Howarth 1997, Miller 2001, Monne 1994, Yu 1994
Adrenal neoplasms	IA	Low levels	Levesque 1995
Renal cell carcinoma	IA	Low levels	Levesque 1995
Lung carcinomas	RT-PCR, IA		Zarghami 1997

IHC = immunohistochemistry; IA = immunoassay of extracts; RT-PCR = reverse transcriptase-polymerase chain reaction; PAP = prostatic acid phosphatase
[1]Including 41% of salivary gland adenocarcinomas (Tazawa 1999)

■ **t13.16 Causes of Elevated Serum PSA**

BPH
Prostatic inflammation
Prostatic carcinoma
Prostatic infarct
Needle biopsy and transurethral resection of prostate

in diagnostic pathology (Chapter 14) and serum PSA measurements in clinical urology.

Serum PSA elevations can be caused by benign prostatic disease and urologic manipulations **t13.16** (Polascik 1999). The most common cause of an elevated PSA is not prostate cancer but BPH. BPH probably accounts for 60% to 70% of cases of an elevated serum PSA. Conversely, 21% to 86% of patients with BPH have an elevated serum PSA (Armbruster 1993, Oesterling 1991, Stamey 1987). Acute urinary retention superimposed on BPH can cause an acute increase in PSA (Tchetgen 1997). Additional benign entities that can cause an elevated serum PSA include prostatic inflammation (Bahnson 1991, Hasui 1994, Nadler 1995, Neal 1992) and infarction (Brawn 1994). We found that ultrasound-determined gland volume (indicative of BPH) and inflammation in needle biopsy were significant factors related to an elevated serum PSA (Nadler 1995). Both acute and chronic inflammation in needle biopsies with benign prostatic tissue were linked to PSA elevation, but inflammation was also present in the needle biopsy cores from some patients without PSA increase, so the presence of inflammation in prostatic needle biopsy does not necessarily account for the abnormal PSA and does not exclude the possibility of unsampled prostatic carcinoma. PIN is not considered a factor in serum PSA elevation (Alexander 1996, Ronnett 1993). Most urologic manipulations such as cystoscopy, urethral catheterization, transrectal ultrasound (TRUS), and DRE do not usually cause a PSA rise (Deliveliotis 1994, Klein 1997, Oesterling 1993, Polascik 1999, Yuan 1992). A small percentage (6% to 15%) of men have a PSA increase after DRE, prostatic massage, and TRUS (Yuan 1992). Needle biopsy and TURP definitely elevate the serum PSA (Deliveliotis 1994, Klein 1997, Oesterling 1993, Yuan 1992).

Serum PSA is clearly the best predictor of a histologic diagnosis of adenocarcinoma in needle biopsy (Catalona 1994B, Klein 1997, Polascik 1999). About 15% of men over 50 have an elevated serum PSA, and 4.6% have a positive biopsy (Catalona 1994B). This detection rate for PSA alone is higher than for DRE alone **t13.12**. A combination of DRE and PSA yields the highest detection rate **t13.12**.

The positive predictive value of a PSA level >4 ng/mL for a histologic diagnosis of carcinoma in needle biopsy is 31% to 51%, with most reports indicating that 1 in 3 men with an elevated serum PSA have a positive biopsy (Catalona 1994B, Humphrey 1998, Polascik 1999). The positive predictive value of a PSA >4.0 ng/mL is increased to 42% to 72% when the DRE is suspicious for malignancy **t13.13** (Catalona 1994B, Polascik 1999). The positive predictive value is also substantially higher for a PSA >10 **t13.17**. Although 4.0 ng/mL is a clinically widely used cutoff, risk of detection exists below 4.0 ng/mL, particularly at 2.0 to 4 ng/mL (Bassler 1999, Catalona 1997, Gann 1995) **t13.13, t13.17**.

A caveat about a negative sextant biopsy in the face of an elevated serum PSA is that this does not provide assurance that the patient does not have carcinoma. The false negative rate of a sextant biopsy is 23% (Rabbani 1998), and in serial screening after a benign diagnosis on the initial set of biopsies, the detection rate

■ **t13.17 Positive Predictive Value of Serum PSA for Histologic Diagnosis of Carcinoma Based on PSA Level**

Serum PSA Level (ng/mL)	Percentage of Patients With Carcinoma
0-2.0	6%
2.0-4.0	25%
4.1-9.9	21%
10.0 and over	42%

[1]In patients with a negative DRE
Data from Catalona 1994, Bassler 1999

■ **t13.18 Types of Serum PSA Protein Measurements**

Type	Definition
Total PSA	Bound and unbound PSA
PSA density	Total serum PSA ÷ prostate volume
PSA velocity	Rate of change of PSA over time (1.5yr-2yr)
Age-specific PSA reference ranges	Increasing cut-off level with age
% Free PSA	Percentage unbound/total PSA
Complexed PSA	Measurement of PSA-ACT complex

ACT = alpha$_1$-antichymotrypsin

was 19% on the second set, 8% on the third, and 7% on the fourth set or later (Keetch 1994).

Variations of serum PSA protein assays have been developed to attempt to increase the positive predictive value of total serum PSA (and decrease the large number of sextant biopsies with benign prostate tissue). These permutations include PSA density, PSA velocity, age-specific PSA reference ranges, free PSA, and complexed PSA **t13.18** (Polascik 1999). PSA in the bloodstream circulation exists in both free (unbound or uncomplexed) and complexed forms. Most PSA (typically 70% to 85%) exists in serum as a protein-protein complex with α_1-antichymotrypsin, with a lesser proportion (of about 5%) bound to α_2-macroglobulin (Sokoll 1998). Total serum PSA immunoassays measure free PSA and PSA bound to α1-antichymotrypsin. PSA density attempts to correct for the contribution of BPH to serum by dividing the total serum PSA level by the volume of the prostate gland, as determined by ultrasound (Beduschi 1997, Polascik 1999). Problems with PSA density that have limited its use include difficulty in obtaining reliable prostate volume measurements, variable amount of epithelium in BPH (which produces the PSA), and failure to detect a substantial percentage of prostate cancers (Catalona 1994C, Polascik 1999). Transition zone PSA density is a modification of whole gland PSA density that suffers from similar drawbacks. PSA velocity or slope is the rate of change of total PSA levels over time (Carter 1997, Polascik 1999). PSA velocity is higher in men with prostate cancer than in men with BPH. Using 3 total PSA measurements over a 2-year period, an increase of 0.75 ng/mL/year or greater is highly suggestive of carcinoma (H Carter 1992B, Smith 1994). The principal disadvantage to PSA velocity in prostate cancer detection is the amount of time needed to generate the velocity figure (Catalona 1994A). A third type of PSA measurement is age-adjusted (specific) reference ranges (Polascik 1999, Richardson 1997). In this approach, younger patients would have a lower cutoff (2.5 ng/mL for men 40 to 49 and 3.5 ng/mL for men 50 to 59) to maximize sensitivity, and older patients would have higher cutoffs (4.5 ng/mL for men 60 to 69 and 6.5 ng/mL for men 70 to 79) to maximize specificity. The main concern in using the higher cutoffs for older men is the failure to detect a substantial number of clinically significant cancers (Bassler 1998).

The estimate of the probability of prostate cancer can be refined by use of percentage of unbound/total PSA or percentage free PSA (Abrahamsson 1997, Catalona 1995, 1997, Polascik 1999), especially in the intermediate elevation range of 4 to 10 ng/mL (Catalona 1995, Polascik 1999). Percentage free PSA values above 18% tend to be associated with BPH, whereas low percentage free PSA is seen more often in men with carcinoma (Catalona 2000, Polascik 1999). Direct measurement of complexed PSA has also been accomplished, but its utility is uncertain and still under investigation (Brawer 1998A, 2002, Djavan 2002, Jung 1999, Rittenhouse 1999).

Total serum PSA has been used to screen for prostate cancer (Arcangeli 1997, Auvinen 1996, Bangma 1997, Catalona 1996, Egawa 1995, Määtänen 2001, Reissigl 1997). Detection rates in screened populations are about 2% to 4.6% (Arcangeli 1997, Catalona 1994B, 1996, Määtänen 2001). PSA outperformed DRE and TRUS in cancer detection (Catalona 1996); again, for early detection of prostate cancer, PSA should be used in conjunction with DRE **t13.12**. Prostate cancer screening is controversial (Catalona 1996), with some professional organizations recommending that PSA screening be offered to men over 50 (ACS 2001, AUA 1999), but not all medical professional societies support this view, and prostate cancer screening has not been widely implemented outside the United States. For men at high risk (African American men and men with a positive family history), it has been suggested that screening begin at a younger age (45 years) (ACS 2001). Suggestive evidence of benefit of early detection has been published (Bartsch 2001), but thus far it has not been proven that PSA screening will reduce cancer-specific mortality. Several larger, prospective randomized trials are under way to address this question (Auvinen 1996, Prorok 2000).

Serum PSA testing has had a profound impact on the clinical and pathologic attributes of detected prostate cancers. The use of serum PSA has even resulted in creation of a new clinical stage category, stage T1c, which is prostatic carcinoma that is nonpalpable and identified by an increased serum PSA level. As indicated earlier, there has been a vast increase in the number of prostate cancers diagnosed between 1987 and 1992 in the United States, with a subsequent decline **f13.2**. This pattern of incidence increase and subsequent decline has been described as one of the characteristics of a successful screening test (Gann 1997). PSA-detected cancers now constitute a significant percentage and often the majority of prostate cancers that are clinically localized and treated by radical prostatectomy (Amling 1998, Mettlin 1996, Stamey 1998A). PSA use has resulted in a trend toward a younger age at diagnosis and a stage migration toward clinically localized malignancy (Farkas 1998, Mettlin 1996, 1997, Rietbergen 1999). Whereas up to one quarter of nonscreened men have presented with metastatic prostatic carcinoma (Rietbergen 1999), 98% of men undergoing PSA-based screening had cancer clinically confined to the prostate (Catalona 1996, D Smith 1997A). There has also been a pathologic stage migration with PSA screening **t13.14**. By histopathologic study of radical prostatectomy specimens, it has been shown that most digitally detected prostatic carcinomas are not organ confined, whereas most PSA-detected carcinomas are confined to the prostate gland (Catalona 1993, Humphrey 1998).

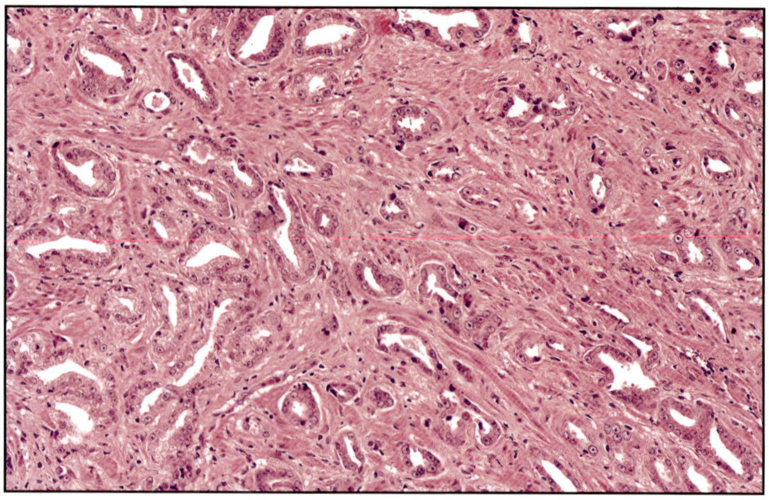

■ i13.9 *Most prostatic carcinomas identified via PSA-screening are intermediate grade Gleason score 6 acinar adenocarcinomas.*

Histopathologically, most PSA-detected carcinomas are of intermediate grade **i13.9** and are organ confined (Humphrey 1998) **t13.14, t13.19**. The Gleason score of PSA-detected carcinomas usually is 5 or 6, but a substantial minority (up to 20%) have a high-grade Gleason pattern 4 component, with a Gleason score of 7. Well-differentiated carcinomas of Gleason score 2 to 4 and high-grade Gleason score 8 to 10 carcinomas are distinctly unusual. Thus, there has been a "grade compression" toward these intermediate-grade carcinomas with PSA testing. Although most PSA-detected carcinomas are organ confined, a substantial minority (30% to 49%) exhibit extraprostatic (extracapsular) extension in the radical prostatectomy specimen and, similarly, a significant minority of patients (10% to 41%) have positive margins. The average size of PSA-detected carcinomas is about 2 cm^3 (Epstein 1994, Humphrey 1996, Stamey 1998B), with 10% of the prostate gland involved by carcinoma (Humphrey 1996). However, the variability in size is substantial, with a range of 0.1% to 36% of gland involvement and with detection of many smaller cancers of <0.5 cm^3 in volume or occupying <5% of the gland.

Most prostatic carcinomas detected by an elevated serum PSA have pathologic characteristics associated with clinically significant disease (Douglas 1997, Elgamal 1997, Humphrey 1996, 1998). These definitions of potential clinical significance of prostatic carcinoma have used tumor size (volume), pathologic stage, and Gleason grade, as determined in radical prostatectomy tissues **t13.20**. "Insignificant" or "clinically unimportant" prostate cancers have been rather arbitrarily defined as organ-confined carcinomas that are <0.2 (Epstein 1994) to 0.5 cm^3 (Ohori 1994A) and that do not have any high-grade elements (no Gleason grade pattern 4 or 5). Using such definitions, the estimates of clinically insignificant prostate cancer detected by PSA elevation have ranged from 5% to 27% (Humphrey 1998). There are caveats about

■ t13.19 Pathologic Characteristics of PSA-Detected (Clinical Stage Tlc) Carcinomas

Most intermediate Gleason score 5 and 6
Average size: 10% of gland involved (but range 0.1 - 36%)
Most organ-confined (but 30-49% exhibit EPE*)
Most margin negative (but 10-41% margin-positive)
Spread to seminal vesicles and lymph nodes uncommon (a few percent)

*EPE = extraprostatic extension of carcinoma

■ **t13.20 Pathologic Features of Potentially Harmless[1] Prostate Cancer[2]**

Tumor volume less than 0.2cc-0.5cc
Organ-confined
No Gleason grade pattern 4 or 5

[1]Also called clinically insignificant or clinically unimportant
[2]As determined in radical prostatectomy specimens

disease classification using these intermediate endpoints of pathologic grade, stage, and tumor size. First, although these morphologic findings are associated with likelihood of outcome, they do not definitively predict outcome for the individual patient. Furthermore, by removal of the prostate gland, the natural history of the disease has obviously been interrupted, such that it is not possible to know with certainty what pathologic features of carcinoma in the whole gland are associated with truly insignificant carcinoma that would not have harmed the patient during his lifetime.

Models have been developed to attempt to predict, before treatment, which PSA-detected prostatic carcinomas have pathologic features of insignificant cancer in the whole gland (Epstein 1998, Humphrey 1998). Most of these incorporate total serum PSA, PSA density or percentage free PSA, Gleason grade on needle biopsy, and amount of tumor in needle biopsy. The most accurate of these models in predicting potentially harmless cancer uses a percentage free PSA >15%, Gleason score <7, and <3 cores involved, with no core having >50% tumor involvement (Epstein 1998). Multi-institutional validation with large numbers of patients will be necessary before this model can be used in routine clinical practice.

Clinical follow-up of patients with PSA-detected (stage T1c) prostatic carcinomas treated with radical prostatectomy has shown that the progression-free survival at 5 years is 70% to 85% (Amling 1998, Ramos 1999, Stamey 1998B). That is, 15% to 30% of patients have a detectable serum PSA after surgery. This rate of failure is lower than for digitally detected carcinomas (at 70%) (Amling 1998). Within the T2 category, patients with T1c carcinomas fail at the same rate as T2a patients but at a lower rate than T2b patients (Ramos 1999, Stamey 1998B). It remains to be determined whether these differences will translate into improved long-term cancer-specific survival due to PSA screening.

Serum PSA is an important component in staging of patients with biopsy-proven prostatic carcinoma. It was initially hoped that total serum PSA level would be sufficiently accurate that clinical staging could be performed using it alone. However, there is substantial overlap of total serum PSA levels between clinical stages, such that PSA level alone does not provide accurate staging information for the individual patient (Hudson 1989, Polascik 1999). Similarly, although there is a trend for increasing total serum PSA with radical prostatectomy–determined pathologic stage **t13.21**, overlap in levels for men with organ-confined and extraprostatic cancer limits its sole use in pretreatment staging.

The pathologic basis for the variable correlation of total serum PSA with stage is the confounding contribution of BPH and histologic grade of carcinoma. Total serum PSA is clearly related to pathologic features of histologic grade, pathologic stage, and tumor volume. The relationship with tumor volume is direct, with increasing PSA with increasing tumor size in the prostate gland, but the correlation is only fair to good (Humphrey 1998, Vollmer 2003). Gleason grade is a confounding factor in the direct linkage of PSA with tumor size and stage because with increasing grade of carcinoma, that is, decreasing differentiation, there is decreased production of PSA per individual carcinoma cell. Thus, although there is a positive correlation between serum PSA and grade, upon correction for tumor volume, there is an inverse relationship between PSA and grade (Aihara 1994, Partin 1990).

Total serum PSA often is used in combination with needle biopsy Gleason grade and DRE-determined local clinical stage to predict pathologic stage. Nomograms based on these 3 parameters have been developed, and these tables provide probabilities for organ-confined disease, seminal vesicle spread, and lymph node metastasis (Partin 1993, 1997, 2001). These probability estimates are not perfect (Kattan 1997, Vollmer 1998B, Penson 2002) but can be helpful in discussions with patients of risk versus benefit considerations for treatment options (Polascik 1998). Other types of PSA measurements such as PSA density, percentage free PSA (Arcangeli 1998, Catalona 2000, Horniger 1999, Pannek 1998, Southwick 1999), and reverse transcriptase–polymerase chain reaction (RT-PCR) for PSA mRNA may be potentially useful in staging (Polascik 1998, 1999), but mixed results have been obtained with these approaches, and they currently remain experimental.

Serum PSA has an extremely important role in monitoring patient response to treatment (Polascik 1999, Pound 1997, Schellhammer 1997, D Smith 1997C). After radical prostatectomy, successful surgical eradication of the cancer should result in an undetectable serum PSA level of <0.2 ng/mL (Pound 1997). (Other cutoffs for persistent carcinoma have been used and range from 0.3 ng/mL [Catalona 1998] to 0.5 ng/mL [Humphrey 1993] and include an extremely low threshold of 0.07 ng/mL [Stamey 1999], with this latter figure generated by an ultrasensitive assay.) Failure of postoperative serum PSA to achieve this level or a rise of postoperative serial PSAs above this level is considered indicative of persistent carcinoma. Rarely, this elevation may be caused by residual benign prostatic tissue (Foster 1993, Fowler 1995, Ravery 1999), which has been detected in a few cases by biopsy of the vesicourethral anastomosis (Foster 1993, Fowler 1995). It is also rare that clinical recurrence of prostate cancer occurs in the absence of a detectable postoperative serum PSA level (Catalona 1998). Roughly one half of men who experience a PSA elevation after radical prostatectomy will do so in the first 1 to 2 years after surgery, but elevations 5 to 10 years after surgery have been reported

■ **t13.21 Relationship of Total Serum PSA to Pathologic Stage of Prostatic Carcinoma**

PSA Level (ng/mL)	Organ-Confined	Seminal Vesicle Positivity	Lymph Node Positivity
0-4	64%	3%	1%
4.1-10	50%	6%	3%
10.1-20	35%	10%	9%
>20	16%	20%	17%

Data from Partin 1997

(Pound 1999). The time from a detectable PSA after surgery to clinically detected recurrence (the lead time) is 3 to 8 years (Abi-Aad 1992, Paulson 1994, Pound 1999), with the latter figure (8 years) representing the time to detection of distant metastasis (Pound 1999).

Preoperative and postoperative clinical and pathologic information can be used to predict the likelihood of a PSA elevation after radical prostatectomy. Preoperative PSA level and pathologic findings in the radical prostatectomy specimen are independent predictors of "PSA failure" after surgery (Arcangeli 1998, Epstein 1996, Han 2001, Humphrey 1993, Kattan 1999, Paulson 1994, Pound 1999, Stamey 1999). (See Chapter 14 for details on the relationship of pathologic findings in radical prostatectomy to clinical outcome.) An estimation of whether a postoperative PSA elevation is likely to represent locally recurrent (or persistent) or metastatic disease can be made. For patients who developed distant metastasis after surgery, the time to the first detectable PSA level after surgery, Gleason histologic grade in the radical prostatectomy specimen, and the PSA doubling time all predicted the probability and time to development of metastatic cancer (Pound 1999). Pathologic stage information from the radical prostatectomy can also help distinguish patients who are likely to have distant metastases from those likely to have local recurrence only (Partin 1994, Roberts 2001). Histopathologic identification of carcinoma in seminal vesicle wall or pelvic lymph nodes is a strong predictor of subsequent development of distant metastases.

Serum PSA has also been widely used to follow disease activity after radiation therapy and androgen deprivation therapy (ASTROCP 1997, Matzkin 1992, Schellhammer 1997, Stamey 1989). Because the prostate gland is still present after radiation therapy, the PSA level after radiation therapy that is indicative of disease-free status is controversial (Polascik 1999, Schellhammer 1997), with variably used nadir cutoffs of 0.5 to 4 ng/mL. Recently, a consensus panel recommended that 3 consecutive increases in PSA after radiation therapy be interpreted as "biochemical failure" (ASTROCP 1997). As for patients treated with radical prostatectomy, clinical stage, Gleason score in needle biopsy, and pretreatment PSA level are predictors of response to radiation therapy. After androgen deprivation therapy for advanced prostate cancer, a fall in PSA without a subsequent rise is a favorable response. Curiously, some patients with progressive metastatic prostate cancer experience a PSA decline with clinical improvement after withdrawal of antiandrogen therapy (Kelly 1997). For patients with hormone-refractory metastatic prostatic carcinoma, log (PSA) and PSA velocity are associated with survival time (Vollmer 1998A, 1999B).

Serum PSA protein is currently a well-established tumor marker for carcinoma of the prostate. Future efforts will be directed toward increasing the sensitivity and specificity of PSA protein measurements in the serum. One approach that holds promise is use of serum human glandular kallikrein 2(hK2), a PSA-like kallikrein (Becker 2000, Partin 1999). Evaluation of serum PSA RNA detection methods, including RT-PCR, will also be important (Chapter 21), as will further development of models that incorporate PSA with clinical, histopathologic, and potentially molecular biologic information (Humphrey 1998, Polascik 1999).

Radiology

Radiologic evaluations are important in diagnosis and staging of prostate cancer. Modalities that have been used include TRUS, computed tomography (CT), magnetic resonance imaging (MRI), bone scintigraphy (bone scan), immunoscintigraphy, and positron emission tomography. TRUS is a commonly used technique in initial diagnosis, where most prostate needle biopsies are performed with ultrasound guidance, to ensure that systematic biopsies widely sample different regions of the gland (Brawer 1998B, Carter 2002, Choyke 1995, Cooner 1990, Terris 2002). TRUS has also been used to identify nonpalpable prostatic lesions, determine gland volume, and stage prostate cancers (Brawer 1998B). However, TRUS is not a primary screening tool (Brawer 1998B, Catalona 1994B, Choyke 1995) because of its relative lack of sensitivity and specificity. Although prostatic carcinoma is characteristically hypoechoic **f2.3**, 20% to 48% of prostate cancers are not visible by ultrasound (Brawer 1998B, Ellis 1994B). The histologic basis for the hypoechoic appearance of some prostate cancers is not clear but may result from sound reflection at the interface of the carcinoma and supporting stroma (Choyke 1995). Ultrasound is best able to visualize well-circumscribed tumor nodules (Hardt 1993), but the common peripheral zone prostatic carcinomas often are infiltrative without formation of such prominent nodularity. TRUS-visible cancers tend to be large, moderately to poorly differentiated, and located in the posterior half of the gland (Ellis 1994B). No clear relationship with histologic grade and echogenicity of prostate cancer has been established (Dahnert 1986, Hardt 1993, Rifkin 1984, Shinohara 1989). Lack of TRUS specificity is indicated by the histopathologic findings of normal prostatic tissue, acute or chronic inflammation, atrophy, infarct, or PIN in needle biopsies of hypoechoic peripheral zone lesions (Lee 1989). Prostate volume measurements can be obtained with TRUS by using formulas that assume the prostate has a prolate ellipsoid or spherical shape (Terris 1991). TRUS volume measurements correlate with weights of prostate glands from radical prostatectomy specimens (Wolff 1995). The TRUS prostate gland volume measurements can be used to calculate PSA density and plan for brachytherapy or cryotherapy (Brawer 1998B). Staging accuracy by TRUS alone varies from 46% to 66% (Perrotti 1999), and, like any other technique that relies on gross architectural changes, TRUS often misses microscopic extraprostatic extension of carcinoma that is detected in radical prostatectomy specimens (J Smith 1997). Therefore, TRUS by itself does not by itself have a useful role in clinical staging.

Computed tomography and MRI, including body coil and endorectal coil MRI, have been evaluated for staging of local disease, but like TRUS they do not currently demonstrate sufficient accuracy for routine use in predicting pathologic stage (Carter 2002, O'Dowd 1997, Perrotti 1999, Rifkin 1990, J Smith 1997). Histopathologic findings in false-positive MRI interpretations include lobular atrophy, cystic hyperplasia, cystic atrophy, florid glandular hyperplasia, and scars with chronic inflammation (Sesterhenn 1992). Pelvic imaging with CT or MRI to detect nodal metastasis is limited by low sensitivity, resulting in part from use of size criteria (such as enlargement of >1cm) in diagnosing metastasis. MRI is rarely used to stage newly diagnosed prostate cancer, and staging CT scans were ordered in 21% of patients in a 1997 survey of urology practice (Gee 1998). Pelvic lymph node imaging may be indicated in patients with high PSA (>20 to 25 ng/mL) or high-grade Gleason score (Carter 2002), but even here CT accuracy can be low (Flanigan 1996). Additionally, most patients in this era have PSA levels between 4 and 10 ng/mL. More recent attempts to image nodal metastasis have used radioimmunoimaging with a monoclonal antibody directed against prostate-specific membrane antigen (Babaian 1994, Perrotti 1999).

Bone scintigraphy (radionuclide bone scan) is commonly used to evaluate for metastatic prostatic carcinoma (Buscombe 1999, Gee 1998),

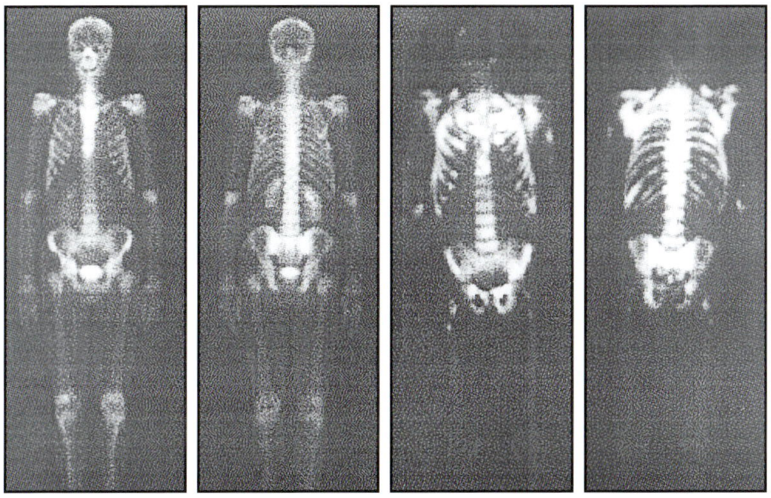

■ **i13.10** *Metastatic prostatic carcinoma as visualized by bone scan (right two panels), compared to normal bone scan (left two panels). Multiple "hot spots" in clavicle, scapula, ribs, spine, pelvis and femur indicate sites of metastatic disease. (Courtesy of Dr. Henry Royal)*

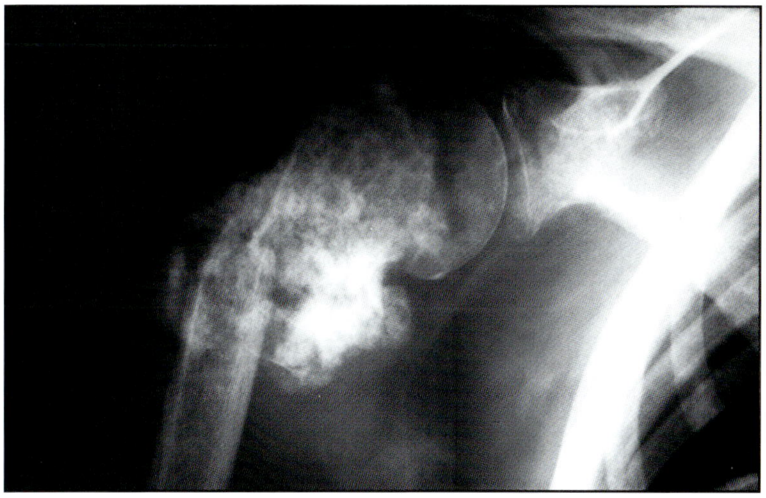

■ **i13.11** *Plain film of osteoblastic metastasis of prostatic carcinoma, with fracture, of humerus.*

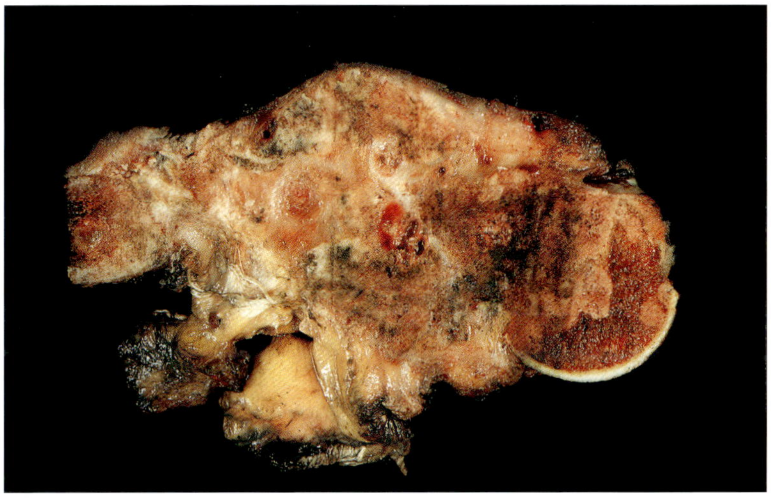

■ **i13.12** *Gross specimen of cross-section of humerus with osteoblastic prostatic carcinoma (same case as shown in* **i13.11***).*

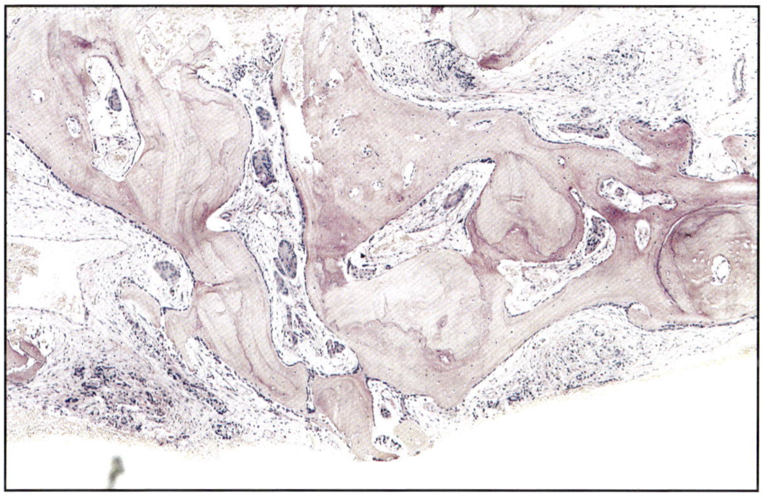

■ **i13.13** *Thickened bony trabeculae in an iliac crest core bone biopsy. There is fibrotic marrow with embedded nests of prostatic carcinoma. This is the histopathologic basis for the radiographic appearance of the bone in* **i13.11**.

especially for intermediate to high-risk patients (Cooperberg 2002) **i13.10**. Bone scans are more sensitive than plain films (radiographs) of bone (also known as bone survey films or skeletal radiography) in detecting bony metastasis (Buscombe 1999). Osteoblastic activity leads to increased uptake ("hot spots") in positive bone scans. Osteoblastic metastasis is classic for prostatic carcinoma spread to bone, as visualized by plain films **i13.11; i13.12**, although a lytic phase can also occur (Choyke 1995). The histopathologic correlate of osteoblastic metastasis is thickened bone trabeculae lined by increased numbers of osteoblasts, with prostatic carcinoma glands in the bone marrow **i13.13**. The chance of a positive bone scan is related to the serum PSA level, and it is extremely rare to find a positive scan in asymptomatic prostate cancer patients with a serum PSA <10 ng/mL (Chybowski 1991, Lee 1997). Accordingly, some have suggested that a bone scan need not be ordered in this circumstance (Lee 1997), but this is controversial, and some physicians request bone scans so as to have a baseline scan. Imaging of soft tissue metastasis or recurrent tumor after surgery has been recently accomplished using TRUS (Foster 1993), radioimmunoscintigraphy (Kahn 1998, Yao 2002), and positron emission tomography (Shreve 1996), with the latter 2 techniques still considered experimental.

[13.3] Natural History and Mortality

The true natural history of prostatic carcinoma is largely uncertain (Ekman 1999). This is so for several reasons. Many studies that have involved "watchful waiting," "surveillance only," or "expectant management" of patients with prostate carcinoma are actually reports of deferred treatment, with therapy instituted on evidence of clinical progression. Another critical point is that all too often, many such studies are of highly selected patients, and therefore the results are difficult to compare with those of other studies. Furthermore, studies that involve watchful waiting typically enroll patients with low-grade and low-stage cancer. Therefore, there are no data on the clinical course of untreated prostatic cancer across the full range of histologic grades and stages. Another difficulty is that to precisely characterize an individual patient's cancer by histopathologic

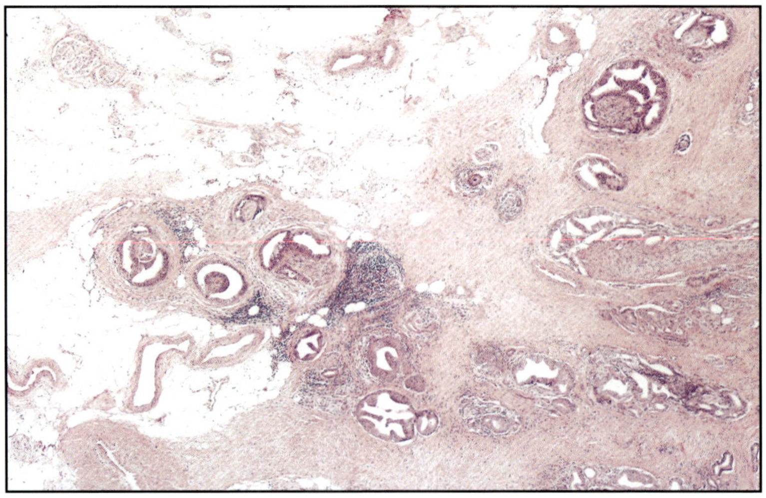

■ **i13.14** *Adenocarcinoma extending into periprostatic adipose tissue via perineural spread.*

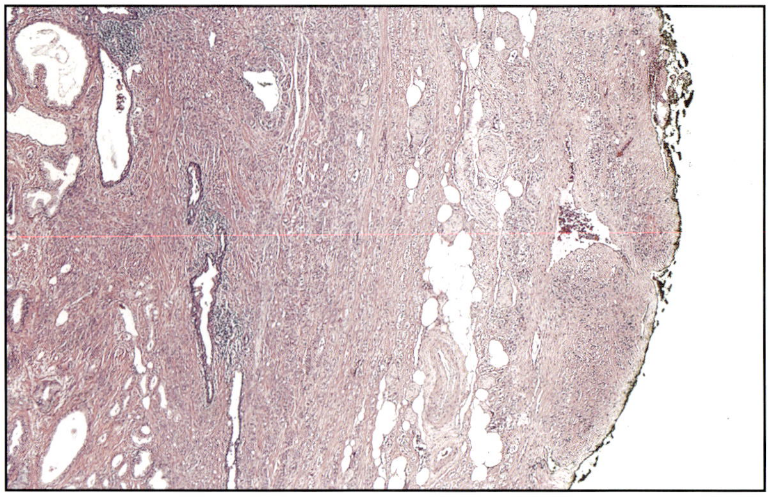

■ **i13.15** *Direct extraprostatic extension of carcinoma through prostatic "capsule", into periprostatic adipose tissue.*

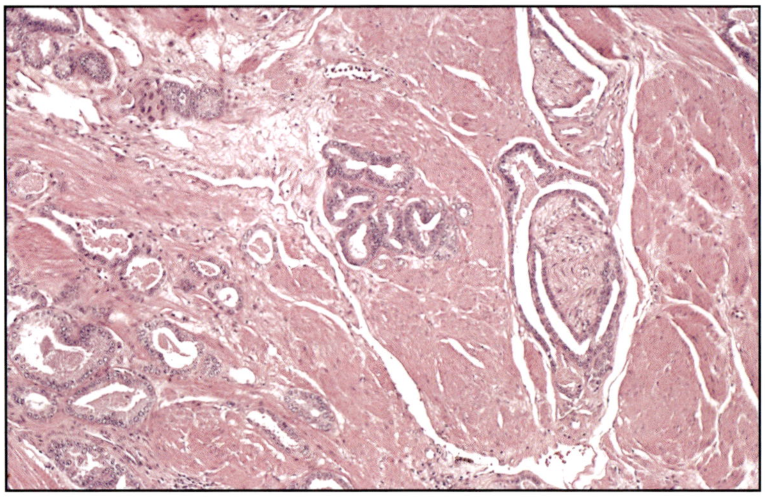

■ **i13.16** *Extension of prostatic adenocarcinoma into thick smooth muscle bundles of bladder neck.*

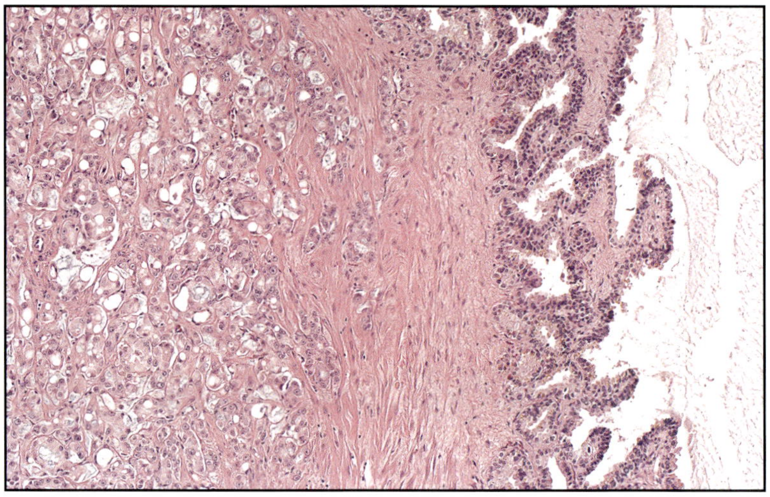

■ **i13.17** *Prostatic adenocarcinoma invading into muscular wall of seminal vesicle.*

examination, it is necessary to excise the primary malignancy by radical prostatectomy. This obviously interrupts the natural history of the disease. Finally, little is known of the phenotypic and genotypic natural progression of prostatic carcinoma over time from detection at the prostate-localized stage because untreated patients are not serially biopsied over time to study possible grade and molecular genetic progression. Even this approach may not yield a definitive knowledge about the natural history of grade and stage progression because biopsy is fraught with potential sampling errors.

The natural history of prostatic carcinoma begins with invasion of prostatic carcinoma cells into stroma. In the peripheral zone, invasive carcinoma probably emanates from high-grade PIN (Chapter 11), but the origin of transition zone carcinomas is not known. It has been suggested that atypical adenomatous hyperplasia might be a precursor for transition zone carcinoma, but this is controversial (Chapter 8). The time from initial invasion of a few carcinoma cells into stroma to clinical detection of carcinoma is unknown but may be years to even decades (Berges 1995), given that PIN can first be detected in the fourth and fifth decades (**f11.2, p 185**). The time from focal invasive carcinoma to clinical detection has been projected to be 11 to 12 years, with the doubling time for clinically localized prostatic carcinoma estimated to be 1 to 2.4 years (Berges 1995, H Carter 1992A). Invasion into periprostatic tissues is the next step in local progression, and this event is more likely to occur if the carcinoma is of higher histologic Gleason grade and larger size. Local extraprostatic extension typically occurs at the apex and anterolaterally for transition zone carcinomas and posterolaterally for the more common peripheral zone carcinomas (McNeal 1990, 2001). The peripheral zone carcinomas may "escape" the prostate gland by invading along nerves **i13.14** (Villers 1989) or by direct penetration through the "capsule" **i13.15**. The perineural permeation appears to be spread along a pathway of least resistance and does not represent perineural lymphatic invasion, as previously thought. Extraprostatic invasion superiorly into the thick smooth bundles of the bladder neck can occur with larger tumors **i13.16** and in advanced cases can eventuate in bladder neck obstruction and ureteral obstruction (Barzell 1977, Michigan 1977). Ureteral obstruction, present in 2% to 10% of patients with extensive local spread, can cause symptoms related to renal failure and uremia, such as anuria, oliguria, edema, fluid retention, pulmonary edema, and electrolyte imbalance symptoms (Kim 1996). Direct extension by carcinoma into the posteriorly situated seminal vesicles can occur by one of several mechanisms (Ohori 1993). The most common type of spread is by invasion of carcinoma into soft tissue at the base of the prostate and then infiltration into the wall of the seminal vesicle **i13.17**. The next most common type of

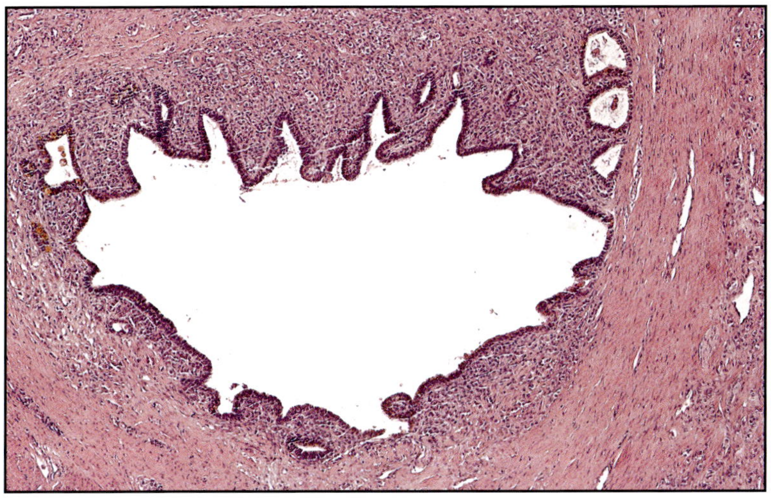

■ **i13.18** *Ejaculatory duct wall and mucosal involvement by prostatic adenocarcinoma.*

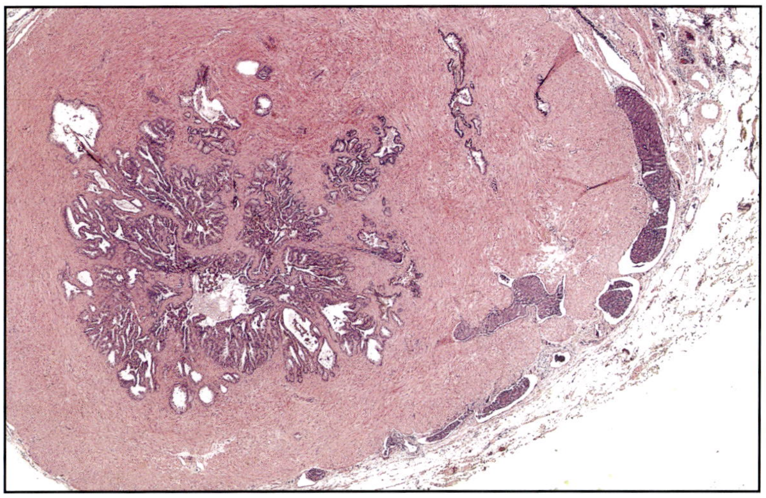

■ **i13.19** *Plugs of carcinoma in seminal vesicle wall and in lymphatic channels just outside seminal vesicle wall.*

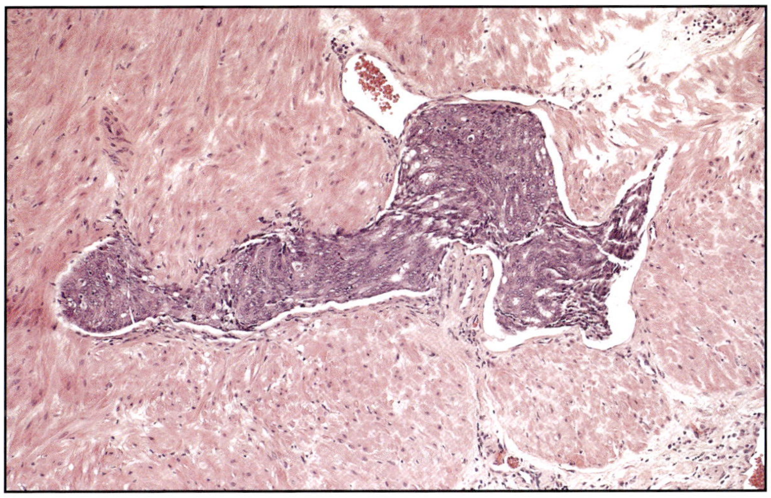

■ **i13.20** *Lymphatic channel invasion by carcinoma in seminal vesicle wall: The carcinoma plug assumes the shape of the channel. (Higher magnification of focus in* **i13.19**.*)*

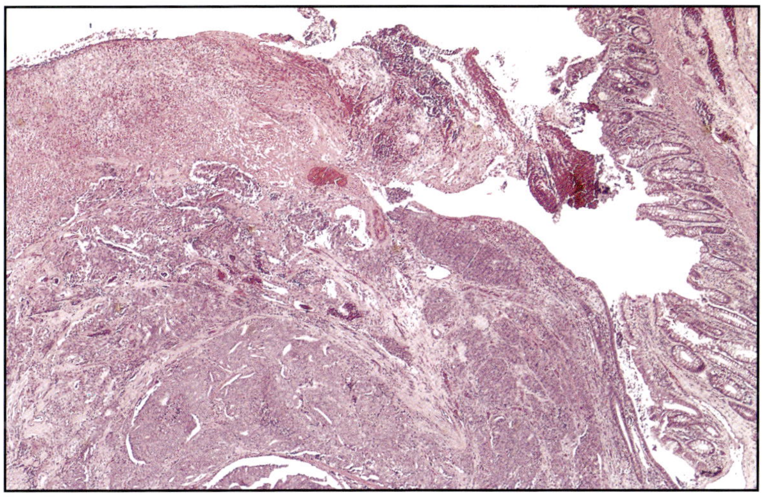

■ **i13.21** *Prostatic carcinoma invasion of rectum, by direct extension, with mucosal ulceration.*

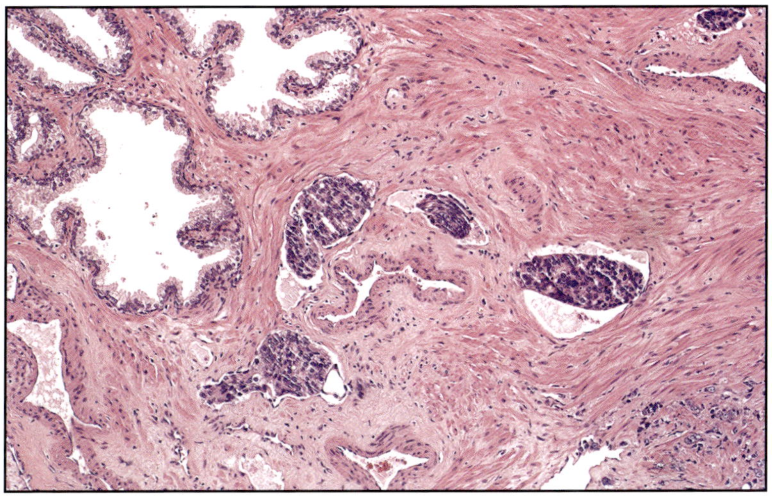

■ **i13.22** *Lymphvascular space invasion by carcinoma within prostate gland.*

involvement is direct spread along the ejaculatory duct complex into the seminal vesicles **i13.18**. Finally, it is possible to find isolated deposits of carcinoma in the seminal vesicle wall, without direct continuity with the prostatic primary **i13.19; i13.20**; these foci can represent lymphvascular spread of carcinoma. Posteriorly, Denonvilliers fascia constitutes an effective physical barrier (Villers 1993), such that direct prostatic carcinoma spread into the rectum is now a rare event **i13.21**. Involvement of the rectum by prostate cancer can produce symptoms similar to those of colon carcinoma, such as constipation, abdominal pain, rectal bleeding, and intermittent diarrhea (Kim 1996). More than 30 years ago, 10% of patients with advanced disease had rectal involvement at autopsy (Rodin 1967). Another unusual late manifestation of extensive local spread is local invasion into penile corporeal bodies, with resultant priapism (Kim 1996). The amount of time needed for those various local invasion events to occur is unknown.

Metastatic spread of prostatic carcinoma begins when carcinoma invades lymphvascular spaces. This can occur within the prostate **i13.22**, in extraprostatic soft tissue, or in seminal vesicles (Graham 1996) **i13.19**. Just as for extraprostatic extension by carcinoma, lymphvascular space invasion is more likely to be found in more aggressive cancers of higher grade, stage, and volume (Bahnson 1989, McNeal 1996, Salomao 1995, van den Ouden 1998). Lymphvascular space invasion is correlated with clinical progression, but not all prostatic carcinoma cells that are found locally in lymphvascular spaces are destined to survive in the bloodstream and implant and grow at sites distant from the prostate. This is

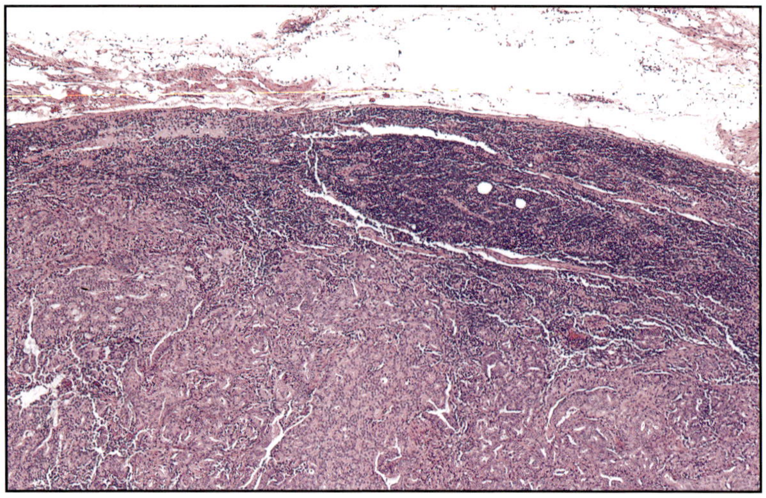

■ **i13.23** *Pelvic lymph node with metastatic prostatic adenocarcinoma, with sheet-like nodal architectural effacement and preservation of a thin rim of subcapsular lymphoid tissue.*

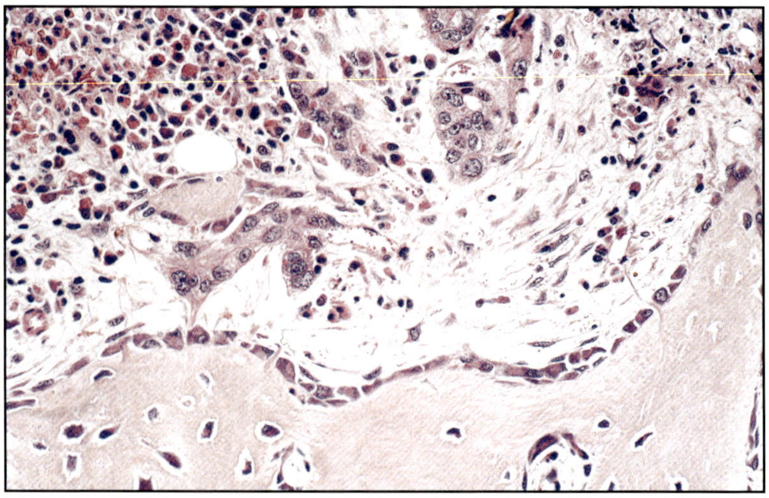

■ **i13.24** *Osteoblastic cell proliferation in response to prostatic adenocarcinoma in bone marrow. Note prominent rim of osteoblasts at bone-marrow interface.*

suggested by RT-PCR detection of circulating prostate cells (presumably carcinoma cells) in a substantial proportion (81%) of patients without evidence of clinical failure (Gao 1999A).

The most common sites of metastatic spread of prostatic carcinoma are the regional pelvic lymph nodes **i13.23** and bones of the pelvis and the axial skeleton **t13.22**. The obturator and hypogastric nodes are the first ones to be involved, followed by external iliac, common iliac, presacral, and presciatic nodes (Golimbu 1979). In a few patients, microscopic periprostatic lymph nodes may be the first ones to be involved, but these nodes are found in <5% of radical prostatectomy specimens (Kothari 2001, Pinto 2000). Although the natural history of metastatic prostatic carcinoma is incompletely understood (Rukstalis 1996), it is clear that the histopathologic detection of metastatic spread is an ominous finding. The doubling time for prostatic carcinoma cells metastatic to lymph nodes is much faster, at 33 days, than that for localized prostatic carcinoma at, ≥475 days (Berges 1995). At 8 years after radical prostatectomy almost all patients with positive pelvic lymph nodes experience "biochemical failure" (an elevated serum PSA) (Pound 1997). More than 75% of untreated patients with lymph node metastasis develop bone metastasis and systemic progression within 5 years, with death due to prostatic carcinoma in 35% to 50% (Rukstalis 1996).

Metastasis to bone marrow is a hallmark of disseminated prostate cancer. The presence of prostatic carcinoma cells in blood vessels in bone marrow or in bone marrow tissue itself can be found early in the natural course of prostate cancer and has been detected by RT-PCR (for PSA) in one half of patients with pathologically organ-confined carcinoma (Gao 1999B, Melchior 1997, Wood 1994). Not all of these cells survive in the marrow, however, and there is only a slight trend toward a positive bone marrow PSA RT-PCR result and clinical progression. Bone metastasis is characteristically osteoblastic **i13.24** and most commonly involves the pelvis, vertebral column, and ribs (Byar 1977, Smith 1990) **t13.22**. Bone pain, bone fractures, and spinal cord compression are among the most disabling symptoms for patients with advanced prostate cancer (Smith 1999). The cellular and molecular basis for the predilection of prostatic carcinoma cells to metastasize to bone is not established but probably relates to the "seed and soil" theory (Paget 1889) that intrinsic factors of the carcinoma cells and host microenvironment play an important role in the growth of cancer cells at specific anatomic sites. Indeed, there is experimental evidence of preferential bidirectional molecular communication between prostatic carcinoma cells and bone marrow stromal cells compared with stromal cells from other sites (Koeneman 1999). The 10-year survival for patients with bony metastasis treated with androgen ablation is 10% (Blackard 1973).

Visceral metastatic deposits in the lung and liver are not often clinically apparent but are common at the end of prostate cancer progression, detected at autopsy **t13.23**. Prostatic carcinoma is capable

■ **t13.22 Most Common Sites of Clinically Detected Prostatic Carcinoma Metastasis**

Regional lymph nodes:	Obturator nodes first, followed by hypogastric, external iliac, common iliac, presacral, presciatic, and inguinal nodes
Axial skeleton:	Pelvis (73%), dorsal and lumbar spine (63%), ribs (61%), cervical spine (51%), femur (40%), skull (28%), sacrum (25%), and humerus (24%)

Golimbu 1979, Smith 1990

■ **t13.23 Most Common Sites of Autopsy-Detected Prostatic Carcinoma Metastasis**

Anatomic Site	Metastasis in Prostate Cancer Cases
Lymph nodes	68%
Bones	67%
Lungs	49%
Bladder	39%
Liver	36%
Adrenals	17%
Kidneys	11%
Peritoneum	10%
Rectum	9%
Ureter	8%
Pleura	8%
Pancreas	5%
Intestines	4%
Spleen	4%
Heart	4%
Skin	3%
Brain	2%
Thyroid	2%

Saitoh 1984

of metastasis to a number of different anatomic sites when the patient has widespread dissemination of cancer late in the course of the disease (Saitoh 1984) **t13.23**.

Overall, the mean time to death after the development of metastatic prostatic carcinoma is 3 to 5 years (Ekman 1999, Pound 1999), with a mean survival of less than 1 year once the patient develops metastatic, hormone-refractory prostate cancer (Ekman 1999).

Carcinoma of the prostate is currently the second-leading killer of American men with cancer (Jemal 2002) and is the sixth leading worldwide killer of men with cancer (Parkin 1999). The 5-year survival rate for men with prostate cancer exhibits substantial worldwide variation (Parkin 1999) **t13.24;** in regions with lower survival rates, it is likely that the disease is being detected at a later stage. The 5-year survival for prostate cancer worldwide is 58% (Parkin 1999). In the United States, the death rate due to prostate cancer was stable from 1950 to 1970, with a slow increase (due to unknown factors) from 1979 to 1990 (Jemal 2002). From 1994 to 1995, there was a decrease in mortality due to prostate cancer of 6.2% (SEERP 1997), again for unknown reasons. A similar trend has been seen in Canada (Meyer 1999) and Austria (Bartsch 2001). It has been hypothesized that prostate cancer death rates are declining in North America because men are increasingly diagnosed when the prostate cancer is localized, possibly through screening (Roberts 1999), and increasingly receive treatments that reduce likelihood of death from the disease (Mettlin 1998, Roberts 1999). The likelihood of death due to prostate cancer is dictated mainly by histologic grade (Chapter 15) and stage (Chapter 16) of the disease (Albertsen 1995, Ekman 1999, Flanigan 1997) **t13.25**. Gleason score 2 to 4 (well-differentiated) carcinomas have little, if any, impact on survival, whereas the estimated lost life expectancy is 4 to 5 years for Gleason score 5 to 7 tumors and 6 to 8 years for Gleason score 8 to 10 tumors (Albertsen 1995). It is clear that once prostate cancer has spread outside the gland, chances for cure are diminished.

■ t13.24 5 Year Survival Rates for Men With Prostate Cancer According to Geographic Region

Region	Five-Year Survival
North America	79%
Australia/New Zealand	63%
Japan	52%
Northwestern Europe	49%
Latin America/Caribbean	43%
Southeast Asia	41%
Sub-Saharan Africa	41%
Middle East/North Africa	40%
China	40%
Eastern Europe	40%
Southern Europe	22%
World Wide	58%

Data from Parkin 1999.

■ t13.25 Prostate Cancer-Specific Survival at 10 years According to Clinical Stage

Clinical Stage	Survival
Tla	98%
Tlb	90%
Tlc	90%
T2, Gleason score 2-6	91%
T2, Gleason score 7-10	66%
T3	60%
N+	40%
M+	10%

Flanigan 1997

[13.4] Treatment

Several treatment options exist for patients with prostate cancer, depending on stage of the cancer, patient age, and competing comorbidities (Catalona 1994D) **t13.26**. In 1993 in the United States, radical prostatectomy and radiation therapy were the most commonly used initial treatments for prostate cancer, followed by no treatment and hormonal therapy (Mettlin 1997) **t13.27**.

For men with clinically localized prostate cancer, curative therapy typically is offered in the United States, whereas elsewhere is the world, physicians more commonly offer expectant management (watchful waiting or surveillance only),which is basically treatment that is deferred until clinical symptoms occur. Expectant management is used in the United States (Catalona 1994D, Steinberg 1998), probably most often for older men with a life expectancy of <10 years and low-grade, low-volume carcinoma detected in TURP chips (stage T1a disease; see Chapter 16). This type of cancer management is controversial for patients, particularly younger men, with carcinoma detected on needle biopsy because it is exceedingly difficult to accurately predict potentially harmless cancer based on pretreatment parameters (Epstein 1998, Humphrey 1998).

■ t13.26 Treatment of Prostate Cancer

Clinical Stage/Qualifying Condition	Recommended Treatment
Tla	
Projected life expectancy < 10 years	Watchful waiting
Projected life expectancy ≥ 10 years	Radical prostatectomy, Radiation therapy, Watchful waiting
Tlb, Tlc, T2	
Projected life expectancy < 10 years	Radiation therapy, Hormonal therapy
Projected life expectancy ≥ 10 years	Radical prostatectomy, Radiation therapy, Hormonal therapy
T3	Radical prostatectomy, Radiation therapy ± Hormonal therapy
N+	Early or delayed Hormonal therapy
M+	Hormonal therapy, Radiation therapy, Corticosteroid therapy, Supportive therapy, Chemotherapy

Modified from Catalona 1994D

■ t13.27 Initial Treatment for Prostate Cancer: 1993

Radiation therapy: 30.1%
Radical prostatectomy: 29.2%
No treatment (watchful waiting): 21.6%
Hormonal therapy: 19.5%

Data from Mettlin 1997

The main therapies offered to patients with clinically localized prostate cancer with intent to cure are radical prostatectomy and radiation therapy. Radical prostatectomy is a mainstay of primary treatment for clinically localized prostate cancer (Catalona 1994D, Eastham 2002, Gibbons 2002, Walsh 2002). Radical prostatectomy can also be performed after hormonal therapy and as salvage treatment after failure of radiation therapy, although in the latter setting there is a high complication rate (Catalona 1994D).

The first radical prostatectomy for prostate cancer was performed in 1904 by Dr. Hugh Hampton Young (Young 1905, 1940). This was actually a radical perineal prostatectomy, but now the retropubic approach is more common. A disadvantage to the radical perineal prostatectomy is that a separate procedure to sample the pelvic lymph nodes must be performed first (Gibbons 2002). The nodes can be sampled by an open procedure or by laparoscopic pelvic lymphadenectomy. In my experience, the perineal surgical specimen has less periprostatic soft (adipose) tissue than the retropubic specimen, such that light microscopic evaluation of extraprostatic extension by carcinoma may be more difficult for the histopathologist in the perineal cases. The nerve-sparing radical retropubic prostatectomy, with preservation of the lateral neurovascular bundles, results in improved potency (Catalona 1989, Walsh 2002) and is a commonly performed surgical operation. Histologic Gleason grade and the presence of perineural invasion in needle biopsy can influence the decision to excise the neurovascular bundle (Walsh 2002). Clinical preoperative and intraoperative findings can also influence this decision (Walsh 2002). Radical prostatectomy has a low mortality rate (0.2%) (Gibbons 1998). Early complications include bleeding, deep venous thrombosis, and pulmonary embolism (Eastham 2002), and late complications include incontinence and impotence (Catalona 1999, Eastham 2002, Gibbons 2002, Walsh 2002). The percentage of patients with incontinence depends in part on the definition and surgeon experience and ranges from 5% to 31% (Eastham 2002). In one series, recovery of urinary continence occurred in 92% of 1870 patients and was correlated with patient age but not pathologic tumor stage (Catalona 1999). In the same series, recovery of erections occurred in 68% of preoperatively potent men treated with bilateral and 47% with unilateral nerve-sparing surgery (Catalona 1999). Overall, the incidence of complications was directly related to patient age and inversely rated to surgeon experience. Excellent prostate cancer control can be achieved with radical prostatectomy performed for clinical T1 to T2 cancers (Catalona 1998, Eastham 2002, Pound 1997). Radical prostatectomy has been performed for clinical T3 cancers and is potentially efficacious in a selected group of men who have been clinically overstaged (Catalona 1994D) or who have low- to intermediate-grade tumor (Gerber 1997). Radical prostatectomy has also been attempted in the face of lymph node metastasis (Seay 1998), although this is not generally done. Tumor progression and patient survival after surgery are independently related to Gleason grade, pathologic stage, and tumor size (percentage carcinoma) in the radical prostatectomy specimen (Carvalhal 2000, Catalona 1998, Eastham 2002, Epstein 1996, Humphrey 1993, Pound 1997, 1999, Stamey 1999) (Chapter 14).

Radiation therapy can be used to primarily treat prostate cancer by external beam radiotherapy or by implantation of radioactive isotopic seeds (brachytherapy) (D'Amico 2002, Porter 1998, 1999). External beam radiotherapy has been used to treat both early-stage (T1 to T2) and locally advanced (T3 to T4) prostate cancer. For some patients with T3 to T4 disease, combination hormonal therapy–radiotherapy has been used. Salvage radiation therapy to the prostatic bed can be used for patients with a detectable or rising serum PSA after radical prostatectomy (Catalona 1994D), although its efficacy is unclear. For patients with disseminated prostate cancer, palliative external beam radiation therapy can help control pain from soft tissue or osseous metastases (Catalona 1994D). Acute complications of external beam radiotherapy include prostatitis, with diarrhea and rectal irritation, and cystitis with dysuria and frequency (Catalona 1994D, D'Amico 2002, Porter 1998, 1999). Chronic complications affect about 5% of patients and include impotence, proctitis, cystitis, urethral stricture, and enteritis (Catalona 1994D). Modifications that can increase the radiation dosage have been developed recently. These approaches include 3-dimensional conformal radiation therapy, proton therapy, and brachytherapy (D'Amico 2002, Porter 1998, 1999). Brachytherapy, or interstitial radiation delivered by implantation of radioactive seeds into the prostate, has a long history in treatment of prostate cancer. Recently, there has been a resurgence of interest in brachytherapy because of the advent of TRUS transperineal implantation, in combination with computer-calculated 3-dimensional dose distributions (Porter 1999, Ragde 2000). Patient outcome in response to radiation therapy can be predicted, just like for surgery, by pretreatment PSA values, Gleason score, and clinical (palpation) stage (Kattan 2001, Shipley 1999), although this predictive capacity harbors much uncertainty (Vollmer 1999A).

Hormonal therapy is the main treatment for men with disseminated prostate cancer (Catalona 1994D). Hormonal therapy for prostate cancer was launched in 1941 by Huggins and Hodges, who won the Nobel Prize for the discovery that prostate cancer growth depended on androgens (Huggins 1941A, 1941B). Endocrine or androgen deprivation therapy is commonly used in both locally advanced and metastatic prostate cancer (Furr 1999, Khoury 1999, Schröeder 2002, Stenner 1999). Neoadjuvant preoperative androgen deprivation therapy has also been used in attempts to downstage clinically localized prostate cancer before radical prostatectomy, but thus far there does not seem to be a benefit for neoadjuvant hormonal therapy in PSA progression rates (Abbas 1996B). Hormonal therapy has also been administered after radical prostatectomy in men with positive lymph nodes (Messing 1999), although the benefits of this approach remain controversial. Methods of endocrine treatment include surgical castration, that is, orchiectomy (because the major source of androgens in males is testicular Leydig cells), and medical castration. Medical castration can be achieved with synthetic estrogens (such as diethylstilbestrol), luteinizing hormone releasing hormone (LHRH) analogs, and antiandrogens (of steroidal and nonsteroidal types [Furr 1999]). These therapies can be used as monotherapies or together in combined androgen blockade, where there is an attempt to block production of testicular androgens and the effect of adrenal androgens. Possible side effects from androgen ablation therapy include hot flashes and decreased libido or potency (in most patients) with orchiectomy and LHRH agonists and gynecomastia, nausea, diarrhea, hepatotoxicity, fluid retention, and thromboembolism with diethylstilbestrol and some of the antiandrogens (Catalona 1994D). Longer term side effects include decreased muscle mass, osteoporosis, and anemia. Endocrine therapy of prostate cancer is viewed as palliative and not curative, although most patients do experience an objective response (Catalona 1994D). Eventually, all stage D2 patients treated with hormonal therapy develop hormone-independent (hormone-refractory or hormone-resistant) prostate cancer, with a rising PSA or other evidence of progression in the presence of androgen blockade. Chemotherapy (Eisenberger 2002, Petrylak 2002, Sternberg 1999), second-line hormonal therapy, and radiotherapy have been used for these patients (Catalona 1994D, Oh 1998), but as mentioned earlier, survival time once this hormone-refractory state is reached typically is around 1 year (Ekman 1999, Smaletz 2002). Serum lactate dehydrogenase, alkaline phosphatase, plasma hemoglobin, performance status, and weight loss are prognostic factors for survival in patients with hormone-refractory prostate cancer (George 1999). A nomogram based on these factors, along with age, PSA, and albumin, can be used to predict 1-year and 2-year survival (Smaletz 2002).

Unproven therapies that have been used in prostate cancer include cryosurgery (Benoit 1999, Long 2001), ultrasound (Gelet 1999), and herbal medicines (DiPaola 1998). These latter over-the-counter herbal substances can contain estrogenic activity or an extract of the ripe berries of the American dwarf palm, saw palmetto, that blocks testosterone metabolism (DiPaola 1998). The phytochemical composition of herbal mixtures, such as PC-SPES, used to manage advanced prostate cancer, can exhibit substantial lot-to-lot variation (Sovak 2002).

Potential future approaches in treatment of prostate cancer include immunotherapy, such as vaccine therapy, gene therapy, new chemotherapeutic agents, growth factor receptor antibodies, and antiangiogenic agents (Crawford 1999, Harrington 2001, Herman 1999, Heston 1999, Murphy 1999, Steiner 2000, Tjoa 1999). Clinical trials evaluating these therapies are in progress, but currently they are experimental.

References

Abbas F, Hochberg D, Civantos F, et al. Incidental prostatic adenocarcinoma in patients undergoing radical cystoprostatectomy for bladder cancer. *Eur Urol* 30:322-326, 1996A.

Abbas F, Scardino PT. Why neoadjuvant androgen deprivation prior to radical prostatectomy is unnecessary. *Urol Clin North Am* 23:587-604, 1996B.

Abi-Aad AS, MacFarlane MT, Stein A, et al. Detection of local recurrence after radical prostatectomy by prostate specific antigen and transrectal ultrasound. *J Urol* 147:952-955, 1992.

Abrahamsson P-A, Lilja H, Oesterling JE. Molecular forms of serum prostate-specific antigen. The clinical value of percent free prostate-specific antigen. *Urol Clin North Am* 24:353-365, 1997.

ACS (American Cancer Society). *Cancer Reference Information. Can Prostate Cancer Be Found Early?* http://www.cancer.org/, 2001.

Adami HO, Bergström R, Engholm G, et al. A prospective study of smoking and risk of prostate cancer. *Int J Cancer* 67:764-768, 1996.

Aihara M, Lebovitz RM, Wheeler TM, et al. Prostate specific antigen and Gleason grade: an immunohistochemical study of prostate cancer. *J Urol* 151:1558-1564, 1994.

Akazaki K, Stemmerman GN. Comparative study of latent carcinoma of the prostate among Japanese in Japan and Hawaii. *J Natl Cancer Inst* 50:1137-1144, 1973.

Albertsen PC, Fryback DG, Storer BE, et al. Long-term survival among men with conservatively treated localized prostate cancer. *JAMA* 274:626-631, 1995.

Alexander EE, Qian J, Wollan PC, et al. Prostatic intraepithelial neoplasia does not appear to raise serum prostate-specific antigen concentration. *Urology* 47:693-698, 1996.

Alexander RB, Maguire MG, Epstein JI, et al. Pathological stage is higher in older men with clinical stage B1 adenocarcinoma of the prostate. *J Urol* 141:880-882, 1989.

Amling CL, Blute ML, Lerner SE, et al. Influence of prostate-specific antigen testing on the spectrum of patients with prostate cancer undergoing radical prostatectomy at a large referral practice. *Mayo Clin Proc* 73:401-406, 1998.

Andrews GS. Latent carcinoma of the prostate. *J Clin Pathol* 2:197-208, 1949.

Aprikian AG, Zhang ZF, Fair WR. Prostate adenocarcinoma in men younger than 50 years. A retrospective review of 151 patients. *Cancer* 74:1768-1777, 1994.

Arcangeli CG, Ornstein DK, Keetch DW, et al. Prostate-specific antigen as a screening test for prostate cancer: the United States Experience. *Urol Clin North Am* 24:299-306, 1997.

Arcangeli CG, Humphrey PA, Smith DS, et al. Percentage of free serum prostate-specific antigen as a predictor of pathologic features of prostate cancer in a screening population. *Urology* 51:558-564, 1998.

Armbruster DA. Prostate-specific antigen: biochemistry, analytical methods, and clinical applications. *Clin Chem* 39: 181-195, 1993.

Aronson WJ, Freeland SJ. Can we lower the mortality rate of black men with prostate cancer [editorial]? *J Urol* 163:150-151, 2000.

ASTROCP (American Society for Therapeutic Radiology and Oncology Consensus Panel). Consensus statement: guidelines for PSA following radiation therapy. *Int J Radiat Oncol Biol Phys* 37:1035-1041, 1997.

AUA (American Urological Association). *Early Detection of Prostate Cancer.* http://www.auanet.org, 1999.

Austin JP, Convery K. Age-race interaction in prostatic adenocarcinoma treated with external beam irradiation. *Am J Clin Oncol* 16:140-145, 1993.

Auvinen A, Rietbergen JB, Denis LJ, et al. Prospective evaluation plan for randomized trials of prostate cancer screening. The International Prostate Cancer Screening Trial Evaluation Group. *J Med Screen* 3:97-104, 1996.

Babaian RJ, Sayer J, Podoloff DA, et al. Radioimmunoscintigraphy of pelvic lymph nodes with 111 indium–labeled monoclonal antibody CYT-356. *J Urol* 152:1952-1955, 1994.

Bahnson RR, Dresner SM, Gooding W, et al. Incidence and prognostic significance of lymphatic and vascular invasion in radical prostatectomy specimens. *Prostate* 15:149-155, 1989.

Bahnson RR. Elevation of prostate specific antigen from bacillus Calmette-Guerin–induced granulomatous prostatitis. *J Urol* 146:1368-1369, 1991.

Bairati I, Meyer F, Fradet Y, et al. Dietary fat and advanced prostate cancer. *J Urol* 159:1271-1275, 1998.

Bangma CH, Rietbergen JBW, Schröder FH. Prostate-specific antigen as a screening test: the Netherlands Experience. *Urol Clin North Am* 24:307-314, 1997.

Baron E, Angrist A. Incidence of occult adenocarcinoma of the prostate. After 50 years of age. *Arch Pathol* 32:787-793, 1941.

Baron JC, Zerbib M, Leveque JM, et al. Detection of a prostatic adenocarcinoma in the cysto-prostatectomy specimens of an invasive tumor of the bladder [in French]. *Ann Urol* (Paris) 23:119-122, 1989.

Bartsch G, Horninger W, Klocker H, et al. Prostate cancer mortality after introduction of prostate-specific antigen mass screening in the federal state of Tyrol, Austria. *Urology* 58:417-424, 2001.

Barzell W, Bean MA, Hilaris BS, et al. Prostatic adenocarcinoma: relationship of grade and local extent to pattern of metastases. *J Urol* 118:278-282, 1977.

Bassler TJ Jr, Orozco R, Bassler IC, et al. Most prostate cancers missed by raising the upper limit of normal prostate-specific antigen for men in their sixties are clinically significant. *Urology* 52:1064-1069, 1998.

Bassler T, Bassler I, Kunnel B, et al. Should the upper limit of normal PSA be lowered [abstract]? *Mod Pathol* 12:89A, 1999.

Bastacky SI, Wojno KJ, Walsh PC, et al. Pathological features of hereditary prostate cancer. *J Urol* 153:987-992, 1995.

Bauer JJ, Sesterhenn IA, Mostofi FK, et al. p53 nuclear protein expression is an independent marker in clinically localized prostate cancer patients undergoing radical prostatectomy. *Clin Cancer Res* 1:1295-1300, 1995.

Bauer JJ, Sesterhenn IA, Mostofi FK, et al. Elevated levels of apoptosis regulator proteins p53 and bcl-2 are independent prognostic biomarkers in surgically treated clinically localized prostate cancer patients. *J Urol* 156:1511-1516, 1996.

Bauer JJ, Connelly RR, Sesterhenn IA, et al. Biostatistical modeling using traditional preoperative and pathological prognostic variables in the selection of men at high risk for disease recurrence after radical prostatectomy for prostate cancer. *J Urol* 159:929-933, 1998.

Becker C, Piironen T, Pettersson K, et al. Discrimination of men with prostate cancer from those with benign disease by measurements of human glandular kallikrein 2 (hK2) in serum. *J Urol* 163:311-316, 2000.

Beduschi MC, Oesterling JE. Prostate-specific antigen density. *Urol Clin North Am* 24:323-332, 1997.

Benoit R, Miller R, Merlotti L, et al. The role of cryosurgery in the treatment of prostate cancer. In: Kaisary AV, Murphy GP, Denis L, et al, eds. *Textbook of Prostate Cancer: Pathology, Diagnosis and Treatment.* London: Martin Dunitz; 261-276, 1999.

Benson MC, Kaplan SA, Olsson CA. Prostate cancer in men less than 45 years old: influence of stage, grade and therapy. *J Urol* 137:888-890, 1987.

Berges RR, Vukanovic J, Epstein JI, et al. Implication of cell kinetic changes during the progression of human prostatic cancer. *Clin Cancer Res* 1:473-480, 1995.

Berthon P, Valeri A, Cohen-Akenine A, et al. Predisposing gene for early-onset prostate cancer, localized on chromosome 1q42.2-43. *Am J Hum Genet* 62:1416-1424, 1998.

Billis A, Souza CAF, Pioresan H. Transitional zone vs. peripheral zone adenocarcinoma of the prostate. An autopsy study [abstract]. *Mod Pathol* 13:94A, 2000.

Blackard CE, Byar DP, Jordan WP Jr. and the Veterans Administration Cooperative Urologic Research Group. Orchiectomy for advanced prostatic carcinoma: a reevaluation. *Urology* 1:553-560, 1973.

Bodie BC. *Lectures on the Diseases of the Urinary Organs.* 3rd rev. ed. London 1842:151-195.

Borek D, Butcher D, Hassanein K, et al. Relationship of age to histologic grade in prostate cancer. *Prostate* 16:305-311, 1990.

Bova GS, Partin AW, Isaacs SD, et al. Biological aggressiveness of hereditary prostate cancer: long-term evaluation following radical prostatectomy. *J Urol* 160:660-663, 1998.

Boyle P, Maisonneuve P, Napalkov P. Geographical and temporal patterns of incidence and mortality from prostate cancer. *Urology* 46:47-55, 1995.

Brasso K, Friis S, Kjaer SK, et al. Prostate cancer in Denmark: a 50-year population-based study. *Urology* 51:590-594, 1998.

Brawer MK. The diagnosis of prostate carcinoma. *Cancer* 71:899-905, 1993.

Brawer MK, Meyer GE, Letran JL, et al. Measurement of complexed PSA improves specificity for early detection of prostate cancer. *Urology* 52:372-378, 1998A.

Brawer MK, Chetner MP. Ultrasonography of the prostate and biopsy. In: Walsh PC, Retik AB, Vaughn ED Jr, et al, eds. *Campbell's Urology.* 7th ed. Philadelphia: WB Saunders; 2506-2517, 1998B.

Brawer MK. Clinical usefulness of assays for complexed prostate-specific antigen. *Urol Clin North Am* 29:193-203, 2002.

Brawley OW, Kramer BS. Epidemiology of prostate cancer. In: Vogelzang NJ, Scardino PT, Shipley WU, et al, eds. *Comprehensive Textbook of Genitourinary Oncology.* Baltimore: Williams & Wilkins; 557-564, 1996.

Brawley OW, Knopf K, Merrill R. The epidemiology of prostate cancer part I: descriptive epidemiology. *Semin Urol Oncol* 16:187-192, 1998.

Brawn PN, Foster DM, Jay DW, et al. Characteristics of prostatic infarcts and their effect on serum prostate-specific antigen and prostatic acid phosphatase. *Urology* 44:71-75, 1994.

Brawn PN, Kuhl D, Speights VO, et al. The incidence of unsuspected metastases from clinically benign prostate glands with latent carcinoma. *Arch Pathol Lab Med* 119:731-733, 1995.

Breslow N, Chan CW, Dhom G, et al. Latent carcinoma of prostate at autopsy in seven areas. *Int J Cancer* 20:680-688, 1977.

Breslow RA, Weed DL. Review of epidemiologic studies of alcohol and prostate cancer: 1971-1996 (review). *Nutr Cancer* 30:1-13, 1998.

Breul J, Pickl U, Hartung R. Prostate-specific antigen in urine. *Eur Urol* 26:18-21, 1994.

Brown L, ed. *The New Shorter Oxford English Dictionary.* Oxford, England: Clarendon Press; 1538, 1993.

Burnett AL, Chan DW, Brendler CB, et al. The value of serum enzymatic acid phosphatase in the staging of localized prostate cancer. *J Urol* 148:1832-1834, 1992.

Buscombe J, Hilson A. Nuclear medicine in prostate cancer. In: Kaisary AV, Murphy GP, Denis L, et al, eds. *Textbook of Prostate Cancer. Pathology, Diagnosis and Treatment.* London: Martin Dunitz; 157-167, 1999.

Bush RB, Bush IM. Early developments in history of prostatic disorders. In: Tannenbaum M, ed. *Urologic Pathology: The Prostate.* Philadelphia: Lea & Febiger; 7-22, 1977.

Butler J, Brunnstein H, Freiman DG, et al. Incidence, distribution, and enzymatic activity of carcinoma of the prostate gland. *Arch Pathol* 68:243-251, 1959.

Byar DP, Mostofi FK. Cancer of the prostate in men less than 50 years old: analysis of 51 cases. *J Urol* 102:726-733, 1969.

Byar DP. VACURG studies on prostate cancer and its treatment. In: Tannenbaum M, ed. *Urologic Pathology: The Prostate.* Philadelphia: Lea & Febiger; 241-268, 1977.

Cannon L, Bishop DT, Skolnick M, et al. Genetic epidemiology of prostate cancer in the Utah Mormon genealogy. *Cancer Surv* 1:49-69, 1982.

Carter BS, Beaty TH, Steinberg GD, et al. Mendelian inheritance of familial prostate cancer. *Proc Natl Acad Sci U S A* 89:3367-3371, 1992.

Carter BS, Bova GS, Beaty TH, et al. Hereditary prostate cancer: epidemiologic and clinical features. *J Urol* 150:797-802, 1993.

Carter HB, Morrell CH, Pearson JD, et al. Estimation of prostatic growth using serial prostate-specific antigen measurements in men with and without prostate disease. *Cancer Res* 52:3323-3328, 1992A.

Carter HB, Pearson JD, Metter EJ, et al. Longitudinal evaluation of prostate-specific antigen levels in men with and without prostate disease. *JAMA* 267:2215-2220, 1992B.

Carter HB, Pearson JD. Prostate-specific antigen velocity and repeated measures of prostate-specific antigen. *Urol Clin North Am* 24:333-338, 1997.

Carter HB, Epstein JI, Partin AW. Influence of age and prostate-specific antigen on the chance of curable prostate cancer among men with nonpalpable disease. *Urology* 53:126-130, 1999.

Carter HB, Partin AW. Diagnosis and staging of prostate cancer. In: Walsh PC, Retik AB, Vaughan ED Jr, et al, eds. *Campbell's Urology.* 8th ed. Philadelphia: Saunders; 3055-3079, 2002.

Carvalhal GF, Smith DS, Mager DE, et al. Digital rectal examination for detecting prostate cancer at prostate specific antigen levels of 4 ng/mL or less. *J Urol* 161:835-839, 1999.

Carvalhal GF, Humphrey PA, Thorson P, et al. Visual estimate of percentage of carcinoma is an independent predictor of prostate carcinoma recurrence after radical prostatectomy. *Cancer* 89:1308-1314, 2000.

Catalona WJ, Bigg SW. Nerve-sparing radical prostatectomy: evaluation of results after 250 patients. *J Urol* 143:538-543, 1989.

Catalona WJ, Smith DS, Ratliff TL, et al. Detection of organ-confined prostate cancer is increased through prostate-specific antigen-based screening. *JAMA* 270:948-954, 1993.

Catalona WJ, Smith DS. Comparison of different serum prostate specific antigen measures for early prostate cancer detection. *Cancer* 74:1516-1518, 1994A.

Catalona WJ, Richie JP, Ahmann FR, et al. Comparison of digital rectal examination and serum prostate specific antigen in the early detection of prostate cancer: results of a multicenter clinical trial of 6,630 men. *J Urol* 151:1283-1290, 1994B.

Catalona WJ, Richie JP, deKernion JB, et al. Comparison of prostate specific antigen concentration versus prostate specific antigen density in the early detection of prostate cancer: receiver operating characteristic curves. *J Urol* 152:2031-2036, 1994C.

Catalona WJ. Management of cancer of the prostate. *N Engl J Med* 331:996-1004, 1994D.

Catalona WJ, Smith DS, Wolfert RL, et al. Evaluation of percentage of free serum prostate-specific antigen to improve specificity of prostate cancer screening. *JAMA* 274:1214-1220, 1995.

Catalona WJ. Prostate cancer. In: Reintgen DS, Clark RA, eds. *Cancer Screening.* St Louis: Mosby; 97-117, 1996.

Catalona WJ, Smith DS, Ornstein DK. Prostate cancer detection in men with serum PSA concentrations of 2.6 to 4.0 ng/mL and benign prostate examination. Enhancement of specificity with free PSA measurements. *JAMA* 277:1452-1455, 1997.

Catalona WJ, Smith DS. Cancer recurrence and survival rates after anatomic radical retropubic prostatectomy for prostate cancer: intermediate-term results. *J Urol* 160:2428-2434, 1998.

Catalona WJ, Carvalhal GF, Mager DE, et al. Potency, continence and complication rates in 1,870 consecutive radical retropubic prostatectomies. *J Urol* 162:433-438, 1999.

Catalona WJ, Partin AW, Slawin KM, et al: Percentage of free PSA in black versus white men for detection and staging of prostate cancer: a prospective multicenter clinical trial. *Urology* 55:372-376, 2000.

Chan JM, Stampfer MJ, Giovannucci E, et al. Plasma insulin-like growth factor-1 and prostate cancer risk: a prospective study. *Science* 279:563-565, 1998A.

Chan JM, Stampfer MJ, Giovannucci EL. What causes prostate cancer? A brief summary of the epidemiology. *Semin Cancer Biol* 8:263-273, 1998B.

Cher ML, Lewis PE, Banjeree M, et al. A similar pattern of chromosomal alterations in prostate cancers from African-Americans and Caucasian Americans. *Clin Cancer Res* 4:1273-1278, 1998.

Chow CH, Liu HW, Lee KW, et al. Carcinoma of the prostate in an 11-year old child with long survival. *Br J Urol* 58:100-101, 1986.

Choyke PL. Imaging of prostate cancer. *Abdom Imaging* 20:505-515, 1995.

Chybowski FM, Larson-Keller JJ, Bergstralh EJ, et al. Predicting radionuclide bone scan findings in patients with newly diagnosed untreated prostate cancer: prostate specific antigen is superior to all other clinical parameters. *J Urol* 145:313-318, 1991.

Clark LC, Combs GF Jr, Turnbull BW, et al. Effects of selenium supplementation for cancer prevention in patients with carcinoma of the skin: a randomized controlled trial. *JAMA* 276:1957-1963, 1996.

Clements J, Mukhtar A. Glandular kallikreins and prostate-specific antigen are expressed in the human endometrium. *J Clin Endocrinol Metab* 78:1536-1539, 1994.

Cochran JS, Kadesky MC. A private practice experience with adenocarcinoma of the prostate in men less than 50 years old. *J Urol* 125:220-221, 1981.

Cook LS, Goldoft M, Schwartz SM, et al. Incidence of adenocarcinoma of the prostate in Asian immigrants to the United States and their descendants. *J Urol* 161:152-155, 1999.

Cooner WH, Mosley BR, Rutherford CL, et al. Prostate cancer detection in a clinical urological practice by ultrasonography, digital rectal examination and prostate specific antigen. *J Urol* 143:1146-1154, 1990.

Cooney KA, McCarthy JD, Lange E, et al. Prostate cancer susceptibility locus on chromosome 1q: a confirmatory study. *J Natl Cancer Inst* 89:955-959, 1997.

Cooperberg MR, Lubeck DP, Grossfeld GD, et al. Contemporary trends in imaging test utilization for prostate cancer staging: data from the cancer of the Prostate Strategic Urologic Research Endeavor. *J Urol* 168:491-495, 2002.

Coptcoat MJ, Darshane A. Laparoscopic pelvic lymphadenectomy for prostate cancer. In: Kaisary AV, Murphy GP, Denis L, et al, eds. *Textbook of Prostate Cancer. Pathology, Diagnosis and Treatment.* London: Martin Dunitz; 220-230, 1999.

Corder EH, Guess HA, Hulka BS, et al. Vitamin D and prostate cancer: a prediagnostic study with stored sera. *Cancer Epidemiol Biomarkers Prev* 2:467-472, 1993.

Crawford ED, Rosenblum M, Ziada AM, et al. Overview: hormone refractory prostate cancer. *Urology* 54(suppl 6A):1-7, 1999.

Culkin DJ, Wheeler JS Jr, Castelli M, et al. Carcinoma of the prostate in a 25-year-old man: a case report and review of the literature. *J Urol* 136:684-685, 1986.

Dahnert WF, Hamper UM, Eggleston JC, et al. Prostatic evaluation by transrectal sonography with histopathologic correlation: the echopenic appearance of early carcinoma. *Radiology* 158:97-102, 1986.

D'Amico AV, Moul JW, Kattan MW. Emerging prognostic factors for outcome prediction in clinically localized prostate cancer: prostate-specific antigen level, race, molecular markers, and neural networks. In: Vogelzang NJ, Scardino PT, Shipley WU, et al, eds. *Comprehensive Textbook of Genitourinary Oncology.* Philadelphia: Lippincott Williams & Wilkins; 680-700, 2000.

D'Amico AV, Covok J, Beard CJ, et al. Radiation therapy for prostate cancer. In: Walsh PC, Retik AB, Vaughan ED Jr, et al. *Campbell's Urology*. 8th ed. Philadelphia: Saunders; 3147-3170, 2002.

DeGuia K, Andea A, Butler C, et al. Small volume prostate cancer (PCA) in patients 50 years or younger treated by radical prostatectomy is more multifocal and associated with more diffuse high grade prostatic intraepithelial neoplasia (HGPIN) (abstract). *Mod Pathol* 14:106A, 2001.

Deliveliotis C, Alivizatos G, Stavropoulos NJ, et al. Influence of digital examination, cystoscopy, transrectal ultrasonography and needle biopsy on the concentration of prostate-specific antigen. *Urol Int* 53:186-190, 1994.

DeVere White RW, Deitch AD, Jackson AG, et al. Racial differences in clinically localized prostate cancers of black and white men. *J Urol* 159:1979-1983, 1998.

Diamandis EP, Yu H. Nonprostatic sources of prostate-specific antigen. *Urol Clin North Am* 24:275-282, 1997.

DiPaola RS, Zhang H, Lambert GH, et al. Clinical and biological activity of an estrogenic herbal combination (PC-SPES) in prostate cancer. *N Engl J Med* 339:785-791, 1998.

Djavan B, Remzi M, Zlotta AR, et al. Complexed prostate-specific antigen, complexed prostate-specific antigen density of total and transition zone, complexed/total prostate-specific antigen ratio, free-to-total prostate-specific antigen ratio, density of total and transition zone prostate-specific antigen: results of the prospective multicenter european trial. *Urology* 80(suppl 1):4-9, 2002.

Douglas TH, McLeod DG, Mostofi FK, et al. Prostate-specific antigen-detected prostate cancer (stage T1c): an analysis of whole-mount prostatectomy specimens. *Prostate* 32:59-64, 1997.

Dunsmuir WD, Edwards SM, Lakhani SR, et al. Allelic imbalance in familial and sporadic prostate cancer at the putative human prostate cancer susceptibility locus, HPC1. The CRC/BPG UK Familial Prostate Cancer Study Collaborators. Cancer Research Campaign/British Prostate Group. *Br J Cancer* 78:1430-1433, 1998.

Eastham JA, Scardino PT. Radical prostatectomy. In: Walsh PC, Retik AB, Vaughan ED Jr, et al, eds. *Campbell's Urology.* 8th ed. Philadelphia: Saunders; 3080-3106, 2002.

Edwards CN, Steinthorsson E, Nicholson D. An autopsy study of latent prostatic cancer. *Cancer* 6:531-554, 1953.

Egawa S, Suyama K, Ohori M, et al. Early detection of prostate cancer. Results of a prostate specific antigen-based detection program in Japan. *Cancer* 76:463-472, 1995.

Eisenberger MA. Chemotherapy for hormone-resistant prostate cancer. In: Walsh PC, Retik AB, Vaughan ED Jr, et al, eds. *Campbell's Urology.* 8th ed. Philadelphia: Saunders; 3209-3226, 2002.

Ekman P, Adolfsson J, Grönberg H. The natural history of prostate cancer. In: Kaisary AV, Murphy GP, Denis L, et al, eds. *Textbook of Prostate Cancer. Pathology, Diagnosis, and Treatment.* London: Martin Dunitz; 1-16, 1999.

Elgamal AA, van de Voorde W, van Poppel H, et al. Immunohistochemical localization of prostate-specific markers within the accessory male sex glands of Cowper, Littre, and Morgagni. *Urology* 44:84-91, 1994.

Elgamal AA, Ectors NL, Sunardhi-Widyaputra S, et al. Detection of prostate specific antigen in pancreas and salivary glands; a potential impact on prostate cancer overestimation. *J Urol* 156:464-468, 1996.

Elgamal AA, van Poppel HP, van de Voorde WM, et al. Impalpable invisible stage T1c prostate cancer: characteristics and clinical relevance in 100 radical prostatectomy specimens—a different view. *J Urol* 157:244-250, 1997.

Ellis WJ, Chetner MP, Preston SD, et al. Diagnosis of prostatic carcinoma: the yield of serum prostate specific antigen, digital rectal examination and transrectal ultrasonography. *J Urol* 52:1520-1525, 1994A.

Ellis JH, Tempany C, Sarin MS, et al. MR imaging and sonography of early prostatic cancer: pathologic and imaging features that influence identification and diagnosis. *Am J Roentgenol* 162:865-872, 1994B.

Ellner HJ, Putra AM, Lecompte I. Prostatic carcinoma in a 17-year-old boy. *J Urol* 94:691-694, 1965.

Epstein JI. PSA and PAP as immunohistochemical markers in prostate cancer. *Urol Clin North Am* 20:757-770, 1993.

Epstein JI, Walsh PC, Carmichael M, et al. Pathologic and clinical findings to predict tumor extent of nonpalpable (stage T1c) prostate cancer. *JAMA* 271:368-374, 1994.

Epstein JI, Partin AW, Sauvageot J, et al. Prediction of progression following radical prostatectomy: a multivariate analysis of 721 men with long-term follow-up. *Am J Surg Pathol* 20:286-292, 1996.

Epstein JI, Chan DW, Sokoll LJ, et al. Nonpalpable stage T1c prostate cancer: prediction of insignificant disease using free/total prostate specific antigen levels and needle biopsy findings. *J Urol* 160:2407-2411, 1998.

Erbersdobler A, Bardenhagen P, Henke RP. Numerical chromosomal anomalies in latent adenocarcinomas of the prostate. *Prostate* 38:92-99, 1999.

Farkas A, Schneider D, Perrotti M, et al. National trends in the epidemiology of prostate cancer, 1973 to 1994: evidence for the effectiveness of prostate-specific antigen screening. *Urology* 52:444-449, 1998.

Flanigan RC, McKay TC, Olson M, et al. Limited efficacy of preoperative computed tomographic scanning for the evaluation of lymph node metastasis in patients before radical prostatectomy. *Urology* 48:428-432, 1996.

Flanigan RC, Shankey TV. The natural history of human prostate cancer. In: Raghaven D, Scher HI, Leibel SA, et al, eds. *Principles and Practice of Genitourinary Oncology.* Philadelphia: Lippincott-Raven; 443-450, 1997.

Fleming ID, Cooper JS, Henson DE, et al, eds. Prostate. In: *AJCC Cancer Staging Manual.* 5th ed. New York: Lippincott-Raven, 1997.

Ford P, Easton DF, Bishop DT, et al. Risks of cancer in BRCA-1 mutation carriers. Breast Cancer Linkage Consortium. *Lancet* 343:692-695, 1994.

Foster LS, Jajodia P, Fournier G Jr, et al. The value of prostate specific antigen and transrectal ultrasound guided biopsy in detecting prostatic fossa recurrences following radical prostatectomy. *J Urol* 149:1024-1028, 1993.

Fowler JE Jr, Brooks J, Pandey P, et al. Variable histology of anastomotic biopsies with detectable prostate specific antigen after radical prostatectomy. *J Urol* 153:1011-1014, 1995.

Fowler JE Jr, Bigler SA, Bowman G, et al. Race and cause specific survival with prostate cancer: influence of clinical stage, Gleason score, age and treatment. *J Urol* 163:137-142, 2000.

Franks LM. Latent carcinoma of the prostate. *J Pathol Bacteriol* 68:603-616, 1954.

Frazier HA, Humphrey PA, Burchette JL, et al. Immunoreactive prostatic specific antigen in male periurethral glands. *J Urol* 147:246-248, 1992.

Freeman VL, Leszczak J, Cooper RS. Race and histologic grade of prostate cancer. *Prostate* 30:79-84, 1997.

Furr BJA, Kaisary AV. Antiandrogens. In: Kaisary AV, Murphy GP, Denis L, et al, eds. *Textbook of Prostate Cancer: Pathology, Diagnosis and Treatment.* London: Martin Dunitz; 277-290, 1999.

Gaddipati JP, McLeod DG, Sesterhenn IA, et al. Mutations of the p16 gene product are rare in prostate cancer. *Prostate* 30:188-194, 1997.

Gann PH, Hennekens CH, Sacks FM, et al. Prospective study of plasma fatty acids and risk of prostate cancer. *J Natl Cancer Inst* 86:281-286, 1994.

Gann PH, Hennekens CH, Stampfer MJ. A prospective evaluation of plasma prostate-specific antigen for detection of prostatic cancer. *JAMA* 273:289-294, 1995.

Gann PH, Ma J, Hennekens CH, et al. Circulating vitamin D metabolites in relation to subsequent development of prostate cancer. *Cancer Epidemiol Biomarkers Prev* 5:121-126, 1996.

Gann PH. Interpreting recent trends in prostate cancer incidence and mortality. *Epidemiology* 8:117-120, 1997.

Gann PH, Ma J, Giovannucci E, et al. Lower prostate cancer risk in men with elevated lycopene levels: results of a prospective analysis. *Cancer Res* 59:1225-1230, 1999.

Gao CL, Maheshwari S, Dean RC, et al. Blinded evaluation of reverse transcriptase-polymerase chain reaction prostate-specific antigen peripheral blood assay for molecular staging of prostate cancer. *Urology* 53:714-721, 1999A.

Gao CL, Dean RC, Pinto A, et al. Detection of circulating prostate specific antigen expressing prostatic cells in the bone marrow of radical prostatectomy patients by sensitive reverse transcriptase polymerase chain reaction. *J Urol* 161:1070-1076, 1999B.

Gaynor EP. Zur Frage des Prostatkrebses. *Virchows Arch Pathol Anat* 301:602-652, 1938.

Gee WF, Holtgrewe HL, Blute ML, et al. 1997 American Urological Association Gallup survey: Changes in diagnosis and management of prostate cancer and benign prostatic hyperplasia, and other practice trends from 1994 to 1997. *J Urol* 160:1804-1807, 1998.

Gelet A, Chapelon JY, Bouvier R, et al. Local control of prostate cancer by transrectal high intensity focused ultrasound therapy: preliminary results. *J Urol* 161:156-162, 1999.

George DJ, Kantoff PW. Prognostic factors in hormone refractory prostate cancer. *Urol Clin North Am* 26:303-310, 1999.

Gerber GS, Thisted RA, Chodak GW, et al. Results of radical prostatectomy in men with locally advanced prostate cancer: multi-institutional pooled analysis. *Eur Urol* 32:385-390, 1997.

Gibbons RP. Radical perineal prostatectomy. In: Walsh PC, Retik AB, Vaughan ED Jr, et al, eds. *Campbell's Urology.* 8th ed. Philadelphia: Saunders; 3131-3146, 2002.

Gibbs M, Stanford JL, McIndoe RA, et al. Evidence for a rare prostate cancer susceptibility locus at chromosome 1p36. *Am J Hum Genet* 64:776-787, 1999.

Giles G, Ireland P. Diet, nutrition and prostate cancer. *Int J Cancer* 10(suppl):13-17, 1997.

Gilliland FD, Hoffman RM, Hamilton A, et al. Predicting extracapsular extension of prostate cancer in men treated with radical prostatectomy. Results from the population based prostate cancer outcomes study. *J Urol* 162:1341-1345, 1999.

Giovannucci E, Rimm EB, Colditz GA, et al. A prospective study of dietary fat and risk of prostate cancer. *J Natl Cancer Inst* 85:1571-1579, 1993.

Giovannucci E. A review of epidemiologic studies of tomatoes, lycopene, and prostate cancer. *Exp Biol Med* 227:852-859, 2002.

Gleaves RC, Militzer RE. Carcinoma of the prostate with metastases. *J Urol* 33:235-251, 1935.

Glover FE Jr, Coffey DS, Douglas LL, et al. The epidemiology of prostate cancer in Jamaica. *J Urol* 159:1984-1987, 1998A.

Glover FE Jr, Coffey DS, Douglas LL, et al. Familial study of prostate cancer in Jamaica. *Urology* 52:441-443, 1998B.

Goldgar DE, Easton DF, Cannon-Albright LA, et al. Systematic population-based assessment of cancer risk in first-degree relatives of cancer probands. *J Natl Cancer Inst* 60:1600-1608, 1994.

Golimbu M, Morales P, Al-Askari S, et al. Extended pelvic lymphadenectomy for prostate cancer. *J Urol* 121:617-620, 1979.

Golz R, Schubert GE. Prostate specific antigen: immunoreactivity in urachal remnants. *J Urol* 141:1480-1482, 1989.

Goode EL, Stanford JL, Peters MA, et al. Clinical characteristics of prostate cancer in an analysis of linkage to four putative susceptibility loci. *Clin Cancer Res* 7:2739-2749, 2001.

Graham SD Jr, Napalkov P, Watts L, et al. Microvascular invasion of the seminal vesicles in adenocarcinoma of the prostate. *Prostate* 28:359-363, 1996.

Grayhack JT, Bockrath JM. Diagnosis of carcinoma of the prostate. *Urology* 17:54-60, 1981.

Grönberg H, Isaacs SD, Smith JR, et al. Characteristics of prostate cancer in families potentially linked to the hereditary prostate cancer 1 (HPC1) locus. *JAMA* 278:1251-1255, 1997A.

Grönberg H, Xu J, Smith JR, et al. Early age at diagnosis in families providing evidence of linkage to the hereditary prostate cancer locus (HPC1) on chromosome 1. *Cancer Res* 57:4707-4709, 1997B.

Grönberg H, Damber L, Tavelin B, et al. No difference in survival between sporadic, familial and hereditary prostate cancer. *Br J Urol* 82:564-567, 1998.

Guileyardo JM, Johnson WD, Welsh RA, et al. Prevalence of latent prostate carcinoma in two U.S. populations. *J Natl Cancer Inst* 65:311-316, 1980.

Han M, Partin AW, Pound CR, et al. Long-term biochemical disease-free and cancer-specific survival following anatomic radical retropubic prostatectomy. *Urol Clin North Am* 28:555-565, 2001.

Hanchette CL, Schwartz GG. Geographic patterns of prostate cancer: evidence for a protective effect of ultraviolet radiation. *Cancer* 70:2861-2869, 1992.

Hanus MC, Zagars GK, Pollack A. Familial prostate cancer: outcome following radiation therapy with or without adjuvant androgen ablation. *Int J Radiat Oncol Biol Phys* 43:379-383, 1999.

Harbitz TB, Haugen OA. Histology of the prostate in elderly men. A study in an autopsy series. *Acta Pathol Microbiol Scand* 80:756-768, 1972.

Hardt NS, Kaude JV, Hackett RL. Prostatic adenocarcinoma. Heterogeneity in sonographic appearance reflects heterogeneity in tumor histology. *J Urol Pathol* 1:173-192, 1993.

Hardy DO, Scher HI, Bogenreider T, et al. Androgen receptor CAG repeat lengths in prostate cancer: correlation with age of onset. *J Clin Endocrinol Metab* 81:4400-4405, 1996.

Harrington KJ, Spitzweg C, Bateman AR, et al. Gene therapy for prostate cancer: current status and future prospects. *J Urol* 166:1220-1233, 2001.

Hasui Y, Marutsuka K, Asada Y, et al. Relationship between serum prostate specific antigen and histological prostatitis in patients with benign prostatic hyperplasia. *Prostate* 25:91-96, 1994.

Heidenberg HB, Moul JW, Mostofi FK, et al. Clinically detected carcinoma of the prostate treated by radical prostatectomy in a 29-year-old man. *J Urol* 152:966-967, 1994.

Heinonen OP, Albanes D, Virtamo J, et al. Prostate cancer and supplementation with α-tocopherol and α-carotene: incidence and mortality in a controlled trial. *J Natl Cancer Inst* 90:440-446, 1998.

Heller JE. Prostatic acid phosphatase: its current clinical status. *J Urol* 137:1091-1103, 1987.

Herman JR, Adler HL, Aguilar-Cordova E, et al. In situ gene therapy for adenocarcinoma of the prostate: a phase I clinical trial. *Hum Gene Ther* 10:1239-1249, 1999.

Herold DM, Hanlon AL, Movsas B, et al. Age-related prostate cancer metastases. *Urology* 51:985-990, 1998.

Heston WDW. Gene therapy. In: Kaisary AV, Murphy GP, Denis L, et al, eds. *Textbook of Prostate Cancer. Pathology, Diagnosis and Treatment.* London: Martin Dunitz; 85-102, 1999.

Hirano D, Werahera PN, Crawford ED, et al. Morphological analysis and classification of latent prostate cancer using a 3-dimensional computer algorithm: analysis of tumor volume, grade, tumor doubling time and life expectancy. *J Urol* 159:1265-1269, 1998.

Hirst AE, Bergman RT. Carcinoma of the prostate in men 80 or more years old. *Cancer* 7:136-141, 1954.

Hoedemaeker RF, Rietbergen JBW, Kranse R, et al. Histopathological prostate cancer characteristics at radical prostatectomy after population based screening. *J Urol* 164:411-415, 2000.

Hølund B. Latent prostatic carcinoma in a consecutive autopsy series. *Scand J Urol Nephrol* 14:29-35, 1980.

Horniger W, Rogatsch H, Reissigl A, et al. Correlation between preoperative predictors and pathologic features in radical prostatectomy specimens in PSA-based screening. *Prostate* 40:56-61, 1999.

Howarth DJ, Aronson IB, Diamandis EP. Immunohistochemical localization of prostate-specific antigen in benign and malignant breast tissues. *Br J Cancer* 75:1646-1651, 1997.

Hudson MA, Bahnson RR, Catalona WJ. Clinical use of prostate specific antigen in patients with prostate cancer. *J Urol* 142:1011-1017, 1989.

Hudson PB, Finkle AL, Trifilio A, et al. Prostatic cancer. VIII. Detection of unsuspected adenocarcinoma in the aging male population. *JAMA* 155:426-429, 1954.

Huggins C, Hodges CV. Studies on prostatic cancer: (I) the effect of estrogen and of androgen injection on serum phosphates in metastatic carcinoma of the prostate. *Cancer Res* 1:293-297, 1941A.

Huggins C, Stevens RE, Hodges CV. Studies on prostatic cancer: (II) the effects of castration on advanced carcinoma of the prostate gland. *Arch Surg* 43:209, 1941B.

Huggins C, Johnson MA. Cancer of the bladder and prostate. *JAMA* 135:1146-1152, 1947.

Humphrey PA, Frazier HA, Vollmer RT, et al. Stratification of pathologic features in radical prostatectomy specimens that are predictive of elevated initial postoperative serum prostate-specific antigen levels. *Cancer* 71:1821-1827, 1993.

Humphrey PA, Keetch DW, Smith DS, et al. Prospective characterization of pathological features of prostatic carcinomas detected via serum prostate specific antigen based screening. *J Urol* 155:816-820, 1996.

Humphrey PA, Vollmer RT. Relationships between serum prostate-specific antigen and histopathologic appearances of prostate carcinoma. In: Foster CS, Bostwick DG, eds. *Pathology of the Prostate.* Philadelphia: WB Saunders; 253-281, 1998.

Immergut M, Flocks RH. Carcinoma of the prostate in patients less than 21-years-old. *J Urol* 95:724-727, 1966.

Ingles SA, Ross RK, Yu MC, et al. Association of prostate cancer risk with genetic polymorphisms in vitamin D receptor and androgen receptor. *J Natl Cancer Inst* 89:166-170, 1997.

Irani J, Millet C, Levillain P, et al. Serum-to-urinary prostate specific antigen ratio: its impact in distinguishing prostate cancer when serum prostate specific antigen level is 4 to 10 ng/mL. *J Urol* 157:185-188, 1997.

Isaacs WB, Bova GS. Prostate cancer. In: Vogelstein B, Kinzler KW, eds. *The Genetic Basis of Human Cancer.* New York: McGraw-Hill; 653-660, 1998.

Iselin CE, Box JW, Vollmer RT, et al. Surgical control of clinically localized prostate carcinoma is equivalent in African-American and white males. *Cancer* 83:2353-2360, 1998.

Iwakiri J, Grandbois K, Wehner N, et al. An analysis of urinary prostate specific antigen before and after radical prostatectomy: evidence for secretion of prostate specific antigen by the periurethral glands. *J Urol* 149:783-786, 1993.

Jadeja NA, Dogra PN, Gupta NP. Carcinoma of the prostate in young patients: a report of two cases. *Urol Int* 52:48-51, 1994.

James GK, Pudek M, Berean KW, et al. Salivary duct carcinoma secreting prostate-specific antigen. *Am J Clin Pathol* 106:242-247, 1996.

Jemal A, Thomas A, Murray T, et al. Cancer statistics 2002. *CA Cancer J Clin* 52:23-47, 2002.

Jewett HJ. Significance of the palpable prostatic nodule. *JAMA* 160:838-839, 1956.

Jung K, Brux B, Lein M, et al. Determination of alpha1-antichymotrypsin-PSA complex in serum does not improve the differentiation between benign prostatic hyperplasia and prostate cancer compared with total PSA and percent free PSA. *Urology* 53:1160-1168, 1999.

Kabalin JN, McNeal JE, Price HM, et al. Unsuspected adenocarcinoma of the prostate in patients undergoing cystoprostatectomy for other causes: incidence, histology and morphometric observations. *J Urol* 141:1091-1094, 1989.

Kahler JE. Carcinoma of the prostate gland: a pathologic study. *J Urol* 41:557-574, 1939.

Kahn D, Williams RD, Manyak MJ, et al. 111-Indium-capromab pendetide in the evaluation of patients with residual or recurrent prostate cancer after radical prostatectomy. *J Urol* 159:2041-2046, 1998.

Kamoshida S, Tsutsumi Y. Extraprostatic localization of prostatic acid phosphatase and prostate specific antigen: distribution in cloacogenic glandular epithelium and sex-dependent expression in human anal gland. *Hum Pathol* 21:1108-1111, 1990.

Karube K. Study of latent carcinoma of the prostate in the Japanese based on necropsy material. *Tohoku J Exp Med* 74:265-285, 1961.

Kattan MW, Stapleton AM, Wheeler TM, et al. Evaluation of a nomogram used to predict the pathologic stage of clinically localized prostate carcinoma. *Cancer* 79:528-537, 1997.

Kattan MW, Eastham JA, Stapleton AM, et al. A preoperative nomogram for disease recurrence following radical prostatectomy for prostate cancer. *J Natl Cancer Inst* 90:766-771, 1998.

Kattan MW, Wheeler TM, Scardino PT. Postoperative nomogram for disease recurrence after radical prostatectomy for prostate cancer. *J Clin Oncol* 17:1499-1507, 1999.

Kattan MW, Potters L, Blasko JC, et al. Pretreatment nomogram for predicting freedom from recurrence after permanent prostate brachytherapy in prostate cancer. *Urology* 58:393-399, 2001.

Keetch DW, Catalona WJ, Smith DS. Serial prostatic biopsies in men with persistently elevated serum prostate specific antigen values. *J Urol* 151:1571-1574, 1994.

Keetch DW, Rice JP, Suarez BK, et al. Familial aspects of prostate cancer: a case control study. *J Urol* 154:2100-2102, 1995.

Keetch DW, Humphrey PA, Smith DS, et al. Clinical and pathological features of hereditary prostate cancer. *J Urol* 155:1841-1843, 1996.

Kelly WK, Slovin S, Scher HI. Steroid hormone withdrawal syndromes. Pathophysiology and clinical significance. *Urol Clin North Am* 24:421-431, 1997.

Khoury S. Testicular androgen ablation. In: Kaisary AV, Murphy GP, Denis L, et al, eds. *Textbook of Prostate Cancer. Pathology, Diagnosis and Treatment.* London: Martin Dunitz; 291-302, 1999.

Kim ED, Grayhack JT. Clinical symptoms and signs of prostate cancer. In: Vogelzang NJ, Scardino PT, Shipley WU, et al, eds. *Comprehensive Textbook of Genitourinary Oncology.* Baltimore: Williams & Wilkins; 557-564, 1996.

Kim JA, Kuban DA, El-Mahdi AM, et al. Carcinoma of the prostate: race as a prognostic indicator in definitive radiation therapy. *Radiology* 194:545-549, 1995.

Kleer E, Larson-Keller JJ, Zinke H, et al. Ability of preoperative serum prostate-specific antigen value to predict pathology stage and DNA ploidy. *Urology* 41:207-216, 1993.

Klein EA, Thompson IM, Lippman SM, et al. SELECT: the next prostate cancer prevention trial. *J Urol* 166:1311-1315, 2001.

Klein LT, Lowe FC. The effects of prostatic manipulation on prostate-specific antigen levels. *Urol Clin North Am* 24:293-297, 1997.

Koeneman KS, Yeung F, Chung LW. Osteomimetic properties of prostate cancer cells: a hypothesis supporting the predilection of prostate cancer metastasis and growth in the bone environment. *Prostate* 39:246-261, 1999.

Kolonel LN, Yoshizawa CN, Hankin JH. Diet and prostatic cancer: a case-control study in Hawaii. *Am J Epidemiol* 127:999-1012, 1988.

Kolonel LN, Nomura AMY, Cooney RV. Dietary fat and prostate cancer: current status. *J Natl Cancer Inst* 91:414-428, 1999.

Konety BR, Tewari A, Howard RJ, et al. Prostate cancer in the post-transplant population. *Urology* 52:428-432, 1998.

Konishi N, Hiasa Y, Tsuzuki T, et al. Comparison of ras activation in prostate carcinoma in Japanese and American men. *Prostate* 30:53-57, 1997.

Kothari PS, Scardino PT, Ohori M, et al. Incidence, location and significance of periprostatic and periseminal vesicle lymph nodes in prostate cancer. *Am J Surg Pathol* 25:1429-1432, 2001.

Kupelian PA, Klein EA, Witte JS, et al. Familial prostate cancer: a different disease? *J Urol* 158:2197-2207, 1997A.

Kupelian PA, Kupelian VA, Witte JS, et al. Family history of prostate cancer in patients with localized prostate cancer: an independent predictor of treatment outcome. *J Clin Oncol* 15:1478-1480, 1997B.

Latil A, Lidereau R. Genetic aspects of prostate cancer. *Virchows Arch* 432:389-406, 1998.

Lee CT, Oesterling JE. Using prostate-specific antigen to eliminate the staging radionuclide bone scan. *Urol Clin North Am* 24:389-394, 1997.

Lee DH, Maru N, Kim I, et al. Racial differences in the size and grade of prostate cancer tumor foci [abstract]. *J Urol* 161(suppl):73, 1999.

Lee F, Torp-Pedersen ST, Carroll JT, et al. Use of transrectal ultrasound and prostate-specific antigen in diagnosis of prostatic intraepithelial neoplasia. *Urology* 34(6 suppl):4-8, 1989.

Lesko SM, Louik C, Vezina R, et al. Vasectomy and prostate cancer. *J Urol* 161:1848-1853, 1999.

Levesque MA, Yu H, D'Costa M, et al. Prostate specific antigen expression by various tumors. *J Clin Lab Anal* 9:123-128, 1995.

Liavåg I. Atrophy and regeneration in the pathogenesis of prostatic carcinoma. *Acta Pathol Microbiol Scand* 73:338-350, 1968.

Linder NM, Greene MH, Mayo Familial Cancer Program. The concise handbook of family cancer syndromes. *J Natl Cancer Inst* 90:1039-1071, 1998.

Long JP, Bahn D, Lee F, et al. Five-year retrospective, multi-institutional pooled analysis of cancer-related outcomes after cryosurgical ablation of the prostate. *Urology* 57:518-523, 2001.

Lowe FC, Trauzzi SJ. Prostatic acid phosphatase in 1993. *Urol Clin North Am* 20:589-595, 1993.

Lumey LH, Pittman B, Zang EA, et al. Cigarette smoking and prostate cancer: no relation with six measures of lifetime smoking habits in a large case-control study among U.S. whites. *Prostate* 33:195-200, 1997.

Lundwall A, Lilja H. Molecular cloning of human prostate specific antigen cDNA. *FEBS Lett* 214:317-322, 1987.

Määtänen L, Auvinen A, Stenman UH, et al. Three-year results of the Finnish prostate cancer screening trial. *J Natl Cancer Inst* 93:552-553, 2001.

Mahadevia PS, Koss LG, Tar IJ. Prostatic involvement in bladder cancer. Prostate mapping in 20 cystoprostatectomy specimens. *Cancer* 58:2096-2102, 1986.

Mannello F, Malatesta M, Luchetti F, et al. Immunoreactivity, ultrastructural localization, and transcript expression of prostate-specific antigen in human neuroblastoma cell lines. *Clin Chem* 45:78-84, 1999.

Matzkin H, Eber P, Todd B, et al. Prognostic significance of changes in prostate-specific markers after endocrine treatment of stage D2 prostatic cancer. *Cancer* 70:2302-2309, 1992.

McCormack RT, Rittenhouse HG, Finlay JA, et al. Molecular forms of prostate-specific antigen and the human kallikrein gene family: a new era. *Urology* 45:729-744, 1995.

McNeal JE. Regional morphology and pathology of the prostate. *Am J Clin Pathol* 49:347-357, 1968.

McNeal JE, Villers AA, Redwine EA, et al. Capsular penetration in prostate cancer. Significance for natural history and treatment. *Am J Surg Pathol* 14:240-247, 1990.

McNeal JE, Yemoto CEM. Significance of demonstrable vascular space invasion for progression of prostatic adenocarcinoma. *Am J Surg Pathol* 20:1351-1360, 1996.

McNeal JE, Haillot O. Patterns of spread of adenocarcinoma in the prostate as related to cancer volume. *Prostate* 49:48-57, 2001.

Melchior SW, Corey E, Ellis WJ, et al. Early tumor cell dissemination in patients with clinically localized carcinoma of the prostate. *Clin Cancer Res* 3:249-256, 1997.

Melegos DN, Yu H, Allen LC, et al. Prostate-specific antigen in amniotic fluid of normal and abnormal pregnancies. *Clin Biochem* 29:555-562, 1996.

Merrill RM, Weed DL, Feuer EJ. The lifetime risk of developing prostate cancer in white and black men. *Cancer Epidemiol Biomarkers Prev* 6:763-768, 1997.

Messing EM, Manola J, Sarosdy M, et al. Immediate hormonal therapy compared with observation after radical prostatectomy and pelvic lymphadenectomy in men with node-positive prostate cancer. *N Engl J Med* 341:1781-1788, 1999.

Mettlin C, Selenskas S, Natarajan N, et al. Beta-carotene and animal fats and their relationship to prostate cancer risk. A case-control study. *Cancer* 64:605-612, 1989.

Mettlin CJ, Murphy GP, Ho R, et al. The National Cancer Data Base report on longitudinal observations on prostate cancer. *Cancer* 77:2162-2166, 1996.

Mettlin C. Changes in patterns of prostate cancer care in the United States: results of American College of Surgeons Commission on Cancer Studies, 1974-1993. *Prostate* 32:221-226, 1997.

Mettlin CJ, Murphy GP. Why is the prostate cancer death rate declining in the United States? *Cancer* 82:249-251, 1998.

Meyer F, Moore L, Bairati I, et al. Downward trend in prostate cancer mortality in Quebec and Canada. *J Urol* 161:1189-1191, 1999.

Michigan S, Catalona WJ. Ureteral obstruction from prostatic carcinoma: response to endocrine and radiation therapy. *J Urol* 118:733-738, 1977.

Miller MK, Unger PD, Bleiweiss IJ. Immunohistochemical analysis of prostate-specific antigen in breast cancer. *Breast Cancer Res Treat* 68:111-116, 2001.

Mills PK, Beeson WL, Phillips RL, et al. Cohort study of diet, lifestyle, and prostate cancer in Adventist men. *Cancer* 64:598-604, 1989.

Monne M, Croce CM, Yu H, et al. Molecular characterization of prostate-specific antigen messenger RNA expressed in breast tumors. *Cancer Res* 54:6344-6347, 1994.

Montie JE, Wood DP Jr, Pontes JE, et al. Adenocarcinoma of the prostate in cystoprostatectomy specimens removed for bladder cancer. *Cancer* 63:381-385, 1989.

Montie JE, Pienta KJ. A unifying model to explain the increased incidence and higher mortality of prostate cancer in black men. *Urology* 53:1073-1076, 1999.

Moore R. The morphology of small prostatic carcinoma. *J Urol* 33:224-234, 1935.

Moul JW, Douglas TH, McCarthy WF, et al. Black race is an adverse prognostic factor for prostate cancer recurrence following radical prostatectomy in an equal access health care setting. *J Urol* 155:1667-1673, 1996.

Moutzouris G, Barbatis C, Plastiras D, et al. Incidence and histological findings of unsuspected prostatic adenocarcinoma in radical cystoprostatectomy for transitional cell carcinoma of the bladder. *Scand J Urol Nephrol* 33:27-30, 1999.

Moyad MA, Pienta KJ, eds. Nontraditional cancer treatments. *Semin Urol Oncol* 17:70-102, 1999.

Muir EG. Carcinoma of the prostate. *Lancet* 1:667-672, 1934.

Murphy GP, Tjoa BA, Simmons SJ, et al. Infusion of dendritic cells pulsed with HLA-A2–specific prostate-specific membrane antigen peptides: a phase II prostate cancer vaccine trial involving patients with hormone-refractory metastatic disease. *Prostate* 38:73-78, 1999.

Nadler RB, Humphrey PA, Smith DS, et al. Effect of inflammation and benign prostatic hyperplasia on elevated serum prostate specific antigen levels. *J Urol* 154:407-413, 1995.

Neal DE Jr, Clejan S, Sarma D, et al. Prostate specific antigen and prostatitis I: effect of prostatitis on serum PSA in the human and nonhuman primate. *Prostate* 20:105-111, 1992.

Nowels K, Kent E, Rinsho K, et al. Prostate specific antigen and acid phosphatase-reactive cells in cystitis cystica and glandularis. *Arch Pathol Lab Med* 112:734-737, 1988.

Öbek C, Louis P, Civantos F, et al. Comparison of digital rectal examination and biopsy results with the radical prostatectomy specimen. *J Urol* 161:494-499, 1999.

O'Dowd GJ, Veltri RW, Orozco R, et al. Update on the appropriate staging evaluation for newly diagnosed prostate cancer. *J Urol* 158:687-698, 1997.

Oesterling JE. Prostate specific antigen: a critical assessment of the most useful tumor marker for adenocarcinoma of the prostate. *J Urol* 145:907-923, 1991.

Oesterling JE, Rice DC, Glenski WJ, et al. Effect of cystoscopy, prostate biopsy, and transurethral resection of prostate on serum prostate-specific antigen concentration. *Urology* 42:276-282, 1993.

Oh WK, Kantoff PW. Management of hormone refractory prostate cancer: current standards and future prospects. *J Urol* 160:1220-1229, 1998.

Ohori M, Scardino PT, Lapin SL, et al. The mechanisms and prognostic significance of seminal vesicle involvement by prostate cancer. *Am J Surg Pathol* 17:1252-1261, 1993.

Ohori M, Wheeler TM, Scardino PT. The new American Joint Committee on Cancer and International Union Against Cancer TNM classification of prostate cancer. Clinicopathologic correlations. *Cancer* 74:101-114, 1994A.

Ohori M, Wheeler TM, Dunn JK, et al. The pathological features and prognosis of prostate cancer detectable with current diagnostic tests. *J Urol* 152:1714-1720, 1994B.

Oota K. Latent carcinoma of the prostate among the Japanese. *Acta Un Int Cancer* 17:952-957, 1961.

Orozco R, O'Dowd G, Del Villar R, et al. Systematic sextant biopsy findings of prostatic adenocarcinoma in US Hispanics and whites. *J Urol Pathol* 6:43-50, 1997.

Page WF, Braun MM, Partin AW, et al. Heredity and prostate cancer: a study of World War II veteran twins. *Prostate* 33:240-245, 1997.

Paget S. The distribution of secondary growths in cancer of the breast. *Lancet* 1:571-573, 1889.

Pannek J, Rittenhouse HG, Evans CL, et al. Molecular forms of prostate-specific antigen and human kallikrein 2 (hK2) in urine are not clinically useful for early detection and staging of prostate cancer. *Urology* 50:715-721, 1997.

Pannek J, Rittenhouse HG, Chan DW, et al. The use of percent free prostate specific antigen for staging clinically localized prostate cancer. *J Urol* 159:1238-1242, 1998.

Parkin DM, Pisani P, Ferlay J. Global cancer statistics. *CA Cancer J Clin* 49:33-64, 1999.

Partin AW, Carter HB, Chan DW, et al. Prostate specific antigen in the staging of localized prostate cancer: influence of tumor differentiation, tumor volume and benign hyperplasia. *J Urol* 143:747-752, 1990.

Partin AW, Steinberg GD, Pitcock RV, et al. Use of nuclear morphometry, Gleason histologic scoring, clinical stage, and age to predict disease-free survival among patients with prostate cancer. *Cancer* 70:161-168, 1992.

Partin AW, Yoo J, Carter HB, et al. The use of prostate specific antigen, clinical stage and Gleason score to predict pathological stage in men with localized prostate cancer. *J Urol* 150:110-114, 1993.

Partin AW, Pearson JD, Landis PK, et al. Evaluation of serum prostate-specific antigen velocity after radical prostatectomy to distinguish local recurrence from distant metastases. *Urology* 43:649-659, 1994.

Partin AW, Kattan MW, Subong ENP, et al. Combination of prostate-specific antigen, clinical stage, and Gleason score to predict pathological stage of localized prostate cancer: a multi-institutional update. *JAMA* 277:1445-1451, 1997.

Partin AW, Catalona WJ, Finlay JA, et al. Use of human glandular kallikrein 2 for the detection of prostate cancer: preliminary analysis. *Urology* 54:839-845, 1999.

Partin AW, Mangold ZA, Lamm DM, et al. Contemporary update of prostate cancer staging nomograms (Partin tables) for the new millenium. *Urology* 58:843-848, 2001.

Paulson DF. Impact of radical prostatectomy in the management of clinically localized disease. *J Urol* 152:1826-1830, 1994.

Penn I. The problem of cancer in organ transplant recipients: an overview. *Transpl Sci* 4:23-32, 1994.

Penson DF, Grossfeld GD, Li YP, et al. How well does the Partin nomogram predict pathological stage after radical prostatectomy in a community based population? Results of the cancer of the prostate strategic urological research endevor. *J Urol* 167:1653-1657, 2002.

Perrotti M, Pantuck A, Rabbani F, et al. Review of staging modalities in clinically localized prostate cancer. *Urology* 54:208-214, 1999.

Petrylak DP. Chemotherapy for hormone refractory prostate cancer. *Semin Urol Oncol* 20:31-35, 2002.

Pettaway CA, Troncoso P, Ramirez EI, et al. Prostate specific antigen and pathological features of prostate cancer in black and white patients: a comparative study based on radical prostatectomy specimens. *J Urol* 160:437-442, 1998.

Philips TH, Thompson IM. Digital rectal examination and carcinoma of the prostate. *Urol Clin North Am* 18:459-465, 1991.

Pienta KJ, Demers R, Hoff M, et al. Effect of age race on the survival of men with prostate cancer in the Metropolitan Detroit tricounty area, 1973 to 1987. *Urology* 45:93-101, 1995.

Pienta KJ. Etiology, epidemiology, and prevention of carcinoma of the prostate. In: Walsh PC, Retik AB, Vaughan ED Jr, et al, eds. *Campbell's Urology.* 7th ed. Philadelphia: WB Saunders; 2489-2496, 1998.

Pinto JE, Babaian RJ, Troncoso P. Prostatic carcinoma metastatic to periprostatic lymph nodes [abstract]. *Mod Pathol* 13:98A, 2000.

Pisani P, Bray F, Parkin DM, et al. Estimates of the worldwide prevalence of cancer in 1990 for 25 sites in the adult population. *Int J Cancer* 97:72-81, 2002.

Polascik TJ, Pearson JD, Partin AW. Multivariate models as predictors of pathological stage using Gleason score, clinical stage, and serum prostate-specific antigen. *Semin Urol Oncol* 16:160-171, 1998.

Polascik TJ, Oesterling JI, Partin AW. Prostate specific antigen: a decade of discovery—what we have learned and where we are going. *J Urol* 162:293-306, 1999.

Pollen JJ, Dreilinger A. Immunohistochemical identification of prostatic acid phosphatase and prostate specific antigen in female periurethral glands. *Urology* 23:303-304, 1984.

Porter AT, Hart KB. Radiation therapy in the treatment of localized/organ-confined prostate cancer. In: Kaisary AV, Murphy GP, Denis L, et al, eds. *Textbook of Prostate Cancer. Pathology, Diagnosis, and Treatment.* London: Martin Dunitz; 231-247, 1999.

Pound CR, Partin AW, Epstein JI, et al. Prostate-specific antigen after anatomic radical retropubic prostatectomy: patterns of recurrence and cancer control. *Urol Clin North Am* 24:395-406, 1997.

Pound CR, Partin AW, Eisenberger MA, et al. Natural history of progression after PSA elevation following radical prostatectomy. *JAMA* 281:1591-1597, 1999.

Pritchett TR, Moreno J, Warner NE, et al. Unsuspected prostatic adenocarcinoma in patients who have undergone radical cystoprostatectomy for transitional cell carcinoma of the bladder. *J Urol* 139:1214-1216, 1988.

Prorok PC, Andriole GL, Bresalier RS, et al. Design of the prostate, lung, colorectal and ovarian cancer screening trial. *Controlled Clin Trials* 21(6 suppl):273S-309S, 2000.

Rabbani F, Stroumbakis N, Kava BR, et al. Incidence and clinical significance of false-negative sextant prostate biopsies. *J Urol* 159:1247-1250, 1998.

Ragde H, Korb L. Brachytherapy for clinically localized prostate cancer. *Semin Surg Oncol* 18:45-51, 2000.

Ramos CG, Carvahal GF, Smith DS, et al. Clinical and pathologic characteristics, and recurrence rates of stage T1c versus T2a or T2b prostate cancer. *J Urol* 161:1525-1529, 1999.

Ravery V. The significance of recurrent PSA after radical prostatectomy: benign versus malignant sources. *Semin Urol Oncol* 17:127-129, 1999.

Reissigl A, Bartsch G. Prostate-specific antigen as a screening test. The Austrian experience. *Urol Clin North Am* 24:315-321, 1997.

Reiter RE, deKernion JB. Epidemiology, etiology, and prevention of prostate cancer. In: Walsh PC, Retik AB, Vaughan ED Jr, et al, eds. *Campbell's Urology*. 8th ed. Philadelphia: Saunders; 3003-3024, 2002.

Rich AR. On the frequency of occurrence of occult carcinoma of the prostate. *J Urol* 33:215-223, 1935.

Richardson TD, Oesterling JE. Age-specific reference ranges for serum prostate-specific antigen. *Urol Clin North Am* 24:339-351, 1997.

Richie JP, Catalona WJ, Ahmann FR, et al. Effect of patient age on early detection of prostate cancer with serum prostate-specific antigen and digital rectal examination. *Urology* 42:365-374, 1993.

Riegman PHJ, Vlietstra RJ, van der Korput JAGM, et al. Characterization of the prostate-specific antigen gene: a novel human kallikrein gene. *Biochem Biophys Res Commun* 159:95-102, 1989.

Ries LAG, Miller BA, Hankey BF, et al, eds. *SEER Cancer Statistics Review, 1973-1991: Tables and Graphs.* NIH publication 94-2789. Bethesda: National Cancer Institute; 11, 1994.

Ries LA, Kosary CL, Hankey BF, et al. *SEER Cancer Statistics Review, 1973-1995.* http://www.seer.ims.nci.nih.gov/publications/CSR7395. Bethesda: National Cancer Institute; 1998.

Rietbergen JBW, Hoedemaeker RF, Kruger AEB, et al. The changing pattern of prostate cancer at the time of diagnosis: characteristics of screen detected cancer in a population based screening study. *J Urol* 161:1192-1198, 1999.

Rifkin MD, McGlynn ET, Choi H. Echogenicity of prostate cancer correlated with histologic grade and stromal fibrosis: endorectal US studies. *Radiology* 170:549-552, 1989.

Rifkin MD, Zerhouni EA, Gatsonis CA, et al. Comparison of magnetic resonance imaging and ultrasonography in staging of early prostate cancer. Results of a multi-institutional cooperative trial. *N Engl J Med* 323:621-626, 1990.

Rittenhouse HG, Chan DW. Can complexed PSA be used as a single test for detecting prostate cancer? *Urology* 54:4-5, 1999.

Roberts RO, Bergstralh EJ, Katusic SK, et al. Decline in prostate cancer mortality from 1980 to 1997, and an update on incidence trends in Olmsted County, Minnesota. *J Urol* 161:529-533, 1999.

Roberts WW, Bergstralh EJ, Blute ML, et al. Contemporary identification of patients at high risk of early prostate cancer recurrence after radical retropubic prostatectomy. *Urology* 57:1033-1037, 2001.

Rodin AE, Larson DL, Roberts DK. Nature of the perineal space invaded by prostatic carcinoma. *Cancer* 20:1772-1779, 1967.

Rodriguez C, Calle EE, Tatham LM, et al. Family history of breast cancer as a predictor for fatal prostate cancer. *Epidemiology* 9:525-529, 1998.

Rohan TE, Hislop TG, Howe GR, et al. Cigarette smoking and risk of prostate cancer: a population-based case-control study in Ontario and British Columbia, Canada. *Eur J Cancer Prev* 6:382-388, 1997.

Romas NA, Kwan DJ. Prostatic acid phosphatase. *Urol Clin North Am* 20:581-538, 1993.

Ronnett BM, Carmichael MJ, Carter HB, et al. Does high-grade prostatic intraepithelial neoplasia result in elevated serum prostate specific antigen levels? *J Urol* 150:386-389, 1993.

Rosai J, ed. *Guiding the Surgeon's Hand. The History of American Surgical Pathology.* Washington, DC: The American Registry of Pathology, 1997.

Rosen G. Beginnings of surgical biopsy. *Am J Surg Pathol* 1:361-64, 1977.

Rukstalis DB, Lawton CA, Brendler CB. Management options for patients with lymph node metastasis from prostate cancer. In: Vogelzang NJ, Scardino PT, Shipley WU, et al, eds. *Comprehensive Textbook of Genitourinary Oncology.* Baltimore: Williams & Wilkins; 557-564, 1996.

Ruska KM, Partin AW, Epstein JI, et al. Adenocarcinoma of the prostate in men younger than 40 years of age: diagnosis and treatment with emphasis on radical prostatectomy findings. *Urology* 53:1179-1183, 1999.

Saitoh H, Hida M, Shimbo T, et al. Metastatic patterns of prostatic cancer. Correlation between sites and number of organs involved. *Cancer* 54:3078-3084, 1984.

Sakr WA, Haas GP, Cassin BF, et al. The frequency of carcinoma and intraepithelial neoplasia of the prostate in young male patients. *J Urol* 150:379-385, 1993.

Sakr WA, Grignon DJ, Crissman JP, et al. High-grade prostatic intraepithelial neoplasia (HGPIN) and prostatic adenocarcinoma between the ages of 20-69: an autopsy study of 249 cases. *In Vivo* 8:439-443, 1994.

Sakr WA, Grignon DJ, Haas GP. Pathology of pre-malignant lesions and carcinoma of the prostate in African-American and white males. *Semin Urol Oncol* 16:214-220, 1998.

Sakr W, Permick N, Butler C, et al. The prevalence of high grade, clinically occult prostatic adenocarcinoma and its relationship to high grade PIN [abstract]. *Mod Pathol* 13:109A, 2000.

Salomao DR, Graham SD, Bostwick DG. Microvascular invasion in prostate cancer correlates with pathologic stage. *Arch Pathol Lab Med* 119:1050-1054, 1995.

Sandhu DP, Munson KW, Benghiat A, et al. Natural history and prognosis of prostate carcinoma in adolescents and men under 35 years of age. *Br J Urol* 69:525-529, 1992.

Scardino PT, Weaver R, Hudson MA. Early detection of prostate cancer. *Hum Pathol* 23:211-222, 1992.

Schaid DJ, McDonnell SK, Blute ML, et al. Evidence for autosomal dominant inheritance of prostate cancer. *Am J Hum Genet* 62:1425-1438, 1998.

Schellhammer PF, El-Mahdi AM, Kuban DA, et al. Prostate-specific antigen after radiation therapy: prognosis by pretreatment level and post-treatment nadir. *Urol Clin North Am* 24:407-414, 1997.

Schröeder FH, Belt E. Carcinoma of the prostate: a study of 213 patients with Stage C tumors treated by total perineal prostatectomy. *J Urol* 114:257-260, 1975.

Schröeder FH, van der Maas P, Beemsterboer P, et al. Evaluation of the digital rectal examination as a screening test for prostate cancer. *J Natl Cancer Inst* 90:1817-1823, 1998.

Schröeder FH. Hormonal therapy of prostate cancer. In: Walsh PC, Retik AB, Vaughan ED Jr, et al, eds. *Campbell's Urology.* 8th ed. Philadelphia: Saunders; 3182-3208, 2002.

Schulman CC, Ekane S, Zlotta AR. Nutrition and prostate cancer: evidence or suspicion? *Urology* 58:318-334, 2001.

Seay TM, Blute ML, Zincke H. Long-term outcome in patients with pTxN+ adenocarcinoma of prostate treated with radical prostatectomy and early androgen ablation. *J Urol* 159:357-364, 1998.

SEERP (Surveillance, Epidemiology, and End Results [SEER] Program). Age-adjusted U.S. cancer death rates. *J Natl Cancer Inst* 89:12, 1997.

Seidman H, Mushinski MH, Gelb SK, et al. Probabilities of eventually developing or dying of cancer: United States, 1985. *CA Cancer J Clin* 35:36-56, 1985.

Serth J, Panitz F, Paeslack U, et al. Increased levels of human papillomavirus type 16 DNA in a subset of prostate cancers. *Cancer Res* 59:823-825, 1999.

Sesterhenn IA, Mostofi FK, Mattrey RR, et al. Preliminary results of three-dimensional reconstruction of previously imaged prostates. Prostate 4(suppl):33-41, 1992.

Shimada H, Misugi K, Sasaki Y, et al. Carcinoma of the prostate in childhood and adolescence: report of a case and review of the literature. *Cancer* 46:2534-2542, 1980.

Shinohara K, Wheeler TM, Scardino PT. The appearance of prostate cancer on transrectal ultrasonography: correlation of imaging and pathological examinations. *J Urol* 142:76-82, 1989.

Shipley WU, Thames HD, Sandler HM, et al. Radiation therapy for clinically localized prostate cancer. A multi-institutional pooled analysis. *JAMA* 281:1598-1604, 1999.

Shiraishi T, Muneyuki T, Fukutome K, et al. Mutations of ras gene genes are relatively frequent in Japanese prostate cancers: pointing to genetic differences between populations. *Anticancer Res* 18:2789-2792, 1998.

Shreve PD, Grossman HB, Gross MD, et al. Metastatic prostate cancer-initial findings of PET with 2-deoxy-2-[F-18] fluoro-D-glucose. *Radiology* 199:751-756, 1996.

Sika JV, Lindquist HD. Relationship of needle biopsy diagnosis of prostate to clinical signs of prostate cancer: an evaluation of 300 cases. *J Urol* 89:737-745, 1963.

Silvestri F, Bussani R, Pavletic N, et al. Neoplastic and borderline lesions of the prostate: Autopsy study and epidemiological data. *Pathol Res Pract* 191:908-916, 1995.

Smith CV, Bauer JJ, Connelly RR, et al. Prostate cancer in men age 50 years or younger: a review of the department of defense center for prostate disease research multicenter prostate cancer database. *J Urol* 164:1964-1967, 2000.

Smith DS, Catalona WJ. Rate of change in serum prostate specific antigen levels as a method for prostate cancer detection. *J Urol* 152:1163-1167, 1994.

Smith DS, Catalona WJ. Interexaminer variability of digital rectal examination in detecting prostate cancer. *Urology* 45:70-74, 1995.

Smith DS, Humphrey PA, Catalona WJ. The early detection of prostate carcinoma with prostate specific antigen: the Washington University experience. *Cancer* 80:1852-1856, 1997A.

Smith DS, Bullock AD, Catalona WJ. Racial differences in operating characteristics of prostate cancer screening tests. *J Urol* 158:1861-1866, 1997B.

Smith DC, Pienta KJ. The use of prostate-specific antigen as a surrogate end point in the treatment of patients with hormone refractory prostate cancer. *Urol Clin North Am* 24:433-437, 1997C.

Smith DS, Carvalhal GF, Mager DF, et al. Use of lower prostate specific antigen cutoffs for prostate cancer screening in black and white men. *J Urol* 160:1734-1738, 1998.

Smith JA Jr, Scardino PT, Resnick MI, et al. Transrectal ultrasound versus digital rectal examination for the staging of carcinoma of the prostate: results of a prospective, multi-institutional trial. *J Urol* 157:902-906, 1997.

Smith JA Jr, Soloway MS, Young MJ. Complications of advanced prostate cancer. *Urology* 54(suppl 6A):8-14, 1999.

Smith JR, Freije D, Carpten JD, et al. Major susceptibility locus for prostate cancer on chromosome l suggested by a genome-wide search. *Science* 274:1371-1374, 1996.

Smith PH, Bono A, Calais da Silva F, et al. Some limitations of the radioisotope bone scan in patients with metastatic prostate cancer. A subanalysis of EORTC trial 30853. The EORTC Urological Group. *Cancer* 66(5 suppl):1009-1016, 1990.

Snowdon DA, Phillips RL, Choi W. Diet, obesity and risk of fatal prostate cancer. *Am J Epidemiol* 120:244-250, 1984.

Sokoll LJ, Chan DW. Total, free, and complexed PSA: analysis and clinical utility. *J Clin Ligand Assay* 21:171-179, 1998.

Southwick PC, Catalona WJ, Partin AW, et al. Prediction of post-radical prostatectomy pathological outcome for stage T1c prostate cancer with percent free prostate specific antigen: a prospective multicenter clinical trial. *J Urol* 162:1346-1351, 1999.

Sovak M, Seligman AL, Konas M, et al. Herbal composition PC-SPES for management of prostate cancer: identification of active principles. *J Natl Cancer Inst* 94:1261-1263, 2002.

Spigelman SS, McNeal JE, Freiha FS, et al. Rectal examination in volume determination of carcinoma of the prostate: clinical and anatomical correlations. *J Urol* 136:1228-1230, 1986.

Spitz MR, Currier RD, Fueger JJ, et al. Familial patterns of prostate cancer: a case-control analysis. *J Urol* 146:1305-1307, 1991.

Stamey TA, Yang N, Hay AR, et al. Prostate-specific antigen as a serum marker for adenocarcinoma of the prostate. *N Engl J Med* 317:909-916, 1987.

Stamey TA, McNeal JE, Freiha FS, et al. Morphometric and clinical studies on 68 consecutive radical prostatectomies. *J Urol* 139:1235-1241, 1988.

Stamey TA, Kabalin JN, Ferrari M, et al. Prostate specific antigen in the diagnosis and treatment of adenocarcinoma of the prostate. IV. Anti-androgen treated patients. *J Urol* 141:1088-1090, 1989.

Stamey TA, Sözen TS, Yemoto CM, et al. Classification of localized untreated prostate cancer based on 791 men treated only with radical prostatectomy: common ground for therapeutic trials and TNM subgroups. *J Urol* 159:2009-2012, 1998A.

Stamey TA, Donaldson AN, Yemoto CE, et al. Histological and clinical findings in 896 consecutive prostates treated only with radical retropubic prostatectomy: epidemiologic significance of annual changes. *J Urol* 160:2412-2417, 1998B.

Stamey TA, McNeal JE, Yemoto CM, et al. Biological determinants of cancer progression in men with prostate cancer. *JAMA* 281:1395-1400, 1999.

Stanford JL, Just JJ, Gibbs M, et al. Polymorphic repeats in the androgen receptor gene: molecular markers of prostate cancer risk. *Cancer Res* 57:1194-1198, 1997.

Stattin P, Bylund A, Rinaldi S, et al. Plasma insulin-like growth factor-I, insulin-like growth factor binding proteins, and prostate cancer risk: a prospective study. *J Natl Cancer Inst* 92:1910-1917, 2000.

Steinberg GD, Carter BS, Beaty TH, et al. Family history and the risk of prostate cancer. *Prostate* 17:337-347, 1990.

Steinberg GD, Bales GT, Brendler CB. An analysis of watchful waiting for clinically localized prostate cancer. *J Urol* 159:1431-1436, 1998.

Steiner MS, Gingrich JR. Gene therapy for prostate cancer: where are we now? *J Urol* 164:1121-1136, 2000.

Stenner J, Crawford ED. Combined androgen blockade. In: Kaisary AV, Murphy GP, Denis L, et al, eds. *Textbook of Prostate Cancer. Pathology, Diagnosis and Treatment.* London: Martin Dunitz; 303-317, 1999.

Stern RC, Hulette CM. Paraneoplastic limbic encephalitis associated with small cell carcinoma of the prostate. *Mod Pathol* 12:814-818, 1999.

Sternberg CN, Ianari A, Newling DWW. Chemotherapy in advanced prostate cancer. In: Kaisary AV, Murphy GP, Denis L, et al, eds. *Textbook of Prostate Cancer. Pathology, Diagnosis and Treatment.* London: Martin Dunitz; 319-330, 1999.

Stone NN, DeAntoni EP, Crawford ED. Screening for prostate cancer by digital rectal examination and prostate-specific antigen: results of prostate cancer awareness week, 1989-1992. *Urology* 44:18-25, 1994.

Takayama TK, Vessella RL, Brawer MK, et al. Urinary prostate specific antigen levels after radical prostatectomy. *J Urol* 151:82-87, 1994.

Tanchou PS. *Recherches sur le Traitement Medical des Tumeurs Cancereuses du Sein. Unknown* 1844:256-261.

Taylor JA, Hirvonen A, Watson M, et al. Association of prostatic cancer with vitamin D receptor gene polymorphism. *Cancer Res* 56:4108-4110, 1996.

Tazawa K, Kurihara Y, Kamoshida S, et al. Localization of prostate-specific antigen–like immunoreactivity in human salivary gland and salivary gland tumors. *Pathol Int* 49:500-505, 1999.

Tchetgen MBN, Oesterling JE. The effect of prostatitis, urinary retention, ejaculation, and ambulation on the serum prostate-specific antigen concentration. *Urol Clin North Am* 24:283-291, 1997.

Tepper SL, Jagirdar J, Heath D, et al. Homology between female paraurethral (Skene's) glands and the prostate. Immunohistochemical demonstration. *Arch Pathol Lab Med* 108:423-425, 1984.

Terris MK, Stamey TA. Determination of prostate volume by transrectal ultrasound. *J Urol* 145:984-987, 1991.

Terris MK. Ultrasonography and biopsy of the prostate. In: Walsh PC, Retik AB, Vaughan ED Jr, et al, eds. *Campbell's Urology.* 8th ed. Philadelphia: Saunders; 3038-3054, 2002.

Thompson H. Cancer of the prostate. In: *The Diseases of the Prostate. Their Pathology and Treatment.* 5th ed. London: J and A Churchill; 119-127, 1883.

Thompson IM, Rounder JB, Teague JL, et al. Impact of routine screening for adenocarcinoma of the prostate on stage distribution. *J Urol* 137:424-426, 1987.

Thompson IM, Zeidman EJ. Presentation and clinical course of patients ultimately succumbing to carcinoma of the prostate. *Scand J Urol Nephrol* 25:111-114, 1991.

Thompson IM, Coltman CA. Screening for prostate cancer: opportunities for prevention. *Semin Urol Oncol* 14:4-11, 1996.

Thompson IM, Tangen CM, Tolcher A, et al. Association of African-American ethnic background with survival in men with metastatic prostate cancer. *J Natl Cancer Inst* 93:219-225, 2001.

Tiguert R, Gheiler EL, Tefilli MV, et al. Racial differences and prognostic significance of tumor location in radical prostatectomy specimens. *Prostate* 37:230-235, 1998.

Tjoa BA, Elgamal AA, Murphy GP. Vaccine therapy for prostate cancer. *Urol Clin North Am* 26:365-374, 1999.

Troncoso P, Babaian RJ, Ro JY, et al. Prostatic intraepithelial neoplasia and invasive adenocarcinoma in cystoprostatectomy specimens. *Urology* 34(6 suppl):52-56, 1989.

Tulinius H, Egilsson V, Olafsdottir GH, et al. Risk of prostate, ovarian, and endometrial cancer among relatives of women with breast cancer. *BMJ* 305:855-857, 1992.

van den Ouden D, Kranse R, Hop WC, et al. Microvascular invasion in prostate cancer: prognostic significance in patients treated by radical prostatectomy for clinically localized carcinoma. *Urol Int* 60:17-24, 1998.

Van Krieken JH. Prostate marker immunoreactivity in salivary gland neoplasms. A rare pitfall in immunohistochemistry. *Am J Surg Pathol* 17:410-414, 1993.

Vatten LJ, Ursin G, Ross RK, et al. Androgens in serum and the risk of prostate cancer: a nested case-control study from the Janus serum bank in Norway. *Cancer Epidemiol Biomarkers Prev* 6:967-969, 1997.

Villers A, McNeal JE, Redwine EA, et al. The role of perineural space invasion in the local spread of prostatic adenocarcinoma. *J Urol* 142:763-768, 1989.

Villers A, McNeal JE, Freiha FS, et al. Invasion of Denonvilliers' fascia in radical prostatectomy specimens. *J Urol* 149:793-798, 1993.

Vollmer RT, Dawson NA, Vogelzang NJ. The dynamics of prostate specific antigen in hormone refractory prostate carcinoma. An analysis of Cancer and Leukemia Group B study 9191 of megestrol acetate. *Cancer* 83:1989-1994, 1998A.

Vollmer RT, Keetch DW, Humphrey PA. Predicting the pathology results of radical prostatectomy from preoperative information. *Cancer* 83:1567-1580, 1998B.

Vollmer RT, Montana GS. Predicting tumor failure in prostate carcinoma after definitive radiation therapy: limitations of models based on prostate-specific antigen, clinical stage, and Gleason score. *Clin Cancer Res* 5:2476-2484, 1999A.

Vollmer RT, Kantoff PW, Dawson NA, et al. A prognostic score for hormone-refractory prostate cancer: analysis of two cancer and leukemia group B studies. *Clin Cancer Res* 5:831-837, 1999B.

Vollmer RT, Humphrey PA. Tumor volume in prostate cancer and serum prostate-specific antigen: analysis from a kinetic viewpoint. *Am J Clin Pathol* 119:80-89, 2003.

Wada T, Ohoishi Y, Tashiro K, et al. Analysis of tumor volume in latent prostatic carcinoma. *Jpn J Urol* (Tokyo) 83:315-320, 1992.

Walsh PC, Partin AW. Family history facilitates the early diagnosis of prostate carcinoma. *Cancer* 80:1871-1874, 1997.

Walsh PC. Anatomic radical retropubic prostatectomy. In: Walsh PC, Retik AB, Vaughan ED Jr, et al, eds. *Campbell's Urology.* 8th ed. Philadelphia: Saunders; 3107-3129.

Watanabe M, Shiraishi T, Yatani R, et al. International comparison on ras gene mutations in latent prostate carcinoma. *Int J Cancer* 58:174-178, 1994.

Watanabe M, Imai H, Kato H, et al. Microsatellite instability in latent prostate cancers. *Int J Cancer* 69:394-397, 1996.

Weitzner S, Sarikaya H, Furness TD. Adenocarcinoma of prostate in a twenty-seven-year-old man. *Urology* 16:286-288, 1980.

West DW, Slattery ML, Robison LM, et al. Adult dietary intake and prostate cancer risk in Utah: a case-control study with special emphasis on aggressive tumors. *Cancer Causes Control* 2:85-94, 1991.

Wiley EL, Davidson P, McIntire DD, et al. Risk of concurrent prostate cancer in cystoprostatectomy specimens is related to volume of high-grade prostatic intraepithelial neoplasia. *Urology* 49:692-696, 1997.

Winfield HN, Reddy PK, Lange PH. Coexisting adenocarcinoma of the prostate in patients undergoing cystoprostatectomy for bladder cancer. *Urology* 30:100-101, 1987.

Wingo PA, Landis S, Ries LA. An adjustment to the 1997 estimate for new prostate cancer cases. *Cancer* 80:1810-1813, 1997.

Wolff JM, Boeckmann W, Mattelaer P, et al. Determination of prostate gland volume by transrectal ultrasound: correlation with radical prostatectomy specimens. *Eur Urol* 28:10-12, 1995.

Wood DP Jr., Banks ER, Humphreys S, et al. Identification of bone marrow micrometastases in patients with prostate cancer. *Cancer* 74:2533-2540, 1994.

Xu J, Meyers D, Freije D, et al. Evidence for a prostate cancer susceptibility locus on the X chromosome. *Nat Genet* 20:175-179, 1998.

Yamamoto S, Senzaki A, Yamagiwa K, et al. Prostatic carcinoma in a young adult: a case report [in Japanese]. *Hinyokika Kiyo* 36:617-622, 1990.

Yao D, Trabulsi EJ, Kostakoglu L, et al. The utility of monoclonal antibodies in the imaging of prostate cancer. *Semin Urol Oncol* 20:211-218, 2002.

Yatani R, Chigusa I, Akazaki K, et al. Geographic pathology of latent prostatic carcinoma. *Int J Cancer* 29:611-616, 1982.

Yatani R, Shiraishi T, Nakakuki H, et al. Trends in frequency of latent prostate carcinoma in Japan from 1965-1979 to 1982 to 1986. *J Natl Cancer Inst* 80:683-687, 1988.

Yoshizawa K, Willet WC, Morris SJ, et al. Study of prediagnostic selenium level in toenails and the risk of advanced prostate cancer. *J Natl Cancer Inst* 90:1219-1224, 1998.

Young H. *A surgeon's autobiography.* New York: Harcourt, Brace & Co; 126-134, 1940.

Young HH. The early diagnosis and radical cure of carcinoma of the prostate: being a study of 40 cases and presentation of a radical operation which was carried out in four cases. *Johns Hopkins Hosp Bull* 16:315-321, 1905.

Young HH. Cancer of the prostate. A clinical, pathological and post-operative analysis of 111 cases. *Ann Surg* 50:1144-1233, 1909.

Young HH, Davis DM. *Young's Practice of Urology.* Philadelphia: WB Saunders: 637, 1926.

Yu H, Diamandis EP, Sutherland DJ. Immunoreactive prostate-specific antigen levels in female and male breast tumors and its association with steroid hormone receptors and patient age. *Clin Biochem* 27:75-79, 1994.

Yu H, Diamandis EP, Levesque M, et al. Expression of prostate specific antigen gene by a primary ovarian carcinoma. *Cancer Res* 55:1603-1606, 1995.

Yuan JJ, Coplen DE, Petros JA, et al. Effects of rectal examination, prostatic massage, ultrasonography, and needle biopsy on serum prostate specific antigen levels. *J Urol* 147:810-814, 1992.

Zarghami N, Levesque M, D'Costa M, et al. Frequency of expression of prostate-specific antigen mRNA in lung tumors. *Am J Clin Pathol* 108:184-190, 1997.

Zhau HE, Zhao LS, Chen BQ, et al. Interracial comparative study of prostate cancer in the United States, China, and Japan. *J Cell Biochem* (suppl 28/29):182-186, 1997.

Zhau HE, Li CI, Yang H, et al. Genotypic comparison of prostate cancers among 161 U.S. whites, U.S. blacks, and mainland Chinese men [abstract]. *J Urol* 161(suppl):70, 1999.

Zhu K, Stanford JL, Daling JR, et al. Vasectomy and prostate cancer: a case-control study in a health maintenance organization. *Am J Epidemiol* 144:717-722, 1996.

Zlotta AR, Schulman CC. Etiology and diagnosis of prostate cancer. What's new? *Eur Urol* 33:351-358, 1998

CHAPTER 14

Adenocarcinoma

[14.1] General Approach **259**

[14.2] Diagnosis of Adenocarcinoma in Needle Core Biopsy **275**

[14.3] Diagnosis of Adenocarcinoma in Transurethral Resections and Open Prostatectomies **289**

[14.4] Diagnosis of Adenocarcinoma in Radical Prostatectomy Specimens **294**

[14.5] Diagnosis of Prostatic Adenocarcinoma in Locally Advanced and Metastatic Disease **311**

[14.1] General Approach

Major and Minor Diagnostic Criteria

A definitive diagnosis of prostate cancer is typically established by histopathologic interpretation of hematoxylin and eosin (H&E)-stained tissue sections. In this chapter the morphologic presentation of prostatic carcinoma in different types of tissue samples and in different anatomic locations is discussed. In all types of tissue samples—needle biopsy, prostatic chips, open and radical prostatectomy—and at all anatomic sites, it is the synthesis of a constellation of histologic attributes that allows a definitive diagnosis.

The foundation for histologic diagnosis of adenocarcinoma of the prostate is the assessment of glandular architecture, arrangement of the glandular epithelium, and cytologic features of the glandular lining cells (Algaba 1996, Mostofi 1993, Totten 1953). For diagnosis of adenocarcinoma in prostatic tissue samples, the classic criteria of Arthur Purdy Stout and colleagues (Totten 1953) are still the most useful **t14.1**. These criteria are nearly equivalent to those that have been recently forwarded as the most critical major criteria **t14.2** (Algaba 1996).

First, prostatic adenocarcinoma exhibits an abnormal architectural glandular pattern, with disturbance of the normal or benign epithelial-stromal relationship. These disturbances are best appreciated at low-power, scanning magnifications. Many of the common growth patterns of prostatic adenocarcinoma are well illustrated by the Gleason pictorial representation of grades of prostatic adenocarcinoma (Gleason 1990) (Chapter 15, **f15.1**). Well-differentiated prostatic adenocarcinoma of Gleason pattern 1 and 2 displays abnormal glandular arrangements in the form of well-circumscribed nodules of closely packed, small acini **i14.1**. The prototypical prostatic adenocarcinoma is a small gland adenocarcinoma, and this is certainly true for many well-differentiated Gleason pattern 1 or 2 and moderately differentiated Gleason pattern 3 adenocarcinomas **i14.2**. For intermediate-grade adenocarcinomas, there is a chaotic dispersion of these small acini. That is, these small, irregular, malignant glands show an infiltrative growth, with a haphazard distribution of the small acini **i14.3**. The infiltrative character of the adenocarcinoma can be appreciated when the malignant glands extend into benign tissues. This invasiveness can manifest itself within the prostate as growth between and around benign glands **i14.3, i14.4**, prostatic intraepithelial neoplasia (PIN) glands **i14.5**, destructive growth **i14.6**, invasion into stroma lacking benign glands **i14.7**, perineural invasion **i14.8**, and lymphvascular space invasion **i14.9**.

■ **t14.1** **Stout Criteria for Prostatic Carcinoma Diagnosis**

Glandular pattern: small irregular glands without any particular relation to the adjacent stroma or normal glands
Arrangement of glandular epithelium: lack of basal cells in cancer
Cellular details: large, deeply staining nucleoli

Totten 1953

■ **t14.2** **Criteria for Diagnosis of Prostatic Adenocarcinoma**

Major Criteria
Architectural: Infiltrative small glands or cribriform glands too large or irregular to represent high-grade PIN
Single cell layer (absence of basal cells)
Nuclear atypia: Nuclear and nucleolar enlargement

Minor Criteria
Intraluminal wispy blue mucin (blue-tinged or basophilic mucinous secretions)
Pink amorphous secretions
Mitotic figures
Intraluminal crystalloids
Adjacent high-grade PIN
Amphophilic cytoplasm

Algaba 1996
PIN = prostatic intraepithelial noeplasia

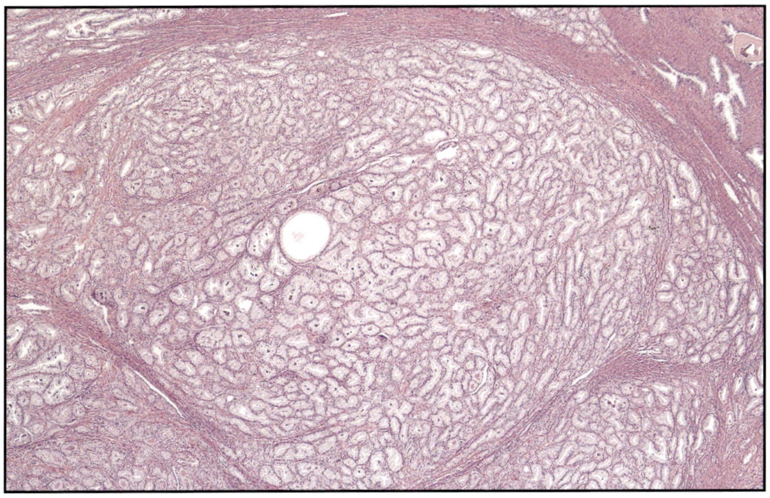

■ **i14.1** *Nodular growth of well-differentiated adenocarcinoma of the prostate: Gleason grade 2+1=score of 3.*

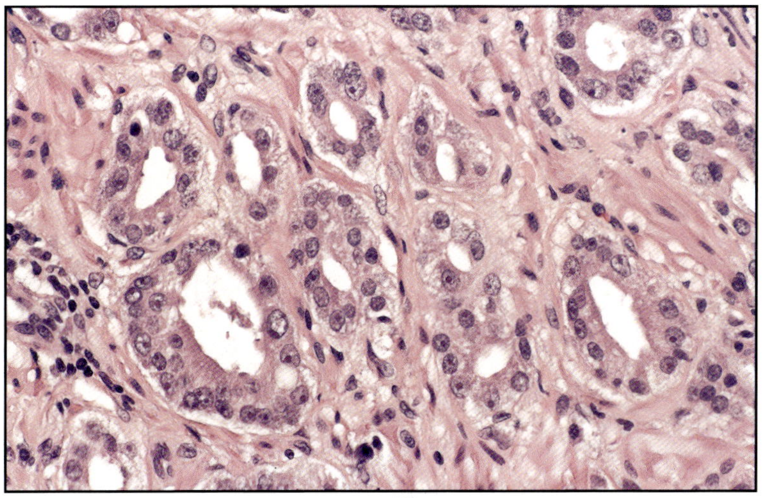

■ **i14.2** *Small acinar prostatic adenocarcinoma.*

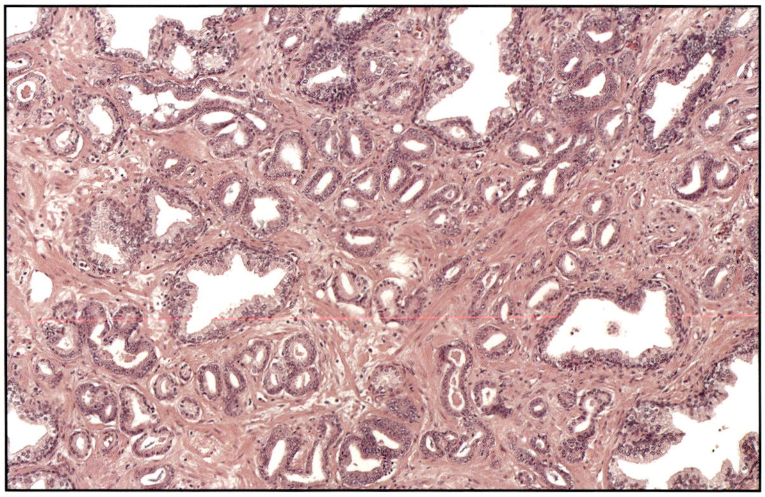

■ **i14.3** *Infiltration of small acinar prostatic adenocarcinoma around and between benign glands: Gleason grade 3+3=score of 6.*

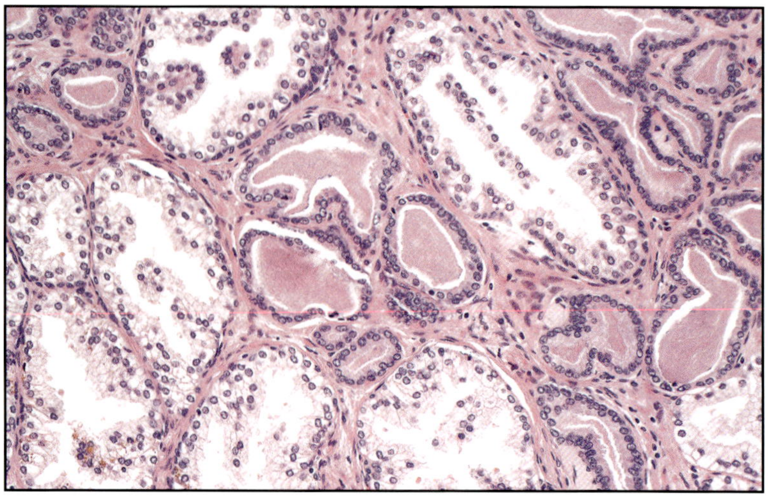

■ **i14.4** *Prostatic adenocarcinoma glands with eosinophilic sections, with insinuation between benign glands: Gleason grade 3+3=score of 6.*

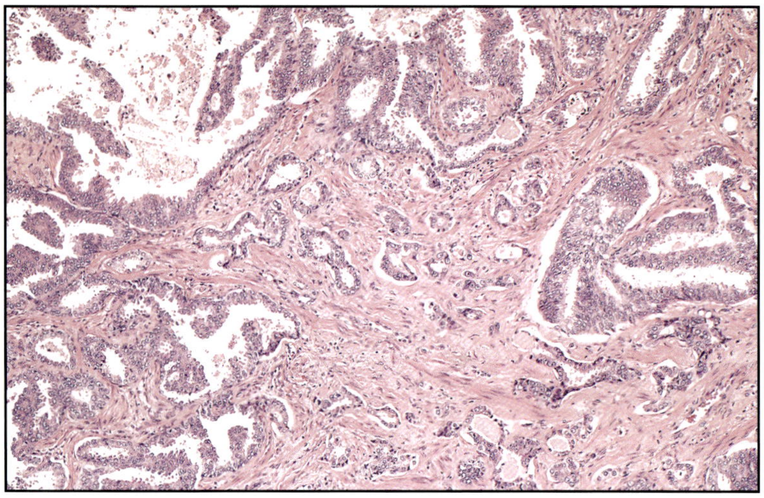

■ **i14.5** *Small acinar prostatic adenocarcinoma adjacent to larger, more complex high-grade PIN glands.*

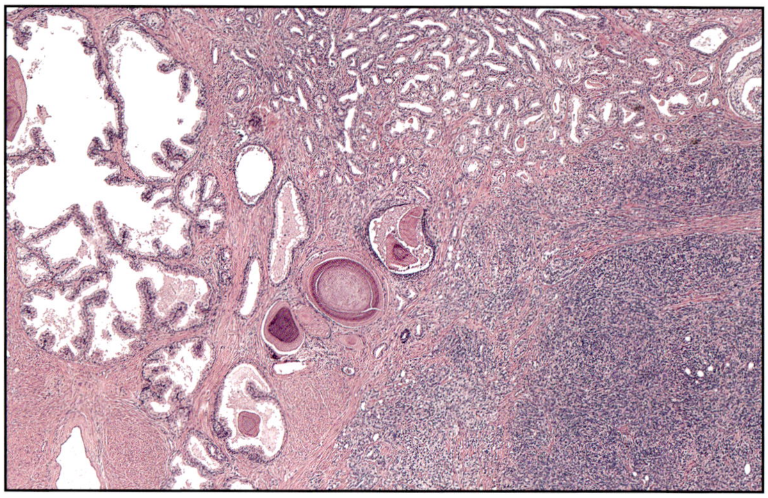

■ **i14.6** *Effacement of benign prostatic tissue (left) by prostatic carcinoma (right): Gleason grade 5+3=score of 8.*

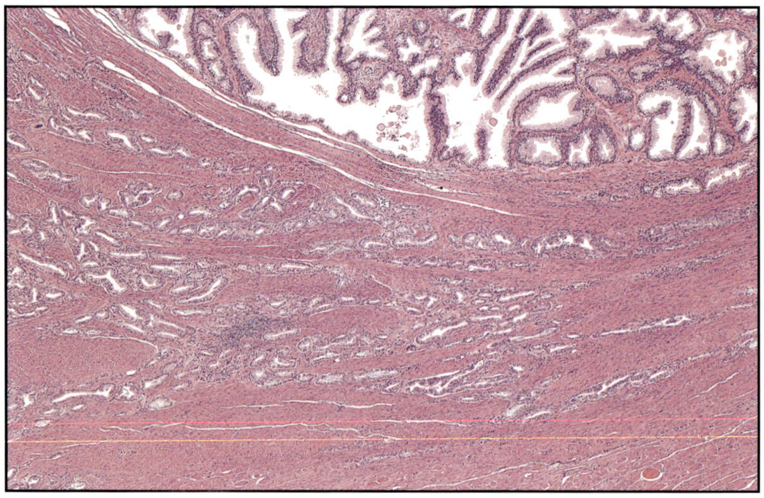

■ **i14.7** *Permeation of prostatic adenocarcinoma into smooth muscle tissue: Gleason grade 3+3=score of 6.*

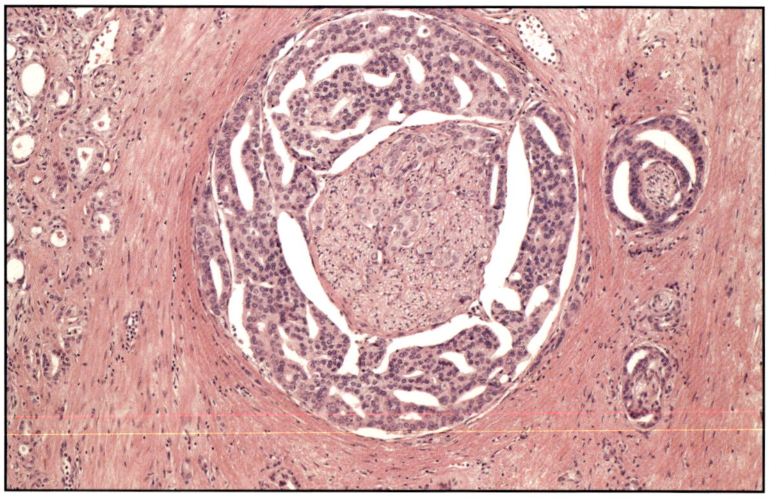

■ **i14.8** *Circumferential extension of prostatic adenocarcinoma around nerves.*

A host response, including a fibrogenic response and inflammatory response, is not often useful in detecting invasion. Most prostatic carcinomas fail to elicit a stromal response, and the malignant glands appear embedded within normal-appearing fibromuscular stroma **i14.10**. Uncommonly, there can be an exuberant sclerotic response to the invading glands **i14.11** or, even more infrequently, an edematous response **i14.12**. An inflammatory response is uncommon, being seen in about 10% of cases, and is usually lymphocytic **i14.13** (see Chapter 4).

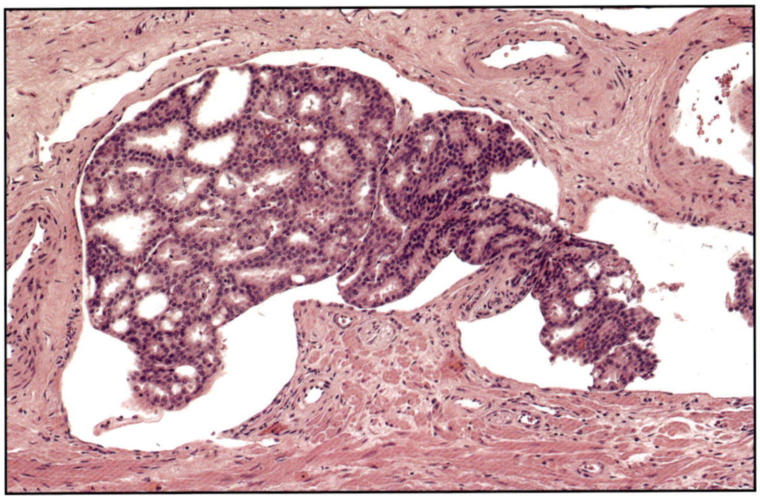

■ **i14.9** *Lymphvascular space invasion by prostatic adenocarcinoma.*

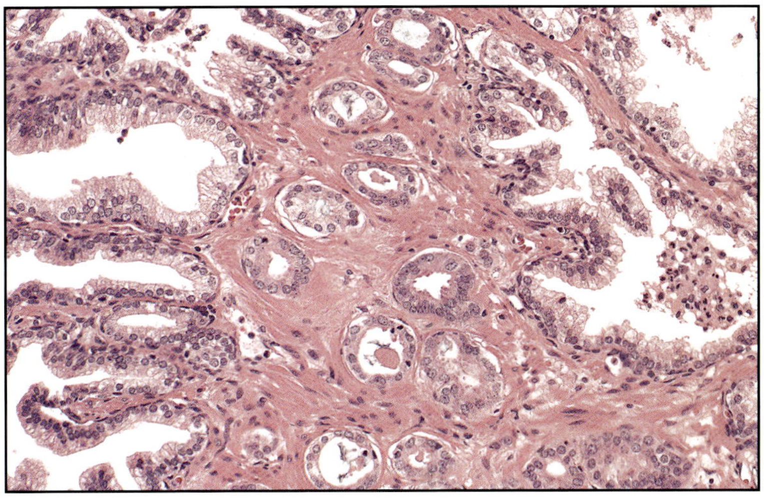

■ **i14.10** *Small acinar prostatic adenocarcinoma invading into fibromuscular stroma between benign glands, without a fibrogeneic or inflammatory cell reposnse.*

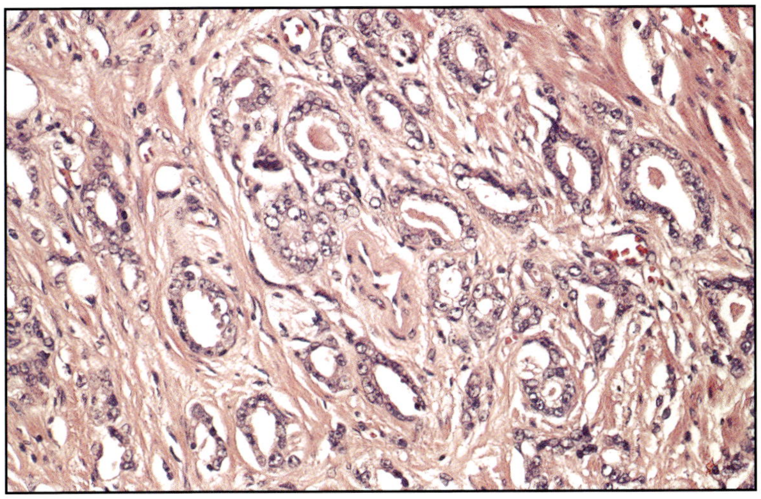

■ **i14.11** *Sclerotic stromal response to invasive prostatic adenocarcinoma.*

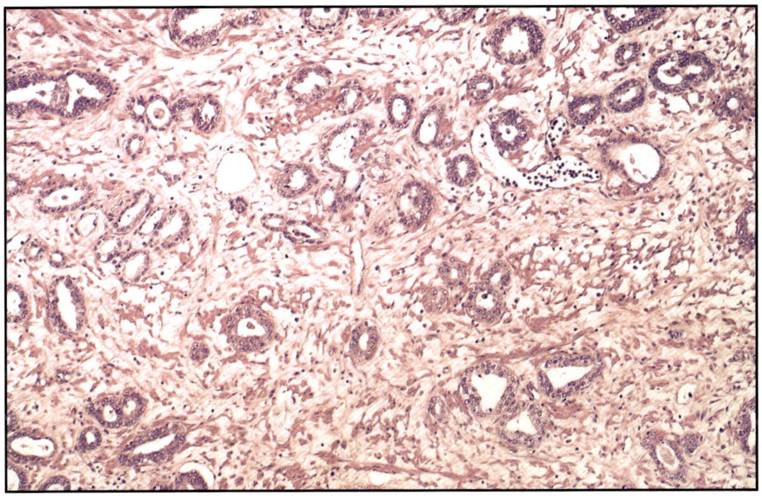

■ **i14.12** *Adenocarcinoma growing within an edematous prostatic stroma.*

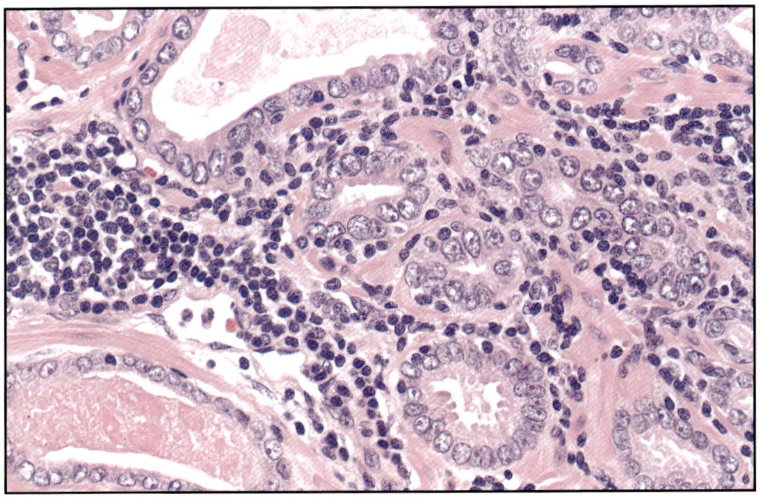

■ **i14.13** *A chronic inflammatory cell infiltrate in stroma around glands of prostatic adenocarcinoma.*

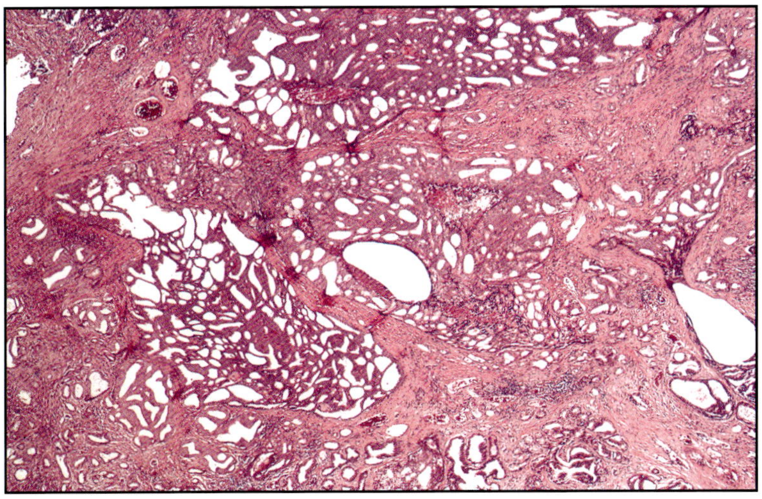

■ **i14.14** *Cribriform prostatic adenocarcinoma.*

Also uncommon are acutely inflamed carcinoma glands, which usually exhibit intraluminal neutrophils. A granulomatous response to invasive prostatic adenocarcinoma is rare, and granulomatous inflammation adjacent to carcinoma typically represents coincidental nonspecific granulomatous inflammation or bacille Calmette-Guérin granulomas (Chapter 4).

Although prostatic adenocarcinoma typically is considered a small acinar malignancy, cribriform **i14.14** and medium-sized,

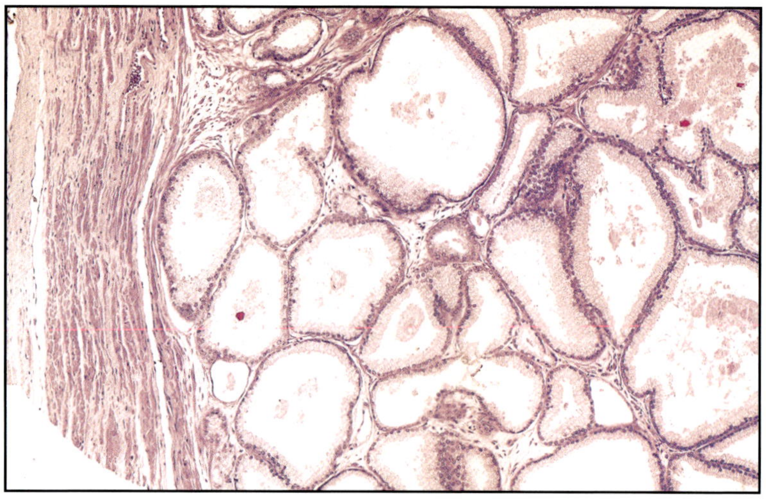

■ **i14.15** *Prostatic adenocarcinoma of intermediate gland size.*

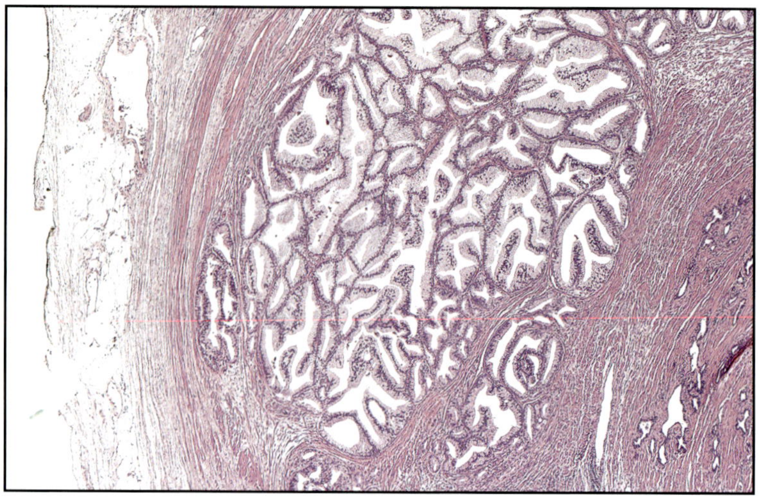

■ **i14.16** *Pseudohyperplastic adenocarcinoma in peripheral zone resembles a nodule of BPH at low-magnification.*

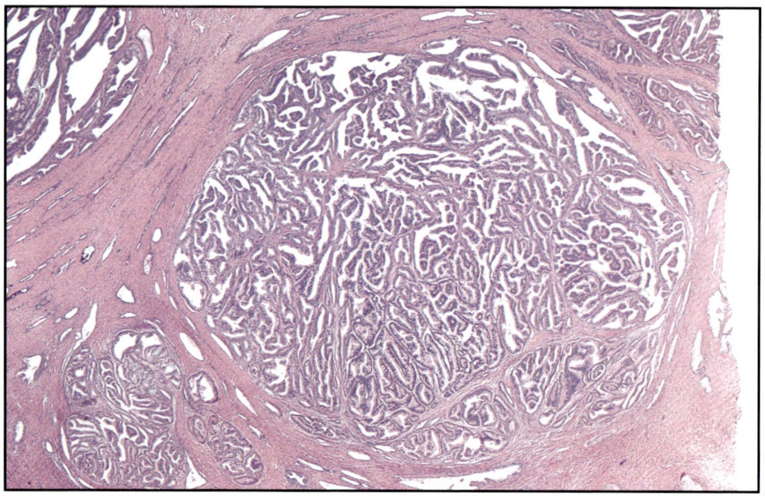

■ **i14.17** *Nodule of ductal adenocarcinoma of prostate, with slit-like spaces indicative of fused papillary growth.*

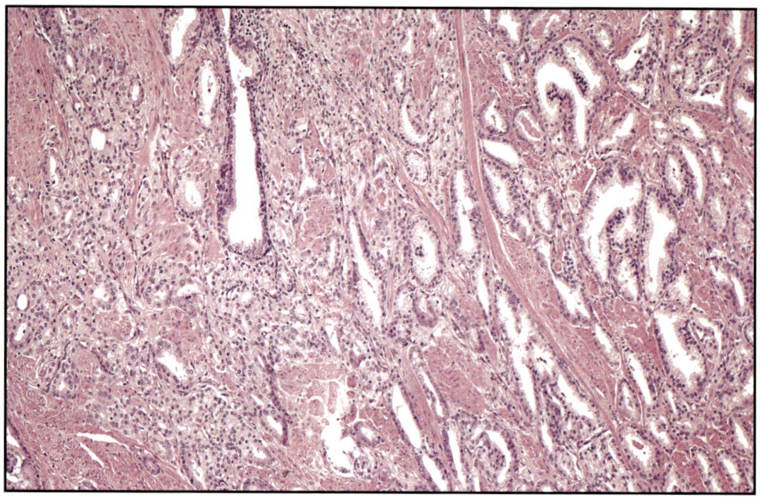

■ **i14.18** *Raggedly infiltrative, high-grade, Gleason pattern 4 adenocarcinoma (left), in continuity with moderately-differentiated pattern 3 (right).*

cystically dilated **i14.15** malignant glands can also be detected (Gleason 1990, Humphrey 1998A, McNeal 1986A, Rubin 1998, Totten 1953). The infiltrative character of these glands can be appreciated by their irregular arrangement. Papillary carcinoma in the prostate can be found in the setting of pseudohyperplastic adenocarcinoma (Humphrey 1998A) and ductal carcinoma (Chapter 17) and can assume abnormal nodular configurations **i14.16, i14.17**. Nodular or well-circumscribed, isolated masses of cribriform and papillary prostatic neoplasia can be difficult to diagnose as invasive carcinoma based on architectural organization alone. Here, absence of a basal cell layer is critical in diagnosing invasion. There is a greater degree of confidence in diagnosing invasion if there are fused masses of cribriform or papillary neoplastic glands **i14.14, i14.17**. High-grade Gleason pattern 4 carcinomas are raggedly infiltrative **i14.18**. These erratically situated structures can be found as fused microacini, chains, cords, cribriform, or papillary growths. The highest grade, Gleason pattern 5, is architecturally distinctive with formation of cylinders with central necrosis: comedocarcinoma **i14.19** and sheets of anaplastic cells with only scattered glandular lumina **i14.20**. This latter growth often is a destructive one, with effacement of normal anatomic structures. A high-grade pattern that can be difficult to identify at scanning magnification is single cell infiltration **i14.21**.

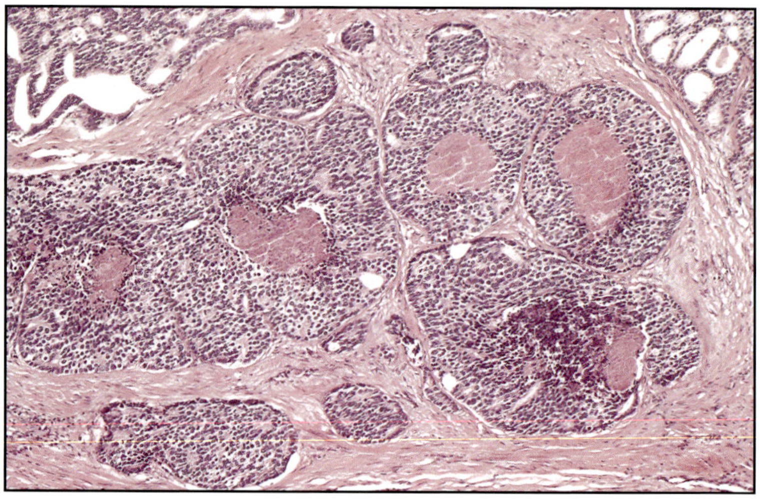

■ **i14.19** *Comedocarcinoma pattern of highest grade prostatic carcinoma — Gleason pattern 5.*

The second major criterion for diagnosis of prostatic adenocarcinoma is absence of basal cells (Algaba 1996, Totten 1953). Basal cells may assume a range of appearances, making careful study of them in glands that are clearly benign a vital exercise to rule out their

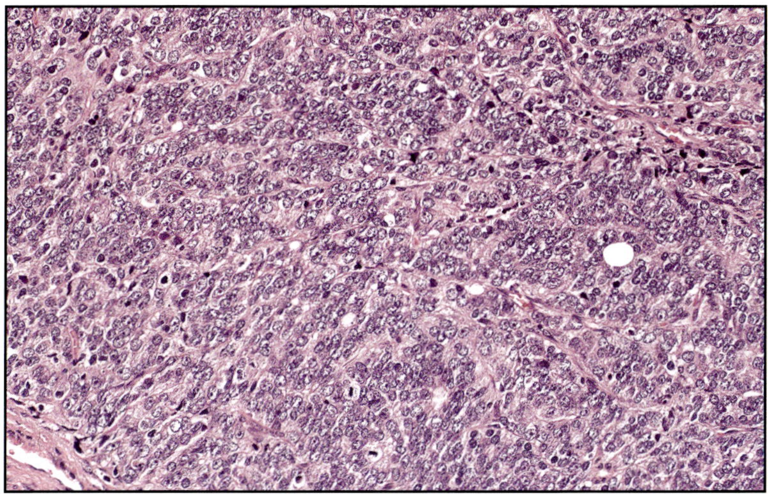

■ **i14.20** *Highest-grade Gleason pattern 5 with nearly solid sheets of carcinoma cells, with only a few, small, glandular lumina.*

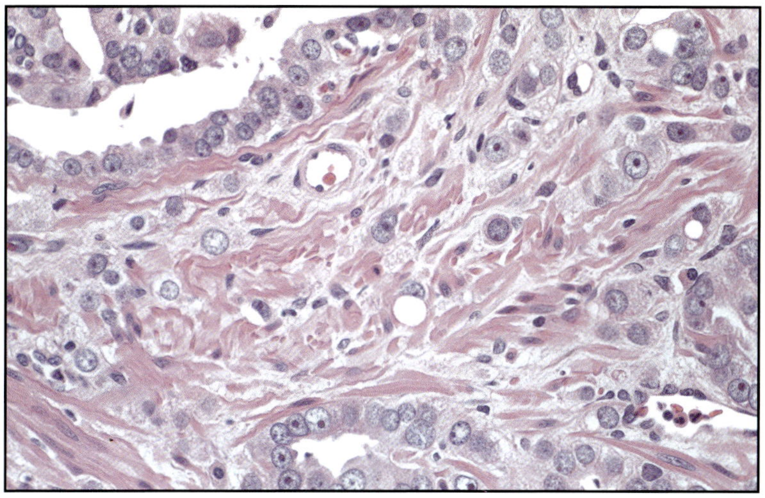

■ **i14.21** *Single cell pattern of prostatic carcinoma infiltration.*

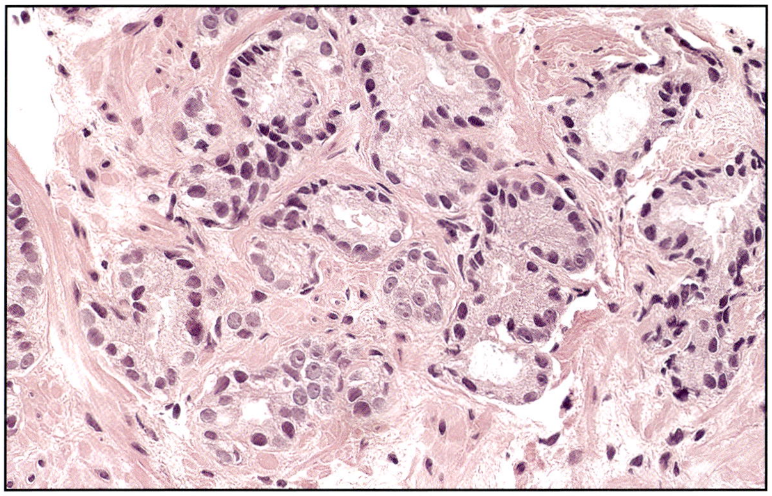

■ **i14.22** *Acinar adenocarcinoma near edge of needle core biopsy-tissue. The darker nuclei in this field do not represent basal cells, but rather, carcinoma cell nuclei with preservation artifact.*

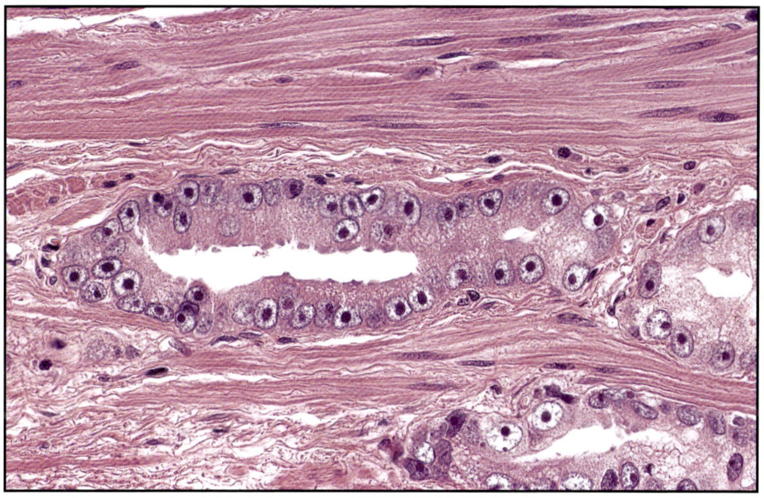

■ **i14.23** *Macronucleoli in prostatic carcinoma nuclei.*

presence in malignant glands. Thin, well-fixed sections with high-quality H&E staining are crucial for the appreciation of a single-cell lining layer in malignant small glands. A historical challenge for the surgical pathologist has been the distinction of periglandular stromal fibroblasts from basal cells. Another common difficulty is that distorted, crushed, or poorly preserved carcinoma cells can mimic basal cells **i14.22**. In cases such as these, application of a basal cell–specific immunohistochemical stain for high-molecular-weight cytokeratin, such as antibody 34βE12, also known as keratin 903, can be diagnostically advantageous. However, this immunostain is not a "malignant stain". Stout and colleagues (Totten 1953) put basal cells in their proper context when they noted the following, based on scrutiny of H&E sections: "This basal cell layer is not always present in benign small glands, so that its absence is not an absolute criterion of carcinoma. Conversely, however, we have not seen it in any case in which the diagnosis was cancer." Thus, absence of basal cells is a key finding in an atypical small acinar proliferation but by itself is not fully diagnostic of carcinoma. Substantiation of absence of basal cells is also important for a diagnosis of invasive cribriform and papillary carcinoma in the prostate.

Nuclear atypia in the form of nuclear enlargement and nucleolar enlargement is the third of the major criteria. Nuclear atypia in malignant glands most often manifests as nuclear enlargement and prominent nucleoli. A classic appearance of a prostatic carcinoma nucleus is a single, large nucleus with chromatin clearing and a deeply staining macronuleolus **i14.23**. The resemblance to an eye is such that it is said that prostatic carcinoma "looks back at you." An eccentrically positioned nucleolus **i14.24** and multiple nucleoli are more often associated with malignant than benign nuclei (Helpap 1988, Hoda 1991, Varma 2002A), but these findings are not specific for carcinoma. Although macronucleoli are characteristic of prostatic carcinoma, not all prostatic carcinomas harbor prominent (>1.5μm) nucleoli (Kramer 1993) **i14.25**. How to define "prominence" is a matter of some debate, and nucleoli anywhere from 1μm to 3μm in diameter have been deemed prominent in the past. Failure to detect prominent nucleoli in prostatic carcinoma nuclei probably is multifactorial; large nucleoli might be present but undetectable because of poor preservation, poor fixation, overstaining, and section thickness. This last factor of overly thick sections is an extremely common problem. Additionally, lack of chromatin clearing might contribute to the inability to detect nucleoli in needle biopsy slides. Lastly, it is certainly possible that some prostate cancers do not harbor macronucleoli. In one study of limited carcinoma in needle biopsy

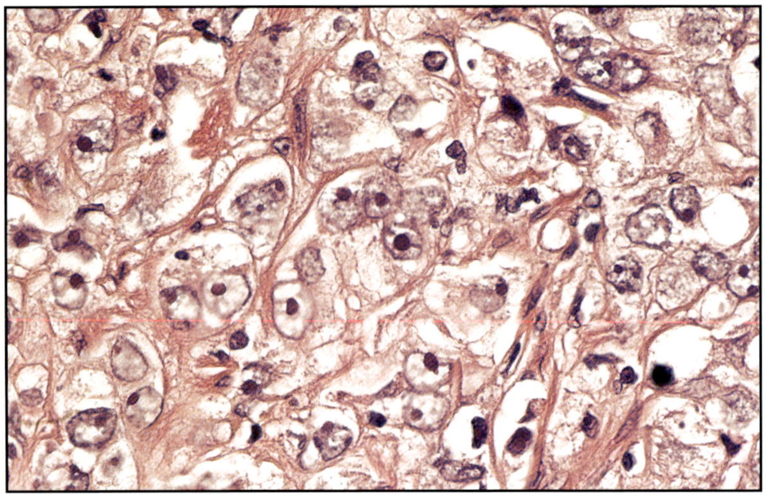

■ **i14.24** *Macronucleoli in prostatic carcinoma cell nuclei: Some are eccentric, abutting the nuclear membrane.*

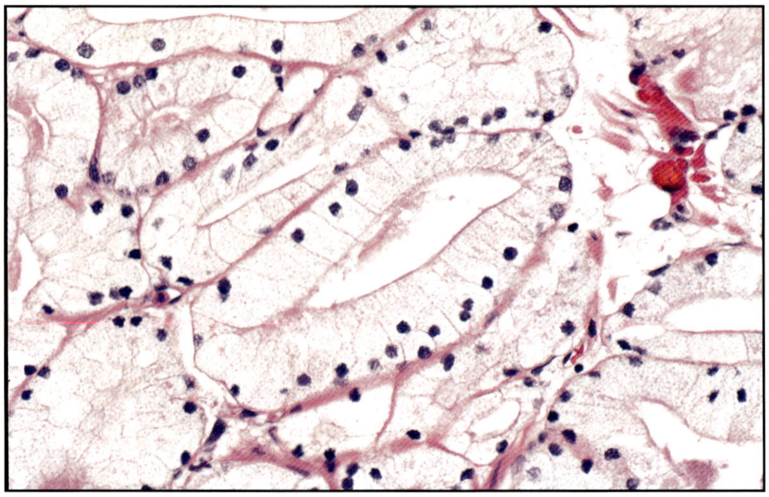

■ **i14.25** *Prostatic adenocarcinoma with small, pyknotic, hyperchromatic nuclei.*

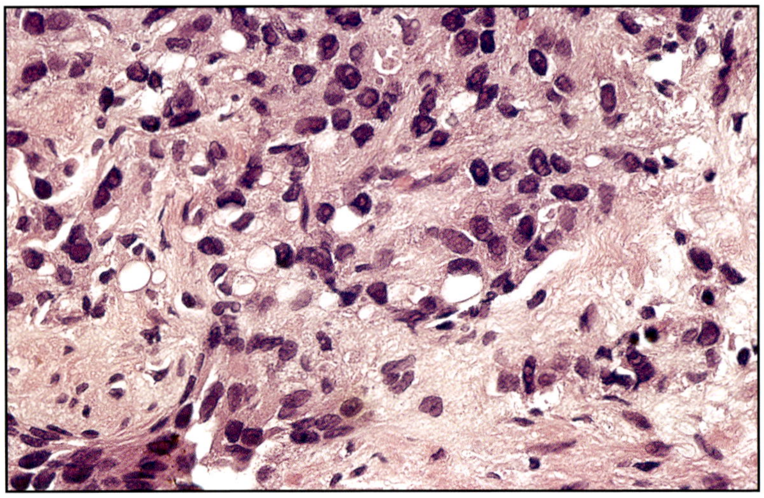

■ **i14.26** *Prostatic carcinoma with hyperchromatic nuclei, with focal signet ring features.*

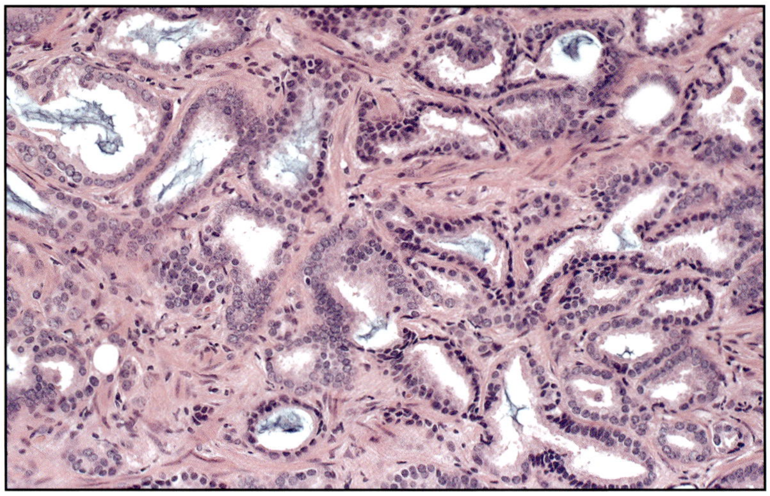

■ **i14.27** *A few strands of wispy blue intraluminal mucin in prostatic adenocarcinoma.*

(Epstein 1995A), fully one quarter of the cases lacked prominent nucleoli, and "nucleolus-poor" carcinoma has been defined in a subset of well-differentiated Gleason score 2 to 4 carcinomas, where 8% of these low-grade adenocarcinomas lacked nucleoli and 20% had only rare prominent nucleoli (Kramer 1993). An important point here is that when macronucleoli are absent, there should be significant nucleomegaly with or without nuclear hyperchromasia **i14.26** to definitively diagnose carcinoma.

Minor, ancillary, or "soft" criteria that can be helpful in diagnosing prostatic adenocarcinoma are listed in **t14.2**. These minor characteristics are not specific for carcinoma but are useful in prompting in-depth study of the glands harboring these changes, with a view toward assessing the aforementioned major diagnostic criteria (Algaba 1996).

Intraluminal wispy blue mucin, also known as basophilic mucin or blue-tinged mucinous secretions, as identified on H&E-stained sections, is more often found in carcinoma than benign epithelial proliferations (Epstein 1992A, 1995A, Kaleem 1998, Thorson 1998, Varma 2002A). The incidence in adenocarcinoma ranges from 18% to 34% in small foci in needle biopsies (Epstein 1995A, Thorson 1998) to 72% in whole (completely embedded) prostate glands at radical prostatectomy (Kaleem 1998). The quantity of intraluminal mucin is variable, from a few thin strands **i14.27** to filling **i14.28** and distention of glands. The mucin often is found in isolated form but can be seen admixed with other ancillary intraluminal materials such as pink, amorphous secretions **i14.29** and crystalloids. This wispy blue mucin corresponds to acidic mucin, as substantiated by Alcian blue histochemical staining at pH 2.5. It is not specific for carcinoma by H&E or Alcian blue staining and can be recognized in mucinous metaplasia, atrophy, basal cell hyperplasia, sclerosing adenosis, atypical adenomatous hyperplasia (AAH), and PIN (Goldstein 1995B, Grignon 1988, 1992, 1993, Humphrey 1991B, Reyes 1997B).

Pink amorphous or acellular intraluminal secretions are also encountered more often in malignant than benign glands (Epstein 1995A, Varma 2002A). These secretions **i14.30** are found in 53% to 72% of minimal or limited adenocarcinomas in needle biopsy (Epstein 1995A, Thorson 1998) and in 84% of adenocarcinomas in the whole gland (Kaleem 1998). They are not related to invasiveness because they can be noted in 62% of high-grade PIN cases (Bostwick 1993A). They are discerned only occasionally in benign glands (Epstein 1995A), including 3% of benign atrophic glands (Kaleem 1998). It is not clear whether this intraluminal material is related to degenerated cellular products, similar to corpora amylacea, which is also usually pink-staining. These pink acellular secretions lack the organized, concentrically

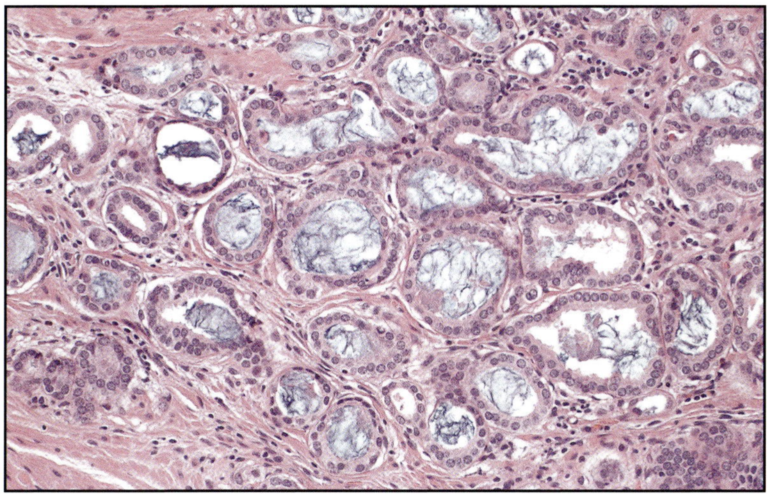

■ **i14.28** *Abundant intraluminal blue mucin in adenocarcinoma of the prostate.*

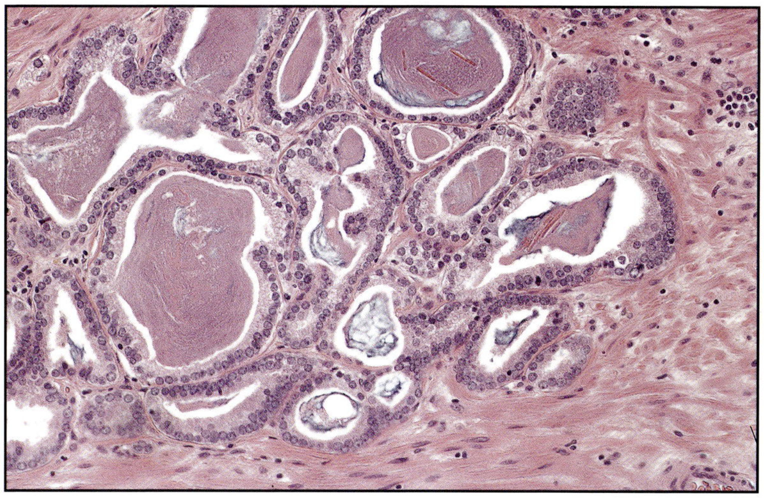

■ **i14.29** *Intraluminal wispy blue mucin mixed with amorphous pink secretions.*

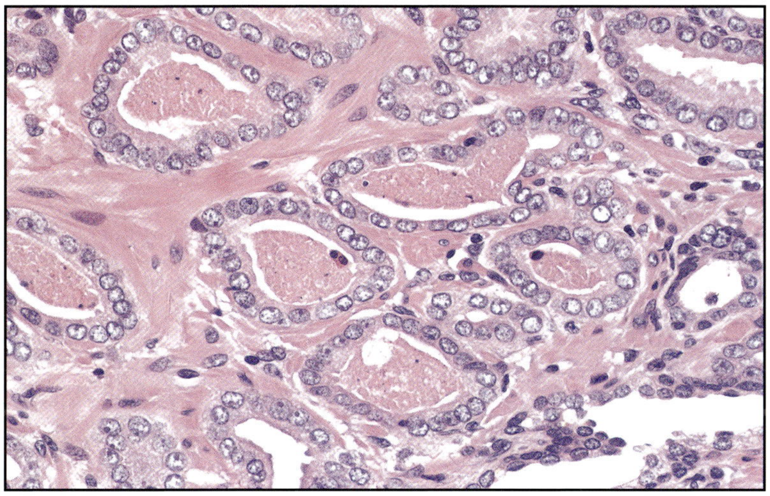

■ **i14.30** *Pink amorphous intraluminal secretions in prostatic adenocarcinoma. These secretions are found more often in neoplastic than benign glands.*

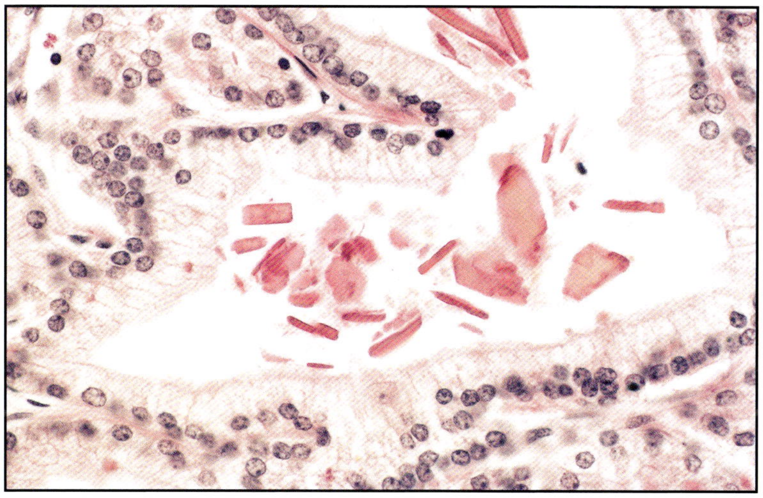

■ **i14.31** *Crystalloids in prostatic adenocarcinoma: These intraluminal structures are discovered more often in neoplastic glands than benign glands.*

layered structure of corpora amylacea. Scattered nuclear debris within the eosinophilic secretions should not be misinterpreted as necrotic tumor debris of comedocarcinoma.

Mitotic figures are an atypical finding in prostatic epithelium, with a trend toward an increased frequency in glands of carcinoma, being detectable in 0.001% of cells in benign glands, 0.1% of cells in high-grade PIN, and 0.06 to 0.15% of adenocarcinoma cells (Giannulis 1993). Given these extremely low percentages, it is not surprising that historically, mitotic figures have been deemed rare in prostatic epithelium (Byar 1972, Totten 1953). Mitotic figures can be identified in 2% to 11% of cases of minimal adenocarcinoma in needle biopsy (Epstein 1995A, Thorson 1998) and 38% of cases of adenocarcinoma in the whole gland (Kaleem 1998). The likelihood of detection of mitotic figures in prostatic adenocarcinoma is related to histologic grade (Eskelinen 1991, Vesalainen 1995). For well-differentiated Gleason score 2 to 4 carcinomas and score 5 to 7 carcinomas, one study found <1 mitotic figure per high-power field, whereas for poorly differentiated Gleason score 8 to 10 carcinomas, 1 to 2 mitoses were found per high-power field (Vesalainen 1995). Most articles in the literature do not attempt quantification of mitotic counts but rather cite detection of any mitotic figures as a rare event. Mitotic figures are not specific for adenocarcinoma and can occur in benign and reactive epithelium, particularly in inflamed, benign epithelium and in benign epithelium adjacent to infarcts. The discovery of atypical mitotic figures is vanishingly rare in primary prostatic carcinoma, except in the anaplastic Gleason grade 5 or neuroendocrine carcinoma. The diagnostic utility of mitoses is diminished because of the lack of specificity, the more common occurrence in readily diagnosed higher-grade carcinoma, and the fact that most prostatic carcinomas in needle biopsy do not harbor mitotic figures.

Prostatic crystalloids are intraluminal, brightly eosinophilic, nonbirefringent structures that often assume striking geometric shapes such as needle-like, triangular, and hexagonal configurations **i14.31, i14.32** (Anton 1998B, Bennett 1980, 1988, Del Rosario 1993, Furusato 1989, Henneberry 1997, Holmes 1977, Jensen 1980, Luna-Moré 1997, Ro 1986, 1988A). They are found more often in adenocarcinoma than in benign glands **t14.3**. The incidence of crystalloids in adenocarcinoma depends on the extent of sampling and the histologic grade of the adenocarcinoma, with the highest likelihood of detection in well-differentiated Gleason score 2 to 4 and Gleason score 5 carcinomas (Epstein 1995A, Holmes 1977, Ro 1986). Crystalloids are rarely found in high-grade, Gleason pattern 4 or 5 adenocarcinomas (Del Rosario 1993), primarily because those carcinomas either do not form glandular luminal spaces at all or the spaces that are formed are small (microacinar).

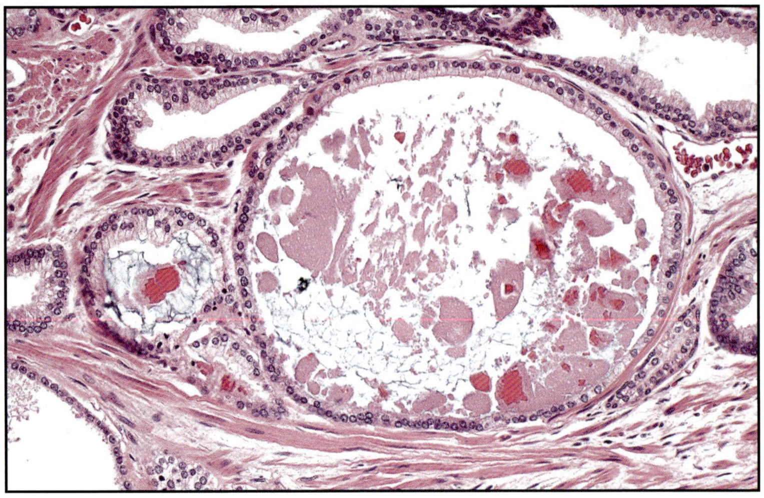

■ **i14.32** *Crystalloids can be seen in intraluminal proteinaceous material and wispy blue mucin.*

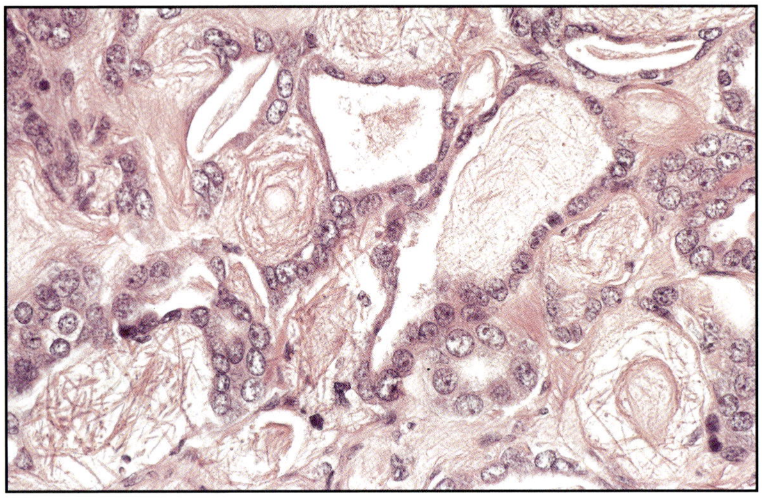

■ **i14.33** *Stromal, needle-like crystalloids. Here they are found in association with atrophic-pattern prostatic adenocarcinoma.*

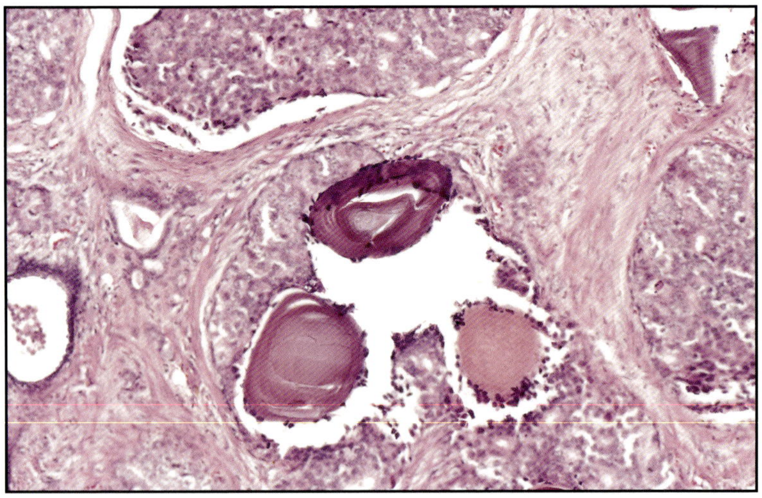

■ **i14.34** *Corpora amylacea within prostatic adenocarcinoma. These intraluminal structures, which may calcify, are more often noted in benign than malignant glands.*

Prostatic crystalloids often are found embedded in intraluminal pink, acellular proteinaceous material **i14.32**. Occasionally, they can be seen in wispy blue mucin **i14.32** or corpora amylacea.

■ **t14.3 Incidence of Prostatic Crystalloids in Various Prostatic Glandular Proliferations**

Epithelial Proliferation	Crystalloid Incidence
Usual hyperplasia/benign glands[1]	1%-5%
High-grade PIN[2]	3%
AAH/adenosis[3]	16%-50%
Carcinoma[4]	10%-75%

PIN = prostatic intraepithelial neoplasia, AAH = atypical adenomatous hyperplasia
[1]Bennett 1980, Anton 1998B, Hu 1998, Varma 2002
[2]Bostwick 1993B
[3]Bostwick 1993A, Hu 1998, Gaudin 1994, Gaudin 1995
[4]Epstein 1995A, Thorson 1998, Kaleem 1998, Ro 1988A, Jensen 1980, Anton 1998B, Bostwick 1993A, Varma 2002

■ **t14.4 Cytoplasmic Appearances of Prostatic Carcinoma Cells**

Common
amphophilic
cleared to granular

Uncommon to Rare
eosinophilic granules
foamy
oncocytic
signet-ring

Crystalloids (especially needle-like ones) can be detected in stroma **i14.33**; the significance of this finding is unknown but may represent a relationship with the formation of collagenous micronodules. Crystalloids should be distinguished from intraluminal corpora amylacea, which are concentrically lamellated bodies that, conversely, are seen more often in benign (78% of cases) than carcinomatous glands (11% to 13% of cases) **i14.34** (Bostwick 1993B, Humphrey 1990A). Little is known of the biochemical composition of prostatic crystalloids other than that they are rich in inorganic sulfur (Del Rosario 1993). The mechanism of their formation is entirely obscure. Diagnostically, the prime advantage to their detection is to direct further scrutiny of the glands that contain the crystalloids.

The diagnostic identification of high-grade PIN should heighten concern for invasive adenocarcinoma, which may be either immediately adjacent to the high-grade PIN or in a separate core (Epstein 1995A, Hu 1998, Weinstein 1993) (Chapter 11). In one large needle biopsy series, 47% of patients with high-grade PIN had prostatic carcinoma on a separate core biopsy, compared with 31% of patients without high-grade PIN (Hu 1998).

The appearance of the cytoplasm in prostatic epithelial cells is of only slight aid in the diagnosis of carcinoma **t14.4**. An amphophilic cytoplasm is more often present in carcinoma cells than benign glandular cells, which tend to have a granular-cleared cytoplasm. However, this is not specific, and a cleared cytoplasm is common in well-differentiated Gleason score 2 to 4 prostatic adenocarcinomas **i14.35**. Cleared cytoplasm can also be found in higher grade prostatic carcinomas **i14.36**, such as the so-called hypernephromatoid variant. Furthermore, benign glands can have amphophilic cytoplasm in an appreciable number of cases (32% in one series [Epstein 1995A]). As for sensitivity, 36% to 60% of prostatic carcinomas in needle biopsy (Epstein 1995A, Thorson 1998) and up to

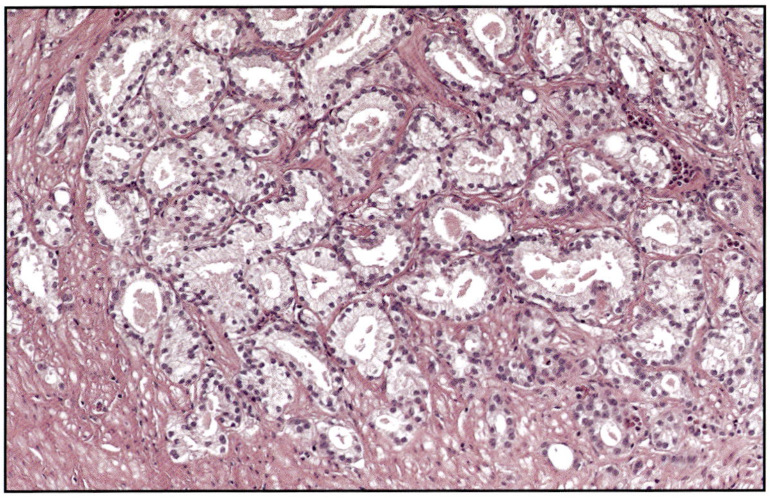

■ **i14.35** *Pale small acinar proliferation: Cleared cytoplasm in well-differentiated, Gleason grade 2 (score 4) adenocarcinoma of the prostate.*

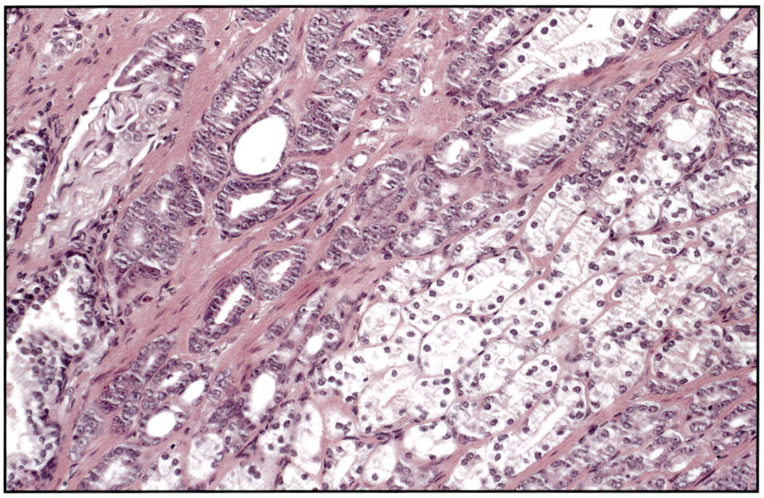

■ **i14.36** *Infiltrative adenocarcinoma with variable amphophilic to cleared cytoplasm.*

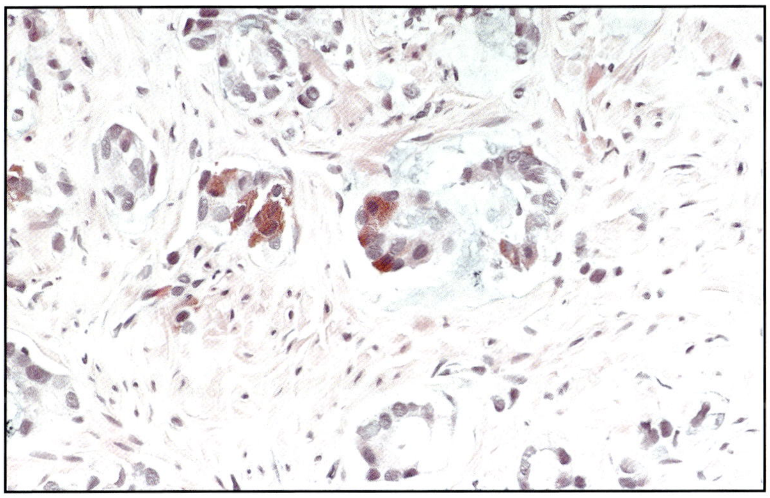

■ **i14.37** *Eosinophilic granules in prostatic adenocarcinoma cytoplasm: A sign of neuroendocrine differentiation.*

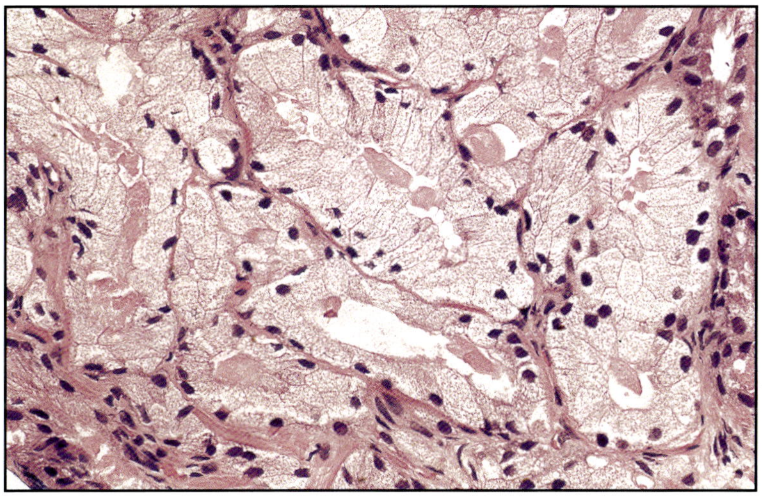

■ **i14.38** *Xanthomatous (foamy) cytoplasm in foamy gland prostatic adenocarcinoma. Despite the bland nuclei, most foamy gland carcinomas are intermediate (Gleason score 5-6) to intermediate-high-grade (Gleason score 7) and seem to be more aggressive, since they often exhibit extraprostatic extension at radical prostatectomy. Foamy cytoplasm is due to the presence of numerous intracytoplasmic vesicles* (Nelson 1996, Tran 2001, Shah 2002).

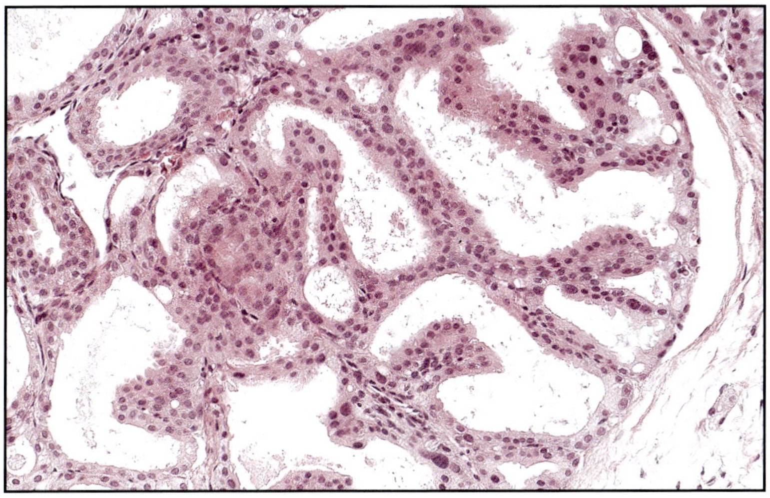

■ **i14.39** *Cribriform carcinoma with eosinophilic cytoplasm consistent with oncocytic features.*

100% of carcinomas in radical prostatectomy specimens (Kaleem 1998) have amphophilic cytoplasm. The tinctorial quality of the prostatic epithelial cell cytoplasm also depends on fixation and staining, which can vary between laboratories; this creates difficulty in uniform application of cytoplasmic amphophilia as an aid in diagnosing malignancy. In addition to being amphophilic or cleared, prostatic carcinoma cytoplasm can uncommonly reveal eosinophilic granules (Paneth cell–like change, a form of neuroendocrine differentiation) **i14.37** (Adlakha 1994, Weaver 1992A, 1992B), xanthomatous cytoplasm (as seen in so-called foamy gland carcinoma) **i14.38** (Nelson 1996, Shah 2002B, Tran 2001), oncocytic cytoplasm **i14.39** (Ordoñez 1992, Pinto 1994), and signet-ring change **i14.40** (Ro 1988B). None of these cytoplasmic changes is specific for malignancy; even signet-ring change can be seen in benign conditions (Alguacil-Garcia 1986, Guerrero-Medrano 1997, Wang 2002).

The amount of cytoplasm can also be somewhat helpful in differential diagnosis of benignancy and malignancy because prostatic carcinoma cells typically have a moderate amount of cytoplasm. In contrast, the benign entity most likely to be misdiagnosed as carcinoma—benign atrophy—has a scanty amount of cytoplasm. Thus, unlike in most malignancies, the nuclear-cytoplasmic (N/C) volume ratio is higher in prostatic epithelium in

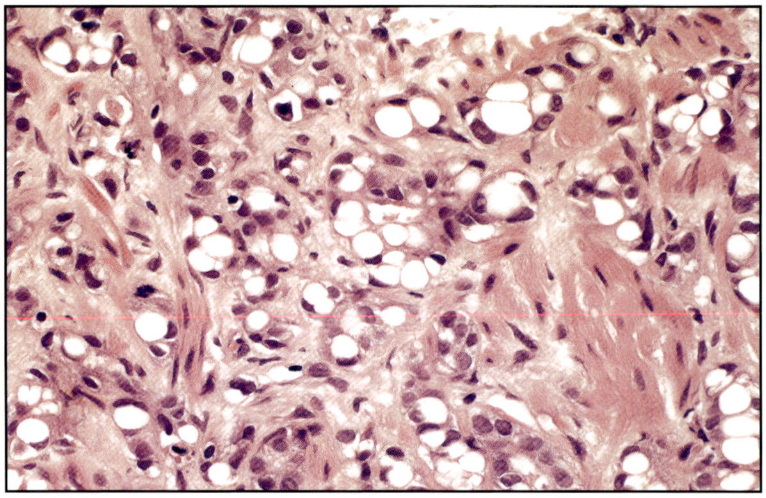

■ **i14.40** *Signet ring cytoplasmic change in prostatic adenocarcinoma.*

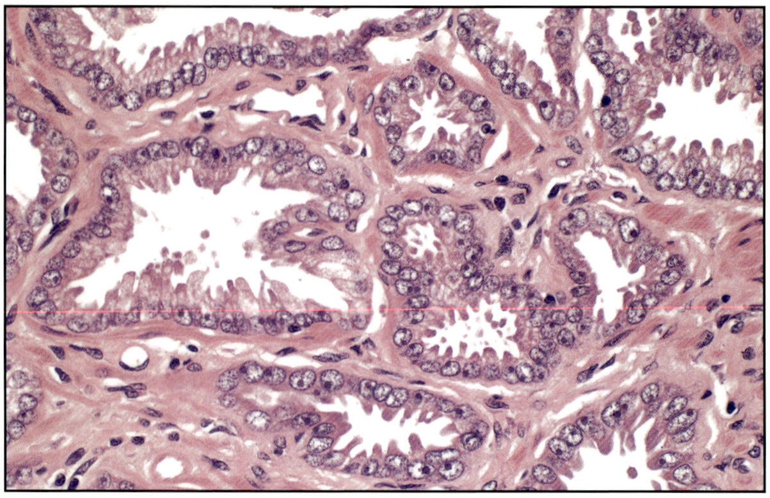

■ **i14.41** *Apocrine-like snout formation along luminal border of prostatic adenocarcinoma glands. This finding is not of diagnostic significance.*

■ **t14.5 Histopathologic Findings Potentially Specific for Prostatic Carcinoma**

Prostatic epithelium outside the prostate gland
Perineural invasion
Collagenous micronodules
Glomerulations

a benign entity, atrophy, than in the malignant proliferation. Amount of cytoplasm is not specific for a particular epithelial proliferation, however, because benign and hyperplastic prostatic epithelial cells often have the same amount of cytoplasm as prostatic carcinoma cells and, moreover, prostatic carcinoma cytoplasm volume is low in small cell carcinoma and atrophic pattern prostatic carcinoma. Atrophic pattern prostatic carcinoma can be found in the setting of androgen deprivation or radiation therapy (Cheng 1999D, Reuter 1997) and in the absence of any therapy (Cina 1997, Egan 1997B, Kaleem 1998).

Cellular characteristics that are not included in the diagnostic criteria checklist include cell size and shape and cytoplasmic borders. Carcinoma cellular borders can be distinct or not, and the luminal border of gland-forming cells, though often flat, can be ruffled, with bleb or snout formation **i14.41**.

Histopathologic Features Considered Specific for Carcinoma

Histologic features that have been considered specific for a diagnosis of prostatic carcinoma include extraprostatic spread of glands and, within the prostate, the findings of perineural invasion, collagenous micronodules, and glomeruloid intraglandular projections **t14.5** (Baisden 1999). The presence of prostatic glands outside the prostate usually indicates malignancy, but it is important to recall that ectopic prostatic glands have been found in many anatomic sites outside the prostate, including testis, epididymis, bladder, penile urethra, seminal vesicle, root of the penis, subvesical space, retrovesical space, pericolonic fat, anal submucosa, perirectal fat, urachal remnant, and spleen (Chapter 1).

■ **t14.6 Perineural Invasion by Prostatic Carcinoma: Incidence**

Tissue Sample Type	Incidence	Comment (reference)
Needle biopsy	37%	n = 326 (Jimenez 2000)
	37%	n = 314 (Bostwick 1996)
	24%	n = 319 (de la Taille 1999)
	22%	n = 250 (Varma 2002)
	20%	n = 302 (Bastacky 1993)
	18%	n = 212 (Stone 1998)
	17%	n = 340 (Vargas 1999)
	16%	n = 651 (Bassily 1999)
	11%	n = 215 (Bismar 2003): a screening population
	11%	"Limited" carcinoma (Epstein 1995A)
	2%	Carcinoma <1 mm (Thorson 1998)
Radical prostatectomy	84%	n = 208 (Byar 1972)
	94%	n = 316 (Bostwick 1994A)

Perineural invasion is a hallmark of prostatic carcinoma (Byar 1972, Kahler 1934, Moore 1935, Totten 1953). In whole prostate glands, perineural invasion can be found in most cases, with the range in the literature being 84% to 94% (Andrews 1949, Bostwick 1994A, Byar 1972, Kahler 1934). In needle core biopsy, 22% of cases on average (of pooled 2929 cases from large contemporary series) exhibit perineural invasion **t14.6**. The likelihood of detection of perineural invasion is related to amount of tumor (Bismar 2002, Rubin 2000B, Thorson 1998, Vargas 1999) and Gleason grade (Vargas 1999) in needle core biopsies. The diagnostic utility of perineural invasion is diminished for a limited (Epstein 1995A) or minimal (Thorson 1998) amount of carcinoma (<1mm in greatest dimension) in needle biopsy tissue because the incidence falls to as low as 2% in this setting.

The significance of perineural invasion for the diagnosis of prostatic carcinomas has long been emphasized (Totten 1953). Patterns of perineural invasion by prostatic carcinoma include "crescentic application" (Andrews 1949) **i14.42**, intraneural invasion **i14.43**, "tracking" along a longitudinally sectioned nerve **i14.44**, and circumferential extension around a nerve **i14.45**. The volume of carcinoma invading around intraprostatic or periprostatic nerves is variable, ranging from a single gland or a few glands to a single layer of perineural glands **i14.45**, to a few perineural gland layers

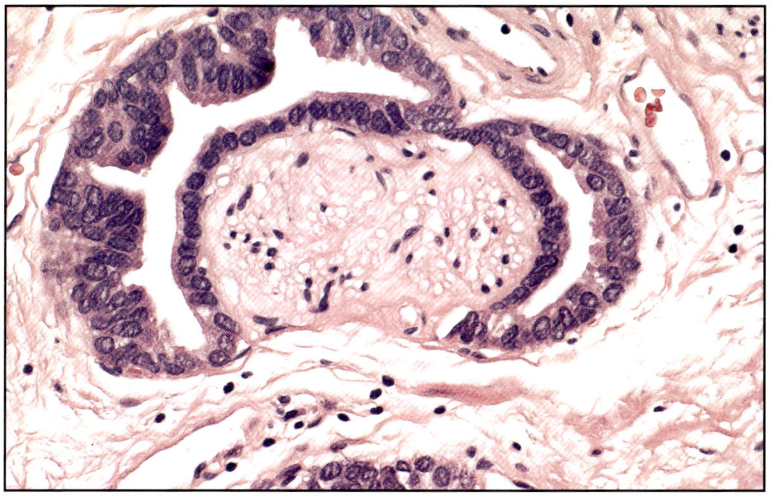

■ **i14.42** *Perineural invasion by prostatic adenocarcinoma: cresentic application.*

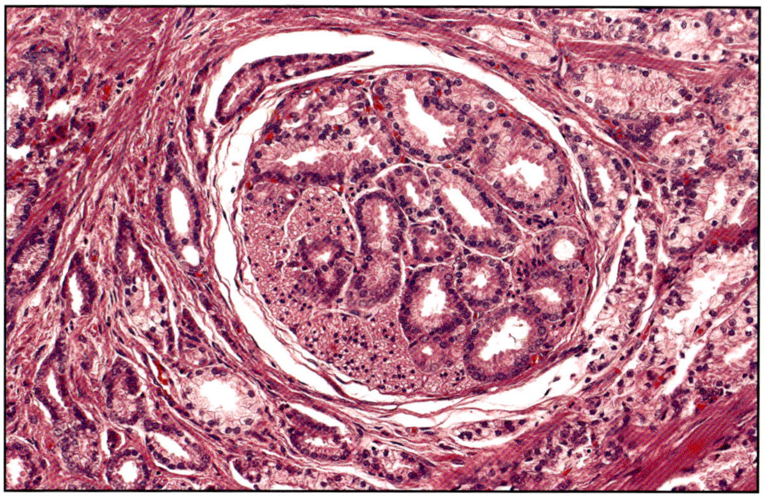

■ **i14.43** *Intraneural invasion by prostatic adenocarcinoma.*

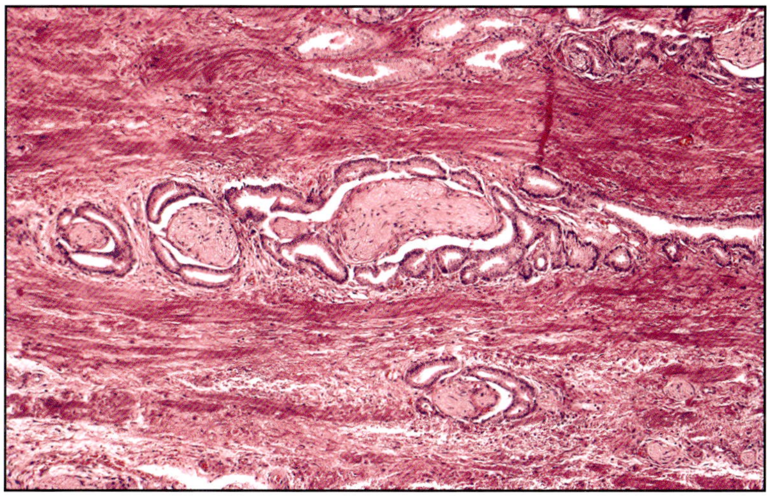

■ **i14.44** *Perineural "tracking" by prostatic adenocarcinoma.*

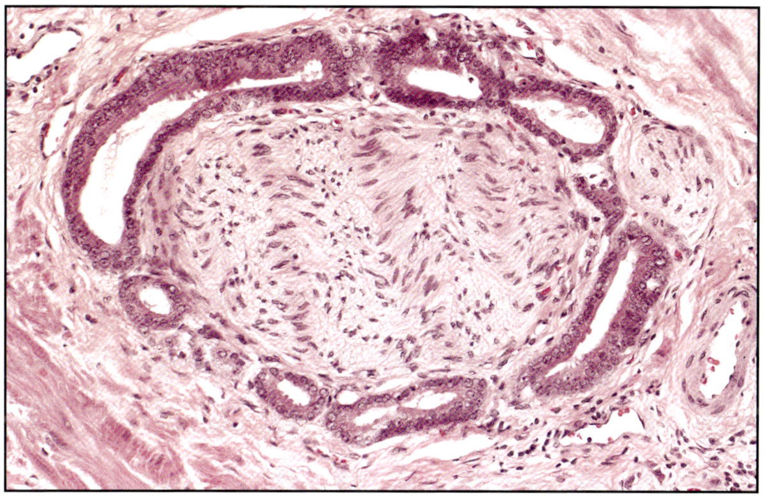

■ **i14.45** *Perineural invasion by prostatic adenocarcinoma, with single-layered circumferential extension.*

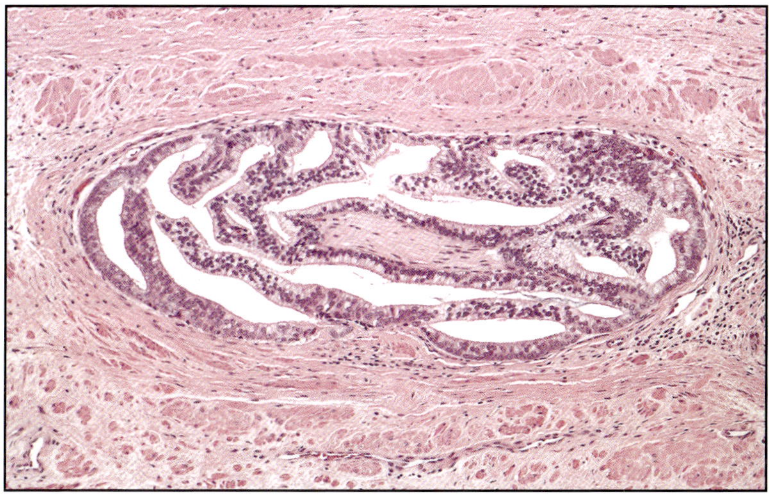

■ **i14.46** *Perineural circumferential extension by small volume of malignant glands with complex architecture.*

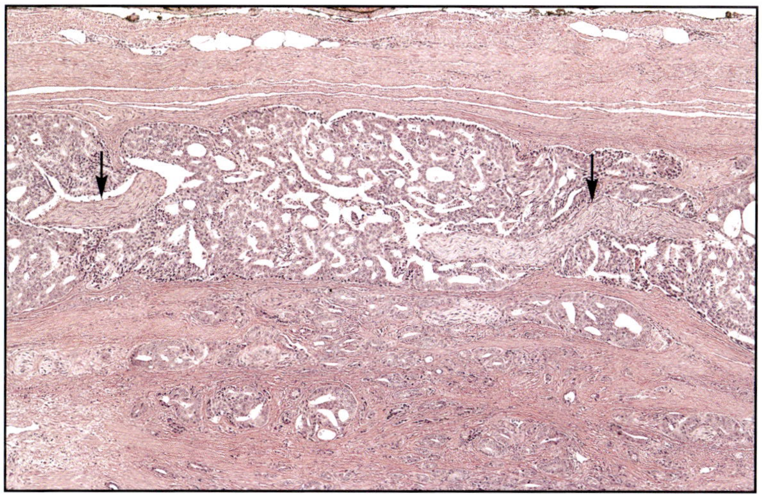

■ **i14.47** *Broad column of carcinoma surrounding several nerve branches (arrows).*

i14.46, to a mass of carcinoma glands surrounding a nerve **i14.47**, where nerve presence may not be immediately apparent **i14.48**. In some cases, the malignant glands surrounding a nerve can show features more often associated with benign glands (Epstein 1996B), such as cystic dilatation and papillary infoldings (Humphrey 1998A) **i14.49**. Here the differential diagnosis encompasses not only benign glands but also high-grade PIN, for the lining cells can be stratified as in PIN. Additional distinctive images of perineural invasion

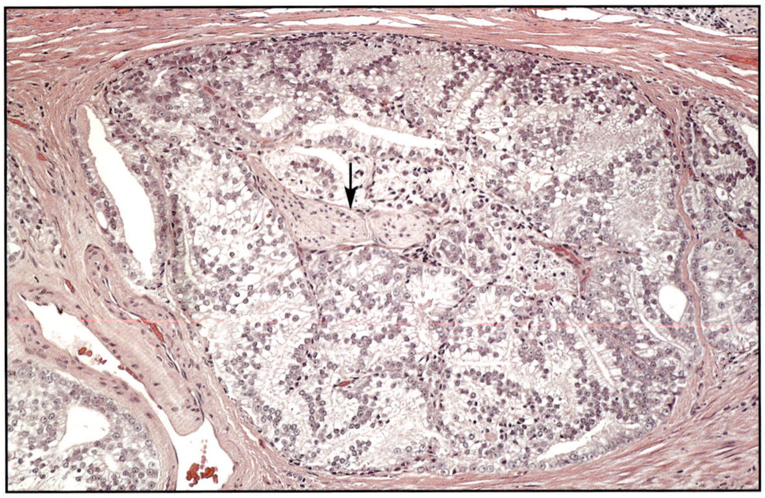

■ **i14.48** *Nodule of prostatic carcinoma surrounding small nerve twig (arrow).*

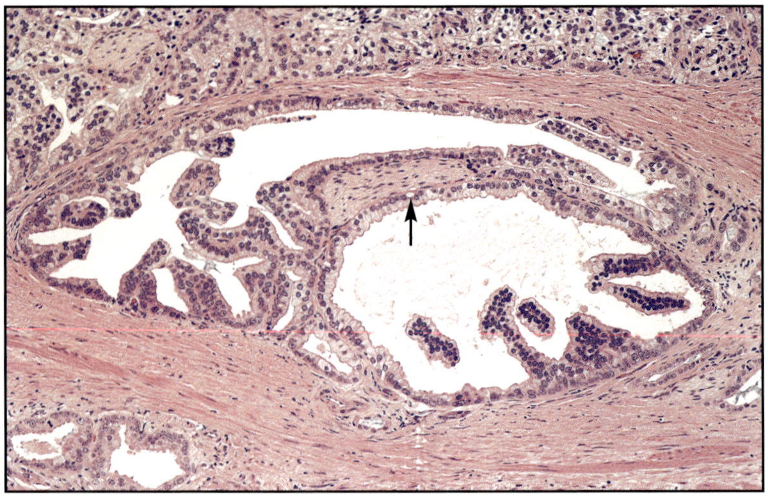

■ **i14.49** *Perineural invasion (arrow) by prostatic carcinoma glands with cystic change and intraluminal micropapillary projections.*

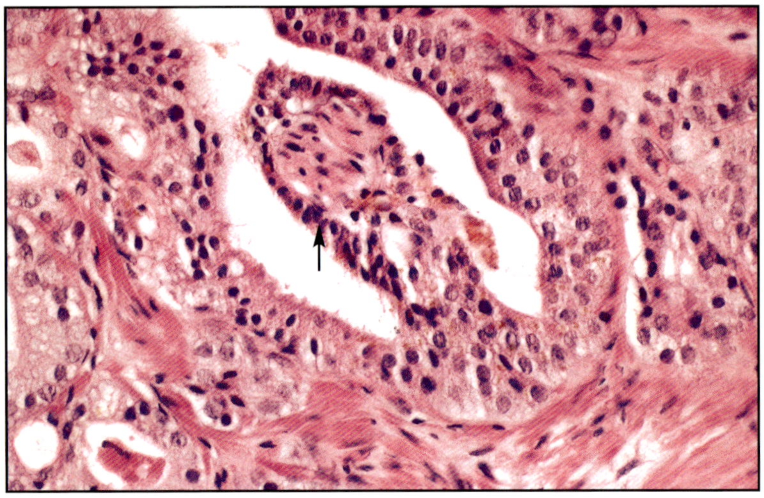

■ **i14.50** *Perineural invasion by carcinoma (arrow), with "peninsula" pattern.*

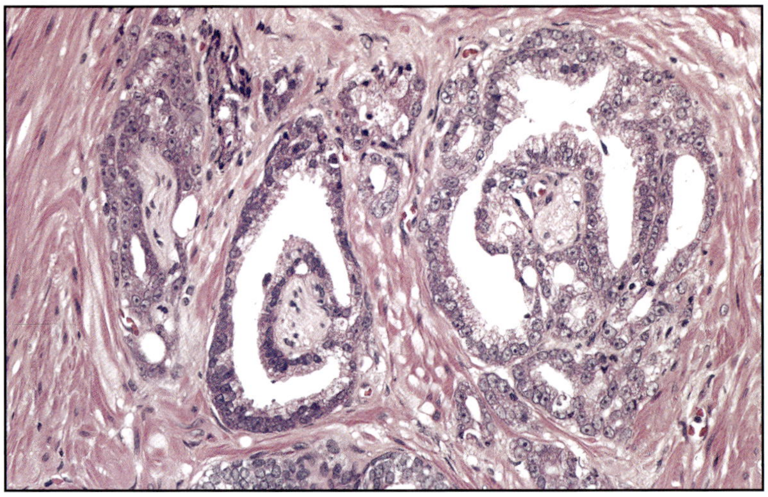

■ **i14.51** *"Knob-like" configurations of perineural invasion by prostatic carcinoma.*

include the "peninsula" formation **i14.50** and knoblike configurations **i14.51**, where a nerve twig can be found encircled at the tip of an intraglandular projection. However, the mere presence of prostatic glands immediately adjacent to nerve is not definitively diagnostic of malignancy. Benign prostatic glands can abut nerves (Carstens 1980, McIntire 1986) and, in extremely rare cases, can be found within nerves (Cramer 1981). Circumferential extension of benign glands around a prostatic nerve has not been reported and appears to be a pattern specific for malignancy. Yet, by itself, architectural pattern of growth in relation to nerve is not sufficient to establish a diagnosis of carcinoma, and other major and minor criteria must be taken into account. A particular diagnostic problem arises when crushed cells are detected around a nerve **i14.52**. In the prostate, lymphocytes can also encircle nerves, so crushed cells rimming a nerve need not necessarily be epithelial. In such cases, one should specifically seek viable, undistorted perineural cells or glands by studying multiple sections, including additional levels, if necessary. Immunohistochemical staining for prostate-specific antigen (PSA) and CD45 (leukocyte common antigen [LCA]) could be carried out in these cases with perineural crushed cells, but even if the PSA immunostain is positive in the crushed cells, a definitive diagnosis of malignancy should not be rendered without evidence of nuclear atypia and basal cell absence. Immunostains for S-100 have been used to highlight small nerve twigs that are enveloped by carcinoma (Aufranc 2000, Zhou 2001), but we have found this necessary only in rare cases.

Perineural invasion was originally thought to represent perineural lymphatic space invasion (Moore 1935, Pennington 1967), but it has been clearly shown that perineural migration of prostatic carcinoma cells reflects growth along a pathway of least resistance (Hassan 1980, Rodin 1967) and intriguingly, possibly a reciprocal biochemical interaction between nerve and carcinoma cells, where the tropism of prostatic carcinoma cells for nerve might be an active process (Ayala 2001, Dalal 1997, Geldof 1997, Yang 1996). Biologically, perineural invasion is a dominant mechanism for spread of cancer outside the prostate glands (Villers 1989).

Lymphvascular space invasion by prostatic epithelial cells can be also viewed as specific for a diagnosis of malignancy, but I have not seen a prostatic tissue sample of any type, including needle core biopsy, with carcinoma in lymphvascular space as the sole finding.

Collagenous micronodules (Bostwick 1995A), also known as mucinous fibroplasia (Baisden 1999), are microscopic aggregates of hyalinized stroma that represent an unusual response to invasive adenocarcinoma of the prostate **t14.7**. They were first described in 1991 in mucinous adenocarcinomas (McNeal 1991) and are often **i14.53**

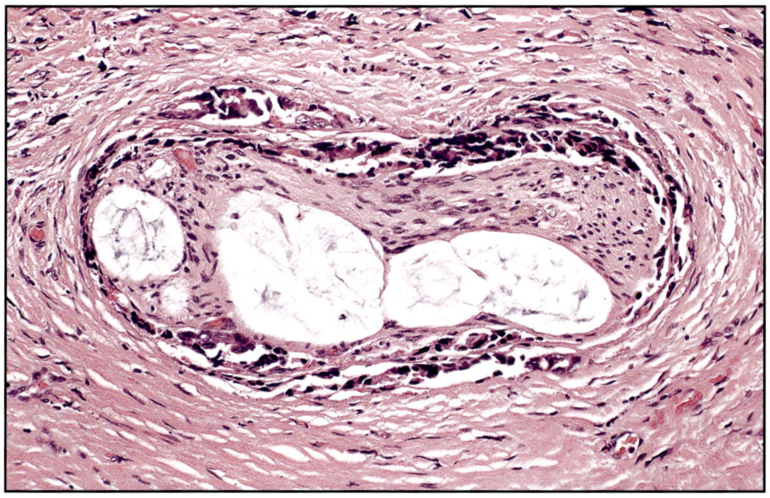

■ **i14.52** *Crushed perineural prostatic carcinoma cells. There is also intraneural mucin. (Such acellular mucinous areas are usually found in the stroma of patients treated with androgen deprivation therapy).*

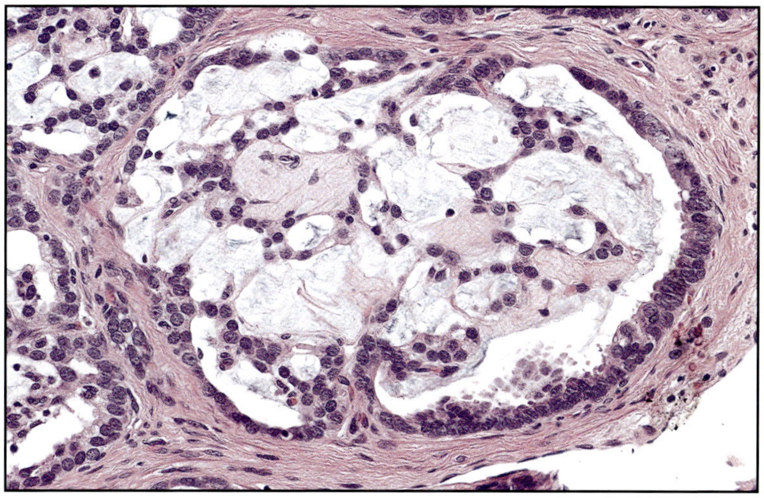

■ **i14.53** *Collagneous micronodules in mucin-producing prostatic adenocarcinoma.*

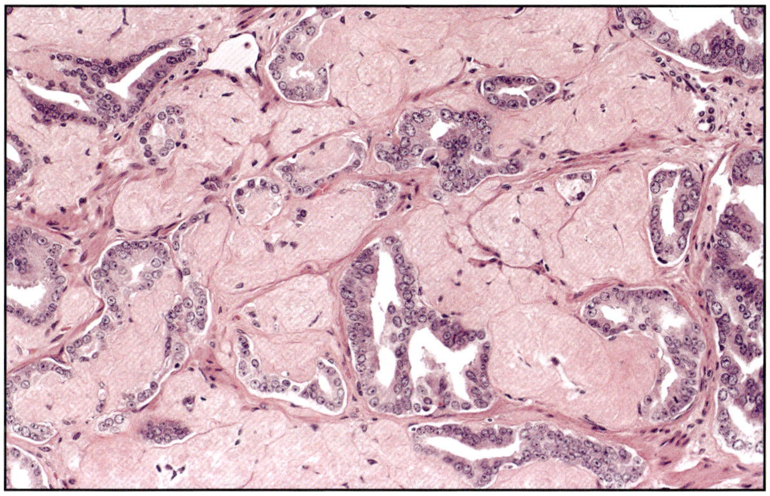

■ **i14.54** *Numerous collagenous micronodules in nonmucinous prostatic adenocarcinoma.*

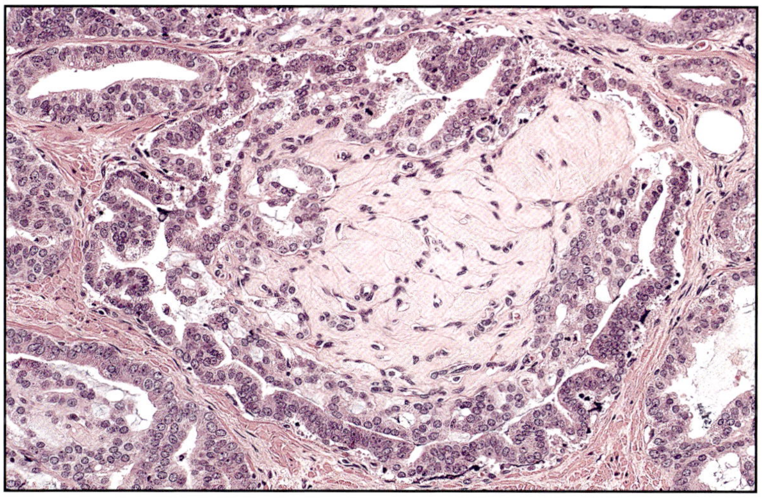

■ **i14.55** *Intraluminal collagenous micronodule of substantial size, with minimal mucin.*

but not invariably **i14.54, i14.55** associated with abundant mucin production (Bostwick 1995A, McNeal 1991). By histochemical and ultrastructural characterization, the micronodules are composed chiefly of collagen and are paucicellular, with a few elongated fibroblastic nuclei seen. These collagen formations can assume a variety of morphologic guises, including true nodules, vaguely lobuled masses, and streaks and strands of the collagenous tissue within mucinous pools **i14.56**. The micronodules can be located in stroma adjacent to adenocarcinomatous glands and also within glandular lumina. The malignant glands can appear to wrap around the micronodules, with glandular indentation **i14.57**.

■ t14.7 **Collagenous Micronodules (Mucinous Fibroplasia)**

Specific for carcinoma
Found in 1%-2% of carcinomas in needle biopsy and 13%-22% of carcinomas in whole prostate
Associated with mucin production (sometimes)
Microscopically: Paucicelllular small nodules to lobular aggregates to thin bands of hyalinized collagen with a few embedded fibroblastic nuclei

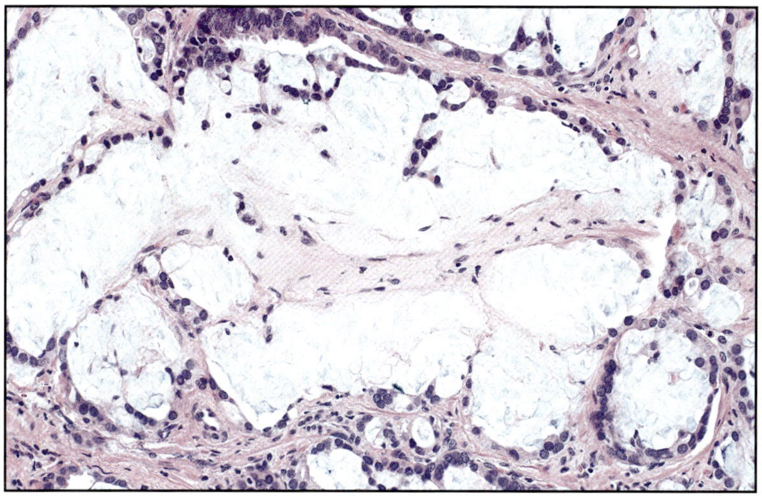

■ **i14.56** *Collagenous strand in mucin-producing prostatic adenocarcinoma.*

For diagnostic purposes, collagenous micronodules seem to be highly specific for carcinoma, but the sensitivity is low, particularly in needle biopsies (Bostwick 1995A, Varma 2002A). Thus far, collagenous micronodules have not been identified in benign prostatic glands,

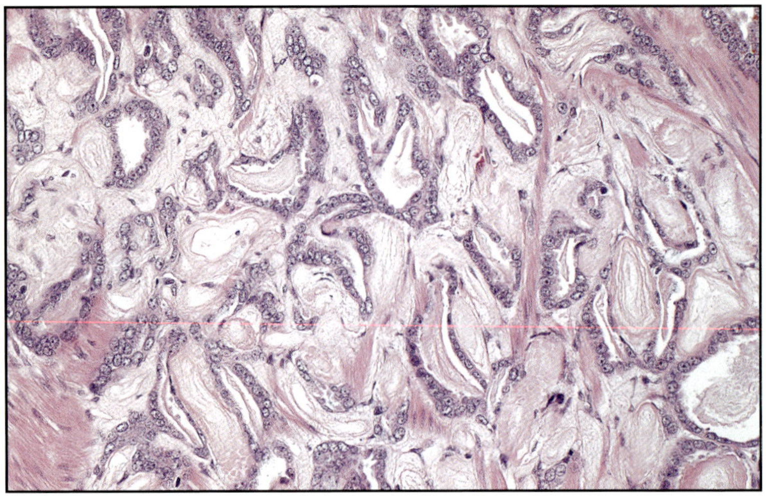

■ **i14.57** *Collagenous micronodules with solid to spiculated appearance, in prostatic adenocarcinoma. The glandular profiles are distorted.*

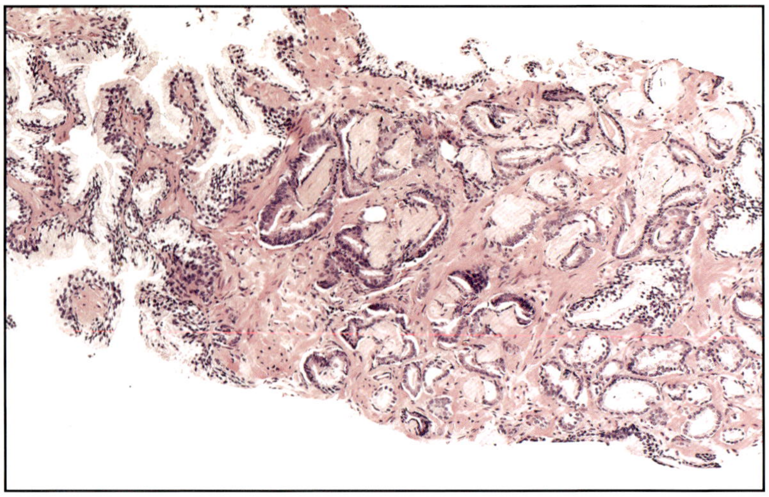

■ **i14.58** *Collagenous micronodules in prostatic carcinoma in needle biopsy tissue.*

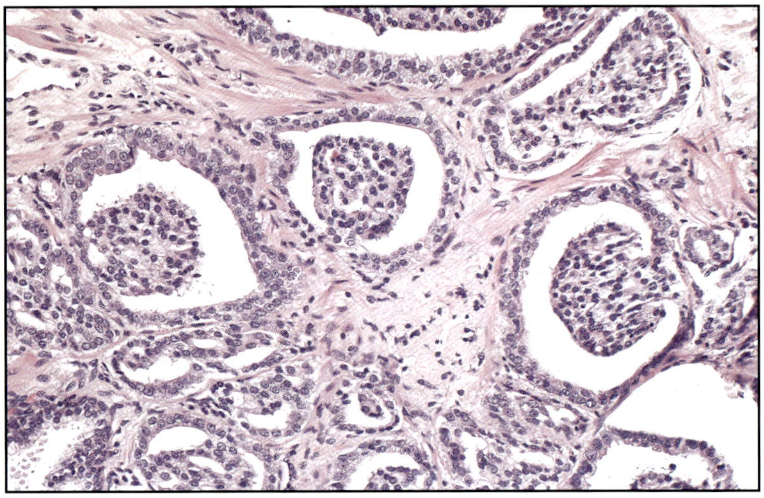

■ **i14.59** *"Glomeruloid" pattern prostatic adenocarcinoma. The intraluminal projections resemble renal glomeruli.*

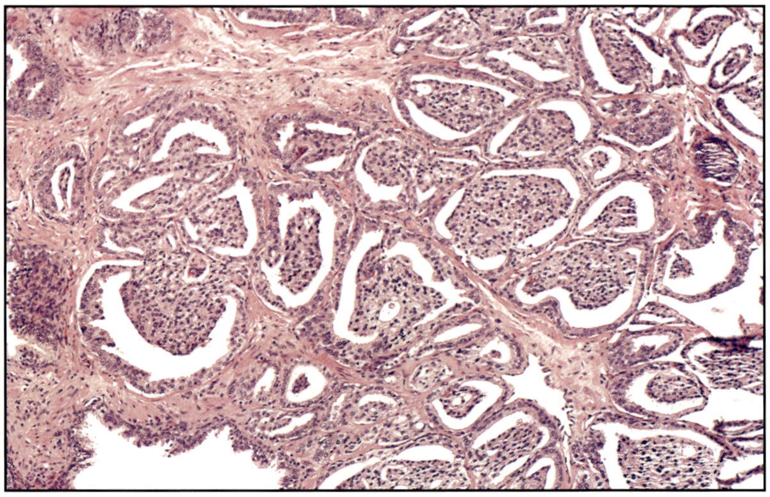

■ **i14.60** *Extensive "glomeruloid" pattern prostatic adenocarcinoma.*

benign prostatic hyperplasia (BPH), or PIN (Bostwick 1995A, Varma 2002A). However, their overall diagnostic utility is somewhat limited because they are found in only 1% to 2% of needle biopsies with carcinoma (Bostwick 1995A, Thorson 1998, Varma 2002A) and 13% to 22% of carcinomas in whole glands in radical prostatectomy specimens (Bostwick 1995A, Kaleem 1998). Moreover, in the small percentage of needle biopsies with collagenous micronodules, the diagnosis usually is straightforward using the classic major criteria. The appearance of collagenous micronodules is so distinctive that their presence can be a low-power diagnostic clue **i14.58**. Collagenous micronodules can simulate perineural invasion, but the micronodules are not as cellular as nerves and the wavy nuclei are not as prevalent in the micronodules as nerves. Collagenous micronodules do not have prognostic significance (Bostwick 1995A).

Glomeruloid structures, or glomerulations (Baisden 1999), are renal glomerulus-like epithelial aggregates within acini of prostatic adenocarcinoma **t14.8; i14.59** (Pacelli 1998). This pattern of intraluminal epithelial growth is thought to be specific for carcinoma (Pacelli 1998, Varma 2002A). The diagnostic value of glomerulations is somewhat limited by their presence in only 3%-15% of needle biopsies with carcinoma and 5% of radical prostatectomies with adenocarcinoma (Pacelli 1998, Varma 2002A). Microscopically, glomeruloid bodies are characterized by rounded to ball-like tufts or buds into small to medium-sized malignant glands. Usually the body appears to be tethered to the outer layer of cells by a single, narrow point of attachment, but several points of connection can be seen occasionally **i14.60** (Pacelli 1998). In about one third of cases, there is a fibrovascular core. The glomeruloid bodies make up only a minority of the carcinoma, ranging from 5% to 10% in needle core tissue to 5% to 20% in the whole gland. The differential diagnosis includes cribriform hyperplasia, but in this proliferation there is a basal cell layer, and the constituent cells are cytologically bland. I have seen rare cases of a benign gland with a glomeruloid

■ t14.8 **Glomeruloid Structures (Glomerulations)**

Highly selective for carcinoma
Found in 3%-15% of carcinomas in needle biopsies and in 5% of carcinomas in whole gland
Microscopically: Ball-like tufts or buds that project into a rounded gland, like a renal glomerulus
Often associated with high-grade carcinoma; recommended Gleason pattern assignment is 3 or 4

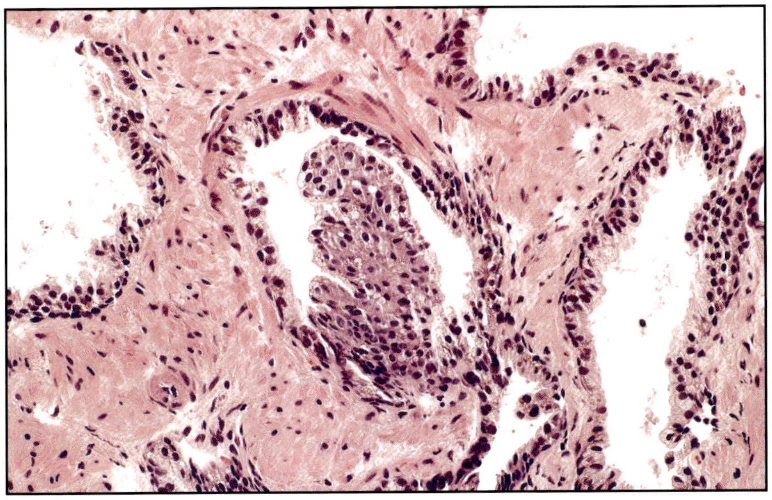

■ **i14.61** *Intraluminal glomeruloid-like projection in a benign gland. The glomeruloid pattern is highly associated with, but is not absolutely specific for, prostatic adenocarcinoma.*

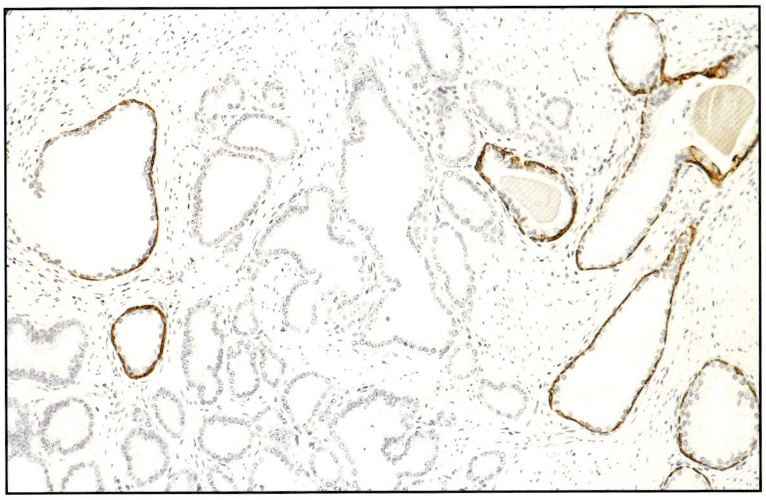

■ **i14.62** *Basal cell absence in malignant glands is substantiated by diffuse absence of 34βE12 immunohistochemical staining, with positive internal control staining of adjacent benign glands.*

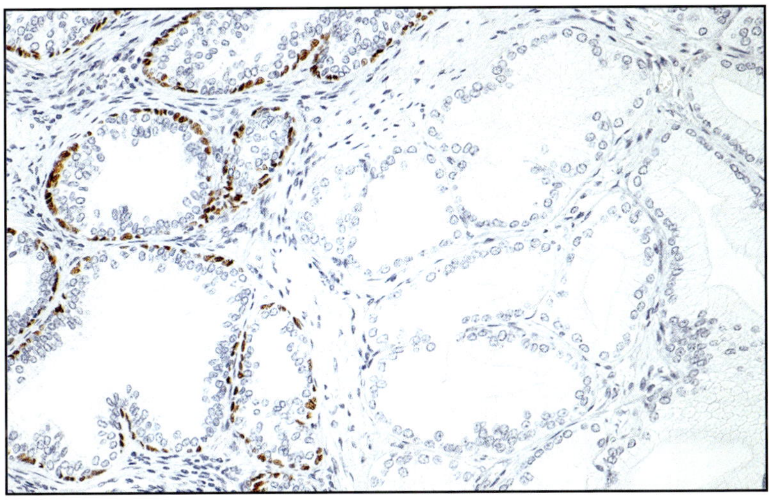

■ **i14.63** *p63 immunostain marks nuclei of basal cells in benign glands (left) compared to absence of staining in carcinoma glands (right).*

projection **i14.61**, so it is unlikely that glomerulations are absolutely specific, and one should again use the major and minor criteria to arrive at a final diagnosis. Glomerulations appear to be associated most often with high-grade (Gleason score 7 or 8), higher-stage (T3) disease, but one recommendation is that these structures be regarded as Gleason grade pattern 3 (Pacelli 1998). Others, including this author, view glomerulations as indicative of Gleason grade pattern 4. The true biologic behavior of this pattern is not known because prostatic adenocarcinoma with pure glomeruloid growth has not been described.

Ancillary Diagnostic Studies

The most valuable adjunctive study for diagnosis of adenocarcinoma of the prostate currently is immunohistochemistry with monoclonal antibody 34βE12 **i14.62**, which binds to high-molecular-weight cytokeratins expressed in basal cells rather than luminal cells (Brawer 1985, Hedrick 1989, Kahane 1995, Shah 1991, Wojno 1995) **t14.9**. (In the future, additional basal cell–specific markers such as p63 **i14.63** (Parsons 2001, Shah 2002A, Signoretti 2000, Weinstein 2002) and cytokeratin 5/6 [Abrahams 2002] may be similarly useful.) The 34βE12 antibody, which has also been identified by its commercial catalog number, CK903, is useful in documenting the absence of basal cells in focal atypical small acinar proliferations, yet there are caveats in the use and interpretation of this immunohistochemical staining reaction. First, basal cell absence is an important criterion for the histologic diagnosis of prostatic carcinoma but is only one of several of the major criteria. That is, this immunostain, like other adjunctive studies, should be interpreted in the context of all histologic findings in the case (Algaba 1996). Also, as Stout noted one half century ago, based on examination of H&E-stained sections, not all benign glands have basal cells (Totten 1953). This has been substantiated by the 34βE12 immunostain because a minority of benign glands can have a discontinuous or absent basal cell layer. Indeed, one of the benign entities most often misdiagnosed as carcinoma, atrophy, can reveal scattered negative glands in 11% to 23% of cases (Amin 1999, Hedrick 1989, Varma 1997). Up to 12% of basal cell hyperplasia glands fail to stain (Hedrick 1989), and 10% to 90% (average = 50%) of glands in AAH do not stain. Furthermore, this immunohistochemical stain is based on a negative result to render a positive diagnosis of malignancy. Many factors can cause failure of immunohistochemical staining, and absence of proof is not proof of absence. Therefore, it is absolutely critical to study the immunostained cores for a positive internal control: benign glands with a strong, positive basal cell signal. Preferably, these benign glands are located near the adjacent carcinoma or, for needle biopsy tissue, are at least in the same core **i14.64**. Finally, despite a single report (Googe 1997) to the contrary, exceedingly few, if any, carcinoma cells are immunoreactive in 34βE12 immunohistochemical staining (Yang 1999).

■ **t14.9 Immunostaining for Basal Cells in the Diagnosis of Prostatic Adenocarcinoma**

Antibody 34βE12 (CK903) often used
Stains high-molecular cytokeratins 1,5,10, and 14 expressed in basal cell, not luminal cell, cytoplasm
p63 immunostain can also be used
Useful in selected cases as a confirmatory tool
Not all glands that are negative are malignant: A minority of atrophic, basal cell hyperplastic and AAH glands can be negative
Incorporate immunostain results into interpretation based on histological context

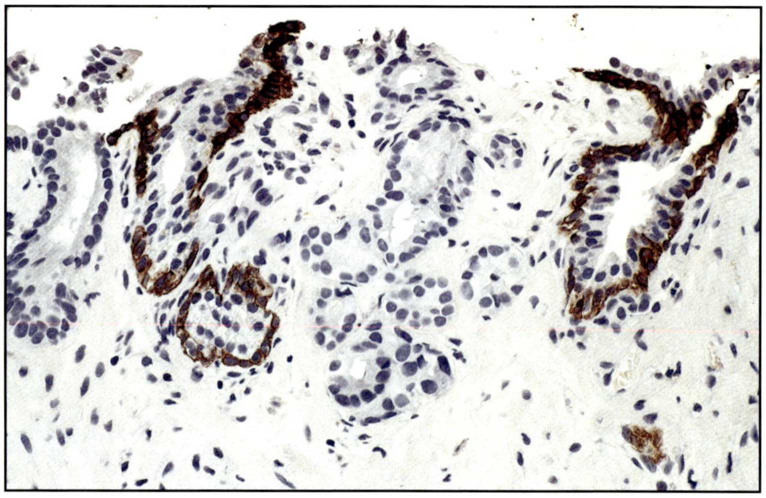

■ **i14.64** *Confirmation of basal cell absence in minimal adenocarcinoma in needle biopsy. Absence of basal cell staining highlights the infiltrative growth between positive-staining benign glands.*

With these pitfalls in mind, the 34βE12 immunostain can be useful as a confirmatory measure in specific circumstances, particularly in the assessment of a focal atypical small acinar proliferation in needle biopsy (Hedrick 1989, Kahane 1995, Shah 1991, Tran 1999, Varma 1997, Wojno 1995). It should not be used as a screening test in all prostate needle biopsies (Algaba 1996) but rather should be specifically applied in selected cases with selection and the differential diagnosis driven by the H&E histologic appearance. It is not necessary to use the 34βE12 immunostain on all carcinomas to confirm basal cell absence; indeed, in our series of 50 minimal carcinomas in needle biopsy, all diagnoses were made on H&E-stained sections alone (Thorson 1998). In a recent large series (Wojno 1995), only 2.8% of all prostate needle biopsies were immunostained with antibody 34βE12. It was most often ordered to evaluate a focus of atypical glands and was also ordered in selected cases where the differential diagnosis encompassed AAH (adenosis), PIN, basal cell hyperplasia, and atrophy (Wojno 1995). The immunostain can also be used to distinguish cribriform high-grade PIN from cribriform invasive carcinoma (Amin 1994). When it was requested to assess a focus of atypical glands, the number of glands per case usually was 4 to 30 (Wojno 1995). Overall, in needle biopsy this immunostain was felt to be confirmatory in 58% of cases, was equivocal in 18% of cases, established the diagnosis in 14% of cases and was of no use in 8% of cases, and changed the favored diagnosis in 2% of cases (Wojno 1995). In needle biopsy cases stained with 34βE12, there was a tendency for cases with fewer glands to be diagnosed as equivocal rather than minimal cancer, but there was extensive overlap in number of glands on which a diagnosis was based, which again speaks to use of this immunostain as a supplementary tool. In another series of needle biopsies, it was concluded that the 34βE12 immunostain substantially reduced the percentage of prostate needle biopsy cases diagnosed as atypical (Kahane 1995).

The 34βE12 immunostain can be particularly valuable when the differential diagnostic consideration is radiation-induced atypia and focal minimal residual carcinoma in patients with prostate cancer treated by radiation therapy (Brawer 1989, Gaudin 1998). In this setting reactive basal cells can cytologically mimic cancer cells in nuclear alterations, and here the 34βE12 immunostain can provide important diagnostic information. Minimal residual carcinoma after hormonal therapy can also pose diagnostic challenges. and positive immunostains for PSA and pan-cytokeratin with a negative 34βE12 immunostain can sometimes be helpful (Gaudin 1998).

The cost and practical methodologic approaches for the 34βE12 immunohistochemical stain should be noted. The estimated cost of performing the immunostain has been estimated at $5.00 per case (Kahane 1995), but the charge to the patient at one hospital was $568.00, including professional fee and all hospital and lab charges (Wojno 1995). This charge is much less than that of rebiopsy (Wojno 1995). There are important technical considerations in performing 34βE12 immunohistochemistry. First, the immunostain works well on formalin-fixed, paraffin-embedded prostate needle biopsies and on Bouin's-fixed needle biopsies (Pins 1999). Second, to optimize the binding reaction, one should use an epitope retrieval technique with protease digestion or heat-induced antigen retrieval (Iczkowski 1999, Kaleem 1998, Varma 1999). Lastly, the immunostain procedure can be carried out on unstained interval sections (on sialiated slides) (Green 1999, Iczkowski 1999), on deeper sections from the block, or even on destained H&E slides (Dardik 2000). For cases with just a few glands on an H&E-stained slide, this latter procedure is feasible in a majority of cases, although the intensity of basal cell staining is, in our experience, sometimes less than that for an immunohistochemical stain performed on an unstained section. In a minority of cases, there is staining failure or the tissue section is lost from the slide during the staining procedure. Accordingly, in our laboratory, we always retain an H&E-stained section or sections with the atypical epithelial proliferation and do not restain the only section of concern with the 34βE12 antibody. The precise conditions that cause staining failure in restaining attempts are not well defined.

An immunostain that can be used as a positive confirmation for prostatic neoplasia is the immunohistochemical reaction for α-methyl-CoA racemase (AMACR), also known as P504S. This marker was discovered to be overexpressed in prostatic adenocarcinoma by cDNA library subtraction using high-throughput RNA microanalysis (Xu 2000). In immunohistochemistry, the protein is selectively expressed in about 80% to 90% of prostatic adenocarninomas (Beach 2002, Jiang 2001, Luo 2002, Zhou 2002), compared to benign glands, but the staining is not specific for carcinoma. Up to 21% of benign prostatic glands can also stain, although the staining signal is usually more focal and weaker compared to carcinoma (Beach 2002, Rubin 2002B). Most high-grade PIN foci stain (Zhou 2002) and a minority of atypical adenomatous hyperplasia cases stain (Yang 2002). The AMACR immunostain is best interpreted only in histologic context and preferably in conjunction with 34βE12 and/or p63 immunostaining.

Finally, in certain cases additional immunohistochemical studies are indicated. For example, in the differential diagnosis of focal granulomatous prostatitis and focal poorly differentiated prostatic adenocarcinoma, a panel of antibodies to cytokeratins (AE1/AE3), PSA, prostate-specific acid phosphatase (PSAP), lysozyme, antimacrophage M, and leukocyte common antigen reliably distinguished the 2 disorders (Presti 1991). As discussed later in this chapter (and highlighted in **t14.16**), the differential diagnostic workup of prostatic carcinoma and transitional cell carcinoma (TCC) can be aided by use of a targeted panel of antibodies, including PSA, PSAP, and 34βE12 (Genega 2000). Immunostains against these same markers can be exceedingly helpful when prostatic carcinoma is the differential diagnosis of a metastatic carcinoma of unknown primary origin. PSA and PSAP are the best prostatic markers in general, but they are not absolutely specific and can stain benign and malignant nonprostatic cells and tissues (Allsbrook 1998, Epstein 1993E). Although usually resolved by examination of H&E slides, the distinction of small seminal vesicle glands and minimal prostatic adenocarcinoma can

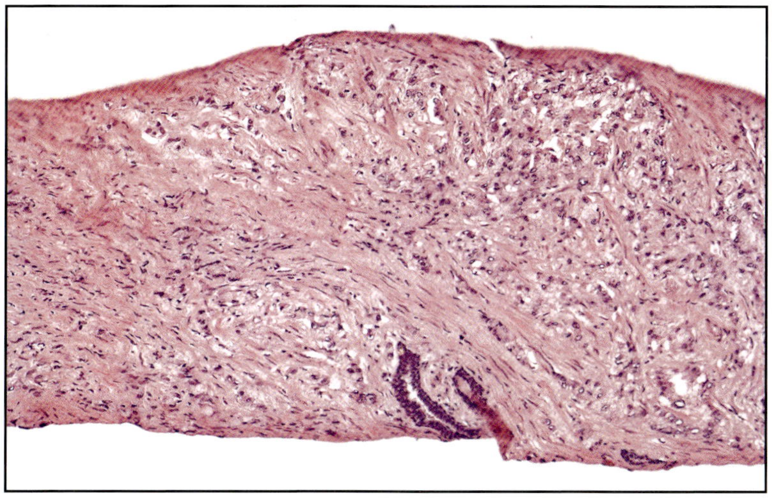

■ **i14.65** *Frozen section of prostate needle biopsy tissue. Increased cellularity due to infiltrative high-grade carcinoma.*

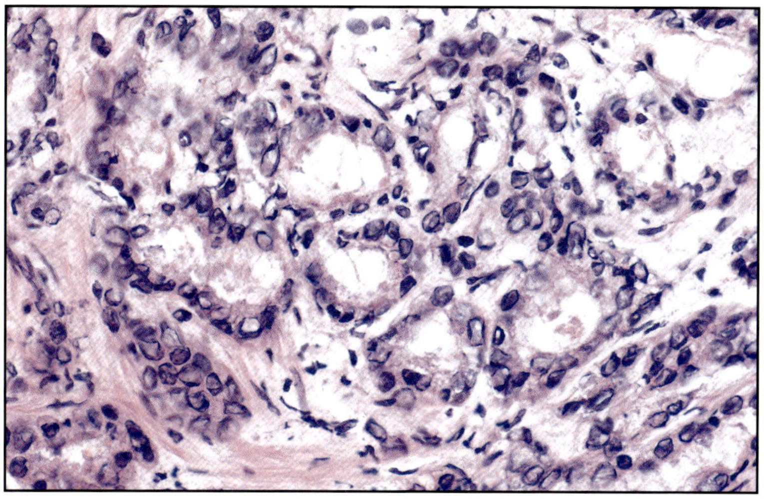

■ **i14.66** *Frozen section of prostatic adenocarcinoma: Intranuclear detail, and especially macronucleoli, can be difficult to appreciate in frozen sections of prostatic adenocarcinoma.*

also be accomplished by PSA (using monoclonal antibody [Varma 2002B]), PSAP, and 34βE12 immunohistochemistry where prostatic carcinoma glands will be positive for the first 2 markers and negative using the latter antibody.

Currently, DNA abnormalities such as DNA ploidy, gain or loss of specific DNA sequences, or specific gene mutations are not used in the diagnosis of carcinoma of the prostate. Clearly, DNA abnormalities that are common in prostatic carcinoma (such as allelic loss on 8p) can also be found in high-grade PIN (Chapter 11) and AAH (Chapter 8), such that current molecular biologic technology does not distinguish between nonmalignant and malignant proliferation in the prostate. Gene expression (RNA transcriptional) profiles, as may be obtained on gene chips, are also not currently used in diagnosis of prostatic carcinoma.

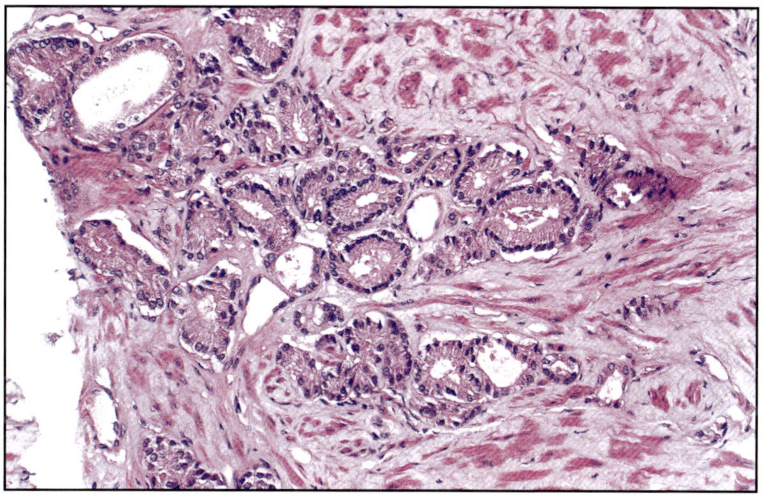

■ **i14.67** *Prostatic adenocarcinoma in prostate needle biopsy tissue fixed in Bouin's solution. The muscular stroma often appears brightly eosinophilic.*

[14.2] Diagnosis of Adenocarcinoma in Needle Core Biopsy

The histopathologic diagnosis of adenocarcinoma of the prostate in needle core biopsy presents a unique set of challenges. First, in the PSA era, the carcinomas that are being detected often are quite small, occupying on average one half as much of the needle core tissue, compared with carcinomas digitally detectable as a mass (Humphrey 1993C, 1998B). Many PSA-detected carcinomas make up <5% to 10% of needle core tissue. Second, it can be difficult to appreciate an infiltrative architectural pattern of growth in the thin 18-gauge needle core biopsies. Lastly, the needle cores can fragment, which can also generate problems in interpretation.

Diagnosis of adenocarcinoma in prostate needle biopsy tissue should, as standard practice, be rendered on fixed, paraffin-embedded tissue sections. In rare cases, frozen sections of needle core tissue from the prostate may be interpreted to establish a diagnosis of malignancy **i14.65, i14.66**. The only valid clinical indication for this is for a man who presents with bony pain and a rock-hard prostate by digital rectal examination (with or without "metastatic" levels of serum PSA), where immediate orchiectomy will be performed to relieve pain. Histologically these cases usually are straightforward, with a large amount of high-grade tumor. However, frozen section artifactual nuclear distortion can be severe, with "blown-out" cleared nuclei, which appear enlarged, without macronuclei **i14.66**. (As a historical note, 40 years ago frozen section diagnosis of needle biopsy or open perineal wedge prostate specimens was commonly performed at the Massachusetts General Hospital, with "good diagnostic success" [Vickery 1963].)

Most needle core biopsy tissue is fixed in neutral buffered formalin, but a few laboratories use Bouin's or Hollande's solution for fixation **i14.67**. These fixatives allow more uniform preservation of nuclear detail, such that benign nuclei in Bouin's-fixed prostate needle core tissue may appear atypical. One should carefully recalibrate one's threshold for nuclear atypia in these cases by study of the appearance of nuclei in clearly benign glands.

To detect carcinoma in prostate needle biopsy, it is best to prepare 3 levels, that is, 3 slides, each with several sections, from each paraffin block (Brat 1999, Lane 1998, Renshaw 1997). Some laboratories save unstained slides with interval sections taken between the 3 levels. These slides can be used for H&E staining or ancillary immunohistochemical staining. It is not necessary to serially section through prostate needle core tissue. We found that this necessitated a mean 30 slides per block, with a mean of 4 sections per slide (Reyes 1998). Additional levels beyond the first 3 standard slides were critical in diagnosing carcinoma only when a diagnosis of focal glandular atypia was rendered in the first 3 slides. In 10% of cases of focal glandular atypia, a single additional level allowed a definitive diagnosis of carcinoma, based on a larger lesional size in the additional level (Reyes 1998). Therefore, for maximal detection of carcinoma in prostate needle biopsy, we recommend obtaining 3 initial levels (H&E-stained slides), with procurement of an additional level (slide) if focal glandular atypia is detected in the initial 3 slides. This additional slide can be stained with H&E or the 34βE12 immunostain.

The initial step in evaluating for the major and minor diagnostic criteria of adenocarcinoma **t14.2** is to study, in the needle biopsy case being examined, glands that one is certain are benign. This is crucial because fixation, staining, and section thickness can affect appearance of the prostatic epithelium. By first inspecting benign glands, one can calibrate one's eye, for each individual case, for the purpose of later comparison with atypical glands. In some cases of very extensive prostatic carcinoma in needle biopsy, normal glands will not be present because of effacement by tumor. It is very important to scan every core section and examine all levels of tissue because different levels may provide additional information. It is also important to appreciate the normal architecture of the prostate gland before diagnosing minimal adenocarcinoma of the prostate. Normal prostate glands are complex and branching, with 2 cell layers: basal cells and luminal cells (Chapter 1).

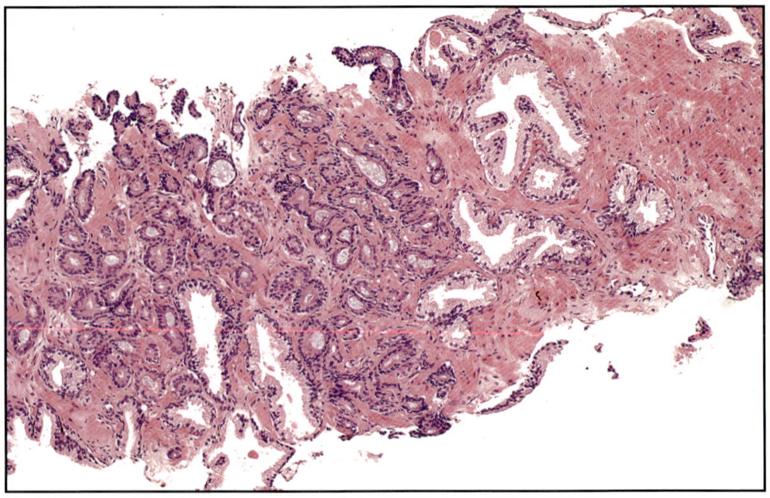

■ **i14.68** *Classical image of small acinar adenocarcinoma infiltrating amongst paler, benign glands in needle biopsy tissue: Gleason grade 3+3=score of 6.*

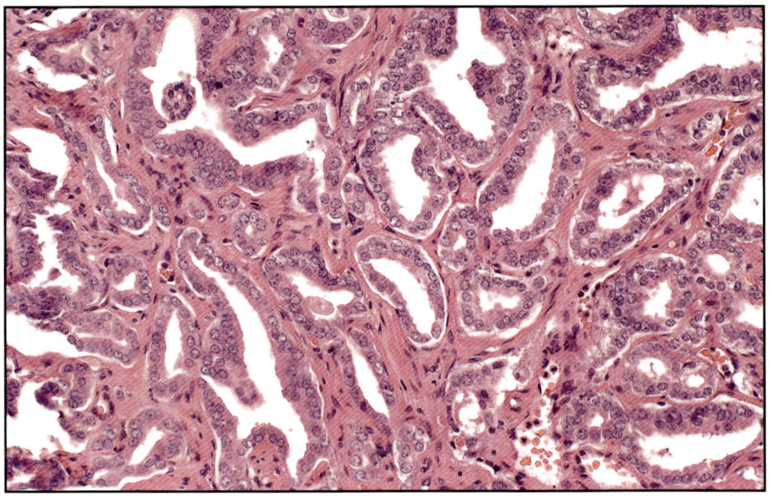

■ **i14.69** *Moderately differentiated Gleason pattern 3 prostatic adenocarcinoma with elongated glandular profiles.*

Application of Major and Minor Diagnostic Criteria

The major and minor criteria and diagnostic attributes of carcinoma **t14.2** should be specifically assessed at both low- and high-power magnifications. Although epithelial-stromal relationships and patterns of carcinoma growth are best surveyed at lower-magnification, high magnification scrutiny is necessary to evaluate for major criteria of basal cell absence and nuclear atypia. Detection of many of the minor diagnostic criteria also necessitates use of high-magnification objectives.

The first assessment one should perform in needle biopsy sections is a search for the first of the major criteria, an infiltrative growth pattern, which often presents as the presence of small malignant glands extending between or around larger, more complex, and often paler benign glands **i14.68; t14.10**. These Gleason grade 3 adenocarcinomas are the most common pattern recognized in needle biopsy (Epstein 1995A, Steinberg 1997, Thorson 1998). They exhibit irregularly distributed small glands of varying size and shape, including angulated, elongated, or "twisted" forms **i14.69** (Allsbrook 1999, Deshmukh 1998, Gleason 1990). There is usually appreciable stromal separation, without back-to-back grouping of malignant glands. In carcinomas that are minimal (<1mm) (Thorson 1998) or limited (Epstein 1995A) in extent in needle biopsy, the presence of a few malignant acini between the benign glands is indicative of invasion even though the glands appear only embedded within the stroma **i14.10**. This deceptive appearance results from the fact that the invading glands do not usually elicit a desmoplastic or inflammatory response, which characterizes many invasive carcinomas at the anatomic sites, and the glands can still appear rounded. Cribriform carcinoma is uncommon in needle biopsy, particularly in pure form **i14.70** and in minimal carcinoma. Here, invasiveness is evident only by complete absence of basal cells because the cribriform masses of neoplastic cells have smooth, rounded outer profiles. An invasive picture can also be difficult to recognize in the rare cases of pseudohyperplastic carcinoma in needle biopsy (Arista-Nasr 1997, Humphrey 1998A, Levi 2000), where the malignant glands display branching **i14.71**, cystic dilatation **i14.72, i14.73**, or papillary structures lined by high columnar cells with cleared cytoplasm. Association with a small acinar carcinoma component and a negative 34βE12 immunostain are useful findings in establishing a diagnosis of malignancy. The infiltrative character of high-grade (Gleason patterns 4 or 5 and score 7 to 10) prostatic carcinoma in needle biopsy is typified by ragged invasion of fused microacinar **i14.74**, cribriform, or papillary masses. Linkage of carcinoma cells into chains and cords **i14.75** also indicates poorly differentiated Gleason pattern 4

■ **t14.10 Patterns of Invasion by Prostatic Carcinoma in Needle Biopsy**

Haphazardly distributed small acini = most common
Rounded cribriform masses without basal cells
Ragged infiltrative, fused microacinar, cribriform or papillary structures
Chains and cords of neoplastic cells
Sheets of anaplastic tumor cells
Comedocarcinoma

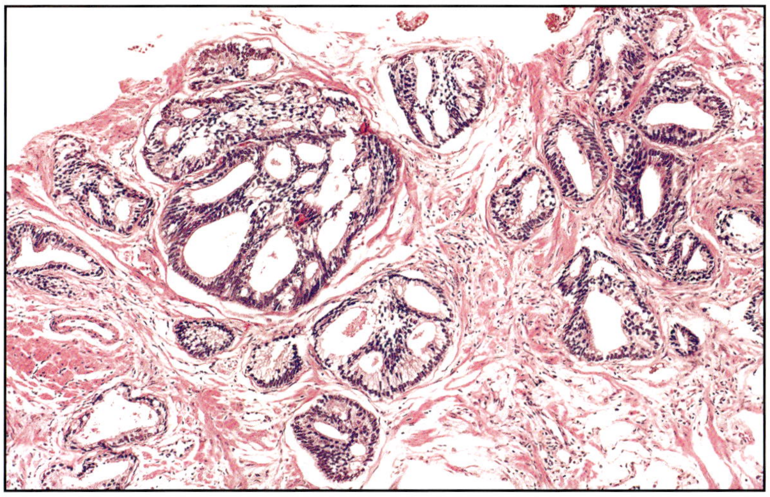

■ **i14.70** *Cribriform prostatic adenocarcinoma (left), adjacent to small acinar adenocarcinoma (right), in prostate needle biopsy tissue.*

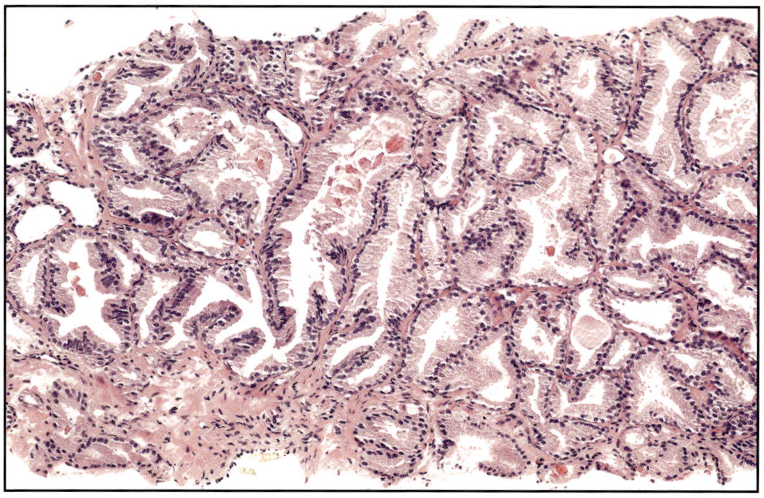

■ **i14.71** *Pseudohyperplastic prostatic adenocarcinoma in needle biopsy tissue: Malignant glands have branches and luminal undulations, simulating hyperplastic glands.*

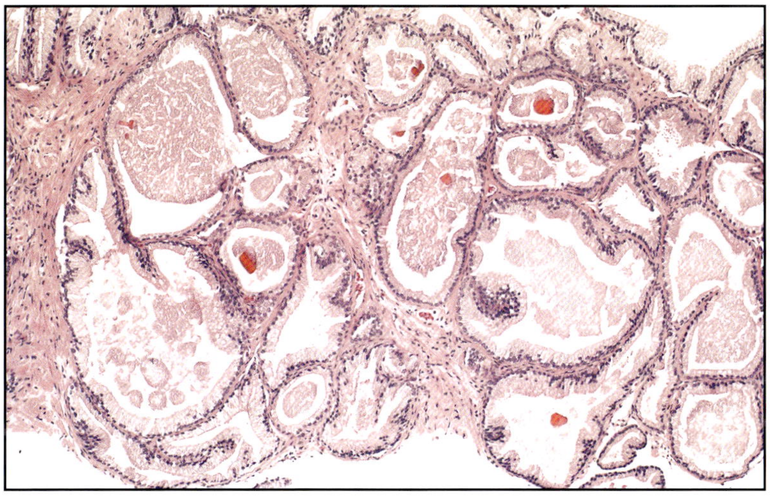

■ **i14.72** *Pseudohyperplastic prostatic adenocarcinoma in needle biopsy tissue: Dilated, intermediate-sized glands.*

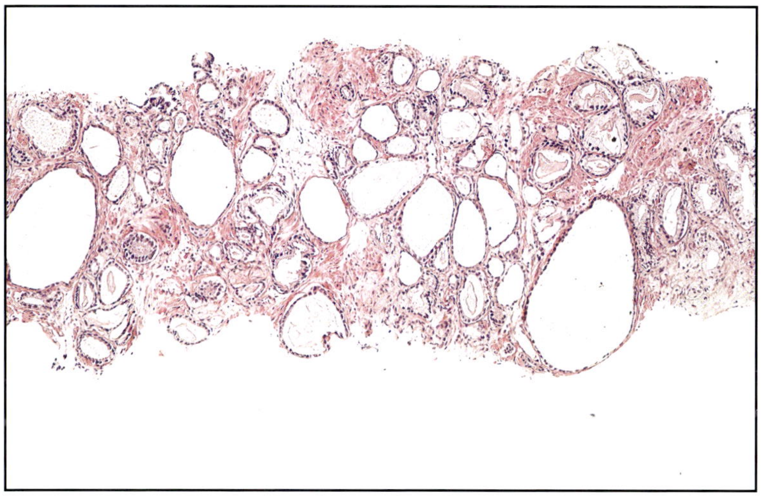

■ **i14.73** *Pseudohyperplastic prostatic adenocarcinoma in prostate needle biopsy tissue: Dilated glands admixed with a few small malignant acini.*

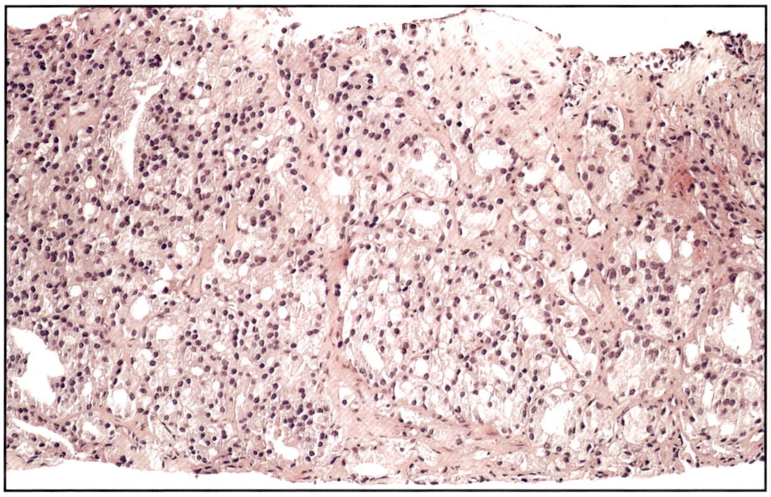

■ **i14.74** *High-grade fused microacinar Gleason grade pattern 4+4 = score of 8 in prostate needle biopsy tissue.*

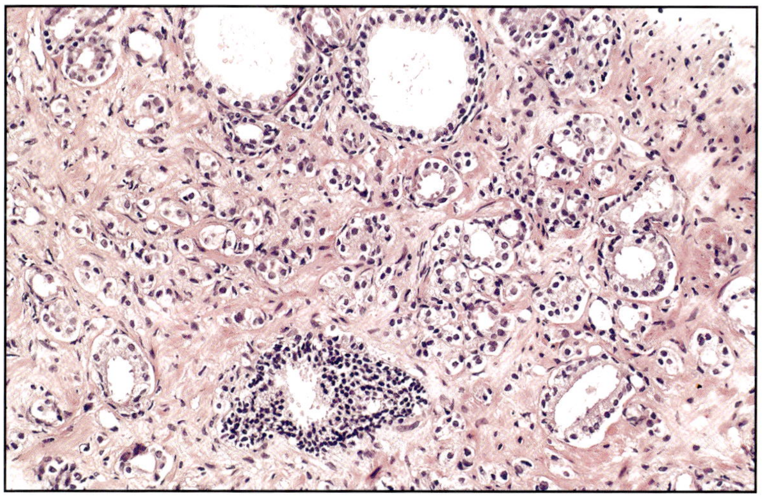

■ **i14.75** *High-grade Gleason pattern 4 prostatic adenocarcinoma in needle biopsy tissue: Short linear arrays of neoplastic cells. There is a minor Gleason pattern 3 element, generating an overall Gleason score of 7.*

adenocarcinoma (Gleason 1990). Gleason pattern 4 is overall a common morphologic manifestation of stromal permeation by carcinoma (Bostwick 1994A) but is not common in minimal carcinomas (Epstein 1995A, Thorson 1998) **i14.76**. High-grade carcinoma can also invade as sheets **i14.77**. This arrangement represents Gleason pattern 5, which is uncommon in needle biopsy (Bostwick 1994A).

In some cases, benign prostate glands are not present to serve as landmarks to evaluate invasion. This can result from destructive

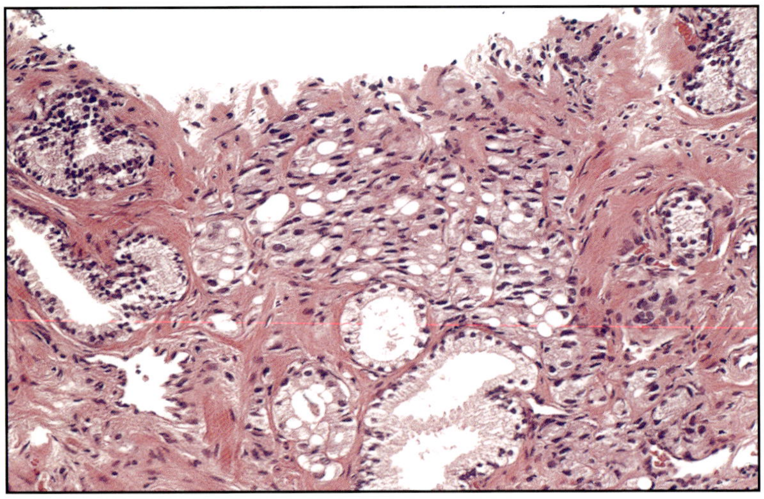

■ **i14.76** *Minimal high-grade fused microacinar adenocarcinoma in prostate needle biopsy tissue. This focus, which measured less than 1mm, was the only area of carcinoma in the needle biopsy tissue.*

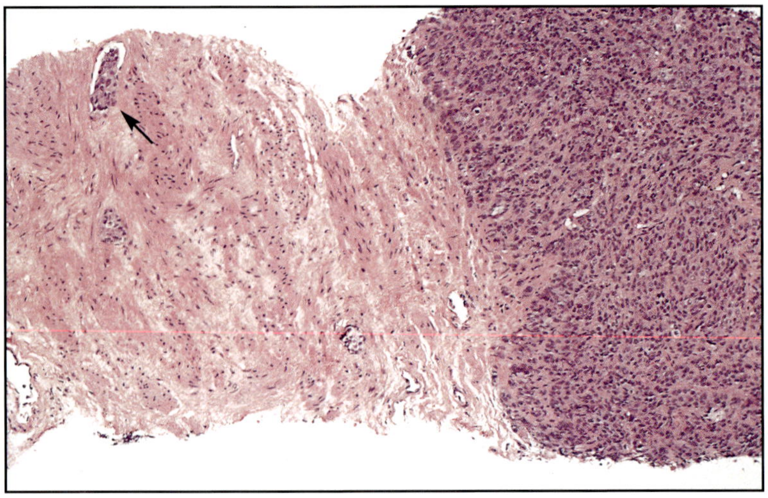

■ **i14.77** *High-grade Gleason pattern 5 in needle core biopsy tissue: Sheet-like growth, with sharp tumoral-stroma interface. Focal lymphovascular space invasion by carcinoma is evident (arrow).*

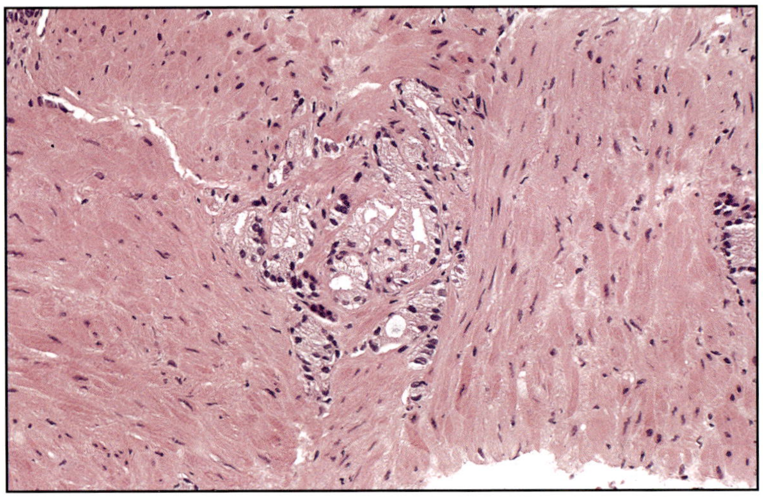

■ **i14.78** *Minimal adenocarcinoma in prostate needle biopsy tissue: Focal carcinoma penetration of smooth muscle stroma.*

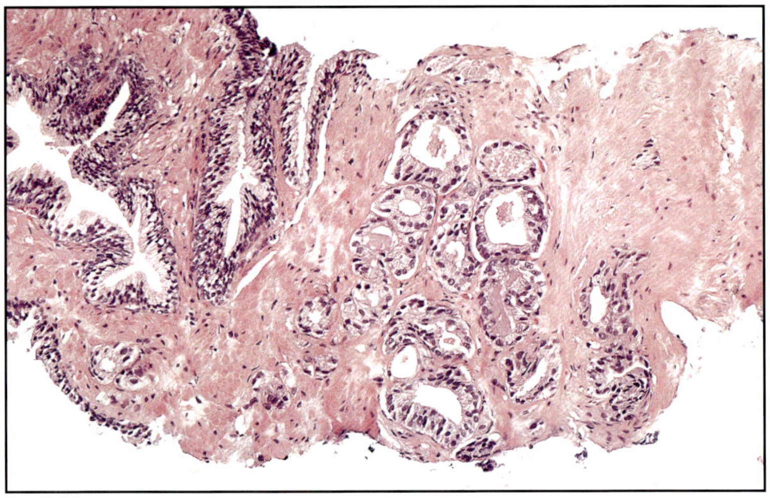

■ **i14.79** *Minimal adenocarcinoma in prostate needle biopsy tissue: Column-like infiltration spans the width of needle core tissue.*

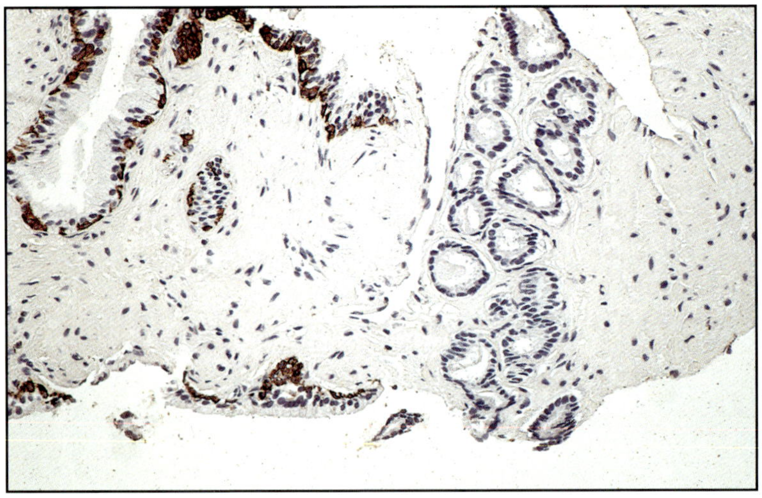

■ **i14.80** *Columnlike invasion of adenocarcinoma across width of prostate needle core tissue, as highlighted by negative 34βE12 immunohistochemical stain, with positive staining of adjacent benign glands with basal cells.*

growth of tumor, invasion into an area of pure fibromuscular stroma, and invasion into extraprostatic tissues, such as periprostatic adipose tissue or seminal vesicle tissue. In limited carcinomas a random dispersion of glands in stroma, without availability of benign glands as a reference point **i14.78**, was the second most common pattern of infiltration (Epstein 1995A). A distinctive pattern of infiltration is a formation of a column of malignant glands spanning the width of the needle core **i14.79, i14.80**. Invasion can also be appreciated when prostatic adenocarcinoma is identified in extraprostatic tissues sampled by needle biopsy. As incidental findings, periprostatic tissue can be found in up to 77% of needle biopsies (Ravery 1994), and seminal vesicle or ejaculatory duct tissue can be seen in up to 20% of needle biopsies (Bostwick 1997B). Periprostatic adipose tissue is most often seen at the tips of the needle cores, and the presence of epithelium in this fat can be a useful diagnostic finding **i14.81**. However, this is rarely an isolated finding and is generally associated with extensive carcinoma in the rest of the needle biopsy tissue. Prostatic carcinoma infiltration into seminal vesicle or ejaculatory duct tissue is an uncommon, incidental discovery, which tends to be more common in more extensive, higher-grade carcinoma in needle biopsy. The diagnosis of carcinoma is substantiated by recognition of infiltration into periprostatic tissues, but extraprostatic extension (EPE) can be diagnosed with certainty only in needle biopsy when malignant glands or cells are present in adipose tissue. Although the seminal vesicle muscle wall is thicker than the ejaculatory duct wall, the

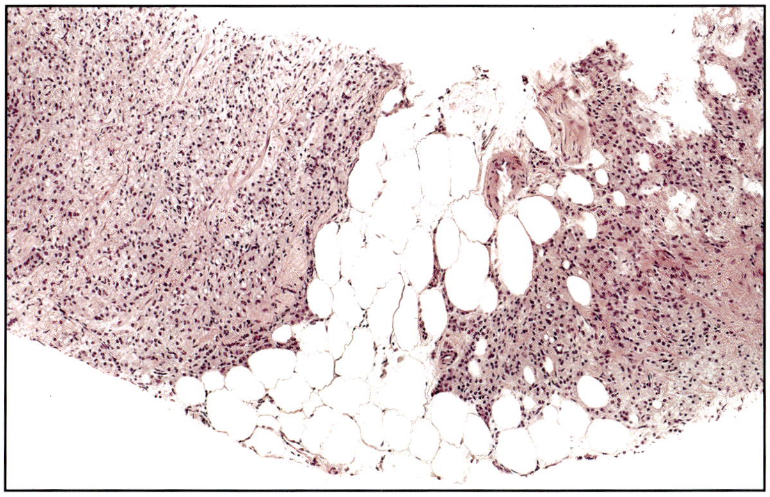

■ **i14.81** *Prostatic adenocarcinoma extension into periprostatic adipose tissue sampled by prostate needle biopsy.*

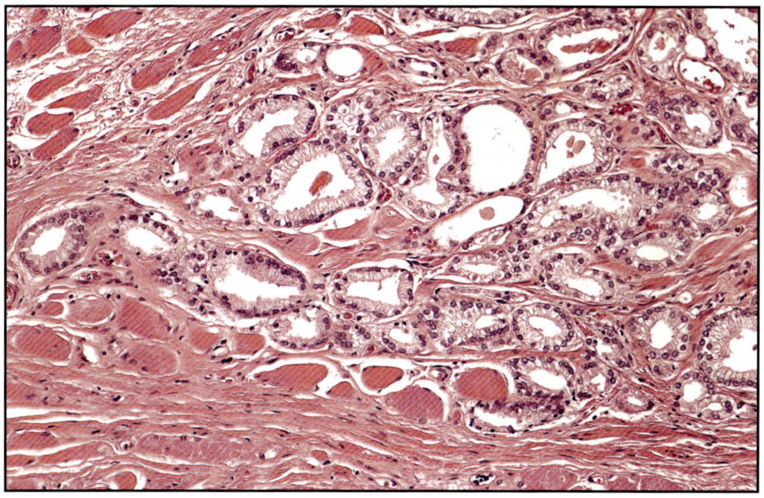

■ **i14.82** *Prostatic adenocarcinoma in skeletal muscle tissue. This finding does not necessarily indicate extraprostatic extension by carcinoma.*

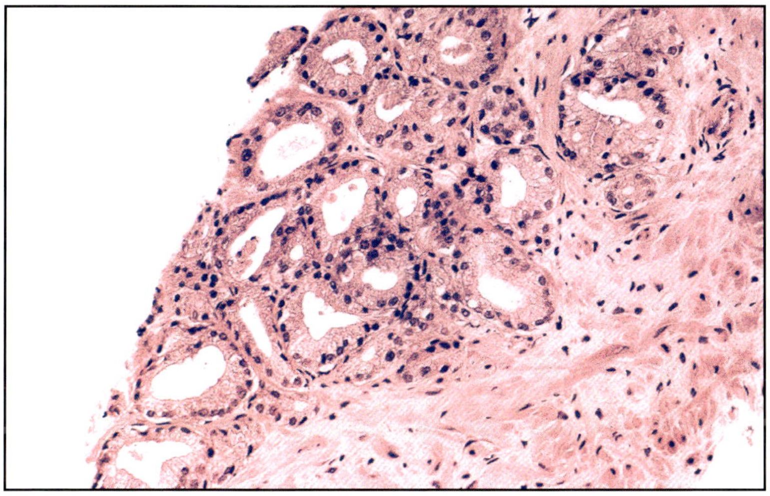

■ **i14.83** *Closely packed pale small acinar adenocarcinoma most consistent with well-differentiated adenocarcinoma. Most of these cases have Gleason pattern 3 elsewhere in the whole gland* (Thorson 1998).

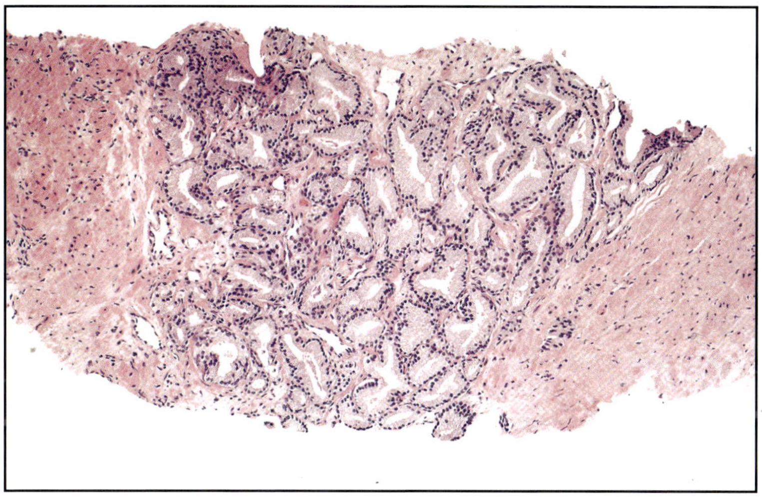

■ **i14.84** *Apparently nodular and well-differentiated adenocarcinoma in prostate needle biopsy tissue, but only a portion of the growth has been sampled.*

epithelium is similar, and the needle biopsy sampling is limited, such that it can be difficult to distinguish carcinoma infiltrating into intraprostatic ejaculatory duct wall from prostatic carcinoma penetrating into extraprostatic seminal vesicle wall. (Note that prostatic carcinoma rarely extends into the ejaculatory duct or seminal vesicle epithelial lining or lumina.) Disordered prostatic glands in thick smooth muscle bundles in needle biopsy can represent invasion of inadvertently sampled extraprostatic bladder neck, but it is difficult to be certain in needle biopsy that this represents extraprostatic spread and not prostatic stroma. Finally, benign or malignant prostatic glands can be observed in skeletal muscle tissue **i14.82** at the apex, where skeletal muscle of the urogenital diaphragm interdigitates into the prostate gland (Chapter 1). The detection of infiltrating carcinoma into skeletal muscle in needle biopsy does not necessarily equate with extraprostatic spread. Thus, in prostatic needle biopsy carcinoma of the prostate can present a range of infiltration images, with invasion into prostatic as well as extraprostatic tissues.

In a minority of needle biopsy cases, an infiltrative pattern is not evident **i14.83–i14.85**. These are well-differentiated, Gleason score 2 to 4 carcinomas that are, by definition, well-circumscribed, with smooth, pushing edges (Gleason 1990). The key low-power recognition clue here is a high density of closely packed, pale, small acini. The entire nodule of well-differentiated carcinoma is rarely sampled by the thin needle core biopsy, such that only a portion of the rim of the stromal-carcinoma interface is seen **i14.83**. In other cases, closely

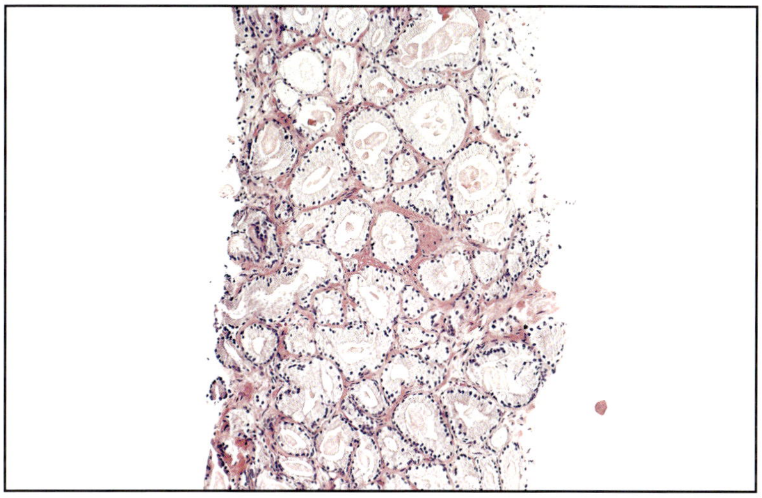

■ **i14.85** *Closely-arranged small pale acini of seemingly well-differentiated adenocarcinoma, but no stromal-adenocarcinoma edges are visualized for evaluation of infiltrative features.*

packed and fairly uniform small glands of carcinoma appear to represent well-differentiated adenocarcinoma **i14.85**, but the center of the nodule has been sampled by the needle, such that the edges of the proliferation and any infiltrative character cannot be evaluated. Well-differentiated Gleason score 2-4 adenocarcinoma in prostate needle biopsy tissue should be rare to nonexistent (Epstein 2000B).

High-power magnifications of atypical glands and cells should be used to assess for absence of a basal cell layer and nuclear atypia. In needle biopsy, thick sections are a major impediment in recognition of a single cell layer. Additional levels from the block cut at 3μm can be most helpful in this situation. Another common problem is nuclear distortion, where it may be difficult to identify elongated dark nuclei as luminal or basal cells **i14.22**. In my experience this quandary is more common in needle biopsy tissue than in carcinoma in whole gland. Why this should be is not established but could be related to shearing forces generated by the spring-loaded needle being driven into the prostate. Immunohistochemical staining using antibody 34βE12 can be useful in this circumstance. This immunostain is also of value in confirming basal cell absence when only a few malignant glands are present in needle biopsy **i14.64**. Nuclear atypia in carcinoma in needle biopsy is present in the form of nucleomegaly or nucleolomegaly. Nucleomegaly can be seen in a minority of cases in association with hyperchromasia and undetectable macronucleoli **i14.26**. No set number of nuclei must have macronucleoli for a diagnosis of carcinoma; this number can range from none to a few to numerous.

Minor diagnostic criteria are present less often in prostate needle biopsy with carcinoma than in whole glands with carcinoma **t14.11**. Abundant intraluminal wispy blue mucin **i14.28** and brightly eosinophilic crystalloids **i14.31** occasionally can be seen at scanning magnification and thereby constitute helpful diagnostic clues in the initial study of prostate needle biopsy sections. The detection of high-grade PIN at low magnifications should also prompt a search for invasive carcinoma. All of the minor findings can be found in nonmalignant prostatic glands and are not specific for carcinoma. If carcinoma is not detected, rebiopsy should be considered only for isolated high-grade PIN.

Features considered specific for carcinoma—perineural invasion, collagenous micronodules, and glomerulations—are also found less often in needle biopsies with carcinoma than in whole glands with carcinoma **t14.12**. The sensitivity of these features is even less in minimal carcinomas in needle biopsy, with only about 2% of cases of minimal carcinoma demonstrating perineural invasion and collagenous micronodules (Baisden 1999, Epstein 1995A, Thorson 1998), with glomerulations being rare (Baisden 1999, Thorson 1998). When deemed a dominant or key feature in the diagnosis of limited carcinoma, their applicability was even further diminished, to 0 to 0.6% of all cases of carcinoma in needle biopsy (Baisden 1999). Another finding specific for carcinoma, lymphvascular space invasion, is vanishingly rare in prostate needle biopsy tissue **i14.77**.

Minimal (Limited) Adenocarcinoma in Needle Biopsy Tissue

One of the major diagnostic challenges confronting the histopathologist in prostate needle biopsy interpretation is the definite in establishment of a malignant diagnosis based on a minimal or limited amount of carcinoma in needle biopsy (Epstein 1995A, Grignon 1998, Thorson 1998, 2000). The major and minor diagnostic criteria should be put into use here, just as for more extensive carcinoma. The presence of a few small malignant glands located between larger, more complex, paler benign glands is the most common pattern of invasion in minimal carcinoma, accounting for fully 80% of cases in one series (Epstein 1995A) **t14.13, i14.86**. The second most common pattern of infiltration of limited carcinoma is a haphazard growth in stroma, without adjacent benign glands **i14.78**. Uncommon patterns of growth that typically accompanied the common patterns are cords of cells, single cells, and cribriform glands (Epstein 1995A). Overall, an infiltrative pattern is found most minimal carcinoma cases (82% to 87%) (Epstein 1995A, Thorson 1998). Most cases are moderately differentiated, Gleason score 6. Basal cell absence usually can be determined using H&E-stained sections (Thorson 1998), with confirmation of absence with 34βE12 immunostain in certain cases **i14.64**. Only 4% of cases have a high-grade element (Gleason score 7 to 10) **i14.87**. Nearly every one of

■ **t14.11 Frequency of Minor Diagnostic Criteria in Adenocarcinoma in Needle Biopsy vs Whole Gland**

Minor Finding	Needle Biopsy	Whole Gland[1]
Intraluminal wispy blue mucin[1]	18%-52%	72%
Pink amorphous secretions[2]	53%-87%	84%
Mitotic figures[3]	Rare	Rare
Intraluminal crystalloids[4]	21%-41%	Up to 75%
Adjacent high-grade PIN[5]	13%-47%	74%[7]
Amphophilic cytoplasm[6]	36%-60%[2]	Up to 100%

[1]Epstein 1992A, Thorson 1998, Kaleem 1998, Varma 2002A
[2]Epstein 1992A, Thorson 1998, Varma 2002A
[3]Epstein 1995A, Thorson 1998, Byar 1972
[4]Epstein 1995A, Kaleem 1998, Anton 1998B, Varma 2002A
[5]Epstein 1995A, Hu 1998
[6]Epstein 1995A, Thorson 1998, Kaleem 1998
[7]See Table **t11.4**

■ **t14.12 Frequency of Features Potentially Specific for Carcinoma in Needle Biopsy With Carcinoma vs Whole Glands With Carcinoma**

Feature	Needle Biopsy	Whole Gland
Perineural invasion[1]	22%[4]	84%-94%
Collagenous micronodules[2]	1%-2%	13%-22%
Glomerulations[3]	3%-15%	5%

[1]Bismar 2003, Byar 1972, Varma 2002A, Andrews 1949, Bostwick 1994A, Bastacky 1993, Bassily 1999, Stone 1998, Bostwick 1996, Vargas 1999, de la Taille 1999, Jimenez 2000
[2]Thorson 1998, Kaleem 1998, Bostwick 1995A, Varma 2002A
[3]Pacelli 1998, Varma 2002A
[4]Range 2%-37%. See **t14.6**

■ **t14.13 Patterns of Invasion by Minimal Prostatic Carcinoma in Needle Biopsy**

Presence of small glands between benign glands—most common
Haphazard growth without adjacent benign glands
Uncommon: Cords of cells, single cells, cribriform structures

Epstein 1995A

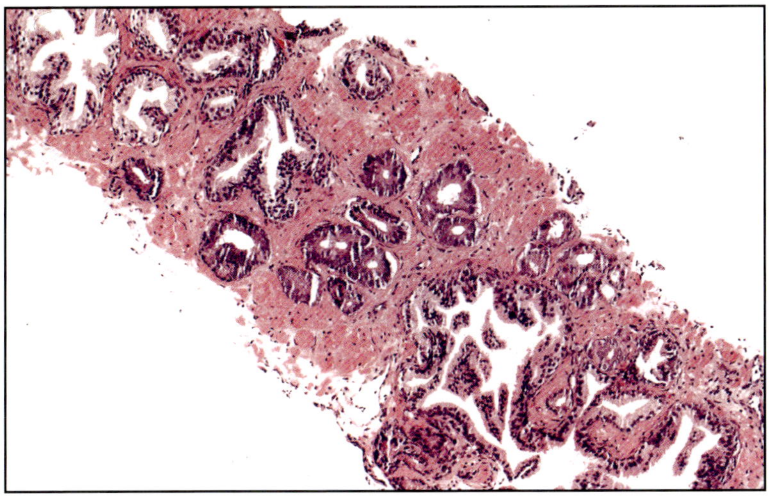

■ **i14.86** *Minimal adenocarcinoma: Several, rounded, small acini course between larger, more complex benign glands.*

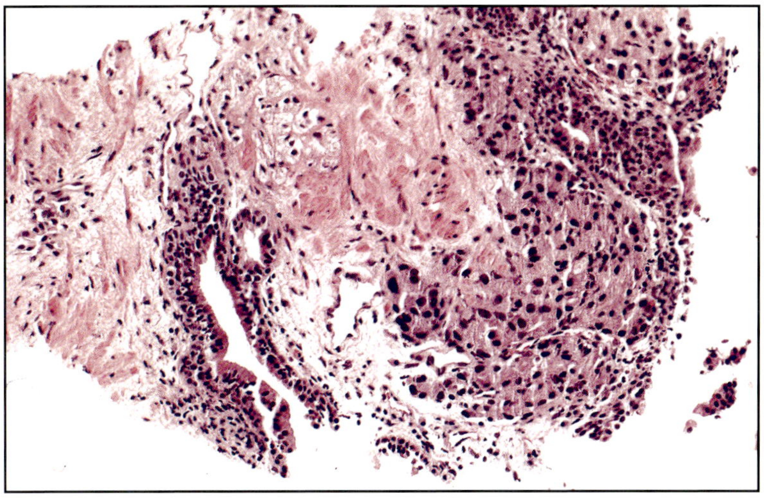

■ **i14.87** *Minimal high-grade adenocarcinoma in prostate needle biopsy, with solid aggregates of malignant tumor cells.*

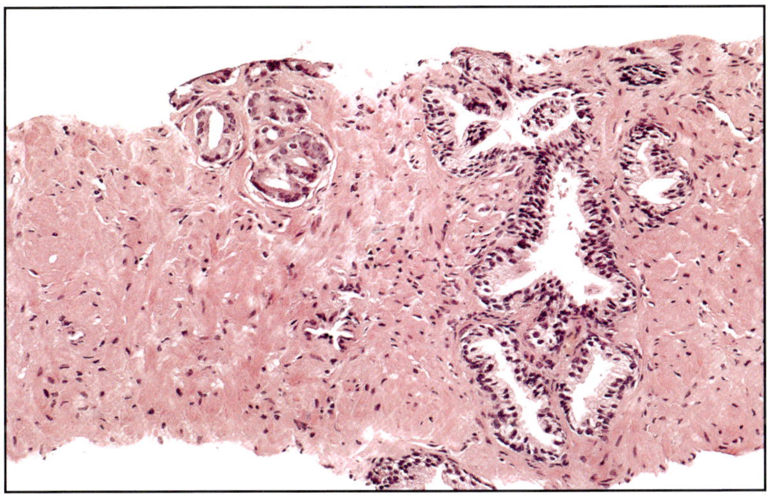

■ **i14.88** *Minimal adenocarcinoma: at edge of needle core.*

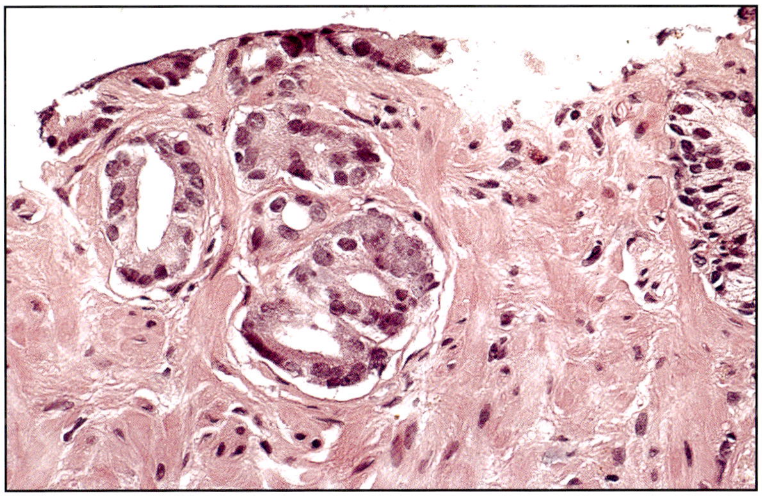

■ **i14.89** *Minimal adenocarcinoma.*

our cases of minimal carcinoma exhibited nucleomegaly, and a majority (64%) had prominent nucleoli (Thorson 1998). In a second series (Epstein 1995A) of minimal (limited) carcinoma in needle biopsy, 24% lacked prominent nucleoli and another 25% had only rare prominent nucleoli.

The major criteria do not include a quantitative threshold for the number of glands needed to establish a diagnosis of malignancy. In our series 80% of minimal carcinoma foci contained >10 glands (Thorson 1998), and in a second series the median number of malignant glands was 20 (Epstein 1995A). It is possible to diagnose invasive carcinoma based on just a few glands **i14.88, i14.89**. In our experience the smallest number of atypical glands that formed the basis for a definitive diagnosis of malignancy was 3 to 4. In these cases, there should be excellent preservation of cellular detail, without tangential sectioning, such that it was clear on the H&E sections that basal cells were absent and that significant nuclear atypia was present. Both of these major criteria are of immense importance for these most minimal of the minimal carcinomas, where architectural abnormalities are difficult or impossible to discern. In another series on minimal (limited) carcinoma, the lowest number of diagnostic glands was 2 (Epstein 1995A). At a recent consensus conference (Algaba 1996), most urologic pathologists felt that 3 glands constituted the typical lowest numerical cutoff, but in rare cases some hold the opinion that carcinoma may be diagnosed by the presence of a single neoplastic gland (Algaba 1996, Grignon 1998). Thus, opinions vary as to the number of glands needed for a definitive diagnosis of malignancy, but 3 glands seem to be the lower limit for many diagnosticians. Different thresholds for establishing a diagnosis of carcinoma do exist (Allam 1996, Amin 1998, Epstein 1995B, Lessels 1997), especially for minimal carcinoma (Amin 1998, Epstein 1995B), but overall there is a high level of interobserver agreement in the diagnosis of adenocarcinoma of the prostate.

To reiterate, it is a combination of features that allows establishment of a diagnosis of prostatic adenocarcinoma based on a minimal amount of tumor. No definite number of criteria must be fulfilled; rather, each case must be individualized and interpreted based on its own unique set of findings.

Differential Diagnosis of Adenocarcinoma in Needle Biopsy

The differential diagnosis of adenocarcinoma in prostate needle biopsy encompasses a long list of benign and malignant entities. Benign conditions include all pseudoneoplasms in the prostate

■ **t14.14 Differential Diagnosis of Prostatic Adenocarcinoma in Needle Biopsy: Most Important Conditions**

Atypical adenomatous hyperplasia[1]
Atrophy[1]
Basal cell hyperplasia
Inflammatory atypia
High-grade PIN
Focal glandular atypia (atypical small acinar proliferation)

[1]Most likely to be misdiagnosed as carcinoma

(Chapter 10, **t10.1**). The most important benign lesions to consider are those that are most often misdiagnosed as carcinoma: AAH (adenosis) and atrophy (Algaba 1996, Epstein 1996A, Gaudin 1997, Young 1997) **t14.14**. AAH, or adenosis, is an atypical small acinar proliferation that can masquerade as well-differentiated adenocarcinoma in needle biopsy (Gaudin 1995). Although both proliferations are characterized by circumscribed, high-density collections of small acini, AAH often is in continuity with larger, more complex glands, AAH exhibits a fragmented basal cell layer, and the luminal cells typically have bland nuclei (Bostwick 1993B, Gaudin 1995). AAH (adenosis) is an uncommon to rare proliferation in needle biopsies, at <1% of all prostate needle biopsy cases (Gaudin 1995, Reyes 1998). Atrophy, on the other hand, is separated from prostatic carcinoma by the presence of basal cells, cytoplasmic volume loss, and typically a lesser degree of nuclear atypia (Billis 1998, Franks 1954, Ruska 1998). However, nuclear enlargement and prominent nucleoli can be observed in atrophy, especially when there is accompanying inflammation (Ruska 1998). A lobular architecture sometimes can be seen in atrophy, but background fibrosis can simulate a fibrogenic response in sclerotic atrophy, with a resultant infiltrative-like picture. Foci of postatrophic hyperplasia (Amin 1999, Anton 1999, Cheville 1995), with its crowded acini, and partial atrophy (Oppenheimer 1998) can also be mistaken for prostatic adenocarcinoma in needle biopsy. One should also be aware that adenocarcinoma of the prostate can have atrophic features, with significant cytoplasmic volume loss (Cina 1997, Egan 1997B, Kaleem 1998). We have seen rare examples of minimal prostatic adenocarcinoma with atrophic features in needle biopsy **i14.90**. In these cases, continuity with usual adenocarcinoma where the cells had a moderate amount of cytoplasm and substantiation of basal cell absence by a 34βE12 immunostain were instrumental in diagnosing malignancy.

Basal cell hyperplasia can generate tubular profiles that can be confused with adenocarcinoma, but basal cell hyperplasia is a multilayered proliferation, whereas small acinar adenocarcinoma typically has a single malignant cell lining layer. Uncommonly, small malignant glands can have more than one layer of malignant cells **i14.91**. Rarely, prominent nucleoli can be found in the nuclei of basal cell hyperplasia, and this finding is commonly associated with inflammation (Devaraj 1993, Epstein 1992B, Thorson 1999). If doubts persist about the type of cell with prominent nucleoli, a 34βE12 immunostain will mark the atypical basal cells.

Caution is advised in diagnosing carcinoma in the setting of inflammation. Inflammation is commonly associated with pseudoneoplastic glands including those with atrophy, basal cell hyperplasia, and reactive nuclear atypia such that if one encounters an inflamed focus of glandular atypia (atypical small acinar proliferation) one should search noninflamed prostatic needle biopsy tissue for unequivocal evidence of carcinoma. Inflammation is more likely to be found with benign than malignant glands (Blumenfeld 1992) but can be found in a small minority of adenocarcinoma cases (Shepherd 1996), where it is predominantly lymphocytic (Blumenfeld 1992, Shepherd 1996) **i14.92**, along with a few macrophages (Shepherd 1996). Inflammatory cells themselves may be misinterpreted as malignant cells if arranged in

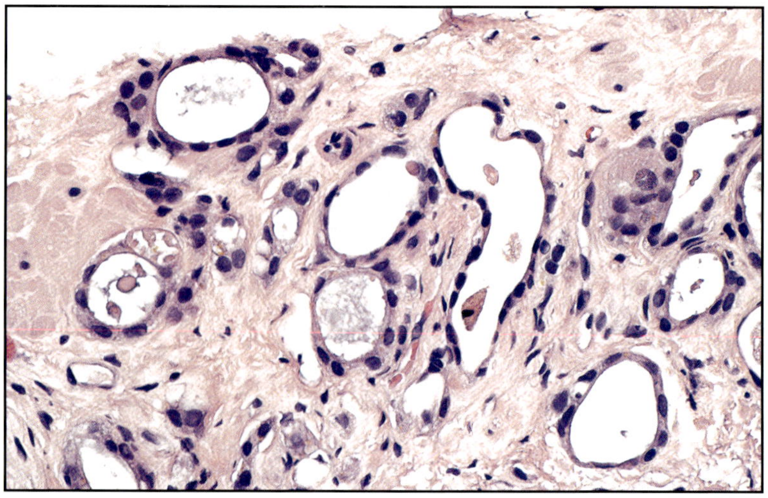

■ **i14.90** *Atrophic pattern prostatic adenocarcinoma with compressed cytoplasm.*

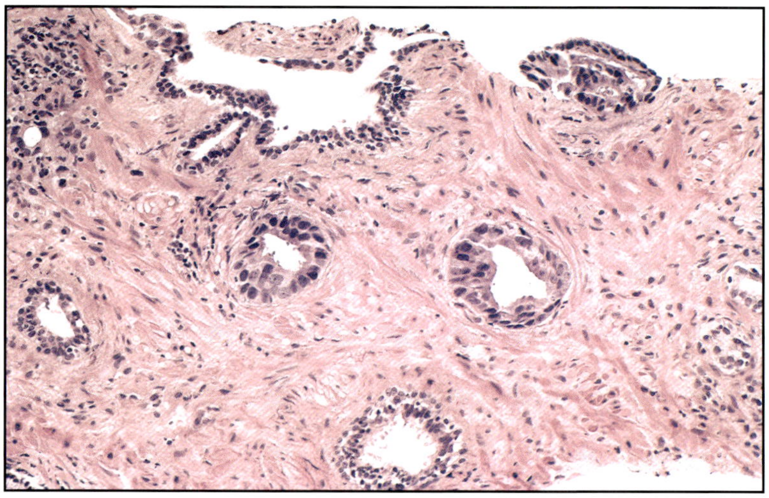

■ **i14.91** *Multilayered small gland prostatic adenocarcinoma in needle biopsy tissue.*

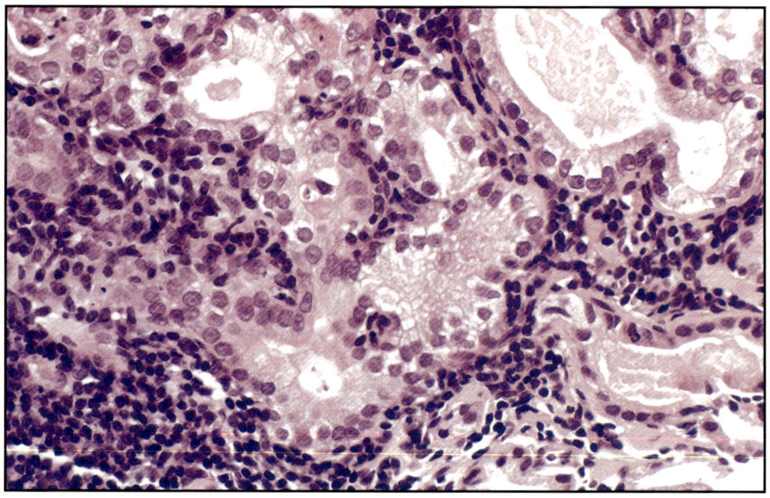

■ **i14.92** *Lymphocytic infiltrate in prostatic adenocarcinoma. Caution is advised in diagnosing malignancy in the setting of admixed inflammation.*

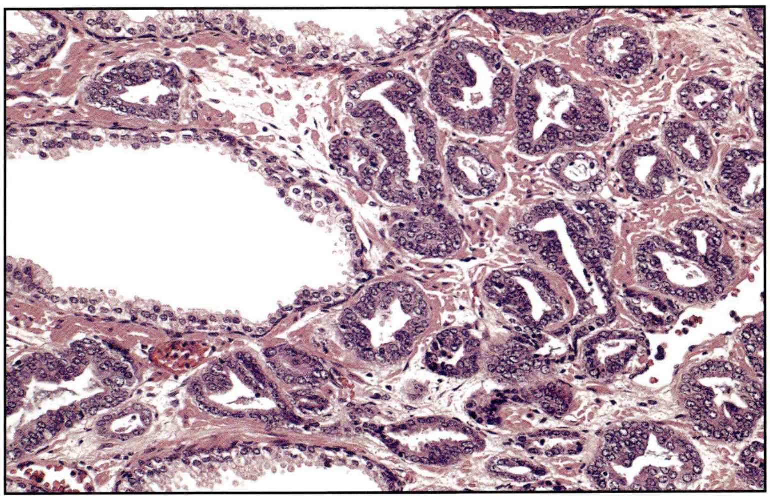

■ **i14.93** *PIN-like invasive adenocarcinoma, with intraluminal tufts.*

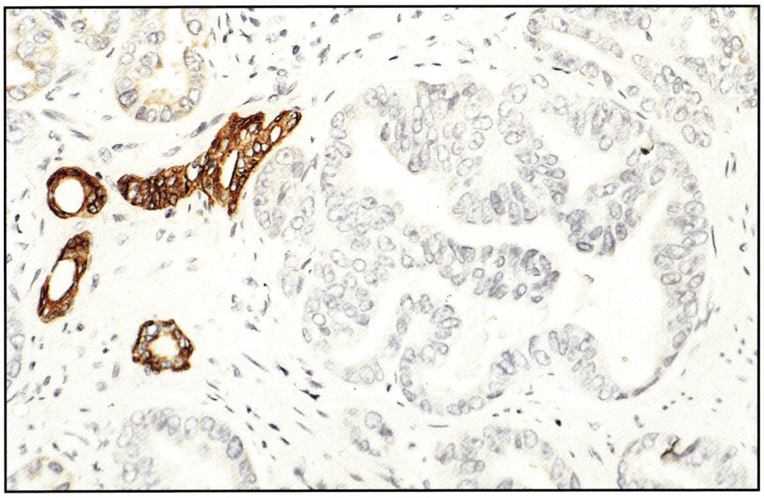

■ **i14.94** *PIN-like invasive adenocarcinoma with absence of basal cells (34βE12 immunohistochemical stain). A few benign, atrophic glands serve as a positive internal control.*

cords or sheets. One form of prostatitis that can readily be mistaken for carcinoma is granulomatous prostatitis (Presti 1991). In particular, sheets or cords of epithelioid histiocytes, which can have prominent nucleoli, could be diagnosed as poorly differentiated carcinoma. Negative immunohistochemical reactions for pan-cytokeratin, PSA, and PSAP, with immunopositivity for CD68 and lysozyme, are useful in establishing a diagnosis of granulomatous prostatitis rather than poorly differentiated prostatic carcinoma (Presti 1991). High-grade PIN figures prominently in the differential diagnosis of adenocarcinoma in needle biopsies. It can be exceedingly difficult to differentiate small foci of cribriform high-grade PIN from cribriform invasive carcinoma in needle biopsy (Davidson 1995, Kronz 2001); the uncommon (2%) cases of minimal carcinoma with cribriform architecture also had a small acinar component (Epstein 1995A). If any basal cells are identified in a pure cribriform proliferation of neoplastic cells on H&E-stained sections or by 34βE12 immunostain, caution is advised, and a diagnosis of high-grade PIN should be rendered. Focal flat high-grade PIN can also be problematic because it can closely resemble small acinar, minimal carcinoma, but it is also uncommon in pure form in needle biopsy (Davidson 1995, Reyes 1997A), and again, basal cell presence excludes invasive carcinoma. It should be noted that small glands of invasive adenocarcinoma can simulate PIN architecturally, with multilayering and tufted intraluminal protrusions **i14.93, i14.94**. Finally, a striking conundrum can be the diagnostic distinction of high-grade PIN with outpouching from high-grade PIN with adjacent invasive glands (Epstein 1995B). One should exercise caution if confronted with a few atypical small acini immediately adjacent to high-grade PIN because these could represent protrusions from the high-grade PIN. Basal cells should be specifically sought in these glands. If there are more than a few atypical small acini and they exhibit a degree of stromal separation from the high-grade PIN and if these small glands lack basal cells, then a diagnosis of carcinoma should be considered. No quantitative criteria exist as to number of glands or amount of stromal distance separation needed to definitely diagnose invasion. In borderline cases, we have used the descriptive diagnosis of "high-grade PIN with associated atypical small acinar proliferation" with a description of the differential diagnosis in a comment.

A descriptive diagnosis of atypia should also be contemplated in the differential diagnosis of carcinoma, particularly minimal carcinoma, in needle biopsy. Recently, diagnoses of atypia have been forwarded as a viable diagnostic category (Chan 1999, Cheville 1997, Iczkowski 1997, 1998, 2000, Renshaw 1998A, Reyes 1998). These terms include "focal glandular atypia" (Reyes 1998), "atypical" (Renshaw 1998A), "atypical suspicious for carcinoma" (Chan 1999), and "atypical small acinar proliferation suspicious for malignancy" (Cheville 1997, Iczkowski 1997, 1998, 2000). This category is undoubtedly a broad diagnostic umbrella and probably encompasses benign and reactive but atypical epithelium to small foci of carcinoma that harbor some but not all of the features needed for a definitive diagnosis of malignancy. Some have suggested 3-tiered stratifications of the atypia into "favor benign," "uncertain," and "highly suspicious" (Iczkowski 1997, 1998) or "favor benign," "favor cancer," and "undetermined" (Chan 1999). We have used a 2-tiered scheme of focal glandular atypia and focal glandular atypia, suspicious for malignancy. Thus far, these stratifications have not been proven to be reproducible (Amin 1998) or clinically significant (Chan 1999, Iczkowski 1997, 1998, Zhang 2000). In our definition of atypia (Reyes 1998), focal glandular atypia was classified as a gland or groups of glands with architectural atypia, cytologic atypia, or both that is atypical but not diagnostic of AAH, high-grade PIN, or carcinoma. Most studies have found that the clinical features such as serum PSA level or digital rectal examination findings are not useful in distinguishing atypia from minimal carcinoma (Chan 1999, Cheville 1997, Iczkowski 1997, 1998, Renshaw 1998A). No set histologic criteria exist to distinguish atypia and, in particular, atypical glands that are suspicious for malignancy from minimal carcinoma. In one study (Iczkowski 2000), minimal carcinoma foci, in comparison with atypical small acinar proliferation, tended to be larger and more infiltrative, with greater nuclear atypia, including nucleomegaly and prominent nucleoli. In the same series, mitotic figures were more often seen in minimal carcinoma (10% of cases) than in atypical small acinar proliferation (Iczkowski 2000), but in our experience, mitoses were found in only 2% of minimal carcinomas, which suggests little diagnostic usefulness. Also more common in focal carcinoma than in atypical small acinar proliferation were luminal blue mucin, concomitant high-grade PIN, and absence of moderate to severe atrophy (Iczkowski 2000). However, there is overlap of all of these features in minimal carcinoma and atypical small acinar proliferation, such that different thresholds exist among histopathologists in the diagnosis of minimal carcinoma and atypia (Amin 1998). Clearly, some cases of atypical, suspicious glands represent prostate cancer that is distorted, poorly preserved, thickly sectioned, or poorly stained. Other cases must represent clinically or histologically undersampled prostate cancer. In 10% of cases of focal glandular atypia, additional sections from the block reveal definitive carcinoma (Reyes 1998). Therefore, we recommend obtaining additional sections after an initial diagnosis of atypia in the first 3 slides. This further sampling can be additional H&E-stained sections, a 34βE12 immunostain, or both. Even after additional levels or a 34βE12 immunostain, some cases are borderline, so a descriptive diagnosis of atypia is warranted.

Additional pseudoneoplastic lesions are rare in needle biopsy but should still be considered before a diagnosis of adenocarcinoma in needle biopsy is rendered. These include sclerosing adenosis (Chapter 8), cribriform hyperplasia (Chapter 7), mesonephric hyperplasia (Chapter 7), nephrogenic metaplasia (Chapter 23), verumontanum mucosal gland hyperplasia (Chapter 7), malakoplakia (Chapter 4), endometriosis (Chapter 9), Cowper's glands (Chapter 9), paraganglia (Chapter 1), and benign glands adjacent to nerves and skeletal muscle (Chapter 1). Squamous metaplasia and transitional cell metaplasia (Chapter 6) can mimic neoplasia but are more likely to be called squamous cell carcinoma and PIN, respectively, than adenocarcinoma.

A classic snare for the histopathologist is the misdiagnosis of seminal vesicle glands as prostatic adenocarcinoma. The small outer tubules of the normal seminal vesicle are alarming because of their large, hyperchromatic atypical nuclei. This cytologic atypia is distinctive in that the chromatin is "smudged," and nuclear pseudoinclusions may be identified. However, there is a uniformity to the nuclear atypia of adenocarcinoma compared with the irregularly dispersed atypical nuclei of the seminal vesicle glands, where these enlarged atypical cells are admixed with small, bland nuclei. The identification of intracytoplasmic golden-brown lipochrome pigment has long been considered useful as a marker of seminal vesicle and ejaculatory duct epithelium, but in fact such pigment can be seen in prostatic epithelium, including adenocarcinoma (Amin 1996, Brennick 1994, Leung 1995, Shidham 1999). Although seminal vesicle and ejaculatory duct epithelial pigment generally is more abundant, coarser, and more refractile, the degree of morphologic overlap precludes diagnostic use of this pigment. Although the distinction between small seminal vesicle and ejaculatory duct glands and prostatic adenocarcinoma usually can be made based on H&E-stained sections, any doubt will be alleviated by negative monoclonal antibody immunolabeling of seminal vesicle glands for PSA and PSAP, in conjunction with positive immunoreaction using 34βE12.

Treatment effects can result in alterations in benign glands such that they mimic prostatic cancer (Bostwick 1982, Gaudin 1998, Goldstein 1998, Grignon 1995, Sheaff 1997, Siders 1992). The most profound of these effects is damage induced in benign glands by radiation therapy for prostate cancer. In particular, nuclear atypia can be marked with nucleomegaly, nuclear pleomorphism, and nucleomegaly. Retention of a lobular architecture is an important finding in favor of benignancy. A critical evaluation is 34βE12 immunohistochemical staining, which demonstrates positivity in the atypical benign glands (Brawer 1989).

Malignant neoplasms, both primary and secondary in the prostate, should be given due consideration in the differential diagnosis of prostatic adenocarcinoma in needle biopsy **t14.15**. Unusual histologic types of carcinoma of the prostate should be considered (Chapter 17) as well as primary mesenchymal and hematolymphoid neoplasms (Chapter 18), which are rare in the prostate. The main secondary malignancy to exclude is TCC originating in the bladder (Oliai 2001). Usually the patient has a history of bladder carcinoma (Esrig 1996, Herr 1999), but this history may not be provided. The prostate is a common site of relapse for bladder cancer, even for patients with superficial bladder tumors. Up to 58% of men with TCC of the bladder have prostatic urethral involvement (Chapter 23, **t23.12**), and of these patients, 70% have prostatic involvement (Esrig 1996). Diagnostic hints at TCC extension into the prostate include presence of a poorly differentiated carcinoma with rounded intraductal profiles and a lymphocytic response. Transitional carcinoma cells are more pleomorphic than poorly differentiated adenocarcinoma cells and often have a squamoid eosinophilic cytoplasm. Focal gland formation is not helpful because high-grade TCCs can show this. Immunostains are extremely valuable in diagnosing TCC involving the prostate. A recommended immunohistochemical marker panel would include PSA, PSAP, and 34βE12, with Leu7, CK7, and p53 as a second marker run if the first 3 are negative or noninformative (Bassily 2000, Chu 2000, Genega 2000, Lindeman 1996) **t14.16**. Of note, although CK7 and CK20 are more often positive in TCC, with a greater percentage of cells staining, focal CK7 and CK20 positivity can be seen in prostatic adenocarcinoma. Potential future markers for distinguishing prostatic adenocarcinoma from poorly differentiated TCC include uroplakin III (Kaufmann

t14.15 Differential Diagnosis of Prostatic Adenocarcinoma in Needle Biopsy: Other Malignant Neoplasms

Direct Extension into Prostate	
Transitional cell carcinoma of bladder or urethra: up to 58% of cases[1]	
Colorectal carcinoma: rare	
Metastatic Spread into Prostate[2]	**% Cases with Prostatic Metastases**
Leukemia/lymphoma	8%-14%
Malignant melanoma	1%
Pancreatic carcinoma	1%
Lung carcinoma	0.6%

[1]See **t23.12**
[2]See expanded **t18.17**

t14.16 Immunophenotype of Prostatic vs Transitional Cell Carcinoma

Marker	Prostatic Carcinoma	Transitional Cell Carcinoma
PSA[1]	94%-100%	0%
PSAP[1]	89%-100%	0%
34βE12[1]	Rare	65%
mCEA	0%-12%	41%
pCEA	47%	63%-68%
LeuM1	32%	30%
Leu7	94%	17%
CK7	0%-12%	83%-100%
CK20	0%-29%	15%-74%
p53 (DO7 antibody)	3%	33%
Thrombomodulin	0%	69%-91%
Uroplakin III	0%	57%

Yang 1999, Genega 2000, Bassily 2000, Lindeman 1996, Goldstein 2002, Ordoñez 1998, Parker 2003
[1]Recommended in a panel. If these three stains are negative or non-informative, Leu7, CK7, and p53 could be used (Genega 2000). The panel should also include a positive control immunostain, such as pan-cytokeratin (cocktail of AE1,AE3 and MAK6 antibodies) and a negative control immunostain such as leukocyte common antigen (LCA, CD45)

t14.17 Prostate Specific Antigen Immunohistochemical Staining Profile in Neoplasms

Neoplasm	% Cases Stained	References
Prostatic Carcinoma	86-100%	Lindeman 1996, Goldstein, 2002, Aihara 1994B, Ford 1985, Nadji 1981, Ellis 1984, Torenbeek 1998
Salivary Gland Neoplasms[1]	0-17%: monoclonal antibody	Tazawa 1999, James 1996, Fan 2000
	33%: polyclonal antibody	Tazawa 1999, Van Krieken 1993, James 1999
Periurethral gland adenocarcinoma	Rare cases positive	Dodson 1994, Zaviacic 1993, Svanholm 1987, Spencer 1990
Bladder adenocarcinoma	0%: monoclonal antibody	Torenbeek 1998,Grignon 1991
	13%: polyclonal antibody	Epstein 1986B,Grignon 1991
Breast carcinoma	0-9%: monoclonal antibody	Papotti 1989, Miller 2001
	0-61%: polyclonal antibody	Allsbrook 1998, Van Krieken 1993, Howarth 1997, Papotti 1989, Gatalica 2000
	0% of male breast carcinoma: monoclonal antibody	Gatalica 2000
Ovarian carcinoma	1 case: polyclonal antibody	Yu 1995
Apocrine sweat gland carcinoma	2 cases: polylonal antibody	Papotti 1989
Pancreatic acinar cell carcinoma	3 cases	Kuopio 1995
Transitional cell carcinoma	0	Lindeman 1996, Genega 2000, Nadji 1981
Colorectal adenocarcinoma	0	Allsbrook 1998, Nadji 1981, Torenbeek 1998, Van Krieken 1993
Other adenocarcinomas: lung, stomach, kidney, testis	0	Allsbrook 1998, Ford 1985, Nadji 1981, Torenbeek 1998, Van Krieken 1993

[1]17% of salivary duct caricnomas can exhibit PSA immunoreactivity, using a monoclonal antibody. Salivary gland neoplasms with PSA immunoreactivity using polyclonal antibody: Warthin's tumor (55%), pleomorphic adenoma (55%), mucoepidermoid carcinoma (43%-66%), adenoid cystic carcinoma (11%-100%), acinic cell carcinoma (50%), adenocarcinoma (41%-100%), adenosquamous carcinoma (50%).

2000, Parker 2003, Yaziji 2001), thrombomodulin (Ordoñez 1998, Parker 2003), and cytokeratin 5 (Yaziji 2001).

In rare cases, colorectal carcinoma can involve the prostate by direct extension (Rub 1999, Yamaguchi 1993). It is almost always clinically recognized that the patient has colon cancer, but in vanishingly rare cases, colonic carcinoma in the prostate can present with hematuria referable to prostatic involvement (Rub 1999). Microscopically, colonic carcinoma can potentially mimic prostatic carcinoma, especially cribriform, ductal, and mucinous prostatic carcinomas, but prostate cancer does not have large malignant glands with large geographic areas of "dirty" necrosis, as may be found in colonic carcinoma. In exceedingly rare cases, secondary involvement of the prostate by colonic carcinoma is detected in needle biopsy (Yamaguchi 1993). In this case PSA and carcinoembryonic antigen (CEA) immunostains were touted as useful in establishing the colon as the primary of origin, although CEA can be seen in prostatic carcinoma, too.

Malignant neoplasms can also secondarily involve the prostate by hematogenous or lymphatic metastatic spread, but these are usually incidentally detected at autopsy in patients with known, widely disseminated disease and not in needle biopsy of prostate (Johnson 1974, Zein 1985). Even at autopsy, the prostate is uncommonly involved by secondary spread of malignancy, with only 1% to 6% of all patients with malignancy of all types having secondary prostatic spread at autopsy (Johnson 1974, Zein 1985) **t14.15**. These figures probably are underestimates because the glands were not completely embedded. Leukemia (and specifically chronic lymphocytic leukemia) is the most common cancer to spread to the prostate, with the most common metastatic solid tumors being malignant melanoma, pancreatic carcinoma, and lung carcinoma (Johnson 1974, Zein 1985). It is only in exceedingly rare cases that needle biopsy of the prostate is performed in patients with metastatic malignancy in the prostate (Bostwick 1998, Madersbacher 1994, Rub 1999).

The diagnostic evaluation of a poorly differentiated carcinoma in prostate needle biopsy usually entails examination of H&E-stained slides only because nearly all cases are classic examples of high-grade Gleason pattern 4 or 5 prostatic adenocarcinoma. If a high-grade neoplasm does not have a typical histologic appearance of poorly differentiated prostatic adenocarcinoma, immunohistochemical markers can be of value in establishing the diagnosis. The most valuable of these immunohistochemical markers are PSA and prostatic acid phosphatase (PAP), also known as PSAP. These are highly sensitive in detecting prostatic differentiation but are not specific for malignant epithelium and are not absolutely specific for prostatic carcinoma, either **t14.17, t14.18**. A few percent of high-grade carcinomas lack PSA **t14.19** and PSAP **t14.20** expression. In these cases, the reactivity profile of additional markers 34βE12, Leu7, CK7, and p53 may be of aid **t14.16** in suggesting a prostatic primary cancer. Positive PSA and PSAP immunoreactions in a carcinoma in prostate needle biopsy are almost always indicative of a primary prostatic carcinoma because those nonprostatic neoplasms that can stain for PSA or PSAP, such as salivary gland neoplasms, periurethral gland adenocarcinoma, breast carcinoma, carcinoids, islet cell tumors, and bladder adenocarcinomas **t14.17, t14.18**, rarely involve the prostate on a secondary basis, with sampling by prostate needle biopsy.

Established Prognostic Attributes and Reporting of Carcinoma in Needle Biopsy

The most important prognostic attributes of adenocarcinoma in prostate needle biopsy that merit reporting are histologic grade and amount of tumor in needle biopsy tissue **t14.21** (Epstein 1996C, Hutter 1996, Wheeler 1998B), with grade being the more significant. The 1999 consensus conferences of the College of American Pathologists (CAP) and the World Health Organization (WHO) recommended reporting Gleason score in needle biopsy (Bostwick 1999B, 2000). The 1999 WHO group further suggested reported of WHO nuclear grade and the relative percentage or proportion of high-grade cancer (percentage Gleason primary patterns 4 or 5), but nuclear grading is not currently used in the United States, and the determinations of the percentage of high-grade disease should be viewed as experimental. The Gleason standard grading is used in the 2003 WHO classification (WHO 2003). Both groups did recommend reporting cancer volume or amount of tumor in needle biopsy specimens.

■ t14.18 Prostatic Specific Acid Phosphatase Immunohistochemical Staining Profile in Neoplasms

Neoplasm	% Cases Stained	References
Prostatic Carcinoma	82%-100%	Genega 2000, Lindeman 1996, Ellis 1984, Nadji 1980, Mahan 1980, Heyderman 1984, Grob 1994, Jobsis 1981, Fishleder 1981
Salivary gland neoplasms	0%-48%: polyclonal antibody[1]	Tazawa 1999, Van Krieken 1993
Periurethral gland adenocarcioma	Rare positive cases	Dodson 1994, Zaviacic 1993, Svanholm 1987, Spencer 1990
Bladder adenocarcinoma	0%: monoclonal, polyclonal antibody	Torenbeek 1998, Grignon 1991, Nadji 1980
	33%: polyclonal	Epstein 1986B
Breast carcinoma	0-28%	Van Krieken 1993, Li 1980, Yam 1981, Jobsis 1981
Carcinoid tumors[2]	27%	Sobin 1986, Kimura 1986B, Azumi 1991, Jobsis 1981, Cohen 1983, Federspiel 1990, Goldblum 1993, Stagno 1987, Sidhu 1993, Fishleder 1981
Islet cell tumors	0%-60%[3]	Mahan 1980, Kimura 1986B, Uribe 1985, Jobsis 1981, Choe 1978, Cohen 1983
Medullary carcinoma	0%-15%	Kimura 1986B,Uribe 1985
Cloacogenic carcinoma	Rare positive cases	Fernandez 1990
Renal cell carcinoma	Rare positive cases	Yam 1981
Transitional cell carcinoma	0	Nadji 1980, Heyderman 1984, Jobsis 1981
Colorectal adenocarcinoma	0	Van Krieken 1993, Nadji 1980, Heyderman 1984, Jobsis 1981
Other adenocarcinomas: lung, stomach, pancreas	0	Dodson 1994, Nadji 1980, Jobsis 1981

[1]Salivary gland neoplasms with PSAP immunoreactivity using polyclonal antibody: Pleomorphic adenoma (64%), mucoepidermoid carcinoma (33%), adenoid cystic carcinoma (66%), adenocarcinoma (66%)
[2]By site: Rectal carcinoids: 67%-83%, colonic/appendix: 25%, stomach/small intestine: 11%, lung: 4%. Negative: Breast, head and neck, liver
[3]60% (6/10) of insulinomas positive (Jobsis 1981)

■ 14.19 PSA Immunohistochemical Staining of Prostatic Adenocarcinoma: Sensitivity

Gleason Primary Grade	Cases Stained	% Acini or Cells Stained
1	100%	100%
2	100%	100%
3	97%	87%
4	94%	79%
5	94%	49%

Genega 2000, Lindeman 1996, Aihara 1994B

■ t14.20 Prostatic-Specific Acid Phosphatase (PSAP) Immunohistochemical Staining of Prostatic Adenocarcinoma: Sensitivity

Gleason Primary Grade	% Cases Stained
1,2	100%
3	94%
4,5	87%

Epstein 1993E

More than 40 grading schemes have been proposed for prostatic carcinoma (Chapter 15). In the United States the Gleason scheme is most widely used and is the grading method that is most often used in research, in the medical literature, and by physicians who see patients with prostate cancer. Gleason grade in needle biopsy has been linked to a large number of pathologic and clinical endpoints such as stage, response to therapy, and survival (Bostwick 1994B, Gleason 1990) (Chapter 15). The pretreatment evaluation of patients with adenocarcinoma in needle biopsy typically entails consideration of histologic grade expressed as Gleason score, clinical stage, and total serum PSA level (Kattan 1998, Partin 1997). Using these 3 pretreatment parameters in combination, one may then predict pathologic endpoints such as risk of carcinoma extension outside the prostate gland and metastatic spread to pelvic lymph nodes (Partin 1997, http://urology.jhu.edu/Partin_tables1) and the chances of failure after radical prostatectomy (Kattan 1998) or radiation therapy (Kattan 2000, Pisansky 1997, http://www.nomograms.org). Thus, histologic grade in needle biopsy is a critical clinical component in stratifying patients into risk categories and treatment plans. Most pathologists (76%) report Gleason grade in needle biopsies (True 1994). Reporting of both Gleason primary and secondary patterns and their sum (Gleason score) is recommend for needle biopsies of the prostate with carcinoma (ADASP 1998, Bostwick 1999B, 2000, Henson 1994, Srigley 2000). When more than 2 patterns are present and the worst grade is neither the predominant nor the secondary pattern, the worst grade is added to the predominant pattern to yield the score (Chapter 15). A Gleason grade should be assigned for all cases, even for minimal or limited adenocarcinoma in needle biopsy (Epstein 1996C, Thorson 1998, 2000). We routinely report Gleason grade for each separately submitted needle core or set of needle cores, designated by the clinically assigned anatomic site of biopsy **t14.22**. When different cores have different Gleason scores, it is controversial whether to assign an overall (composite) score or whether the highest score for any one core should be considered the patient's grade (WHO 2003).

■ t14.21 Established Prognostic Attributes of Prostatic Adenocarcinoma in Needle Biopsy

Histological grade: report Gleason grade
Amount of tumor in needle biopsy: report visual estimate of percentage tissue involved, number of positive cores out of total number of cores, and linear mm of tumor

The amount of tumor in prostate needle core biopsies should also be provided in surgical pathology reports (Bostwick 1999B, 2000, Henson 1994, Srigley 2000) because this parameter correlates, albeit imperfectly, with tumor volume **f14.1**, **f14.2**, margins, and stage in radical prostatectomy specimens **t14.23**. Amount of carcinoma in

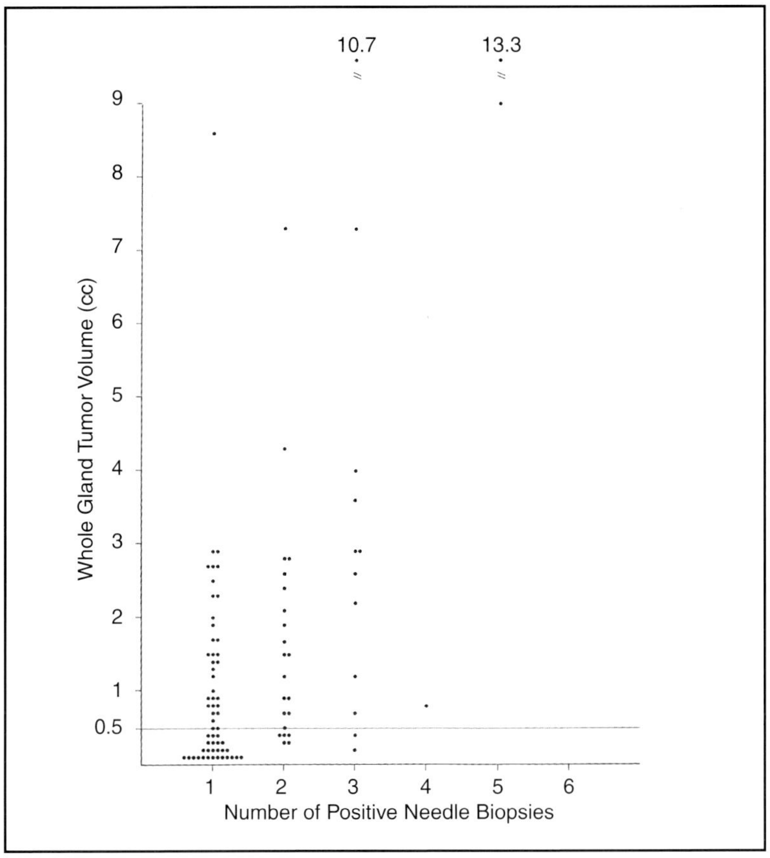

■ **f14.1** *Relationship of number of positive needle cores and total tumor volume in the whole gland. Data from 150 patients from the Washington University Medical Center PSA-screening program.*

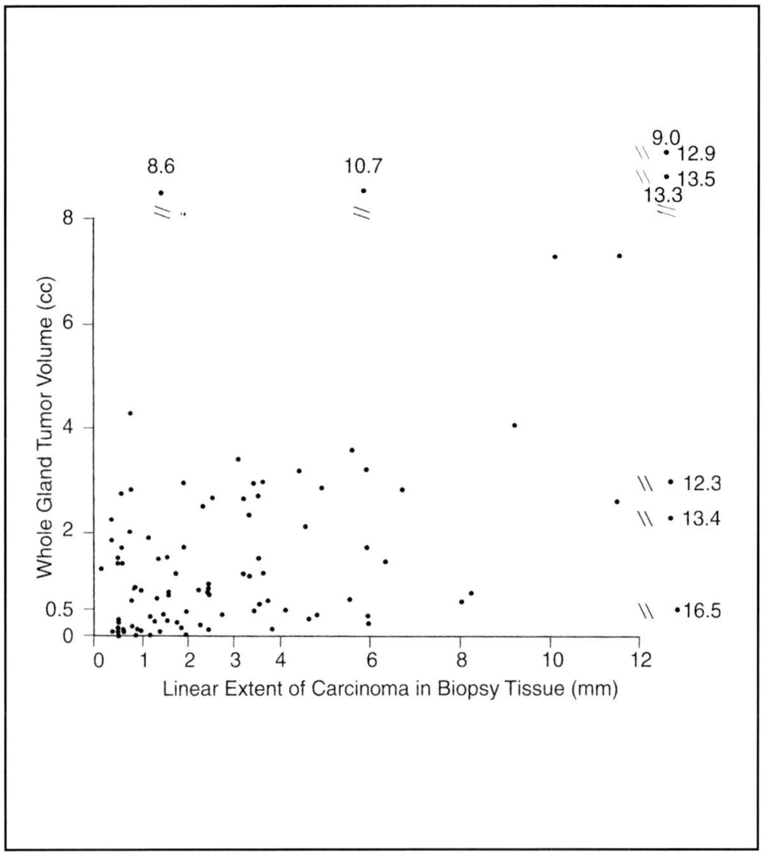

■ **f14.2** *Relationship between total linear mm of carcinoma in needle biopsy tissue and total tumor volume in the whole gland. Data from 150 patients from the Washington University Medical Center PSA-screening program.*

needle biopsy also predicts response to radical prostatectomy and radiation therapy (D'Amico 1997, 2002, Freedland 2002, Gardner 1998, Grann 1998, Huland 1996, Presti 1998, Ravery 1994). In sextant biopsy tissue, measures of tumor extent in needle biopsy include number of positive needle cores, percentage of positive needles, percentage of tissue involved by carcinoma as determined by visual inspection, tumor area, and linear millimeters of tumor extent as quantified using an ocular micrometer. It is likely that all these measures provide nearly equivalent information, such that there is not a standard method of appraising needle biopsy tumor extent. Indeed, several measures should be given for the same set of needle biopsies **t14.22**. Currently, we routinely report number of positive cores out of total number of cores examined, with a visual inspection estimate of total percentage of tissue involved. In cases in which it is unclear how many cores are involved because of core fragmentation, we specify number of core fragments rather than number of cores involved. Based on emerging data (Bismar 2003, Lewis 2002), consideration should also be given to reporting total linear millimeters of carcinoma. It is important to recognize that in a although a large amount of tumor in needle core tissue often (but not always) is associated with a large tumor in the whole gland, a small focus of carcinoma in needle biopsy does not reliably predict a small amount of clinically insignificant tumor in the entire prostate gland (Cupp 1995, D'Amico 2000, Epstein 1994A, Humphrey 1995, Rubin 2001, Thorson 1998, 2000).

It is also worthwhile to report, for needle core biopsies, the presence of extraprostatic carcinoma in adipose tissue or seminal vesicle (although, as previously mentioned, seminal vesicle can be difficult to distinguish from intraprostatic ejaculatory duct) and lymphvascular space invasion. Perineural invasion often is noted in needle biopsy reports, but it is unsettled whether this finding is of independent prognostic significance (Algan 1999, Anderson 1998, Bismar 2003, D'Amico 2001, de la Taille 1999A, 1999B, Egan 1997A, Jimenez 2000, O'Malley 2002, Rubin 2000B, Sebo 2002, Vargas 1999). Perineural invasion in needle biopsy lacks independent ability to predict radical prostatectomy stage once Gleason grade and amount of tumor in needle biopsy are known (Bismar 2003, Egan 1997A, Rubin 2000B). The data on perineural invasion in needle biopsy as a predictor of response to therapy are mixed. According to the 1999 CAP and WHO conferences, perineural invasion is classified as a category III prognostic factor that is not currently recommended for routine reporting (Bostwick 1999B, 2000).

Currently, special studies of prostatic carcinoma in needle biopsy are not established prognostic indicators. Some laboratories report DNA ploidy status of prostatic carcinoma in needle biopsy, but the data on ploidy as a prognosticator in needle cores are mixed (Brinker 1999, Ross 1994, 1999, Sebo 2002, Stamey 1995), and the consensus view is that the data are insufficient or inconclusive to recommend its use in prostate needle biopsies (Hutter 1996). Once accurate Gleason grading is provided in needle biopsy, determination of DNA ploidy is not necessary in needle biopsy of prostatic carcinoma. Sampling error and tumor

■ **t14.22 Reporting of Prostate Adenocarcinoma in Needle Biopsy: Sample Format**

PROSTATE, LEFT SIDE, NEEDLE BIOPSY
ADENOCARCINOMA, GLEASON GRADE 3+3 = SCORE OF 6, IN ONE OF THREE CORES, INVOLVING 10% OF TISSUE

PROSTATE, RIGHT SIDE, NEEDLE BIOPSY
ADENOCARCINOMA, GLEASON GRADE 3+4 = SCORE OF 7, IN TWO OF THREE CORES, INVOLVING 40% OF TISSUE

■ t14.23 Extent of Carcinoma in Prostate Needle Biopsy in Relation to Radical Prostatectomy and Clinical Endpoints

Study (Reference)	No. Biopsy Cores	Endpoint	Comment
Terris 1992	6 (sextant)	Tumor volume	<3 mm cancer in needle biopsies was associated with small (0.5cc) tumors
Ackerman 1993	6 (sextant)	Margins, node status	Number of positive cores associated with positive margins, positive nodes
Ravery 1994	6	Extracapsular disease	More than 66% positive cores had 87% positive predictive value
Häggman 1994	10	Tumor volume, margins, stage	Percentage carcinoma in biopsy tissue correlated with tumor volume and positive margins
Irwin 1994	NG	Low grade (Gleason score ≤4) and tumor volume (≤0.5cc)	≤3 mm carcinoma in needle biopsy linked to low-grade, small-volume tumor
Epstein 1994A	5	Tumor volume, grade, stage	Less than 3 cores positive or 50% core involvement with low PSAD[1] and grade related to "insignificant" tumor[2]
Terris 1995	6	Tumor volume	Cancer length in needle core tissue used with serum PSA and ultrasound to predict volume
Humphrey 1995	4	Tumor volume	Number of positive biopsies significant
Cupp 1995	6	Tumor volume	Percentage cancer, percentage cores, and mm cancer in needle core tissue nearly equivalent in predicting volume
Dietrick 1995	6	Tumor volume	Greater than 3mm cancer predicted volume greater than 0.5cc
Peller 1995	6	Tumor volume, stage	Number of positive cores predictive
Bostwick 1996	6	Tumor stage	Percentage cancer in needle core tissue significant
Ravery 1996	6	Stage, margins, PSA failure after radical prostatectomy	Percentage cancer related to all three
Lee 1996	6	PSA failure after radiation therapy	Percentage cancer and % biopsies not significant
Goto 1996	6	"Unimportant" tumor[3]	Maximum length of cancer in any core significant
Badalament 1996	6	Stage	Percentage cancer and number positive cores important in predicting organ-confined cancer
Huland 1996	6	Stage, margins, PSA failure after radical prostatectomy	Number of positive biopsies correlated with stage, margins, and failure
Egan 1997A	6	Stage	Proportion of biopsy involved by cancer significant in multivariate analysis
Borirakchanyavat 1997	6	Stage	Number of positive cores correlated with extraprostatic extension
D'Amico 1997	6	Stage and PSA failure after radical prostatectomy	Percent positive cores helped predict stage and failure
Bassily 1999	NG	Stage	Greatest percentage of cancer in one core significant in multivariate analysis
Grann 1998	6	Failure after brachytherapy analysis	Tumor length and percentage tumor in needle biopsy not significant in multivariate
Wills 1998	6	Stage	Number of positive cores predicted stage
Gardner 1998	NG	Stage, margins, PSA failure after radical prostatectomy	Tumor ≤3 mm in a single core biopsy predicted lower stage, fewer positive margins and decreased failure
Egevad 1998	6-10	Tumor volume	Total cancer length in mm correlates better with 10 vs 6 cores
Presti 1998	6	PSA failure after radical prostatectomy	Fraction of positive biopsies was related to failure
Egawa 1998	6	Stage	Number of positive cores and maximum cancer length useful
Conrad 1998	6	Lymph node metastasis	Number of cores with predominantly high grade (Gleason pattern 4 or 5) important
Arcangeli 1998	6	Stage, margins, tumor volume related to all three parameters	Percentage of positive biopsies and percentage of tumor in cores both significantly
Sanwick 1998	6-8	Stage	Number of positive cores not predictive
Vargas 1999	6	Stage	Number of positive cores predictive in multivariate analysis
Tigrani 1999	6	Margins	Number of positive cores best predictor of margins
Sebo 2000	6	Stage, tumor volume	Percent of positive cores significant
Rubin 2000	NG	Stage, margins	Greatest percentage of any single biopsy involved by prostate carcinoma predictive of pT3 disease in multivariate analysis
Rubin 2001	6	Tumor volume	Weak correlation of biopsy tumor area and radical prostatectomy total tumor volume
Lewis 2002	6 (mean)	Tumor volume	Total linear mm of carcinoma and number of positive cores most strongly related to total tumor volume in a screening population
Bismar 2003	6	Pathologic stage	Total linear mm and total percentage of carcinoma significantly linked to extraprostatic extension by carcinoma and positive margins; fraction of positive cores linked to positive margins or pT3 disease

[1]PSAD = Prostate specific antigen density
[2]Insignificant tumor = Tumor volume <0.2 cc, organ-confined, and not Gleason pattern 4 or 5
[3]Unimportant tumor = Tumor volume <0.5 cc, organ-confined, and not Gleason pattern 4 or 5

heterogeneity hinder use of ploidy (Greene 1991C, O'Malley 1993, Reiter 1999) and molecular markers in needle biopsy of prostate cancer. It may be anticipated that gene expression profiling may yield important markers in the future. Examples of such candidate markers include hepsin (Chapter 21), Pim-1 kinase (Rubin 2002A), and EZH2 (Varambally 2002). There are many promising potential molecular biologic and genetic prognostic markers for prostate cancer (Chapter 21), but thus far not a single one has yet entered routine clinical practice (Reiter 1999).

[14.3] Diagnosis of Adenocarcinoma in Transurethral Resections and Open Prostatectomies

The histologic diagnosis of adenocarcinoma in transurethral resection of the prostate (TURP) and open or simple (that is, enucleation) prostatectomies usually is incidental and clinically unexpected because these procedures typically are performed to treat BPH. In about 10% of cases, histologic detection of carcinoma is clinically anticipated because the TURP is done for palliative purposes to relieve obstruction in a patient with known prostatic carcinoma (Mebust 1989). Diagnostic difficulties encountered in these tissue samples relate to a higher proportion of low-grade carcinomas of transition zone origin because it is mainly transition zone tissue that is removed by these surgical procedures and because well-differentiated carcinomas have a propensity to arise in the transition zone. Also, cautery artifact in TURP chips can create diagnostic problems.

t14.24 Clinical Aspects of Incidental Prostatic Carcinoma in TURP Chips

Patients in their 60s or 70s present with symptoms of BPH
Digital rectal examination not suspicious for malignancy
PSA generally not elevated
Clinical stage is Tla or b (stage A1 or A2) (see **t2.7**)

Clinical, Gross, and Microscopic Features of Carcinoma in TURP Chips and Open Prostatectomies

Clinically, incidentally discovered prostatic carcinoma in TURP chips or open prostatectomy tissue is by definition not palpable by digital rectal examination **t14.24**. Serum PSA levels generally are not able to distinguish BPH from these incidental carcinomas (Cohen 1993, Monda 1994), although for T1b (A2) carcinoma with a Gleason score >7, the median serum PSA was slightly higher at 5.9 ng/mL (range 2.7 to 25.9) than in BPH, with a median of 3.4 (range 0.1 to 61.0).

The frequency of diagnosis of incidental prostatic adenocarcinoma in TURP chips and open prostatectomy specimens ranges from 1% to 26% **t14.25**, with an average of about 10% to 16% often

t14.25 Frequency of Detection of Incidental Adenocarcinoma in TURP Chips and Open Prostatectomy Specimens

Study (reference)	Year	Sampling Method	Frequency (%)
TURP Chips			
Bergman	1955	Not given	31/1,000 (3.1%)
Greene	1955	"Multiple sections"	83/2,090 (4%)
Denton	1965	1-3 cassettes	30/500 (6%)
		Completely embedded	21/100 (21%)
Melchior	1974	Not given	44/644 (7%)
Newman	1982	Partial sampling[1]	43/500 (8.6%)
		Completely embedded	71/500 (14.2%)
Moore	1986	Completely embedded	39/151 (26%)
Murphy	1986	Completely embedded	66/383 (17%)
Yamabe	1986-Japan	Completely embedded	24/191 (13%)
	1986-Netherlands	Completely embedded	57/452 (13%)
Eble	1986	Some (432) completely embedded	132/700 (19%)
Rohr	1987	Completely embedded	65/457 (14.2)
Asakawa	1988-Japan	Not known	9/108 (8.3%)
Masuda	1989-Japan	Not known	38/461 (8.2%)
Chang	1991-Taiwan	Partial[2]	49/5,529 (0.9%)
Tombal	1995-Belgium	Completely embedded	56/449 (12%)
TOTAL			**858/14,215 (6%)[3]**
Open (Enucleation) Prostatectomy Specimens			
Wade	1914	Not given	14/134 (10%)
Treiger	1948	Not given	15/108 (14%)
Smith	1950	Not given	62/648 (9.6%)
Labess	1952	Not given	9/98 (9.2%)
Bauer	1960	Mean of 3.6 sections	55/847 (6.5%)
Delides	1976	Not given	144/3,072 (5%)
Battaglia	1979	Completely embedded	86/100 (86%)
Yamabe	1986-Japan	Completely embedded	21/152 (14%)
	1986-Netherlands	Completely embedded	14/64 (22%)
Stillwell	1989	At least 8 slides	28/468 (6%)
Change	1991-Taiwan	Not given	4/346 (1.2%)
Vecchioli	1992-Italy	Sections every5 mm	82/683 (12%)
Tombal	1999-Belgium	Not given	56/449 (12%)
TOTAL			**590/7,169 (8%)**

[1]Protocol in this study = All tissue submitted if less than 10g of chips; if >10g, 1 cassette submitted for each 5g of chips
[2]Protocol in this study = Chips less than 8g completely-embedded, then 1 block for each additional 10 gm of tissue
[3]Minus Chang 1991 data, the frequency = 9%

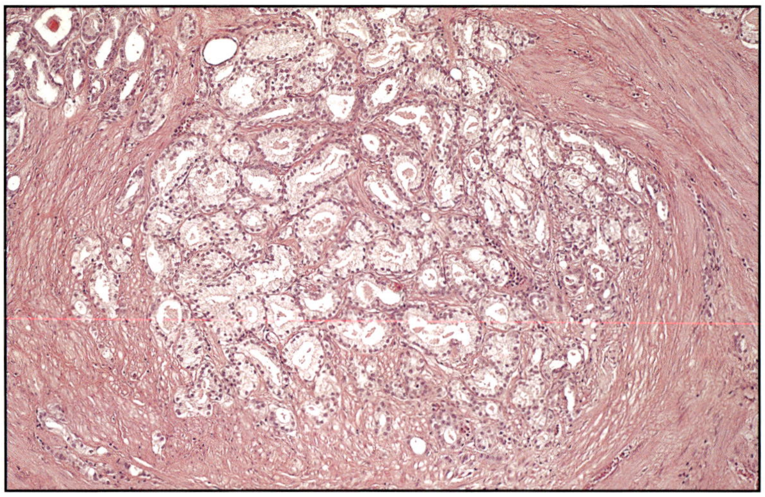

■ **i14.95** *Nodule of well-differentiated adenocarcinoma of Gleason score 3 in TURP chip.*

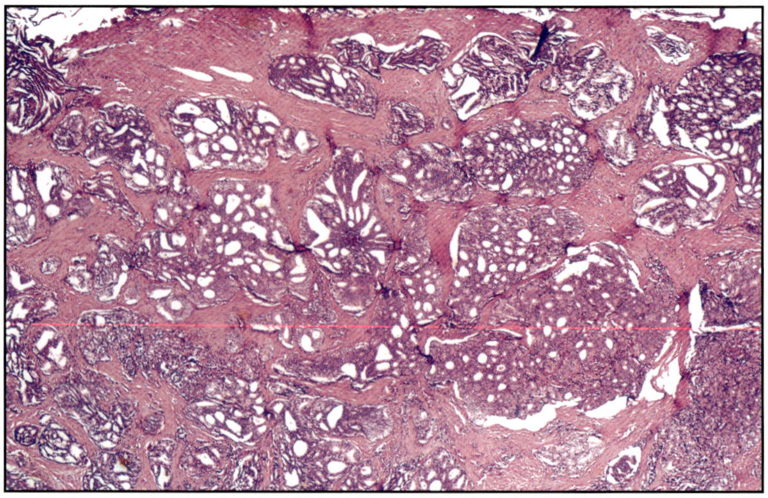

■ **i14.96** *Prostatic adenocarcinoma, with high-grade Gleason pattern 4 (and score of 7) in TURP chip.*

cited (Eble 1990, Epstein 1992C, Petersen 1992). The detection rate increases with increasing age of the patient population and with increasing extent of gross tissue sampling. The incidence does not seem to exhibit significant worldwide variation.

Grossly, it is not possible to definitively diagnose prostatic carcinoma in TURP chips (Mills 1990, Murphy 1989) **t14.26**. Yellow and indurated chips may suggest malignancy (Geddy 1996), but the coloration correlates with cellular and epithelial proliferation in general, not carcinoma specifically (Mills 1990). In open prostatectomy specimens, firm, yellow nodules may be suspicious for carcinoma, but often this finding is not specific for carcinoma (Murphy 1989), and many such masses turn out to be BPH nodules. For both types of tissue specimens, the detection rate of prostatic carcinoma depends on the extent of gross sampling.

Microscopically, incidental prostatic carcinoma in TURP chips often is well-differentiated and focal (Bostwick 1995B, Sheldon 1980), necessitating careful low-magnification surveys for circumscribed, densely packed prostatic acini **i14.95**. About 60% of incidental carcinomas are well differentiated (Gleason score 2 to 4), but intermediate and high-grade carcinomas **i14.96** can also be seen in TURP chips. For patients with known prostatic cancer who undergo TURP to relieve obstruction ("channel" TURPs), the carcinoma often is high-grade and diffuse.

The major and minor diagnostic criteria for carcinoma are applied to TURP chips and open (enucleation) prostatectomies, just as for needle biopsies **t14.2**. One major difference is that architectural abnormalities of most carcinomas in TURP chips and open prostatectomy specimens are typified by transition zone nodular growths of malignant prostatic acini **i14.97** rather than infiltrative small acini. These nodules can be made up of back-to-back or closely arranged small acini **i14.95, i14.97** or nodules with

■ **t14.26 Gross and Microscopic Features of Incidental Carcinoma in TURP Chips and Open (Enucleation) Prostatectomy Specimens**

Grossly, firm yellow nodules may be suspicious for carcinoma
Microscopically, many are focal and well differentiated (Gleason score 2-4)

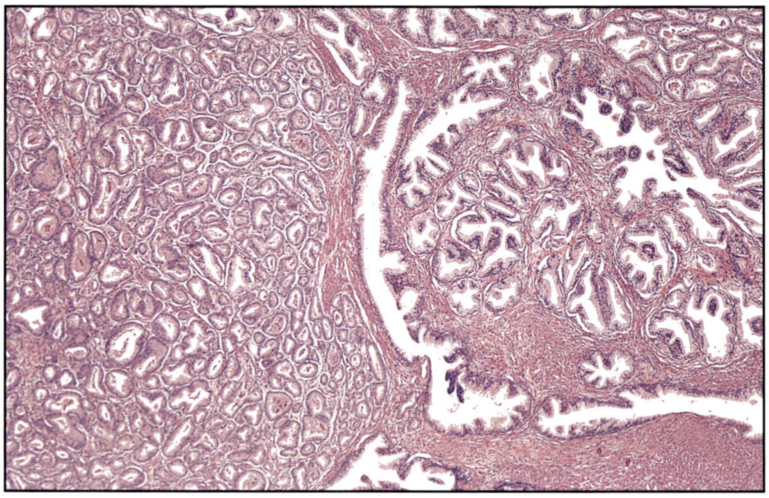

■ **i14.97** *Nodule of well-differentiated Gleason score 3 adenocarcinoma (left) in transition zone, adjacent to BPH nodule (right).*

cystically dilated or complex glands, with a pseudohyperplastic pattern **i14.98, i14.99** (Humphrey 1998A, Levi 2000). In this diagnostically treacherous grouping of glands, one can visualize complex papillary growths **i14.99**, with luminal undulations and branching, just as in BPH nodules. Cystic change can also be found in both pseudohyperplastic prostatic adenocarcinoma (Humphrey 1998A) and BPH nodules. These pseudohyperplastic malignant glands often exhibit basally situated nuclei and columnar cytoplasm with clearing **i14.100**. For all nodular, well-differentiated carcinomas the findings of nuclear atypia and a diffuse lack of basal cells are critical. Ideally, the nuclear atypia should manifest itself as both diffuse nucleomegaly and nucleolomegaly. However, there are cases in which prominent (>1.6μm) nucleoli are rare to absent **i14.25**. In one series, fully one quarter of low-grade adenocarcinomas in TURP chips fell into this category (Kramer 1993). For these "nucleolus-poor" adenocarcinomas, one should observe substantial nuclear enlargement. Diffuse basal cell absence is almost always evident on H&E-stained sections. In contrast to needle biopsies, only in rare cases is a 34βE12 immunostain necessary as a confirmatory measure to diagnose adenocarcinoma in TURP chips and open prostatectomy cases **i14.101**. One source of diagnostic difficulty with TURP

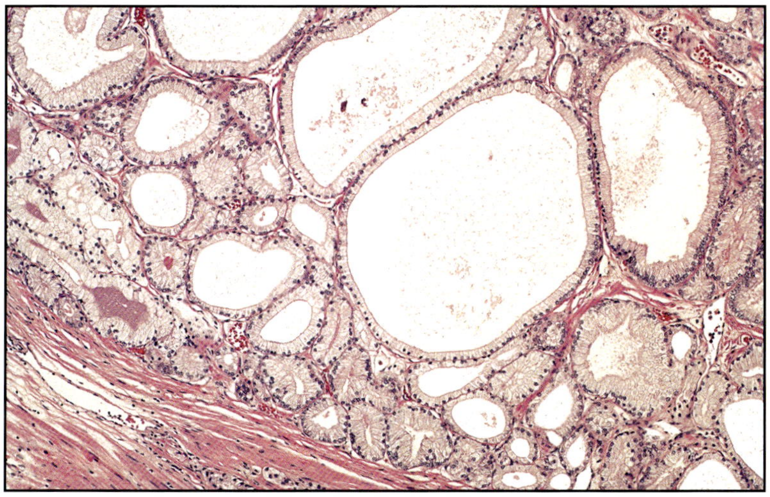

■ **i14.98** *Dilated, pseudohyperplastic prostatic adenocarcinoma glands in a TURP chip.*

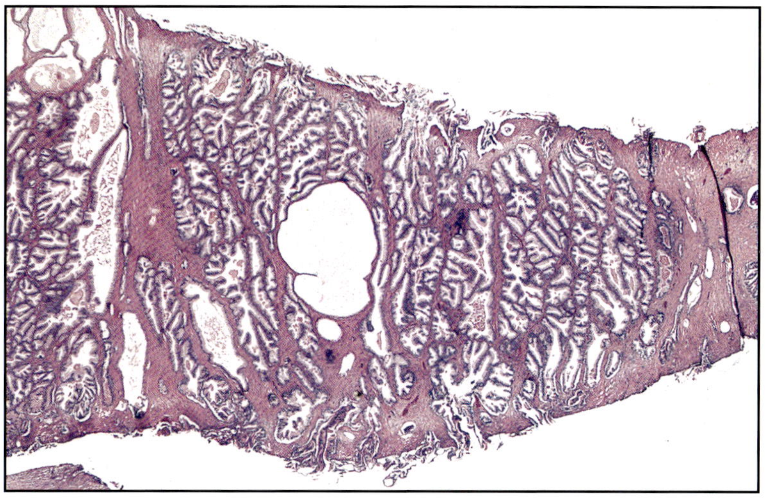

■ **i14.99** *Pseudohyperplastic adenocarcinoma in TURP chip.*

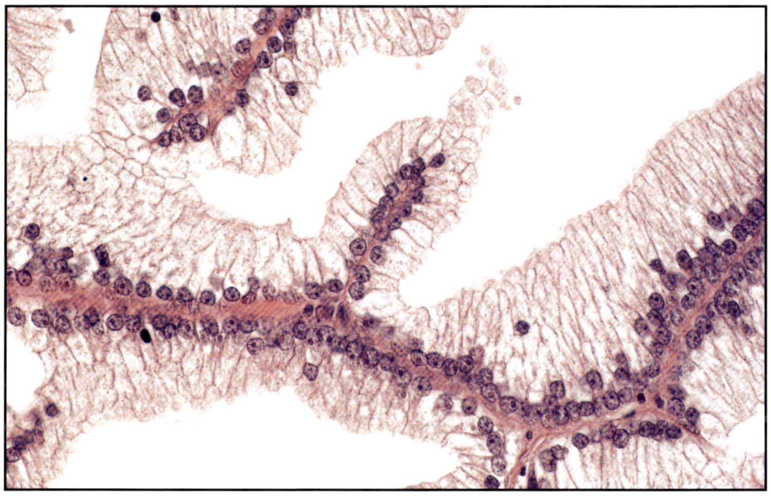

■ **i14.100** *Pseudohyperplastic prostatic adenocarcinoma comprised of malignant columnar cells with basally situated nuclei.*

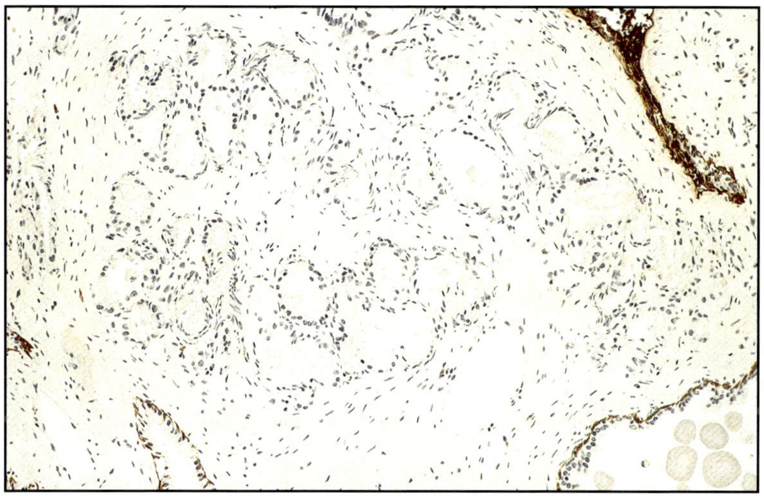

■ **i14.101** *Adenocarcinoma with lack of basal cells, by 34βE12 immunohistochemical staining. Positive internal control staining is evident (especially in benign upper right gland).*

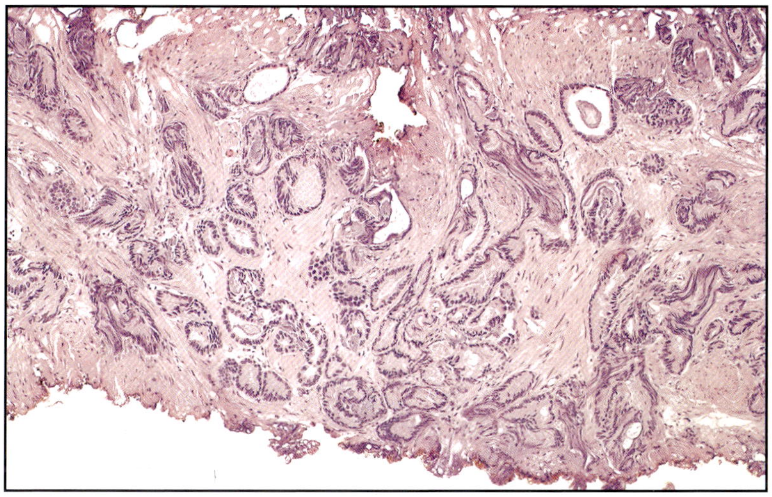

■ **i14.102** *Cautery artifact in adenocarcinoma in TURP chip.*

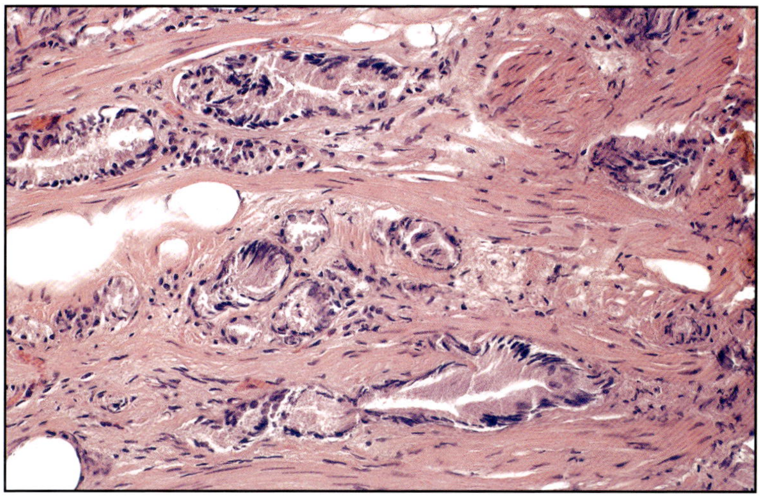

■ **i14.103** *Cautery artifact in adenocarcinoma in TURP chip: Nuclear elongation and smudged chromatin are characteristic (higher power of* **i14.102***).*

chips is cautery artifact at the edges of the chips. It is possible to diagnose carcinoma with cautery artifact **i14.102, i14.103**, but one should do so only if there is continuity of artifactually distorted cells with well-preserved cells. Additional levels, 34βE12 immunostains, or submission of additional tissue may be helpful in cases of atypical glands with cautery artifact.

Differential Diagnosis

The main diseases that are likely to be misdiagnosed as adenocarcinoma in TURP chips include AAH (adenosis), basal cell hyperplasia, atrophy, sclerosing adenosis, high-grade PIN, xanthogranulomatous prostatitis, florid cribriform hyperplasia, and postatrophic hyperplasia (Bostwick 1999A) **t14.27**. Just as for needle biopsies, benign entities in the differential diagnosis should encompass all prostatic pseudoneoplasms **t10.1**. The most common problem is distinguishing AAH, basal cell hyperplasia, atrophy, and usual hyperplasia from adenocarcinoma. Unlike needle biopsies, AAH figures more prominently in the differential diagnosis because it is more common in the transition zone sampled by TURP and open (enucleation) prostatectomy than in peripheral zone tissues typically sampled by needle biopsy. Most TURP chip cases of AAH (adenosis) can be distinguished from adenocarcinoma by a constellation of morphologic features, including nuclear atypia, intraluminal crystalloids and wispy blue mucin, and basal cell layer presence or absence. Architectural abnormalities are not of great utility here (Bostwick 1993B, Gaudin 1994) **t14.28**. In a few borderline cases, a descriptive diagnosis of focal glandular atypia or atypical small acinar proliferation of uncertain significance (Bostwick 1993B) may be rendered. Basal cell hyperplasia and cystic atrophy are also common in the transition zone and should be excluded before adenocarcinoma is diagnosed. Usual epithelial hyperplasia can mimic pseudohyperplastic prostatic adenocarcinoma, which can be found in transition and peripheral zones. Here, nuclear atypia and diffuse lack of basal cells are pivotal findings in favor of carcinoma. For poorly differentiated carcinoma in TURP chips and open prostatectomy specimens, the main malignancy to rule out (or rule in) is TCC. An immunohistochemical marker panel can be of substantial value in addressing this differential diagnosis **t14.16**. Rarely, both prostatic adenocarcinoma and TCC can be encountered in the same TURP chip (Kunze 1994).

■ t14.27 Differential Diagnosis of Prostatic Adenocarcinoma in TURP Chips and Open (Enucleation) Prostatectomies

Atypical adenomaotus hyperplasia (adenosis)
Basal cell hyperplasia
Cribriform hyperplasia
Usual hyperplasia
Atrophy (including postatrophic hyperplasia)
Sclerosing adenosis
High-grade PIN
Inflammatory atypia
Transitional cell carcinoma

Established Prognostic Attributes and Reporting for TURP Chips and Open Prostatectomy

Extent of carcinoma and histologic grade of carcinoma in TURP chips and open (enucleation) prostatectomies are crucial to report because these 2 parameters are related to staging, patient prognosis, and treatment. Carcinoma that is incidentally detected by light microscopic examination of sections from TURPs and open (enucleation) prostatectomies performed for clinically benign disease is classified as stage T1a/b or stage A in the older literature, using the Whitmore-Jewett scheme (Fleming 1997) **t2.7**. Stage T1 disease is further subclassified into substages T1a (A1) and T1b (A2) cancer. Variable definitions have been used to distinguish T1a and T1b carcinoma, with the most widely accepted one being based on percentage of prostatic tissue involved by carcinoma. In stage T1a cancer, 5% or less of the tissue is involved by tumor. This percentage carcinoma determination is made by simple visual inspection of the surface area of the chips involved by carcinoma. Circling of the area of carcinoma or morphometric measurements (including use of an image analyzer) are not necessary. (However, it should be noted that in the original study [Cantrell 1981] that formed the basis for the current subclassification of stage T1a and T1b, percentage carcinoma was estimated after circling areas of cancer on the slides with a marking pen.) Other measures of tumor extent in TURP chips include number of foci involved, diameter of largest focus, number of blocks involved, percentage of blocks involved, number of chips involved, and percentage (ratio) of chips involved (reviewed in Eble 1990, Humphrey 1988). Recommendations for reporting amount of tumor in TURP chips and open (enucleation) prostatectomy specimens include percentage of tissue that contains tumor and number of positive chips or microscopic foci of carcinoma (ADASP 1998, Henson 1994, Srigley 2000). We routinely report percentage of tissue involved by carcinoma, as determined by visual inspection, without circling of foci, and number of positive chips out of the total number of chips counted **t14.29**.

Histologic grade should also be reported in TURP chips and open (enucleation) prostatectomy specimens, with the Gleason system recommended (ADASP 1998, Henson 1994, Srigley 2000). Primary and secondary patterns and the score (sum) should be recorded. Low-grade carcinoma occupying <5% of tissue is deemed T1a (A1) disease, and any high-grade carcinoma is T1b (A2) disease (ADASP 1998). What constitutes "low-grade" carcinoma has been a source of controversy (Epstein 1992C, Humphrey 1993A). Low-grade carcinoma has been variously defined as Gleason score 2 to 4, 2 to 6, or even 2 to 7. Gleason score 7 carcinoma should be viewed as high-grade carcinoma. In the future, it may be important to report percentage Gleason grade 4/5 (Egevad 2002).

It is not necessary to report surgical margin status in enucleation prostatectomies or approach of tumor to the edge of

■ t14.28 Most Useful Features in Differential Diagnosis of Atypical Adenomatous Hyperplasia (Adenosis) vs Adenocarcinoma in TURP Chips

Feature	AAH (Adenosis)	Well-differentiated Adenocarcinoma
Nucleolar size	Usually less than 1μm	Most greater than 1μm
Nuclear size variation	Less variable	Variable
Crystalloids	Infrequent (16%)	Frequent (75%)
Intraluminal wispy blue mucin	Infrequent	Frequent
Basal cell layer	Fragmented	Absent

Bostwick 1993A

■ **t14.29 Reporting of Prostatic Adenocarcinoma in TURP Chips: Sample Format**

PROSTATE, TRANSURETHRAL RESECTION
ADENOCARCINOMA, GLEASON GRADE 2+3 = SCORE OF 5, IN TEN OF SIXTY CHIPS, INVOLVING 10% OF TISSUE

TURP chips because these are not radical surgeries intended to completely excise carcinoma.

Follow-up by examination of radical prostatectomy specimens and clinical progression rates highlight the importance of the separation of T1a and T1b clinical stage categories, as generated by histologic grade and tumor extent. At radical prostatectomy after a histopathologic diagnosis of T1a or T1b carcinoma, the majority (75% to 100%) of patients have residual carcinoma in the prostate, when the gland is completely embedded **t14.30**. Moreover, this carcinoma often is multifocal and peripheral, such that a restaging by repeat TURP would not have sampled the residual carcinoma (Epstein 1988, Greene 1991B). T1b disease definitely indicates much more ominous findings in radical prostatectomy tissues than does T1a disease **t14.30**, with a higher likelihood of EPE, seminal vesicle invasion, and lymph node metastasis. However, for the individual patient, it is difficult to precisely predict radical prostatectomy tumor extent based on TURP chip histologic grade and tumor extent (Eble 1990, Epstein 1992C). These radical prostatectomy studies indicate that the greatest threat to patients with T1a/b carcinoma discovered in TURP chips is the associated separate peripheral zone carcinoma. Carcinomas in TURP chips tend to be lower-grade adenocarcinomas of transition zone origin, whereas peripheral zone carcinomas typically are of a higher grade and more aggressive (Blute 1985, Colombo 2001, Crundwell 1997, Erbersdobler 1997, 2002, Greene 1991A, 1991D, Grignon 1994, McNeal 1988A, 1988B, 1990A, Van de Voorde 1995) **t14.31**. Clinical follow-up studies indicate progression rates of 8% to 27% for untreated T1a carcinoma at 7 to 10 years (Amakasu 1995, Blute 1985, Cheng 1999E, Epstein 1986, Lowe 1988, Roy 1990, Thompson 1989, Tombal 1999, Zhang 1991)

■ **t14.30 Radical Prostatectomy Findings After a Diagnosis of Carcinoma in TURP Chips**

TURP Chip Stage	% Cases With Residual Tumor	Gleason Score[1]	TV	EPE	SV Invasion	LN Metastasis
Tla	75%-94%	5	0.4cc-0.6cc	8%-14%	0%-8%	Rare
Tlb	91%-100%	5.4	1.6cc-2.7cc	12%-48%	4%-22%	5%-38%

[1]Histologic grade expressed as mean Gleason Score (Greene 1991D)
TV = mean tumor volume (range for Tla disease = 0cc-2.6cc; range for Tlb disease = 0.02cc-24cc [Greene 1991D, Christensen 1990, Larsen 1991]); EPE = extraprostatic extension by carcinoma; SV = seminal vesicle; LN = pelvic lymph nodes
Paulson 1988, Epstein 1988, Greene 1991D, Voges 1992, Elder 1985, Parfitt 1983B, Fowler 1985, Oesterling 1987, Christensen 1990, Golimbu 1978, Donohue 1982, Smith 1983, Larsen 1991, Zincke 1991

■ **t14.31 Transition Zone Versus Peripheral Zone Carcinoma**

	Anatomic Zone of Carcinoma	
Parameter	**Transition**	**Peripheral**
% of all carcinomas	20%	75%
Sampling procedure	TURP, Open prostatectomy[1]	Needle core biopsy[2]
Typical histological grade	Low; mean Gleason score = 5	Intermediate to high; mean Gleason score = 6-7
Typical invasion pattern	Into anterior fibromuscular stroma and BPH nodules	Into posterolateral extraprostatic soft tissue, seminal vesicles
Tumor volume (mean)		
Clinical stage Tla/b	2.5cc	1.9cc
Clinical stage T2	0.7cc	4.0cc
Multicentricity	62%	49%
Association with high-grade PIN	No	Yes
Proliferation index	1.6%	5%
DNA ploidy	6%-13% aneuploid	51%-53% aneuploid
Extraprostatic extension[3]	25%	51%
Seminal vesicle invasion	Rare	~5%
Biochemical failure at 5 years years after radical prostatectomy[4]	29%	51%
Genetic changes	Common, including allelic loss on 8p (37%), and 11q (50%), and microsatellite instability (MSI) (31%)[5]	Common[6]

[1]TURP = transurethral resection of prostate; open = simple or enucleation prostatectomy. The transition zone can also targeted by needle core biopsies, although this is not standard.
[2]Peripheral zone tissue can also be sampled by aggressive TURP.
[3]McNeal 1990A
[4]Noguchi 2000
[5]Crundwell 1997, Crundwell 1999. Recent data suggest that TZ and PZ carcinomas exhibit genetic alterations in different chromosomes (Colombo 2001). Allelic losses on chromosome 11 were higher in TZ carcinomas and MSI was significantly higher in TZ carcinomas compared to PZ carcinomas (Colombo 2001).
[6]See Chapter 21

compared with 25% to 33% of T1b carcinomas at 3 to 4 years (Blute 1985, Cantrell 1981, Tombal 1999).

Reporting of perineural and vascular invasion, as well as carcinoma invasion of periprostatic tissues, such as adipose tissue and seminal vesicle tissue, has also been recommended (Henson 1994, Srigley 2000). High-grade PIN should definitely be reported when found in isolated form, but it is not know whether its presence in the setting of invasive carcinoma has any impact on the patient's future risk of progression.

Special studies are not currently of established value as prognostic indicators in carcinoma diagnosed in TURP chips or enucleation specimens. Proposed indicators include DNA ploidy (McIntire 1988), nuclear roundness (Mohler 1992), nucleolar organizing regions (Amakasu 1995), p21 (Amakasu 1995) and α-catenin (Crundwell 1997). Weight of resected chips at ≥30g has also been forwarded as a favorable prognosticator (Cheng 1999E). Preliminary findings suggest that allelic loss at 8p and 13q, p53, Rb, and microsatellite instability are not related to progression of incidentally detected transition zone carcinomas (Crundwell 1997, 1999).

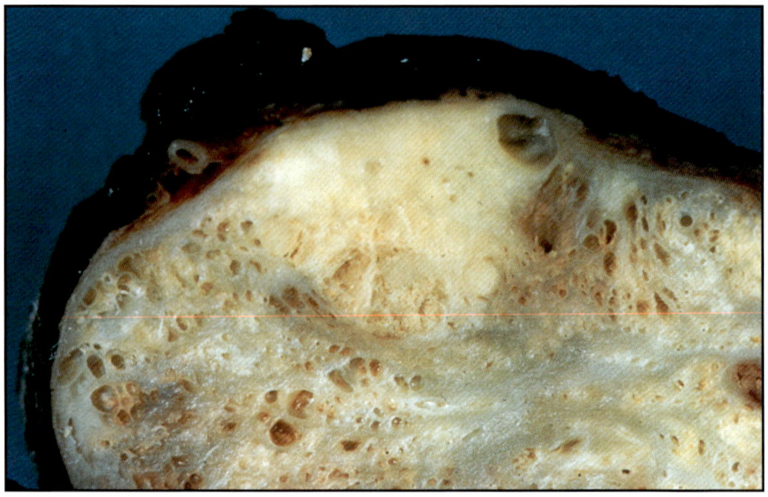

■ **i14.104** *Nodule of peripheral zone adenocarcinoma in radical prostatectomy specimen: Solid and white cancer, compared to surrounding benign prostatic tissue with cystic change.*

[14.4] Diagnosis of Adenocarcinoma in Radical Prostatectomy Specimens

Histopathologic characterization of adenocarcinoma in radical prostatectomy is important because this assessment provides the patient and doctor with a snapshot of disease status at that time. Specifically, the features of histologic grade, tumor size, margin status, and pathologic stage in radical prostatectomy tissues allow prognostic and therapeutic stratification for the individual patient. The pathologic findings in the radical prostatectomy specimen and the pelvic lymph nodes that are often excised at the same surgery often influence the clinical decision of whether to treat the patient after surgery with radiation therapy or androgen deprivation or to monitor the patient. Histologic detection of adenocarcinoma in radical prostatectomy tissues often is more straightforward than in smaller tissue samples, such as needle core biopsies or TURP chips, because anatomic landmarks are present, it is easier to appreciate architectural abnormalities at scanning magnifications, and a greater amount of carcinoma is present. Distinctive challenges in radical prostatectomy specimen samples include assessments of tumor size, EPE of carcinoma, and margins.

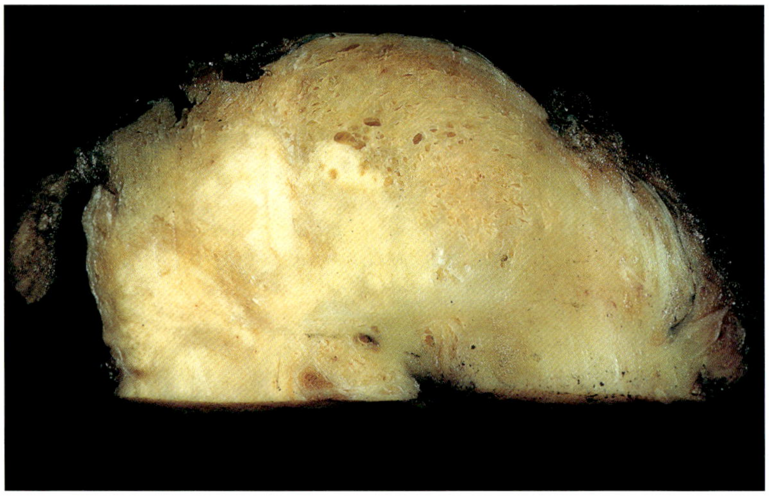

■ **i14.105** *Irregular, yellow-white adenocarcinoma in radical prostatectomy tissue.*

Gross and Microscopic Features of Carcinoma in Radical Prostatectomy Specimens

Grossly, it can be difficult or impossible to recognize prostatic carcinoma (Bostwick 1997A, Renshaw 1998B), even with the whole gland available. Palpation of the excised, intact prostate glands can be helpful in a minority of cases in delineating the sites of nodularity, but in the PSA-screening era, most carcinomas are clinically impalpable and are also impalpable at the surgical pathology cutting bench (Renshaw 1998B). When visible on cut sections, carcinoma can appear nodular and white **i14.104** to irregular, gray or white-yellow **i14.105, i14.106**, compared with adjacent benign prostatic tissue, which is tan, spongy, and often cystic **i14.104; t14.32**. Macroscopically recognizable carcinoma tends to be, not surprisingly, of higher grade, stage, and size (Renshaw 1998B). The lower limit of size detection of gross carcinoma is about 0.5cm (Bostwick 1997A). More often, no gross lesion is evident, or a lesion only suggestive of

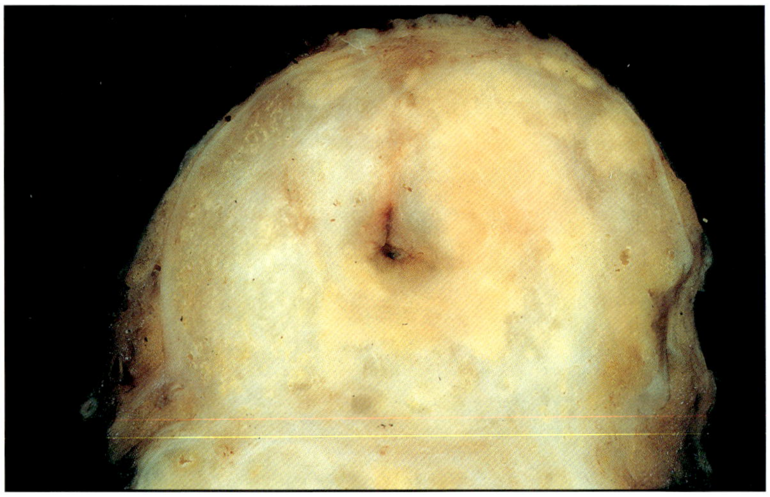

■ **i14.106** *Extensive, yellow to white adenocarcinoma in radical prostatectomy tissue. Central slit-like structure is prostatic urethra.*

carcinoma is visualized (Renshaw 1998B). Subtle gross changes in cut sections are best appreciated by comparing right and left halves of the prostate with each other (Hall 1992); they include ill-defined, asymmetric, firm, yellow-white areas in the peripheral zone. These alterations are

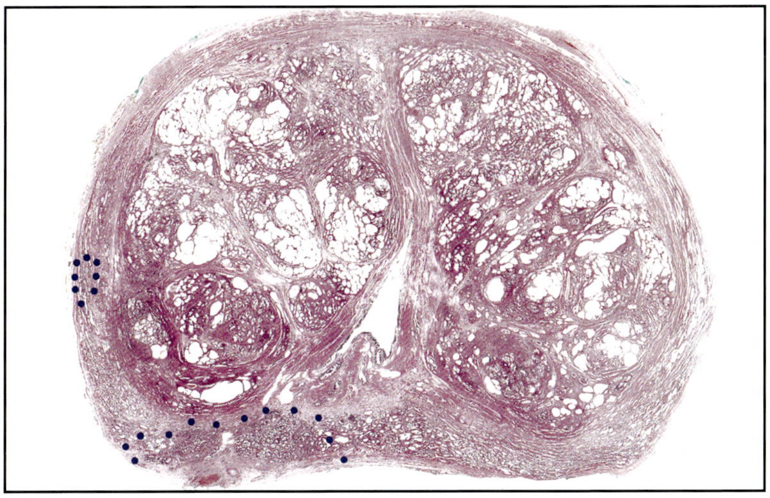

■ **i14.107** *Whole-mount section of radical prostatectomy specimen showing two separate peripheral zone carcinomas (delineated by black dots). This is also extensive transition zone BPH. (Courtesy of Dr Patricia Troncoso).*

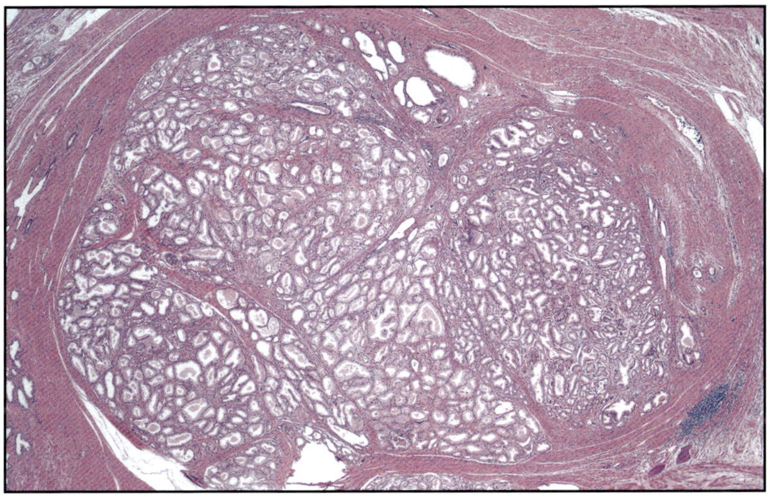

■ **i14.108** *Nodular well-differentiated Gleason score 4 adenocarcinoma in radical prostatectomy tissue.*

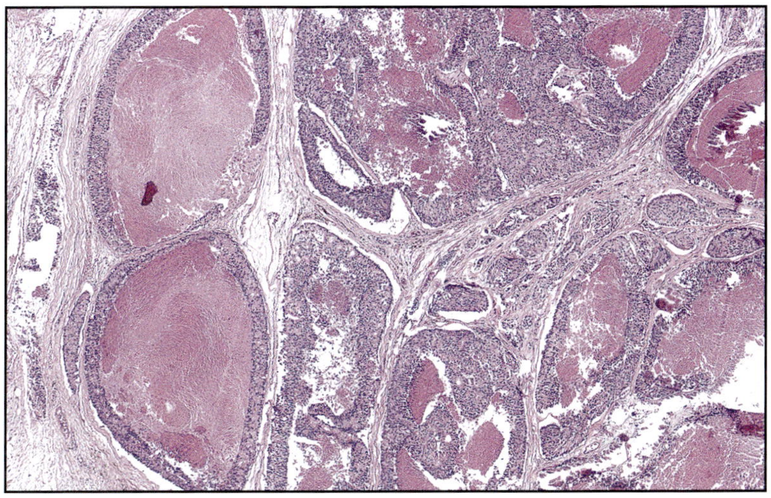

■ **i14.109** *Gleason pattern 5 (score 10) comedocarcinoma in radical prostatectomy tissue.*

more readily found in fixed than in fresh tissues (Hall 1992, Renshaw 1998B). The more centrally located transition zone carcinomas are characteristically nodular, solid, and bright yellow (Sakr 1999), but BPH nodules can precisely simulate this guise. Attempts to recognize gross extension of carcinoma into extraprostatic tissues and surgical margins in radical prostatectomy specimens can also be a futile exercise. Even if there is a grossly identifiable lesion, in only about one half of cases will EPE by carcinoma and positive margins be microscopically present at that site (Renshaw 1998B).

■ **t14.32 Gross Features of Prostatic Carcinoma in Radical Prostatectomy Specimens**

Gross recognition difficult to impossible
Most impalpable
Cut sections: Solid, white, grey or yellow nodules to ill defined, asymmetrical firm yellow-white areas

■ **t14.33 Microscopical Features of Prostatic Adenocarcinoma in Radical Prostatectomy Specimens**

95% acinar type
Usually multifocal
Most Gleason score 5-7
Variable size; current average size = 10% of gland (range 0.1%-80%)
Extraprostatic extension in 43% (PSA-detected) to 66% (DRE-detected) of cases
Invasion of seminal vesicle uncommon (~ 6%-21% of cases)
Positive margins in 28% of cases

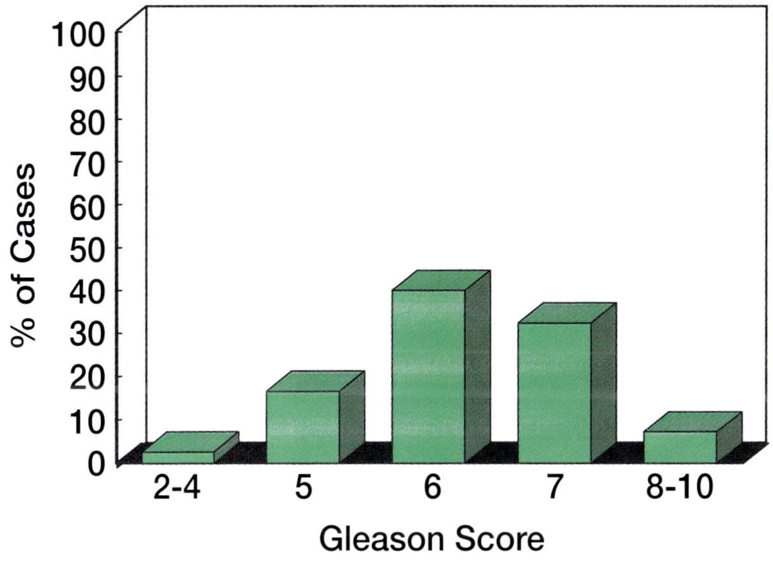

■ **f14.3** *Gleason score distribution of adenocarcinoma in contemporary radical prostatectomy specimens. Most are of Gleason score 5-7 (pooled data from Pound 1997 and Carvalhal 2000).*

Microscopically, adenocarcinoma in the whole prostate gland typically is a multifocal acinar malignancy that is most common in the peripheral zone **t14.33, i14.107**. Multifocality is present in 60% to 97% of cases (Aihara 1994A, Byar 1972, Djavan 1999, Feng 2000, Miller 1994, Pinto 2000B, Ruijter 1996, Wise 2002), with an average of 2 or 3 separate cancers per gland, with the range extending up to 10 separate tumors per prostate gland (Aihara 1994A, Douglas 1997, Hoedemaker 2000, Miller 1994, Ruijter 1996). Most prostatic carcinomas in radical prostatectomy specimens (80% to 90%) are located in the peripheral zone and are of Gleason score 5 to 7, that is, moderately (Gleason score 5 and 6) to moderately poorly (Gleason score 7) differentiated (Catalona 1998, Pound 1999) **f14.3**. Well-differentiated (Gleason score 2 to 4) adenocarcinomas **i14.1; i14.108**, which tend to be found in the transition zone, and poorly differentiated (Gleason score 8 to 10) adenocarcinomas **i14.109** are uncommon in contemporary

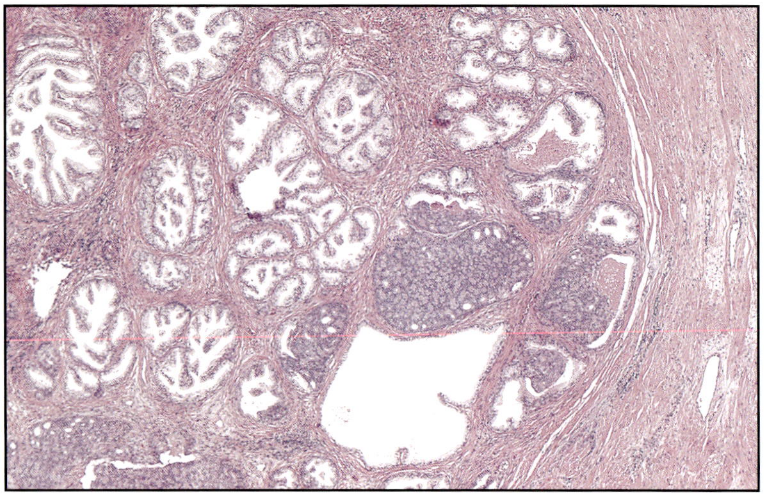

■ **i14.110** *Focal, high-grade Gleason pattern 4 adenocarcinoma in BPH nodule.*

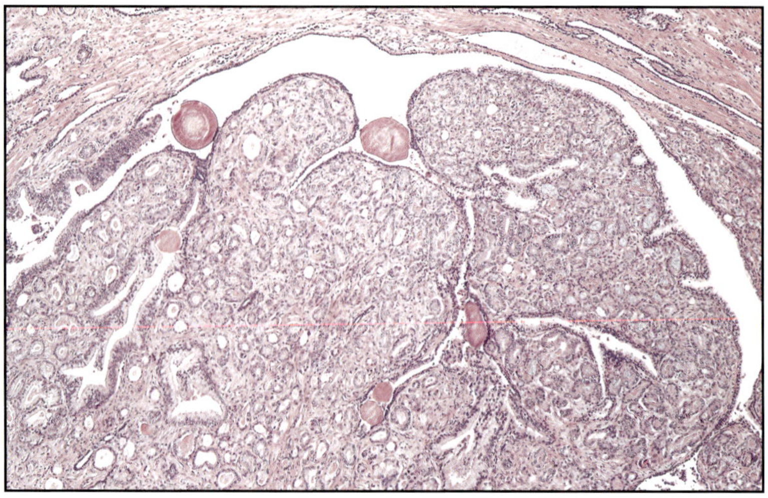

■ **i14.111** *Prostatic adenocarcinoma, with Gleason patterns 3 and 4, involving BPH nodule, generating a phyllodes-like pattern.*

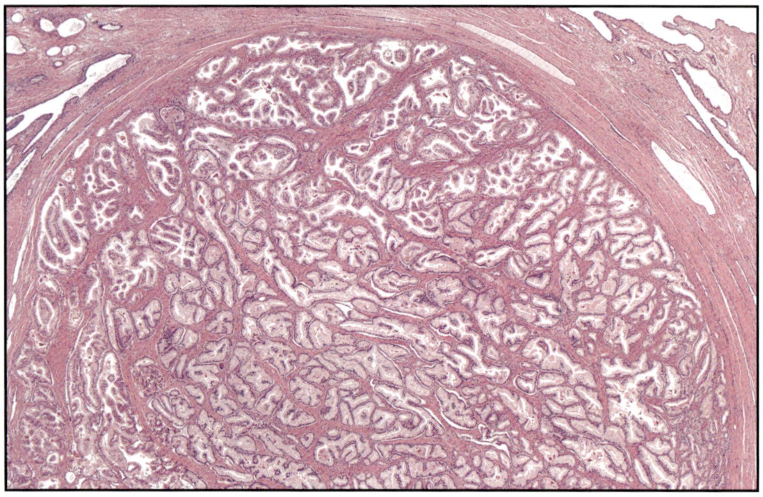

■ **i14.112** *Pseudohyperplastic pattern prostatic adenocarcinoma in radical prostatectomy tissue. The carcinoma simulates a BPH nodule at low-power magnification. This was the index case* (Humphrey 1998A).

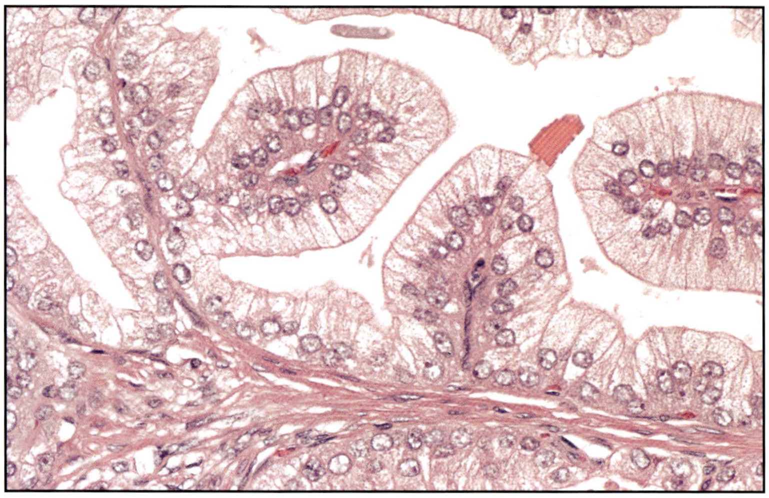

■ **i14.113** *Pseudohyperplastic pattern prostatic adenocarcinoma: Nuclear atypia and complete absence of basal cells.*

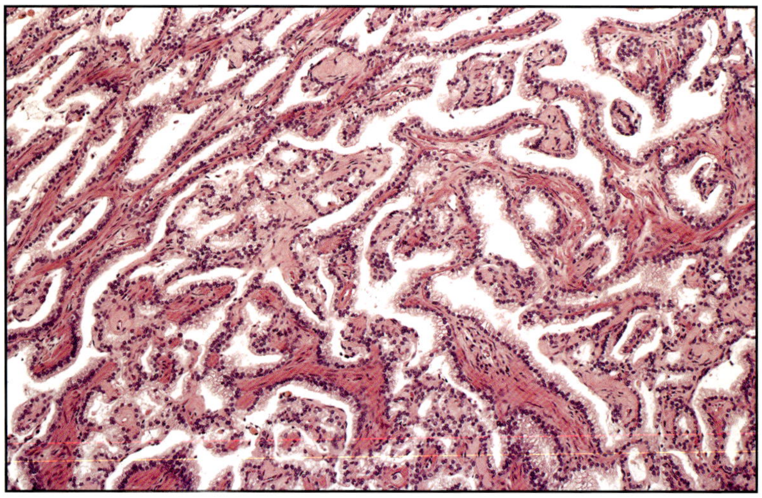

■ **i14.114** *Complex, interanastomosing, branching architecture of prostatic adenocarcinoma.*

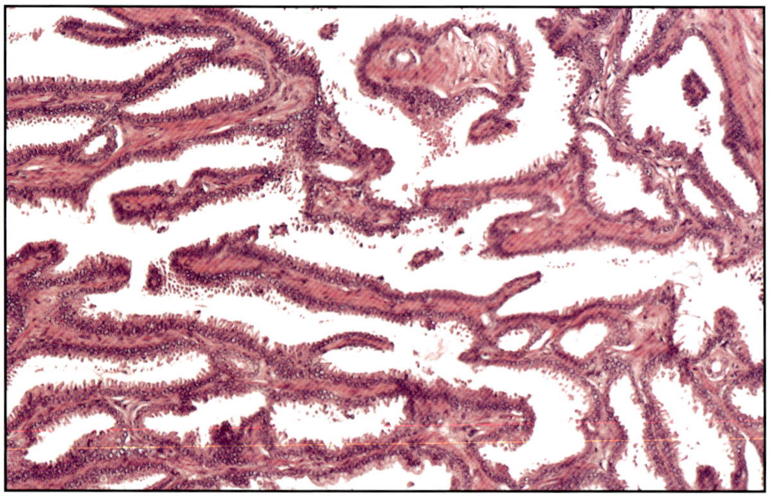

■ **i14.115** *Channel-like arrangement of prostatic adenocarcinoma glands.*

series **f14.3**. Nodular, well-differentiated Gleason score 2 to 4 adenocarcinoma in the transition zone is almost always associated with multifocal peripheral zone carcinoma, even when the dominant cancer is in the transition zone (Chen 2000, Noguchi 2000). Transition zone location does not automatically indicate a well-differentiated carcinoma. High-grade, peripheral zone carcinomas can extend into the transition zone and can even involve BPH nodules **i14.110, i14.111**. The patterns of growth and stromal-epithelial relationships of prostatic carcinoma in the whole gland are reasonably but not fully represented by the pictorial Gleason grading scheme.

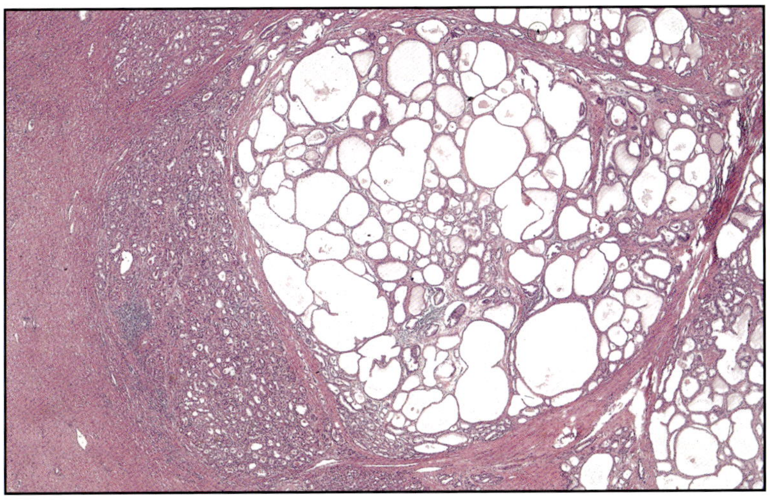

■ **i14.116** *Nodulocystic prostatic adenocarcinoma.*

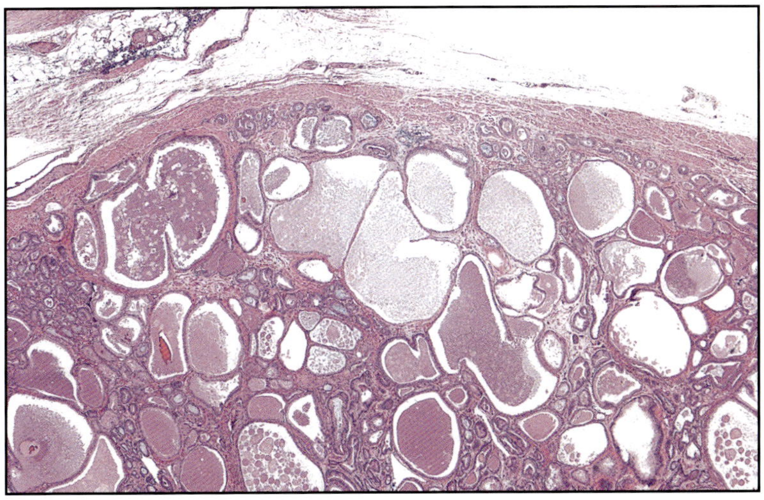

■ **i14.117** *Peripheral zone adenocarcinoma in radical prostatectomy tissue, with cystic dilatation of malignant glands.*

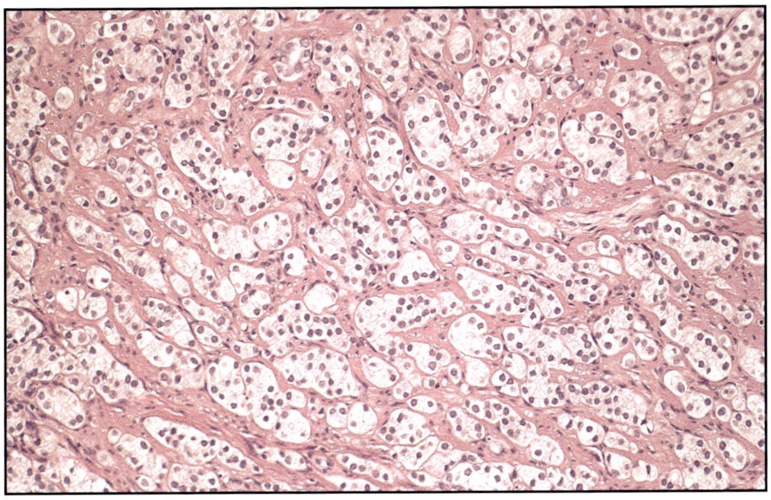

■ **i14.118** *Nested pattern of prostatic adenocarcinoma growth.*

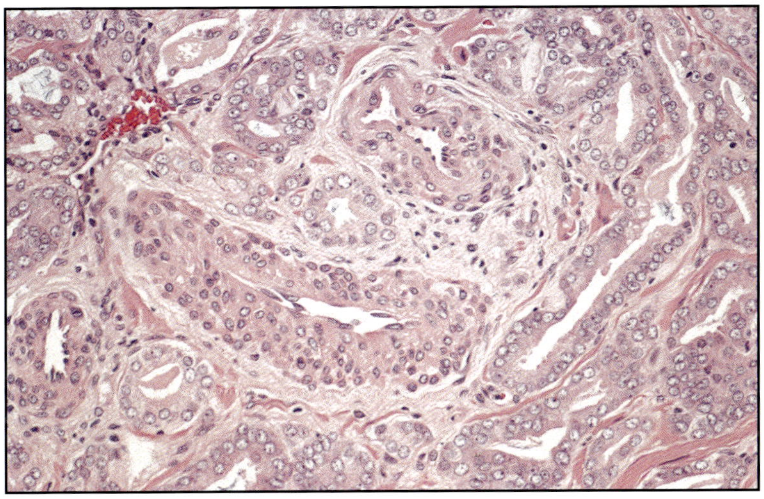

■ **i14.119** *Prostatic adenocarcinoma encircling small blood vessels. (Note the vascular media hypercellularity, a finding associated with adjacent adenocarcinoma* [Garcia 2000]*).*

Uncommon patterns of carcinoma glands seen in radical prostatectomy tissues and not depicted by Gleason include pseudohyperplastic configurations (Humphrey 1998A, Levi 2000), which we have defined as complex glands with intraluminal papillary projections **i14.16; i14.112, i14.113**, undulating luminal surfaces and branching patterns **i14.114, i14.115**, and cystic dilatation **i14.116, i14.117**. A rare pattern I have seen that has not been characterized is a high-grade nested arrangement **i14.118**. Moreover, the Gleason scheme does not depict modes of prostatic adenocarcinoma invasion in relation to benign prostatic glands **i14.3, i14.4; i14.10**, PIN glands **i14.5**, intraprostatic nerves **i14.42–i14.52**, intraprostatic vessels **i14.9; i14.119**, intraprostatic ejaculatory duct **i14.120**, intraprostatic apical skeletal muscle **i14.121**, the prostatic urethra **i14.122, i14.123**, and the prostatic fibromuscular sling (capsule) **i14.124**.

Diagnosis of adenocarcinoma in radical prostatectomy tissue sections uses the major and minor diagnostic criteria **t14.2**, just as for smaller tissue samples. The confirmation of the presence of carcinoma, previously established by needle biopsy, TURP, or open prostatectomy, usually is straightforward, where the disordered arrangement of the typical case of moderately differentiated small malignant acini is readily appreciated at scanning magnification, because the large tissue sections allow evaluation of the architec-

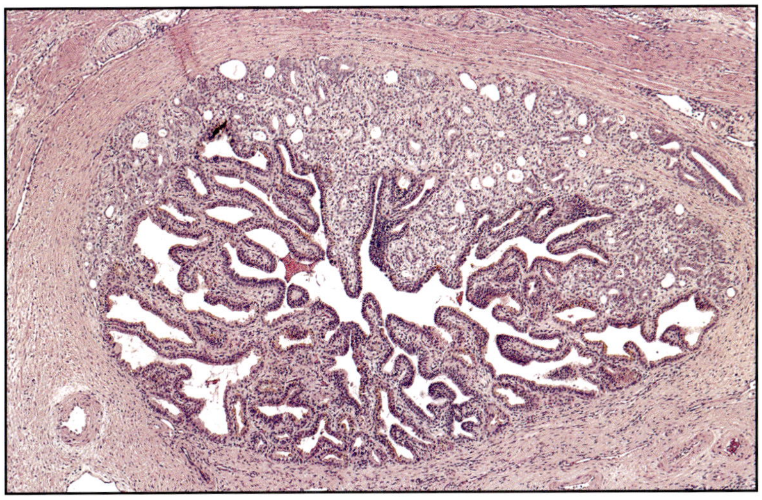

■ **i14.120** *Prostatic adenocarcinoma surrounding ejaculatory duct.*

tural relationship of the malignant acini and the nonneoplastic prostatic tissues.

Differential diagnostic difficulties in detecting carcinoma can arise if the carcinoma mimics benign proliferations (Chapter 20), if pseudoneoplasms are misdiagnosed as carcinoma (Chapter 10), or,

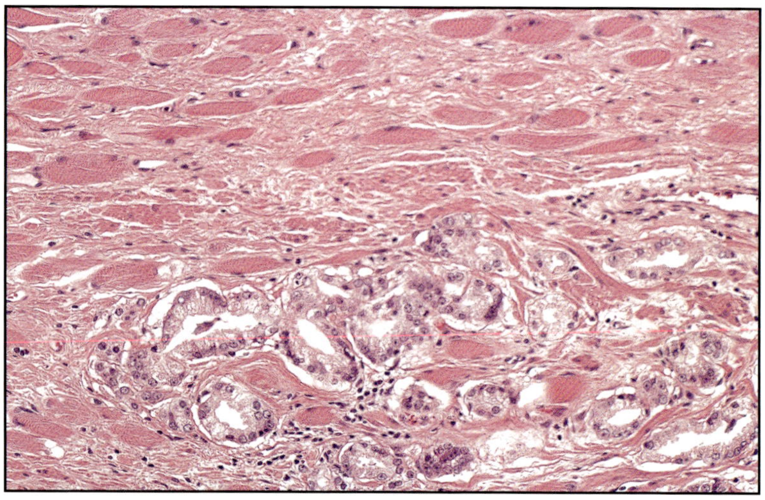

■ **i14.121** *Adenocarcinoma of prostate extending into apical skeletal muscle.*

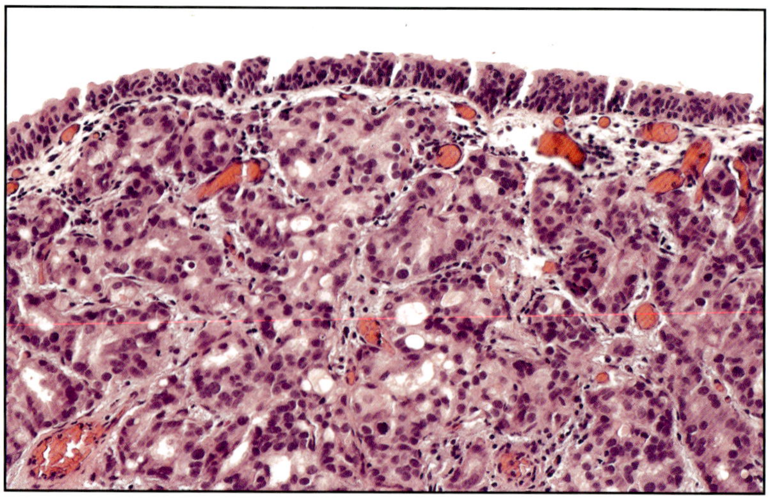

■ **i14.122** *Prostatic adenocarcinoma, with invasion to, but not into, prostatic urethral urothelium.*

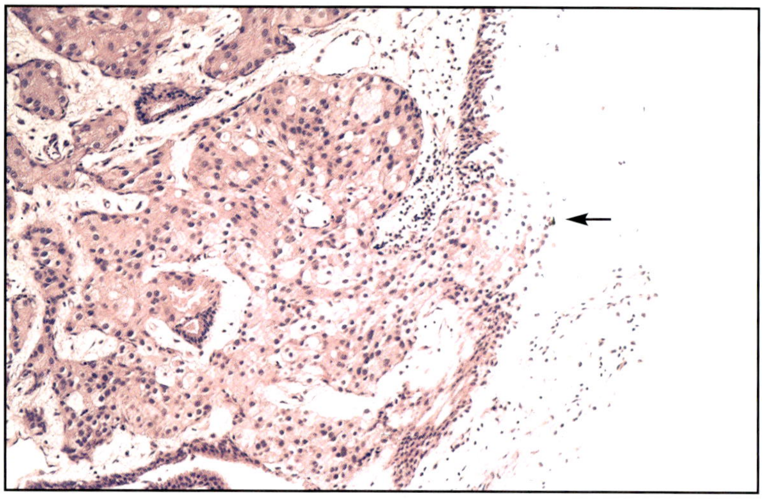

■ **i14.123** *Penetration and focal rupture of prostatic adenocarcinoma throughout prostatic urethral urothelium (arrow).*

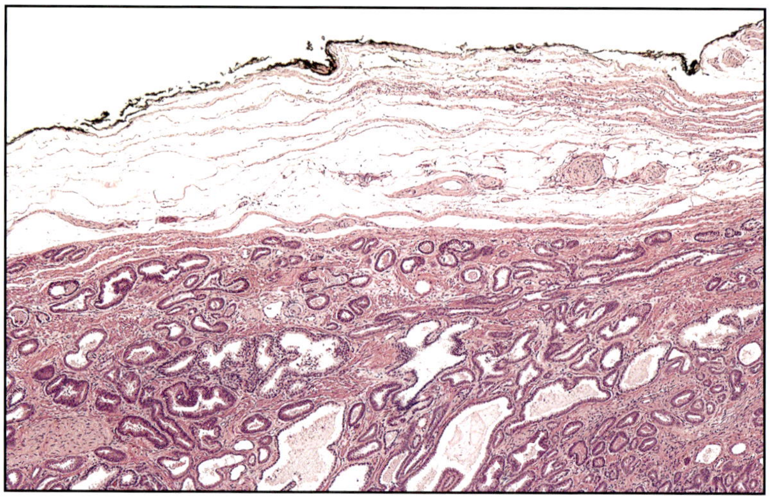

■ **i14.124** *Prostatic adenocarcinoma invasion of prostatic "capsule" (fibromuscular sling), without extraprostatic extension into periprostatic soft tissue or to inked margin.*

most commonly, if only a small amount of carcinoma is present in the whole gland.

Tumor size in radical prostatectomy specimens is quite variable, ranging from just a few malignant glands **i14.125** to large, bulky tumors that occupy most of the entire prostate gland. Tumor size must be determined by microscopy because unlike in other common malignancies such as breast, lung, and colon cancer, it is not possible to obtain accurate gross size estimates from radically excised prostate cancer. We estimate tumor size in radical prostatectomy specimens by providing, after light microscopic examination of routine sections, a visual inspection estimate of the percentage of the prostatic parenchyma that is involved by carcinoma. This method is simple and practical and does not necessitate extra time, complete embedding of the prostate glands, circling of carcinomatous foci, or morphometric measurements such as that needed for volumetric determinations. Currently, the average tumor size is about 10% of the prostate gland involved by carcinoma, but the range is extremely wide at 0.1% to 80% (Carvalhal 2000, Humphrey 1996).

Uncommonly, initial sections from a radical prostatectomy may reveal minimal or no carcinoma, which has been deemed of "vanishing cancer phenomenon" (Goldstein 1995A) or "minimal residual carcinoma" (DiGiuseppe 1997). These minute cancers are defined as those

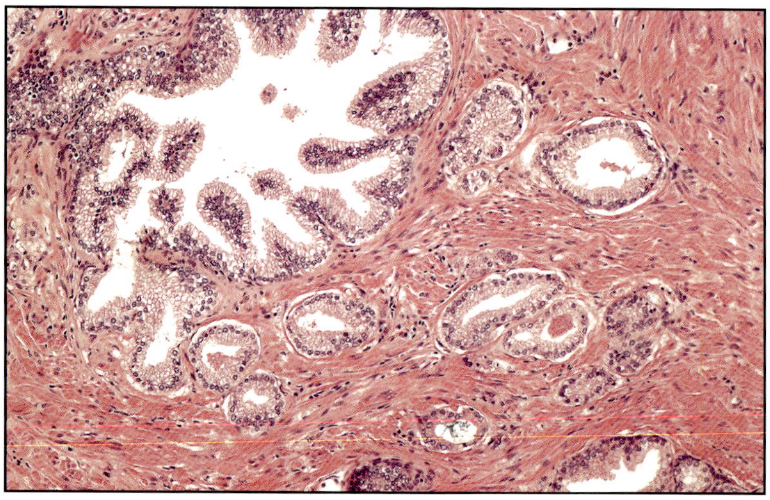

■ **i14.125** *Minimal adenocarcinoma in radical prostatectomy tissue. This was the only focus in the entire, completely embedded gland.*

of <0.1cm^3 in volume (range 0.01cm^3 to 0.13cm^3) or 3mm in greatest dimension **i14.125**. With increasing use of serum PSA screening, the incidence of these tiny cancers in patients not treated with preoperative or neoadjuvant therapy has increased from 0.5%

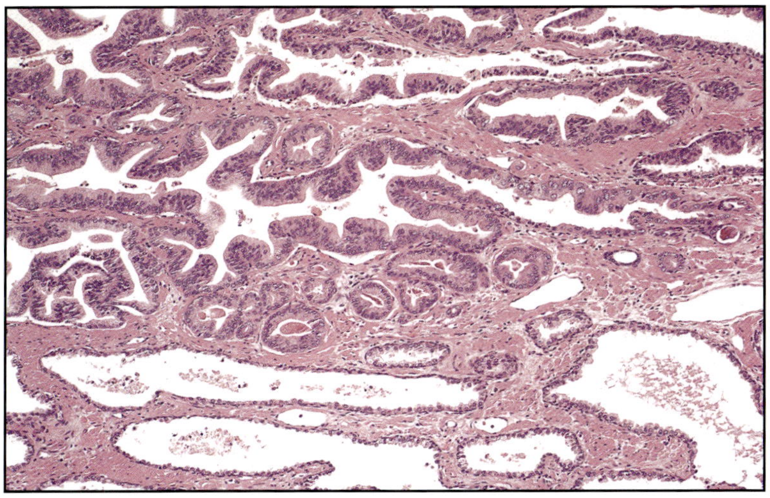

■ **i14.126** *Small focus of invasive adenocarcinoma (Gleason grade 3+3=score of 6) adjacent to high-grade PIN.*

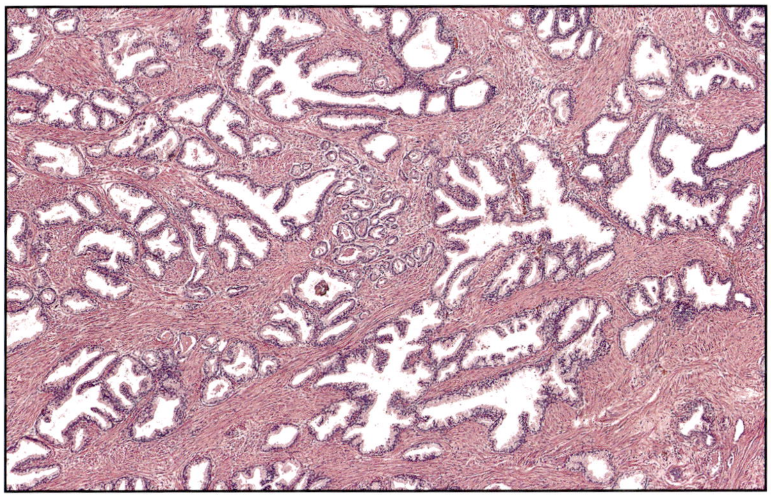

■ **i14.127** *Focal cluster of small prostatic adenocarcinoma glands in center of field.*

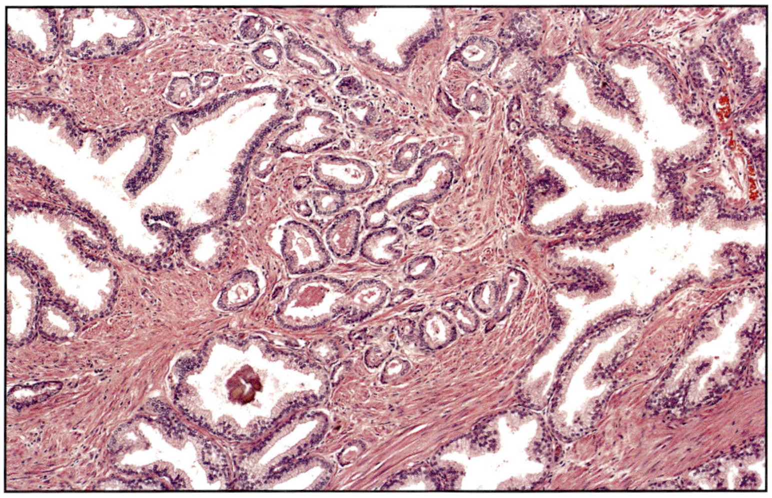

■ **i14.128** *Focal cluster of small prostatic adenocarcinoma glands, with infiltration between benign glands at periphery: Higher magnification of* **i14.127**.

in 1988 to the current level of 3% to 4% (DiGiuseppe 1997). There may also be failure to find carcinoma in radical prostatectomy specimens when patients have undergone preoperative hormonal therapy (Chapter 19) or after TURP (in up to 25% of cases; **t14.30**). It can be difficult to detect these small foci of carcinoma at low-power magnifications. Diagnostic clues include small acini immediately adjacent to high-grade PIN **i14.126** or clustered small acini **i14.127, i14.128**. In some cases, the minute foci of carcinoma are represented by haphazardly scattered small acini. The prevalence of no tumor at radical prostatectomy in previously untreated patients is <0.1% (DiGiuseppe 1997). (For suggested sampling maneuvers in this setting, see Chapter 2.)

Increasing tumor size in radical prostatectomy specimens correlates with increasing histologic grade in radical prostatectomy specimens, an increased risk of positive margins, and higher pathologic stage (reviewed in Humphrey 1997). Therefore, many small tumors tend to be lower-grade (McNeal 1993) and organ confined, whereas larger carcinomas are of the higher grade, with a higher percentage of Gleason patterns 4 and 5 and with a greater likelihood of EPE. These larger, high-grade carcinomas can grow as sheets, with effacement of normal glands or with only a few residual benign glands remaining in a sea of poorly differentiated carcinoma. However, exceptions do occur (Epstein 1994B, Miller 1994), and it is possible to identify peripheral zone low-volume, high-grade carcinoma (Epstein 1994B, Miller 1994) and transition zone high-volume, low-grade carcinoma.

Invasion of prostatic adenocarcinoma into tissue outside the prostate gland has been given a number of names, including "capsular penetration," "capsular perforation," "capsular transgression," and "EPE by carcinoma" **t14.34**. Given that the prostate does not have a true capsule but rather an incomplete fibromuscular sling, this latter designation is most appropriate (Sakr 1996). EPE by carcinoma is most likely to occur with high-grade, high-volume carcinomas and is associated with positive margins in most cases (although a substantial minority of men with EPE have negative margins). EPE is a common finding in radical prostatectomy specimens, ranging from 43% of PSA-detected (clinical stage T1c) carcinomas to 66% of digitally detected (clinical stage T2) carcinomas (Chapter 13, **t13.14**).

The anatomic site of carcinoma permeation into periprostatic tissues depends on zone of origin of the carcinoma **t14.31**. Low-grade transition zone carcinomas tend to invade into the anterior and apical fibromuscular stroma and only rarely breach the posterolateral periphery to spread into soft tissues and seminal vesicles (Blute 1985, Greene 1991A, 1991D, Grignon 1994, McNeal 1988A, 1988B, 1990A, Van de Voorde 1995). The boundary between the transition zone and peripheral zone may constitute a barrier for posterolateral spread of transition zone carcinoma. It can be difficult microscopically to evaluate EPE in the anterior and apical portion of the radical prostatectomy specimen. Invasion of carcinoma into adipose tissue is the most definitive sign of EPE, yet adipose tissue is absent anteriorly and apically. Moreover, anteriorly, prostatic stroma merges imperceptibly with external

■ t14.34 **Extraprostatic Extension (EPE) by Carcinoma in Radical Prostatectomy Specimens**

Capsular penetration, perforation, or transgression
Most clear-cut when carcinoma invades periprostatic adipose tissue
EPE by transition zone cancers into anterior and apical soft-tissue does not involve invasion of fat
EPE posterolaterally by peripheral zone carcinomas can occur by perineural invasion, by fat infiltration, and by pushing (bulging) patterns of spread

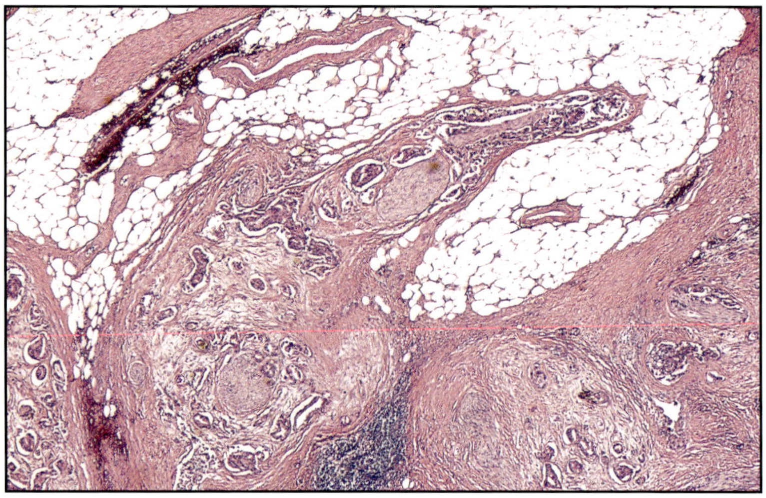

■ **i14.129** *Extraprostatic extension of adenocarcinoma via perineural tracking into periprostatic soft (adipose) tissue.*

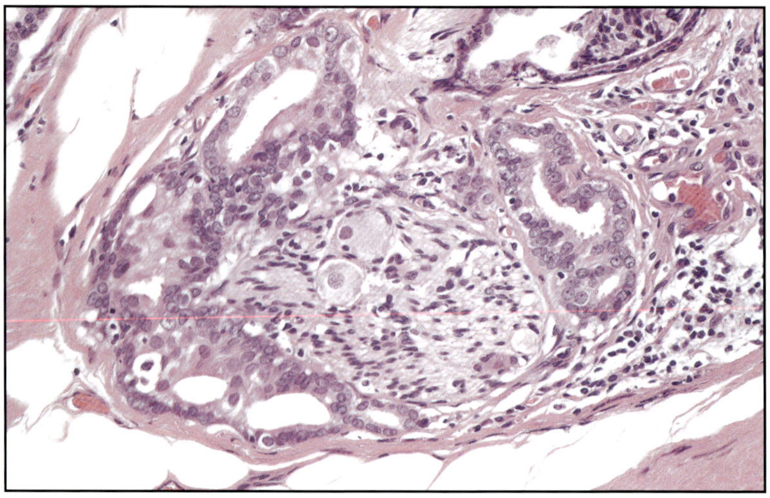

■ **i14.130** *Extraprostatic extension of adenocarcinoma via perineural tracking into periprostatic soft (adipose) tissue.*

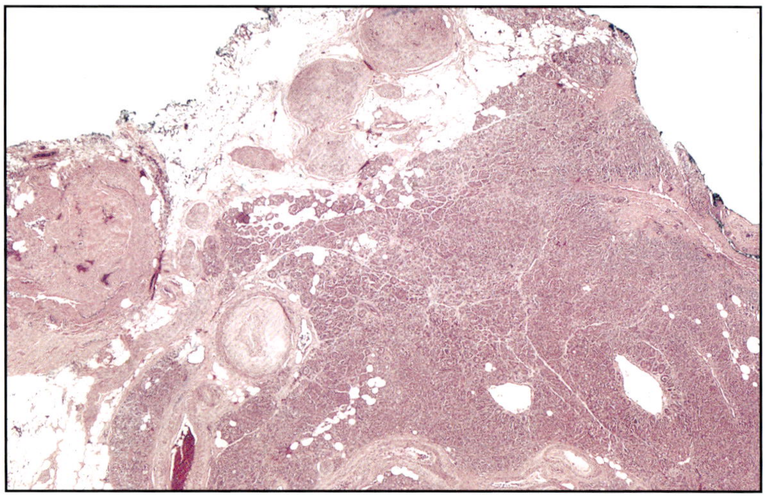

■ **i14.131** *Direct extension of prostatic adenocarcinoma into periprostatic adipose tissue.*

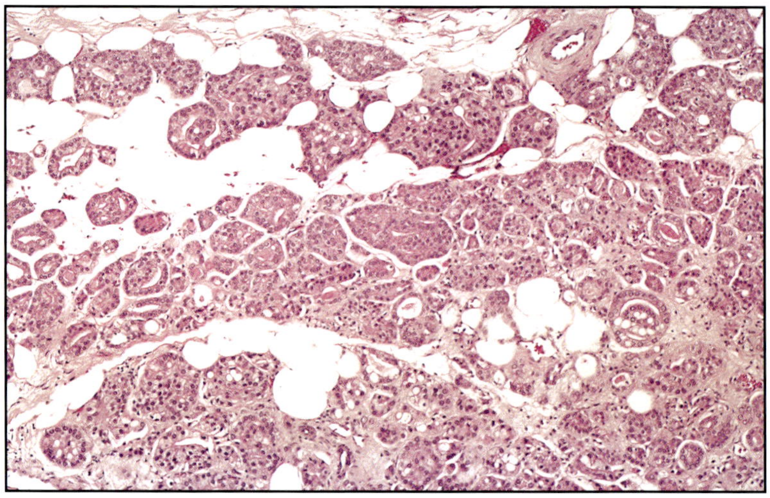

■ **i14.132** *Direct extension of prostatic adenocarcinoma into periprostatic adipose tissue (higher magnification of* **i14.131**).

smooth muscle, whereas apically, skeletal muscle of the urogenital diaphragm interdigitates with the prostate. Therefore, one must mentally draw a rounded boundary line or arc at the outer edge of benign prostatic glands and consider all malignant glands outside this arc as extraprostatic. Difficulties can arise when the malignant glands have destroyed the reference benign glands and when the outer aspect of the benign glands is not rounded. A caveat about the apex is that carcinoma glands in skeletal muscle do not necessarily equate with EPE. Posterolaterally, prostatic carcinoma can violate the capsule by invasion along perineural sheaths **i14.129, i14.130**, by insinuation of glands into or adjacent to adipose tissue **i14.131, i14.132**, and by nodular, pushing advancement **i14.133**. This EPE can occur with or without a fibrogenic response. In the bulging type of EPE, adipose tissue can be replaced by fibrous tissue so that EPE can be diagnosed when such nodules or bands of carcinomas are clearly present in or adjacent to adipose tissue. A potential problem in diagnosis of EPE is recognition of carcinoma cells outside the prostate after androgen deprivation therapy (Reuter 1997). In some cases, after such hormonal therapy the tumor cells may appear to be lymphocytes or histiocytes, where single-cell tumor infiltration into periprostatic soft tissues can be difficult to discern. Immunostains for pan-cytokeratin and PSA may be useful in these cases.

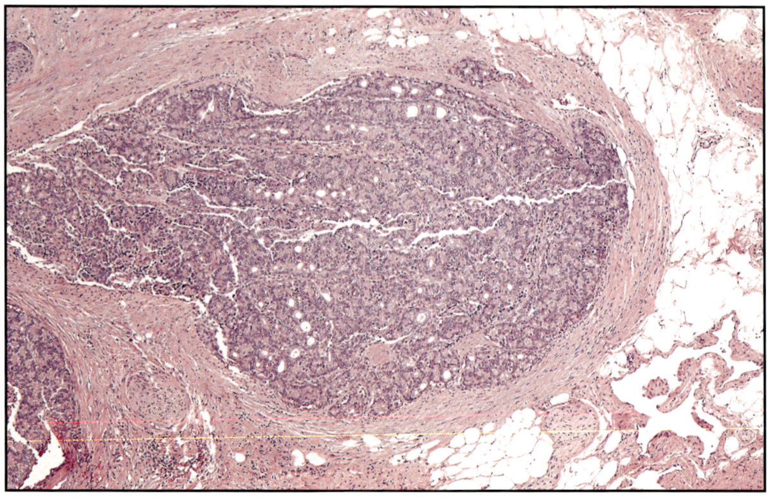

■ **i14.133** *Nodular mass of high-grade prostatic adenocarcinoma with pushing invasion into periprostatic adipose tissue.*

Capsular invasion or carcinoma invasion into the poorly defined fibromuscular sling of the prostate should be distinguished from the bulging type of EPE. In some cases the fibromuscular sling constitutes an anatomic blockade to EPE, and carcinoma can be

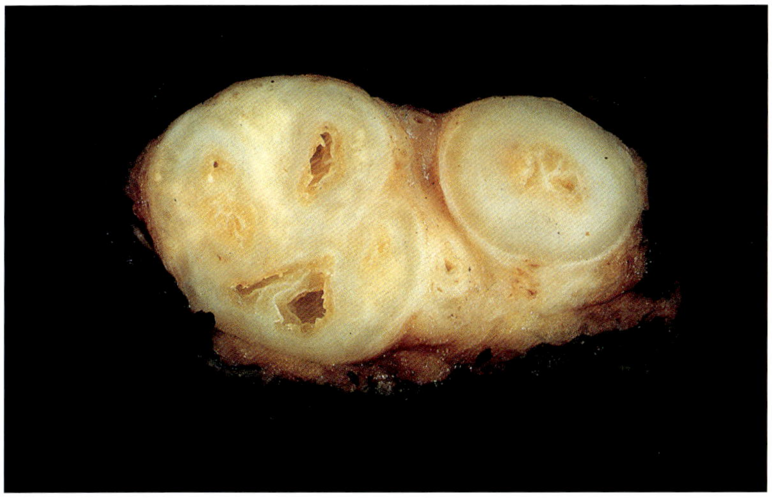

■ **i14.134** *Seminal vesicle invasion by yellowish areas of prostatic adenocarcinoma.*

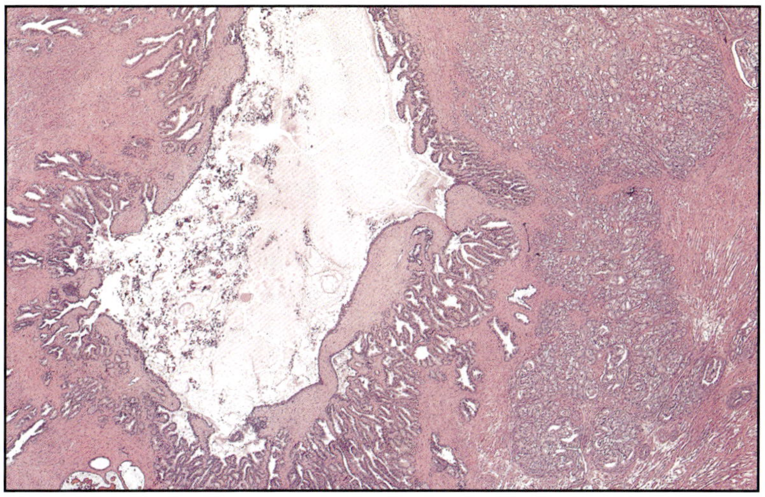

■ **i14.135** *Seminal vesicle wall invasion by prostatic adenocarcinoma.*

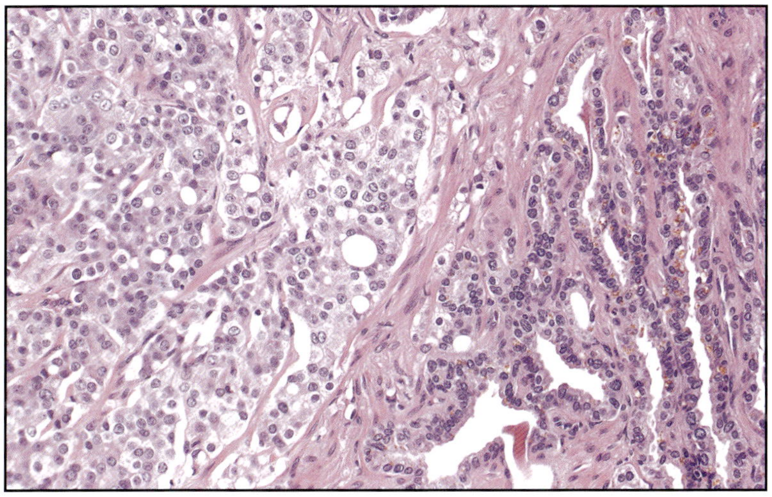

■ **i14.136** *Prostatic adenocarcinoma (left) infiltrating seminal vesicle wall, adjacent to benign seminal vesicle epithelium (right).*

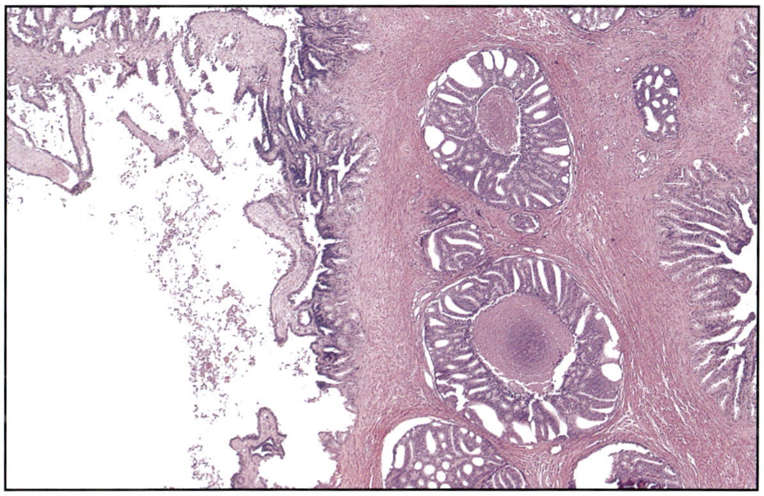

■ **i14.137** *Seminal vesicle wall invasion by prostatic comedocarcinoma.*

found growing as bands, columns, or masses immediately underneath or within **i14.124** the ill-defined fibromuscular band.

Perineural invasion and even invasion around ganglia can be seen within the prostate and do not automatically signal EPE. Lymphvascular space invasion in periprostatic tissue is hardly ever an isolated finding but is most often found with high-grade, high-volume cancer with extensive EPE. Another probable pathway for EPE is retrograde spread along the intraprostatic ejaculatory duct sheath into soft tissue at the base of the prostate.

The seminal vesicles are excised in the radical prostatectomy procedure, and microscopic evaluation for carcinoma spread into these paired structures is vital. Seminal vesical invasion is found less often in the PSA-screening era, with a current incidence of around 6% **t13.14**; the incidence in clinically palpable (stage T2) disease is 14% to 21% (Byar 1972, Epstein 1994A, Ohori 1993), and for palpable disease clinically outside the prostate (clinical stage T3) the incidence is 67% (Ohori 1993). Seminal vesicle invasion by carcinoma usually is diagnosed in prostatic carcinoma cases that are high grade and high volume, with EPE elsewhere and a high incidence of lymph node metastasis **t14.35** (McNeal 1986B, 1990A, Ohori 1993, Stamey 1988, Villers 1990).

Grossly, it is usually impossible to diagnose prostatic carcinoma in seminal vesicles, although in exceptional, advanced cases there can be nodules, diffuse thickening of the seminal vesicle muscular wall, or a yellowish-white, irregular infiltrate **i14.134**. To diagnose seminal vesicle invasion, carcinoma should be seen by light microscopy within the smooth muscle wall of the seminal vesicle **i14.135–i14.137** (Epstein 1993A). Invasion of soft tissue surrounding the seminal vesicle does not count. Seminal vesicle invasion by prostatic carcinoma usually is found in the proximal portion near the base of the prostate, although isolated deposits can be found in the tip. Involvement can be focal, with just a few malignant glands in the wall, or diffuse, with thickening of the seminal vesicle wall by carcinoma. Extent of seminal vesicle involvement is directly related to cancer volume within the prostate (Villers 1990). Spread of prostatic carcinoma into

■ **t14.35 Seminal Vesicle Invasion by Prostatic Carcinoma**

Most common in high-grade, high-volume cancers
Spread occurs by invasion into wall from periprostatic soft tissue, by penetration along ejaculatory duct sheath, or by lymphvascular invasion
Intraluminal spread and involvement of ejaculatory duct or seminal vesicle epithelium rare

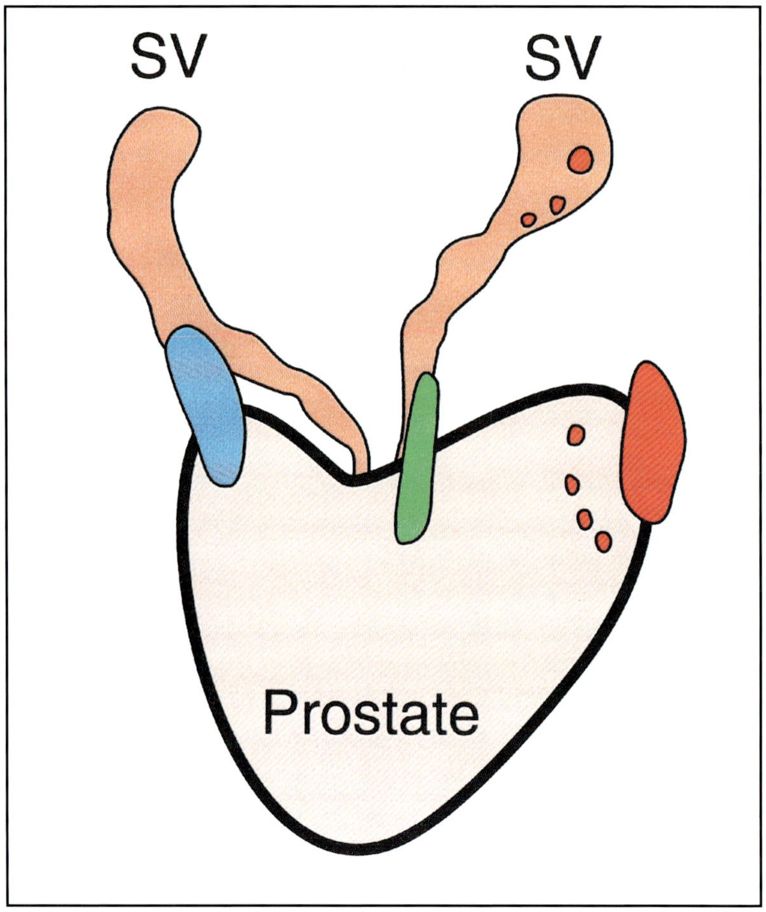

■ **f14.4** *Pathways of spread of prostatic carcinoma into seminal vesicle (SV) tissue. 1: Direct extension from prostate into periprostatic soft tissue, with penetration of seminal vesicle wall (blue nodule). 2: Direct extension along ejaculatory duct sheath (green nodule). 3: Lymphvascular space invasion from noncontiguous prostatic carcinoma (red).*

seminal vesicles occurs by several mechanisms **f14.4** (Byar 1972, Epstein 1991, 1993A, Graham 1996, Ohori 1993, Villers 1990), with several different resultant histomorphologic appearances. The most common type is EPE by carcinoma into periprostatic soft tissue at the base of the prostate, with penetration into the seminal vesicle wall **f14.4**. The second most common form of involvement is direct tracking along the ejaculatory duct complex into the seminal vesicles **f14.4**. The third kind of involvement is characterized by isolated deposits of cancer in the seminal vesicle, without contiguous spread from the prostate. This represents lymphvascular space invasion in seminal vesicle wall **i14.138** (Graham 1996, Villers 1990) and correlates with lymphvascular space invasion in the prostate itself (Graham 1996). Finally, it is notable that prostate cancer does not appear to spread within the lumen of the ejaculatory duct and seminal vesicle. Like the urothelium, the ejaculatory duct and seminal epithelium seem resistant, for unknown reasons, to invasion by prostatic carcinoma **i14.139-i14.141**. In rare cases we have seen intraluminal extension by prostatic carcinoma in seminal vesicles **i14.142**, but only with bulky prostate cancer in the seminal vesicle. Perineural invasion by carcinoma can be identified within the seminal vesicle wall **i14.143**, and this is another potential avenue of prostate cancer reach into the seminal vesicles, resulting from extension along nerves in the periprostatic and periseminal vesicular adipose tissue (Ohori 1993).

The differential diagnosis of prostatic carcinoma invasion into the seminal vesicle wall is centered mainly on outpouching of seminal vesicle glands into the wall, which can be disturbing if oblique sections of the wall are taken. Usually the diagnosis of prostatic carcinoma involvement of the wall is straightforward, based on the presence of numerous malignant prostatic glands in the wall and on the uniform nuclei of prostatic carcinoma in comparison to seminal vesicle glands, which have randomly dispersed giant

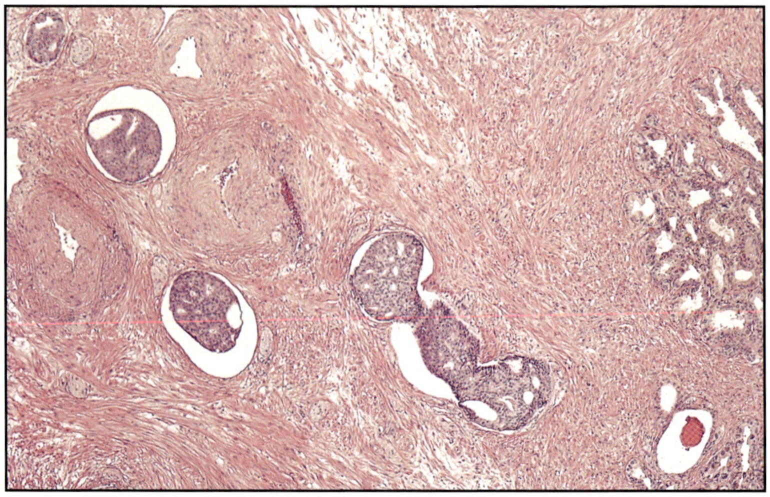

■ **i14.138** *Lymphvascular space invasion by prostatic carcinoma in seminal vesicle wall.*

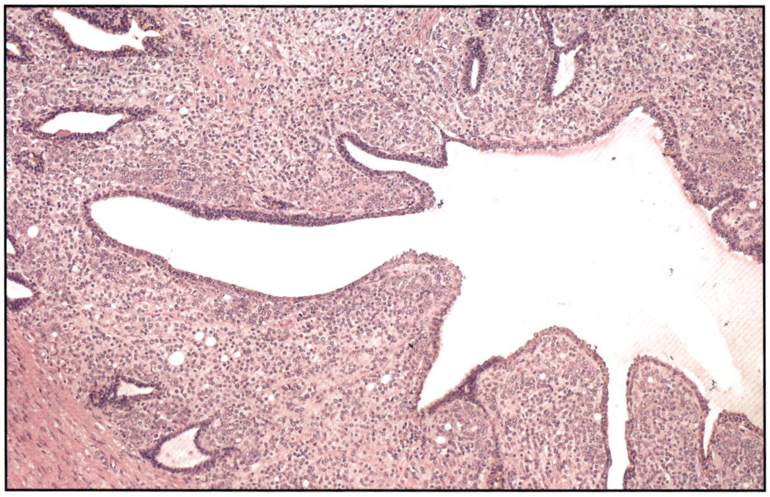

■ **i14.139** *Extensive seminal vesical involvement by prostatic adenocarcinoma, with sparing of seminal vesicle glands.*

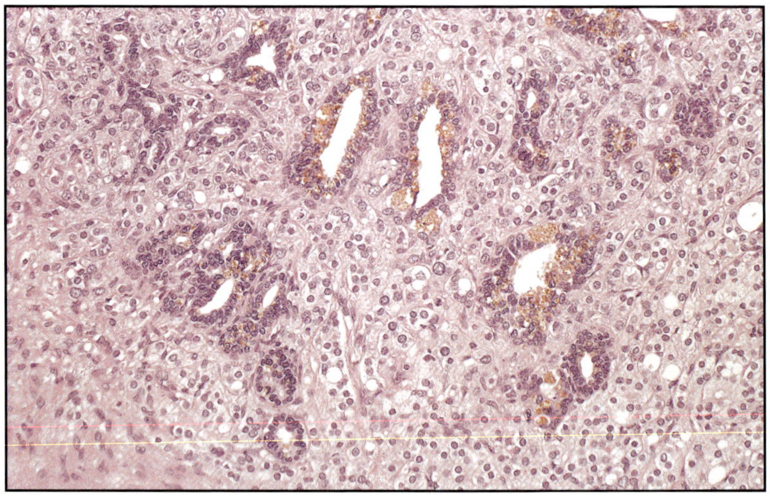

■ **i14.140** *High-grade prostatic carcinoma growing between and around seminal vesicle glands, which contain brown pigment.*

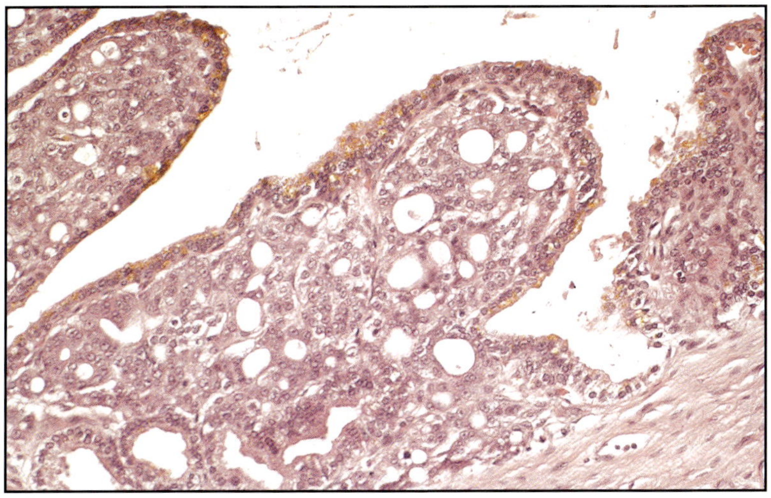

■ **i14.141** *Encroachment of prostatic adenocarcinoma, with invasion to, but not into, seminal vesicle epithelium.*

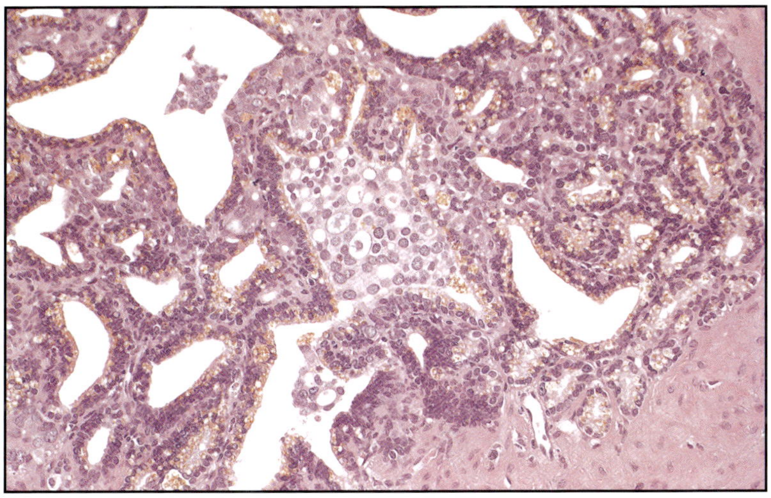

■ **i14.142** *Prostatic adenocarcinoma (pale glands in center) inside seminal vesicle lumen (a rare finding).*

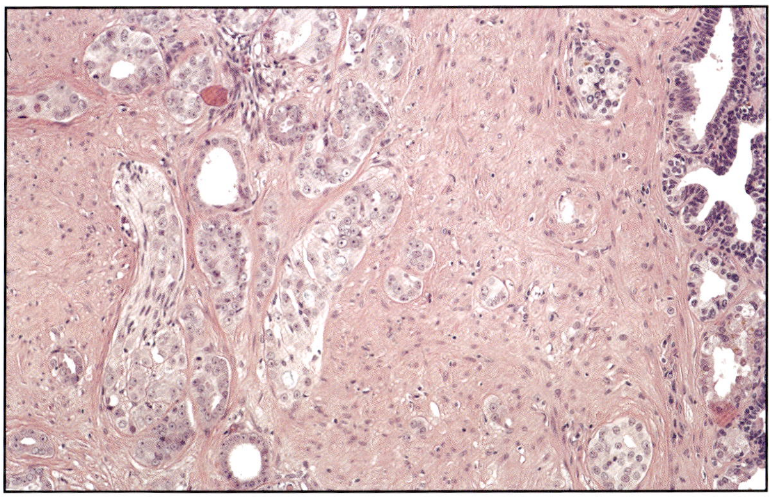

■ **i14.143** *Perineural invasion by carcinoma in wall of seminal vesicle. Perineural invasion can also be seen in soft tissue surrounding the seminal vesicle.*

smudged nuclei. As discussed earlier, positive immunostaining using monoclonal antibodies reactive against PSA and negative 34βE12 immunostaining (Chapter 22) can be of diagnostic aid in establishing a diagnosis of prostatic carcinoma invasion in seminal vesicle, although we have not had to resort to the immunostains in seminal vesicle sections from radical prostatectomy specimens. Other malignancies can involve the seminal vesicle, such as carcinoma of the bladder (Ro 1987), and are in the differential diagnosis, but these patients usually have known primary malignancies elsewhere.

■ **t14.36 Positive Surgical Margins in Radical Prostatectomy Specimens**

Increasing incidence with higher grade, volume, and stage of carcinoma
Peripheral margin positivity = ink on tumor cells
Positivity of distal urethral (apical) and bladder neck shave margins = tumor anywhere in tissue
Positivity of coned apical margin = ink on tumor cells
Can have positive margin, particularly at apex, without demonstrable EPE due to surgical incision into gland (17% of all positive margins)

Surgical margin status of the radical prostatectomy is crucial because completeness of cancer excision relates to prognosis and consideration for additional therapy (Cheng 1999B, Epstein 1996D, Öbek 1999, Ohori 1999, Wieder 1998). A positive radical prostatectomy margin might seem to suggest that residual tumor is left behind in the patient, but actually positive margins represent a risk factor for subsequent failure and do not automatically mean that the patient will experience disease progression. The incidence of positive surgical margins in radical prostatectomy specimens depends on many factors. First, it varies according to clinical stage of the prostate cancer, with an overall mean of 28% (and range of 0% to 71%) based on a literature survey of 12 056 patients (Wieder 1998). The incidence also depends on the intrinsic characteristics of the cancer, where increasing tumor size, grade, and stage are associated with an increasing risk of a positive margin **t14.36**. Furthermore, the positive margin rate changes in relation to thoroughness of sampling of the radical prostatectomy specimen and the definition of surgical margin (Epstein 1996D, Wieder 1998). Preoperative neoadjuvant hormonal therapy affects incidence (decreases it [Wieder 1998]), as does surgeon experience. There does not appear to be a statistically significant difference in the rate of positive surgical margins between perineal and retropubic radical prostatectomy and between nerve-sparing and non–nerve-sparing radical retropubic prostatectomy (Wieder 1998). However, the bladder neck–sparing modification of radical retropubic prostatectomy may increase the positive margin rate (Marcovich 2000). It is too soon to tell how laparoscopic radical prostatectomy positive margin incidence compares with open radical prostatectomy, although in one report of 120 laparoscopic radical prostatectomies only 15% of patients had positive margins (Guillonneau 2000).

The histopathologic definition of a positive surgical margin has varied in the literature (Epstein 1996D, Wieder 1998). Some histopathologists have considered tumor that closely approaches an inked margin **i14.144, i14.145** to represent a positive margin, but clinical follow-up data indicate that only ink on tumor cells **i14.146** is significant as a risk factor for subsequent failure (Epstein 1997). For thin 2mm distal urethral (apical) and bladder neck shave margins, carcinoma presence anywhere in this tissue indicates a positive margin. For those who prefer to amputate the distal 5mm of the prostate and essentially generate conization sections (see Chapter 2), ink on tumor cells equates with a positive margin.

The most common sites for a positive margin in the radical prostatectomy specimen are, in order, the apex, the posterolateral or posterior region, and the bladder neck **t14.37** (Epstein 1996D, Wieder 1998). The apex is most frequently involved because there is only a scant

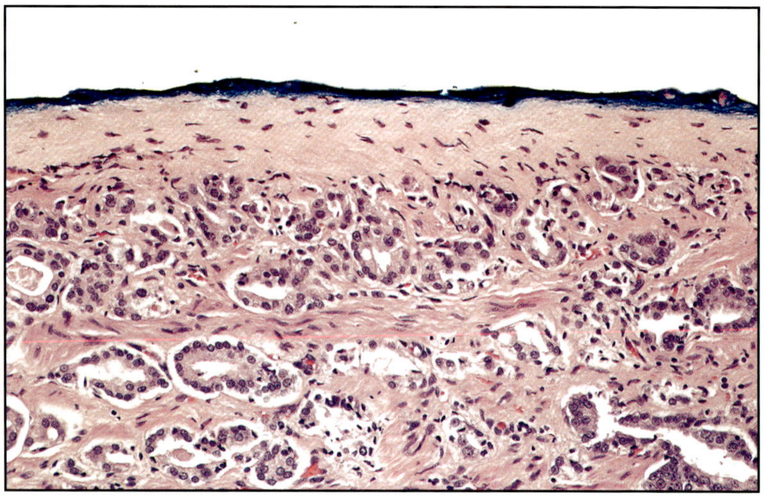

■ **i14.144** *Close approach of prostatic adenocarcinoma to inked peripheral surgical margin of resection.*

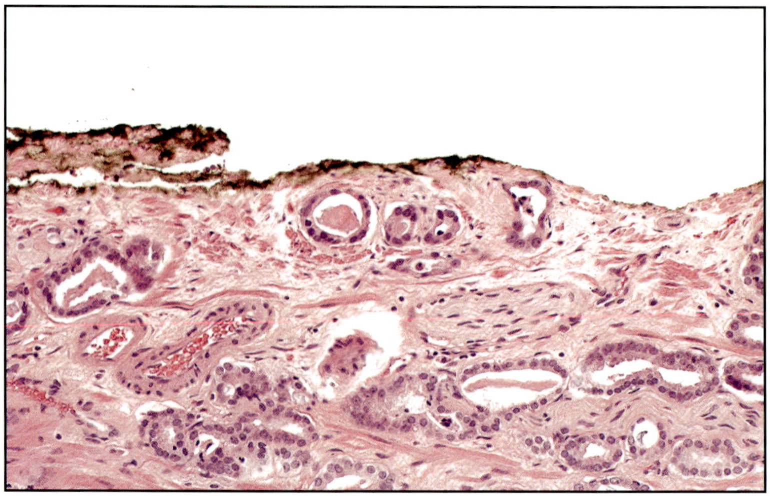

■ **i14.145** *Extremely close approach of adenocarcinoma to margin.*

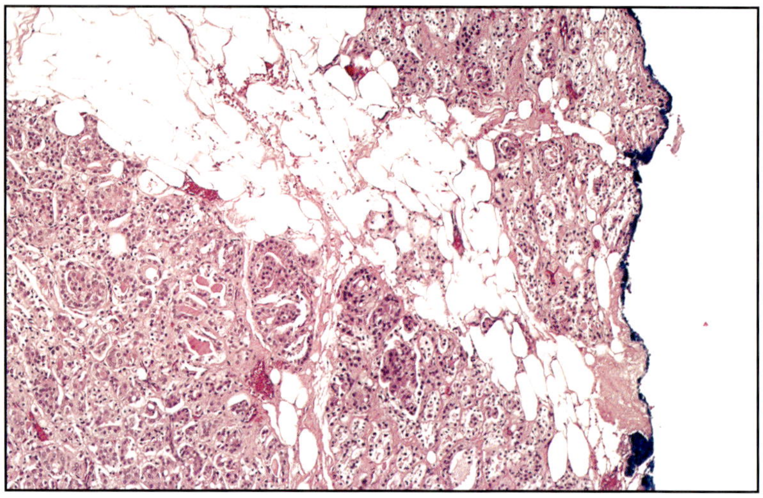

■ **i14.146** *Positive surgical margin. Prostatic adenocarcinoma with extraprostatic extension into periprostatic adipose tissue, and with ink on tumor.*

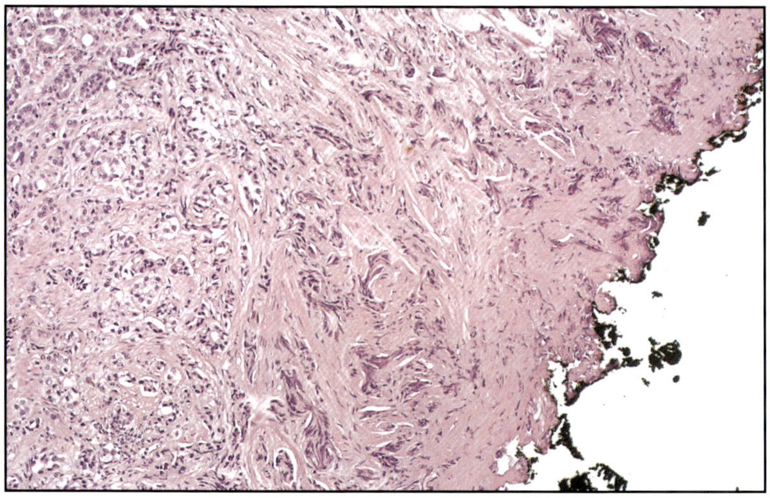

■ **i14.147** *Cauterized adenocarcinoma extending to inked peripheral surgical margin of resection in radical prostatectomy tissue.*

■ **t14.37 Anatomic Sites of Positive Surgical Margins in Radical Prostatectomy Specimens**

Apex /anterior: most common = 22%-38% of positive margins
Posterolateral/posterior = 14%-33% of positive margins
Bladder neck = 7%-19% of positive margins

amount of tissue surrounding the prostate at this site and because surgically the apex can be difficult to visualize and expose, and surgical attempts to preserve continence include dividing the urethra close to the apex (Wieder 1998). The posterolateral and posterior sites are common locations of EPE of peripheral zone carcinoma, which can then extend to the margin here. Involvement of the bladder neck usually is seen in large tumors.

The apex is also the most common site of a positive margin produced by inadvertent, intraoperative incision into the prostate (iatrogenic positive margins) (Epstein 1996D, Wieder 1998). Overall, 17% of positive margins (range, 9% to 71%) are "incisional," without evidence of EPE (Cheng 1999B, Ohori 1995, Wieder 1998). Microscopically, these margins are most easily recognized when ink representing a true surgical margin is present on adjacent benign and malignant epithelium. At this site, the presence or absence of EPE by carcinoma cannot be determined, and thus the stage is T2 at least or, in one proposal (Sakr 1996), T2+.

Evaluating margin status can be difficult if there is crush or cautery artifact **i14.147** or poor tissue preservation near the margin. Continuity of distorted atypical cells at the margin with clear-cut carcinoma more distant from the margin can be sufficient for a diagnosis of a positive margin. Additional levels into the block in an effort to "step out" of the crushed area occasionally are of value. Disruption of the capsule during surgery, during harvest of tissue for research purposes, and during inking and sectioning can all hinder appraisal of margins. This is particularly so when there is "running ink," with ink extending into tissue cracks and crevices or along knife cut surfaces. Here, judgment is needed and one should be certain that ink on tumor cells is a true positive margin before diagnosing definitive margin involvement. Indeterminate cases, which are uncommon, should be described in a comment. Lastly, recognition of positive margins can be exceptionally difficult in patients treated preoperatively with hormonal therapy because tumor cells may be present as single cells that can mimic lymphocytes or histiocytes. Again, immunostains for pan-cytokeratin or PSA can be useful in identifying such cells at the margin.

The standard of practice in determining surgical margin status is histologic examination of permanent radical prostatectomy tissue sections. Frozen sections of posterolateral margins have been performed as an aid in the intraoperative decision to excise or not excise neurovascular bundles (Cangiano 1999), but from a practical standpoint it is not feasible to sample, at frozen section, the entire margin. Moreover, frozen sections of prostatic tissue can be challenging to interpret because presentation of nuclear detail is suboptimal and determination of number of glandular cell layers can also be a problem. Some urologists may request frozen sections of the apical margin, but this is also to be discouraged (Epstein 1996D) because in most cases no further tissue can be excised, and thus the frozen section result does not change intraoperative management. Proposals exist to evaluate adequacy of surgical excision by use of margin cytologic touch preparations or washings (Brannigan 1998, Pearle 1994, Ward 2001) and by use of reverse transcriptase–polymerase chain reaction (RT-PCR) for PSA or prostate-specific membrane antigen (PSMA) in prostatic fossa biopsies (Theodorescu 1999) or intraoperative field blood (Oefelein 1996) after removal of the prostate gland, but these are currently experimental.

Established Prognostic Attributes and Reporting for Radical Prostatectomy

The most important prognostic attributes of prostate cancer in radical prostatectomy specimens that warrant reporting are histologic type, histologic grade, tumor size, pathologic stage, and margin status (ADASP 1998, Bostwick 1999B, 2000, Henson 1994, Humphrey 1993A, Hutter 1996, Srigley 2000) **t14.38**. We report these features, and a number of others, using a standardized synoptic form **t14.39**, which is printed at the end of each radical prostatectomy report. This synoptic reporting does not replace diagnostic field reporting **t14.40**, nor does it replace the gross and microscopic or comment fields. The attending pathologist still has the freedom to generate a radical prostatectomy report in the manner she or he desires. This synoptic reporting has been extremely well-received by urologists and oncologists and generates important database information for our cancer center. Also, the pathologic stage assignment is important documentation for the patient's medical record chart.

The first synoptic field is simply whether a neoplasm is present. As previously noted, there are several reasons why residual carcinoma may not be present in the radical prostatectomy specimen. For example, all tumor may have been previously excised by TURP **t14.30**. After needle biopsy diagnosis, no detectable cancer in the whole gland from untreated patients should be extremely rare (DiGiuseppe 1997). Finally, identification of residual carcinoma in patients treated with preoperative neoadjuvant hormonal therapy can be difficult on occasion (Reuter 1997). Although no residual carcinoma (pT0) has been reported in 4% to 15% of such cases, with complete embedding of the prostate gland and knowledge of androgen deprivation therapy effects on prostatic carcinoma (see Chapter 19), the pT0 rate in this setting should be well below 5% (Reuter 1997). If no residual carcinoma is detected after thorough workup, probably one should document in a comment the nature of the evaluation to rule out residual carcinoma and state the probable basis for failure to detect carcinoma in the radical prostatectomy specimen.

The second field is histologic type of the carcinoma, which in 95% of cases is a conventional acinar type. Unusual histologic types of carcinoma, including ductal, mucinous, signet-ring, neuroendocrine, squamous cell, adenosquamous, transitional cell, and sarcomatoid carcinomas should be reported because they typically harbor a worse prognosis (Chapter 17).

Tumor size is reported in the third field. Tumor size, as measured by a variety of techniques in the whole prostate gland, is an important prognostic indicator, where prostatic carcinoma size has been linked to a number of pathologic and clinical endpoints such as grade, stage, PSA level, response to therapy, and risk of death due to prostatic carcinoma (Byar 1972, review in Humphrey 1997, Carvalhal 2000, Eastham 1998, Renshaw 1998C, Stamey 1999, Vollmer 2001) **t14.41**. Moreover, all definitions of clinically significant and clinically unimportant prostatic carcinomas **t13.20** based on radical prostatectomy findings incorporate tumor size measurements (Dugan 1996, Epstein 1994A, Humphrey 1996, Irwin 1994, Ohori 1994, Terris 1995,). Some debate has centered on whether tumor size is an independent predictor of failure after surgery when grade, stage, and margins are included in multivariate analysis. In our experience, percentage carcinoma in radical prostatectomy specimens independently predicts prostate cancer recurrence after surgery (Carvalhal 2000, Humphrey 1991A, 1993D) and patient survival (Vollmer 2001).

A number of methods are available for quantitating tumor size in radical prostatectomy specimens, including visual inspection, measurement of the diameter of the largest tumor focus, counting of the number of blocks involved by tumor, 3-dimensional estimates, grid morphometric analysis, and computer-assisted image analysis (reviewed in Humphrey 1997). The last approach is widely viewed as the most rigorous and quantitative method, but it is impractical because of the time-intensive and labor-intensive nature of mapping and the cost of image analyzers. For research purposes we use completely embedded glands with grid morphometric analysis to determine percentage carcinoma (Humphrey 1990B) and image analysis to calculate total tumor volume (Humphrey 1996). For routine daily practice one may use a simple, light microscopic, visual inspection estimate of the percentage of the prostatic parenchyma that is involved by carcinoma, without circling foci of carcinoma. Capture of this percentage figure, which is reported in 5% to 10% increments, is made without additional time or expense and without complete embedding of the prostate glands, which is not standard of practice, being performed in only 12% of laboratories nationwide (True 1994). Reporting tumor size in radical prostatectomy specimens as percentage of the prostate involved by carcinoma is recommended by the CAP (Bostwick 1999B, 2000, Henson 1994, Srigley 2000) and the Association of Directors of Anatomic and Surgical Pathology (ADASP 1998) **t14.42**.

Histologic grade in the whole gland is one of the most powerful markers of prostatic carcinoma biologic aggressiveness (Chapter 15). The 1999 CAP and WHO conferences and the 2003 WHO classification (WHO 2003) recommended routine reporting of

■ 14.38 Most Important Histopathologic Features to Report in Radical Prostatectomy Specimens

Histological grade (Gleason grade)
Tumor size (percentage carcinoma)
TNM stage
Surgical margin status

■ **t14.39 Sample Synoptic Report Form: Radical Prostatectomy**

Synoptic Report Form for Prostate Carcinoma

1. _____ A neoplasm is PRESENT
_____ There is no residual neoplasm

2. _____ The TUMOR TYPE is:
_____ Adenocarcinoma, acinar (conventional) type
_____ OTHER: (specify)

3. _____ The INTRAGLANDULAR TUMOR VOLUME = (reported as percent of prostate gland involved by carcinoma ________________)

4. _____ The GLEASON GRADE is: ___ + ___ = SCORE OF _____

5. _____ The LOCATION OF THE TUMOR involves:
_____ The tumor involves the right base
_____ The tumor involves the right apex
_____ The tumor involves the left base
_____ The tumor involves the left apex

6. _____ PERINEURAL INVASION
_____ Is not identified
_____ Is identified

7. _____ VASCULAR INVASION
_____ Is not identified
_____ Is identified

8. _____ EXTRAPROSTATIC EXTENSION (EPE)
_____ Absent
_____ Present
_____ The tumor extends into the periprostatic soft tissue
(specify site) ________________________________
Extent of EPE is focal (less than or equal to two 400X fields)/non-focal (circle one)

9. _____ SEMINAL VESICLES
_____ The seminal vesicles are free of tumor
_____ The tumor extends into the right seminal vesicle wall
_____ The tumor extends in to the left seminal vesicle wall
_____ The tumor involves the right seminal vesicle lumen
_____ The tumor involves the left seminal vesicle lumen
_____ The tumor involves perivesicular fascia

10._____ SURGICAL MARGINS
_____ All surgical margins are free of tumor
_____ Tumor is present at the apical (urethral) margin of resection
_____ Tumor is present at the peripheral margin of resection
(specify site)____________________, with/without EPE (circle one)
_____ Tumor is present at the bladder neck margin of resection

11._____ The NON-NEOPLASTIC PROSTATE
_____ Shows no abnormalities
_____ Shows nodular hyperplasia
_____ Shows inflammation
_____ Shows infarction
_____ Shows prostatic intraepithelial neoplasia, focal, high-grade
_____ Shows prostatic intraepithelial neoplasia, diffuse, high-grade
_____ Shows: ______________________ (specify)

12._____ LYMPH NODES: Regional lymph nodes show:
(expressed as the number of nodes containing metastases in relation to the total number of nodes examined)
Right pelvic: ____________________________
Right internal iliac: ____________________________
Right external iliac: ____________________________
Right periaortic: ____________________________
Left pelvic: ____________________________
Left internal iliac: ____________________________
Left external iliac: ____________________________
Left periaortic: ____________________________
______ extranodal extension by tumor is NOT APPLICABLE; no nodal metastases are present
______ extranodal extension by tumor metastases is PRESENT
______ extranodal extension by tumor metastases is ABSENT
______ greatest dimension of metastatic deposit (cm)

13. The "T" Sub-Stage of the Tumor is:
_____ TX = Primary tumor cannot be assessed
_____ T0 = No evidence of primary tumor
_____ T2 = Tumor confined within the prostate
_____ T2a = Tumor involves one half of one lobe or less
_____ T2b = Tumor involves more than one half of one but not both lobes
_____ T2c = Bilateral carcinoma
_____ T3 = Tumor extends through the prostatic capsule
_____ T3a = Unilateral or bilateral extracapsular extension
_____ T3b = Tumor invades seminal vesicles
_____ T4 = Tumor is fixed or invades adjacent structures other than the seminal vesicles: bladder neck, external sphincter, rectum, levator muscles and/or pelvic wall
Note: There is no pathologic T1 classification

14. The "N" Sub-Stage of the Tumor is:
_____ NX = Regional lymph nodes cannot be assessed
_____ N0 = No regional lymph node metastasis
_____ N1 = Metastasis in regional lymph node or nodes

15. The "M" Sub-Stage of the Tumor is:
_____ MX = Presence of distant metastasis cannot be assessed
_____ M0 = No distant metastasis
_____ M1 = Distant metastasis
_____ M1a = Nonregional lymph notde(s)
_____ M1b = Bone(s)
_____ M1c = Other site(s)

16. Based on this information, the overall AJCC/UICC stage of the tumor is:
_____ Stage X = Insufficient data to assign stage
_____ Stage II = T2/N0/M0/Any Gleason score
_____ Stage III = T3/N0/M0/Any Gleason score
_____ Stage IV = T4/N0/M0 Any Gleason score or
Any T/N1/M0/Any Gleason score or
Any T/Any N/M1/Any Gleason score

The stage assigned should be viewed as provisional, and may change with additional clinical information not provided with this specimen.

the Gleason grade **t14.43** (Bostwick 1999B, 2000, Srigley 2000). Some have provided the Gleason score only for the "dominant nodule" (Sakr 1999), but because a dominant nodule or index tumor often cannot be recognized in the PSA-screening era (Feng 2000), we recommend reporting Gleason grade on the entire tumor in radical prostatectomy specimens. Both primary and secondary Gleason grade patterns should be recorded, along with the sum (score). Scant data exist on how to deal with tertiary patterns, but any high-grade (pattern 4 or 5) carcinoma should be recorded, even if it is a minor component and the third most common pattern (Pan 2000) (see

■ **t14.40 Reporting of Prostatic Adenocarcinoma in Radical Prostatectomy Specimens: Sample Diagnostic Field Format**

PROSTATE, RADICAL PROSTATECTOMY
ADENOCARCINOMA, GLEASON GRADE 3 + 3 = SCORE OF 6 (SEE SYNPOSIS)
TEN PERCENT OF PROSTATE GLAND INVOLVED BY CARCINOMA
LEFT BASE, RIGHT BASE, AND LEFT APEX ARE INVOLVED BY CARCINOMA
LEFT APEX IS FREE OF TUMOR
EXTRAPROSTATIC EXTENSION BY CARCINOMA IS IDENTIFIED AT RIGHT BASE
BLADDER NECK AND DISTAL URETHRAL (APICAL) SURGICAL MARGINS OF RESECTION ARE FREE OF TUMOR
PERIPHERAL SURGICAL MARGINS ARE FREE OF TUMOR

SEMINAL VESICLES, RIGHT AND LEFT, RADICAL PROSTATECTOMY
NO EVIDENCE OF MALIGNANCY

LYMPH NODES, RIGHT PELVIC, DISSECTION
NO EVIDENCE OF MALIGNANCY IN TWO LYMPH NODES (0/2)

LYMPH NODES, LEFT PELVIC, DISSECTION
NO EVIDENCE OF MALIGNANCY IN THREE LYMPH NODES (0/3)

■ **t14.41 Tumor Size in Radical Prostatectomy in Specimens in Relation to Pathologic and Clinical Endpoints**

Increasing tumor size in the prostate gland is related to these endpoints:
Increasing preoperative total serum PSA
Lower preoperative percent free PSA
Increased DNA aneuploidy in carcinoma
Increased surface area of extraprostatic extension
Higher pathologic stage
Increased risk of positive surgical margins
Increased incidence of pelvic lymph node metastasis
Increased risk of failure after therapy
Increased risk of death due to prostate cancer

■ **t14.42 Recommended Reporting of Tumor Size in Radical Prostatectomy Specimens: Percentage Carcinoma**

Percentage carcinoma determined by simple microscopical visual inspection (eyeball estimate)
Report % involvement of prostatic parenchyma on glass slides
Complete embedding of prostate gland not required
Report in 5%-10% increments

■ **t14.43 Recommended Reporting of Histological Grade in Radical Prostatectomy Specimens**

Report primary (most common) Gleason pattern and secondary pattern to yield score (sum)
Other grading schemes may be used in addition to Gleason grade, if desired

■ **t14.44 Recommended Reporting of Extraprostatic Extension (EPE) by Carcinoma in Radical Prostatectomy Specimens**

Report presence or absence of EPE, location of EPE, and extent of EPE
Quantitate extent of EPE as focal (tumor outside the prostate equals to, or is less than two high-power (40X) microscopic fields) or extensive[1]

[1]WHO recommendation (Bostwick 1999B)

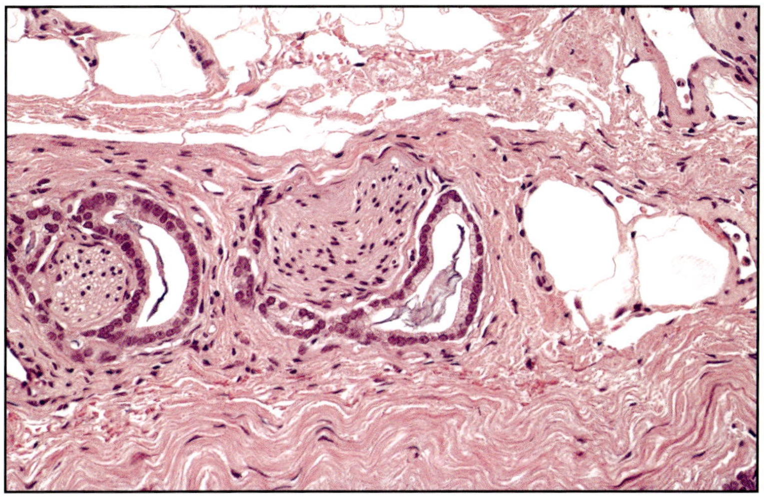

■ **i14.148** *Focal extraprostatic extension by carcinoma, with only a few perineural carcinoma glands adjacent to adipose cells.*

Chapter 15). Evidence exists that the percentage of high-grade carcinoma may be prognostically significant (Herman 1999, McNeal 1990B, Skacel 2000, Stamey 1999), and in the future consideration may be given to reporting this parameter, although reproducibility and interobserver agreement remain to be demonstrated (Herman 1999).

Location of tumor within the prostate should also be specified, based on light microscopic evaluation of radical prostatectomy tissue sections (Bostwick 1999B, Henson 1994). We specify location by quadrant **t14.40**. Another approach, listed as optional by one group (ADASP 1998), would be to provide location of the carcinoma in relation to the anatomic zones of the prostate, which could be done with a diagram (ADASP 1998, True 1994). In practice, however, anatomic boundaries between the transition zone and peripheral zone are not often well defined; moreover, it is not established that zone origin, independent of grade, is of prognostic significance.

Invasion into the vague fibromuscular sling that is called the prostatic capsule has historically not been associated with patient survival (Byar 1972). It is not likely to be a reproducibly definable finding, and need not be reported. In large series from multiple hospitals, EPE is associated with an increased risk of recurrence at 5 to 15 years (Carvalhal 2000, Catalona 1998, Eastham 1998, Epstein 1996E, Han 2001, Myers 1983, Paulson 1990, Pound 1997, 1999, Stamey 1999, Wheeler 1998A) and death from prostate cancer at 5 and 10 years (Byar 1972, Gerber 1996). After radical prostatectomy, the 10-year prostate cancer–specific survival was 91% for men with organ-confined carcinoma, compared with 77% from men with non–organ-confined disease (Gerber 1996).

EPE should be designated in surgical pathology reports as present or absent, and if present, the anatomic site should be given **Field 8, t14.39; t14.44** (ADASP 1998, Bostwick 2000). Data suggest that the extent of EPE is related to patient outcome (Davis 1999, Epstein 1993C, 1996E, Pound 1997, Stamey 1988, Wheeler 1998A), but exactly how to measure the amount of EPE is not settled. Various measures have been used, including linear centimeters (McNeal 1990A, Stamey 1988), which can be either greatest linear dimension or radial dimension (Davis 1999, Sohayda 2000), cubic centimeters, or focal versus nonfocal, extensive, or established (Bostwick 1999B, Epstein 1993C, Wheeler 1998A). Focal EPE has been defined as a few neoplastic glands exterior to the prostate (Epstein 1993C) or where tumor outside the prostate equals or is less than 2 high-power (40×) microscopic fields (Bostwick 1999B, Wheeler 1998A) **i14.148**. The WHO recommends application of this latter definition (Bostwick 1999B), but thus far quantitation of EPE is not a part of

International Union Against Cancer (UICC) and American Joint Committee on Cancer (AJCC) staging schemes (Chapter 16).

Seminal vesicle invasion by prostatic carcinoma is associated with a worse prognosis than EPE alone, with a 60% to 85% chance of progression by 10 to 15 years after surgery (Han 2001, Myers 1983, Pound 1997). This invasion is not uniformly associated with a poor prognosis, and identification of a subgroup with slow progression can be accomplished based on Gleason score, margin status, and vascular invasion status (Epstein 2000A) or serum PSA, percentage carcinoma in the radical prostatectomy, and age (Sofer 2003). Presence or absence of seminal vesicle wall invasion should be reported **Field 9, t14.39**. If invasion is present, unilateral or bilateral involvement should be noted, but otherwise quantitation of amount of tumor in the seminal vesicles is not necessary. Lymphvascular space invasion in the seminal vesicle wall probably should also be recorded because in one series (Graham 1996) (but not a second [Ohori 1993]), this finding was associated with a higher risk of progression and lymph node metastasis.

Surgical margin status of the radical prostatectomy specimen is linked to patient outcome after surgery. By 5 years 26% to 65% of men with positive margins had PSA failure (reviewed in Wieder 1998) and a 45% to 70% probability of PSA failure by 10 years (Epstein 1996E, Han 2001, Paulson 1990). In one series (Iselin 1999), this failure preceded cancer-associated death by 5 to 12 years, depending on Gleason score. At 13.5 years after surgery, 40% of men with positive margins died of prostate cancer, compared with 10% of patients with negative margins (Paulson 1994). Therefore, although it is a high-risk factor, a positive margin does not always mean inexorable progression or a death sentence. A positive margin with lack of clinical progression could result from insufficient length of clinical follow-up, artifactual creation of a positive margin by margin disruption at surgery or in tissue processing, destruction of a few residual tumor cells by ischemia or granulation tissue (Epstein 1996D), intrinsic lack of aggressive infiltrative behavior, as in lower-grade tumors, and gross and histologic sampling error, where all positive margins will not be detected unless the prostate gland is completely embedded and all blocks serially sectioned (Humphrey 1993B). Conversely, a negative margin, just as for pathologically organ-confined cancer, does not always signify that the patient is definitely cured because prostate cancer that is completely excised or prostate-confined can still spread by lymphvascular space invasion. It is not known whether a positive margin is associated more closely with local or distant failure (Epstein 1996D). Also unknown is the best treatment for a positive margin (Wieder 1998). Management options include adjuvant external beam radiation, adjuvant androgen ablation, and surveillance with delayed radiation or hormone therapy for recurrence (Wieder 1998).

Conflicting data exist as to whether surgical margin status is an independent predictor of outcome after grade, tumor volume, and pathologic stage are known (Ohori 1995, Sanda 2001, Stamey 1999, Wieder 1998). Generally, a positive margin appears to have greater significance in the absence of seminal vesicle or lymph node spread (Epstein 1996E, Ohori 1995). For patients with a positive margin due to incision into the gland (pT2+), progression occurred at a much lower rate than for patients with EPE and a positive margin (Cheng 1999B, Herman 2000). Furthermore, pT2+ patients had significantly higher progression rates than patients with EPE and negative margins (Herman 2000). Surgical margin status has been shown in some series to be of prognostic value in both lower-grade (Gleason score 2 to 6) (Ohori 1995) and higher-grade (Gleason score 7 or greater) (Epstein 1998A, Pound 1997, Tefilli 1999) carcinomas.

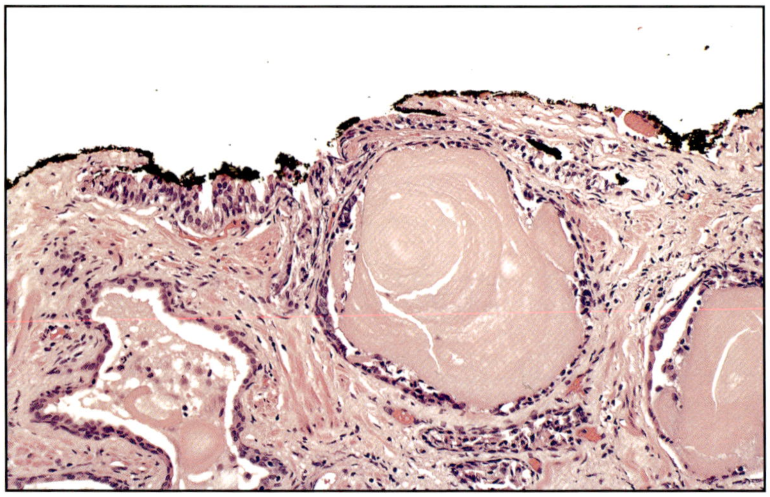

■ **i14.149** *Benign prostatic glands at inked peripheral surgical margin. This may be associated with increased risk of residual benign glands that could potentially cause an elevated post-operative serum PSA.*

Surgical margin status should be reported separately from pathologic stage because a positive margin does not necessarily indicate EPE. Location and extent of margin positivity should also be recorded **Field 10, t14.39; t14.45**. The impact of margin location on clinical progression is not clear (Wieder 1998) because the data are mixed as to whether location relates to subsequent failure after surgery. Most series do report that the greater the extent of margin positivity, the higher the likelihood of carcinoma progression (D'Amico 1996, Epstein 1993B, Paulson 1990, Troncoso 1999, Watson 1996, Weldon 1995). Certainly, multiple positive margins increase the risk of postoperative failure, but beyond counting of number of positive sites, the method of quantitating extent of margin positivity is not set (Bostwick 1999B). Finally, the WHO recommends reporting ink on benign prostatic glands (Bostwick 1999B) **i14.149** because this could result in residual benign prostate tissue that could elevate the postoperative serum PSA (Djavan 2000, Pansare 2001, Shah 2000) and falsely indicate residual prostatic carcinoma.

Additional features in radical prostatectomy specimens that merit reporting include perineural invasion **Field 6, t14.39; t14.46**, vascular invasion **Field 7**, and abnormalities in nonneoplastic prostatic tissues

■ **t14.45 Recommended Reporting of Surgical Margins in Radical Prostatectomy Specimens**

Report presence or absence of margin positivity, and location of positive margins[1]
Report margin status independent of stage, since positive margins can be seen with or without EPE
Report ink on benign prostatic glands (indicating surgical incision into prostate)[2]

[1]Extent of margin positivity can be quantitated, if desired, but no consensus exists on how to measure this
[2]Recommended by WHO (Bostwick 1999B)

■ **t14.46 Perineural Invasion by Carcinoma in Radical Prostatectomy Specimens**

Very common: 90% of cases exhibit perineural invasion
Report presence or absence
Presence not independently related to progression or patient survival
"Large volume" = large nodule of tumor around nerve may indicate a worse prognosis

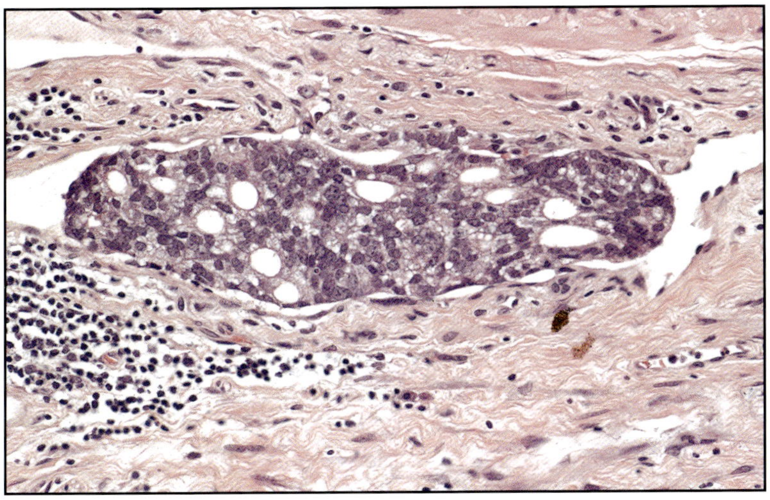

■ **i14.150** *Lymphvascular space invasion by prostatic adenocarcinoma.*

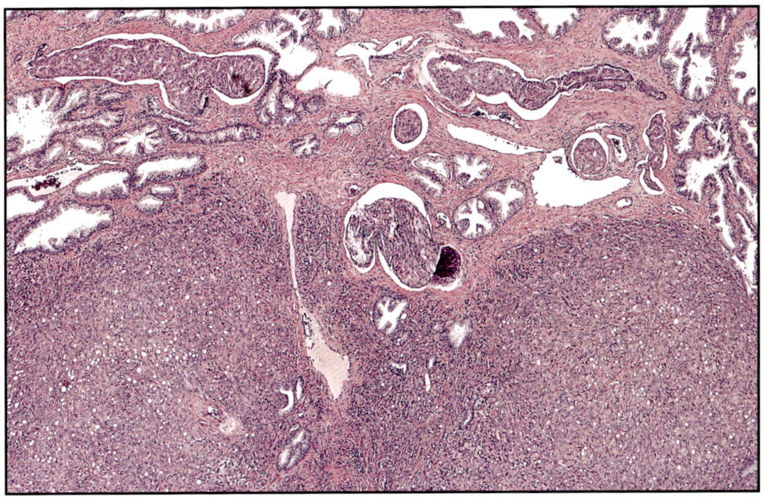

■ **i14.151** *"Worm-like" plugs of prostatic carcinoma in several lymphvascular spaces (top), adjacent to mainly solid growth of high-grade carcinoma (below).*

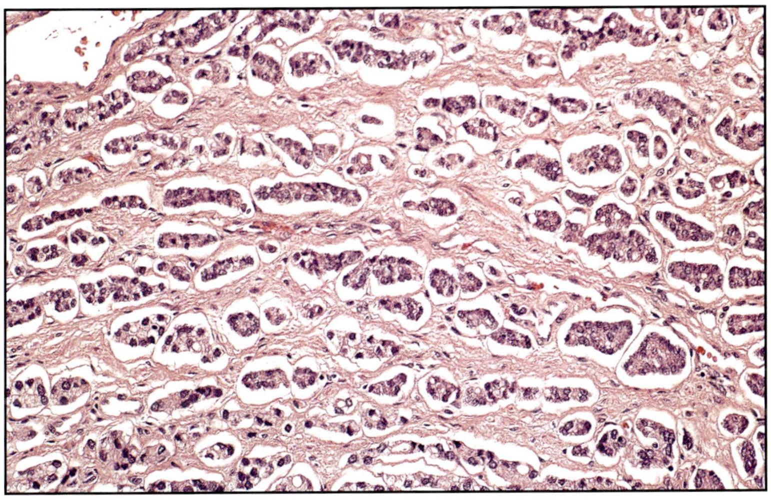

■ **i14.152** *Pseudo-LVI (lymphvascular space invasion): Diffuse artifactual separation of carcinoma aggregates from stroma.*

Field 11. (Reporting of pelvic lymph nodes **Field 12** is discussed later in this chapter.) Perineural invasion by carcinoma is extremely common in radical prostatectomy specimens, with an incidence of about 90% (Bostwick 1994A, Byar 1972). Its presence predicted progression in univariate but not multivariate analysis (van den Ouden 1997), and it was not related to patient survival (Byar 1972). In a recent study, the amount (greatest diameter) of perineural invasion was a predictor of disease progression (Maru 2001), but this measurement is not routinely made.

Lymphvascular space invasion absence or presence should be noted **t14.47**. (Tumor cell emboli in lymphatic channels can be difficult to distinguish from small blood vessels. The terms *vascular, microvascular, lymphvascular,* and *angiolymphatic invasion* can be used when this distinction is not made.) Lymphvascular space invasion by carcinoma is present in 12% to 53% of radical prostatectomy specimens (Bahnson 1989, McNeal 1996, Salomao 1995, van den Ouden 1998) by examination of H&E-stained slides **i14.9; i14.150-i14.151**. In my experience, only a few percent of cases exhibit lymphvascular space invasion. The foci are most often localized to the perimeter of the carcinomatous area (McNeal 1996). Small (0.05mm to 0.3mm) vessels invaded by carcinoma are simple endothelial-lined spaces with no evidence of underlying fibrous or muscular wall (McNeal 1996). Adherence of tumor cell emboli to the vascular lining, assumption of the shape of the vascular space by the tumor cell mass, and the presence of endothelial cells are features that help distinguish true vascular invasion from pseudoemboli that are tumor cell nests with artifactual separation from stroma **i14.152**. Also, true emboli tend to be solitary within a given field and tend not to show shreds of torn cytoplasm, as seen with pseudoemboli. Although more extensive vascular invasion is seen in higher-stage and higher volume cancers, it is not necessary to quantitate vascular invasion. It is also not necessary to perform immunostains for endothelial cell markers, such as factor VII–related antigen, CD31, and CD34, to define vascular invasion. If uncertain about lymphvascular invasion, one should use the descriptor "equivocal." Intraprostatic lymphvascular space invasion is associated with higher-grade, higher-volume, and high-stage prostatic cancers (Bahnson 1989, McNeal 1996, van den Ouden 1998) and appears to be independently predictive of cancer progression after surgery (McNeal 1996, Stamey 1999, van den Ouden 1998).

■ **t14.47 Lymphvascular Space Invasion by Carcinoma in Radical Prostatectomy Specimens**

Tumor emboli in small intraprostatic vessels = vascular, microvascular, lymphvascular or angiolymphatic invasion
Found in 12%-53% of cases
Presence related to high-grade, high-volume, and high-stage tumors, and clinical progression
Report as present or absent

Treatment effects should also be included in the surgical pathology report on radical prostatectomy specimens (Bostwick 1999B, Srigley 2000). Therefore, if the patient received any sort of preoperative therapy, such as hormonal (androgen deprivation) or radiation therapy, the specific effects of the therapy on neoplastic and nonneoplastic tissue (see Chapter 19) should be noted. However, exactly how to quantitate the extent and severity of such changes is uncertain (Bostwick 1999B). We include a description of such alterations in a comment. One proposal to quantitate extent of residual tumor is as follows: RX, residual tumor cannot be assessed; RO, no residual tumor; R1, microscopic residual tumor; and R2, macroscopic residual tumor (Srigley 2000). Additionally, the standard TNM classification (T = primary tumor, N = regional lymph nodes, M = distant metastases) **t14.39** should be used.

Of lesser importance is reporting abnormalities in the noncancerous prostate **Field 11, t14.39**. Nodular hyperplasia, inflammation, and high-grade PIN are seen in most cases and do not affect clinical progression after surgery.

Pathologic staging is critical and should be performed using the TNM system **t14.39** (Chapter 16). We report staging information, including T (primary tumor) status, N (lymph node) status (see below), and M status. The M status should be presumed to be MO (no distant metastasis) because patients who undergo radical prostatectomy should have a negative clinical metastatic workup. An overall AJCC and UICC stage assignment should be given **Field 16, t14.39**, which we usually follow with a comment stating that the stage assignment is provisional and may change upon inclusion of clinical information not provided with this specimen.

There are a multitude of experimental prognosticators in radical prostatectomy tissues that are not currently recommended for routine reporting (Bostwick 2000). These include histopathologic, morphometric, histochemical, immunophenotypic, and genotypic markers (Chapter 21). Histopathologically, a high-grade inflammatory cell response in carcinoma in radical prostatectomy sections has been associated with a higher risk of progression (Irani 1999), but this is only one study, and the findings must be validated at additional hospitals. Quantification of tumoral mitotic counts, apoptotic body counts, and necrosis in histologic sections also are not of proven prognostic utility. Morphometric analysis of tumor cell nuclei, including nuclear size, nuclear roundness, nucleolar size, and chromatin texture are potentially useful, but this evaluation is time-consuming and expensive, and suffers from difficulties in lack of standardized methods and reproducibility (Bostwick 1999B). Histochemical staining (such as argyrophilic silver staining) has been used to detect nucleolar organizer regions in relation to prognosis (Bostwick 1999B), but this is not a standard prognostic tool. Promising immunophenotypic prognostic markers include Ki-67 (for proliferation index), p53, cell death–related proteins (such as bcl-2), cell cycle regulators (such as $p27^{Kip1}$), neuroendocrine proteins (such as chromogranin), cell adhesion molecules (such as E-cadherin), and polypeptide growth factors and growth factor receptors (reviewed in Bostwick 1999B and Chapter 21). Immunostaining for the androgen receptor does not appear to provide practical information on prognosis or response to hormonal therapy. Genetic abnormalities are of potential utility, especially measurement of tumor cell DNA content (DNA ploidy). The data on use of DNA ploidy in radical prostatectomy specimens are mixed. We did not find DNA ploidy to be of independent prognostic significance in carcinoma in radical prostatectomy tissues (Humphrey 1991A), a finding that was recently corroborated in a large series of 966 radical prostatectomies (Ostrowski 2000). Reporting of DNA ploidy in radical prostatectomy cases should be considered optional. Gains or loss of specific chromosomal regions and genes and mutations in specific oncogenes, tumor suppressor genes, and cell cycle and androgen receptor genes are potential prognostic indicators in the future (see Chapter 21) but are not currently analyzed on a routine basis. Similarly, gene expression profiles, using microarrays or gene chips to assess the expression status of thousands of genes at once, holds potential promise but is also experimental.

Lastly, histologic features of prostatic adenocarcinoma have been used in combinations with or without serum PSA levels to generate risk categories that can be used to stratify patients for consideration of adjuvant therapy. One approach has been to classify prostatic carcinomas based on tumor size (volume), pathologic stage, and Gleason grade **t14.48**. A disadvantage to these schemes is that they were derived based on complete embedding of prostate glands and calculation of tumor volumes, which are not routine daily practices. A commonly used clinical approach is to use nomograms that provide a measure of recurrence based on preoperative PSA level and to use radical prostatectomy findings including Gleason score (sum), EPE, surgical margin status, seminal vesicle invasion, and lymph node status (D'Amico 1998, Kattan 1999). Other models calculate risk of recurrence using preoperative PSA as a sigmoidal transformation (PSA_{ST}) with (Bauer 1998) or without (Partin 1995) race, and radical prostatectomy findings:

t14.48 Definition of Potential Clinical Behavior of Prostate Cancer Based on Combination of Radical Prostatectomy Findings

I. Johns Hopkins Criteria (Epstein 1994A)
   Insignificant = TV[1] smaller than 0.2 cc, organ-confined, Gleason score < 7
   Minimal = TV 0.2-0.5 cc, organ-confined, Gleason score < 7
   Moderate = TV > 0.5 cc or EPE, with Gleason score < 7
   Advanced = EPE, with Gleason score ≥ 7 or positive margins, seminal vesicles, or lymph nodes

II. Baylor Criteria (Ohori 1994)
   Clinically unimportant = TV < 0.5 cc, organ-confined, no Gleason pattern 4 or 5*

III. Mayo Clinic Criteria (Dugan 1996)
   Clinically insignificant cancer = a tumor that would give rise to no more than 20 cm^3 of cancer within the prostate by the time of expected patient death and where Gleason score was less than 4 in 40 to 49-year-olds, 5 in 50 to 59-year-olds, 6 in 60 to 69-year-olds, and 7 in 70 to 79-year-olds.

[1]TV = tumor volume
*This is currently the most widely used pathologic definition of an insignificant prostate cancer.

Relative risk of recurrence = Rr

$$Rr = \exp(0.51 \times race) + (0.12 \times PSA_{ST}) + (0.25 \times \text{postoperative Gleason sum}) + (0.89 \times \text{organ confined})$$

(where race=1 if the patient is African-American and 0 if white or other, and organ-confined cancer is 0, and non-organ confined is 1)

Log relative risk = Rw

$$Rw = (PSA_{ST} \times 0.006) + (\text{Gleason score} \times 0.54) + (\text{pathologic stage} \times 1.87)$$

A recently published model for weighted risk of recurrence, Rw', based on a large series of 904 men, with validation in a series of 901 men from a second hospital, used this equation (Roberts 2001):

$$Rw' = \text{lymph node involvement } (0/1) \times 1.43 + \text{surgical margin status } (0/1) \times 1.5 + \text{modified Gleason score } (0 \text{ to } 4) \times 0.71 + \text{seminal vesicle involvement } (0/1) \times 0.51$$

Postoperative PSA has been also used in conjunction with radical prostatectomy Gleason score and pathologic stage to try to distinguish local recurrence from distant metastasis after surgery (Partin 1994). Finally, computerized neural networks could be used in the future to predict prostate cancer progression after radical prostatectomy (Potter 1999). Histopathologists need not calculate and report these categories of risk but should be aware that Gleason grade, pathologic stage, and surgical margin status from radical prostatectomy reports are clinically used to stratify patients for treatment options.

[14.5] Diagnosis of Prostatic Adenocarcinoma in Locally Advanced and Metastatic Disease

Locally Advanced Prostatic Carcinoma

Locally advanced prostatic carcinoma can manifest as permeation into periprostatic fat, pelvic soft tissue, or seminal vesicles, and as extension into the rectum or bladder **t14.49**. Extensive local spread of prostatic adenocarcinoma with rectal involvement is a clinically rare, late event in prostate cancer growth and usually is associated with widespread metastatic disease (Chapter 13). Rectal involvement at autopsy of men with metastatic prostate cancer is not rare, with an incidence of 9% (Saitoh 1984). Rectal involvement by prostate cancer can mimic the symptoms of rectosigmoid carcinoma. It can occur via direct extension or lymphvascular space invasion. Confirmation of prostatic origin may necessitate use of an immunophenotypic marker panel **t14.50**, especially in small biopsies. The best antibodies to distinguish prostatic from colorectal carcinoma are those reactive against the prostate-associated proteins PSA and PSAP. Markers associated with colorectal carcinoma, such as CEA, CK20, and CA19-9, are more often present in colorectal adenocarcinoma but can also be found in prostatic carcinoma **t14.50**.

Prostatic carcinoma invasion into the urinary bladder is uncommon in low-stage disease detected in the PSA-screening era but is common in advanced cases. Therefore, in patients with metastatic prostate cancer at autopsy, 39% had bladder involvement (Saitoh 1984). In one series (Bates 2000), prostatic carcinoma represented 14% of all secondary neoplasms of the bladder. The presence of prostatic carcinoma in the bladder signals a high chance of dissemination, as in about one half of these cases there is metastatic disease elsewhere (Bates 2000, Saitoh 1984). Rarely, patients with prostatic carcinoma involving the bladder can clinically present with urinary obstruction or hematuria, an exophytic bladder mass, and low or undetectable serum PSA, thereby simulating a primary bladder tumor (Reyes 2000). Bladder involvement by prostatic carcinoma can occur by direct extension **i14.153** or by lymphvascular invasion. Direct infiltration into the bladder typically is seen as large, bulky tumors, with the bladder neck and trigone most often involved. In one series (Bates 2000), these two sites comprised 87% of bladder locations involved by prostatic carcinoma, whereas anterior, posterior, and lateral walls constituted 8% and fundus and multiple sites were a few percent. Histopathologically, prostatic carcinoma dispersion into the bladder is most often a high-grade malignancy with growth in sheets and cords **i14.154**. Glandular luminal space formation is variable, but when it is diffuse, in conjunction with uniform nuclei, a prostatic primary is likely. In contrast, high-grade TCC of the bladder is exemplified by greater nuclear pleomorphism, sometimes with a more squamoid appearance of the cytoplasm. TCC can exhibit glandular differentiation, and adenocarcinomas can be primary in the bladder, so the mere presence of glandular spaces does not prove prostate or bladder origin of a carcinoma. For all poorly differentiated carcinomas in the bladder, one should include prostatic carcinoma in the differential diagnosis. Ductal prostatic carcinomas in the bladder are most likely to be misdiagnosed as TCC, where the prostatic carcinoma exhibits papillary or solid patterns (Reyes 2000). Thus, not all bladder tumors with papillary fronds are primary in the bladder. Just as for needle biopsies of prostate that contain a poorly differentiated carcinoma of uncertain origin, an immunophenotypic marker panel can be of great utility here **t14.16**.

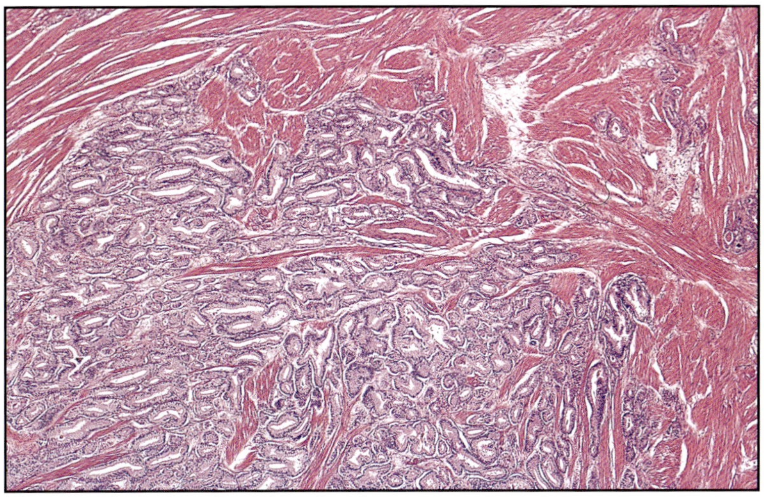

■ **i14.153** *Bladder neck involvement by prostatic adenocarcinoma, with infiltration of smooth muscle bundles.*

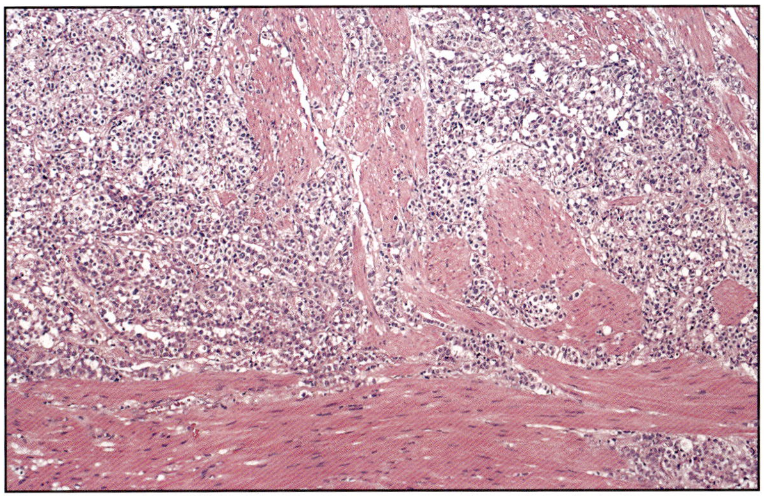

■ **i14.154** *High-grade prostatic carcinoma invading smooth muscle bundles of bladder neck.*

Prostatic carcinoma can grow as locally advanced disease after treatment. After radical prostatectomy, recurrent or persistent carcinoma can be found at the vesicourethral anastomotic site or in the prostatic bed (Abi-Aad 1992, Foster 1993, Fowler 1995, Ripple 2000, Saleem 1998, Shekarriz 1999). Here, the diagnosis of recurrence usually is based on an elevated serum postoperative PSA. Commonly used clinical modalities to evaluate this recurrence include digital rectal examination, transrectal ultrasonography (TRUS) with biopsy, pelvic computed tomography, serum PAP, and bone scan. In one survey (Ornstein 1998), about one half of men with an elevated serum

■ **t14.49 Locally Advanced Prostatic Carcinoma**

Extensive disease in periprostatic soft tissue
Spread into seminal vesicles
Posterior growth into rectum by direct extension or lymphvascular invasion
Direct expansion superiorly into bladder neck
Growth in prostatic fossa or into vesicourethral anastamosis after radical prostatectomy

t14.50 Diagnostic Immunophenotype of Prostatic Carcinoma[1,2]

Marker (reference)	% Cases Positivity	Comment
PSA[3]	86%-100%	Expression usually maintained in mets
PSAP[4]	82%-100%	
Pan-cytokeratin[6] (Nagle 1996)	100%	Using antibody cocktail[5]
High molecular weight cytokeratin[6]	0%-5%	Rare expression using 34βE12[16]
CK5/6 (Goldstein 2002)	0%	
CK7[7]	5%-19%	
CK17 (Goldstein 2002)	0%	
CK20[8]	2%-32%	2%-10% in 1° tumors, 27% in mets
EMA[9]	15%-80%	
TAG-72[10]	63%-80%	Detection with B72.3 or CC49 antibody
CEA[11]	0%-86%	Lower % with monoclonal antibody
Leu7 (Lindeman 1996, May 1987)	96%-100%	Not specific for prostatic carcinoma
CA125 (Torenbeek 1998, Loy 1992)	2%-5%	
CA19-9 (Loy 1993, Gatalica 1994)	3%-13%	
Ber-EP4 (Gaffey 1992)	89%	
CA15-3 (Gatalica 1994)	78%	
LCA (CD45)	0%	
LeuM1 (CD15) (Lindeman 1996)	4%	
CD30 (Millward 1998)	0%	Only 5 cases tested
Vimentin[12]	0%-60%	
Muscle-specific actin	0%[17]	
Smooth-muscle actin	0%[17]	
Desmin	0%[17]	
PLAP (Wick 1987)	0	
AFP (Ellis 1984)	0%	
hCG (Ellis 1984, Bostwick 1994C)	0%-22%	
S-100 (Hancock 1991, Howat 1988)	0%-50%	
HMB-45 (Hancock 1991)	0%	
Chromogranin A[13]	20%-100%	Staining of non-small cell carcinomas[18]
Synaptophysin (Speights 1997)	50%	Staining of non-small cell carcinoma[18]
NSE[14]	20%-46%	Staining of non-small cell carcinoma[18]
Endocrine peptide hormones[15]	0%-100%	Serotonin: 54%-100%; somatostatin: 5% to 28%; thyroid stimulating hormone: 0-85%; ACTH: < 5% to 20%; parathormone: 16%; parathormone-related protein: few %; leu-enkephalin: 13%, β-endorphin: 8%; glucagon: 0-3%; calcitonin: 5%; prolactin: 0%. Expression also reported for bombesin/gastrin-related peptide and insulin-like growth factor (IGF)-II.
Villin (Goldstein 2002)	0%	
Thyroid transcription factor-1 (Goldstein 2002)	0%	
Thrombomodulin (Ordoñez 1998)	0%	
Uroplakin III (Parker 2003)	0%	

[1]Immunophenotype of malignant epithelial cells
[2]Abbreviations: mets = metastases; PSA = prostate specific antigen; PSAP = prostate specific acid phosphatase; CK =cytokeratin; EMA = epithelial membrane antigen; TAG = tumor-associated glycoprotein; LCA = leukocyte common antigen; PLAP = placental alkaline phosphatase; AFP = alpha feto protein; hCG = human chorionic gonadotropin; NSE = neuron-specific enolase
[3]Lindeman 1996, Genega 2000, Aihara 1994B, Ford 1985, Nadji 1981, Ellis 1984, Torenbeek 1998
[4]Lindeman 1996, Genega 2000, Ellis 1984, Torenbeek 1998, Lippert 1982, Nadji 1980, Mahan 1980, Heyderman 1984, Grob 1994, Jobsis 1981, Fishleder 1981
[5]Pan-cytokeratin antibody cocktail such as AE1, AE3, and CAM 5.2 detects high and low molecular weight cytokeratins. All carcinomas express cytokeratins 8 and 18, and most 19 (Nagle 1996). Cytokeratin expression does not vary with Gleason grade (Nagel 1991)
[6]Antibody 34βE12 (reactive against cytokeratins 1,5,10, and 14) most often used to detect high molecular weight cytokeratins in basal cells. Antibodies CK8.12 (vs cytokeratins 13 and 16) and 312C8-1 (versus cytokeratin 14) have also been used (Oakda 1992). (See **t1.4** for expression distribution of cytokeratins in normal basal cells.) Brawer 1985, Hedrick 1989, Shah 1991, Wojno 1995, Kahane 1995, Varma 1997, Googe 1997, Yang 1999, Tran 1999, Amin 1994, Brawer 1989, Okada 1992
[7]Bassily 2000, Lindeman 1996, Goldstein 2002, Genega 2000, Chu 2000, Torenbeek 1998, Wang 1995
[8]Bassily 2000, Lindeman 1996, Goldstein 2002, Genega 2000, Chu 2000, Torenbeek 1998, Wang 1995
[9]Ellis 1984, Torenbeek 1998, Thomas 1987
[10]Myers 1994, Myers 1995, Brenner 1995
[11]Lindeman 1996, Genega 2000, Ellis 1984, Torenbeek 1998, Ghazizadeh 1984
[12]Nagle 1991, Ghazizadeh 1984, Heatley 1995, Leong 1988
[13]Bonkhoff 1994, Faris 1995, McWilliam 1997, Krijnen 1997, Schmid 1994, Nakopoulou 1996, Aprikian 1993, Speights 1997, Allen 1995, Aprikian 1994, Noodzij 1995, MK Cohen 1994, Speights 1994, Weinstein 1996, Krijnen 1993, Cansella 1998
[14]Bostwick 1994C, Faris 1995, McWilliam 1997, Aprikian 1997, Speights 1997, Allen 1995, Cohen 1994B, Speights 1994, Berner 1993, Abrahamson 1987
[15]Bostwick 1994C, Aprikian 1993, Aprikian 1994, Abrahamsson 1987, Aprikian 1998, Iwamura 1994, Li 1998
[16]2% of cases of metastatic carcinoma in lymph nodes showed strong staining in less than 0.2% of tumor cells (Yang 1999)
[17]Excluding cases of sarcomatoid carcinoma
[18]Staining is focal and minimal in most cases, and extensive and multifocal in about 10% of cases

PSA >1 year after surgery underwent TRUS with biopsy; this is an uncommon procedure in our experience. Physicians often treat the rising postoperative serum PSA rather than obtain a tissue diagnosis. This is so because only one half of men with presumed local recurrence have positive biopsies, several biopsy sessions may be needed to procure a positive biopsy (Foster 1993, Fowler 1995), and a negative biopsy does not have meaning because it may be negative due to sampling error or the fact that distant metastasis, not local

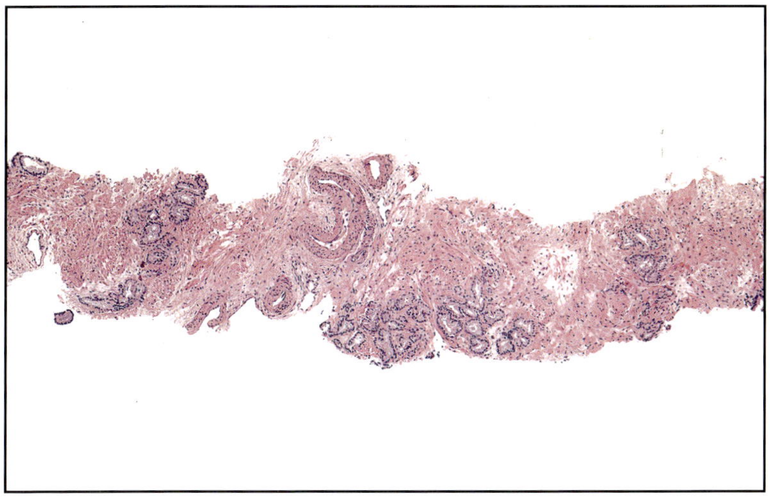

■ **i14.155** *Vesicourethral anastomotic site biopsy tissue with several foci of prostatic adenocarcinoma embedded in smooth muscle tissue.*

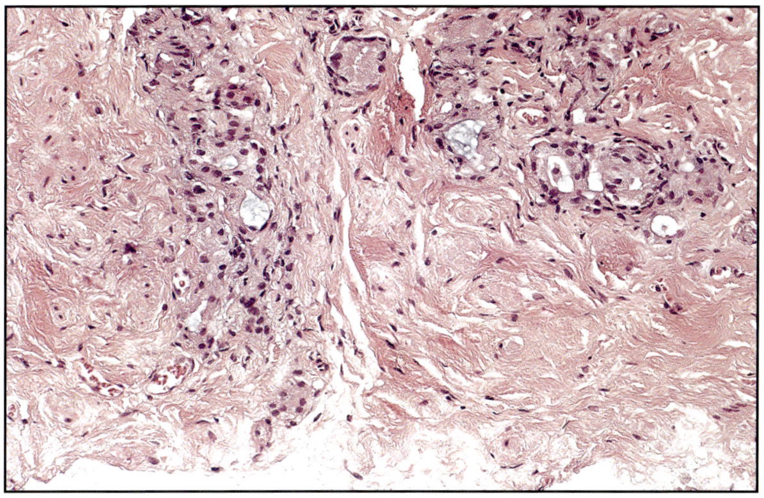

■ **i14.156** *Vesicourethral anastomotic site biopsy tissue with prostatic adenocarcinoma infiltrating fibromuscular tissue (higher-power view of* **i14.155***).*

recurrence, as the basis for the elevated PSA after surgery. A positive digital rectal examination or TRUS enhances the likelihood of a positive biopsy. Pathologic stage and Gleason grade of the carcinoma in the radical prostatectomy were not predictive of a positive anastomotic or fossa biopsy in 2 studies (Fowler 1995, Saleem 1998), whereas in a third, PSA level and pathologic stage were the strongest determinants of a positive biopsy (Shekarriz 1999). Microscopically, needle core biopsies of the anastomotic site or prostatic fossa (bed) show a fibrous and smooth muscle tissue background **i14.155, i14.156**, usually without accompanying benign prostatic glands. The amount of tumor in core biopsy tissue is highly variable (ranging from 0.1 to 18mm), with a mean size of 3mm (Ripple 2000). The glands of adenocarcinoma are irregularly dispersed and demonstrate nuclear atypia and a single cell lining layer. The malignant glandular proliferation usually is small acinar, although a cribriform pattern is not uncommon (Ripple 2000). The diagnosis usually is straightforward except when only a few glands are present or there is distortion artifact. In a minority of cases, the diagnosis of malignancy can be challenging because of minimal nuclear atypia, including rare to absent nucleoli (Ripple 2000). For differential diagnosis purposes, one should be aware that benign prostatic tissue can be left behind after radical prostatectomy and that there are reported instances of benign prostatic tissue in needle biopsy of the anastomotic site or prostatic fossa (Foster 1993, Fowler 1995, Ripple 2000). Such a diagnosis of benign prostatic tissue on initial needle biopsy does not rule out recurrence because repeat biopsy in some of these patients showed carcinoma (Foster 1993, Fowler 1995). Gleason grading has been performed on these anastomotic biopsies (Ripple 2000), even though technically this is not valid because Gleason grading should be done only on intraprostatic tumor. A mean Gleason score of 6.5 was given in one series (Ripple 2000).

Lymph Node Prostatic Carcinoma Metastasis

Metastatic prostatic carcinoma clinically is discovered most often in lymph nodes **t14.51**. The lymph nodes most often examined by histopathologists for metastatic prostatic carcinoma are the pelvic lymph nodes removed before or during radical prostatectomy. In the past (in the 1970s) the incidence of histologically diagnosed metastatic prostatic carcinoma in pelvic lymph nodes was 20% to 40% (Fowler 1981A, Smith 1983), while in this PSA screening era 1% to 6% of patients have metastatic disease in these lymph nodes (reviewed in Humphrey 1998B).

A pathologic diagnosis of metastatic prostatic carcinoma in pelvic lymph nodes can be established at frozen section or on permanent sections. Some urologists no longer request frozen sections of pelvic lymph nodes because of the low incidence of positive nodes. When a frozen section of pelvic nodes is requested as part of an intraoperative consultation, one should probably select palpable nodes for sectioning while recognizing several caveats pertaining to lymph node sampling and detection of metastatic disease. First, gross examination of lymph nodes is of limited value because of low sensitivity and specificity. In one study (Sgrignoli 1994), frozen sections of grossly suspicious nodes resulted in detection of only 34% of microscopically positive nodes; furthermore, 82% of all nodes that grossly appeared suspicious were negative on frozen and permanent, deeper sections. Second, in another study lymph node size did not correlate with the presence of prostate cancer metastasis (Tiguert 1999), so nodes of all sizes should be examined by frozen section. Third, a low sensitivity of 58% to 73% for identifying lymph node metastasis has been reported in the literature (Catalona 1982, Davis 1995, Epstein 1986A, Fowler 1981B, Kramolowsky 1984, Saltzstein 1977, Sgrignoli 1994, Young 1999). This usually represent micrometastases diagnosed in permanent sections of tissue used for frozen sections (that represent additional sampling) and in additionally submitted tissue that did not contain grossly evident lymph nodes. Microscopically, the fatty nature of pelvic nodes can cause difficulty in the preparation of

■ **t14.51 Lymph Node Metastasis of Prostatic Carcinoma**

First site of metastatic spread of prostate cancer; pelvic obturator and hypogastric nodes usually involved first[1]
In clinically localized disease, metastasis discovered in 1%-6% of pelvic nodes by histologic diagnosis
Gross examination of limited value
Microscopically, most cases are moderately poorly differentiated adenocarcinoma
Immunohistochemical marker panel of PSA, PSAP, pan-cytokeratin, CK7, and CK20 can be helpful in selected cases of metastatic carcinoma in lymph nodes.
Detection of "micrometastasis" by immunohistochemistry or RT-PCR is currently experimental

[1]In rare cases, periprostatic and periseminal vesicle lymph nodes may be involved first

intact, thin, nonfolded frozen sections. The carcinoma can be focal or diffuse in the nodal tissue; when focal, the standard presentation is a few neoplastic glands in the subcapsular sinus. Tumor can also be found in perinodal soft tissue (adipose tissue), but this is typically in association with nodal-based metastasis. Cytologic touch imprints can be used in conjunction with frozen sections but are insensitive (Bastacky 1994) and should not be used alone.

Permanent section histologic diagnosis of pelvic lymphadenectomy specimens should be based on complete submission and microscopic examination of all tissue, including all nodes and, if possible, perinodal soft tissue. This is so for several reasons. First, the number of nodes examined is directly related to detection of metastatic disease (Barth 1999). Second, in about 10% of cases, the only microscopically visualized metastatic deposits will be in soft tissue (Sgrignoli 1994) or small, grossly invisible lymph nodes or soft tissue (Bastacky 1994). These soft tissue metastatic deposits probably are plugs of carcinoma in lymphvascular spaces.

Initial lymph node spread of prostatic carcinoma is primarily to the pelvic obturator and hypogastric nodes, although in rare cases periprostatic or periseminal vesicle lymph node may be involved first (Kothari 2001, Pinto 2000A). (Such lymph nodes are seen in <5% of radical prostatectomy specimens, and in only about 0.5% of patients is metastasis to these lymph nodes detected [Kothari 2001, Pinto 2000A].) Later, involvement of external iliac, common iliac, presacral, and presciatic nodes is observed **t13.22**. With widely disseminated prostate cancer, patients can have positive nodes in the retroperitoneum, para-aortic region, neck, pelvic cavity, lung hilus, and inguinal region (Bubendorf 2000, Mintz 1934, Saitoh 1984) **t14.52**. Rarely (in <1% of cases of metastatic prostate cancer), prostatic carcinoma can involve distant lymph nodes only, without metastatic deposits elsewhere (Saitoh 1984). Another rarity is the clinical presentation of prostatic carcinoma as lymphadenopathy, such as cervical lymphadenopathy (Cho 1987).

Microscopically, prostatic carcinoma in lymph nodes usually resembles one of the patterns in the primary tumor and is usually moderately or poorly differentiated **i14.157–i14.163** (Brawn 1990A, 1990B, Cheng 1999C, Kramer 1981). The pattern of growth often resembles fused microacinar Gleason pattern 4 or sheets of Gleason pattern 5 tumor (Note, however, that one should not apply the Gleason grading system to metastatic carcinoma; it was designed to portray prostatic stromal-carcinoma cell relationships). Ductal-type differentiation with papillary structures can also be seen. The metastatic tumor can elicit an intranodal fibrogenic reaction **i14.158** or may "sit" within the lymphoid tissue without an apparent response **i14.160**. The amount of intranodal tumor is quite variable, with just a few subcapsular cancerous glands within the sinus space **i14.161** to complete or near-complete nodal effacement and replacement **i14.162**. In a few cases, sinusoidal expansion growth pattern can be seen **i14.163**. Extranodal extension by prostatic carcinoma through the lymph node capsule into perinodal soft tissue has been reported in 60% to 70% of cases of lymph node metastasis (Cheng 2000, Griebling 1997) and was associated with number of positive nodes and increasing size of the nodal metastatic deposit (Cheng 2000). Cytologically, the uniformity of the neoplastic nuclei is striking and is useful in identifying the metastasis as prostatic.

The differential diagnosis of metastatic prostatic carcinoma in lymph node tissue should include benign and malignant conditions. Pseudoneoplastic benign nodal entities that can be confused with carcinoma include benign glandular inclusions, usual histiocytosis, foreign body histiocytosis, signet-ring histiocytosis, nodal nevi, and extramedullary hematopoiesis (see Chapter 10). Malignant neoplasms of all types should be differentiated from prostatic carcinoma in lymph nodes. With regard to pelvic lymph nodes removed before radical prostatectomy, it should first be

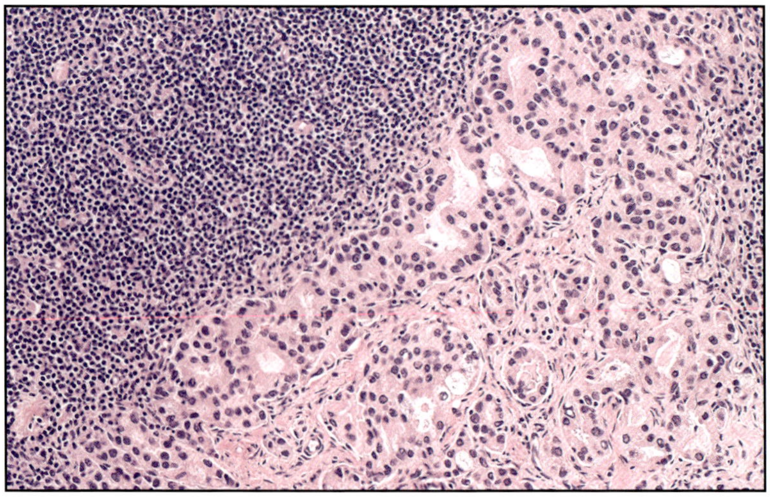

■ **i14.157** *Lymph node metastasis of small acinar prostatic adenocarcinoma.*

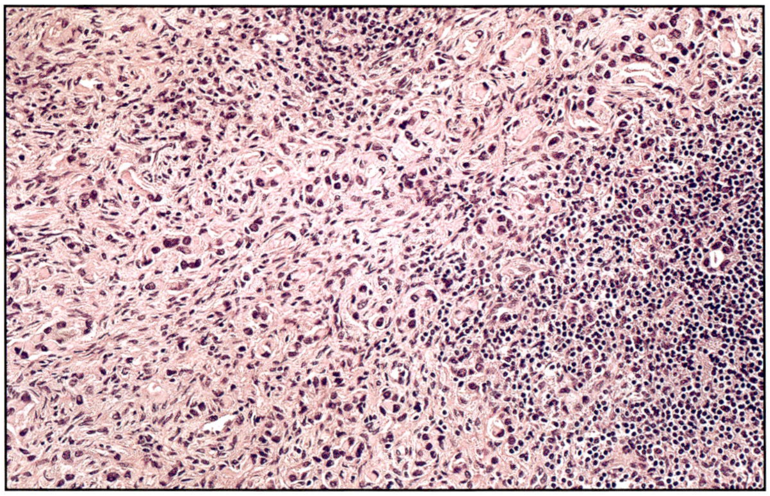

■ **i14.158** *High-grade prostatic carcinoma in pelvic lymph node, with minimal gland formation, and a sclerotic response.*

■ **t14.52 Anatomic Sites of Prostatic Carcinoma Lymph Node Metastasis in Widely-Disseminated Disease**

Lymph Node Site	% of Cases
Retroperitoneum	30%
Para-aortic	22%
Neck	18%
Lung hilus	15%
Pelvic cavity	12%
Inguinal	11%
Para-tracheal	9%
Mesenteric	7%
Mediastinum	3%
Axilla	2%

Saitoh 1984

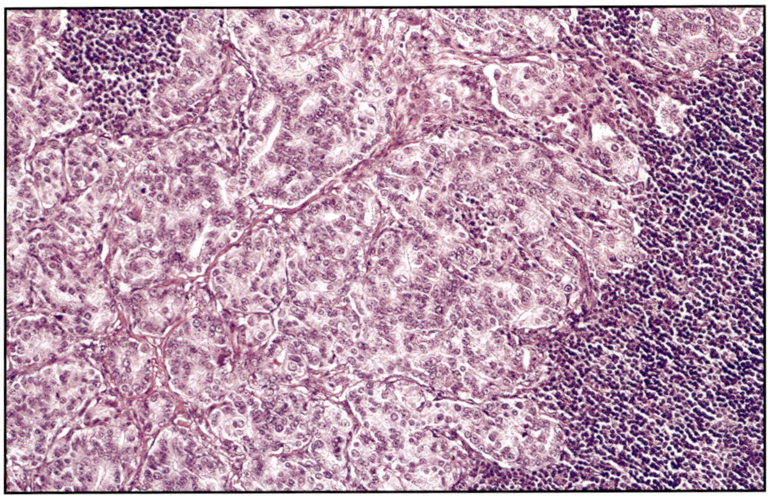

■ **i14.159** *Fused microacinar prostatic adenocarcinoma in pelvic lymph node.*

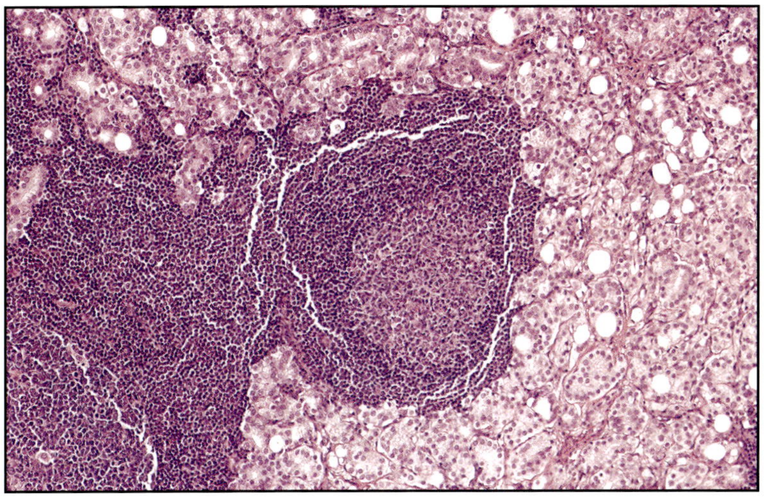

■ **i14.160** *Prostatic adenocarcinoma lymph node metastasis, without fibrogenic response.*

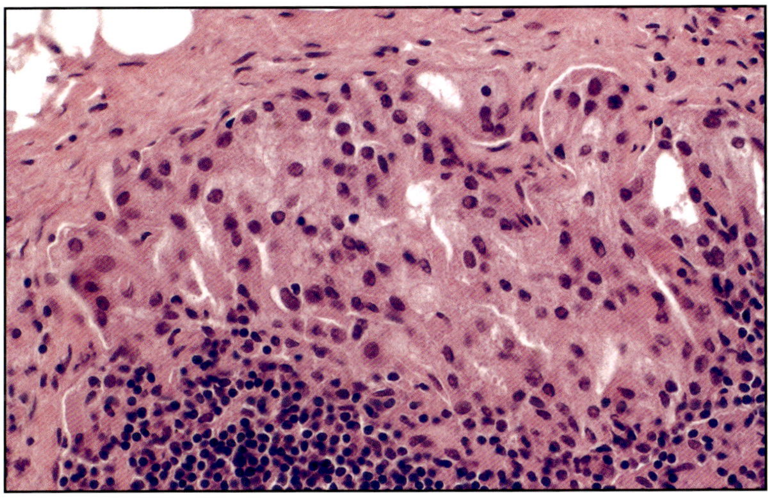

■ **i14.161** *Small subcapsular deposit of prostatic adenocarcinoma in lymph node.*

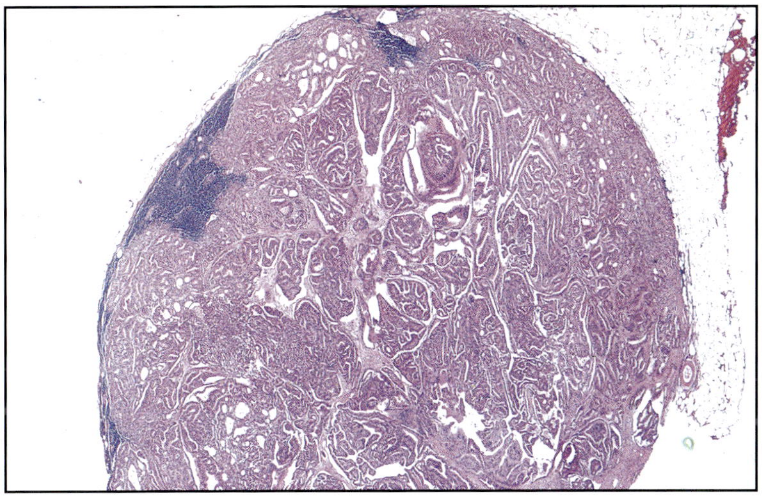

■ **i14.162** *Near complete effacement of pelvic lymph node by prostatic adenocarcinoma.*

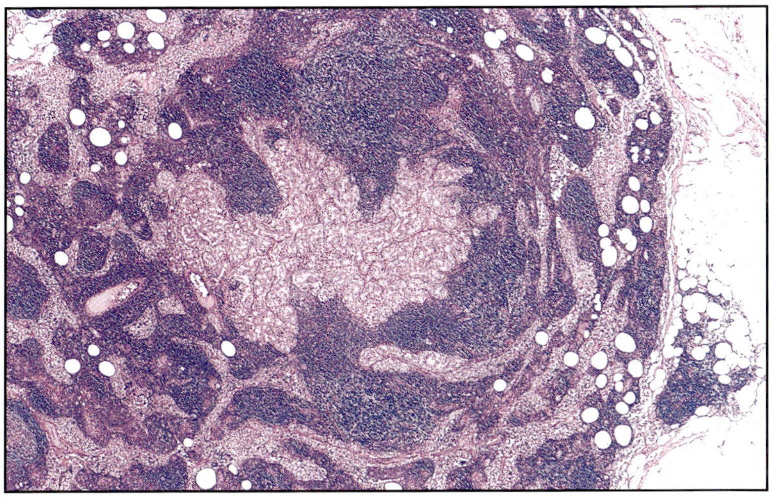

■ **i14.163** *Sinusoidal pattern of lymph node infiltration by prostatic adenocarcinoma, including larger central growth of tumor.*

noted that in about 1% of cases (13 of 1092), there was an incidentally discovered hematolymphoid malignancy (Terris 1997), including small lymphocytic lymphoma (6 patients), chronic lymphocytic leukemia (3 cases), Hodgkin lymphoma (3 cases), and hairy cell leukemia (1 case). In addition to these hematolymphoid malignancies, poorly differentiated malignant neoplasms of all types should enter into the differential diagnosis of poorly differentiated prostatic carcinoma in a lymph node. Therefore, the broad categories of poorly differentiated carcinoma, poorly differentiated hematolymphoid malignancy, malignant melanoma, high-grade sarcoma, and germ cell tumor should be given due consideration if a question exists as to the primary site. For metastatic prostatic carcinoma in pelvic lymph node, removed before radical prostatectomy, the diagnosis usually is straightforward at the level of examination of H&E-stained sections. One should be aware of the possibility of a second carcinoma metastatic to pelvic lymph nodes. For example, 3% to 4% of patients with prostate cancer also have bladder cancer (Androulakakis 1986, Chun 1997, Kim 1994, Konski 1991). In rare cases, coexistent bladder carcinoma and prostatic carcinoma can "collide" in the same pelvic lymph node (Ergen 1995, Gohji 1997). For difficult cases at the H&E level, the immunohistochemical marker panel in **t14.16** can be used to help separate metastatic prostatic carcinoma from metastatic TCC. In distant lymph nodes, metastatic prostatic carcinoma usually is suspected clinically because of a rising serum PSA level in a patient with a history of prostate cancer. (In rare cases, clinically advanced prostatic adenocarcinoma may not be

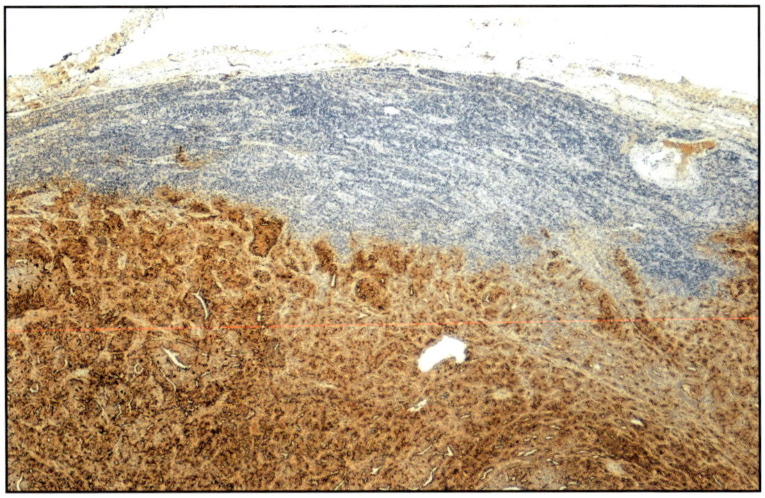

■ **i14.164** *PSA immunoreactivity in metastatic deposit of prostatic carcinoma.*

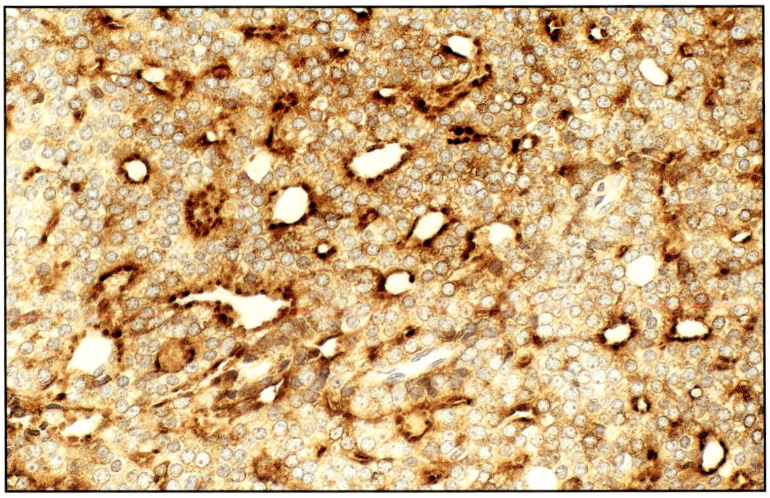

■ **i14.165** *Luminal accentuation of PSA immunostaining of metastatic prostatic adenocarcinoma.*

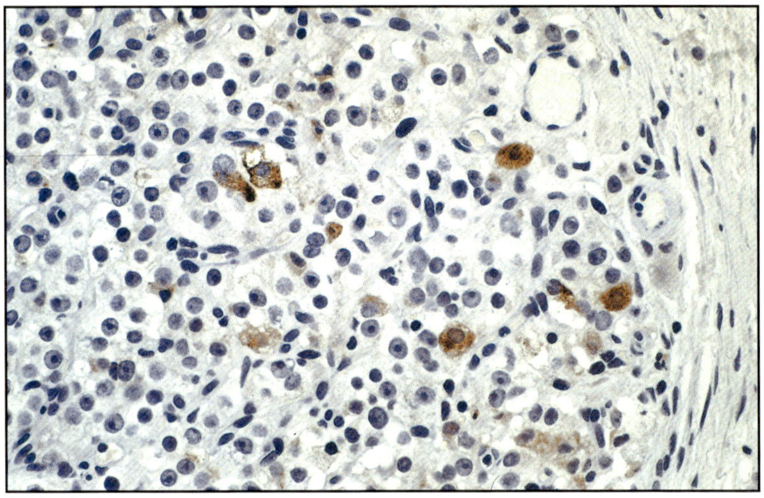

■ **i14.166** *Focal PSA expression in metastatic prostatic adenocarcinoma deposit, as detected by immunohistochemical stain.*

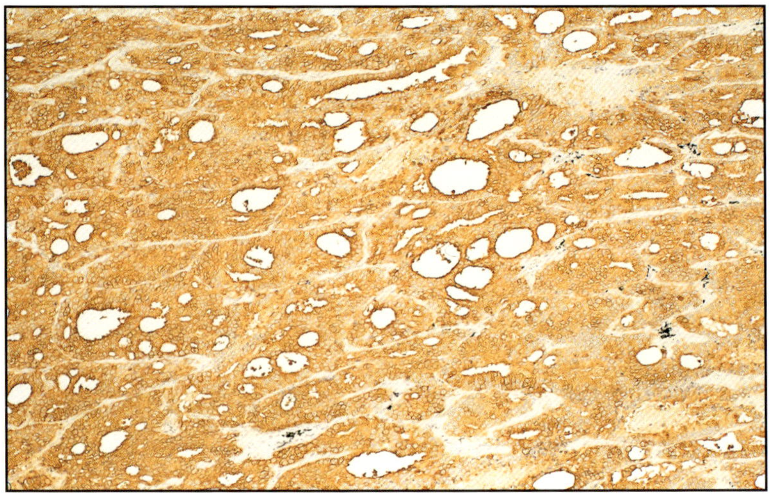

■ **i14.167** *Diffuse PSA expression in metastatic deposit of prostatic adenocarcinoma.*

associated with an elevated serum PSA [R Cohen 1994, Leibman 1995]. Also, there may be clinical progression without a rising serum PSA if there is expansion of a neuroendocrine line of differentiation, which may occur in a minority of patients after hormonal therapy [Logothetis 1996].)

It is rare for prostatic carcinoma to present as a neoplasm of unknown primary site (Mayordomo 1993). One should always rule in or out prostatic adenocarcinoma in a man presenting with a carcinoma of unknown primary in a lymph node or other metastatic site. This can be accomplished by including PSA and PSAP in an immunohistochemical marker panel (DeYoung 2000) **t14.50**. PSA and PSAP expression usually is maintained by prostatic carcinoma cells in metastatic sites (Bates 1982, Bentz 1982, Bovenberg 1993, Cho 1987, Ford 1985, Jöbsis 1981, Li 1980, Lippert 1982, Nadji 1980, Stein 1984) **i14.164, i14.165**, although the number of cells staining can be quite variable **i14.166, i14.167**, as can staining intensity. A small percentage (8% to 14%) of high-grade prostatic carcinomas fail to stain for PSA, so a negative result does not completely exclude a prostatic primary. In such cases, PSAP positivity or correlations of the histomorphologic appearance of the tumor, results of the other tissue immunomarkers, the serum PSA level, and clinicoradiologic findings are needed to suggest a prostatic primary. CK7 and CK20 immunostains can be of some utility **t14.50** but are not uniformly negative in prostatic carcinoma, as suggested by some reports (Chu 2000). CK7 and CK20 staining, when present in prostatic carcinoma, usually is focally positive. Additional carcinoma markers such as EMA, TAG-72, CEA, Leu-7, CA-125, CA19-9, Ber-EP4, and CA15-3 are less useful **t14.50**, but one should be aware of the immunoreactivity profile of these markers in prostatic carcinoma when they are used in a panel. Pertinent negative immunostains in prostatic carcinoma include hematolymphoid markers CD45 (LCA) and CD30, melanocytic markers, the muscle markers desmin, SMA and MSA, and the germ cell tumor markers PLAP and AFP **t14.50**. Neuroendocrine markers and endocrine peptides can be found in a substantial percentage of usual prostatic adenocarcinomas **t14.50**. As always, the immunostain results should be interpreted in the context of the histomorphologic, radiologic, and clinical findings.

The parameters recommended for pelvic lymph node reporting include clinically designated anatomic site of pelvic lymph nodes, number of nodes examined, number involved by carcinoma and greatest dimension of the largest metastatic deposit, and extranodal extension, if present (ADASP 1998, Bostwick 1999B, Srigley 2000) **t14.53**. Sample synoptic and diagnostic formats are given in **t14.39** and **t14.40**. We report anatomic site by container submission, which is almost always "right pelvic" and "left pelvic" in site designation. One should probably report extranodal extension by carcinoma into perinodal soft tissue, although the data are conflicting as to whether this is an independent prognosticator (Cheng 2000, Griebling 1997).

The amount of prostatic carcinoma in pelvic lymph nodes does appear to carry prognostic weight. Historically, extent of nodal prostatic carcinoma has been defined by the number of positive nodes, but the value of this measure as an independent prognostic indicator is controversial (reviewed in Cheng 1998, Lawton 2000). When the nodal tumor burden is quantified as cancer volume, using the grid method (Humphrey 1990B), independent prognostic significance was achieved in one study (Cheng 1998). These authors suggest reporting nodal cancer volume or a surrogate, the diameter of the largest metastasis (Cheng 1998). One should note that no accepted nodal cancer size cutoffs exist for distinguishing low-risk and high-risk patient groups. In particular, no "micrometastatic" nodal prostate cancer size has been established, although a size of <2mm (Srigley 2000) or =2mm (Bostwick 2000) has been recommended as a definition of micrometastasis. Additional potential but currently experimental prognosticators include nodal histologic grade (moderately vs poorly differentiated) (Brawn 1990A, 1990B), RT-PCR for PSA or PSMA (Okegawa 2000), DNA ploidy (Bazinet 1992, Peters-Gee 1992) and proliferation (MIB-1 immunolabeling) index of the metastatic carcinoma deposits (Cheng 1999A).

Experimental diagnostic tools for detecting prostate carcinoma in lymph nodes include immunohistochemical stains for PSA, PSAP, and cytokeratin (Freeman 1995, Gomella 1993, Köllermann 1999, Moul 1994). Occult pelvic nodal metastatic carcinoma was found by immunostains of additional sections in 3% to 18% of all patients who had undergone radical prostatectomy (Freeman 1995, Gomella 1993, Köllermann 1999, Moul 1994). Thus far, detection of occult metastatic prostatic carcinoma cells in lymph nodes does not affect prognosis (PSA failure after surgery [Köllermann 1999]). Moreover, the additional sections used for immunostaining represented additional node sampling, and it was not tested in these studies whether H&E-staining of the additional sections would have resulted in detection of the carcinoma cells. Use of these stains to detect micrometastases is not currently standard practice. Rather, examination of a single H&E-stained section of completely embedded lymph node tissue is. Enhanced detection of prostatic carcinoma cells in lymph nodes by RT-PCR for PSA or PSMA has also been observed (Deguchi 1993, Edelstein 1996, Mao 1998, Okegawa 2000, Takahashi 1996), but the possibility exists that the detected cells could be in blood in the nodes and not actually infiltrative into nodal tissue. Also, the additional lymph node tissue used for the PCR reactions may have harbored detectable carcinoma cells detectable by light microscopy if H&E sections had been prepared from this tissue.

t14.53 Recommended Reporting of Pelvic Node Status

Report number of lymph nodes microscopically examined for each location
Report number of lymph nodes involved by carcinoma for each location
Report greatest dimension of largest metastatic deposit[1]
Report soft tissue extranodal extension by carcinoma

[1]Less than 2 mm = micrometastasis

t14.54 Bone Metastasis of Prostatic Carcinoma

A hallmark of disseminated prostate cancer
Pelvis, vertebral column, and ribs most frequently involved
Can be diagnosed by bone scan in patients with known prostate cancer and a rising serum PSA
Classically, osteoblastic by plain films and microscopic examination of tissue sections
Microscopically, the adenocarcinoma is typically high-grade and can replace marrow cavity and/or grow in a fibrogenic background in the marrow space

Finally, antibodies have been generated that may be useful in an immunohistochemical panel to substantiate prostatic origin of a poorly differentiated carcinoma in lymph nodes. These include antibodies directed against PSMA (Horoszewicz 1987, Maraj 1998, Roberts 2001, Silver 1997, Sweat 1998) and human glandular kallikrein 2 (hK2) (Silver 1997), a protein related to PSA (which is human glandular kallikrein 3). Further characterization of the specificity and sensitivity of these 2 antibodies will be necessary before implementation in diagnostic immunohistochemical marker panels.

Bony Prostatic Carcinoma Metastasis

A characteristic feature of distant prostate cancer spread is metastatic disease in the bone marrow, with an osteoblastic response **t14.54**. Bones are involved in widely disseminated prostatic carcinoma in 70% of cases (Bubendorf 2000, De La Monte 1986, Elkin 1954, Saitoh 1984, True 2000), with pelvic bones, dorsal and lumbar spine, ribs, cervical spine, femur, skull, sacrum, and humerus being most commonly affected, in decreasing order **t13.22**. Bony metastasis is usually (in 92% of cases) associated with metastatic deposits elsewhere (Mintz 1934). High-grade and diffuse bone metastases typically are found in patients who have not responded to radiation and hormonal therapy and died of prostate cancer (True 2000).

Bony metastases of prostate cancer usually are diagnosed by radiologic means in patients with biopsy-proven prostate cancer, in the setting of an elevated serum PSA. (To reiterate, it is rare, but possible, for a patient to have distant metastatic spread of prostatic adenocarcinoma without an elevated serum PSA [R Cohen 1994, Leibman 1995].) Radionuclide bone scans **i13.10**, which are much more sensitive than plain films, are particularly useful (Buscombe 1999). However, because of specificity problems with bone scintigraphy, positive findings may need to be compared with radiographs of the abnormal area (Buscombe 1999). In rare cases with a solitary hot spot on bone scan that is also suspicious by skeletal radiography, bone biopsy or excision of the lesion may be contemplated. However, if the serum PSA is <10 ng/mL and there is an asymptomatic, solitary hot spot on bone scan, most lesions will prove to be benign reparative fibro-osseous proliferations (McDermott 1999). These patients could be followed radiographically. In general, bone biopsies to confirm metastatic prostatic carcinoma are not performed.

Grossly, metastatic prostatic carcinoma may be encountered in large portions of bone removed because of pathologic fractures (**i13.12, p 241**) or at autopsy **i14.168**. Here, prostatic carcinoma metastatic deposits appear as gray, tan, or white irregular, solid masses that replace the red-tan spongelike bone marrow. Microscopically, prostatic adenocarcinoma in the bone marrow is

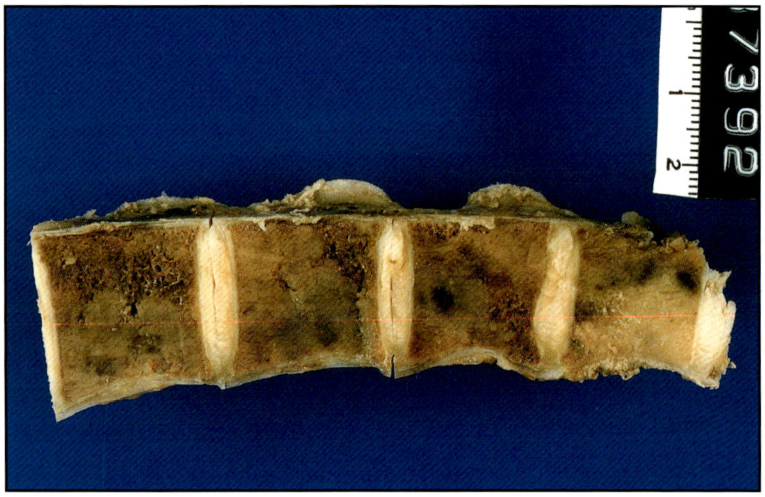

■ **i14.168** *Vertebral bony metastasis of prostatic carcinoma (arrow).*

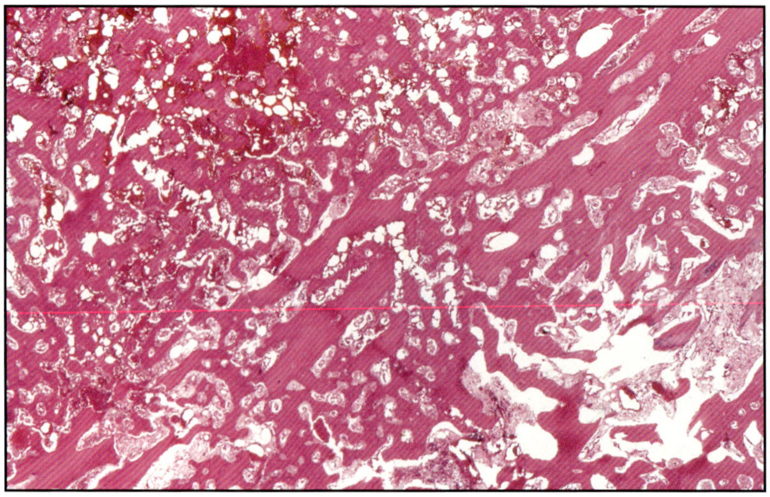

■ **i14.169** *Thickened bony trabeculae typify the response of bone to metastatic prostatic carcinoma. (Courtesy of Dr. Michael Kyriakos).*

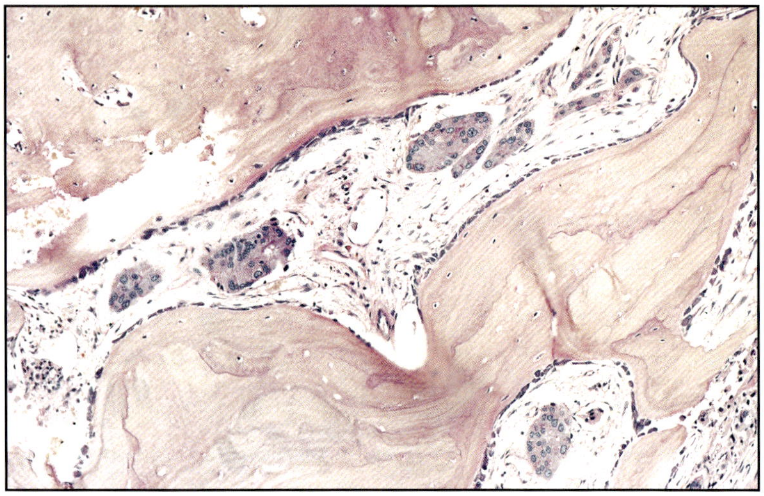

■ **i14.170** *Metastatic prostatic carcinoma in fibrogenic bone marrow, with associated osteoblastic proliferation rimming thickened bony trabeculae.*

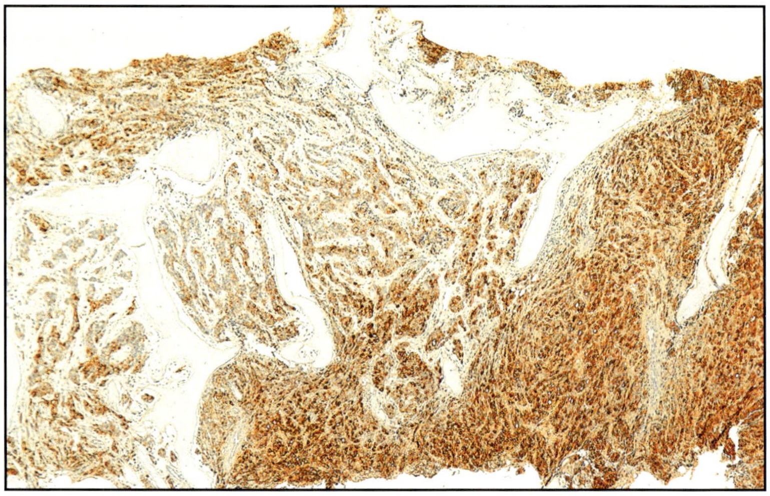

■ **i14.171** *Replacement of iliac crest core bone marrow biopsy tissue by sheets of prostatic carcinoma, as highlighted by PSA immunostain.*

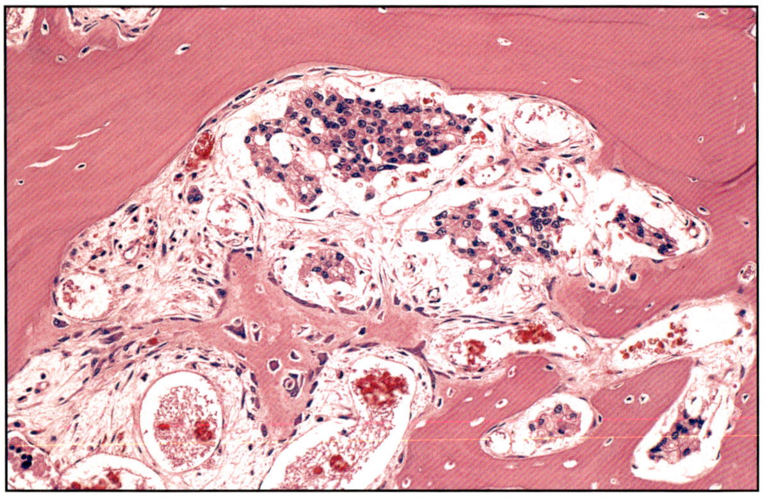

■ **i14.172** *Nests of metastatic prostatic carcinoma in fibrogenic bone marrow, with focal osteoblastic response.*

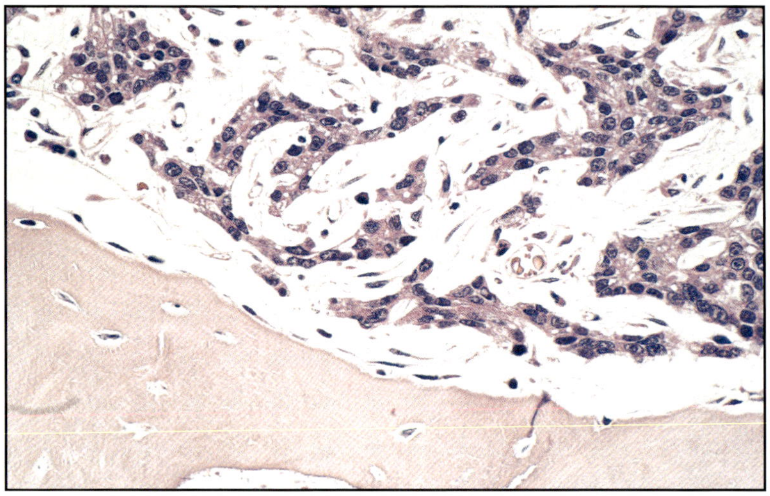

■ **i14.173** *Cords of metastatic prostatic carcinoma in fibrogenic bone marrow.*

classically osteoblastic, with thickened trabeculae lined by numerous osteoblasts **i14.169, i14.170**. The carcinoma, which is high grade, can grow as sheets, with complete replacement of the marrow space **i14.171**, or as individual glands, fused glands, or cords and nests embedded in a fibrotic marrow **i14.170; i14.172, i14.173**. Not always is there a fibrogenic response **i14.174**. Diagnostic difficulty may be faced when the carcinoma cells show hormonal therapy effect, which is often manifested in the form of cytoplasmic

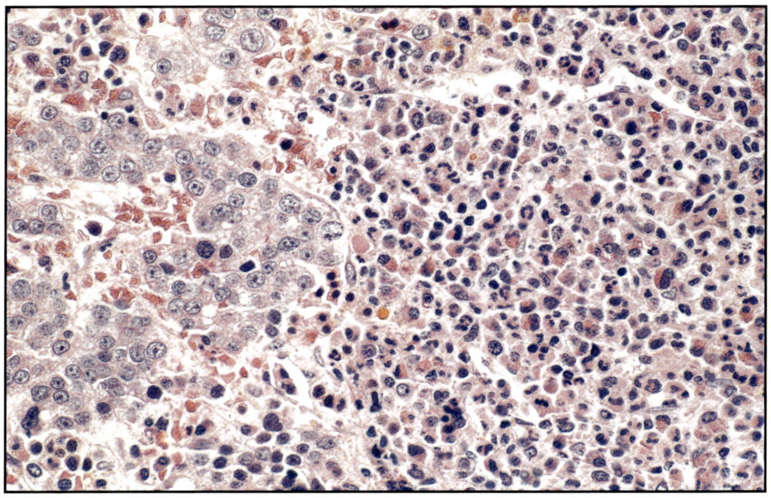

■ **i14.174** *Metastatic prostatic carcinoma (left) in cellular bone marrow (right), without a fibrogenic response.*

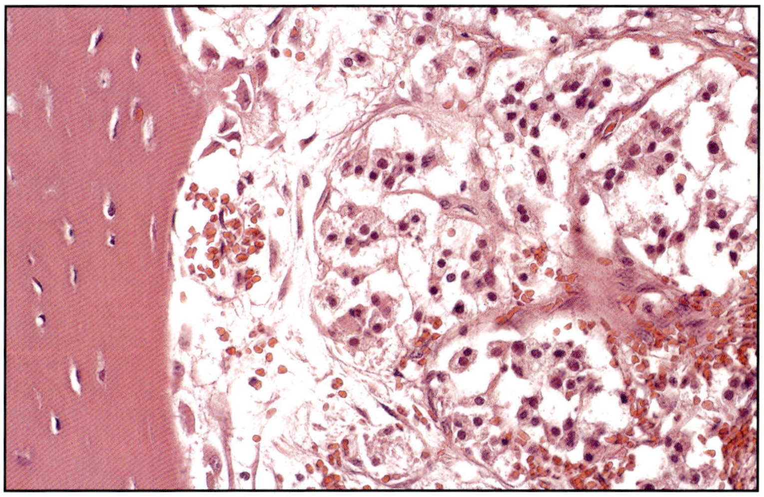

■ **i14.175** *Metastatic prostatic carcinoma in bone marrow, with androgen deprivation therapy effect, including nuclear pyknosis and cytoplasmic vacuolization.*

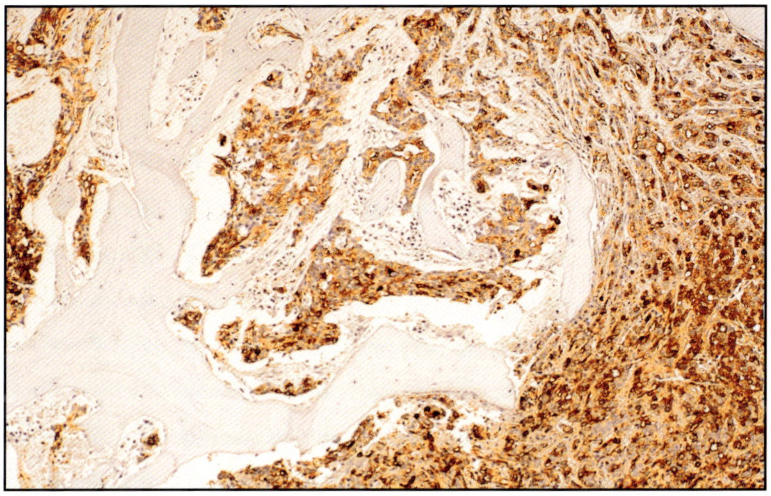

■ **i14.176** *Strong and diffuse PSA immunoreactivity in prostatic carcinoma in decalcified bone marrow biopsy tissue.*

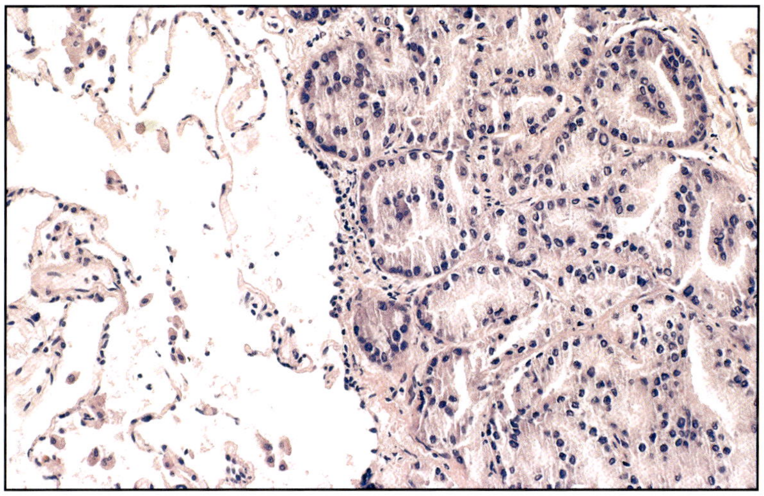

■ **i14.177** *Prostatic adenocarcinoma metastatic to lung.*

vacuolization and nuclear pyknosis **i14.175**. The treated carcinoma cells may then be mistaken for histiocytes. The differential diagnosis also includes carcinoma from other sites. A directed marker panel, using immunostains for PSA, PSAP, and pan-cytokeratin **t14.50**, is of aid in cases of unknown primary. Importantly, immunostains for PSA work well in bone marrow biopsies fixed in mercuric Zenkers solution and decalcified in concentrated formic acid (Shah 1985) **i14.176**. Of note, loss of PSAP immunoreactivity in prostatic carcinoma biopsies decalcified with nitric or formic acid has been reported (Allsbrook 1998, Shah 1985).

Experimental methods for detecting prostatic carcinoma cells in bone marrow include immunohistochemistry for cytokeratins or PSA (Bretton 1994, Hochtlen-Vollmar 1997, Köllermann 1999, Pantel 1994, Riesenberg 1993, Wood 1994B, 1997) and RT-PCR for PSA mRNA (Gao 1999, Melchior 1997, Wood 1994A, 1994B, 1997). Although there is some evidence suggesting a worse outcome when the bone marrow is RT-PCR positive for PSA mRNA (Wood 1997), the patient number is low and the results are preliminary. Currently, these techniques should not be used for routine management (Slovin 1998).

Reports on prostatic carcinoma in bone excisions or needle core biopsies of bone should include mainly the presence or absence of tumor and any treatment effect. There is no evidence that histologic grading of the bony metastatic deposit is of prognostic value. Although the overall extent of skeletal involvement by prostatic carcinoma, as determined by bone scan, may be related to survival (Eisenberger 1994, Sabbatini 1999), there are no data on whether the amount of tumor in bone specimens is linked to patient outcome. A simple description of tumor amount (such as focal vs extensive involvement) would seem to suffice.

Distant Nonbony Prostatic Carcinoma Metastasis

Clinically detectable metastatic prostatic carcinoma in organs other than lymph nodes and bone is uncommon and typically is found late in the course of known, widespread disease (Saitoh 1984). At autopsy, in addition to lymph nodes and bone, anatomic sites commonly involved in late-stage, metastatic prostatic carcinoma include lung **i14.177**, soft tissue, liver **i14.178**, serosal surfaces, adrenals, and kidneys **t13.23** (Bubendorf 2000, De La Monte 1986, Elkin 1954, Mintz 1934, Saitoh 1984). Less common sites, at <10% of cases of widely disseminated prostate cancer at autopsy, are gastrointestinal tract, ureter, pancreas, spleen, heart, brain or dura (Pfister 1995), thyroid, and skin **i14.179** (Allan 1998, Segal 1994). Cutaneous involvement usually is

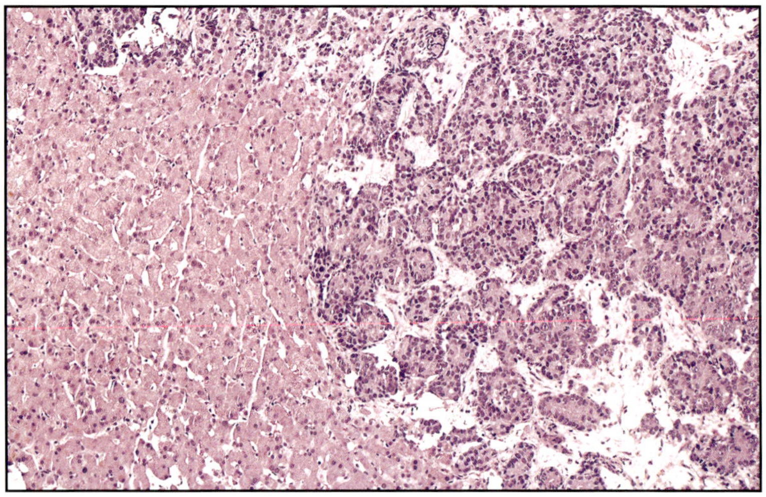

■ **i14.178** *Prostatic adenocarcinoma metastatic to liver.*

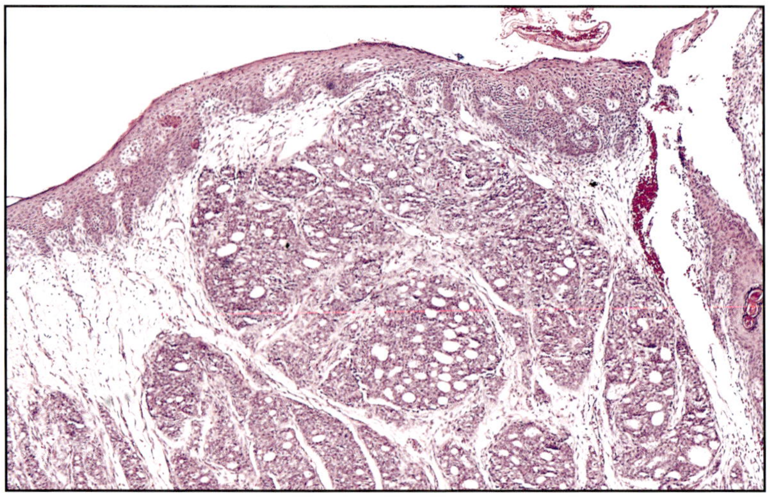

■ **i14.179** *Prostatic adenocarcinoma metastatic to dermis of skin.*

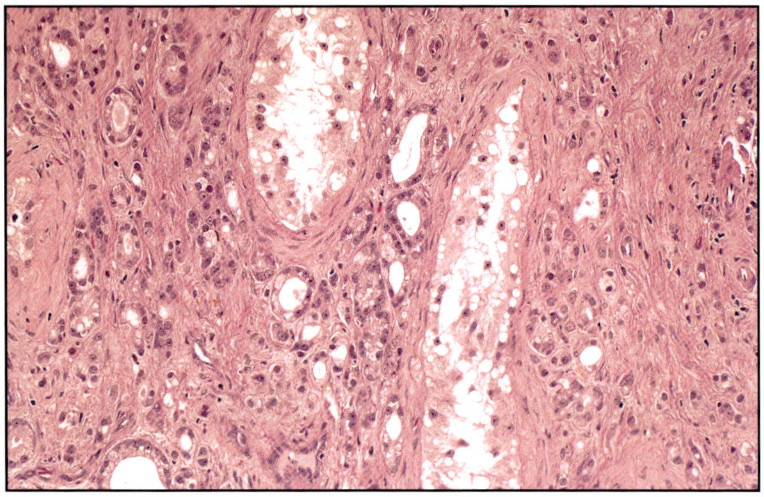

■ **i14.180** *Prostatic adenocarcinoma metastatic to testis.*

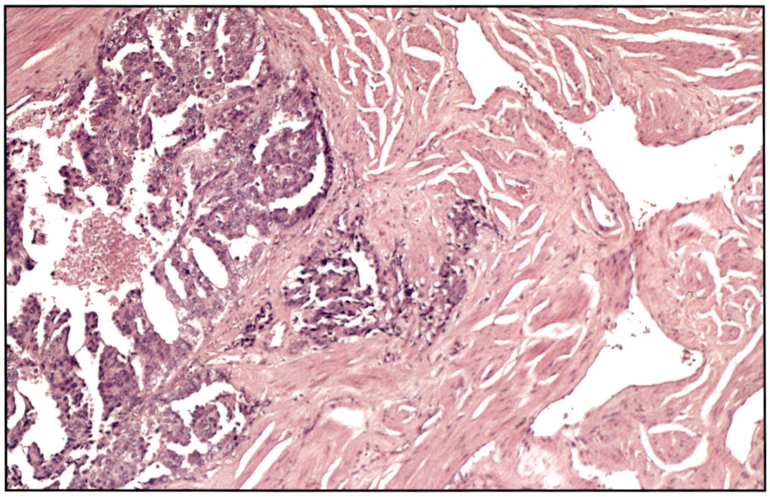

■ **i14.181** *Prostatic adenocarcinoma of ductal type, metastatic to penis.*

deep and dermal, although prostatic carcinoma cells have produced an extramammary Paget's disease picture in a few cases (Allan 1998). Examples of unusual or rare locations for metastatic prostatic carcinoma are testis (Tu 2002, Young 1987) **i14.180**, epididymis (Rizk 1990), penis (Celebi 1997, Osther 1991, Tu 2002) **i14.181**, salivary gland (Hrebinko 1993, Moul 1989, Simpson 1997), breast (Salyer 1973, Soda 1999), hernia sac (Bostwick 1993C, Liu 2000), and eye or orbit (Gonzalez 1997, Wiegel 1998). Rare cases of prostatic carcinoma metastatic to a pulmonary hamartoma have been reported (King 1995, Kuo 1978).

Clinically detectable lung involvement by metastatic prostatic carcinoma is uncommon or rare (Apple 1985, Arnheim 1948, Copeland 2002, Gentile 1988, Heffner 1982, Lalli 1983, Lindell 1982, Mestitz 1989, Petras 1983, Scherz 1986, Smith 1999, Speiler 1985), whereas metastatic prostatic carcinoma in the lungs at autopsy is common at around 40% to 50% (range 23% to 74%) (Bubendorf 2000, Elkin 1954, Mintz 1934, Saitoh 1984, Scheidemandel 1972, Varkarakis 1974) **t14.55**. This discrepancy apparently is based on the tendency of metastatic deposits in the lung to be microscopic and intralymphatic (Varkarakis 1974), without substantial nodule formation that could be detected by radiologic means. Chest radiographs in patients with autopsy-proven metastatic prostatic carcinoma in the lung often are interpreted as normal or as demonstrating an interstitial pattern, which correlates with lymphatic spread (Elkin 1954, Mintz 1934, Varkarakis 1974). Discrete nodules on chest radiograph are seen in a minority of patients (Elkin 1954), and rarely, a single mass is seen that can be confused with primary adenocarcinoma of the lung (Scoggins 1978, Varkarakis 1974). Pleural involvement is uncommon (at about 15% to 20% of cases with pulmonary metastasis), and endobronchial spread and malignant effusions of prostatic carcinoma are rare (Apple 1985, Arnheim 1948, Heffner 1982, Lalli 1983, Lindell 1982, Renshaw 1996, Scheidemandel 1972, Scherz 1986, Scoggins 1978, Sears 1987, Spieler 1985, Varkarakis 1974). The percentage of all malignant pleural effusions caused by prostatic carcinoma is only 1% to 2% (Renshaw 1996, Sears 1987, Speiler 1985).

■ **t14.55 Lung Metastasis of Prostatic Carcinoma**

- Uncommon to rare clinically, but common (40%-50%) at autopsy of patients with prostate cancer
- Chest x-ray normal or demonstrates interstitial pattern, consistent with lymphatic spread
- Nodules in parenchyma uncommon radiographically or at gross examination
- Microscopically, multiple small, discrete nodules and intralymphatic spread often seen
- Immunohistochemical marker panel, including PSA and PSAP, is valuable when adenocarcinoma of unknown primary is found in lungs of men

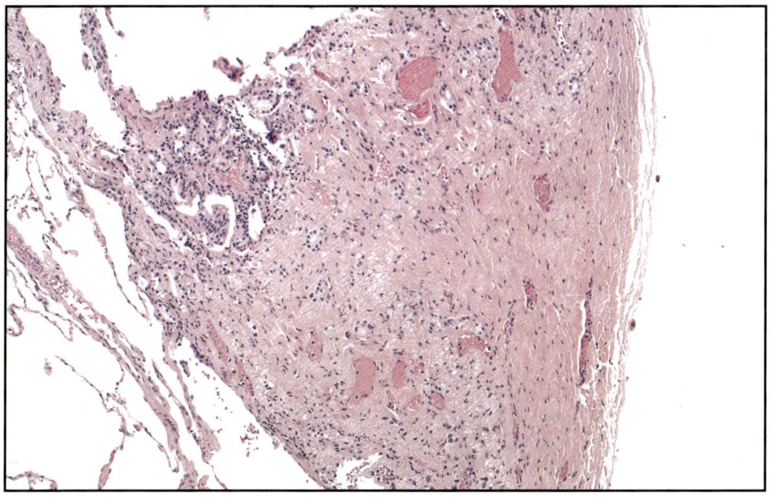

■ **i14.182** *Pleural metastatic deposit of prostatic adenocarcinoma.*

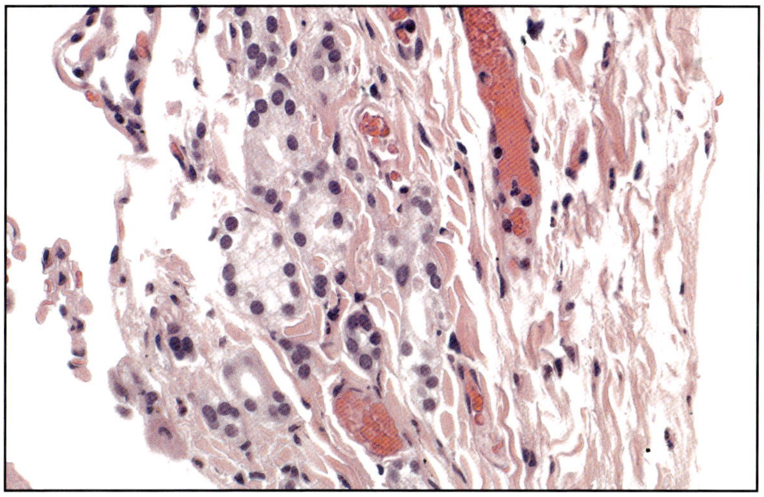

■ **i14.183** *Subtle small acinar proliferation of pleural metastatic prostatic adenocarcinoma depicted in* **i14.182**.

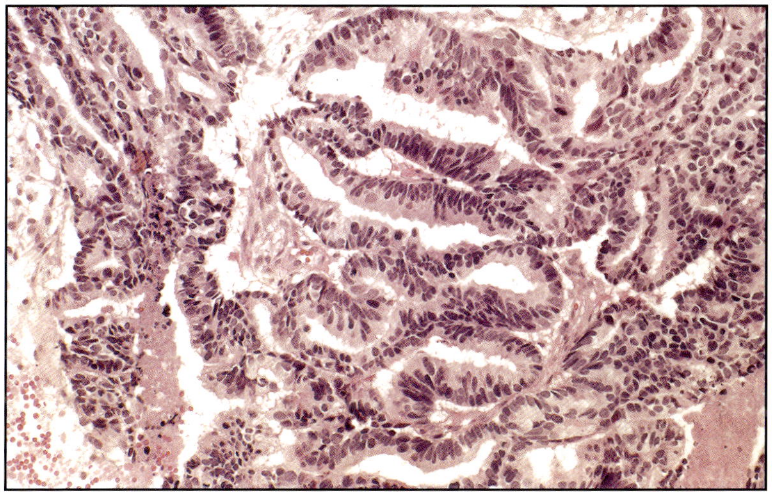

■ **i14.184** *Prostatic carcinoma of ductal type metastatic to lung, simulating enteric-type primary lung cancer or metastatic carcinoma of enteric origin.*

Clinically, metastatic prostatic carcinoma in the lungs is most often associated with bony metastasis. Correspondingly, at postmortem examination, the lung is seldom the sole site of metastatic spread (5% of cases) of prostatic carcinoma (Mintz 1934).

Grossly, at autopsy, lung metastases are not evident 75% of the time (Elkin 1954). Even when macroscopically apparent, the metastatic tumor nodules tend to be small (up to 7mm [Elkin 1954]), firm, and discrete (Mintz 1934). They vary from single to numerous (Elkin 1954, Mintz 1934). Exceptionally, large nodules can be seen. Microscopically, metastatic prostatic carcinoma in the lung usually is parenchymal-based, with lymphatic infiltration commonly identified. Small pleural or subpleural nodules with fibrous thickening and embedded prostatic carcinoma can be seen **i14.182, i14.183**. Most metastatic deposits are moderately to poorly differentiated. The morphologic presentation can range from the more common small acinar malignant glands, with or without cribriform structures, that resemble primary prostatic carcinoma due to nuclear monotony with nucleomegaly and abundant cytoplasm to monomorphous-appearing, sheetlike growth of a poorly differentiated carcinoma that has a carcinoid-like appearance (Anton 1998A, Copeland 2002). Ductal carcinomas of the prostate can metastasize as a papillary carcinoma and simulate a primary lung neoplasm **i14.184**. Metastatic ductal carcinomas with columnar cells can mimic an enteric-type carcinoma primary in or metastatic to the lung. For all men who present with metastatic adenocarcinoma of the lung without a known primary, the immunohistochemical marker panel should always include PSA and PSAP (Gentile 1988). These same immunostains should also be performed when there is a past history of prostatic carcinoma and the patient undergoes excision of a mass that clinically and radiologically appears to be a lung primary because in rare cases pulmonary metastasis of prostatic carcinomas can be solitary (Elkin 1954, Scoggins 1978, Smith 1999, Varkarakis 1974).

Liver metastases of prostatic carcinoma are also uncommon clinically but are found in 20% to 36% of cases at autopsy (Bubendorf 2000, Elkin 1954, Mintz 1934, Saitoh 1984). Similar to that in the lung, metastatic prostatic carcinoma in the liver most often forms small, multiple firm and discrete nodules (Mintz 1934). In the past, massive liver nodules caused by prostatic carcinoma have been reported as rare (Mintz 1934), although in a recent small series of patients with hormone-refractory disease, a large mass in the liver was depicted, and the metastatic deposits in the liver were characterized as the largest metastatic tumors anywhere in the body (Rubin 2000A).

Metastatic deposits of prostatic carcinoma usually are not biopsied in patients with known disseminated disease. Biopsy has been performed in rare cases in which prostatic carcinoma clinically presented as a metastasis in patients without a previous diagnosis of prostate cancer (Petersen 1992, Saitoh 1984) or in rare instances when, in the setting of known prostate cancer, there is clinical detection of solitary mass that turns out to be metastatic prostatic carcinoma rather than a second primary. In the former setting, the most common distant sites for initial presentation of metastatic carcinoma, were, in one review (Petersen 1992), supraclavicular lymph node ($n = 31$), lung ($n = 14$), skin ($n = 4$), brain ($n = 3$), abdomen ($n = 2$), orbit ($n = 1$), pleura ($n = 1$), and esophagus ($n = 1$). Clinically solitary prostatic carcinoma metastatic deposits, in patients with or without a history of prostate cancer, can mimic another primary cancer. For example, metastatic prostatic carcinoma has been reported to simulate lung cancer (Copeland 2002, Elkin 1954, Scoggins 1978, Smith 1999, Varkarakis 1974), primary testicular tumor (Young 1987), epididymal adenomatoid tumor (Rizk 1990), primary cutaneous malignant melanoma (Segal 1994), primary penile tumor (Celebi 1997), and primary parotid tumors (Moul 1989, Simpson 1997). (One should be cautious in diagnosing prostatic carcinoma metastatic to salivary glands [Hrebinko 1993, Moul 1989, Simpson 1997], based on PSA immunoreactivity in carcinoma cells, because PSA can be present in salivary gland tumors **t14.17**.)

The diagnosis in these cases of metastatic disease is correctly made when the histopathologist is aware of the potential for prostatic carcinoma to initially present at distant sites. A clinical history of previous prostatic carcinoma, which may or may not be transmitted, is helpful. To reiterate, whenever a man (usually over 50 years of age) presents with a metastatic monotonous-appearing adenocarcinoma or poorly differentiated carcinoma of unknown primary, immunostains for PSA and PSAP should be included in the marker panel.

Reporting of metastatic prostatic carcinoma at distant sites should include the number and size of the tumoral deposits in the tissue submitted, presence of absence of treatment effect, and degree of glandular differentiation. Neuroendocrine differentiation, if present, should also be noted because this may be indicative of evolution of an androgen-independent clone. Finally, histomorphologic comparison of the tumor in the prostatic primary and the metastatic sites would be desirable. The established prognostic indicators for patients with widely disseminated prostate cancer are almost exclusively clinical and include anemia, anorexia, weight loss, pain, number of lesions on bone scan, diabetes mellitus, and elevated alkaline phosphatase, serum lactate dehydrogenase, and performance status (Chodak 1991, De Voogt 1989, Fujikawa 1995, George 1999, Ishikawa 1989, Jørgensen 1995, 1997, Kato 1993, Matzkin 1993, Mulders 1990). Tissue-based prognostic markers in widely metastatic prostatic carcinoma are experimental and include histologic grade of primary or metastatic disease, morphometric analyses of nuclear volume and chromatin texture, DNA ploidy, immunophenotype, RT-PCR detection of carcinoma in metastatic sites, genotype, and gene expression profile by DNA microarray (Latulippe 2002). In the future, such markers could be important because they could help in stratification in prospective, controlled, randomized clinical trials comparing treatments and could also aid in counseling patients with regard to prognosis and in selecting treatment choices.

References

Abenoza P, Manivel C, Fraley EE. Primary adenocarcinoma of urinary bladder. Clinicopathologic study of 16 cases. *Urology* 29:9-14, 1987.

Abi-Aad AS, MacFarlane MT, Stein A, et al. Detection of local recurrence after radical prostatectomy by prostate specific antigen and transrectal ultrasound. *J Urol* 147:952-955, 1992.

Abrahams NA, Ormsby AH, Brainard J. Validation of cytokeratin 5/6 as an effective substitute for keratin 903 in the differentiation of benign from malignant glands in prostate needle biopsies. *Histopathology* 41:35-41, 2002.

Abrahamsson PA, Wadström LB, Alumets J, et al. Peptide-hormone and serotonin-immunoreactive tumour cells in carcinoma of the prostate. *Pathol Res Pract* 182:298-307, 1987.

Ackerman DA, Barry JM, Wicklund RA, et al. Analysis of risk factors associated with prostate cancer extension to the surgical margin and pelvic node metastasis at radical prostatectomy. *J Urol* 150:1845-1850, 1993.

ADASP (Association of Directors of Anatomic and Surgical Pathology). Recommendations for the reporting of resected prostate carcinoma. *Am J Clin Pathol* 105:667-670, 1998.

Adlakha H, Bostwick DG. Paneth cell–like change in prostatic adenocarcinoma represents neuroendocrine differentiation: report of 30 cases. *Hum Pathol* 25:135-139, 1994.

Aihara M, Wheeler TM, Ohori M, et al. Heterogeneity of prostate cancer in radical prostatectomy specimens. *Urology* 43:60-67, 1994A.

Aihara M, Lebovitz RM, Wheeler TM, et al. Prostate specific antigen and Gleason grade: an immunohistochemical study of prostate cancer. *J Urol* 151:1558-1564, 1994B.

Algaba F, Epstein JI, Aldape HC, et al. Assessment of prostate carcinoma in core needle biopsy: definition of minimal criteria for the diagnosis of cancer in biopsy material. *Cancer* 78:376-381, 1996.

Algan O, Pinover WH, Hanlon AL, et al. Is there a subset of patients with PSA > or = 20 ng/mL who do well after conformal beam radiotherapy? *Radiat Oncol Investig* 7:106-110, 1999.

Alguacil-Garcia A: Artifactual changes mimicking signet ring cell carcinoma in transurethral prostatectomy specimens. *Am J Surg Pathol* 10:795-800, 1986.

Allam CK, Bostwick DG, Hayes JA, et al. Interobserver variability in the diagnosis of high-grade prostatic intraepithelial neoplasia and adenocarcinoma. *Mod Pathol* 9:742-751, 1996.

Allan SJR, McLaren K, Aldridge RD. Paget's disease of the scrotum: a case exhibiting positive prostate-specific antigen staining and associated prostatic adenocarcinoma. *Br J Dermatol* 138:689-691, 1998.

Allen FJ, van Velden DJJ, Heyns CF. Are neuroendocrine cells of practical value as an independent prognostic parameter in prostate cancer? *Br J Urol* 75:751-754, 1995.

Allsbrook WC Jr, Pfeifer EA. Histochemistry of the prostate. In: Foster CS, Bostwick DG, eds. *Pathology of the Prostate.* Philadelphia: WB Saunders; 282-303, 1998.

Allsbrook WC Jr, Mangold KA,Yang X, Epstein JI: The Gleason grading system. An overview. *J Urol Pathol* 10:141-157, 1999.

Amakasu M, Akimoto S, Akakura K, et al. Disease progression in stage A prostate cancer. *Int J Urol* 2:39-43, 1995.

Amin MB, Schultz DS, Zarbo RJ. Analysis of cribriform morphology in prostatic neoplasia using antibody to high-molecular-weight cytokeratins. *Arch Pathol Lab Med* 118:260-264, 1994.

Amin MB, Bostwick DG. Pigment in prostatic epithelium and adenocarcinoma: a potential source of diagnostic confusion with seminal vesicular epithelium. *Mod Pathol* 9:791-795, 1996.

Amin MB, Bostwick DG, Epstein JI, et al. Interobserver reproducibility in the diagnosis of small foci of prostatic adenocarcinoma in needle biopsies [abstract]. *Mod Pathol* 11:76A, 1998.

Amin MB, Tamboli P, Varma M, et al. Postatrophic hyperplasia of the prostate gland. A detailed analysis of its morphology in needle biopsy specimens. *Am J Surg Pathol* 23:925-931, 1999.

Anderson PR, Hanlon AL, Patchefsky A, et al. Perineural invasion and Gleason 7-10 tumors predict increased failure in prostate cancer patients with pretreatment PSA <10 ng/mL treated with conformal external beam radiation therapy. *Int J Radiat Oncol Biol Phys* 41:1087-1092, 1998.

Andrews GS. Latent carcinoma of the prostate. *J Clin Pathol* 2:197-208, 1949.

Androulakakis PA, Schneider HM, Jacobi GH, et al. Coincident vesical transitional cell carcinoma and prostatic carcinoma: clinical features and treatment. *Br J Urol* 58:153-156, 1986.

Anton RC, Schwartz MR, Kessler ML, et al. Metastatic carcinoma of the prostate mimicking primary carcinoid tumor of the lung and mediastinum. *Pathol Res Pract* 194:753-758, 1998A.

Anton RC, Chakraborty S, Wheeler TM. The significance of intraluminal prostatic crystalloids in benign needle biopsies. *Am J Surg Pathol* 22:446-449, 1998B.

Anton RC, Kattan MW, Chakraborty S, et al. Postatrophic hyperplasia of the prostate. Lack of association with prostate cancer. *Am J Surg Pathol* 23:932-936, 1999.

Apple JS, Paulson DF, Baber C, et al. Advanced prostatic carcinoma: pulmonary manifestations. *Radiology* 154:601-604, 1985.

Aprikian AG, Cordon-Cardo C, Fair WR, et al. Characterization of neuroendocrine differentiation in human benign prostate and prostatic adenocarcinoma. *Cancer* 71:3952-3965, 1993.

Aprikian AG, Cordon-Cardo C, Fair WR, et al. Neuroendocrine differentiation in metastatic prostatic adenocarcinoma. *J Urol* 151:914-919, 1994.

Aprikian AG, Han K, Guy L, et al. Neuroendocrine differentiation and the bombesin/gastrin-releasing peptide family of neuropeptides in the progression of human prostate cancer. *Prostate* 8(suppl):52-61, 1998.

Arcangeli CG, Humphrey PA, Smith DS, et al. Percentage of free serum prostate-specific antigen as a predictor of pathologic features of prostate cancer in a screening population. *Urology* 51:558-564, 1998.

Arista-Nasr J, Cortés E, Pichardo R. Low grade adenocarcinoma simulating benign glandular lesions in needle prostatic biopsy. *Rev Invest Clin* 49:37-40, 1997.

Arnheim FK. Carcinoma of the prostate: a study of the postmortem findings in one hundred and seventy-six cases. *J Urol* 60:599-603, 1948.

Asakawa M, Yasumoto R, Kamizuru M, et al. Transurethral resection of the prostatic gland (TUR-P) and incidental carcinoma [in Japanese]. *Acta Urol Jpn* 34:1003-1005, 1988.

Aufranc ST, Rosen S, Li T, et al. Unrecognized perineural invasion in prostate needle biopsy is revealed by staining for S-100 protein [abstract]. *Mod Pathol* 13: 92A, 2000.

Ayala GE, Wheeler TM, Shine HD, et al. In vitro dorsal root ganglia and human prostate cell line interaction: redefining perineural invasion in prostate cancer. *Prostate* 49:213-223, 2001.

Azumi N, Traweek ST, Battifora H. Prostatic acid phosphatase in carcinoid tumors. Immunohistochemical and immunoblot studies. *Am J Surg Pathol* 15:785-790, 1991.

Babaian RJ, Troncoso P, Steelhammer LC, et al. Tumor volume and prostate-specific antigen: implications for early detection and defining a window of curability. *J Urol* 154:1808-1812, 1995.

Badalament RA, Miller MC, Peller PA, et al. An algorithm for predicting nonorgan confined prostate cancer using the results obtained from sextant core biopsies with prostate specific antigen level. *J Urol* 156:1375-1380, 1996.

Bahnson RR, Dresner SM, Gooding W, et al. Incidence and prognostic significance of lymphatic and vascular invasion in radical prostatectomy specimens. *Prostate* 15:149-155, 1989.

Baisden BL, Kahane H, Epstein JI. Perineural invasion, mucinous fibroplasia, and glomerulations. Diagnostic features of limited cancer on prostate needle biopsy. *Am J Surg Pathol* 23:918-924, 1999.

Barth PJ, Gerharz EW, Rawaswamy A, et al. The influence of lymph node counts on the detection of pelvic lymph node metastasis in prostate cancer. *Pathol Res Pract* 195:633-636, 1999.

Bass RB Jr, Barrett DM. Radical retropubic prostatectomy after transurethral prostatic resection. *J Urol* 124:495-497, 1980.

Bassily NH, Manley SC, Wojno KJ, et al. Perineural invasion on prostate needle biopsy independent predictor of stage T3-T4 disease [abstract]. *Mod Pathol* 12:89A, 1999.

Bassily NH, Vallorosi CJ, Akdas G, et al. Coordinate expression of cytokeratins 7 and 20 in prostate adenocarcinoma and bladder urothelial carcinoma. *Am J Clin Pathol* 113:383-388, 2000.

Bastacky SI, Walsh PC, Epstein JI. Relationship between perineural tumor invasion on needle biopsy and radical prostatectomy capsular penetration in clinical stage B adenocarcinoma of the prostate. *Am J Surg Pathol* 17:336-341, 1993.

Bastacky S, Silver SA, Epstein JI. Composite cytological smears of pelvic lymph nodes at the time of radical prostatectomy to identify nodal metastases. *Hum Pathol* 25:1352-1359, 1994.

Bates AW, Baithun SI. Secondary neoplasms of the bladder are histological mimics of nontransitional cell primary tumours: clinicopathological and histological features of 282 cases. *Histopathology* 36:32-40, 2000.

Bates RJ, Chapman CM, Prout GR Jr, et al. Immunohistochemical identification of prostatic acid phosphatase: correlation of tumor grade with acid phosphatase distribution. *J Urol* 127:574-580, 1982.

Battaglia S, Barbolini G, Botticelli AR. Early (stage A) prostatic cancer. IV. Methodological criteria for histopathological diagnosis. *Virchows Arch* [A] 382:245-249, 1979.

Bauer JJ, Connelly RR, Sesterhenn IA, et al. Biostatistical modeling using traditional preoperative and pathological prognostic variables in the selection of men at high risk for disease recurrence after radical prostatectomy for prostate cancer. *J Urol* 159:929-933, 1998.

Bauer WC, McGavran MH, Carlin MR. Unsuspected carcinoma of the prostate in suprapubic prostatectomy specimens. *Cancer* 13:370-378, 1960.

Bazinet M, Hamdy SM, Begin LR, et al. Prognostic significance of antigenic heterogeneity, Gleason grade, and ploidy of lymph node metastases in patients with prostate cancer. *Prostate* 20:311-326, 1992.

Beach R, Gown AM, Ue Peralta-Venturina MN, et al. P504S immunohistochemical detection in 405 prostatic specimens including 376 18-gauge needle biopsies. *Am J Surg Pathol* 26:1588-1596, 2002.

Bennett B, Gardner WA Jr. Crystalloids in prostatic hyperplasia. *Prostate* 1:31-35, 1980.

Bennett BD, Gardner WA Jr. Prostatic crystalloids. *JAMA* 260:2287, 1988.

Bentz MS, Cohen C, Demers LM, et al. Immunohistochemical demonstration of prostatic origin of metastases. *Urology* 19:584-586, 1982.

Bergman RT, Turner R, Barnes RW, et al. Comparative analysis of one thousand consecutive cases of transurethral prostatic resection. *J Urol* 74:533-548, 1955.

Berner A, Nesland JM, Waehre H, et al. Hormone resistant prostatic adenocarcinoma. An evaluation of prognostic factors in pre- and post-treatment specimens. *Br J Cancer* 68:380-384, 1993.

Billis A. Prostatic atrophy: an autopsy study of a histologic mimic of adenocarcinoma. *Mod Pathol* 11:47-54, 1998.

Bismar TA, Lewis JS Jr, Vollmer RT, et al. Multiple measures of carcinoma extent vs perineural invasion in prediction of pathologic stage in a screening population. *Am J Surg Pathol, 2003* (in press).

Blackwell KL, Bostwick DG, Myers RP, et al. Combining prostate-specific antigen with cancer and gland volume to predict more reliably pathological stage: the influence of prostate specific antigen cancer density. *J Urol* 151:1565-1570, 1994.

Blumenfeld W, Tucci S, Narayan P. Incidental lymphocytic prostatitis. Selective involvement with nonmalignant glands. *Am J Surg Pathol* 16:975-981, 1992.

Blute ML, Zinke H, Farrow GM. Long-term follow-up of young patients with stage A adenocarcinoma of the prostate. *J Urol* 136:840-843, 1986.

Blute ML, Bostwick DG, Seay TM, et al. Pathologic classification of prostate carcinoma: the impact of margin status. *Cancer* 82:902-908, 1998.

Bolton BH. Pulmonary metastases from carcinoma of the prostate: incidence and case report of a long remission. *J Urol* 94:73-77, 1965.

Bonkhoff H, Stein U, Remberger K. Multidirectional differentiation in the normal, hyperplastic and neoplastic human prostate: simultaneous demonstration of cell-specific epithelial markers. *Hum Pathol* 25:42-46, 1994.

Borirakchanyavat S, Bhargava V, Shinohara K, et al. Systematic sextant biopsies in the prediction of extracapsular extension at radical prostatectomy. *Urology* 50:373-378, 1997.

Bostwick DG, Egbert BM, Fajardo LF. Radiation injury of the normal and neoplastic prostate. *Am J Surg Pathol* 6:541-551, 1982.

Bostwick DG, Amin MB, Dundore P, et al. Architectural patterns of high-grade prostatic intraepithelial neoplasia. *Hum Pathol* 24:298-310, 1993A.

Bostwick DG, Srigley J, Grignon D, et al. Atypical adenomatous hyperplasia: morphologic criteria for its distinction from well-differentiated carcinoma. *Hum Pathol* 24:819-832, 1993B.

Bostwick DG, Eble JN. Prostatic adenocarcinoma metastatic to inguinal hernia sac. *J Urol Pathol* 1:193-199, 1993C.

Bostwick DG, Graham SD Jr, Napalkov P, et al. Staging of early prostate cancer: a proposed tumor volume-based prognostic index. *Urology* 41:403-411, 1993D.

Bostwick DG. Gleason grading of prostatic needle biopsies. Correlation with grade in 316 matched prostatectomies. *Am J Surg Pathol* 18:796-803, 1994A.

Bostwick DG. Grading prostate cancer. *Am J Clin Pathol* 102(suppl) S38-S56, 1994B.

Bostwick DG, Dousa MK, Crawford BG, et al. Neuroendocrine differentiation in prostatic intraepithelial neoplasia and adenocarcinoma. *Am J Surg Pathol* 18:1240-1246, 1994C.

Bostwick DG, Wollan P, Adlakha K. Collagenous micronodules in prostate cancer. A specific but infrequent diagnostic finding. *Arch Pathol Lab Med* 119:444-447, 1995A.

Bostwick DG. The pathology of incidental carcinoma. *Cancer Surv* 23:7-18, 1995B.

Bostwick DG, Qian J, Bergstralh E, et al. Prediction of capsular perforation and seminal vesicle invasion in prostate cancer. J Urol 155:1361-1367, 1996.

Bostwick DG, Montironi R. Evaluating radical prostatectomy specimens: therapeutic and prognostic importance. *Virchows Arch* 430:1-16, 1997A.

Bostwick DG, Dundore PA. Normal anatomy and histology. In: *Biopsy Pathology of the Prostate.* London: Chapman & Hall, 1997B:12.

Bostwick DG, Iczkowski KA, Amin MB, et al. Malignant lymphoma involving the prostate. Report of 62 cases. *Cancer* 83:732-738, 1998.

Bostwick DG, Cheng L. Overdiagnosis of prostatic adenocarcinoma. *Semin Urol Oncol* 17:199-205, 1999A.

Bostwick DG, Foster CS. Predictive factors in prostate cancer: current concepts from the 1999 College of American Pathologists Conference on Solid Tumor Prognostic Factors and the 1999 World Health Organization Second International Consultation on Prostate Cancer. *Semin Urol Oncol* 17:222-272, 1999B.

Bostwick DG, Grignon DJ, Hammond EH, et al. Prognostic factors in prostate cancer. College of American Pathologists Consensus Statement 1999. *Arch Pathol Lab Med* 124:995-1000, 2000.

Bovenberg SA, van der Zwet CJJ, van der Kwast TH, et al. Prostate-specific antigen expression in prostate cancer and its metastases. *J Urol Pathol* 1:55-61, 1993.

Brannigan RE, Shin E, Rademaker A, et al. The usefulness of touch preparation cytological evaluation and prostatic capsule involvement in prediction of prostate cancer recurrence. *J Urol* 160:1741-1747, 1998.

Brat DJ, Wills ML, Lecksell KL, et al. How often are diagnostic features missed with less extensive histologic sampling of prostate needle biopsy specimens? *Am J Surg Pathol* 23:257-262, 1999.

Brawer MK, Peehl DM, Stamey TA, et al. Keratin immunoreactivity in the benign and neoplastic human prostate. *Cancer Res* 45:3663-3667, 1985.

Brawer MK, Nagle RB, Pitts W, et al. Keratin immunoreactivity as an aid to the diagnosis of persistent adenocarcinoma in irradiated human prostates. *Cancer* 63:454-460, 1989.

Brawn PN. Histologic features of metastatic prostate cancer. In: Bostwick DG, ed. *Pathology of the Prostate.* New York: Churchill Livingstone; 83-903, 1990A.

Brawn P, Kuhl D, Johnson C III, et al. Stage D1 prostate carcinoma. The histologic appearance of nodal metastases and its relationship to survival. *Cancer* 65:538-543, 1990B.

Brenner PC, Rettig WJ, Sanz-Moncasi MP, et al. TAG-72 expression in primary, metastatic and hormonally treated prostate cancer as defined by monoclonal antibody CC49. *J Urol* 153:1575-1579, 1995.

Brennick JB, O'Connell JX, Dickersin GR, et al. Lipofuscin pigmentation (so-called "melanosis") of the prostate. *Am J Surg Pathol* 18:446-454, 1994.

Bretton PR, Melamed MR, Fair WR, et al. Detection of occult micrometastases in the bone marrow of patients with prostate carcinoma. *Prostate* 25:108-114, 1994.

Brinker DA, Ross JS, Tran TA, et al. Can ploidy of prostate carcinoma diagnosed in needle biopsy predict radical prostatectomy stage and grade? *J Urol* 162:2036-2039, 1999.

Bubendorf L, Schöpfer A, Wagner U, et al. Metastatic patterns of prostate cancer: an autopsy study of 1,589 patients. *Hum Pathol* 31:578-583, 2000.

Buscombe J, Hilson A. Nuclear medicine in prostate cancer. In: Kaisary AV, Murphy GP, Denis L, et al, eds. *Textbook of Prostate Cancer.* London: Martin Dunitz; 157-168, 1999.

Byar DP, Mostofi FK. Carcinoma of the prostate: prognostic evaluation of certain pathologic features in 208 radical prostatectomies. Examined by the step-section technique. *Cancer* 30:5-13, 1972.

Cangiano TG, Litwin MS, Naitoh J, et al. Intraoperative frozen section monitoring of nerve-sparing radical retropubic prostatectomy. *J Urol* 162:655-658, 1999.

Cansella R, Bubendorf L, Sauter G, et al. Focal neuroendocrine differentiation lacks prognostic significance in prostate core needle biopsies. *J Urol* 160:406-410, 1998.

Cantrell BB, DeKlerk DP, Eggleston JC, et al. Pathological factors that influence prognosis in stage A prostatic cancer: the influence of extent versus grade. *J Urol* 125:516-520, 1981.

Carstens PH. Perineural glands in normal and hyperplastic prostate. *J Urol* 123:686-688, 1980.

Carvalhal GF, Humphrey PA, Thorson P, et al. Visual estimate of percentage carcinoma is an independent predictor of prostate cancer recurrence after radical prostatectomy. *Cancer* 89:1308-1314, 2000.

Catalona WJ, Stein AJ. Accuracy of frozen section detection of lymph node metastases in prostatic carcinoma. *J Urol* 127:460-461, 1982.

Catalona WJ, Smith DS. Cancer recurrence and survival rates after anatomic radical retropubic prostatectomy for prostate cancer: intermediate-term results. *J Urol* 160:2428-2434, 1998.

Celebi MM, Venable DD, Nopajaroonsri C, et al. Prostate cancer metastatic only to the penis. *South Med J* 90:959-961, 1997.

Chan TY, Epstein JI. Follow-up of atypical prostate needle biopsies suspicious for cancer. *Urology* 53:351-355, 1999.

Chang CP, Chang YH, Chiang-H, et al. Incidental adenocarcinoma of the prostate: a retrospective analysis. *Eur Urol* 20:282-286, 1991.

Chang SS, Reuter VE, Heston WDW, et al. Comparison of anti-prostate-specific membrane antigen antibodies and other immunomarkers in metastatic prostate carcinoma. *Urology* 57:1179-1183, 2001.

Chen ME, Johnston DA, Tang K, et al. Detailed mapping of prostate carcinoma foci. *Cancer* 89:1800-1809, 2000.

Cheng L, Bergstralh EJ, Cheville JC, et al. Cancer volume of lymph node metastasis predicts progression in prostate cancer. *Am J Surg Pathol* 22:1491-1500, 1998.

Cheng L, Pisansky TM, Sebo TJ, et al. Cell proliferation in prostate cancer patients with lymph node metastasis: a marker for progression. *Clin Cancer Res* 5:2820-2823, 1999A.

Cheng L, Darson MF, Bergstralh EJ, et al. Correlation of margin status and extraprostatic extension with progression of prostate carcinoma. *Cancer* 86:1775-1782, 1999B.

Cheng L, Slezak J, Bergstralh EJ, et al. Dedifferentiation in the metastatic progression of prostate carcinoma. *Cancer* 86:657-663, 1999C.

Cheng L, Cheville JC, Bostwick DG. Diagnosis of prostate cancer in needle biopsies after radiation therapy. *Am J Surg Pathol* 23:1173-1183, 1999D.

Cheng L, Bergstralh EJ, Scherer BG, et al. Predictors of cancer progression in T1a prostate adenocarcinoma. *Cancer* 85:1300-1304, 1999E.

Cheng L, Pisansky TM, Ramnani DM, et al. Extranodal extension in lymph node-positive prostate cancer. Mod Pathol 13:113-118, 2000.

Cheville JC, Bostwick DG. Postatrophic hyperplasia of the prostate. A histologic mimic of prostatic adenocarcinoma. *Am J Surg Pathol* 19:1068-1076, 1995.

Cheville JC, Reznicek MJ, Bostwick DG. The focus of atypical glands suspicious for malignancy in prostatic needle biopsy specimens: incidence, histologic features, and clinical follow-up of cases diagnosed in a community practice. *Am J Clin Pathol* 108:633-640, 1997.

Cho KR, Epstein JI. Metastatic prostatic carcinoma to supradiaphragmatic lymph nodes. A clinicopathologic and immunohistochemical study. *Am J Surg Pathol* 11:457-463, 1987.

Chodak GW, Vogelzang NJ, Caplan RJ, et al. Independent prognostic factors in patients with metastatic (stage D2) prostate cancer. The Zoladex Study Group. *JAMA* 265:618-621, 1991.

Choe B-K, Pontes E, Rose NR, et al. Expression of human prostatic acid phosphatase in a pancreatic islet cell carcinoma. *Invest Urol* 15:312-318, 1978.

Christensen WN, Partin AW, Walsh PC, et al. Pathologic findings in clinical stage A2 prostate cancer. Relation of tumor volume, grade, and location to pathologic stage. *Cancer* 65:1021-1027, 1990.

Chu P, Wu E, Weiss LM. Cytokeratin 7 and cytokeratin 20 expression in epithelial neoplasms: a survey of 435 cases. *Mod Pathol* 13:962-972, 2000.

Chun TY. Coincidence of bladder and prostate cancer. *J Urol* 157:65-67, 1997.

Cina SJ, Epstein JI. Adenocarcinoma of the prostate with atrophic features. *Am J Surg Pathol* 21:289-295, 1997.

Cohen C, Bentz MS, Budgeon LR. Prostatic acid phosphatase in carcinoid and islet cell tumors [letter]. *Arch Pathol Lab Med* 107:277, 1983.

Cohen MK, Riggs MW, Brawn PN, et al. Serum prostate-specific antigen levels in stage A1 prostatic cancer. *Am J Clin Pathol* 100:127-129, 1993.

Cohen MK, Arber DA, Coffield KS, et al. Neuroendocrine differentiation in prostatic adenocarcinoma and its relationship to tumor progression. *Cancer* 74:1899-1903, 1994.

Cohen RJ, Haffejee Z, Steele GS, et al. Advanced prostate cancer with normal serum prostate-specific antigen values. *Arch Pathol Lab Med* 118:1123-1126, 1994.

Colombo P, Patriarca C, Alfano RM, et al. Molecular disorders in transitional vs peripheral zone adenocarcinoma. *Int J Cancer* 94:383-389, 2001.

Conrad S, Graefen M, Pichlmeier U, et al. Systematic sextant biopsies improve preoperative prediction of pelvic lymph node metastases in patients with clinically localized prostatic carcinoma. *J Urol* 159:2023-2029, 1998.

Copeland JN, Amin MB, Humphrey PA, et al. The morphologic spectrum of metastatic prostatic adenocarcinoma to the lung. Special emphasis on histologic features overlapping with other pulmonary neoplasms. *Am J Clin Pathol* 117:552-557, 2002.

Cramer SF. Benign glandular inclusion in prostatic nerve. *Am J Clin Pathol* 75:854-855, 1981.

Crundwell MC, Arkell DG, Gearty J, et al. Genetic alterations in incidentally diagnosed, transitional zone prostate cancer: a seven year follow-up. *J Urol* 158:1568-1575, 1997.

Crundwell MC, Morton DG, Arkell DG, et al. Genetic instability in incidentally discovered and advanced prostate cancer. *BJU Int* 84:123-127, 1999.

Cupp MR, Bostwick DG, Myers RP, et al. The volume of prostate cancer in the biopsy specimen cannot reliably predict the quantity of cancer in the radical prostatectomy specimen on an individual basis. *J Urol* 153:1543-1548, 1995.

Dalal R, Djakiew D. Molecular characterization of neurotrophin expression and the corresponding tropomyosin receptor kinases (TRKs) in epithelial and stromal cells of the human prostate. *Mol Cell Endocrinol* 134:15-22, 1997.

D'Amico AV, Whittington R, Malkowicz SB, et al. An analysis of the time course of postoperative prostate-specific antigen failure in patients with positive surgical margins: implications on the use of adjuvant therapy. *Urology* 47:538-547, 1996.

D'Amico AV, Whittington R, Malkowicz SB, et al. Combined modality staging of prostate carcinoma and its utility in predicting pathologic stage and postoperative prostate specific antigen failure. *Urology* 49(3A suppl):23-30, 1997.

D'Amico AV, Whittington R, Malkowicz SB, et al. The combination of preoperative prostate specific antigen and postoperative pathological findings to predict prostate specific antigen outcome in clinically localized prostate cancer. *J Urol* 160:2096-2101, 1998.

D'Amico AV, Wu Y, Chen MH, et al. Pathologic findings and prostate specific antigen outcome after radical prostatectomy for patients diagnosed on the basis of a single microscopic focus of prostate carcinoma with a Gleason score ≤7. *Cancer* 89:1810-1817, 2000.

D'Amico AV, Wu Y, Chen MH, et al. Perineural invasion as a predictor of biochemical outcome following radical prostatectomy for select men with clinically localized prostate cancer. *J Urol* 165:126-129, 2001.

D'Amico AV, Whittington R, Malkowicz SB, et al. Biochemical outcome after radical prostatectomy or external beam radiation therapy for patients with clinically localized prostate carcinoma in the prostate specific antigen era. *Cancer* 95:281-286, 2002.

Dardik M, Epstein JI. Efficacy of restaining prostate needle biopsies with high molecular weight cytokeratin. *Hum Pathol* 31:1155-1161, 2000.

Darson MF, Pacelli A, Roche P, et al. Human glandular kallikrein 2 expression in prostate adenocarcinoma and lymph node metastases. *Urology* 53:939-944, 1999.

Davidson D, Bostwick DG, Qian J, et al. Prostatic intraepithelial neoplasia is a risk factor for adenocarcinoma: predictive accuracy in needle biopsies. *J Urol* 154:1295-1299, 1995.

Davis BJ, Pisansky TM, Wilson TM, et al. The radial distance of extraprostatic extension of prostate carcinoma: implications for prostate brachytherapy. *Cancer* 85:2630-2637, 1999.

Davis G. Sensitivity of frozen section examination of pelvic lymph node for metastatic prostate carcinoma. *Cancer* 76:661-668, 1995.

De La Monte SM, Moore GW, Hutchins GM. Metastatic behavior of prostate cancer. Cluster analysis of patterns with respect to estrogen treatment. *Cancer* 58:985-993, 1986.

de la Taille A, Rubin MA, Bagiella E, et al. Can perineural invasion on prostate needle biopsy predict prostate specific antigen recurrence after radical prostatectomy? *J Urol* 162:103-106, 1999A.

de la Taille A, Katz A, Bagiella E, et al. Perineural invasion on prostate needle biopsy: an independent predictor of final pathologic stage. *Urology* 54:1039-1043, 1999B.

De Voogt HJ, Suciu S, Sylvester R, et al. Multivariate analysis of prognostic factors in patients with advanced prostatic cancer: results from 2 European Organization for Research on Treatment of Cancer trials. *J Urol* 141:883-888, 1989.

Deguchi T, Doi T, Ehara H, et al. Detection of micrometastatic prostate cancer cells in lymph nodes by reverse transcriptase-polymerase chain reaction. *Cancer Res* 53:5350-5354, 1993.

Del Rosario AD, Bui HX, Abdulla M, et al. Sulfur-rich prostatic intraluminal crystalloids: a surgical pathologic and electron probe x-ray microanalytic study. *Hum Pathol* 24:1159-1167, 1993.

Delides GS, Baltopoulos G, Papaharalampous NX. Latent carcinoma of the prostate: the probability of identifying small lesions in routine histology. *Br J Urol* 48:207-209, 1976.

Denton SE, Choy SH, Valk WL. Occult prostatic carcinoma diagnosed by the step-section technique of the surgical specimen. *J Urol* 93:296-298, 1965.

Deshmukh N, Foster CS. Grading prostate cancer. In: Foster CS, Bostwick DG, eds. *Pathology of the Prostate.* Philadelphia: WB Saunders; 191-227, 1998.

Devaraj LT, Bostwick DG. Atypical basal cell hyperplasia of the prostate. Immunophenotypic profile and proposed classification of basal cell proliferations. *Am J Surg Pathol* 17:645-659, 1993.

DeYoung BR, Wick MR. Immunohistologic evaluation of metastatic carcinomas of unknown origin: an algorithmic approach. *Semin Diagn Pathol* 17:184-193, 2000.

Dietrick DD, McNeal JE, Stamey TA. Core cancer length in ultrasound-guided systematic sextant biopsies: a preoperative evaluation of prostate cancer volume. *Urology* 45:987-992, 1995.

DiGiuseppe JA, Sauvageot J, Epstein JI. Increasing incidence of minimal residual cancer in radical prostatectomy specimens. *Am J Surg Pathol* 21:174-178, 1997.

Djavan B, Susani M, Bursa B, et al. Predictability and significance of multifocal prostate cancer in the radical prostatectomy specimen. *Tech Urol* 5:139-142, 1999.

Djavan B, Sesterhenn I, Hruby S, et al. Benign prostatic glands in the surgical margin of radical retropubic prostatectomies: redefining PSA nadir [abstract]. *J Urol* 163(suppl):142, 2000.

Dodson MK, Cliby WA, Keeney GL, et al. Skene's gland adenocarcinoma with increased serum level of prostate-specific antigen. *Gynecol Oncol* 55:304-307, 1994.

Donohue RE, Mani JH, Whitesel JA, et al. Pelvic lymph node dissection. Guide to patient management in clinically locally confined adenocarcinoma of prostate. *Urology* 20:559-565, 1982.

Douglas TH, McLeod DG, Mostofi FK, et al. Prostate-specific antigen-detected prostate cancer (stage T1c): an analysis of whole-mount prostatectomy specimens. *Prostate* 32:59-64, 1997.

Dugan JA, Bostwick DG, Myers RP, et al. The definition and preoperative prediction of clinically insignificant prostate cancer. *JAMA* 275:288-294, 1996.

Eastham JA, Scardino PT. Radical prostatectomy. In: Walsh PC, Retik AB, Vaughan ED Jr, et al, eds. *Campbell's Urology.* 7th ed. Philadelphia: WB Saunders; 2552-2553, 1998.

Eble JN, Tejada E. Cost implications of sampling strategies for prostatic transurethral resection specimens: analysis of 549 cases [abstract]. *Am J Clin Pathol* 85:382, 1986.

Eble JN, Epstein JI. Stage A carcinoma of the prostate. In: Bostwick DG, ed. *Pathology of the Prostate.* New York: Churchill Livingstone; 61-72, 1990.

Edelstein RA, Zietman AL, de las Morenas A, et al. Implications of prostatic micrometastases to the pelvic lymph nodes: an archival tissue study. *Urology* 47:370-375, 1996.

Egan AJM, Bostwick DG. Prediction of extraprostatic extension of prostate cancer based or needle biopsy findings: perineural invasion lacks significance on multivariate analysis. *Am J Surg Pathol* 21:1496-1500, 1997A.

Egan AJ, Lopez-Beltran A, Bostwick DG. Prostatic adenocarcinoma with atrophic features: malignancy mimicking a benign process. *Am J Surg Pathol* 21:931-935, 1997B.

Egawa S, Suyama K, Matsumoto K, et al. Improved predictability of extracapsular extension and seminal vesicle involvement based on clinical and biopsy findings in prostate cancer in Japanese men. *Urology* 52:443-440, 1998.

Egevad L, Norberg M, Mattson S, et al. Estimation of prostate cancer volume by multiple core biopsies before radical prostatectomy. *Urology* 52:653-658, 1998.

Egevad L, Granfors T, Karlberg L, et al. Percent Gleason grade 4/5 as prognostic factor in prostate cancer diagnosed at transurethral resection. *J Urol* 168:509-513, 2002.

Eisenberger MA, Crawford ED, Wolf M, et al. and Investigators of the National Cancer Institute Intergroup Study #0036. Prognostic factors in stage D2 prostate cancer; important implications for future trials: results of a cooperative intergroup study. *Semin Oncol* 1:613-619, 1994.

Elder JS, Gibbons RP, Correa RJ Jr, et al. Efficacy of radical prostatectomy for stage A2 carcinoma of the prostate. *Cancer* 56:2151-2154, 1985.

Elkin M, Mueller HP. Metastases from cancer of the prostate. Autopsy and roentgenological findings. *Cancer* 6:1246-1248, 1954.

Ellis DW, Leffers S, Davies JS, et al. Multiple immunoperoxidase markers in benign hyperplasia and adenocarcinoma of the prostate. *Am J Clin Pathol* 81:279-284, 1984.

Epstein JI, Paull G, Eggleston JC, et al. Prognosis of untreated stage A1 prostate carcinoma: a study of 94 cases with extended follow-up. *J Urol* 136:837-839, 1986.

Epstein JI, Oesterling JE, Eggleston JC, et al. Frozen section detection of lymph node metastases in prostatic carcinoma: accuracy in grossly uninvolved pelvic lymphadenectomy specimens. *J Urol* 136:1234-1237, 1986A.

Epstein JI, Kuhajda FP, Lieberman PH. Prostate-specific acid phosphatase immunoreactivity in adenocarcinomas of the urinary bladder. *Hum Pathol* 17:939-942, 1986B.

Epstein JI, Oesterling JE, Walsh PC. The volume and anatomical location of residual tumor in radical prostatectomy specimens removed for stage A1 prostate cancer. *J Urol* 139:975-979, 1988.

Epstein JI. The evaluation of radical prostatectomy specimens. Therapeutic and prognostic implications. *Pathol Ann* 26:159-210, 1991.

Epstein JI, Fynheer J. Acidic mucin in the prostate: can it differentiate adenosis from adenocarcinoma? *Hum Pathol* 23:1321-1325, 1992A.

Epstein JI, Armas OA. Atypical basal cell hyperplasia of the prostate. *Am J Surg Pathol* 16:1205-1214, 1992B.

Epstein JI. Cancer detected incidental to simple prostatectomy (stage A1). *J Cell Biochem* 16H(Suppl):78-82, 1992C.

Epstein JI, Carmichael M, Walsh PC. Adenocarcinoma of the prostate invading the seminal vesicle: definition and relation of tumor volume, grade and margins of resection to prognosis. *J Urol* 149:1040-1045, 1993A.

Epstein JI, Pizov G, Walsh PC. Correlation of pathologic findings with progression after radical retropubic prostatectomy. *Cancer* 71:3582-3593, 1993B.

Epstein JI, Carmichael MJ, Pizov G, et al. Influence of capsular penetration on progression following radical prostatectomy: a study of 196 cases with long-term followup. *J Urol* 150:135-141, 1993C.

Epstein JI, Carmichael M, Partin AW, et al. Is tumor volume an independent predictor of progression following radical prostatectomy? A multivariate analysis of 185 clinical stage B adenocarcinomas of the prostate with 5 years of follow-up. *J Urol* 149:1478-1481, 1993D.

Epstein JI. PSA and PAP as immunohistochemical markers in prostate cancer. *Urol Clin North Am* 20:757-770, 1993E.

Epstein JI, Walsh PC, Carmichael M, et al. Pathologic and clinical findings to predict tumor extent of nonpalpable (stage T1c) prostate cancer. *JAMA* 271:368-374, 1994A.

Epstein JI, Carmichael MJ, Partin AW, et al. Small high grade adenocarcinoma of the prostate in radical prostatectomy specimens performed for nonpalpable disease: pathogenetic and clinical implications. *J Urol* 151:1587-1592, 1994B.

Epstein JI. Diagnostic criteria of limited adenocarcinoma of the prostate on needle biopsy. *Hum Pathol* 26:223-229, 1995A.

Epstein JI, Grignon DJ, Humphrey PA, et al. Interobserver reproducibility in the diagnosis of prostatic intraepithelial neoplasia. *Am J Surg Pathol* 19:873-886, 1995B.

Epstein JI, Walsh PC, Sanfilippo F. Clinical and cost impact of second-opinion pathology. Review of prostate biopsies prior to radical prostatectomy. *Am J Surg Pathol* 20:851-857, 1996A.

Epstein JI. Diagnosing adenocarcinoma of the prostate on needle biopsy. In: *Prostate Biopsy Interpretation.* New York: Raven Press, 1996B:75-98.

Epstein JI. The diagnosis and reporting of adenocarcinoma of the prostate in core needle biopsy specimens. *Cancer* 78:350-356, 1996C.

Epstein JI. Incidence and significance of positive margins in radical prostatectomy specimens. *Urol Clin North Am* 23:651-663, 1996D.

Epstein JI, Partin AW, Sauvageot J, et al. Prediction of progression following radical prostatectomy: a multivariate analysis of 721 men with long-term follow-up. *Am J Surg Pathol* 20:286-292, 1996E.

Epstein JI, Sauvageot J. Do close but negative margins in radical prostatectomy specimens increase the risk of postoperative progression? *J Urol* 157:241-243, 1997.

Epstein JI, Pound CR, Partin AW, et al. Disease progression following radical prostatectomy in men with Gleason score 7 tumor. *J Urol* 160:97-101, 1998A.

Epstein JI. The role of perineural invasion and other biopsy characteristics as prognostic markers for localized prostate cancer. *Semin Urol Oncol* 16:124-128, 1998B.

Epstein JI, Partin AW, Potter SR, et al. Adenocarcinoma of the prostate invading the seminal vesicle. Prognostic stratification based on pathologic parameters. *Urology* 56:283-288, 2000A.

Epstein JI. Gleason score 2-4 adenocarcinoma of the prostate on needle biopsy. a diagnosis that should not be made. *Am J Surg Pathol* 24:477-478, 2000B.

Erbersdobler A, Hammerer P, Huland H, et al. Numerical chromosomal aberrations in transition-zone carcinomas of the prostate. *J Urol* 158:1594-1598, 1997.

Erbersdobler A, Fritz H, Schroger S, et al. Tumor grade, proliferation, apoptosis, microvessel density, p53, and hol-2 in prostate cancers: differences between tumors located in the transition zone and in the peripheral zone. *Eur Urol* 41:40-46, 2002.

Ergen A, Balbay MD, Irwin M, et al. Collision metastasis of bladder and prostate carcinoma to a single pelvic lymph node. *Int Urol Nephrol* 27:743-745, 1995.

Eskelinen M, Lipponen P, Majapuro R, et al. Prognostic factors in prostatic adenocarcinoma assessed by means of quantitative histology. *Eur Urol* 19:274-278, 1991.

Esrig D, Freeman JA, Elmajian DA, et al. Transitional cell carcinoma involving the prostate with a proposed staging classification for stromal invasion. *J Urol* 156:1071-1076, 1996.

Fan CY, Wang J, Barnes EL. Expression of androgen receptor and prostatic specific markers in salivary duct carcinoma. An immunohistochemical analysis of 13 cases and review of the literature. *Am J Surg Pathol* 24:579-586, 2000.

Faris G, Stein A, Sova Y, et al. Chromogranin is a marker for neuroendocrine differentiation in prostate carcinoma of various grades and stages. *J Urol Pathol* 3:29-36, 1995.

Federspiel BH, Burke AP, Sobin LH, et al. Rectal and colonic carcinoids. A clinicopathologic study of 84 cases. *Cancer* 65:135-140, 1990.

Feng J, de Guia K, Gharibian A, et al. Changes in the frequency and volume of "index" tumors and HGPIN in radical prostatectomy specimens (RPS) in the 1990s [abstract]. *Mod Pathol* 13:99A, 2000.

Fernandez P, Gomez M, Caballero T, et al. Prostatic acid phosphatase in cloacogenic carcinoma. *Acta Oncol* 29:776-777, 1990.

Fesseha T, Sakr W, Grignon D, et al. Prognostic implications of a positive apical margin in radical prostatectomy specimens. *J Urol* 158:2176-2179, 1997.

Fishleder A, Tubbs RR, Levin HS. An immunoperoxidase technique to aid in the differential diagnosis of prostatic carcinoma. *Cleve Clin Q* 48:331-335, 1981.

Fleming ID, Cooper JS, Henson DE, et al, eds. *Cancer Staging Manual (American Joint Committee on Cancer).* 5th ed. Philadelphia: Raven-Lippincott; 1997.

Ford TF, Butcher DN, Masters JRW, et al. Immunocytochemical localisation of prostate-specific antigen: specificity and application to clinical practice. *Br J Urol* 57:50-55, 1985.

Foster LS, Jajodia P, Fournier G Jr, et al. The value of prostate specific antigen and transrectal ultrasound guide biopsy in detecting prostatic fossa recurrences following radical prostatectomy. *J Urol* 149:1024-1028, 1993.

Fowler JE, Whitmore WF. The incidence and extent of pelvic lymph node metastases in apparently localized prostatic cancer. *Cancer* 47:2941-2945, 1981A.

Fowler JE Jr, Torgerson L, McLeod DG, et al. Radical prostatectomy with pelvic lymphadenectomy: observations on the accuracy of staging with lymph node frozen sections. *J Urol* 126:618-619, 1981B.

Fowler JE Jr, Mills SE. Operable prostatic carcinoma: correlations among clinical stage, pathologic stage, Gleason histological score and early disease-free survival. *J Urol* 133:49-52, 1985.

Fowler JE Jr, Brooks J, Pandey P, et al. Variable histology of anastomotic biopsies with detectable prostate specific antigen after radical prostatectomy. *J Urol* 153:1011-1014, 1995.

Franks LM. Atrophy and hyperplasia in the prostate proper. *J Pathol Bacteriol* 68:617-621, 1954.

Freedland SJ, Csathy GS, Dorey F, et al. Percent prostate needle biopsy tissue with cancer is more predictive of biochemical failure or adverse pathology after radical prostatectomy than prostate specific antigen of Gleason score. *J Urol* 167:516-520, 2002.

Freeman JA, Esrig D, Grossfeld GD, et al. Incidence of occult lymph node metastases in pathological stage C (pT2NO) prostate cancer. *J Urol* 154:474-478, 1995.

Fujikawa K, Sasaki M, Aoyama T, et al. Prognostic criteria in patients with stage D2 prostate cancer. Correlation with mean nuclear volume. *Cancer* 76:91-95, 1995.

Furusato M, Kato H, Takahashi H, et al. Crystalloids in latent prostatic carcinoma. *Prostate* 15:259-262, 1989.

Gaffey MJ, Mills SE, Swanson PE, et al. Immunoreactivity for BER-EP4 in adenocarcinomas, adenomatoid tumors, and malignant mesotheliomas. *Am J Surg Pathol* 16:593-599, 1992.

Gao CL, Dean RC, Pinto A, et al. Detection of circulating prostate-specific antigen expressing prostatic cells in the bone marrow of radical prostatectomy patients by sensitive reverse transcriptase polymerase chain reaction. *J Urol* 161:1070-1076, 1999.

Garcia FU, Taylor CA, Hou JS, et al. Increased cellularity of tumor-encased native vessels in prostate carcinoma is a marker for tumor progression. *Mod Pathol* 13:717-722, 2000.

Gardner TA, Lemer ML, Schlegel PN, et al. Microfocal prostate cancer: biopsy cancer volume does not predict actual tumor volume. *Br J Urol* 81:839-843, 1998.

Gatalica Z, Miettinen M. Distribution of carcinoma antigens CA19-9 and CA15-3. An immunohistochemical study of 400 tumors. *Appl Immunohistochem* 2:205-211, 1994.

Gatalica Z, Norris BA, Kovatich AJ. Immunohistochemical localization of prostate-specific antigen in ductal epithelium of male breast. Potential diagnostic pitfall in patients with gynecomastia. *Appl Immunohistol Mol Morphol* 8:158-161, 2000.

Gaudin PB, Epstein JI. Adenosis of the prostate. Histologic features in transurethral resection specimens. *Am J Surg Pathol* 18:863-870, 1994.

Gaudin PB, Epstein JI. Adenosis of the prostate. Histologic features in needle biopsy specimens. *Am J Surg Pathol* 19:737-747, 1995.

Gaudin PB, Reuter VE. Benign mimics of prostatic adenocarcinoma on needle biopsy. In: Fechner RE, Rosen PP, eds. *Anatomic Pathology 1997.* Vol 2. Chicago: American Society of Clinical Pathologists; 111-134, 1997.

Gaudin PB. Histopathologic effects of radiation and hormonal therapies on benign and malignant prostate tissues. *J Urol Pathol* 8:55-67, 1998.

Geddy PM, Reid IN. Selective sampling of yellow prostate chips: a specific method for detecting prostatic adenocarcinoma. *Urol Int* 56:33-35, 1996.

Geldof AA, De Kleijn MA, Rao BR, et al. Nerve growth factor stimulates in vitro invasive capacity of DU145 human prostatic cancer cells. *J Cancer Res Clin Oncol* 123:107-112, 1997.

Genega EM, Hutchinson B, Reuter VE, et al. Immunophenotype of high grade prostatic and urothelial carcinoma. *Mod Pathol* 13:1186-1191, 2000.

Gentile PS, Carloss HW, Huang TY, et al. Disseminated prostatic carcinoma simulating primary lung cancer. Indications for immunodiagnostic studies. *Cancer* 62:711-715, 1988.

George DJ, Kantoff PW. Prognostic indicators in hormone refractory prostate cancer. *Urol Clin North Am* 26:303-310, 1999.

Gerber GS, Thisted RA, Scardino PT, et al. Results of radical prostatectomy in men with clinically localized prostate cancer. Multi-institutional pooled analysis. *JAMA* 276:615-619, 1996.

Ghazizadeh M, Kagawa S, Izumi K, et al. Immunohistochemical detection of carcinoembryonic antigen in benign hyperplasia and adenocarcinoma of the prostate with monoclonal antibody. *J Urol* 131:501-503, 1984.

Giannulis I, Montironi R, Galluzzi CM, et al. Frequency and location of mitoses in prostatic intraepithelial neoplasia (PIN). *Anticancer Res* 13:2447-2451, 1993.

Gleason DF. Histologic grading of prostatic carcinoma. In: Bostwick DG, ed. *Pathology of the Prostate.* New York: Churchill Livingstone; 83-93, 1990.

Gohji K, Nomi M, Kizaki T, et al. "Collision phenomenon" of prostate and bladder cancers in lymph node metastases. *Int J Urol* 4:222-224, 1997.

Goldblum JR, Lloyd RV. Primary renal carcinoid: Case report and literature review. *Arch Pathol Lab Med* 117:855-858, 1993.

Goldstein NS, Bégin LR, Grody WW, et al. Minimal or no cancer in radical prostatectomy specimens: report of 13 cases of the "vanishing cancer phenomenon." *Am J Surg Pathol* 19:1002-1009, 1995A.

Goldstein NS, Qian J, Bostwick DG. Mucin expression in atypical adenomatous hyperplasia of the prostate. *Hum Pathol* 26:887-891, 1995B.

Goldstein NS, Martinez A, Vicini F, et al. The histology of radiation therapy effect on prostate adenocarcinoma as assessed by needle biopsy after brachytherapy boost. Correlation with biochemical failure. *Am J Clin Pathol* 110:765-775, 1998.

Goldstein NS. Immunophenotypic characterization of 225 prostate adenocarcinomas with intermediate or high Gleason scores. *Am J Clin Pathol* 117:471-477, 2002.

Golimbu M, Schinella R, Morales P, et al. Differences in pathological characteristics and prognosis of clinical A2 prostatic cancer from A1 and B disease. *J Urol* 119:618-622, 1978.

Gomella LG, White JL, McCue PA, et al. Screening for occult nodal metastasis in localized carcinoma of the prostate. *J Urol* 149:776-778, 1993.

Gonzalez CM, Kuzel T, Carter MA. Metastatic adenocarcinoma of the prostate to the orbit as a presenting symptom. *J Urol* 157:625, 1997.

Googe PB, McGinley KM, Fitzgibbon JF. Anticytokeratin antibody 34βE12 staining in prostate carcinoma. *Am J Clin Pathol* 107:219-223, 1997.

Goto Y, Ohori M, Arakawa A, et al. Distinguishing clinically important from unimportant prostate cancers before treatment: value of systematic biopsies. *J Urol* 156:1059-1063, 1996.

Graefen M, Hammerer P, Michl U, et al. Incidence of positive surgical margins after biopsy-selected nerve-sparing radical prostatectomy. *Urology* 51:437-442, 1998.

Graham SD Jr, Napalkov P, Watts L, et al. Microvascular invasion of the seminal vesicles in adenocarcinoma of the prostate. *Prostate* 28:359-363, 1996.

Grann A, Gaudin PB, Raben A, et al. Pathologic features from prostate needle biopsy and prognosis after I-125 brachytherapy. *Radiol Oncol Investig* 6:170-174, 1998.

Green R, Epstein JI. Use of intervening unstained slides for immunohistochemical stains for high molecular weight cytokeratin on prostate needle biopsies. *Am J Surg Pathol* 23:567-570, 1999.

Greene DR, Wheeler TM, Egawa S, et al. A comparison of the morphological features of cancer arising in the transition zone and in the peripheral zone of the prostate. *J Urol* 146:1069-1076, 1991A.

Greene DR, Egawa S, Neerhut G, et al. The distribution of residual cancer in radical prostatectomy specimens in stage A prostate cancer. *J Urol* 145:324-328, 1991B.

Greene DR, Taylor SR, Wheeler TM, et al. DNA ploidy by image analysis of individual foci of prostate cancer: a preliminary report. *Cancer Res* 51:4084-4089, 1991C.

Greene DR, Wheeler TM, Egawa S, et al. Relationship between clinical stage and histological origin in early prostate cancer: morphometric analysis. *Br J Urol* 68:499-509, 1991D.

Greene LF, Simon HB. Occult carcinoma of the prostate. Clinical and therapeutic study of eighty-three cases. *JAMA* 17:1494-1498, 1955.

Griebling TL, Özkutlu D, See WA, et al. Prognostic implications of extracapsular extension of lymph node metastases in prostate cancer. *Mod Pathol* 10:804-809, 1997.

Grignon DJ, Ro JY, Ordonez NG, et al. Basal cell hyperplasia, adenoid basal cell tumor, and adenoid cystic carcinoma of the prostate gland: an immunohistochemical study. *Hum Pathol* 19:1425-1433, 1988.

Grignon DJ, Ro JY, Ayala AG, et al. Primary adenocarcinoma of the urinary bladder. A clinicopathologic analysis of 72 cases. *Cancer* 67:2165-2172, 1991.

Grignon DJ, Ro JY, Srigley JR, et al. Sclerosing adenosis of the prostate gland: a lesion showing myoepithelial differentiation. *Am J Surg Pathol* 16:383-391, 1992.

Grignon DJ, O'Malley FP. Mucinous metaplasia in the prostate gland. *Am J Surg Pathol* 17:287-290, 1993.

Grignon DJ, Sakr WA. Zonal origin of prostatic adenocarcinoma: are there biologic differences between transition zone and peripheral zone adenocarcinomas of the prostate gland. *J Cell Biochem* 19(suppl):267-269, 1994.

Grignon DJ, Sakr WA. Histologic effects of radiation therapy and total androgen blockade on prostate cancer. *Cancer* 75:1837, 1995.

Grignon DJ. Minimal diagnostic criteria for adenocarcinoma of the prostate. *J Urol Pathol* 8:31-43, 1998.

Grob BM, Schellhammer PF, Brassil DN, et al. Changes in immunohistochemical staining of PSA, PAP, and TURP-27 following irradiation therapy for clinically localized prostate cancer. *Urology* 44:525-529, 1994.

Guerrero-Medrano J, Delgado R, Albores-Saavedra J. Signet-ring histiocytosis. A reactive disorder that mimics metastatic adenocarcinoma. *Cancer* 80:277-285, 1997.

Guillonneau B, Vallancien G. Laparoscopic radical prostatectomy: the Montsouris experience. *J Urol* 163:418-422, 2000.

Häggman M, Nybacka O, Nordin B, et al. Standardized in vitro mapping with multiple core biopsies of total prostatectomy specimens: localization and prediction of tumor volume and grade. *Br J Urol* 74:617-625, 1994.

Hall GS, Kramer CE, Epstein JI. Evaluation of radical prostatectomy specimens: a comparative analysis of sampling methods. *Am J Surg Pathol* 16:315-324, 1992.

Han M, Partin AW, Pound CR, et al. Long-term biochemical disease-free and cancer-specific survival following anatomic radical retropubic prostatectomy. The 15-year Johns Hopkins Experience. *Urol Clin North Am* 28:555-565, 2001.

Hancock C, Allen BC, Herrera GA. HMB-45 in adenocarcinomas. *Arch Pathol Lab Med* 115:886-890, 1991.

Hassan MO, Maksem J. The prostatic perineural space and its relation to tumor spread: an ultrastructural study. *Am J Surg Pathol* 4:143-148, 1980.

Heatley M, Maxwell P, Whiteside C, et al. Vimentin and cytokeratin expression in nodular hyperplasia and carcinoma of the prostate. *J Clin Pathol* 48:1031-1034, 1995.

Hedrick L, Epstein JI. Use of keratin 903 as an adjunct in the diagnosis of prostate carcinoma. *Am J Surg Pathol* 13:389-396, 1989.

Heffner JE, Duffey DJ, Schwarz MI. Massive pleural effusions from prostatic lymphangitic carcinomatosis. Resolution with endocrine therapy. *Arch Intern Med* 142:375-376, 1982.

Helpap B. Observations on the number, size and location of nucleoli in hyperplastic and neoplastic prostatic disease. *Histopathology* 13:203-211, 1988.

Henneberry JM, Kahane H, Humphrey PA, et al. The significance of intraluminal crystalloids in benign prostatic glands on needle biopsy. *Am J Surg Pathol* 21:725-728, 1997.

Henson DE, Hutter RVP, Farrow G, for members of the Cancer Committee and the Task Force on the Examination of Specimens Removed from Patients with Prostate Cancer. Practice protocol for the examination of specimens removed from patients with carcinoma of the prostate gland. *Arch Pathol Lab Med* 118:779-783, 1994.

Herman CM, Kattan MW, Scardino PT, et al. Quantification of high grade tumor is a predictor of disease progression in pT3N0 prostate cancer [abstract]. *Mod Pathol* 12:97A, 1999.

Herman CM, Kattan MW, Scardino PT, et al. Pathologic stage influences the significance of positive surgical margins in prostate cancer [abstract]. *Mod Pathol* 13:101A, 2000.

Herr HW, Donat SM. Prostatic tumor relapse in patients with superficial bladder tumors: 15-year outcome. *J Urol* 161:1854-1857, 1999.

Heyderman E, Brown BM, Richardson TC. Epithelial markers in prostatic, bladder, and colorectal cancer: an immunoperoxidase study of epithelial membrane antigen, carcinoembryonic antigen, and prostatic acid phosphatase. *J Clin Pathol* 37:1363-1369, 1984.

Hochtlen-Vollmar W, Gruber R, Bodenmuller H, et al. Occult epithelial tumor cells detected in bone marrow by an enzyme immunoassay specific for cytokeratin 19. *Int J Cancer* 70:396-400, 1997.

Hoda SA, Reed RJ. Morphologic characteristics of nucleoli in the differential diagnosis of well-differentiated prostatic adenocarcinoma [abstract]. *Am J Clin Pathol* 95:271, 1991.

Hoedemaeker RF, Rietbergen JBW, Kranse R, et al. Histopathological prostate cancer characteristics at radical prostatectomy after population based screening. *J Urol* 164:411-415, 2000.

Holmes EJ. Crystalloids of prostatic carcinoma: relationship to Bence-Jones crystals. *Cancer* 39:2073-2080, 1977.

Horoszewicz JS, Kawinski E, Murphy GP. Monoclonal antibodies to a new antigenic marker in epithelial prostatic cells and serum of prostatic cancer patients. *Anticancer Res* 7:927-935, 1987.

Howarth DJ, Aronson IB, Diamandis EP. Immunohistochemical localization of prostate-specific antigen in benign and malignant breast tissues. *Br J Cancer* 75:1646-1651, 1997.

Howat AJ, Mills PM, Lyons TJ, et al. Absence of S-100 protein in prostatic glands. *Histopathology* 13:468-470, 1988.

Hrebinko R, Taylor SR, Bahnson RR. Carcinoma of prostate metastatic to parotid gland. *Urology* 41:272-273, 1993.

Hu JC, Palapattu GS, Kattan MW, et al. The association of selected pathological features with prostate cancer in a single needle biopsy accession. *Hum Pathol* 29:1536-1538, 1998.

Huland H, Hammerer P, Henke RP, et al. Preoperative prediction of tumor heterogeneity and recurrence after radical prostatectomy for localized prostatic carcinoma with digital rectal examination, prostate specific antigen and the results of 6 systematic biopsies. *J Urol* 155:1344-1347, 1996.

Humphrey P, Vollmer RT. The ratio of prostate chips with cancer: a new measure of tumor extent and its relationship to grade and prognosis. *Hum Pathol* 19:411-418, 1988.

Humphrey PA, Vollmer RT. Corpora amylacea in adenocarcinoma of the prostate: prevalence in 100 prostatectomies and clinicopathologic correlations. *Surg Pathol* 3:133-141, 1990A.

Humphrey PA, Vollmer RT. Intraglandular tumor extent and prognosis in prostatic carcinoma: application of a grid method to prostatectomy specimens. *Hum Pathol* 21:799-804, 1990B.

Humphrey PA, Walther PJ, Currin SM, et al. Histologic grade, DNA ploidy, and intraglandular tumor extent as indicators of tumor progression of clinical stage B prostatic carcinoma. A direct comparison. *Am J Surg Pathol* 15:1165-1170, 1991A.

Humphrey PA. Mucin in severe dysplasia in the prostate. *Surg Pathol* 4:137-143, 1991B.

Humphrey PA, Walther PJ. Adenocarcinoma of the prostate. Part II. Tissue prognosticators. *Am J Clin Pathol* 100:256-269, 1993A.

Humphrey PA. Complete histologic serial sectioning of a prostate gland with adenocarcinoma. *Am J Surg Pathol* 17:468-472, 1993B.

Humphrey PA, Geary WA, Catalona WJ. Prostate specific antigen-detected versus digitally-detected prostatic adenocarcinoma: comparative pathologic features in needle biopsies [abstract]. *Mod Pathol* 6:61A, 1993C.

Humphrey PA, Frazier HA, Vollmer RT, et al. Stratification of pathologic features in radical prostatectomy specimens that are predictive of elevated initial postoperative serum prostate-specific antigen levels. *Cancer* 71:1821-1827, 1993D.

Humphrey PA, Baty J, Keetch D. Relationship between serum prostatic specific antigen, needle biopsy findings, and histopathologic features of prostatic carcinoma in radical prostatectomy tissues. *Cancer* 75:1842-1849, 1995.

Humphrey PA, Keetch DW, Smith DS, et al. Prospective characterization of pathologic features of prostatic carcinomas detected via serum prostate specific antigen-based screening. *J Urol* 155:816-820, 1996.

Humphrey PA, Vollmer RT. Percentage carcinoma as a measure of prostatic tumor size in radical prostatectomy tissues. *Mod Pathol* 10:326-333, 1997.

Humphrey PA, Kaleem Z, Swanson PE, et al. Pseudohyperplastic adenocarcinoma. *Am J Surg Pathol* 22:1239-1246, 1998A.

Humphrey PA, Vollmer RT. Relationships between serum prostate-specific antigen and histopathologic appearances of prostate carcinoma. In: Foster CS, Bostwick DG, eds. *Pathology of the Prostate.* Philadelphia: WB Saunders; 282-303, 1998B.

Hutter RVP, Montie JE, Busch C, et al. Current prognostic factors and their relevance to staging. *Cancer* 78:369-371, 1996.

Iczkowski KA, MacLennan GT, Bostwick DG. Atypical small acinar proliferation suspicious for malignancy in prostate needle biopsies: clinical significance in 33 cases. *Am J Surg Pathol* 21:1489-1495, 1997.

Iczkowski KA, Bassler JT, Schwob VS, et al. Diagnosis of "suspicious for malignancy" in prostate biopsies: predictive value for cancer. *Urology* 51:749-758, 1998.

Iczkowski KA, Cheng L, Crawford BG, et al. Steam heat with an EDTA buffer and protease digestion optimizes immunohistochemical expression of basal cell-specific antikeratin 34βE12 to discriminate cancer in prostatic epithelium. *Mod Pathol* 12:1-4, 1999.

Iczkowski KA, Bostwick DG. Criteria for biopsy diagnosis of minimal volume prostatic adenocarcinoma: analytic comparison with nondiagnostic but suspicious atypically small acinar proliferation. *Arch Pathol Lab Med* 124:98-107, 2000.

Irani J, Goujon JM, Ragni E, et al. High-grade inflammation in prostate cancer as a prognostic factor for biochemical recurrence after radical prostatectomy. *Urology* 54:467-472, 1999.

Irwin MB, Trapasso JG. Identification of insignificant prostate cancers: analysis of preoperative parameters. *Urology* 44:862-868, 1994.

Iselin CE, Robertson JE, Paulson DF. Radical perineal prostatectomy: oncological outcome during a 20-year period. *J Urol* 161:163-168, 1999.

Ishikawa S, Soloway MS, Van der Zwaag R, et al. Prognostic factors in survival free of progression after androgen deprivation therapy for treatment of prostate cancer. *J Urol* 141:1139-1142, 1989.

Iwamura M, Wu G, Abrahamsson PA, et al. Parathyroid hormone-related protein is expressed by prostatic neuroendocrine cells. *Urology* 43:667-674, 1994.

James GK, Pudek M, Berean KW, et al. Salivary duct carcinoma secreting prostate-specific antigen. *Am J Clin Pathol* 106:242-247, 1996.

Jensen PE, Gardner WA Jr, Piserchia PV. Prostatic crystalloids: association with adenocarcinoma. *Prostate* 1:25-30, 1980.

Jiang Z, Woda BA, Rock KL, et al. P504S: a new molecular marker for the detection of prostatic carcinoma. *Am J Surg Pathol* 25:1397-1404, 2001.

Jimenez RE, Lu JD, Mesic J, et al. Perineural invasion as a prognostic marker in patients treated by radiation therapy (RT): a radiation therapy oncology group (RTOG) study [abstract]. *Mod Pathol* 13:103A, 2000.

Jöbsis AC, De Vries GP, Meijer AEFH, et al. The immunohistochemical detection of prostatic acid phosphatase: its possibilities and limitations in tumor histochemistry. *Histochem J* 13:961-973, 1981.

Johnson DE, Chalbaud R, Ayala AG. Secondary tumors of the prostate. *J Urol* 112:507-508, 1974.

Jones EC. Resection margin status in radical retropubic prostatectomy specimens: relationship to type of operation, tumor size, tumor grade and local tumor extension. *J Urol* 144:89-93, 1990.

Jørgensen T, Yogesan K, Skjørten F, et al. Histopathological grading and DNA ploidy as prognostic markers in metastatic prostatic cancer. *Br J Cancer* 71:1055-1060, 1995.

Jørgensen T, Kanagasingam Y, Kaalhus O, et al. Prognostic factors in patients with metastatic (stage D2) prostate cancer: experience from the Scandinavian Prostatic Cancer Group Study-2. *J Urol* 158:164-170, 1997.

Kahane H, Sharp JW, Shuman GB, et al. Utilization of high molecular weight cytokeratin on prostate needle biopsies in an independent laboratory. *Urology* 45:981-986, 1995.

Kahler JE. Carcinoma of the prostate gland: a pathologic study. *J Urol* 41:557-574, 1934.

Kaleem Z, Swanson PE, Vollmer RT, et al. Prostatic adenocarcinoma with atrophic features. A study of 202 consecutive completely-embedded radical prostatectomy specimens. *Am J Clin Pathol* 109:695-703, 1998.

Kato M, Okada K, Yamashina M, et al. Clinical assessments on pre-treatment prognostic factors in 138 patients with advanced prostatic carcinoma (stage D2). *Acta Urol Jpn* 39:131-134, 1993.

Kattan MW, Eastham JA, Stapleton AMF, et al. A preoperative nomogram for disease recurrence following radical prostatectomy for prostate cancer. *J Natl Cancer Inst* 90:766-771, 1998.

Kattan MW, Wheeler TM, Scardino PT. Postoperative nomogram for disease recurrence after radical prostatectomy for prostate cancer. *J Clin Oncol* 17:1499-1507, 1999.

Kattan MW, Zelefsky MJ, Kupelian PA, et al. Pretreatment nomograms for predicting the outcome of three-dimensional conformal radiotherapy in prostate cancer. *J Clin Oncol* 18:3352-3359, 2000.

Kaufmann O, Volmerig J, Dietel M. Uroplakin III is a highly specific and moderately sensitive immunohistochemical marker for primary and metastatic urothelial carcinoma. *Am J Clin Pathol* 113:683-687, 2000.

Keetch DW, Humphrey PA, Smith DS, et al. Clinical and pathologic features of hereditary prostate cancer. *J Urol* 155:1841-1843, 1996.

Kim ED, Ignatoff JM. Unsuspected bladder carcinoma in patients undergoing radical prostatectomy. *J Urol* 152:397-400, 1994.

Kimura N, Sasano N, Namiki T. Evidence of hybrid cell of thyroid follicular cell and carcinoid cell in stromal carcinoid. *Int J Gynecol Pathol* 5:269-277, 1986A.

Kimura N, Sasano N. Prostate-specific acid phosphatase in carcinoid tumors. *Virchows Arch [A] Pathol Anat Histopathol* 410:247-251, 1986B.

King TC, Meyers J. Isolated metastasis to a pulmonary hamartoma. *Am J Surg Pathol* 19:472-475, 1995.

Köllermann J, Heseding B, Helpap B, et al. Comparative immunocytochemical assessment of isolated carcinoma cells in lymph nodes and bone marrow of patients with clinically localized prostate cancer. *Int J Cancer* 84:145-149, 1999.

Konski A, Rubin P, DiSantagnese PA, et al. Simultaneous presentation of adenocarcinoma of prostate and transitional cell carcinoma of bladder. *Urology* 37:202-206, 1991.

Kothari PS, Scardino PT, Ohori M, et al. Incidence, location and significance of periprostatic and periseminal vesicle lymph nodes in prostate cancer. *Am J Surg Pathol* 25:1429-1432, 2001.

Kramer CE, Epstein JI. Nucleoli in low-grade prostate adenocarcinoma and adenosis. *Hum Pathol* 24:618-623, 1993.

Kramer SA, Farnham R, Glenn JF, et al. Comparative morphology of primary and secondary deposits of prostatic adenocarcinoma. *Cancer* 48:271-273, 1981.

Kramolowsky EV, Narayana AS, Platz CE, et al. The frozen section in lymphadenectomy for carcinoma of the prostate. *J Urol* 131:899-900, 1984.

Krijnen JLM, Janssen PJA, Ruizeveld de Winter JA, et al. Do neuroendocrine cells in human prostate cancer express in androgen receptor? *Histochemistry* 100:393-398, 1993.

Krijnen JLM, Bogdanowicz JFAT, Seldenrijk CA, et al. The prognostic value of neuroendocrine differentiation in adenocarcinoma of the prostate in relation to progression of disease after endocrine therapy. *J Urol* 158:171-174, 1997.

Kronz JD, Shaikh AA, Epstein JI. Atypical cribriform lesions on prostate biopsy. *Am J Surg Pathol* 25:147-155, 2001.

Kunze E, Weidhase A, Schulz H. Incidence and morphology of concurrent primary carcinomas of the urinary bladder and prostate in transurethral resection specimens. *Zentralbl Pathol* 140:113-122, 1994.

Kuo T. Cancer to hamartoma metastasis. *Arch Pathol Med* 102:658, 1978.

Kuopio T, Ekfors TO, Nikkanen V, et al. Acinar cell carcinoma of the pancreas: report of three cases. *APMIS* 103:69-78, 1995.

Labess M. Occult carcinoma in clinically benign hypertrophy of the prostate: a pathological and clinical study. *J Urol* 68:893-902, 1952.

Lalli C, Gogia H, Raju L. Multiple endobronchial metastases from carcinoma of the prostate. *Urology* 21:164-165, 1983.

Lane RB Jr, Lane CG, Mangold KA, et al. Needle biopsies of the prostate: what constitutes adequate histologic sampling? *Arch Pathol Lab Med* 122:833-835, 1998.

Larsen MP, Carter HB, Epstein JI. Can stage A1 tumor extent be predicted by transurethral resection, tumor volume, percent, or grade? A study of 64 stage A1 radical prostatectomies with comparison to prostates removed for stage A2 and B disease. *J Urol* 146:1059-1063, 1991.

Lattanzi JP, Hanlon AL, Hanks GE. Early stage prostate cancer treated with radiation therapy: stratifying an intermediate risk group. *Int J Radiat Oncol Biol Phys* 38:569-573, 1997.

Latulippe E, Satagopan J, Smith A, et al. Comprehensive gene expression analysis of metastatic prostate cancer reveals distinct transcriptional programs associated with metastatic disease. *Cancer Res* 62:4499-4506, 2002.

Lawton CA, Steinberg GD. Management options for patients with lymph node metastases from prostate cancer. In: Vogelzang N, Scardino PT, Shipley WU, et al, eds. *Comprehensive Textbook of Genitourinary Oncology.* 2nd ed. Baltimore: Williams & Wilkins; 761-773, 2000.

Lee WR, Hanlon A, Hanks GE. Do the results of systematic biopsies predict outcome in patients with T1-T2 prostate cancer treated with radiation therapy alone? *Urology* 47:704-707, 1996.

Legge DA, Good CA, Ludwig J. Roentgenologic features of pulmonary carcinomatosis from carcinoma of the prostate. *Am J Roentgenol* 111:360-364, 1971.

Leong AS, Gilham P, Milios J. Cytokeratins and vimentin intermediate filament proteins in benign and neoplastic prostatic epithelium. *Histopathology* 13:435-442, 1988.

Lessels AM, Burnett RA, Howatson SR, et al. Observer variability in the histopathological reporting of needle biopsy specimens of the prostate. *Hum Pathol* 28:646-649, 1997.

Leung CS, Srigley JR. Distribution of lipochrome pigment in the prostate gland: biologic and diagnostic implications. *Hum Pathol* 26:1302-1307, 1995.

Levi AW, Epstein JI. Pseudohyperplastic prostatic adenocarcinoma on needle biopsy and simple prostatectomy. *Am J Surg Pathol* 24:1039-1048, 2000.

Lewis JS Jr, Vollmer RT, Humphrey PA. Carcinoma extent in prostate needle biopsy tissue in the prediction of whole gland tumor volume in a screening population. *Am J Clin Pathol* 118:442-450, 2002.

Li CY, Lam WKW, Yam LT. Immunohistochemical diagnosis of prostatic cancer with metastasis. *Cancer* 46:706-712, 1980.

Li SL, Goko H, Xu ZD, et al. Expression of insulin-like growth factor (IGF)-II in human prostate, breast, bladder, and paraganglioma tumors. *Cell Tissue Res* 291:469-479, 1998.

Leibman BD, Dillioglugil O, Wheeler TM, et al. Distant metastasis after radical prostatectomy in patients without an elevated serum prostate specific antigen level. *Cancer* 76:2530-2534, 1995.

Lindell MM, Doubleday LC, von Eschenbach AC, et al. Mediastinal metastases from prostatic carcinoma. *J Urol* 128:331-334, 1982.

Lindeman N, Weidner N. Immunohistochemical profile of prostatic and urothelial carcinoma. Impact of heat-induced epitope retrieval and presentation of tumors with intermediate features. *Appl Immunohistochem* 4:264-275, 1996.

Lippert MC, Bensimon H, Javadpour N. Immunoperoxidase staining of acid phosphatase in human prostatic tissue. *J Urol* 128:1114-1116, 1982.

Liu L, Devine P, Einhorn E, et al. Incidental finding of an isolated prostate cancer metastasis in an inguinal hernia sac. *J Urol* 164:457-458, 2000.

Lo J, Kerns BJ, Amling CL, et al. Correlation of DNA ploidy and histologic diagnosis from prostate core-needle biopsies: is DNA ploidy more sensitive than histology for the diagnosis of carcinoma in small specimens? *J Surg Oncol* 63:41-45, 1996.

Logothetis CJ, Hossien NM, Ro J. Neuroendocrine progression. In: Vogelzang N, Scardino PT, Shipley WU, et al, eds. *Comprehensive Textbook of Genitourinary Oncology.* Baltimore: Williams & Wilkins; 914-919, 1996.

Lowe BA, Listrom MB. Incidental carcinoma of the prostate: an analysis of the predictors of progression. *J Urol* 140:1340-1344, 1988.

Loy TS, Quesenberry JT, Sharp SC. Distribution of CA 125 in adenocarcinomas. An immunohistochemical study of 481 cases. *Am J Clin Pathol* 98:175-179, 1992.

Loy TS, Sharp SC, Andershock CJ, et al. Distribution of CA19-9 in adenocarcinomas and transitional cell carcinomas. An immunohistochemical study of 527 cases. *Am J Clin Pathol* 99:726-728, 1993.

Luna-Moré S, Florez P, Ayala A, et al. Neutral and acid mucins and eosinophil and argyrophil crystalloids in carcinoma and atypical adenomatous hyperplasia of the prostate. *Pathol Res Pract* 193:291-298, 1997.

Luo J, Zha S, Gage WR, et al. Alpha-methylacyl-CoA racemose: a new molecular marker for prostate cancer. *Cancer Res* 82:2220-2226, 2002.

Madersbacher S, Schatzl G, Susani M, et al. Prostatic metastasis of a small cell lung cancer in a young male. *Eur Urol* 26:267-269, 1994.

Mahan DE, Bruce AW, Manley PN, et al. Immunohistochemical evaluation of prostatic carcinoma before and after radiotherapy. *J Urol* 124:488-491, 1980.

Manseck A, Wirth M, Theiss M, et al. Radical prostatectomy in patients with incidental prostate carcinoma. *Urol Int* 53:196-208, 1994.

Mao H, Hoshi S, Takahashi T, et al. Detection of PSA mRNA from the peripheral blood and pelvic lymph nodes in patients with prostatic cancer by means of reverse transcription-polymerase chain reaction (RT-PCR) [in Japanese]. *Jpn J Urol* 89:596-603, 1998.

Maraj BH, Whelan P, Markham AF. Prostate-specific membrane antigen. *Br J Urol* 81:523-528, 1998.

Marcovich R, Wojno KJ, Wei JT, et al. Bladder neck–sparing modification of radical prostatectomy adversely affects surgical margins in pathologic T3a prostate cancer. *Urology* 55:904-908, 2000.

Maru N, Ohori M, Kattan MW, et al. Prognostic significance of the diameter of perineural invasion in radical prostatectomy specimens. *Hum Pathol* 32:828-833, 2001.

Masuda M, Ishibashi Y, Fukuoka H, et al. Incidental prostatic carcinoma obtained from the tissue by transurethral resection [in Japanese]. *Acta Urol Jpn* 35:403-407, 1989.

Matzkin H, Soloway MS, Schellhammer PF, et al. Prognostic factors in stage D2 prostate cancer treated with a pure non-steroidal antiandrogen. *Cancer* 72:1286-1290, 1993.

May EE, Perentes E. Anti-Leu 7 immunoreactivity with human tumours: its value in the diagnosis of prostatic adenocarcinoma. *Histopathology* 11:295-304, 1987.

Mayordomo JI, Guerra JM, Guijarro C, et al. Neoplasms of unknown primary site: a clinicopathological study of autopsied patients. *Tumori* 79:321-324, 1993.

McDermott MB, Kyriakos M, Flanagan FL. Posttraumatic fibro-osseous lesion of rib. *Hum Pathol* 30:770-780, 1999.

McIntire TL, Franzini DA. The presence of benign prostatic glands in perineural spaces. *J Urol* 135:507-509, 1986.

McIntire TL, Murphy WM, Coon JS, et al. The prognostic value of DNA ploidy combined with histologic substaging of incidental carcinoma of the prostate gland. *Am J Clin Pathol* 89:370-373, 1988.

McNeal JE, Reese JH, Redwine EA, et al. Cribriform adenocarcinoma of the prostate. *Cancer* 58:1714-1719, 1986A.

McNeal JE, Bostwick DG, Kindrachuk RA, et al. Patterns of progression in prostate cancer. *Lancet* 1:60-63, 1986B.

McNeal JE, Price HM, Redwine EA, et al. Stage A versus stage B adenocarcinoma of the prostate: morphological comparison and biological significance. *J Urol* 139:61-65, 1988A.

McNeal JE, Redwine EA, Freiha FS, et al. Zonal distribution of prostatic adenocarcinoma: correlation with histologic pattern and direction of spread. *Am J Surg Pathol* 12:847-906, 1988B.

McNeal JE, Villers AA, Redwine EA, et al. Capsular penetration in prostate cancer. Significance for natural history and treatment. *Am J Surg Pathol* 14:240-247, 1990A.

McNeal JE, Villers AA, Redwine EA, et al. Histologic differentiation, cancer volume, and pelvic lymph node metastasis in adenocarcinoma of the prostate. *Cancer* 66:1225-1233, 1990B.

McNeal JE, Alroy J, Villers A, et al. Mucinous differentiation in prostatic adenocarcinoma. *Hum Pathol* 22:979-988, 1991.

McNeal JE. Prostatic microcarcinomas in relation to cancer origin and the evolution to clinical cancer. *Cancer* 71 (3 suppl):984-991, 1993.

McNeal JE, Yemoto CEM. Significance of demonstrable vascular space invasion for the progression of prostatic adenocarcinoma. *Am J Surg Pathol* 20:1351-1360, 1996.

McWilliam LJ, Manson C, George NJR. Neuroendocrine differentiation and prognosis in prostatic adenocarcinoma. *Br J Urol* 80:287-290, 1997.

Mebust WK, Holtgrewe HL, Cockett ATK, et al. Transurethral prostatectomy: immediate and postoperative complications. A comparative study of 13 participating institutions evaluating 3,885 patients. *J Urol* 141:243-247, 1989.

Melchior J, Valk WL, Foret JD, et al. Transurethral resection of the prostate via perineal urethrostomy: complete analysis of 7 years of experience. *J Urol* 111: 640-643, 1974.

Melchior SW, Corey E, Ellis WJ, et al. Early tumor cell dissemination in patients with clinically localized carcinoma of the prostate. *Clin Cancer Res* 3:249-256, 1997.

Mestitz H, Pierce RJ, Holmes PW. Intrathoracic manifestations of disseminated prostatic adenocarcinoma. *Respir Med* 83:161-166, 1989.

Miller GJ, Cygan JM. Morphology of prostate cancer: the effects of multifocality on histological grade, tumor volume and capsule penetration. *J Urol* 152:1709-1713, 1994.

Miller MK, Unger PD, Bleiweiss IJ. Immunohistochemical analysis of prostate specific antigen in breast cancer. *Breast Cancer Res Treat* 68:111-116, 2001.

Mills SE, Bostwick DG, Murphy WM, et al. A symposium on the surgical pathology of the prostate. *Pathol Annu* 25:109-158, 1990.

Millward C, Weidner N. CD30 (Ber-H2) expression in nonhematopoietic tumors. *Appl Immunohistochem* 6:164-168, 1998.

Mintz ER, Smith GG. Autopsy findings in 100 cases of prostatic cancer. *N Engl J Med* 211:479-487, 1934.

Mohler JL, Partin AW, Epstein JI, et al. Prediction of prognosis in untreated stage A2 prostatic carcinoma. *Cancer* 69:511-519, 1992.

Monda JM, Barry MJ, Oesterling JE. Prostate specific antigen cannot distinguish stage T1a (A1) prostate cancer from benign prostatic hyperplasia. *J Urol* 151:1291-1295, 1994.

Moore GH, Lawshe B, Murphy J. Diagnosis of adenocarcinoma in transurethral resectates of the prostate gland. *Am J Surg Pathol* 10:165-169, 1986.

Moore R. The morphology of small prostatic carcinoma. *J Urol* 33:224-234, 1935.

Mostofi FK, Sesterhenn IA, Davis CJ Jr. A pathologist's view of prostatic carcinoma. *Cancer* 71 (3 suppl):906-932, 1993.

Moul JW, Lewis DJ, Ross AA, et al. Immunohistologic detection of prostate cancer pelvic lymph node micrometastases: correlation to preoperative serum prostate-specific antigen. *Urology* 43:68-73, 1994.

Moul JW, Paulson DF, Fuller G, et al. Prostate cancer with solitary parotid metastasis correctly diagnosed with immunohistochemical stains. *J Urol* 142:1328-1329, 1989.

Mulders PF, Dijkman GA, Fernandez del Moral P, et al. Analysis of prognostic factors in disseminated prostatic cancer. An update. Dutch Southeastern Urological Cooperative Group. *Cancer* 65:2758-2761, 1990.

Murphy WM, Dean PJ, Brasfield JA, et al. Incidental carcinoma of the prostate. How much sampling is adequate? *Am J Surg Pathol* 10:170-174, 1986.

Murphy WM, Gaeta JF. Diseases of the prostate gland and seminal vesicles. In: Murphy WM, ed. *Urological Pathology.* Philadelphia: WB Saunders; 170-202, 1989.

Myers RB, Meredith RF, Schlom J, et al. Tumor-associated glycoprotein-72 is highly expressed in prostatic adenocarcinomas. *J Urol* 152:243-246, 1994.

Myers RB, Schlom J, Srivastava S, et al. Expression of tumor-associated glycoprotein 72 in prostatic intraepithelial neoplasia and prostatic adenocarcinoma. *Mod Pathol* 8:260-265, 1995.

Myers RP, Fleming TR. Course of localized adenocarcinoma of the prostate treated by radical prostatectomy. *Prostate* 4:461-472, 1983.

Nadji M, Tabei SZ, Castro A, et al. Prostatic origin of tumors. An immunohistochemical study. *Am J Clin Pathol* 73:735-739, 1980.

Nadji M, Tabei SZ, Castro A, et al. Prostate-specific antigen: an immunohistologic marker for prostatic neoplasms. *Cancer* 48:1229-1232, 1981.

Nagle RB, Brawer MK, Kittelson J, et al. Phenotypic relationships of prostatic intraepithelial neoplasia to invasive prostatic carcinoma. *Am J Pathol* 138:119-128, 1991.

Nagle RB. Intermediate filament expression in prostate cancer. *Cancer Metastasis Rev* 15:473-482, 1996.

Nakopoulou L, Stefanafi K, Deliveliotis C, et al. Neuroendocrine differentiation and proliferation state estimation in the hyperplastic and neoplastic human prostate. *J Urol Pathol* 4:239-251, 1996.

Nelson RS, Epstein JI. Prostatic carcinoma with abundant xanthomatous cytoplasm. Foamy gland carcinoma. *Am J Surg Pathol* 20:419-426, 1996.

Newman AJ Jr, Graham MA, Carlton CE Jr, et al. Incidental carcinoma of the prostate at the time of transurethral resection: importance of evaluating every chip. *J Urol* 128:948-950, 1982.

Nichols RT, Barry JM, Hodges C. The morbidity of radical prostatectomy for multifocal stage I prostatic carcinoma. *J Urol* 117:83-84, 1977.

Noguchi M, Stamey TA, McNeal JE, et al. An analysis of 148 consecutive transition zone cancers: clinical and histological characteristics. *J Urol* 163:1751-1755, 2000.

Noordzij MA, van der Kwast TH, van Steenbrugge GJ, et al. The prognostic influence of neuroendocrine cells in prostate cancer: results of a long-term follow-up study with patients treated by radical prostatectomy. *Int J Cancer* 62:252-258, 1995.

Öbek C, Sadek S, Lai S, et al. Positive surgical margins with radical retropubic prostatectomy: anatomic site-specific pathologic analysis and impact on prognosis. *Urology* 54:682-688, 1999.

Oefelein MG, Kaul K, Herz B, et al. Molecular detection of prostate epithelial cells from the surgical field and peripheral circulation during radical prostatectomy. *J Urol* 155:238-242, 1996.

Oesterling JE, Brendler CB, Epstein JI, et al. Correlation of clinical stage, serum prostatic phosphatase and preoperative Gleason grade with final pathological stage in 275 patients with clinically localized adenocarcinoma of the prostate. *J Urol* 138:92-98, 1987.

Ohori M, Scardino PT, Lapin SL, et al. The mechanisms and prognostic significance of seminal vesicle involvement by prostate cancer. *Am J Surg Pathol* 17:1252-1261, 1993.

Ohori M, Wheeler TM, Dunn JK, et al. The pathological features and prognosis of prostate cancer detectable with current diagnostic tests. *J Urol* 152:1714-1720, 1994.

Ohori M, Wheeler TM, Kattan MW, et al. Prognostic significance of positive surgical margins in radical prostatectomy specimens. *J Urol* 154:1818-1824, 1995.

Ohori M, Abbas F, Wheeler TM, et al. Pathological features and prognostic significance of prostate cancer in the apical section determined by whole mount histology. *J Urol* 161:500-504, 1999.

Okada H, Tsubura A, Okamura A, et al. Keratin profiles in normal/hyperplastic prostates and prostate carcinoma. *Virchows Arch A Pathol Anat Histopathol* 421:157-161, 1992.

Okegawa T, Nutahara K, Higashihara E. Detection of micrometastatic prostate cancer cells in the lymph nodes by reverse transcriptase polymerase chain reaction is predictive of biochemical recurrence in pathological stage T2 prostate cancer. *J Urol* 163:1183-1188, 2000.

Oliai BR, Kahane H, Epstein JI. A clinicopathologic analysis of urothelial carcinomas diagnosed on prostate needle biopsy. *Am J Surg Pathol* 25:794-801, 2001.

O'Malley FP, Grignon DJ, Keeney M, et al. DNA heterogeneity in prostatic adenocarcinoma. A DNA flow cytometric mapping study with whole organ sections of prostate. *Cancer* 71:2797-2802, 1993.

O'Malley KJ, Pound CR, Walsh PC, et al. Influence of perineural invasion on long-term biochemical disease-free survival after radical prostatectomy. *Urology* 59:85-90, 2002.

Oppenheimer JR, Wills ML, Epstein JI. Partial atrophy in prostate needle cores. Another diagnostic pitfall for the surgical pathologist. *Am J Surg Pathol* 22:440-445, 1998.

Ordoñez NG, Ro JY, Ayala AG. Metastatic prostatic carcinoma presenting as an oncocytic tumor. *Am J Surg Pathol* 16:1007-1012, 1992.

Ordoñez NG: Thrombomodulin expression in transitional cell carcinoma. *Am J Clin Pathol* 110:385-390, 1998.

Ornstein DK, Colberg JW, Virgo KS, et al. Evaluation and management of men whose radical prostatectomies failed: results of an international survey. *Urology* 52:1047-1054, 1998.

Osther PJ, Lontoft E. Metastasis to the penis. Case reports and review of the literature. *Int Urol Nephrol* 23:161-167, 1991.

Ostrowski ML, Chakroborty S, Wheeler TM. DNA ploidy, Gleason grade, and percentage of intraglandular tumor correlate with non-organ-confined prostatic adenocarcinoma [abstract]. *Mod Pathol* 9:80A, 1996.

Ostrowski ML, Chakraborty S, Wheeler TM. DNA ploidy lacks independent prognostic significance in prostate cancer in patients treated by radical prostatectomy [abstract]. *Mod Pathol* 13:112A, 2000.

Pacelli A, Lopez-Beltran A, Egan AJM, et al. Prostatic adenocarcinoma with glomeruloid features. *Hum Pathol* 29:543-546, 1998.

Palken M, Cobb OE, Warren BH, et al. Prostate cancer: correlation of digital rectal examination, transrectal ultrasound and prostate-specific antigen levels with tumor volumes in radical prostatectomy specimens. *J Urol* 143:1155-1162, 1990.

Pan CC, Potter SR, Partin AW, et al. The prognostic significance of tertiary Gleason patterns of higher grade in radical prostatectomy specimens: a proposal to modify the Gleason grading system. *Am J Surg Pathol* 24:563-569, 2000.

Pansare V, Andea A, Ward C, et al. Correlation of benign epithelium at the resection margins of organ confined prostate cancer (PCA) with PSA recurrence [abstract]. *Mod Pathol* 14:120, 2001.

Pantel K, Schlimok G, Angstwurm M, et al. Methodological analysis of immunocytochemical screening for disseminated epithelial tumor cells in bone marrow. *J Hematoth* 3:165-173, 1994.

Papotti M, Paties C, Peveri V, et al. Immunocytochemical detection of prostate-specific antigen (PSA) in skin adnexal and breast tissues and tumors. *Basic Appl Histochem* 33:25-29, 1989.

Parfitt HE Jr, Smith JA Jr, Gliedman JB, et al. Accuracy of staging in A1 carcinoma of the prostate. *Cancer* 51:2346-2350, 1983A.

Parfitt HE Jr, Smith JA Jr, Seaman JP, et al. Surgical treatment of stage A2 prostatic carcinoma: significance of tumor grade and extent. *J Urol* 129:763-765, 1983B.

Parker DC, Folpe AL, Bell J, et al. Potential utility of uroplakin III, thrombomodulin, high molecular weight cytokeratin, and cytokeratin 20 in noninvasive, invasive, and metastatic urothelial (transitional cell carcinomas). *Am J Surg Pathol* 29:1-10, 2003.

Parsons JK, Gage WR, Nelson WG, et al. P63 protein expression is rare in prostate adenocarcinoma: implications for cancer diagnosis and carcinogenesis. *Urology* 58:619-624, 2001.

Partin AW, Epstein JI, Cho KR, et al. Morphometric measurement of tumor volume and percent of gland involvement as predictors of pathologic stage in clinical stage B prostate cancer. *J Urol* 141:341-345, 1989.

Partin AW, Carter HB, Chan DW, et al. Prostate-specific antigen in the staging of localized prostate cancer: influence of tumor differentiation, tumor volume and benign hyperplasia. *J Urol* 143:747-752, 1990.

Partin AW, Pearson JD, Landis PK, et al. Evaluation of serum prostate specific antigen velocity after radical prostatectomy to distinguish local recurrence from distant metastases. *Urology* 43:649-659, 1994.

Partin AW, Piantadosi S, Sanda MG, et al. Selection of men at high risk for disease recurrence for experimental adjuvant therapy following radical prostatectomy. *Urology* 45:831-888, 1995.

Partin AW, Kattan MW, Subong EN, et al. Combination of prostate-specific antigen, clinical stage, and Gleason score to predict pathological stage of localized prostate cancer: a multi-institutional update. *JAMA* 277:1445-1451, 1997.

Paulson DF, Robertson JE, Daubert LM, et al. Radical prostatectomy in stage A prostatic adenocarcinoma. *J Urol* 140:535-539, 1988.

Paulson DF, Moul JW, Walther PJ. Radical prostatectomy for clinical stage T1-2NOMO prostatic adenocarcinoma: long-term results. *J Urol* 144:1180-1184, 1990.

Paulson DF. Impact of radical prostatectomy in the management of clinically localized disease. *J Urol* 152:1826-1830, 1994.

Pearle MS, Oyasu R, Hidvegi D, et al. Touch preparation cytological evaluation of radical prostatectomy specimens. *J Urol* 152:124-128, 1994.

Peller PA, Young DC, Marmaduke DP, et al. Sextant prostate biopsies. A histopathologic correlation with radical prostatectomy specimens. *Cancer* 75:530-538, 1995.

Pennington JW, Prentiss RJ, Howe G. Radical prostatectomy for cancer: significance of perineural lymphatic invasion. *J Urol* 97:1075-1077, 1967.

Peters-Gee JM, Miles BJ, Cerny JC, et al. Prognostic significance of DNA quantitation in stage D1 prostate carcinoma with the use of image analysis. *Cancer* 70:1159-1165, 1992.

Petersen RO. *Urologic Pathology.* 2nd ed. Philadelphia: JB Lippincott; 623, 633, 1992.

Petras AF, Wollett FC. Metastatic prostatic pulmonary nodules with normal bone image. *J Nucl Med* 24:1026-1027, 1983.

Pfister S, Kleinschmidt-DeMasters BK. Dural metastases from prostatic adenocarcinoma. Report of five cases and review of the literature. *J Urol Pathol* 3:119-127, 1995.

Pins MR, Okonkwo AM. High molecular weight cytokeratin (HMWCK) epitope stability in prostate needle cores as a function of fixation time, fixative type, and duration of slide storage [abstract]. *Mod Pathol* 12:104A 1999.

Pinto JA, González JE, Granadillo MA. Primary carcinoma of the prostate with diffuse oncocytic change. *Histopathology* 25:286-288, 1994.

Pinto JE, Babaian RJ, Troncoso P. Prostatic carcinoma metastatic to periprostatic lymph nodes [abstract]. *Mod Pathol* 13:98A, 2000A.

Pinto JE, Pettaway CA, Babaian RJ, et al. Racial differences in prostate cancer foci distribution in radical prostatectomy specimen [abstract]. *Mod Pathol* 13:98A, 2000B.

Pisansky TM, Kahn MJ, Rasp GM, et al. A multiple prognostic index predictive of disease outcome after irradiation for clinically localized prostate carcinoma. *Cancer* 79:337-344, 1997.

Potter SR, Miller MC, Mangold LA, et al. Genetically engineered neural networks for predicting prostate cancer progression after radical prostatectomy. *Urology* 54:791-795, 1999.

Pound CR, Partin AW, Epstein JI, et al. Prostate-specific antigen after anatomic radical retropubic prostatectomy. *Urol Clin North Am* 24:395-406, 1997.

Pound CR, Partin AW, Eisenberger MA, et al. Natural history of progression after PSA elevation following radical prostatectomy. *JAMA* 281:1591-1597, 1999.

Presti B, Weidner N. Granulomatous prostatitis and poorly differentiated prostate cancer. Their distinction with use of immunohistochemical methods. *Am J Clin Pathol* 95:330-334, 1991.

Presti JC Jr, Shinohara K, Bacchetti P, et al. Positive fraction of systematic biopsies predicts risk of relapse after radical prostatectomy. *Urology* 52:1079-1084, 1998.

Rabbani F, Bastar A, Fair WR. Site specific predictors of positive margins at radical prostatectomy: an argument for risk based modification of technique. *J Urol* 160:1727-1733, 1998.

Ravery V, Boccon-Gibod LA, Dauge-Geffroy MC, et al. Systematic biopsies accurately predict extracapsular extension of prostate cancer and persistent/recurrent detectable PSA after radical prostatectomy. *Urology* 44:371-376, 1994.

Ravery V, Schmid HP, Toublanc M, et al. Is the percentage of cancer in biopsy cores predictive of extracapsular disease in T1-T2 prostate carcinoma? *Cancer* 78:1079-1084, 1996.

Reiter RE. Editorial: Prostate cancer diagnostics: obstacles and opportunities. *J Urol* 162:2046-2047, 1999.

Renshaw AA, Nappi D, Cibas ES. Cytology of metastatic adenocarcinoma of the prostate in pleural effusions. *Diagn Cytopathol* 15:103-107, 1996.

Renshaw AA. Adequate tissue sampling of prostate core needle biopsies. *Am J Clin Pathol* 107:26-29, 1997.

Renshaw AA, Santis WF, Richie JP. Clinicopathologic characteristics of prostatic adenocarcinoma in men with atypical prostate needle biopsies. *J Urol* 159:2018-2022, 1998A.

Renshaw AA. Correlation of gross morphologic features with histologic features in radical prostatectomy specimens. *Am J Clin Pathol* 110:38-42, 1998B.

Renshaw AA, Richie JP, Loughlin KR, et al. The greatest dimension of prostate carcinoma is a simple, inexpensive predictor of prostate specific antigen failure in radical prostatectomy specimens. *Cancer* 83:748-752, 1998C.

Reuter VE. Pathological changes in benign and malignant tissue following androgen deprivation therapy. *Urology* (3Asuppl) 49:16-22, 1997.

Reyes AO, Tu S, Ruiz C, et al. Prostate cancer clinically and histologically mimicking primary bladder carcinoma [abstract]. *Mod Pathol* 13:110A, 2000.

Reyes AO, Humphrey PA. Flat high-grade prostatic intraepithelial neoplasia (HGPIN) in needle biopsy [abstract]. *Mod Pathol* 10:86A 1997A.

Reyes AO, Swanson PE, Carbone JM, et al. Unusual histologic types of high-grade prostate intraepithelial neoplasia. *Am J Surg Pathol* 21:1215-1222, 1997B.

Reyes AO, Humphrey PA. Diagnostic effect of complete histologic sampling of prostate needle biopsy specimens. *Am J Clin Pathol* 109:416-422, 1998.

Riesenberg R, Oberneder R, Kreigmair M, et al. Immunocytochemical double staining of cytokeratin and prostate-specific antigen in individual prostate tumor cells. *Histochemistry* 99:61-66, 1993.

Ripple MG, Potter SR, Partin AW, et al. Needle biopsy of recurrent adenocarcinoma of the prostate after radical prostatectomy. *Mod Pathol* 13:521-527, 2000.

Rizk CC, Scholes J, Chen SK, et al. Epididymal metastasis from prostatic adenocarcinoma mimicking adenomatoid tumor. *Urology* 36:526-530, 1990.

Ro JY, Ayala AG, Ordonez NG, et al. Intraluminal crystalloids in prostatic adenocarcinoma: Immunohistochemical, electron microscopic, and x-ray microanalytic studies. *Cancer* 57:2397-2407, 1986.

Ro JY, Ayala AG, el-Naggar A, et al. Seminal vesicle involvement by in situ and invasive transitional cell carcinoma of the bladder. *Am J Surg Pathol* 11:951-958, 1987.

Ro JY, Grignon DJ, Troncoso P, et al. Intraluminal crystalloids in whole-organ sections of prostate. *Prostate* 13:233-239, 1988A.

Ro JY, El-Naggar A, Ayala AG, et al. Signet-ring cell carcinoma of the prostate. Electron-microscopic and immunohistochemical study of eight cases. *Am J Surg Pathol* 12:453-460, 1988B.

Roberts WW, Bergstralh EJ, Blute ML, et al. Contemporary identification of patients at high risk of early prostate cancer recurrence after radical retropubic prostatectomy. *Urology* 57:1033-1037, 2001.

Rodin AE, Larson DL, Roberts DK. Nature of the perineural space invaded by prostatic carcinoma. *Cancer* 20:1772-1779, 1967.

Rohr LR. Incidental adenocarcinoma in transurethral resections of the prostate. Partial versus complete microscopic examination. *Am J Surg Pathol* 11:53-58, 1987.

Ross JS, Figge H, Bui HX, et al. Prediction of pathologic stage and postprostatectomy disease recurrence by DNA ploidy analysis of initial needle biopsy specimens of prostate cancer. *Cancer* 74:2811-2818, 1994.

Ross JS, Sheehan CE, Ambros RA, et al. Needle biopsy DNA ploidy status predicts grade shifting in prostate cancer. *Am J Surg Pathol* 23:296-301, 1999.

Roy CR, Horne D, Raife M, et al. Incidental carcinoma of the prostate: long term follow-up. *Urology* 36:210-213, 1990.

Rub R, Jossiphov J, Avidor Y. Macroscopic hematuria as an initial manifestation of carcinoma of the colon. *J Urol* 161:922, 1999.

Rubin MA, de La Taille A, Bagiella E, et al. Cribriform carcinoma of the prostate and cribriform prostatic intraepithelial neoplasia: incidence and clinical implications. *Am J Surg Pathol* 22:840-848, 1998.

Rubin MA, Putzi M, Mucci N, et al. Rapid ("warm") autopsy study for procurement of metastatic prostate cancer. *Clin Cancer Res* 6:1038-1045, 2000A.

Rubin MA, Bassily N, Sanda M, et al. Relationship and significance of greatest percentage of tumor and perineural invasion on needle biopsy in prostatic adenocarcinoma. *Am J Surg Pathol* 24:183-189, 2000B.

Rubin MA, Dunn R, Kambham N, et al. Should a Gleason score be assigned to a minute focus of carcinoma on prostate biopsy? *Am J Surg Pathol* 24:1634-1640, 2000.

Rubin MA, Mucci NR, Manley S, et al. Predictors of Gleason pattern 4/5 prostate cancer on prostatectomy specimens: can high grade tumor be predicted preoperatively? *J Urol* 165:114-118, 2001.

Rubin MA, Dhanasekaran SM, Barrette TR, et al. Pim-1 kinase: prognostic biomarker in prostate cancer identified by cDNA and tissue microarray analysis [abstract]. *Mod Pathol* 15:179A, 2002A.

Rubin MA, Zhou M, D'hanasekaran SM, et al. (alpha)-methylacyl coenzyme A racemase as a tissue biomarker for prostate cancer. *JAMA* 287:1662-1670, 2002B.

Ruijter ET, van de Kaa CA, Schalken JA, et al. Histological grade heterogeneity in multifocal prostate cancer. Biological and clinical implications. *J Pathol* 180:295-299, 1996.

Ruska KM, Sauvageot J, Epstein JI. Histology and cellular kinetics of prostatic atrophy. *Am J Surg Pathol* 22:1073-1077, 1998.

Sabbatini P, Larson SM, Kremer A, et al. Prognostic significance of extent of a disease in bone patients with androgen-independent prostate cancer. *J Clin Oncol* 17:948-957, 1999.

Safa AA, Reese DM, Carter DM, et al. Undetectable serum prostate-specific antigen associated with metastatic prostate cancer: a case report and review of the literature. *Am J Clin Oncol* 21:323-326, 1998.

Saitoh H, Hida M, Shimbo T, et al. Metastatic patterns of prostatic carcinoma. Correlation between sites and number of organs involved. *Cancer* 54:3078-3084, 1984.

Sakr WA, Wheeler TM, Blute M, et al. Staging and reporting of prostate cancer: sampling of the radical prostatectomy specimen. *Cancer* 78:366-368, 1996.

Sakr WA, Grignon DJ. Prostate. Practice parameters, pathologic staging and handling radical prostatectomy specimens. *Urol Clin North Am* 26:453-463, 1999.

Saleem MD, Sanders H, Abu El Naser M, et al. Factors predicting cancer detection in biopsy of the prostatic fossa after radical prostatectomy. *Urology* 51:283-286, 1998.

Salomao DR, Graham SD, Bostwick DG. Microvascular invasion in prostate cancer correlates with pathologic stage. *Arch Pathol Lab Med* 119:1050-1054, 1995.

Saltzstein SL, McLaughlin AP. Clinicopathologic features of unsuspected regional lymph node metastases in prostatic adenocarcinoma. *Cancer* 40:1212-1221, 1977.

Salyer WR, Salyer DC. Metastases of prostatic carcinoma to the breast. *J Urol* 109:671-675, 1973.

Sanda M, Manley S, Rubin MA. Surgical margin status adds predictive value to prostate cancer staging: single institution study of 1050 radical prostatectomy cases [abstract]. *Mod Pathol* 14:122A, 2001.

Sanwick JM, Dalkin BL, Nagle RB. Accuracy of prostate needle biopsy in predicting extracapsular tumor extension at radical retropubic prostatectomy: application in selecting patients for nerve-sparing surgery. *Urology* 52:814-819, 1998.

Scheidemandel V, Salisbury B, Tate CF Jr. Pleural effusion: unusual presentation of prostatic cancer. *Chest* 61:686-689, 1972.

Scherz H, Schmidt JD. Endobronchial metastasis from prostate carcinoma. *Prostate* 8:319-324, 1986.

Schmid KW, Helpap B, Tötsch M, et al. Immunohistochemical localization of chromogranins A and B secretogranin II in normal, hyperplastic and neoplastic prostate. *Histopathology* 24:233-239, 1994.

Scoggins WG, Witten JA Jr, Texter JH Jr, et al. Endobronchial metastasis from prostatic carcinoma in patient with renal cell carcinoma. *Urology* 12:207-209, 1978.

Sears D, Hajdu SK. The cytologic diagnosis of malignant neoplasms in pleural and peritoneal effusions. *Acta Cytol* 31:85-97, 1987.

Sebo TJ, Bock BJ, Cheville JC, et al. The percent of cores positive for cancer in prostate needle biopsy specimens is strongly predictive of tumor stage and volume at radical prostatectomy. *J Urol* 163:174-178, 2000.

Sebo TJ, Cheville JC, Riehle DL, et al. Perineural invasion and MIB-1 positivity in addition to Gleason score are significant preoperative predictors of progression after radical retropubic prostatectomy for prostate cancer. *Am J Surg Pathol* 26:431-439, 2002.

Segal R, Penneys NS, Nahass G. Metastatic prostatic carcinoma histologically mimicking malignant melanoma. *J Cutan Pathol* 21:280-282, 1994.

Sesterhenn IA, Mostofi FK, Mattrey RR, et al. Preliminary results of three-dimensional reconstruction of previously imaged prostates. Prostate 4(suppl):33-41, 1992.

Sgrignoli AR, Walsh PC, Steinberg GD, et al. Prognostic factors in men with stage D1 prostate cancer: identification of patients less likely to have prolonged survival after radical prostatectomy. *J Urol* 152:1077-1081, 1994.

Shah IA, Schlageter MO, Stinnett P, et al. Cytokeratin immunohistochemistry as a diagnostic tool for distinguishing malignant from benign epithelial lesions of the prostate. *Mod Pathol* 4:220-224, 1991.

Shah NT, Tuttle SE, Strobel SL, et al. Prostatic carcinoma metastatic to bone: sensitivity and specificity of prostate-specific antigen and prostatic acid phosphatase in decalcified material. *J Surg Oncol* 29:265-268, 1985.

Shah R, Bassily N, Wei J, et al. Benign prostatic glands at surgical margins of radical prostatectomy specimens: frequency and associated risk factors. *Urology* 56:721-725, 2000.

Shah RB, Zhou M, LeBlanc M, et al. Comparison of the basal cell-specific markers, p63 and 34βE12, in the diagnosis of prostate cancer. *Am J Surg Pathol* 26:1161-1168, 2002A.

Shah R, Ingold C, Rubin MA. Prostate adenocarcinoma with foamy gland features diagnosed on needle biopsies: prevalence and clinico-pathologic associations [abstract]. *Mod Pathol* 15:181A, 2002B.

Sheaff MT, Baithun SI. Effects of radiation on the normal prostate gland. *Histopathology* 30:341-348, 1997.

Shekarriz B, Upadhyay J, Wood PD Jr, et al. Vesicourethral anastomosis biopsy after radical prostatectomy: predictive value of prostate specific antigen and pathologic stage. *Urology* 54:1044-1048, 1999.

Sheldon CA, Williams RD, Fraley EE. Incidental carcinoma of the prostate: a review of the literature and critical reappraisal of classification. *J Urol* 124:626-631, 1980.

Shepherd DS, Humphrey PA, Swanson PE, et al. Tumor-infiltrating lymphocytes in prostatic carcinoma [abstract]. *Urology* 155:514A, 1996.

Shidham VB, Lindholm PF, Kajdacsy-Balla A, et al. Prostate specific antigen expression and lipochrome pigment granules in the differential diagnosis of prostatic adenocarcinoma versus seminal vesicle-ejaculatory duct epithelium. *Arch Pathol Lab Med* 123:1093-1097, 1999.

Siders DB, Lee F. Histologic changes of irradiated prostatic carcinoma diagnosed by transrectal ultrasound. *Hum Pathol* 23:344-351, 1992.

Sidhu J, Sánchez RL. Prostatic acid phosphatase in stromal carcinoids of the ovary. An immunohistochemical study. *Cancer* 72:1673-1678, 1993.

Signoretti S, Waltregny D, Dilks J, et al. p63 is a prostate basal cell marker and is required for prostate development. *Am J Pathol* 157:1769-1775, 2000.

Silver DA, Pellicer I, Fair WR, et al. Prostate-specific membrane antigen expression in normal and malignant human tissues. *Clin Cancer Res* 3:81-85, 1997.

Simpson RH, Skalova A. Metastatic carcinoma of the prostate presenting as parotid tumor. *Histopathology* 30:70-74, 1997.

Skacel M, Ormsby AH, Abrahams NX, et al. The relative amount of Gleason pattern (GP) 4 tumor and surgical margin status are independent prognostic factors in Gleason score (GS) 7 prostate carcinoma treated by radical prostatectomy [abstract]. *Mod Pathol* 13:108A, 2000.

Slovin SF, Scher HI. Detectable tumor cells in the blood and bone marrow. Smoke or fire? *Cancer* 83:394-398, 1998.

Smith CP, Sharma A, Ayala G, et al. Solitary pulmonary metastasis from prostate cancer. *J Urol* 162:2102, 1999.

Smith GG, Woodruff LM. The development of cancer of the prostate after subtotal prostatectomy. *J Urol* 63:1077-1080, 1950.

Smith JA Jr, Seaman JP, Gleidman JB, et al. Pelvic lymph node metastasis from prostatic cancer: influence of tumor grade and stage in 452 consecutive patients. *J Urol* 130:290-292, 1983.

Sobin LH, Hjermstad BM, Sesterhenn IA, et al. Prostate acid phosphatase activity in carcinoid tumors. *Cancer* 58:136-138, 1986.

Soda T, Onishi H, Terachi T, et al. Bilateral breast metastases from prostatic carcinoma: a case report [in Japanese]. *Acta Urol Jpn* 45:269-271, 1999.

Sofer M, Savoie M, Kim SS, et al. Biochemical and pathological predictors of the recurrence of prostatic adenocarcinoma with seminal vesicle invasion. *J Urol* 169:153-156, 2003.

Sohayda C, Kupelian PA, Levin HS, et al. Extent of extracapsular extension in localized prostate cancer. *Urology* 55:382-386, 2000.

Speights VO Jr, Cohen MK, Coffield KS, et al. Neuroendocrine staining in malignant, hyperplastic, and atrophic prostate tissue. *Appl Immunohistochem* 2:212-217, 1994.

Speights VO Jr, Cohen MK, Riggs MW, et al. Neuroendocrine stains and proliferative indices of prostatic adenocarcinoma in transurethral resection samples. *Br J Urol* 80:281-286, 1997.

Spencer JR, Brodin AG, Ignatoff JM. Clear cell adenocarcinoma of the urethra: evidence for origin within paraurethral ducts. *J Urol* 143:122-125, 1990.

Spieler P, Gloor F. Identification of types and primary sites of malignant tumors by examination of exfoliated tumor cells in serous fluids. Comparison with the diagnostic accuracy on small histologic biopsies. *Acta Cytol* 29:753-767, 1985.

Srigley JR, Amin MB, Bostwick DG, et al. Updated protocol for the examination of specimens from patients with carcinomas of the prostate gland. A basis for checklists. *Arch Pathol Lab Med* 124:1034-1037, 2000.

Stagno PA, Petras RE, Hart WR. Stromal carcinoids of the ovary. An immunohistologic and ultrastructural study. *Arch Pathol Lab Med* 111:440-446, 1987.

Stamey TA, Yang N, Hay AR, et al. Prostate-specific antigen as a serum marker for adenocarcinoma of the prostate. *N Engl J Med* 317:909-916, 1987.

Stamey TA, McNeal JE, Freiha FS, et al. Morphometric and clinical studies on 68 consecutive radical prostatectomies. *J Urol* 139:1235-1241, 1988.

Stamey TA, Villers AA, McNeal JE, et al. Positive surgical margins at radical prostatectomy: importance of the apical dissection. *J Urol* 143:1166-1173, 1990.

Stamey TA. DNA ploidy status. *Urology* 45:563-565, 1995.

Stamey TA, McNeal JE, Yemoto CM, et al. Biological determinants of cancer progression in men with prostate cancer. *JAMA* 281:1395-1400, 1999.

Stein BS, Vangore S, Petersen RO. Immunoperoxidase localization of prostatic antigens. Comparison of primary and metastatic sites. *Urology* 24:146-152, 1984.

Steinberg DM, Sauvageot J, Piantodosi S, et al. Correlation of prostate needle biopsy and radical prostatectomy Gleason grade in academic and community settings. *Am J Surg Pathol* 21:566-576, 1997.

Stillwell TJ, Malek RS, Engen DE, et al. Incidental adenocarcinoma after open prostatic adenectomy. *J Urol* 141:76-78, 1989.

Stone NN, Stock RG, Parikh D, et al. Perineural invasion and seminal vesicle involvement predict pelvic lymph node metastasis in men with localized carcinoma of the prostate. *J Urol* 160:1722-1726, 1998.

Svanholm H, Andersen OP, Rohl H. Tumour of female paraurethral duct. Immunohistochemical similarity with prostatic carcinoma. *Virchows Arch [A] Pathol Anat Histopathol* 411:395-398, 1987.

Sweat SD, Pacelli A, Murphy GP, et al. Prostate-specific membrane antigen expression is greatest in a prostate adenocarcinoma and lymph node metastases. *Urology* 52:637-640, 1998.

Takahashi T, Hoshi S, Kaneda T, et al. Genetic diagnosis of pelvic lymph node metastasis in prostate cancer using aspiration biopsy samples [in Japanese]. *Jpn J Clin Pathol* 44:1183-1188, 1996.

Tazawa K, Kurihara Y, Kamoshida S, et al. Localization of prostate-specific antigen–like immunoreactivity in human salivary gland and salivary gland tumors. *Pathol Int* 49:500-505, 1999.

Tefilli MV, Gheiler EL, Tiguert R, et al. Role of radical prostatectomy in patients with prostate cancer of high Gleason score. *Prostate* 39:60-66, 1999.

Terris MK, McNeal JE, Stamey TA. Detection of clinically significant prostate cancer by transrectal ultrasound-guided systematic biopsies. *J Urol* 148:829-832, 1992.

Terris MK, Haney DJ, Johnstone IM, et al. Prediction of prostate cancer volume using prostate specific antigen levels, transrectal ultrasound, and systematic sextant biopsies. *Urology* 45:75-80, 1995.

Terris MK, Hausdorff J, Freiha FS. Hematolymphoid malignancies diagnosed at the time of radical prostatectomy. *J Urol* 158:1457-1459, 1997.

Theodorescu D, Frierson HF Jr, Sikes RA. Molecular determination of surgical margins using fossa biopsies at radical prostatectomy. *J Urol* 161:1442-1448, 1999.

Thomas P, Battifora H. Keratins versus epithelial membrane antigen in tumor diagnosis: an immunohistochemical comparison of five monoclonal antibodies. *Hum Pathol* 18:728-734, 1987.

Thompson IM, Zeidman EJ. Extended followup of stage A1 carcinoma of the prostate. *Urology* 33:455-458, 1989.

Thorson P, Vollmer RT, Arcangeli C, et al. Minimal carcinoma in prostate needle biopsy specimens: diagnostic features and radical prostatectomy follow-up. *Mod Pathol* 11:543-551, 1998.

Thorson P, Swanson PE, Humphrey PA. Basal cell proliferations of the peripheral zone of the prostate gland [abstract]. *Mod Pathol* 12:108A, 1999.

Thorson P, Humphrey PA. Minimal adenocarcinoma in prostate needle biopsy tissue. *Am J Clin Pathol* 114:896-909, 2000.

Tigrani VS, Bhargava V, Shinohara K, et al. Number of positive systematic sextant biopsies predicts surgical margin status at radical prostatectomy. *Urology* 54:689-693, 1999.

Tiguert R, Gheiler EL, Tefilli MV, et al. Lymph node size does not correlate with the presence of prostate cancer metastasis. *Urology* 53:367-371, 1999.

Tombal B, De Visocher L, Cosyns JP, et al. Assessing the risk of unsuspected prostate cancer in patients with benign prostatic hypertrophy: a 13-year retrospective study of the incidence and natural history of T1a-T1b prostate cancers. *BJU Int* 84:1015-1020, 1999.

Torenbeek R, Lagendijk JH, van Diest PJ, et al. Value of a panel of antibodies to identify the primary origin of adenocarcinomas presenting as bladder carcinoma. *Histopathology* 32:20-27, 1998.

Totten RS, Heinemann MW, Hudson PB, et al. Microscopic differential diagnosis of latent carcinoma of prostate. *Arch Pathol* 55:131-141, 1953.

Tran TA, Ayala AG, Amin MB, et al. Utility of high-molecular weight cytokeratin 34βE12 in atypical small acinar proliferations in prostatic needle biopsies. *Appl Immunol Mol Morphol* 7:186-192, 1999.

Tran TT, Sengupta E, Yang XY. Prostatic foamy gland carcinoma with aggressive behavior. Histologic, immunohistochemical, and ultrastructural analysis. *Am J Surg Pathol* 25:618-623, 2001.

Trieger P, Welfeld J, Marx J. Suprapubic prostatectomy: a review of 108 cases. *Urol Cutan Rev* 52:8-9, 1948.

Troncoso P, Johnston D, Babaian RJ. Extent of margin positivity in radical prostatectomy specimens predicts prostate cancer recurrence [abstract]. *Mod Pathol* 12:108A, 1999.

True LD. Surgical pathology examination of the prostate gland. Practice survey by American Society of Clinical Pathologists. *Am J Clin Pathol* 102:572-579, 1994.

True LD, Felice D, Vessela R, et al. Grade progression in lethal prostate carcinoma [abstract]. *Mod Pathol* 13:105A, 2000.

Tu SM, Reyes A, Maa A, et al. Prostate carcinoma with testicular or penile metastases, clinical, pathologic, and immunohistochemical features. *Cancer* 94:2610-2617, 2002.

Uribe M, Fenoglio-Preiser CM, Grimes M, et al. Medullary carcinoma of the thyroid gland. Clinical, pathological, and immunohistochemical features with review of the literature. *Am J Surg Pathol* 9:577-594, 1985.

Van de Voorde WM, van Poppel HP, Verbeken EK, et al. Morphologic and neuroendocrine features of adenocarcinoma arising in the transition zone and in the peripheral zone of the prostate. *Mod Pathol* 8:591-598, 1995.

van den Ouden D, Bentvelsen FM, Boeve ER, et al. Positive margins after radical prostatectomy: correlation with local recurrence and distant progression. *Br J Urol* 72:489-494, 1993.

van den Ouden D, Hop WCJ, Kranse R, et al. Tumor control according to pathological variables in patients treated by radical prostatectomy for clinically localized carcinoma of the prostate. *Br J Urol* 79:203-211, 1997.

van den Ouden D, Kranse R, Hop WC, et al. Microvascular invasion in prostate cancer: prognostic significance in patients treated by radical prostatectomy for clinically localized carcinoma. *Urol Int* 60:17-24, 1998.

Van Krieken JHJM. Prostate marker immunoreactivity in salivary gland neoplasms. A rare pitfall in immunohistochemistry. *Am J Surg Pathol* 17:410-414, 1993.

Varambally S, Dhanasekaran SM, Zhou M, et al. The polycomb group protein EZH2 is involved in progression of prostate cancer. *Nature* 419:624-629, 2002.

Vargas SO, Jiroutek M, Welch WR, et al. Perineural invasion in prostate needle biopsy specimens. Correlation with extraprostatic extension at resection. *Am J Clin Pathol* 111:223-228, 1999.

Varkarakis MJ, Winterberger AR, Gaeta J, et al. Lung metastases in prostatic carcinoma. Clinical significance. *Urology* 3:447-452, 1974.

Varma M, Amin MB, Linden MD, et al. Discriminant staining patterns of small glandular and preneoplastic lesions of the prostate using high molecular weight cytokeratin (HMCK): a study of 301 consecutive needle biopsies [abstract]. *Mod Pathol* 10:93A 1997.

Varma M, Linden MD, Amin MB. Effect of formalin fixation and epitope retrieval techniques on antibody 34βE12 immunostaining of prostatic tissues. *Mod Pathol* 12:472-478, 1999.

Varma M, Lin MW, Tamboli P, et al. Morphologic criteria for the diagnosis of prostatic adenocarcinoma in needle biopsy specimens: a study of 250 consecutive cases in routine surgical pathology practice. *Arch Pathol Lab Med* 126:554-561,2002A.

Varma M, Morgan M, Jasani B, et al. Polyclonal anti-PSA is more sensitive but less specific than monoclonal anti-PSA. *Am J Clin Pathol* 118:202-207,2002B.

Vecchioli Scaddazza C. Incidental carcinoma of the prostate. Study of 683 patients operated upon for benign prostatic hypertrophy [in Italian]. *Minerva Urol Nefrol* 44:109-112, 1992.

Vesalainen S, Lipponen P, Talja M, et al. Mitotic activity and prognosis in prostatic adenocarcinoma. *Prostate* 26:80-86, 1995.

Vickery AL Jr, Kerr WS Jr. Carcinoma of the prostate treated by radical prostatectomy. A clinicopathological survey of 187 cases followed for 5 years and 148 cases followed for 10 years. *Cancer* 12:1598-1608, 1963.

Villers A, McNeal JE, Redwine EA, et al. The role of perineural space invasion in the local spread of prostatic adenocarcinoma. *J Urol* 142:763-768, 1989.

Villers AA, McNeal JE, Redwine EA, et al. Pathogenesis and biological significance of seminal vesicle invasion in prostatic adenocarcinoma. *J Urol* 143:1183-1189, 1990.

Voges GE, McNeal JE, Redwine EA, et al. The predictive significance of substaging stage A prostate cancer (A1 versus A2) for volume and grade of total cancer in the prostate. *J Urol* 147:858-863, 1992.

Vollmer RT, Humphrey PA. The relative importance of anatomic and PSA factors to outcomes after radical prostatectomy for prostate cancer. *Am J Clin Pathol* 118:864-870, 2001.

Wade H. Prostatism. *Ann Surg* 59:321-359, 1914.

Wang HL, Humphrey PA. Exaggerated signet-ring cell change in stromal nodule of prostate: a pseudoneoplastic proliferation. *Am J Surg Pathol* 26:1066-1070, 2002.

Wang NP, Zee S, Zarbo RJ, et al. Coordinate expression of cytokeratins 7 and 20 defines unique subsets of carcinomas. *Appl Immunohistochem* 3:99-107, 1995.

Ward JF, Sands JP, Nowacki M, et al. Malignant cytological washings from prostate specimens: an independent predictor of biochemical progression after radical prostatectomy. *J Urol* 165:469-473, 2001.

Watson RB, Civantos F, Soloway MS. Positive surgical margins with radical prostatectomy: detailed pathological analysis and prognosis. *Urology* 48:80-90, 1996.

Weaver MG, Abdul-Karim FW, Srigley J, et al. Paneth cell–like change of the prostate gland. A histological, immunohistochemical, and electron microscopic study. *Am J Surg Pathol* 16:62-68, 1992A.

Weaver MG, Abdul-Karim FW, Srigley JR. Paneth cell–like change and small cell carcinoma of the prostate. Two divergent forms of prostatic neuroendocrine differentiation. *Am J Surg Pathol* 16:1013-1016, 1992B.

Weinstein MH, Epstein JI. Significance of high grade prostatic intraepithelial neoplasia (PIN) on needle biopsy. *Hum Pathol* 24:624-629, 1993.

Weinstein MH, Partin AW, Veltri MW, et al. Neuroendocrine differentiation in prostate cancer: enhanced prediction of progression after radical prostatectomy. *Hum Pathol* 27:683-687, 1996.

Weinstein MH, Signoretti S, Loda M. Diagnostic utility of immunohistochemical staining for p63, a sensitive marker of prostatic basal cells. *Mod Pathol* 15:1302-1308, 2002.

Weldon VE, Tavel FR, Neuwirth H, et al. Patterns of positive specimen margins and detectable prostate specific antigen after radical perineal prostatectomy. *J Urol* 153:1565-1569, 1995.

Wheeler TM, Dillioglugil O, Kattan MW, et al. Clinical and pathological significance of the level and extent of capsular invasion in clinical stage T1-2 prostate cancer. *Hum Pathol* 29:856-862, 1998A.

Wheeler TM. Prediction of pathologic stage and patient outcome from prostate biopsy findings. *J Urol Pathol* 8:45-53, 1998B.

WHO. World health organization classification of tumours. In: *Tumours of the Urinary System and Male Genital Organs*. Lyon, France: IARC Press; in press, 2003.

Wick MR, Swanson PE, Manivel JC. Placental-like alkaline phosphatase reactivity in human tumors: an immunohistochemical study of 520 cases. *Hum Pathol* 18:946-954, 1987.

Wieder JA, Soloway MS. Incidence, etiology, location, prevention and treatment of positive surgical margins after radical prostatectomy for prostate cancer. *J Urol* 160:299-315, 1998.

Wiegel T, Kreusel KM, Heicapell R, et al. Metastatic adenocarcinoma of the prostate to the choroid with loss of visual acuity as a presenting symptom. *J Urol* 160:2158-2159, 1998.

Wills ML, Sauvageot J, Partin AW, et al. Ability of sextant biopsies to predict radical prostatectomy stage. *Urology* 51:759-764, 1998.

Wise AM, Stamey TA, McNeal JE, et al. Morphologic and clinical significance of multifocal prostate cancers in radical prostatectomy specimens. *Urology* 60:264-269, 2002.

Wojno KJ, Epstein JI. The utility of basal cell–specific anti-cytokeratin antibody (34βE12) in the diagnosis of prostate cancer. A review of 228 cases. *Am J Surg Pathol* 19:251-260, 1995.

Wood DP Jr, Banks ER, Humphreys S, et al. Identification of bone marrow micrometastases in patients with prostate cancer. *Cancer* 74:2533-2540, 1994A.

Wood DP Jr, Banks ER, Humphreys S, et al. Sensitivity of immunohistochemistry and polymerase chain reaction in detecting prostate cancer cells in bone marrow. *J Histochem Cytochem* 42:505-511, 1994B.

Wood DP Jr, Banerjee M. Presence of circulating prostate cells in the bone marrow of patients undergoing radical prostatectomy is predictive of disease-free survival. *J Clin Oncol* 15:3451-3457, 1997.

Xu J, Stolk JA, Zhang X, et al. Identification of differentially expressed genes in human prostate cancer using subtraction and microarray. *Cancer Res* 60:1677-1682, 2000.

Yam LT, Janckila AJ, Lam WK, et al. Immunohistochemistry of prostatic acid phosphatase. *Prostate* 2:97-107, 1981.

Yamabe H, ten Kate FJW, Gallee MPN, et al. Stage A prostatic cancer: a comparative study in Japan and the Netherlands. *World J Urol* 4:136-140, 1986.

Yamaguchi S, Hashimoto H, Kaneko S, et al. Secondary mucinous adenocarcinoma of the prostate in a patient with ulcerative colitis. *Urol Int* 50:231-233, 1993.

Yang G, Wheeler TM, Kattan MW, et al. Perineural invasion of prostate carcinoma cells is associated with reduced apoptotic index. *Cancer* 78:1267-1271, 1996.

Yang XJ, Wu CL, Woda B, et al. Expression of alpha-methylacyl-CoA racemase (P504S) in atypical adenomatous hyperplasia of the prostate. *Am J Surg Pathol* 26:921-925, 2002A.

Yang XJ, Lecksell K, Gaudin P, et al. Rare expression of high-molecular weight cytokeratin in adenocarcinoma of the prostate gland. A study of 100 cases of metastatic and locally advanced prostatic cancer. *Am J Surg Pathol* 23:147-152, 1999.

Yaziji H, Davie PL, Gown AM. Use of cytokeratins 7 and 20 in the differentiation between transitional cell carcinoma and prostate adenocarcinoma [letter]. *Am J Clin Pathol* 115:159-160, 2001.

Young MPA, Kirby RS, O' Donoughue EPN, et al. Accuracy and cost of intraoperative lymph node frozen sections at radical prostatectomy. *J Clin Pathol* 52:925-927, 1999.

Young RH, Talerman A. Testicular tumors other than germ cell tumors. *Semin Diagn Pathol* 4:342-360, 1987.

Young RH. Pseudoneoplastic lesions of the urinary bladder, prostate gland, and urethra. In: Wick MR, Humphrey PA, Ritter JR, eds. *Pathology of Pseudoneoplastic Lesions.* New York: Lippincott-Raven; 223-235, 1997.

Yu H, Diamandis EP, Levesque M, et al. Expression of the prostate specific antigen gene by a primary ovarian carcinoma. *Cancer Res* 55:1603-1606, 1995.

Zaviacic M, Šidlo J, Borovský M. Prostate specific antigen and prostate specific acid phosphatase in adenocarcinoma of Skene's paraurethral glands and ducts. *Virchows Arch [A] Pathol Anat Histopathol* 423:503-505, 1993.

Zein TA, Huben R, Lane W, et al. Secondary tumors of the prostate. *J Urol* 133:615-616, 1985.

Zhang G, Wasserman NF, Sidi AA, et al. Long-term follow-up results after expectant management of stage A1 prostatic carcinoma. *J Urol* 146:99-103, 1991.

Zhang PL, Shuffler SH, Bihrle W III, et al. Subclassification of small atypical glands in prostate biopsies provides a clearer indication for re-biopsies [abstract]. *Mod Pathol* 13:105A, 2000.

Zhou M, Patel A, Rubin MA. Prevalence and location of peripheral nerve found on prostate needle biopsy. *Am J Clin Pathol* 115:39-43, 2001.

Zhou M, Chinnaiyan AM, Kleer CG, et al. Alpha-methylacyl-CoA racemase: a novel tumor marker overexpressed in several human cancers and their precursor lesions. *Am J Surg Pathol* 26:926-931, 2002.

Zincke H, Blute ML, Fallen MJ, et al. Radical prostatectomy for stage A adenocarcinoma of the prostate: staging errors and their implications for treatment recommendations and disease outcome. *J Urol* 146:1053-1058, 1991.

Grading of Prostatic Carcinoma

[15.1] History **339**

[15.2] World Health Organization (Mostofi) System **340**

[15.3] Gleason System **340**

[15.4] Grading in Metastatic Deposits **355**

[15.5] Grading After Radiation and Hormonal Therapy **355**

[15.6] Grade Progression **356**

[15.7] Prognosis and Grade **356**

CHAPTER 15

"Malignity only differs in degree."

—Rudolph Virchow, 1860

"Some cancers grow slowly and closely imitate normal cells while others grow with extreme rapidity and depart markedly from the structure of the normal cell."

—Albert Broders, 1926

[15.1] History

Grade may be as defined as a step in a process (Brown 1993). The histologic grade of a neoplastic process often is equated with the degree of differentiation of the neoplastic cells. Since the time of Virchow, it has been recognized that the grade of neoplasm is related to its malignant potential (Gardner 1982). It was not until 1920, however, that Broders, in his seminal study of 537 squamous cell carcinomas of the lip, devised a scheme that stratified malignant neoplasms based on the degree of differentiation (Broders 1920). This was a 4-tiered system, with grades 1 through 4, that used cellular keratinization, nuclear cytologic features, and mitotic counts. Grading schemes for neoplasms have used a number of tiers, with the more common general approaches being either 2-tiered (low-grade vs. high-grade) and 3-tiered (well-differentiated vs. moderately differentiated vs. poorly differentiated). Specific grading systems have been developed for tumors arising at different anatomic sites, and often numerous grading techniques have been applied to a single type of malignancy.

In the last three quarters of the twentieth century, >40 histologic grading systems for prostatic carcinoma have been proposed **t15.1**. The systems typically have used differentiation capacity, architectural growth patterns, mitotic activity, and nuclear abnormalities to derive a histologic grade assignment.

Currently, the most widely used grading scheme in the United States (True 1994) and worldwide (Deshmukh 1998) is the Gleason system (Gleason 1966, 1974, 1977, Mellinger 1967), whereas other grading methods, such as the World Health Organization (WHO) system (Dhom 1977, Utz 1969), are applied in some laboratories (Miller 1990). Both of these grading methods are based on standard light microscopic interpretation of hematoxylin and eosin (H&E)-stained tissue sections. The Gleason grading system is based entirely on architectural growth patterns of prostatic carcinoma, whereas the WHO scheme incorporates both gland-forming ability and nuclear anaplasia.

■ **t15.1 Grading Schemes for Prostatic Carcinoma: Selected Approaches**

Study	Characteristics
Young 1926	Four groups (1-4) based on gland appearance.
Muir 1934	Three groups (I-III) based on differentiation and ability to form "tubules".
Kahler 1938	Grades 1-4; grade related to presence of metastasis, but criteria for grading not given.
Evans 1942	Grade I-IV, using composite grade for three criteria; ability to form acini, cell shape, and nuclear characteristics.
Pool 1956	Grade on 1-4 scale but grade definition not given.
Shelley 1956	Class I-IV, based on "degree of cytologic atypism and anaplasia".
Bauer 1960	Three grades - well, moderate, and poor, "depending upon the retention of the glandular pattern."
Vickery 1963	Two grades: well-differentiated and poorly differentiated.
Gleason 1966-1974	Five patterns and their combination as most common and second most common pattern (score).
Jewett 1968	Three grades of well-, moderately, and poorly differentiated cancer.
Mobley 1968	Grades 1-3, using gland forming ability and nuclear features.
Utz 1961	Grades 1-4, based on architecture, cytology, and mitoses.
Hohbach 1972,1977	Four groups based on histologic pattern, in order from best to worst prognosis: well-differentiated, poorly-differentiated, cribriform, solid-anaplastic.
Mostofi 1975,1980 (WHO)	Grade I-III, using capacity to form glandular spaces and nuclear atypia.
Gaeta 1980	Grades I-IV, defined by gland formation and organization, amount of stroma, nuclear atypia, and mitotic count.
Böcking 1980,1982	Grade of 1-3 based on differentiation pattern and nuclear anaplasia, using highest grade.
Brawn 1982	MDAH System: Grade 1-4, depending on % tumor that is gland-forming or non-gland-forming.
Myers 1982	Nucleolar prominence correlated with progression in very small series (n=13).
Tannenbaum 1982	Measurement of nucleolar surface area.
Diamond 1982	Relative nuclear roundness used.
Schroeder 1985	Scoring system with 5 prognostic groups, based on architecture, nuclear anaplasia, mitoses.
Uchida 1988	Japanese General Rules of Prostatic Cancer: Well-, moderately, and poorly differentiated.
Robutti 1989	Morphometric nuclear grading related to clinical stage.
Bibbo 1991,1993	Automated histometric and Bayesian belief network grading.
Eskelinen 1991	Morphometric nuclear perimeter and mitotic activity used with or without WHO grade in predicting progression.
Nielsen 1992	Mean nuclear volume predicted survival.
Irinopoulou 1993	Grading by image analysis of chromatin texture linked to metastasis.
Bostwick 1994	Nuclear grade on a 1-3 scale not useful in predicting pathologic stage: almost all cases were grade 2.
Jorgensen 1996	Image analysis of nuclear texture features used to predict tumor progression and survival.
Fujikawa 1995, 2000	Mean nuclear volume correlated with pathologic stage and survival.
Arima 1997	Mean nuclear volume predicted survival.
Hurwitz 1999	Nuclear morphometry predicted disease-free interval after radiation therapy.

[15.2] World Health Organization (Mostofi) System

In 1975, Mostofi devised a histopathologic grading method that combined light microscopic evaluation of differentiation and the degree of nuclear anaplasia (Mostofi 1975, 1980) **t15.2**. *Differentiation* here indicates the ability of the carcinoma cells to form glands. However, the characteristics of "well-differentiated" glands in grade I carcinoma are not specified (Mostofi 1975). Nuclear grade is based on variation from normal nuclei: slight anaplasia is seen in grade I, moderate variation and moderate anaplasia characterize grade II, and marked variation and marked anaplasia are present in grade III (Mostofi 1975). One problem with this system, as is true for all 3-tiered grading approaches, is the tendency to place most cases in the middle, grade II bin (Lilleby 2001).

[15.3] Gleason System

General Approach

The Gleason grading system for prostatic carcinoma is the dominant method around the world in research and in daily practice. This technique was developed by Dr. Donald F. Gleason, a pathologist in Minnesota, and members of the Veterans Administration Cooperative Urological Research Group (VACURG). From 1960 to 1975 the VACURG enrolled roughly 5000 patients with prostate cancer in prospective randomized clinical trials (Gleason 1966, 1974, 1977, 1990, 1992, Mellinger 1967). One of the outstanding strengths of the Gleason grading system is that it was tested in this large patient population, with long-term follow-up that included use of survival as an endpoint. The first article on the Gleason grading system was published in 1966 (Gleason 1966), and the last review written by Gleason was published in 1992 (Gleason 1992).

The Gleason grading system is based entirely on the histologic pattern of arrangement of carcinoma cells in H&E-stained prostatic tissue sections **t15.3**. Specifically, the method is one of categorization of histologic patterns "at relatively low magnification (×10-40) by the extent of glandular differentiation and the pattern of growth of the tumor in the prostatic stroma" (Gleason 1990). Nine growth patterns were consolidated into 5 grades, and these were illustrated in a drawing by Dr. Gleason **f15.1**. These 5 basic grade patterns are used to generate a histologic score, which can range from 2 to 10, by adding the primary grade pattern and the secondary grade pattern.

■ t15.2 World Health Organization (Mostofi) Grading System

Grade	Definition
I	Well-differentiated glands with nuclei that show slight nuclear anaplasia
II	Gland formation but the nuclei show moderate nuclear anaplasia
III	Glands with marked nuclear anaplasia or tumors that are undifferentiated (do not form glands)

Mostofi 1980

■ t15.3 Gleason Grading System for Prostatic Carcinoma

Developed from 1960-1975 and based on follow-up of 5,000 patients
Employs extent of glandular differentiation and pattern of growth
Nuclear atypia not used
Five basic grade patterns, which are well-described
Patterns are illustrated in a standard and simple drawing
Primary grade pattern (predominant by area) and secondary grade pattern added to yield histologic score, which can range from 2-10
Nine scores of 2-10 are correlated with numerous prognostic, pathologic and clinical endpoints, including patient survival

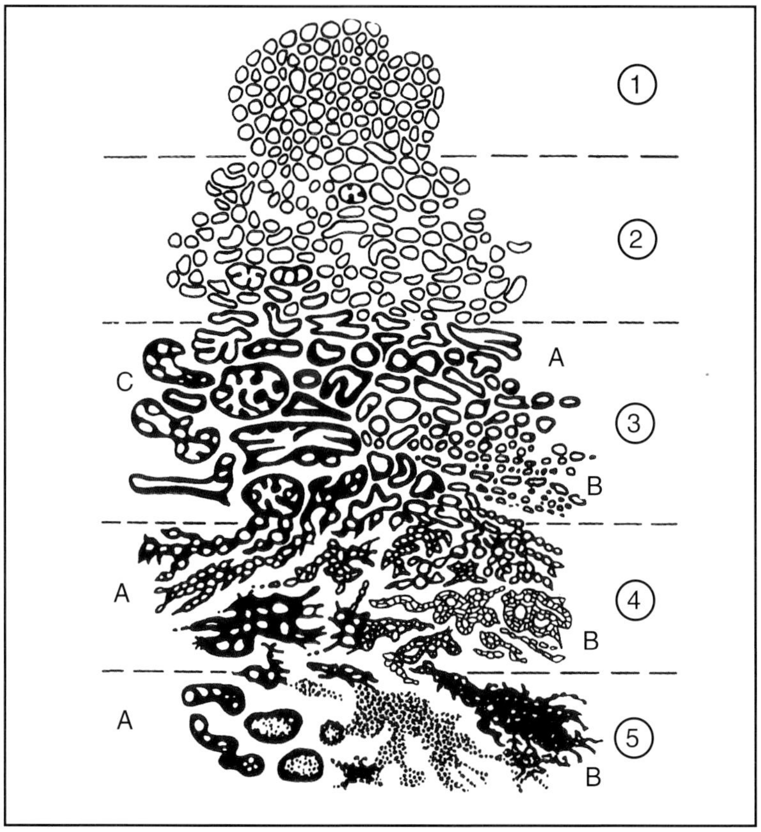

■ f15.1 *Gleason grades: Standard drawing (Reproduction of Fig. 6-1 from "Histologic grading of prostatic carcinoma"* [Gleason 1990]*).*

The primary pattern is the one that is predominant in area, by simple visual inspection. The secondary pattern is the second most common pattern. If only 1 grade is in the tissue sample, that grade is multiplied by 2 to give the score. According to the Gleason approach of 1990, if the second grade is <3% of the total tumor, it is ignored, and the primary grade is again doubled to give the Gleason score (Gleason 1990). Currently, this cutoff is not commonly used.

Gleason sum, Gleason grade, combined Gleason grade, and *category score* have been used as synonyms for *Gleason score,* but "histological pattern score" was the initial 1974 designation for the sum of the 2 patterns (Mellinger 1967). and "histologic score" has endured in usage in the writings of Gleason (Gleason 1974, 1977, 1990, 1992).

The assignment of a Gleason score, which is the addition of the 2 most common patterns, essentially averages the primary and secondary grades. This procedure appears to be unique in grading of human cancers, where, for other malignancies, it is the worst grade that determines patient outcome. Peculiarly, for prostatic carcinoma, when there are 2 different Gleason grade patterns, the cancer death rates are intermediate between the rates for patients with only the pure form of each of those 2 grades (Gleason 1977, 1990, 1992).

The Gleason grading system allows 2 separate grade patterns in an individual tissue sample, but the histomorphologic appearance of prostatic carcinoma is more heterogeneous than this. Indeed, in one study (Aihara 1994), an average of 2.7 Gleason grade patterns (range 1 to 5) was found in carcinomas in whole prostate glands. Two additional articles reported that 14% to 18% of patients had more than 2 grades in sections of their prostatic carcinoma (McGowan 1983, Ruijter 1996). In one of these reports (Ruijter 1996), 3% of cases had 4 different Gleason patterns. The number of grades assigned depends on tumor sample size and size of the tumor in the whole gland (Aihara 1994, McGowan 1983, Ruijter 1996). Therefore, more than 2 grades is more often observed in transurethral resection of the prostate (TURP) chips (28% of cases) than in needle biopsies (4% of cases) (McGowan 1983), and tumors >1cm^3 in size tended to have more than 2 grades (Aihara 1994, Ruijter 1996).

There are limited data on how to grade carcinomas with more than 2 grades. Gleason wrote that the VACURG was unable to acquire enough 3-grade tumors to evaluate their behavior but has proposed an algorithm to provide a Gleason score in cases with more than 2 grades (Gleason 1990). Recent data on radical prostatectomy specimens indicate that a high-grade Gleason pattern 4 or 5 that is a tertiary component occupying <5% of the tumor influences pathologic stage and progression rates (Pan 2000). Therefore, any tertiary high-grade pattern should be mentioned in surgical pathology reports on radical prostatectomy specimens. In needle biopsies, Gleason has recommended that the 2 highest grades be recorded (Gleason 1990). (This is a contradiction of Gleason's own system, which was devised in large part [60% of cases] on needle biopsies.) The 2003 WHO recommendation for needle biopsy tissue with three grades, where the highest grade is the least common, is to in corporate the highest grade as the secondary pattern (WHO 2003).

"Lumping" or "grade compression" by combining Gleason scores in attempts to translate to other grading systems should be avoided. Such grouping often results in loss of information, with the risk of combining grades of different biologic aggressiveness into one larger category. Many different approaches to lumping Gleason scores have been published **t15.4** (Bagshaw 1990, Catalona 1994, Epstein 1993, 1996, Gleason 1977, Green 1998, Hanks 1995, Ohori 1994A, Pilepich 1987, Russell 1991, Tefilli 1999, Zagars 1995). As compared with the 9 groups of Gleason score 2 to 10, groupings of 2, 3, and 4 categories have been used **t15.4**. A common practice has been to translate Gleason score 2 to 4 carcinoma as well-differentiated, Gleason score 5 to 7 as moderately differentiated, and Gleason score 8 to 10 as poorly differentiated. Yet Gleason score 7 carcinoma harbors an element of high-grade pattern carcinoma and is intermediate in clinical aggressiveness between patterns 5 to 6 and 8 to 10 (Epstein 1996, Zagars 1995) and should not be included in a moderately differentiated category. If lumping is necessary because of low patient numbers in a research setting, the 2 to 6 vs 7 vs 8 to 10 lump or 2 to 4 vs 5 to 6 vs 7 vs 8 to 10 lump seems most appropriate.

Gleason Pattern 1 (Grade 1)

This is a rare pattern of very well-differentiated growth of closely packed but separate, uniform, rounded to oval, medium-sized acini **t15.5**. Of the original 2911 cases of prostatic carcinoma in the VACURG series, this pattern was found in 3.5% of cases

■ t15.4 Lumping of Gleason Scores

Lumping Approach	Reference
2-6 vs 7-10	Hanks 1995, Epstein 1993
2-5 vs 6-7 vs 8-10	Pilepich 1987
2-4 vs 5-7 vs 8-10	Catalona 1994, Russell 1991
2-4 vs 5-6 vs 7-10	Freedland 2000
2-6 vs 7 vs 8-10	Tefilli 1999
2-5 vs 6 vs 7 vs 8-10	Bagshaw 1990
2-3 vs 4-6 vs 7 vs 8-10	Zagars 1995
2-4 vs 5-6 vs 7 vs 8-10	Epstein 1996, Ohori 1994A, Green 1998
2-3 vs 4-5 vs 6 vs 7-8 vs 9-10	Gleason 1977

■ t15.5 Gleason Grading System for Prostatic Adenocarcinoma

Pattern	Tumor Shape and Borders	Stromal Invasion	Tumor Cell Arrangements	Gland Size
1	Nodular, well-defined and smooth edges	Pushing	Single, round to oval, closely-packed, but separate glands	Medium
2	Masses less well-defined and less well-circumscribed	Some gland separation at tumor edge	Single, separate, round to oval glands, with more variation in gland size and shape, and loosely-packed with stromal separation (up to one gland diameter, on average)	Medium
3A	Ill-defined infiltrating edges	Irregular extension	Single separate glands of variable shape and size, with elongated, angular and twisted forms, usually with wide stromal separation	Medium
3B	Ill-defined infiltrating edges	Irregular extension	Same as 3A but glands are smaller	Small to very small
3C	Masses and cylinders with smooth rounded edges	Expansile	Papillary and cribriform epithelium, without necrosis	Medium to large
4A	Raggedly infiltrative	Diffusely permeative	Fused glands, creating masses, cords, or chains	Small, medium, or large
4B	Raggedly infiltrative	Diffusely permeative	Similar to 4A, but cells have cleared cytoplasm = hypernephromatoid variant	Small, medium, or large
5A	Smooth, rounded cylinders	Expansile	Papillary, cribriform or solid masses with central necrosis = comedocarcinoma	Variable
5B	Raggedly infiltrative	Diffusely permeative	Masses and sheets of anaplastic carcinoma, with a few tiny glands or signet ring cells	Small

■ t15.6 Gleason Pattern 1 (Grade 1): Mixture With Other Patterns[1]

Pattern 1 is Primary Grade	% of Cases[2]
1+1	0.5%
1+2	1.1%
1+3	0.1%[3]
1+4	0.03%[4]
1+5	0%
Pattern 1 is Secondary Grade	**% of Cases**
1+1	0.5%
2+1	1.8%
3+1	0%
4+1	0%
5+1	0%

[1]Data from original Gleason series of 2,911 prostate cancer patients (Gleason 1977)
[2]% of all 2,911 cases
[3]3 cases
[4]1 case

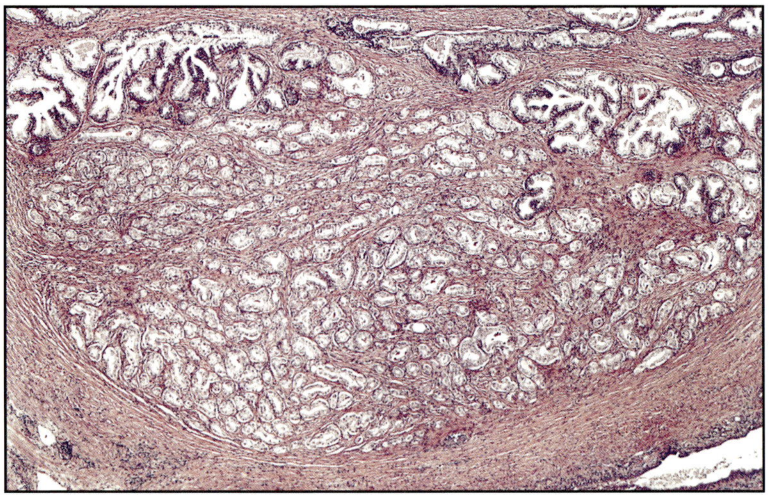

■ **i15.1** *Gleason pattern 1 admixed with 2 = score of 3. Nodule of fairly uniform small malignant acini, with a smooth outer contour. (Courtesy of Dr. Allan Tucker).*

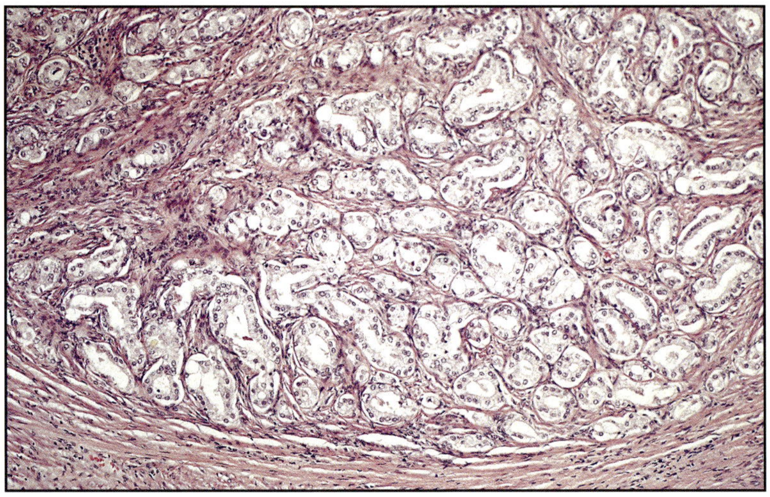

■ **i15.2** *Gleason score 3 adenocarcinoma: Higher power view of* **i15.1.**

(Gleason 1977), usually admixed with pattern 2 **t15.6; i15.1**. Of critical importance, this is a nodular and circumscribed mass of glands with a rounded border of tumoral-stromal interface **i15.2**.

Although the Gleason grading system is supposed to be based solely on gland pattern and differentiation (Gleason 1990), the original article (Gleason 1966) and a subsequent publication (Gleason 1990), both written by Gleason, incorporate cytologic features in diagnosis of Gleason pattern 1, also called grade 1 carcinoma. The tumor cells were portrayed as being of uniform size, with pale cytoplasm and uniform small nuclei (Gleason 1966) but with at least a few cells containing prominent nucleoli (>1μm in diameter) (Gleason 1990). The latter criterion was added in 1990 to address the differential diagnosis with atypical adenomatous hyperplasia (adenosis), yet nucleolomegaly is not always detected in well-differentiated adenocarcinoma.

Infiltration of malignant acini into surrounding stroma, including encirclement of benign glands or penetration between benign glands, is indicative of a higher-grade carcinoma. Also, the back-to-back glands should be separated by thin stromal rims. If tumor cells form back-to-back glands, without intervening stroma, then the Gleason pattern is high-grade 4, not pattern 1 or 2.

Pattern 1 is most often admixed with pattern 2 to yield a Gleason score of 3 (Gleason 1977) **t15.6**. A pure pattern 1 adenocarcinoma, with Gleason grade 1 + 1 = score of 2 is rare or nonexistent (McNeal 2001). In the VACURG series, score 2 adenocarcinomas made up <1% of all cases **t15.6**. This author has never diagnosed a pure pattern 1; one must wonder whether these cases represent atypical adenomatous hyperplasia (adenosis) because Gleason score 2 carcinomas were defined before the availability of high-molecular-weight cytokeratin immunostains and use of standardized definitions of atypical adenomatous hyperplasia (adenosis) (Chapter 8). Combinations of pattern 1 with intermediate-grade Gleason pattern 3 and high-grade Gleason patterns 4 and 5 are vanishingly rare **t15.6**. Before diagnosing a pure Gleason pattern 1 adenocarcinoma, one should exclude atypical adenomatous hyperplasia (adenosis).

Pattern 1 carcinoma is most often an incidental finding in transition zone tissue, diagnosed in TURP chips resected because of a clinical diagnosis of benign prostatic hyperplasia (BPH) or in radical prostatectomies performed because an associated, peripheral zone, intermediate- to high-grade carcinoma was detected. It has been argued that well-differentiated Gleason pattern 1 and 2 adenocarcinomas should not be diagnosed in peripheral zone needle biopsies because a diagnosis of Gleason score 2 to 4 carcinoma in needle biopsy almost always represents undergraded intermediate-grade carcinoma (Epstein 2000B).

Pattern scores are strongly correlated with tumor extent, expressed as the percentage area of prostate tissue in TURP chips or radical prostatectomy specimens (Gleason 1977, Humphrey 1990). Therefore, pattern 1 in scores of 2 and 3 usually is a focal finding, involving <10% of prostatic tissue (Gleason 1977, Humphrey 1990).

Gleason Pattern 2 (Grade 2)

This well-differentiated pattern forms less well-defined masses that are not as circumscribed as pattern 1, with a tumor-stromal boundary that is not as rounded as pattern 1 (Gleason 1966, 1977, 1990) **i15.3–i15.5**. Compared to pattern 1, the carcinomatous glands of pattern 2 display a degree of separation by stroma, with an average of partial separation distance of less than one gland diameter **i15.5**. Another distinctive characteristic of pattern 2 adenocarcinoma is the increase in variability

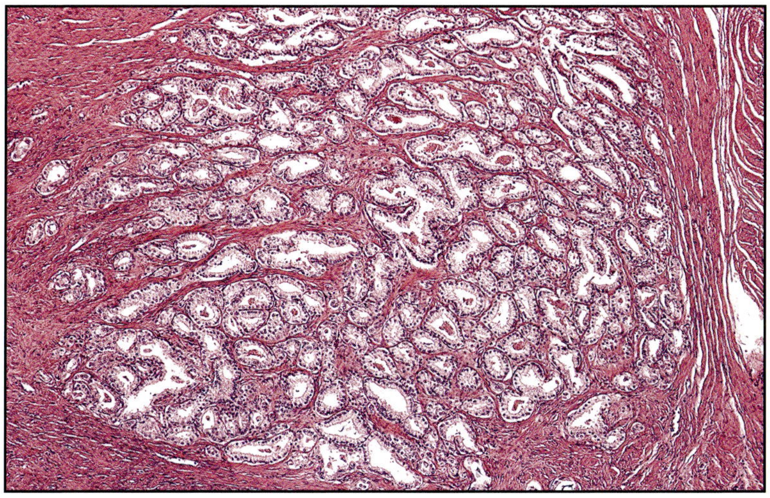

■ **i15.3** *Gleason pattern 2, with score of 4. There is greater variability in gland size and shape.*

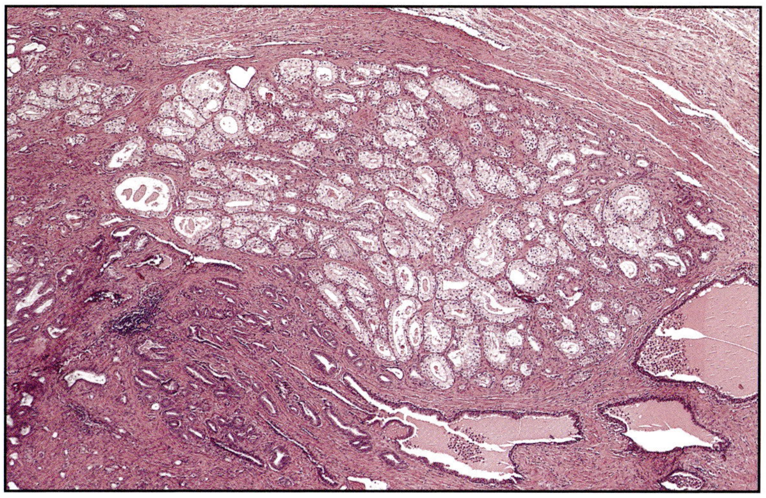

■ **i15.4** *Pale nodule of well-differentiated prostatic adenocarcinoma, Gleason grade 2+2 = score of 4.*

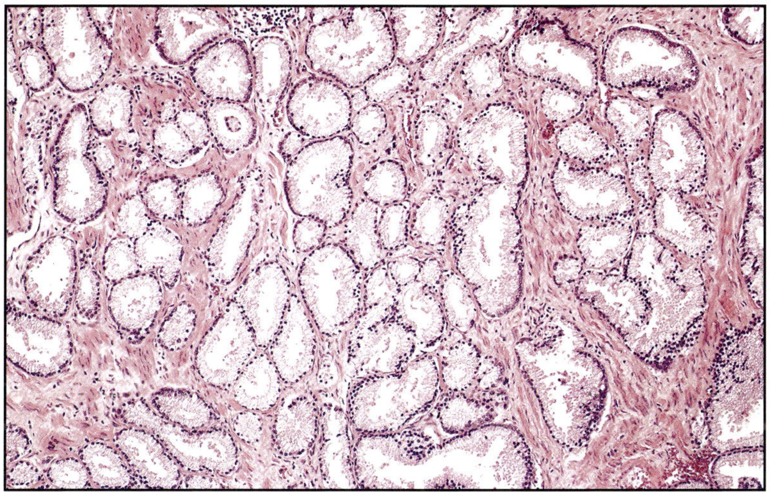

■ **i15.5** *Stromal separation in Gleason pattern 2 adenocarcinoma.*

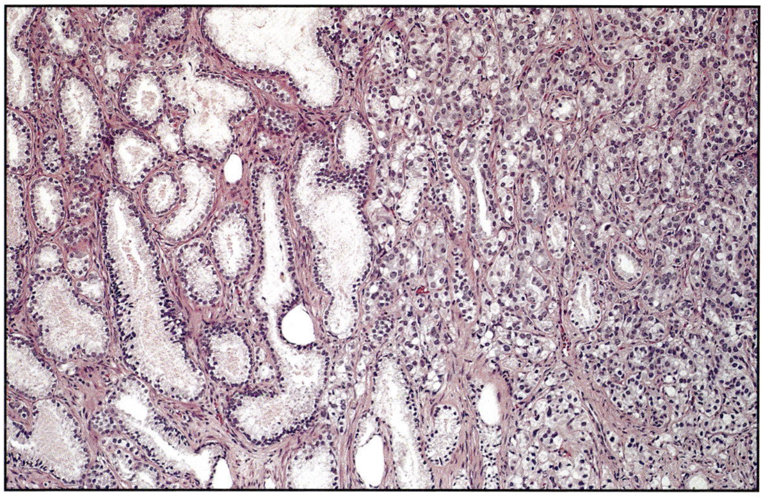

■ **i15.6** *Pattern 2 (left) merging with pattern 4 (right) = score of 6.*

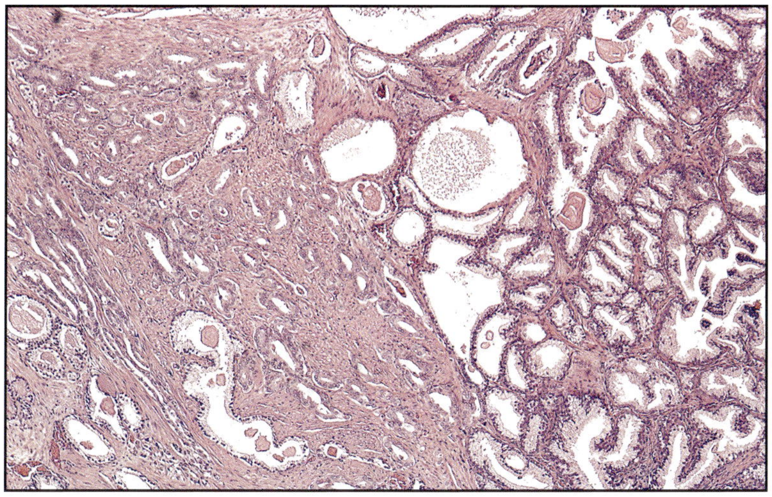

■ **i15.7** *Pattern 3 (left) adenocarcinoma, with score of 6, infiltrating adjacent to hyperplasia (right).*

in gland size and shape. However, there is only a limited capacity to infiltrate into stroma, as suggested by some gland separation at the periphery of the tumor mass. The original description of pattern 2 (Gleason 1966) and the standardized drawing of pattern 2 indicate that focal cribriform structures might be present, but cribriform arrangements are most characteristic of intermediate- to high-grade disease.

Pattern 2 usually is found admixed with pattern 3 to yield a Gleason score of 5 (Gleason 1977) **t15.7**. In a small percentage of cases pattern 2 is pure (such that the score is 2 + 2 = 4) or is intermingled with pattern 1. A composite of pattern 2 with high-grade patterns 4 or 5 is extremely uncommon **i15.6; t15.7**.

Pattern 2 adenocarcinoma, like pattern 1, often is an incidental finding in transition zone carcinomas and therefore is typically seen in TURP chips. Pattern 2 as a component of Gleason score 5 can also be found fairly commonly in radical prostatectomy specimens. In needle biopsy, one should diagnose pattern 2 in a Gleason score of 3 or 4 either rarely or not at all (Epstein 2000B).

Pattern 2 in the score setting of 4 to 5 often is focal (<10% of tissue [Humphrey 1990]) but can be extensive, involving 20% to 50% of TURP chips or prostatectomy tissue (Gleason 1977).

Gleason Pattern 3 (Grade 3)

This moderately differentiated grade is the most common pattern of growth of prostatic adenocarcinoma, both in the pre-PSA

■ **t15.7 Gleason Pattern 2 (Grade 2): Mixture With Other Patterns**[1]

Pattern 2 is Primary Grade	**% of Cases**[2]
2+1	1.8%
2+2	2.2%
2+3	8.6%
2+4	0.03%[3]
2+5	0.03%[3]
Pattern 2 is Secondary Grade	**% of Cases**
1+2	1.1%
2+2	2.2%
3+2	10.5%
4+2	0%
5+2	0.03%[3]

[1]Data from original Gleason series of 2,911 prostate cancer patients (Gleason 1977)
[2]% of all 2,911 cases
[3]1 case

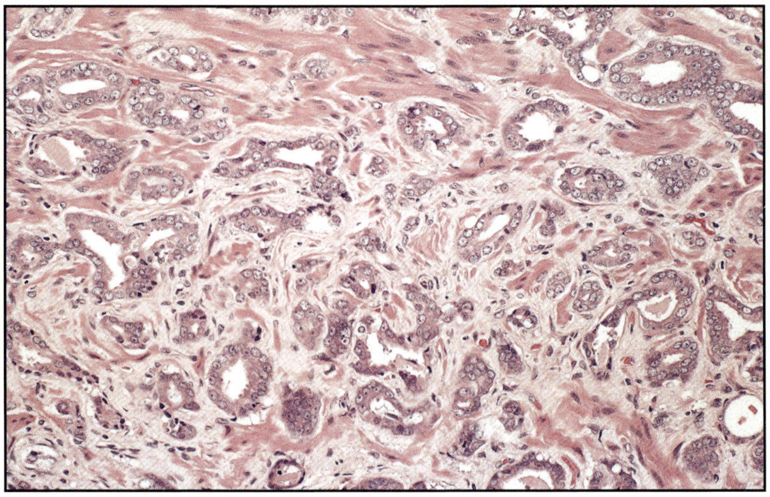

■ **i15.8** *Gleason pattern 3 (and score of 6) with separation of variable, single, small, malignant acini.*

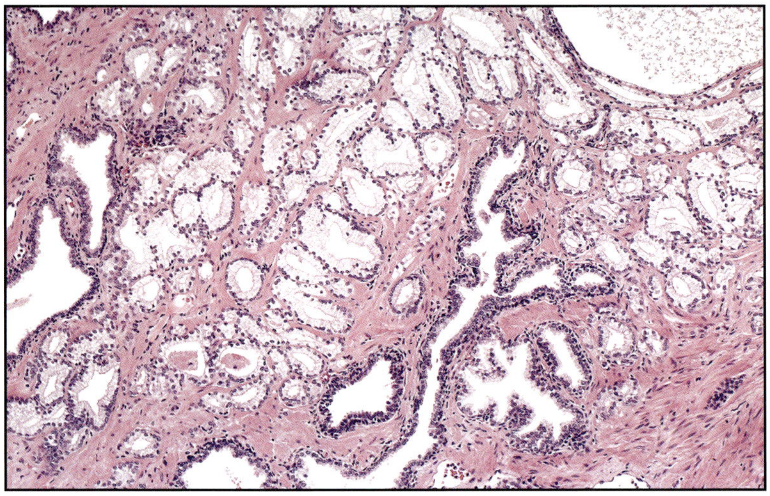

■ **i15.9** *Pattern 3 (and score of 6), with invasion of pale small acini between and around benign glands. Due to lack of nodularity, with infiltrative growth pattern, this is pattern 3, not 2.*

era (Gleason 1977) and in the PSA screening era (Epstein 1994A, Humphrey 1996). Pattern 3 has been characterized as having 3 distinctive appearances, designated patterns 3A, 3B, and 3C **f15.1; t15.5**. It has been suggested that there is increased aggressiveness of pattern 3 carcinoma in proceeding from pattern 3A to 3B to 3C (Gleason 1990), but no data have been published in support of this notion. Accordingly, it is not necessary to specify pattern 3A, 3B, or 3C. Rather, these different subpatterns within the range of pattern 3 images serve a role in recognition of grade 3 disease.

Gleason grade pattern 3A is characterized by infiltrating, medium-sized, single glands of irregular shape and spacing and haphazard, irregular extension of glands into stroma **i15.7**. There is typically appreciable, stromal separation of glands, where the intervening stroma usually is greater than 1 gland diameter. Densely packed gland arrangements are allowable in pattern 3, but there should be attendant evidence of infiltrative growth. The shape of the glands is quite variable **i15.8**, with angular, elongated, and "twisted" forms described (Gleason 1990). The angular glands can have sharp corners or points (Gleason 1990). Pattern 3 adenocarcinoma glands generally are darker than well-differentiated patterns 1 and 2, which results in part from cytoplasmic basophilia (Gleason 1990), but again, cytoplasmic features should not be used in Gleason grading; it is possible to detect Gleason pattern 3 glands with cytoplasmic clearing **i15.9**.

Pattern 3B is essentially the same as 3A except that the glands are smaller **f15.1** (Gleason 1990). These glands should still have the capability of forming glandular luminal spaces. If cords or chains without glandular lumina are seen, this is indicative of high-grade Gleason pattern 4, not intermediate-grade pattern 3.

Pattern 3C consists of expanded cylinders or ducts with masses of cribriform or papillary tumor **f15.1** (Gleason 1990, 1992). Consistent with the possibility that this pattern actually represents intraductal growth, the tumor masses should have smooth, rounded edges, like expanded duct profiles. However, the Gleason grading scheme does not distinguish in situ growth from invasive carcinoma, such that it is possible that some of these 3C patterns may be ducts with basal cells present. Therefore, some pattern 3C cribriform proliferations represent cribriform high-grade prostatic intraepithelial neoplasia (Rubin 1998). Another view (McNeal 1986A, 1996) is that these duct lumen–spanning cribriform masses are intraductal carcinoma (carcinoma in situ), but this is not currently an accepted diagnostic entity. The papillary pattern 3C carcinomas may, in similar fashion, represent in situ spread of the ductal variant of prostatic carcinoma.

Cribriform masses can also present in high-grade Gleason pattern 4, but the edges of these masses are ragged and infiltrative, not smooth. Necrosis should not be seen in pattern 3C; if necrosis is visible, pattern 5, not pattern 3, should be diagnosed.

In most cases Gleason grade pattern 3 is found in pure form, such that the most common Gleason score is 3 + 3 = 6 **t15.8**. It is also fairly common to identify Gleason pattern 3 in combination with low-grade pattern 2 for a score of 5 or in conjunction with pattern 4 to yield a score of 7. In Gleason's series, a composite with pattern 5 to give a score of 8 **i15.10** was more common than a mingling with 4 to produce a score of 7 (Gleason 1977) **t15.8**, but today Gleason score 7 **i15.11** is more common than 8 **i15.10** (Bostwick 1994A, Humphrey 1996, Pound 1997). Overall, Gleason scores of 5 to 7 with embedded pattern 3 are the most common histologic grades of prostatic adenocarcinoma **t15.8, t15.9**.

Gleason Pattern 4 (Grade 4)

This is a high-grade and poorly differentiated carcinoma growth, with raggedly infiltrative masses or chains or cords of malignant

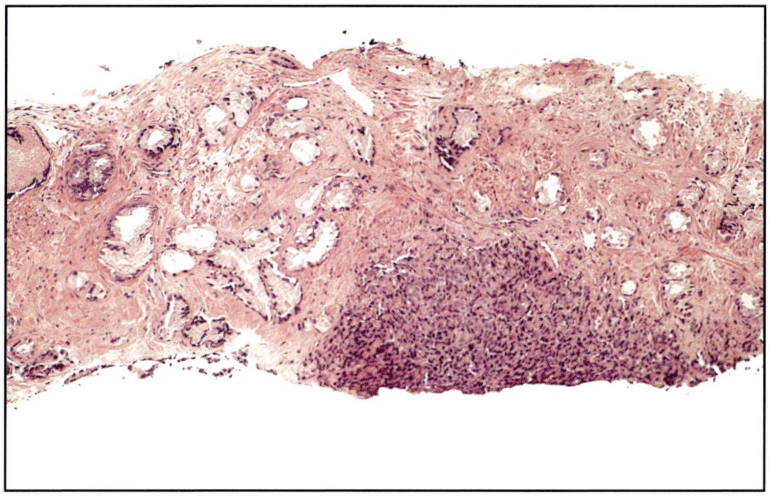

■ **i15.10** *Gleason grade 3 (small pale acini) plus 5 (solid sheet) = score of 8 in needle biopsy tissue.*

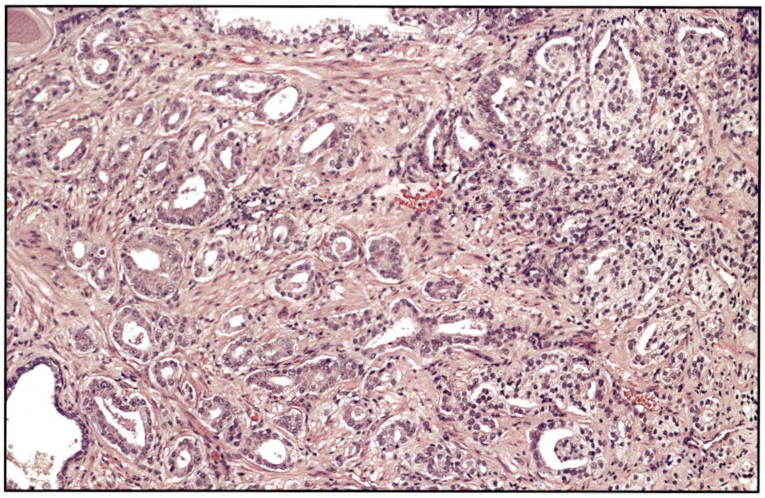

■ **i15.11** *Gleason grade 3 (left) plus 4 (right) = score of 7.*

■ **t15.8 Gleason Pattern 3 (Grade 3): Mixture With Other Patterns**[1]

Pattern 3 is Primary Grade	% of Cases[2]
3+1	0%
3+2	10.5%
3+3	42.6%
3+4	6.1%
3+5	12%
Pattern 3 is Secondary Grade	**% of Cases**
1+3	0.1%[3]
2+3	8.6%
3+3	42.6%
4+3	2.6%
5+3	5.3%

[1]Data from original Gleason series of 2,911 prostate cancer patients (Gleason 1977)
[2]% of all 2,911 cases
[3]3 cases

epithelial cells **i15.12–i15.15**. The cellular arrangements can be fused microacinar **i15.15**, cribriform **i15.13**, or papillary. Cribriform and papillary pattern 4 carcinomas can resemble cribriform and papillary pattern 3 carcinomas in gland formations and papillary projections, but pattern 4 is recognized by the ragged edges or outlines of the invasive periphery compared with the smooth, pushing borders of pattern 3C. Carcinoma growing in this manner, but with cleared cytoplasm, is deemed pattern 4B and can simulate renal cell carcinoma of clear cell type (hypernephroma). Therefore, this variant has been called the hypernephroid (Gleason 1977) or hypernephromatoid pattern. The nuclei in pattern 4 may be deceptively bland, with little nucleomegaly and no nucleolomegaly. In these cases, highly infiltrative small, fused glands should be a clue as to the high-grade nature of the carcinoma.

Pattern 4 is most often combined with pattern 3 to yield a score of 7 **i15.11, i15.16**, which is currently one of the most commonly assigned Gleason scores **t15.9**. Pure high-grade disease, where there is pure pattern 4 or mingling with pattern 5 to produce scores of 8 and 9, is less common. Gleason score 8 is more common in series, such as the VACURG series (Gleason 1977), that include higher-stage, clinically non–organ-confined prostate cancer. Pattern 4 is hardly ever found with well-differentiated patterns 1 and 2 **t15.10**.

■ **t15.9 Gleason Score Distribution**

Gleason Score	Original Gleason/ VACURG Series, 1977[1] (N = 2,911)	Needle Biopsies[2] (N = 965)	Radical Prostatectomy[3] (N = 1,623)
2	0.5%	0%	2-4: 4%
3	3%	0.3%	2-4: 4%
4	2%	6%	2-4: 4%
5	19%	15%	19%
6	43%	48%	35%
7	9%	24%	33%
8	18%	6%	8-10: 9%
9	2%	5%	8-10: 9%
10	3%	0.4%	8-10: 9%

[1]Based on examination of needle biopsies (60% of cases), TURP chips and prostatectomies (Gleason 1977). Clinical stages: I: 10.2%; II: 8.3%; III: 45.6%; IV: 35.9%
[2]Pooled contemporary data from three centers (Bostwick 1994A, Steinberg 1997, Narain 2001). These are patients with clinically localized disease who were candidates for radical prostatectomy
[3]Based on examination of radical prostatectomy specimens (Pound 1997)

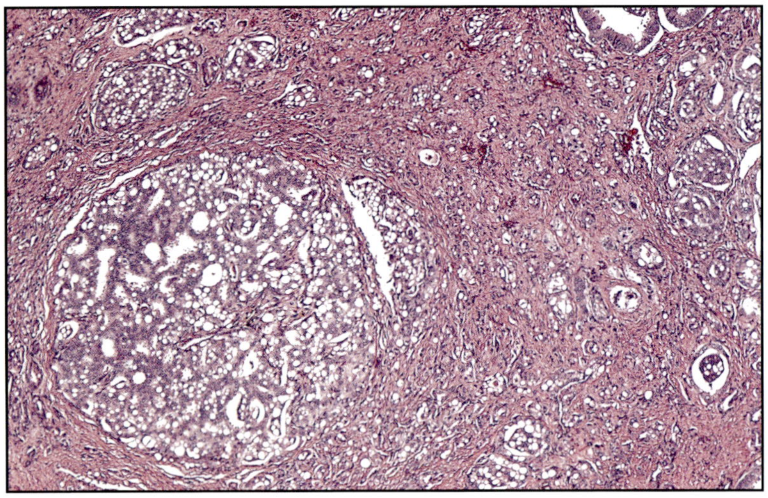

■ **i15.12** *Pattern 4 with nodular mass and surrounding raggedly infiltrative cords of cells.*

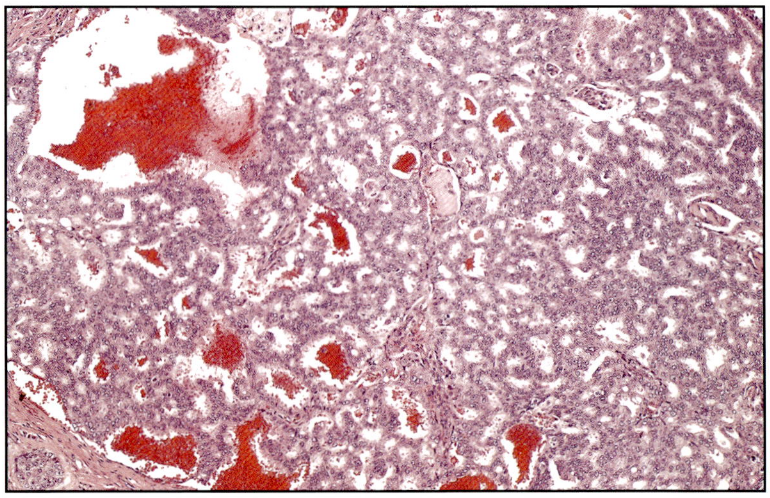

■ **i15.13** *Mass of cribriform pattern 4.*

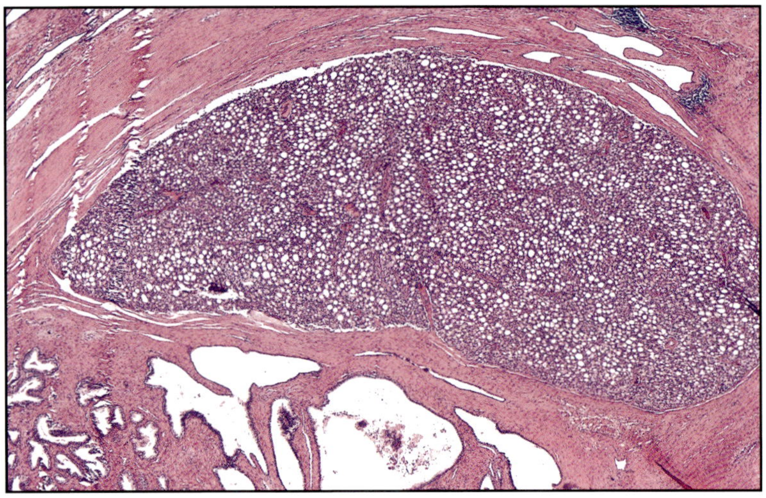

■ **i15.14** *Nodule of fused microacinar pattern 4.*

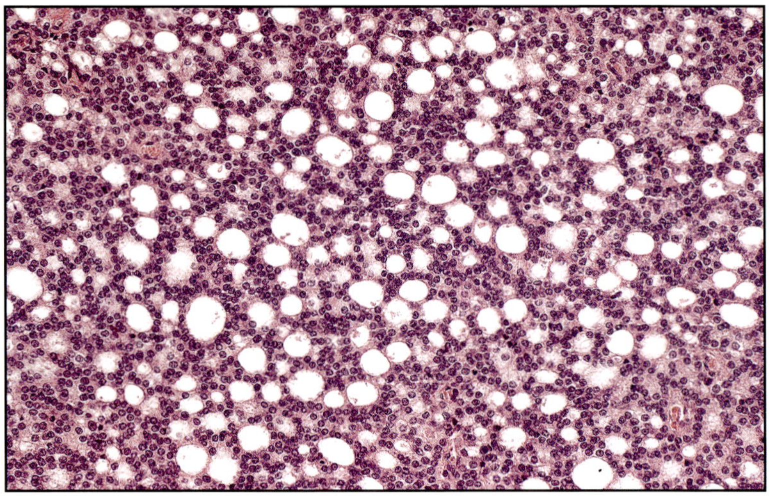

■ **i15.15** *Fused microacinar adenocarcinoma: Higher magnification of* **i15.14**.

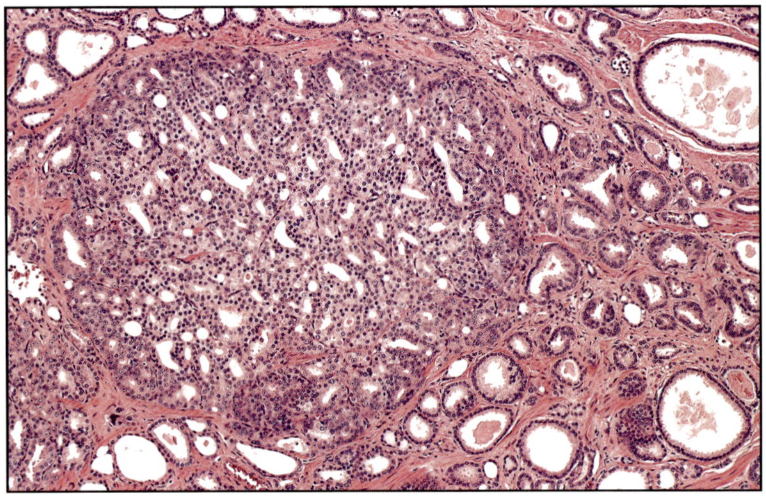

■ **i15.16** *Nodular pattern 4, with surrounding pattern 3 = score of 7.*

■ t15.10 **Gleason Pattern 4 (Grade 4): Mixture With Other Patterns**[1]

Pattern 4 is Primary Grade	% of Cases[2]
4+1	0%
4+2	0%
4+3	2.6%
4+4	1.2%
4+5	1.1%
Pattern 4 is Secondary Grade	**% of Cases**
1+4	0.03%[3]
2+4	0.03%[3]
3+4	6.1%
4+4	1.2%
5+4	1%

[1]Data from original Gleason series of 2,911 prostate cancer patients (Gleason 1977)
[2]% of all 2,911 cases
[3]1 case

Gleason Pattern 5 (Grade 5)

This is the most poorly differentiated pattern of prostatic carcinoma, which presents in two forms: 5A and 5B **f15.1, t15.5**. There is no need to specify 5A or 5B; the distinction is solely for the purpose of grade 5 diagnostic recognition. Pattern 5A resembles the

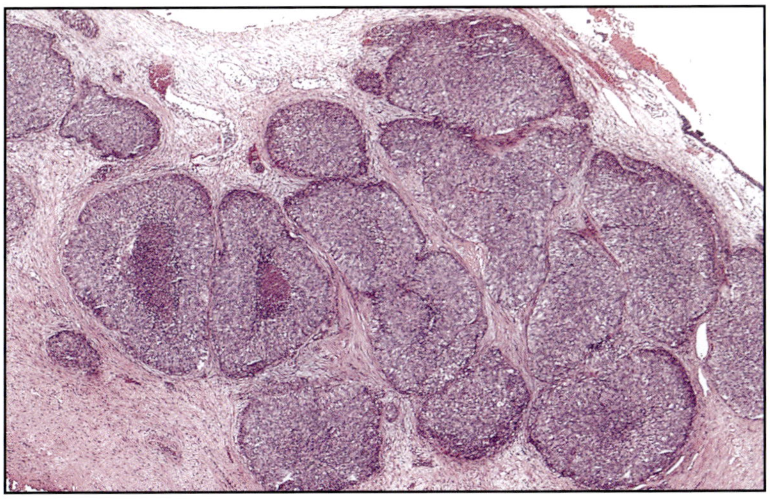

■ **i15.17** *Solid cylinders, with focal comedocarcinoma of Gleason pattern 5 (and score of 10).*

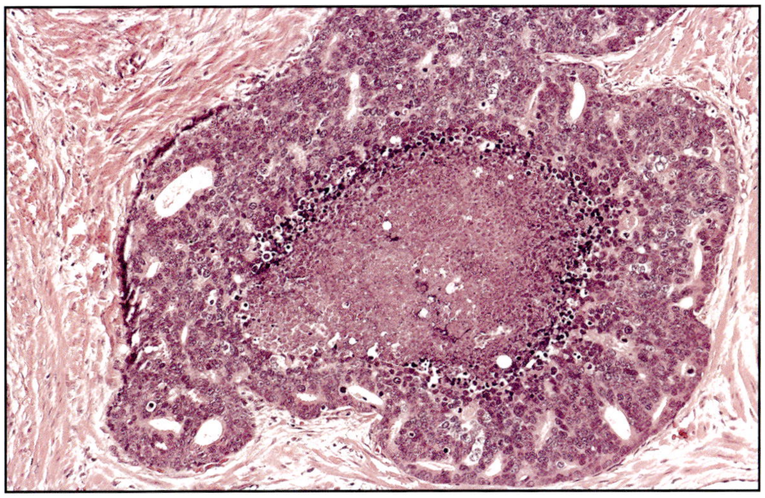

■ **i15.18** *Comedocarcinoma = pattern 5.*

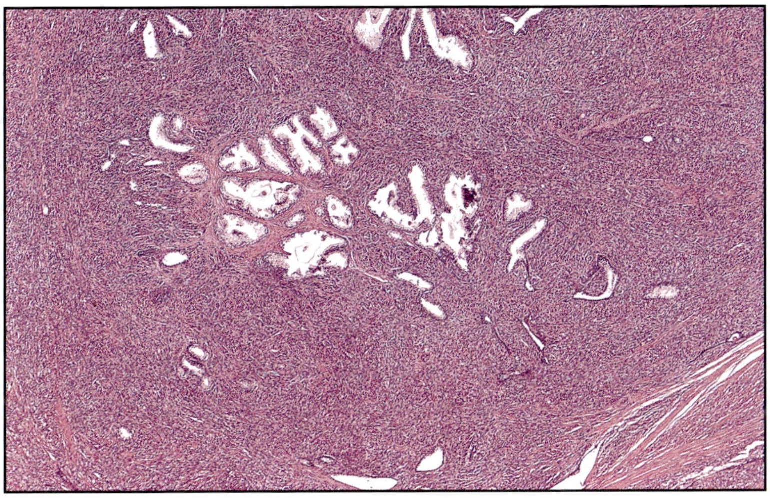

■ **i15.19** *Sheetlike, destructive growth of pattern 5.*

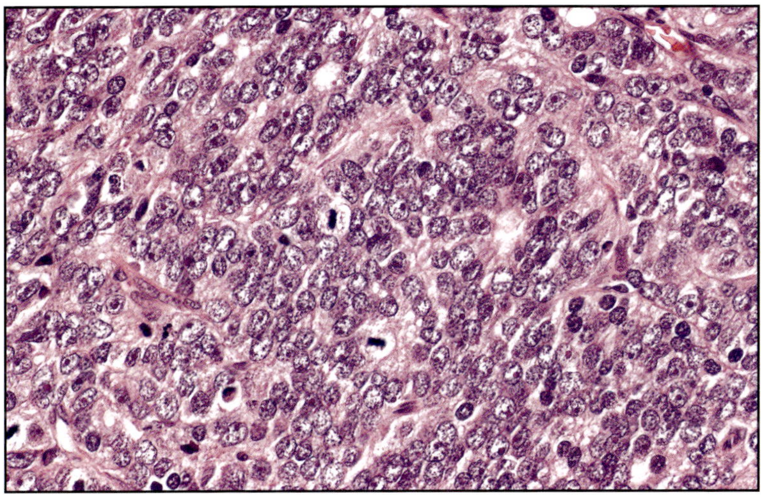

■ **i15.20** *Pattern 5 adenocarcinoma: High magnification view of* **i15.19**.

comedo type of intraductal carcinoma of the breast, with smooth, rounded masses, cords, or cylinders of carcinoma **i15.17**. The necrosis typically is central, being surrounded by papillary, cribriform, or solid masses of carcinoma **i15.17, i15.18**. The appearance can be similar to pattern 3C except for the presence of necrosis. Proteinaceous secretions in prostate carcinoma should not be mistaken for the tumoral cell necrosis of comedocarcinoma, where one can visualize ghostlike outlines of dead carcinoma cells, particularly at the interface of the central necrosis and the viable epithelium. Some cases of pattern 5A actually represent comedo intraductal prostatic carcinoma or in situ spread of ductal adenocarcinoma because basal cells can be observed, but in the Gleason scheme, these designations are not used, and this pattern 5A is just called a Gleason pattern 5 adenocarcinoma.

Pattern 5B consists of ragged sheets of anaplastic adenocarcinoma cells **i15.19-i15.21**. This form is so poorly differentiated that only a few small glandular lumina or signet-ring cells may be present to indicate adenocarcinoma rather than a poorly differentiated malignant neoplasm of unknown cell type.

In summary, raggedly infiltrative sheetlike growth and comedo necrosis are the hallmarks of Gleason pattern 5. Single cell tumor growth often is assumed to be high-grade carcinoma, but this pattern

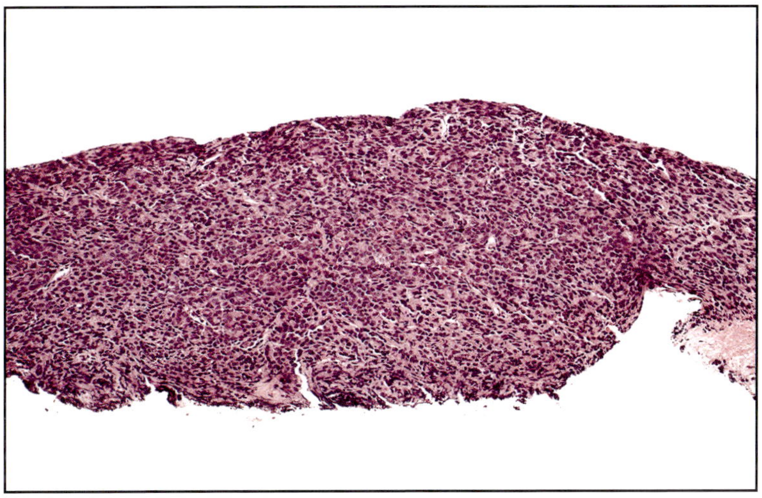

■ **i15.21** *Gleason pattern 5 (and score of 10) carcinoma in needle biopsy tissue: sheetlike growth.*

is not formally recognized in the Gleason system. Indeed, the only time single cells are mentioned in the Gleason publications is in the original 1966 description (Gleason 1966), where single cells are discussed under patterns 2 and 3. Still, if the single cells are raggedly infiltrative

■ **t15.11 Gleason Pattern 5 (Grade 5): Mixture With Other Patterns[1]**

Pattern 5 is Primary Grade	% of Cases[2]
5+1	0%
5+2	0.03%
5+3	5.2%
5+4	1%
5+5	3.2%
Pattern 5 is Secondary Grade	**% of Cases**
1+5	0%
2+5	0.03%[3]
3+5	12%
4+5	1.1%
5+5	3.2%

[1]Data from original Gleason series of 2,911 prostate cancer patients (Gleason 1977)
[2]% of 2,911 cases
[3]1 case

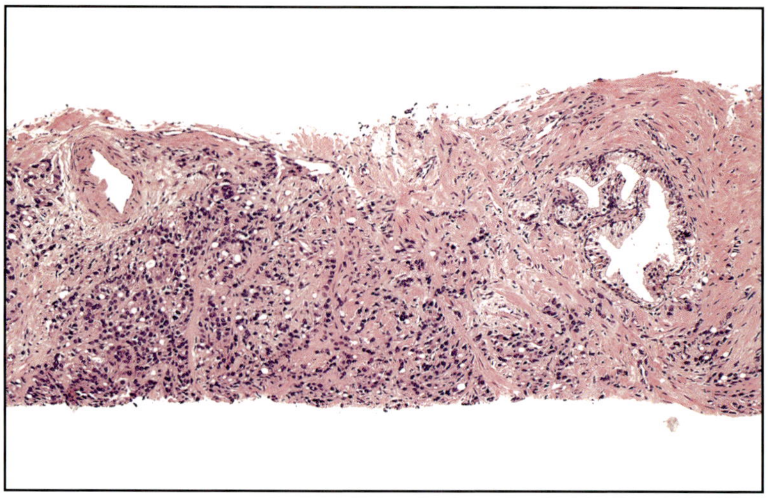

■ **i15.22** *High-grade prostatic carcinoma: Gleason grade 5 + 4 = score of 9.*

or of signet-ring type, then assignment of pattern 5 seems reasonable (Allsbrook 1999, Bostwick 1994A).

Pattern 5 is most often found with pattern 3, with a resultant score of 8 **i15.10; t15.11**. Less common is pure pattern 5 **i15.17–i15.21** or commingling with pattern 4 to yield scores of 10 and 9 **i15.22**, respectively. Gleason scores 9 and 10 are often seen associated with high clinical stage disease, with clinically detectable cancer outside the prostate, either locally or in the form of metastatic disease (Gleason 1977). In only 2 of 2911 cases in the Gleason/VACURG study was pattern 5 detected with patterns 1 or 2 (Gleason 1977) **t15.11**.

Gleason Grade of Histologic Variants of Prostatic Carcinoma

The Gleason system is designed for application in grading of all untreated prostatic glandular carcinomas. Histomorphologic variants of prostatic carcinoma are uncommon, accounting for <10% of all prostatic carcinoma cases (Chapter 17). The Gleason approach specifically addresses 3 variants: ductal (called endometrioid in the past), signet-ring cell, and prostatic carcinoma resembling small cell carcinoma (Gleason 1977, 1990) **t15.12**. A number of additional histologic variants are not explicitly discussed by Gleason; these include mucinous (colloid) carcinoma, sarcomatoid carcinoma (carcinosarcoma), adenoid basal cell tumor or adenoid cystic carcinoma, and lymphoepithelioma-like carcinoma **t15.12**. Growth or cytologic variants including atrophic pattern carcinoma, pseudo-hyperplastic carcinoma, foamy gland carcinoma, carcinoma with Paneth-like (neuroendocrine) cells, and carcinoma with oncocytic cells, were also not graded in the original Gleason system. One growth or cytologic variant, the hypernephroid pattern, has been given a specific pattern, that of 4.

Recommendations have been published on grade assignments for specific histologic variants (Bostwick 1994A, 1997B) **t15.12**, although it is controversial as to whether to assign a Gleason grade to morphological variants of prostatic carcinoma (WHO 2003). Conventional adenocarcinoma mixed with a morphological variant should be assigned a standard Gleason grade (WHO 2003). For the growth or cytologic variants, most can be graded using the standard Gleason approach. An exception is the pseudohyperplastic variant. It is not clear how to grade these glandular arrangements because they are not illustrated in the Gleason standardized drawing. In our experience, this variant is most often associated with Gleason patterns 2 and 3 (Humphrey 1998A). In a second series, the association usually was with Gleason pattern 3 (Levi 2000).

Squamous cell carcinomas and transitional cell (urothelial) carcinomas primary in the prostate should not be graded by the Gleason method. Squamous cell carcinomas of the prostate have been graded using the 4-tiered Broders scheme (Kahler 1939) or, more commonly, with the 3-step approach of well-differentiated, moderately differentiated, and poorly differentiated (Mai 1996, Mott 1979, Wang 1996). Most cases are moderately to poorly differentiated. In cases of adenosquamous carcinoma (Devaney 1991, Okamoto 1996) the squamous cell carcinoma component was graded separately from the adenocarcinoma component, which was assigned a Gleason grade. In the past, primary transitional cell (urothelial) carcinomas of the prostatic urethra or central prostatic ducts have been graded

■ **t15.12 Gleason Grade of Histologic Variants of Prostatic Carcinoma**

Histologic Variant	Gleason Pattern (Grade)
Ductal (endometrioid) carcinoma	3-4: without necrosis 5: with necrosis
Signet-ring cell carcinoma	5
Mucinous (colloid) carcinoma	4
Sarcomatoid carcinoma (carcinosarcoma)	5 (glands graded separately)
Lymphoepithelioma-like	5
Squamous cell carcinoma	Not applicable
Transitional cell carcinoma	Not applicable
Small cell carcinoma	Not applicable
Basaloid/adenoid cystic "carcinomas"	Not applicable
Growth/Cytologic Variants	**Gleason Pattern (Grade)**
Hypernephroid (hypernephromatoid) pattern	4
Atrophic pattern	Variable (most 3)
Pseudohyperplastic pattern	Most 2-3
Foamy gland carcinoma	Variable (most 3-4)
Carcinoma with Paneth-like cells	Variable
Carcinoma with oncocytic cells	Variable

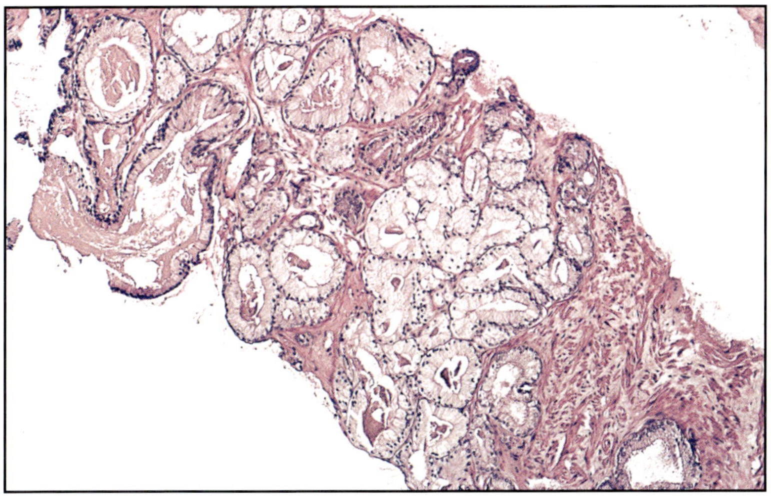

■ **i15.23** *Apparently well-differentiated Gleason grade 2+2 = score of 4 in needle biopsy. Most such cases turn out to be moderately differentiated Gleason pattern 3 adenocarcinoma when the whole gland is examined.*

according to the 1973 3-step WHO method (Chibber 1981, Goebbels 1985, Johnson 1972, WHO 1973) or by the 4-tiered Broders technique (Greene 1976). Currently, concomitant application of the 1998 WHO/International Society of Urological Pathologists scheme (Epstein 1998C) is recommended (Chapter 23). Urothelial carcinomas in the prostate usually are high grade, with most being grade III/III in WHO classification (Goebbels 1985, Johnson 1972) and 3 to 4 of 4 in the Broders scheme (Greene 1976). Noninvasive papillary tumors in or near the urethra can be low grade (well differentiated) (Chibber 1981).

Grading in Fine Needle Aspirates

Attempts have been made to apply Gleason grading to fine needle aspiration biopsy samples of prostatic carcinoma (DeMay 1996, Jacobs 1989, Layfield 1987, Maksem 1987, 1988), but because epithelial-stromal relationships are not preserved in these specimens, this is not advisable. Rather, traditional cytologic grading as well, moderately, or poorly differentiated is recommended (DeMay 1996) (Chapter 3).

Grading in Needle Core Biopsy Tissue

Gleason grading should be performed in all prostatic tissue samples, including needle core biopsy specimens. Indeed, of Gleason's original series of 2911 patients, 60% were graded solely on the basis of a needle biopsy (Gleason 1977). One unique aspect of Gleason grading of carcinoma in needle biopsy is that, in the uncommon event that >2 Gleason patterns are found in needle biopsy, and the highest grade in the least common, it should be incorporated as the secondary pattern (WHO 2003). As previously noted, >2 Gleason patterns are found in only 4% of all needle biopsy cases with carcinoma (McGowan 1983).

The most common Gleason scores in contemporary prostate core needle biopsy tissue procured in patients with clinically localized carcinomas are 5, 6, and 7 **t15.9**. This distribution is similar to that of Gleason's original series **t15.9**, 60% of which were needle biopsies, although today Gleason score 7 is much more common than Gleason score 8.

Well-differentiated Gleason score 2 to 4 adenocarcinoma in prostate needle biopsy (Chapter 14, **i14.83-i14.85, p 279**) **i15.23** should be a rare or nonexistent grade assignment (Epstein 2000B, Iczkowski 1998, Steinberg 1997) **t15.13**. However, 22% (Steinberg 1997) to 56% (Iczkowski 1998) of needle biopsy cases referred to tertiary care medical centers were originally designated as well-differentiated at the contributing hospital. It has also been our experience that almost all referred needle biopsy cases with an assigned Gleason score of 2 to 4 are upgraded, upon review, to a moderately differentiated (Gleason score 6, usually) adenocarcinoma.

■ **t15.13 Well-differentiated Gleason Score 2-4 Adenocarcinoma in Prostate Needle Biopsy**

- Should be a rare or nonexistent grade assignment
- Most cases are moderately differentiated (Gleason score 5 or 6) in whole gland
- A substantial percentage of patients [55% in one series (Steinberg 1997)] have carcinoma outside the prostate in radical prostatectomy specimens
- Poor interobserver reproducibility
- Should not be assigned based solely on a minimal amount of carcinoma in needle biopsy
- Cleared carcinoma cytoplasm does not necessarily equal well-differentiated carcinoma

Well-differentiated Gleason score 2 to 4 adenocarcinoma should rarely be diagnosed in prostate needle biopsy, if at all, because it is poorly predictive of well-differentiated carcinoma in the whole gland, does not predict organ-confined prostate cancer, and is not a reproducible grade assignment, even among urologic pathologists (Allsbrook 2001B). Follow-up comparison with matched whole prostate glands in radical prostatectomy specimens has demonstrated that most prostatic carcinomas deemed well-differentiated in needle biopsy turn out to be higher-grade and usually moderately differentiated Gleason score 5 or 6 in the whole gland (Bostwick 1994A, Cecchi 1998, Fernandes 1997, Humphrey 1995, Kojima 1995, Narain 2001, Steinberg 1997). This is so for several reasons. First, most transrectal needle biopsies are directed toward the peripheral zone of the prostate, where well-differentiated Gleason score 2 to 4 carcinomas are rarely found. Also, it is not possible to visualize an entire well-differentiated prostatic adenocarcinoma nodule in the small needle biopsy sample, and so the only way to be certain that a small gland adenocarcinoma with close-packed acini is well circumscribed, without an infiltrative periphery, is to examine larger tissue samples such as TURP chips and radical prostatectomy specimens.

Radical prostatectomy follow-up after a diagnosis of Gleason score 2 to 4 carcinoma in needle biopsy has also demonstrated that a large number are aggressive, with extraprostatic extension, seminal vesicle invasion, or lymph node involvement in up to 55% of cases (Steinberg 1997). It is of concern, then, that a grade of well-differentiated Gleason score 2 to 4 in prostate needle biopsy has the potential to create, for the patient and physician, a misleading impression of a low-grade and indolent tumor. A common problem that leads to undergrading is the false assumption that a small focus of adenocarcinoma in prostate needle biopsy tissue must represent low-grade or well-differentiated prostate cancer. Yet in our series of 50 prostatic adenocarcinomas <1mm in size in needle biopsy, only 3 (or 6%) were well-differentiated Gleason score 4 in the whole gland (Thorson 1998).

Another false impression that can produce undergrading is the assumption that because carcinoma cell cleared cytoplasm resembles benign epithelial cell cytoplasm, this must indicate low-grade disease. Again, the Gleason grading system is based on pattern of growth, not cytoplasmic tinctorial characteristics. Therefore, cleared cytoplasm, though characteristic of well-differentiated Gleason score 2 to 4 adenocarcinoma, is not specific for low-grade prostate cancer. An outstanding example of this is high-grade hypernephroid Gleason pattern 4 carcinoma, which has cleared cytoplasm.

The rare Gleason score 2 to 4 adenocarcinomas in prostate needle biopsy that are truly representative of low-grade carcinoma in the whole gland may be found in transition zone–directed needle biopsies. Well-differentiated adenocarcinomas typically are found in this zone, but this zone usually is not sampled clinically. These adenocarcinomas are characterized by a nodular proliferation of closely packed small malignant acini. Only 1 or 2 edges of the nodule can be seen because of the small size of the needle core.

Moderately differentiated adenocarcinomas of Gleason score 5 or 6 make up the majority of adenocarcinomas currently diagnosed in prostate needle biopsy, with Gleason score 6 being by far the dominant grade **t15.9; t15.14**. These are infiltrative carcinomas, where the invasive character of the carcinoma is best assessed by noting the relationship of the malignant glands and benign glands. Gleason score 6 carcinoma glands grow between and around benign glands (**i14.68, p 276**). For a large amount of tumor in needle biopsy, there may be effacement of all benign tissue. Here, reliance on the Gleason pictorial representation, which depicts only carcinoma and not admixture with benign glands, is useful. At the other end of the spectrum of tumor extent in needle biopsy, minimal or limited invasion can be manifested as the mere presence of a few malignant glands between benign glands (**i14.86, p 281**) (Epstein 1995, Thorson 1998) or linear columns or arrays of adenocarcinoma (**i14.79, p 278**). This latter pattern of streaming glands is useful in recognition of infiltrative Gleason pattern 3 when no adjacent benign glands are available as anatomic landmarks. An admixed group of closely arranged glands with a rounded profile may suggest a component of pattern 2 and a score of 5. Of Gleason score 5 carcinomas in needle biopsy, 50% to 76% are undergraded and are Gleason score 6 to 7 in the whole gland (Bostwick 1994A, Narain 2001, Steinberg 1997). This may be a function of inability to appreciate infiltrative architecture or tissue sampling error, where the higher-grade component in the whole gland is not sampled by the needle biopsy. Gleason score 6 in needle biopsy is most often score of 6 in the matched whole gland (Narain 2001, Steinberg 1997), but often scores of 5 or 7 can also be seen in the matched radical prostatectomy (Bostwick 1994A, Narain 2001, Steinberg 1997). The distinction between Gleason score 5 and 6 in needle biopsy is not crucial, but the difference between score 6 and 7 is important because a 7 score has an element of high-grade carcinoma. Gleason score 6 adenocarcinoma in needle biopsy can be misinterpreted as Gleason score 7 or higher when there is artifactual glandular compression ("squeeze artifact") or distortion that produces apparent cords of cells.

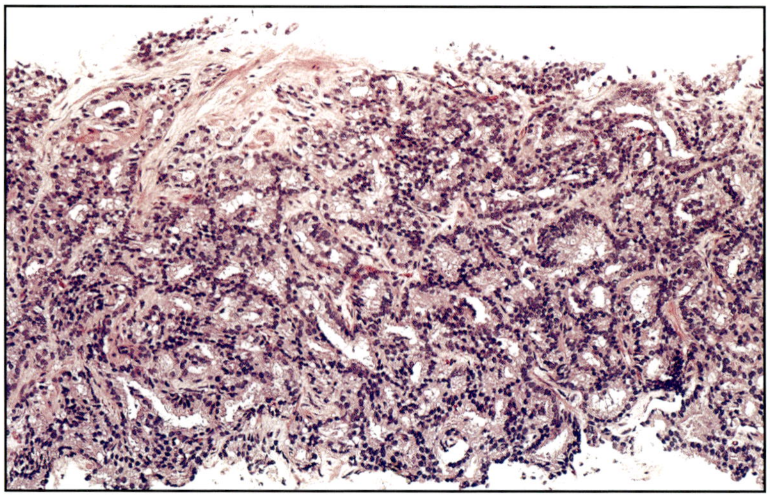

■ **i15.24** *Gleason pattern 4 (and score of 8) in core needle biopsy tissue.*

Gleason score 7 (moderately to poorly differentiated) adenocarcinoma in needle biopsy is also a common grade assignment (**i14.75, p 277**) (Bostwick 1994A, Narain 2001, Steinberg 1997) **i15.11; t15.9, t15.15**. Fused small acini and chains or cords of malignant cells in conjunction with pattern 3 are diagnostic of Gleason score 7 in needle biopsy. Gleason score 7 is most often fairly extensive in needle core tissue but on a few occasions can be detected in cases with minimal carcinoma (<1mm in greatest dimension) (Epstein 1995, Thorson 1998).

Gleason score 8 to 10 (poorly differentiated) carcinoma is an uncommon grade in needle biopsy performed in the clinical stage scenario of localized cancer **t15.9, t15.16**. These are usually destructive and sweeping growths in needle biopsy **i15.21; i15.24** and constitute only a small percentage (2%) of minimal carcinomas (<1mm in size) (**i14.76, i14.89, pp 278, 281**) (Thorson 1998). Gleason score 8 fused small acini with cleared cytoplasm should not be confused with low-grade Gleason score 4 adenocarcinomas. The hypernephromatoid variant is deceptively bland in appearance, often with shrunken nuclei. In these cases the small acini are back to back but without intervening stroma. Sheets of prostatic carcinoma cells **i15.21** and comedo necrosis of Gleason scores 9 and 10 are readily recognized in needle biopsy.

■ **t15.14 Moderately Differentiated Gleason Score 5 and 6 Adenocarcinoma in Prostate Needle Biopsy**

Most common grade of prostate carcinoma in needle biopsy
Most cases of minimal carcinoma (less than 1mm in greatest dimension) in needle biopsy are score 6
Infiltration can be manifested as destructive growth, as penetration between and/or around benign glands, and as linear columns extending across the core
Do not confuse crushed/distorted areas with high-grade carcinoma

■ **t15.15 Moderately to Poorly Differentiated Gleason Score 7 Adenocarcinoma in Prostate Needle Biopsy**

A common grade in needle biopsy
Fused small acini, cords, and chains are common pattern 4 components that merge with pattern 3
Rarely less than 1mm in size (minimal carcinoma)

■ **t15.16 Poorly Differentiated Gleason Score 8-10 Adenocarcinoma in Prostate Needle Biopsy**

Uncommon grade in needle biopsy
Raggedly infiltrative, fused small acini, cords, chains, sheets and comedo carcinoma are common patterns
Usually effaces a large amount of needle biopsy tissue
Rarely less than 1mm in size (minimal carcinoma)
Do not confuse hypernephromatoid Gleason score 8 with low-grade carcinoma

Proteinaceous secretions in Gleason pattern 3 adenocarcinoma should not be mistaken for the comedo necrosis of pattern 5, as seen in Gleason score 9 and 10 carcinomas in needle biopsy. The former intraluminal material is smooth, pink, and homogenous, without necrotic tumor cells, whereas abundant carcinoma cell debris and ghostlike outlines should be found in the comedo carcinoma pattern.

Grading in core needle biopsies presents a unique set of potential difficulties compared with larger tissue samples **t15.17**. One glaring problem is the struggle to assign an architectural growth pattern (Gleason pattern) based on such a thin core of tissue. The inability to appreciate an infiltrative pattern has led to a historical tendency toward undergrading of prostate needle biopsies relative to the matched whole prostate **t15.18, t15.19**. Another confounding factor in the assignment of an accurate Gleason grade is that such grading in the PSA-screening era often is based on only a limited amount of tumor, compared with the digitally detected carcinomas of the era when the

■ t15.17 Sources of Error in Gleason Grading of Prostatic Carcinoma in Prostate Needle Biopsy

Difficulty in identification of infiltrative growth pattern (undergrading)
Grading of minimal amount of carcinoma
Tissue sampling error (related to small amount of tissue sampled by needle biopsy and prostatic carcinoma grade heterogeneity)
Pathologist education and experience
Intraobserver and interobserver variability

■ t15.18 Comparison of Needle Biopsy Gleason Grade and Matched Radical Prostatectomy Gleason Grade

Study	No. of Patients	Size of Needle	Mean No. Cores/Case	Correlation Exact	Correlation ± 1 Unit	Needle Higher	Needle Lower	Comment
Tannenbaum 1982	52	NG[1]	NG	20%	NG	NG	NG	Most cases had greater than 30% change in score.
Lange 1983	72	NG	NG	47%	68%	39%	14%	Grading error highest with lower grade.
Garnett 1984	111	NG	3 ½	30%	72%	32%	38%	Concordance improved with increasing grade.
Babaian 1985	31	–	–	39%	87%	26%	35%	Amount of tumor did not influence error.
Mills 1986	38	NG	NG	44%	74%	50%	5%	Degree of correlation related to amount of cancer in biopsy.
Spires 1994	70	18G(gauge)	NG	58%	94%	15%	27%	Small amount of cancer (≤ 10%) in needle did not influence grading error.
Bostwick 1994	316	18G	6 (median)	35%	74%	25%	40%	Greatest grading error with low-low-grade carcinoma and small amount of cancer.
Paulson 1994	734	NG	NG	41%	72%	14%	45%	Of 118 patients with Gleason score 2-4 on biopsy, only 29 had score 2-4 in prostatectomy.
Humphrey 1995	50	18G	4	26%	86%	26%	48%	High correlation in PSA-screening population.
Kojima 1995	135	NG	NG	48%	89%	5%	47%	Grading errors more likely with increasing serum PSA and PSA density.
Thickman 1996	124	NG	6 (mode)	28%	62%	14%	57%	Improved correlation with increase in # biopsy cores, up to 4-6 cores.
Cookson 1997	226	18G	NG	31%	74%	15%	54%	Lowest accuracy when Gleason score 2-4 diagnosed in needle biopsy.
Fernandes 1997	446	14G	NG	59%	NG	9%	31%	Comparison made using three broad categories.
Steinberg 1997	499[2]	NG	NG	58%	93%	6%	36%	Sampling error was the major source of discrepancy.
	390[3]	NG	NG	34%	67%	6%	60%	
Danziger 1997	100[4]	NG	6 (at least)	34%	68%	17%	49%	Higher correlation for single, uro-pathologist vs multiple observers.
	100[5]	NG	6 (at least)	42%	84%	22%	36%	
Djavan 1998	415	NG	NG	37%	74%	13%	50%	Kappa statistics used to indicate poor correlation.
Thorson 1998	50	18G	6	46%	96%	30%	24%	Study on minimal carcinoma <1mm in size in needle biopsy.
Carlson 1998	106	NG	NG	68%	97%	8%	25%	Higher serum PSA level (> 11ng/mL) was associated with lower correlation.
Cecchi 1998	72	18G	NG	47%	83%	15%	38%	Correlation called poor.
Rubin 2000	963	18G	"variable"	57%	92%	9%	26%	Subset of patients with minimal carcinoma (n = 108) exhibited similar results.
Humphrey 2003[6]	150	18G	6	43%	93%	23%	35%	High correlation in PSA-screening population.
San Francisco 2003	340	18G	6	63%	98%	12%	25%	Extended biopsy protocol with 12 cores/patient resulted in higher correlation.
	126	18G	12	76%	98%	10%	14%	

[1]NG = not given
[2]Academic hospital biopsy grade series
[3]Community hospital biopsy grade series
[4]Multiple observers
[5]Single uropathologist
[6]Unpublished data

■ t15.19 Summary of Literature on Comparison of Needle Biopsy Gleason Grade with Radical Prostatectomy Gleason Grade

Exactly equal = 43% of cases
±1 Gleason score unit = 77%
Needle biopsy overgrading = 15% of cases
Needle biopsy undergrading = 42% of cases

[1]Based on a compilation of 3,789 patients from 18 studies (Lange 1983, Garnett 1984, Babaian 1985, Mills 1986, Spires 1994, Paulson 1994, Humphrey 1995, Kojima 1995, Thickman 1996, Cookson 1997, Fernandes 1997, Djavan 1998, Thorson 1998, Carlson 1998, Cecchi 1998, Iczkowski 1998, Allsbrook 2001B, Epstein 1995)

■ t15.20 Grading of Minimal (< 1mm) Carcinoma in Prostate Needle Biopsy

Gleason grading can be just as accurate for minimal vs larger amount of carcinoma
Most common grades are Gleason scores 5 and 6
A common mistake is to assume a minimal amount of carcinoma in needle biopsy is equivalent to low-grade tumor

Gleason grading system was devised (Humphrey 1998B). Additional sources of potential grading error in needle biopsy include tissue sampling error, prostatic carcinoma heterogeneity, pathologist education and experience, and pathologist interobserver and intraobserver variability.

Comparisons of Gleason grade in needle biopsy with Gleason grade in the matched whole prostate gland indicate exact correlation in 43% of cases (range 20% to 88%) and agreement to within 1 score unit in 77% of 3789 cases (range 62% to 97%) **t15.18, t15.19**. Undergrading of tumor in the needle biopsy, with a higher Gleason score in the matched whole gland, is the most common problem, occurring, on average, in 42% of all cases. Overgrading of carcinoma in needle biopsy tissue also takes place, but with a much lower mean of 15% of all cases **t15.18, t15.19**. Similar needle biopsy–radical prostatectomy carcinoma grade correlations have been obtained using other grading schemes (Catalona 1982, Kojima 1995, Müller 1980).

Gleason grading of a minimal or limited amount of carcinoma in needle biopsy, defined as <1mm of carcinoma (Steinberg 1997, Thorson 1998) or <5% (Rubin 2000) or 10% of needle core tissue involvement by carcinoma, can be just as accurate as for a large amount of tumor in needle biopsy (Rubin 2000, Spires 1994, Steinberg 1997, Thorson 1998) **t15.20**. A small amount of carcinoma in needle biopsy does not correlate with well-differentiated cancer on needle biopsy and is usually of Gleason score 5 or 6 (Thorson 1998).

Tissue sampling error is unavoidable with prostate needle biopsy, even with multiple prostate needle biopsy samples, because an 18-gauge needle biopsy samples only 3/10 000 of all tissue in prostate gland (Humphrey 1995) and because there are typically multiple grades of carcinomas in the whole gland (Aihara 1994, Gleason 1990, McGowan 1983). Undergrading can occur when a higher-grade component in the whole gland is not sampled by the needle. Overgrading can result from so-called reverse sampling error (Steinberg 1997), in which high-grade carcinoma in the needle biopsy sample represents only a small proportion of the cancer in the whole gland, such that historically this high-grade component was not incorporated into the overall Gleason score. Recent data (Pan 2000) suggest that this reverse sampling error can be avoided by taking into account small tertiary high-grade (pattern 4 or 5) components.

The Gleason grading system, like all histologic grading methods, entails an inherent degree of subjectivity. Intraobserver and interobserver variability does exist **t15.21**. Very few studies have focused solely on interobserver variability of Gleason grading of carcinoma in needle biopsy **t15.21**. Recent data suggest that for needle biopsy grading, pathologist training (Allsbrook 2001A) and experience, with subspecialty expertise in urologic pathology (Allsbrook 2001B) can influence the degree of interobserver agreement. In one study, 41 general pathologists exhibited moderate agreement, with a kappa coefficient of .435 (Allsbrook 2001A). For general pathologists, the main difficulty was undergrading. Pathologists with better interobserver agreement had learned the Gleason grading system at a meeting or course (Özdamar 1996). Experience and interest in urologic pathology resulted in enhanced interobserver agreement, with kappa coefficients of .6 to .7, indicating substantial agreement, for 9 of 10 urologic pathologists. In this investigation (Allsbrook 2001B), several (8 of 46) cases were problematic in that a consensus could not be reached on grade assignment. These cases included low-grade tumors, tumors with small cribriform proliferations, and borderline cases that exhibited structures at the border between 2 patterns.

Other grading systems have been compared with the Gleason system (Cintra 1991, De Las Morenas 1988, Harada 1977, Svanholm 1985, Ten Kate 1986), with only 1 of 4 studies showing superior interobserver agreement for the Gleason system. However, no study has compared reproducibility of the different grading systems in application specifically to carcinoma in needle biopsy.

Pathologists can improve their Gleason grading of carcinoma in needle biopsy by using tutorial programs including Web site programs (at http://www.pathology.jhu.edu/prostate [Kronz 2000] and http://www.pathology.ks.se/egevad/gleason.html [Egevad 2001]). Clinically, attempts to improve Gleason grading in needle biopsy have included increasing number of cores taken clinically (King 2000, San Francisco 2003, Thickman 1996), repeat biopsy (Fleshner 1998), use of total serum prostate-specific antigen (PSA) level (Carlson 1998, Kojima 1995) and PSA density (Kojima 1995), and combinations of prostate gland size, total serum PSA level, and clinical stage (D'Amico 1999).

Grading in TURP Chips

A distinctive characteristic of carcinoma grade in TURP chips is that well-differentiated Gleason score 2 to 4 adenocarcinomas are much more common in TURP chips and open (simple) enucleation prostatectomy specimens than in needle biopsies and radical prostatectomy specimens **t15.22, t15.23**. These are typically transition zone, incidental clinical stage T1a/b or A carcinomas microscopically detected by histopathologists after prostatic tissue resection for a clinical diagnosis of BPH. An average of 60% (with a range of 40% to 92%) of incidental carcinomas were deemed well-differentiated in 8 studies published before widespread use of Gleason grading (Blackard 1971, Golimbu 1978, Heaney 1977, Khalifa 1976, Lehman 1968, Munsie 1968, Scott 1969, Sheldon 1980), compared with 41% of incidental carcinomas classified in 5 more recent studies as well-differentiated Gleason score 2 to 4 (Christensen 1990, Elder 1985, Fujita 1991, Greene 1991, Thompson 1989). This roughly 40% to 60% incidence of Gleason score 2 to 4 carcinomas in TURP chips is 10 times higher than the incidence of Gleason score 2 to 4 carcinomas in needle biopsies and radical

t15.21 Reproducibility of Gleason Grading

Study	No. of Patients	Type Tissue/Sample	Intraobserver Variability	Interobserver Variability	Comment
Harada 1977	584-772	NG	71% exact agreement for Gleason score; 91% ± 1 unit.	38% exact agreement for Gleason Score; 82% ± 1 unit.	Reasonable accuracy
Guileyardo 1982	143	Autopsy prostates		81% exact agreement for Gleason score.	2 observers (pathologists).
Bain 1982	58	49: TURP chips 9: needle biopsies	1 pathologist with correlations of 0.86, 0.93, and 0.94 three occasions	55% exact agreement on consensus score; 86% ± 1 unit	7 pathologists self-taught Gleason system; agreement level viewed as satisfactory
Babaian 1985	31	13: TURP chips 17: needle biopsies 1 both	Difference for 1 observer: 0.63 Gleason units, correlation coefficient = 0.89		Suggested accurate reproducibility
Svanholm 1985	31-91	96% TURP chips	42%-65% exact agreement; 87% ± 1 unit	36% exact agreement; 69% ± 1 unit	For 2 observers, Böcking system more reproducible than Gleason system.
Ten Kate 1986	50	radical prostatectomy		36% exact agreement among 5 observers	Low reproducibility, with weighted kappa = 0.3, for three Gleason score tiers: 2-4, 5-7, and 8-10.
Humphrey 1988	118	TURP chips		Median difference for 2 observers = 1 score unit	Determining extent of tumor showed better interobserver agreement than Gleason grade.
De las Morenas 1988	100	NG		66% exact agreement for 3 pathologists	MDAH (88%) and Böcking (75%) systems exhibited better agreement.
Di Loreto 1991	41	14 needle biopsy, 12 TURP chips, 15 radical prostatectomy		68%-73% perfect agreement for 3 pathologists; 71-83% ±1 score unit	Study restricted to Gleason patterns 1-3.
Cintra 1991	139	TURP chips and open prostatectomy cases	63% exact agreement; 72% ± 1 unit		WHO (Mostofi) (80%) and Böcking (78%) systems had better agreement.
Gleason 1992	NG	NG	~ 50% exact agreement; 85% ± 1 unit.		Data not provided
Ozdamar 1996	96	NG	78% agreement	71% for 2 observers	Intraobserver agreement for WHO system similar at 75%; WHO interobserver agreement was 60%
McLean 1997	71	NG		Kappa values 0.16 to 0.29	Low reproducibility
Lessels 1997	100	needle biopsies		Kappa values 0.37-0.54 for 12 observers	Overall satisfactory or adequate level of agreement.
Allsbrook 2001	46	needle biopsies		70% agreement among 10 urologic pathologists for 4 broad categories with kappa values of 0.56-0.70	Substantial agreement for exact Gleason scores for 9/10 urologic pathologists
Allsbrook 2001	38	needle biopsies		Kappa coefficient 0.435 for 41 general pathologists	Barely moderate agreement. Better agreement for pathologists who took a grading course.
Freeman 2001	12	needle biopsies		Kappa values 0.13-0.33	"Generally high" level of agreement in Gleason scores assigned by pathologists from three different continents.

NG = not given
MDAH = MD Anderson Hospital

t15.22 Well-differentiated Gleason Score 2-4 Prostatic Adenocarcinoma in Different Tissue Samples

Tissue Sample	% Cases with Gleason Score 2-4
Prostate needle biopsy	6%
TURP/Simple prostatectomy	40%-60%
Radical prostatectomy	4%

Needle biopsy and radical prostatectomy data from Table 15-9. TURP/Simple prostatectomy data from Bauer 1960, Khalifa 1976, Golimbu 1978, Scott 1969, Blackard 1971, Lehman 1968, Munsie 1968, Heaney 1977, Sheldon 1980, Elder 1985, Thompson 1989, Christensen 1990, Fujita 1991

t15.23 Gleason Grades in TURP Chips

Most common Gleason score = 5

Well-differentiated Gleason score 3 and 4 carcinomas also common as incidental, clinically unsuspected finding

Gleason score 6-10 carcinomas can be detected in a minority of patients with clinical diagnosis of BPH

High-grade and hormonally treated carcinomas common in chips resected due to obstruction in patients with known prostatic carcinoma prostatectomies. This high incidence of low-grade adenocarcinomas in TURP chips and simple prostatectomy specimens results from the fact that these tissue samples consist mainly of transition zone prostatic tissue, which is the anatomic site of origin of most low-grade prostate cancers.

Well-differentiated adenocarcinomas in TURP chips (Chapter 14, **i14.95, p 290**) and open enucleation prostatectomies **i15.1, i15.2** are commonly focal, involving a few chips and <5% of chip surface area (stage T1a or A1), but can be extensive. In fact, in 2 series (Christensen 1990, Greene 1991) of stage T1b (A2) carcinomas that involve >5% of chip tissue, fully 40% of the cases were Gleason score 2 to 4.

Moderately and poorly differentiated carcinomas can be an incidental, clinically unsuspected finding in TURP chips. Most often, a Gleason pattern 3 component is admixed with a well-differentiated pattern 2, yielding a score of 5. Indeed, in one series (Cheng 1999D) of T1a carcinomas, the median Gleason score was 5, and in 2 series (Christensen 1990, Greene 1991) of T1b (A2) carcinoma, a score of 5 was the most common grade assignment. So overall, Gleason scores of 3 to 5 are the most common grades for incidental, T1a/b or A carcinomas of the prostate in TURP chips and open, enucleation prostatectomies.

Gleason score 7 to 10 adenocarcinomas, which harbor a high-grade component, can occasionally be a histologic diagnosis in TURP chips and open end enucleation specimens from patients with a clinical diagnosis of BPH (Chapter 14, **i14.96, p 290**) (Christensen 1990, Greene 1995). With increasing grade of carcinoma in TURP chips, there is increasing extent, such that these poorly differentiated carcinomas usually are extensive, involving multiple chips (Humphrey 1988). When a channel TURP is performed to relieve obstruction in patients with known prostatic carcinoma, numerous chips usually are permeated with poorly differentiated carcinoma. In these cases there is often evidence of androgen deprivation therapy effect, which, as we shall see, precludes assignment of a Gleason grade.

A unique challenge for grading of carcinoma in TURP chips is generated by cautery artifact (Chapter 14, **i14.102, p 291**). This heat-induced tissue damage is seen at the edges of the chips, with variable extension into the substance of the chip. When carcinoma is located near the periphery of a chip with cautery damage, there can be nuclear elongation and compression of glandular luminal spaces. This artifactual distortion can thereby yield an impression of a higher-grade carcinoma. To accurately grade carcinoma with areas of cautery damage, one should study only nondamaged fields; if most of the carcinoma is cautery-damaged, additional levels should be obtained or additional chips submitted, if any remain.

The Gleason grade of clinically unsuspected stage T1a/b (A) carcinoma in TURP chips tends to be somewhat less than the grade in the whole gland **t15.24** (Christensen 1990, Greene 1991, 1995). This is so because the transition zone cancer in TURP chips often is low grade and because transition zone carcinomas are a marker for the presence of associated, higher-grade peripheral zone carcinomas (Greene 1995). In one series (Greene 1991), 90% of whole glands had a peripheral zone carcinoma associated with a transition zone carcinoma detected in TURP chips. These peripheral zone carcinomas are of a median Gleason score of 6 (range 5 to 10) compared with median score of 5 for transition zone carcinomas (Greene 1995). Therefore, although about one half of cases exhibit equal grades in TURP chips and matched radical prostatectomy specimens (Larsen 1991), upgrading is fairly common when one compares TURP Gleason grade with the corresponding whole gland (radical prostatectomy) grade. This upgrading results from the nature of the selective transition zone sampling by the TURP.

■ t15.24 Gleason Grade in TURP Chips Compared With Matched Whole Gland (Radical Prostatectomy Specimen)

TURP chip carcinoma grade lower (median = 5) compared with corresponding radical prostatectomy grade (median = 6)
Lower grade in TURP chips due to transition zone sampling by TUR, whereas associated, unsampled peripheral zone carcinoma is higher grade

Reproducibility of Gleason grading in TURP chips has been addressed mainly by studies that evaluated TURP chips along with other tissue samples (Babaian 1985, Bain 1982, Cintra 1991, di Loreto 1991, Humphrey 1988, Svanholm 1985) **t15.21**. Intraobserver and interobserver variability in grading of carcinoma in TURP chips should be less than that for needle biopsies because a larger amount of is tissue available for examination, where specific Gleason architectural patterns should be more readily appreciated. Yet intraobserver and interobserver exact agreement was only 42% to 65% (Cintra 1991, Svanholm 1985) and 36% to 55% (Bain 1982, Svanholm 1985), respectively. In the majority (69% to 87%) of cases, the assigned Gleason score was within 1 score unit, indicating a satisfactory level of agreement (Bain 1982) and supporting application of the Gleason grading system to carcinoma in TURP chips.

Grading in Radical Prostatectomy Specimens

The assignment of a Gleason grade in radical prostatectomy tissues should be more straightforward than that in the aforementioned tissue samples because a larger amount of tissue is available for evaluation **t15.25**. However, in one interobserver variability study exclusively on radical prostatectomy specimens (Ten Kate 1986), there was only 36% exact agreement and low reproducibility.

In this era, the most commonly assigned Gleason scores in radical prostatectomy specimens are 5 to 7 (Carvalhal 2000, Humphrey 1996, Pound 1997) **t15.9**. Well-differentiated Gleason score 2 to 4 adenocarcinoma, at about 1% to 6%, and poorly differentiated Gleason score 8 to 10 carcinomas, at 2% to 9%, are uncommon (Carvalhal 2000, Humphrey 1996, Pound 1997). This dominance of moderately differentiated (Gleason score 5 and 6) and moderately to poorly differentiated adenocarcinoma (Gleason score 7) results from needle biopsy diagnosis of these peripheral zone carcinomas, whereas lower-grade carcinomas are sampled by TURP chips. Gleason score 8 to 10 carcinomas are more likely to have clinically spread beyond the prostate, such that many of these patients would not be surgical candidates.

Several grading challenges are more likely to be encountered in radical prostatectomy specimens. Because prostatic carcinomas typically are multifocal, with an average >2 (2.7) Gleason patterns per whole gland (Aihara 1994), selecting the 2 most voluminous Gleason

■ t15.25 Gleason Grading in Radical Prostatectomy Specimens

Most common Gleason scores: 5-7
Gleason scores 2-4 uncommon: 1%-6% of cases
Gleason score 8-10 uncommon: 2%-9% of cases
Grade based on all carcinoma foci, not just largest focus or nodule
Note high-grade pattern 4 and 5 carcinoma in report even if it is focal

patterns can be difficult. Although it has been suggested that one should assign a Gleason score to the dominant (index) tumor in radical prostatectomy specimens (Allsbrook 1999), this approach was not a part of the original Gleason proposal. This author assigns a Gleason score based on all carcinoma foci because a dominant tumor nodule does not always exist (Feng 2000) and because small high-grade foci distant from a larger nodule can be found. As noted earlier, scant data exist on how to handle 3 or more grades in radical prostatectomy specimens. If 3 Gleason patterns of equal volume are visualized, one should include the 2 higher grades in the Gleason score and mention that there is a tertiary pattern. A tertiary high-grade pattern 4 or 5 adversely affects prognosis, but the prognosis is not necessarily equated with the addition of the primary Gleason pattern and the tertiary highest Gleason pattern (Pan 2000). When there is a tertiary pattern 4 or 5, it should be noted in addition to the standard Gleason score (WHO 2003). These data (Pan 2000) suggest that a modification of the Gleason system may be necessary in the future, when there is a tertiary high-grade pattern 4 or 5.

[15.4] Grading in Metastatic Deposits

Grading in metastatic sites has been attempted using both the Gleason system and a 3-tiered scheme **t15.26** (Bazinet 1992, Brawn 1989, 1990, Cheng 1999B, Kramer 1981, McCullough 1974, Prout 1980). The Gleason grading system is based on epithelial (carcinoma)-stromal architectural relationships within the prostate and therefore should not be applied to prostatic carcinoma locally outside the prostate or in metastatic sites. Nevertheless, there are several reports of Gleason grading of carcinoma in pelvic lymph nodes (Bazinet 1992, Cheng 1999B, Kramer 1981). Three-tiered grades of well-differentiated, moderately differentiated, and poorly differentiated have also been applied to metastatic deposits of prostatic carcinoma in lymph nodes (Brawn 1990). Well-differentiated and Gleason score 2 to 4 prostatic carcinoma in pelvic lymph nodes is rare (Brawn 1990, McCullough 1974) or nonexistent (Cheng 1999B, Kramer 1981, Prout 1980). Well-differentiated adenocarcinoma of the prostate in lymph nodes has been equated with M.D. Anderson Hospital (MDAH) Grade 1, in which 75% to 100% of the tumor forms glands (Brawn 1982, 1990). Mixed findings exist as to whether moderately differentiated or poorly differentiated prostatic carcinomas predominate in nodal metastatic deposits (Bazinet 1992, Brawn 1990, Cheng 1999B, Kramer 1981). Moderately differentiated (MDAH Grade 2 to 3) metastatic deposits were those in which 25% to 75% of the tumor forms glands or where cribriform or papillary carcinoma is the predominant pattern (Brawn 1990). In poorly differentiated metastatic nodal disease, 0% to 25% of the carcinoma forms glands (Brawn 1990).

Comparison of histologic grade in lymph node metastasis with that of the primary carcinoma in the prostate has demonstrated either a similar histologic pattern (Brawn 1990, Kramer 1981, McCullough 1974, Prout 1980), or a trend toward a higher grade in the lymph node metastasis (Cheng 1999B). This latter tendency has been called "dedifferentiation," but this suggests reversion of a differentiated cell, whereas "clonal or genetic divergence, progression, and expansion" would be a preferable description of this process.

Grading of prostatic carcinoma in distant metastatic sites (abdominal lymph nodes, bone, and viscera) has also been performed (Brawn 1989). Most patients with widely disseminated prostatic adenocarcinoma had undifferentiated metastatic deposits, compared with regional lymph node metastatic deposits, which prompted the proposal that metastases disseminate as they "dedifferentiate" (Brawn 1990), that is, undergo clonal evolution. However, the patients in this series (Brawn 1989) had received hormonal therapy, which can induce histologic changes that mimic high-grade carcinoma. This theory of dedifferentiation remains unproven.

t15.26 Grade of Metastatic Prostatic Carcinoma

Gleason system has been used but is not appropriate
Three-tiered system of well-, moderately, and poorly differentiated carcinoma also used
Most metastatic deposits moderately-to-poorly differentiated; well-differentiated metastases rare to nonexistent
Histologic grade of metastatic deposits usually similar to or higher than primary

[15.5] Grading After Radiation and Hormonal Therapy

In general, the Gleason grading system should be applied only to tumor that shows no evidence of treatment effect **t15.27**. This is so because the Gleason system was originally devised based on untreated prostatic carcinomas and because both radiation and hormonal therapies can induce histologic alterations in prostatic carcinoma that simulate high-grade disease.

Radiation therapy effect on prostatic carcinoma is variable, with individual cases demonstrating no effect, partial effect with admixed affected and unaffected areas, or complete effect. Where there is no evidence or minimal evidence of therapy effect (see Chapter 19), Gleason grading may be used. In a number of studies, however, Gleason grading was performed in all cases of irradiated prostatic carcinoma (Ahlering 1992, Bostwick 1982, Cheng 1998B, Cheng 1999C, Moul 1991, Pontes 1993, Prestidge 1997, Rogers 1995, Siders 1992, 1998, Wheeler 1993). The effect of radiation on Gleason grade is controversial, with some studies (Ahlering 1992, Pontes 1993, Siders 1992, Wheeler 1993) showing increased Gleason grade, whereas others reported no change (Bostwick 1982, Goldstein 1998) or even a trend toward lower Gleason scores (Crook 1997). For patients with a higher grade after radiation therapy, it has been suggested that there may be grade progression or "dedifferentiation" related to radiation treatment, but this probably is an artifact of treatment effect that results in patterns of high-grade carcinoma (Grignon 1995). Just as for untreated prostatic carcinoma, Gleason scores of irradiated prostatic carcinoma in needle biopsy tend to underestimate the Gleason score in the whole gland excised in a salvage radical prostatectomy procedure.

t15.27 Gleason Grading After Radiation and/or Hormonal Therapy

Should not be performed when there is evidence of such treatment effect
Treatment effect can induce pattern alterations mimicking high-grade carcinoma
Effect of radiotherapy on Gleason grade controversial with most studies showing an increase in grade after irradiation—this is likely an artifact
Similarly, hormonal therapy can cause changes simulating poorly-differentiated carcinoma

Hormonal therapy is similarly variable in effect and can cause pattern alterations resembling poorly differentiated carcinoma (Grignon 1995, Montironi 1998, Reuter 1997) (Chapter 19). In particular, in areas affected by androgen deprivation, a decrease in gland size, compressed or absent glandular lumens, single cell formation, and increased stromal separation of glands result in the appearance of a higher Gleason grade (Abbas 1996, Armas 1994, Ferguson 1994, Grignon 1995, Hugosson 1996, Murphy 1991, Ohki 1996, Tran 1998, Vaillancourt 1996). An increase in grade after hormonal therapy has also been observed using other grading systems (Fergusson 1953, Hellström 1993, Voges 1994). This upgrading has been observed after a number of different forms of androgen deprivation therapy, including estrogen (or diethylstilbestrol) administration, luteinizing hormone–releasing hormone agonists such as leuprolide, with or without an antiandrogen (such as flutamide or bicalutamide), and estramustine. Androgen deprivation by surgical castration (orchiectomy) should produce a similar effect on grade, whereas androgen deprivation induced by the 5α-reductase inhibitor finasteride seems, in preliminary data, to show a minimal to modest effect on prostatic carcinoma (Bostwick 1997A, Civantos 1997, Yang 1999).

The apparent increase in histologic grade after hormonal therapy probably is artifactual, as opposed to outgrowth of higher-grade hormone-resistant tumor cells. Modified Gleason scoring, with adjustment for small glands and increased stroma after hormonal therapy (Civantos 1995), has been proposed but has not been validated (Reuter 1997). Overall, the consensus view is that one should not report histologic grade after hormonal therapy (Algaba 1996).

[15.6] Grade Progression

Is it possible for histologic grade progression to occur with time, with development of higher-grade prostatic carcinomatous components in the primary tumor or metastatic sites? Or does the hypothesis of "histologic determinism" apply to prostate cancer, where prostatic carcinomas have an inherent, fixed degree of biologic malignancy (Gleason 1992)? Ultimately, these questions are difficult or impossible to definitely address in men because thorough characterization of grade in the primary tumor of the prostate requires its complete removal, which obviously interrupts the natural history of the disease. If one samples the primary cancer by needle biopsy or even TURP, one can never be certain that this tissue sample is representative of carcinoma grade in the whole gland. The limited information published in follow-up biopsy studies is not conclusive on this question. In the VACURG study, Gleason reported "only a mild increase in average histologic scores with time" (Gleason 1992). In a more recent needle biopsy study (Epstein 2001), over a 1 to nearly 2-year period, only 13% of men experienced a significant change in Gleason score (from ≤6 to ≥7) in follow-up biopsies. These findings could be related to sampling error and suggest minimal, if any, potential for an increase in grade of men with clinically localized, lower-grade prostatic carcinoma.

Another complicating factor is that grade of untreated, clinically progressing and spreading prostate cancer is not known because these men are treated. The reported "dedifferentiation" after radiation therapy (Wheeler 1993) and with metastatic spread (Brawn 1989, Cheng 1999B) could represent selection, under therapeutic pressure, of a high-grade clone that was not sampled in the initial biopsy.

The concept that histologic grade is established initially at an early phase in the life history of prostatic carcinoma is attractive because it is possible to detect small primary prostatic carcinomas that are well-differentiated, moderately differentiated, and poorly differentiated (Epstein 1994B). In animal models, prostatic carcinoma can be high grade from the inception of tumorigenesis, with maintenance of the poorly differentiated phenotype throughout the course of neoplastic growth, from prostatic intraepithelial neoplasia through local invasion and distant metastasis (Garabedian 1998). It is also likely that over time progression to higher-grade disease could occur in a subset of untreated patients with prostate cancer. This latter proposal is in line with the known genetic instability of neoplasia, with clonal evolution and selection of neoplastic cells that are more likely to survive, grow, and spread. In this model, high-grade Gleason pattern 4 carcinoma would evolve from low-grade carcinomas as tumor volume increased (McNeal 1993).

[15.7] Prognosis and Grade

Relationship of Histologic Grade and Pathologic Endpoints

Increasing histologic grade, including Gleason grade, is directly related to a number of histopathologic endpoints, including perineural invasion by carcinoma, lymphvascular space invasion by carcinoma, tumor size, and pathologic stage **t15.28**. In needle biopsy, Gleason score is related to the presence of perineural invasion and amount of tumor in needle core tissue (Orozco 1998, Vargas 1999). In one series (Vargas 1999) the mean Gleason score for prostate needle cores with perineural invasion was significantly higher, at 6.6, compared with 6.1 for cases without perineural invasion.

Needle biopsy Gleason score is also related to histopathologic findings in the whole prostate gland. Numerous studies have linked needle biopsy Gleason grade to tumor size, and pathologic stage in radical prostatectomy tissues **t15.29**. Most models incorporate Gleason grade with tumor extent in needle biopsy to predict tumor volume (Chan 1998, Cupp 1995, D'Amico 1997A, Egevad 1998, Noguchi 2001) **t15.29**. Increasing Gleason grade in needle biopsy has been shown in numerous studies to be related to an increasing likelihood of extraprostatic extension by carcinoma and seminal vesicle invasion **t15.29, t15.30**. Surprisingly, in several studies needle biopsy Gleason score did not predict positive margins in radical prostatectomy

■ t15.28 Gleason Grade in Needle Biopsy: Relationship to Pathologic Endpoints

Increasing grade related to increasing tumor size, and increased likelihood of positive margins, extraprostatic extension, seminal vesicle invasion in whole prostate gland; also related to increased likelihood of pelvic lymph node metastasis.
Prior to treatment usually combined with serum PSA level and local clinical T stage to predict pathologic stage and likelihood of response to therapy[1].
Can be used with % free PSA or PSA density and amount of tumor in needle biopsy to attempt to predict "insignificant" cancer in whole prostate gland.

[1]Radical prostatectomy and radiation therapy.

■ **t15.29 Correlation of Gleason Histologic Grade in Prostate Needle Biopsy with Pathologic Endpoints in Radical Prostatectomy Specimens and Pelvic Lymph Nodes**

Study	Pathologic Endpoint	Findings
D'Amico 1997	Tumor volume	Needle biopsy Gleason weighted average (based on number of cores with tumor), PSA and ultrasound gland volume used to predict prostate cancer volume
Chan 1998	Tumor volume	Predictive value of D'Amico calculated prostate cancer volume not confirmed
Egevad 1998	Tumor volume	Men with needle biopsy Gleason score < 7 and < 3mm tumor had tumor volume < 1mL(but n = only 6 patients.)
Oesterling 1987	Extraprostatic extension Seminal vesicle invasion Lymph node spread	Gleason grade highly correlated (p <0.0002) with all three endpoints
Wolf 1993	Extraprostatic extension	Combination of Gleason score, PSA, and transrectal ultrasound used
Partin 1993	Extraprostatic extension Seminal vesicle invasion Lymph node spread	Combination in nomograms with clinical stage and serum PSA best
Ravery 1994	Extraprostatic extension	Gleason score was not predictive
Zietman 1994	Extraprostatic extension	Any Gleason pattern 4 or 5 in needle biopsy was predictive
Peller 1995	Extraprostatic extension(EPE)	Only Gleason score and number of positive cores predicted EPE in logistic regression model
Bostwick 1996	Extraprotatic extension Seminal vesical invasion	Gleason score, PSA, and percent cancer in needle core tissue together provided best model in multivariate analysis
Huland 1996	Extraprostatic extension(EPE)	Significantly higher Gleason score in men with (mean = 6.5) vs without (mean = 5.7) EPE
Badalament 1996	Extraprostatic extension(EPE)	Gleason score predictive in univariate analysis
Puppo 1997	Extraprostatic extension Lymph node involvement	Nomograms using Gleason score, PSA, and clinical stage used for 1,738 patients from 34 Italian Urology Departments
D'Amico 1999	Extraprostatic extension Seminal vesicle invasion	Combined modality staging using Gleason score, percent positive biopsies, PSA, and endorectal coil MRI
Partin 1997	Extraprostatic extension Seminal vesicle involvement Lymph node involvement	Confirmation and extension of Partin 1993 above, with 4,133 patients
Steinberg 1997	Extraprostatic extension	Weak correlation between needle biopsy Gleason score and pathologic stage (r = 0.274)
Wills 1998	Extraprostatic extension (EPE)	High Gleason score (≥7) and more than one positive core correlated with high (90%) likelihood of EPE
Arcangeli 1998	Extraprostatic extension (EPE)	Weak (r = 0.16), non-significant correlation of Gleason score and EPE
Rabbani 1998	Extraprostatic extension Seminal vesicle involvement Lymph node involvement	Model with Gleason score, PSA density and clinical stage predicted EPE with, but not without, neoadjuvant androgen withdrawal therapy
Egawa 1998	Extraprostatic extension Seminal vesicle involvement	Best model: Gleason score with PSA, clinical stage, number of positive cores, and maximum core length
De la Taille 1999	Extraprostatic extension Seminal vesicle involvement	Gleason score independently predicted stage in multivariate analysis
Vargas 1999	Extraprostatic extension (EPE)	Gleason score not predictive of EPE in multivariate analysis
Southwick 1999	Extraprostatic extension	Gleason score used with % free PSA
Makarov 2002	Extra-prostatic extension	Needle biopsy Gleason grade 4+3 associated with higher pathologic stage than grade 3+4.
Ackerman 1993	Margins	Gleason score not predictive of positive margins
Watson 1996	Margins	Margin-positive patients had a significantly higher biopsy tumor grade
Arcangeli 1998	Margins	Needle biopsy score not predictive of positive margins (r = 0.09)
Rabbini 1998	Margins	Needle biopsy Gleason grade not correlated with margin status
Huland 1996	Margins	Needle biopsy Gleason score significantly (p = 0.0008) higher for men with positive margins (mean = 6.6) vs negative margins (mean = 6.1)
Kramer 1980	Positive pelvic lymph nodes	Gleason score 2-4: 0% metastasis; 8-10: 93% metastasis
Paulson 1980	Positive pelvic lymph nodes	Gleason scores 2-4 and 9-10 patients had a 13% and 100% chance of lymph node metastasis, respectively. These numbers are the highest reported
Sagalowsky 1982	Positive pelvic lymph nodes	Gleason score 2-4: 0% positive nodes; scores 7-9: 44%-60%
Arai 1990	Positive pelvic lymph nodes	Gleason score 8-10 and PSA > 10: 71% of men had positive nodes
Roach 1993	Positive pelvic lymph nodes	Risk of positive nodes N = 2/3 (PSA) + (Gleason score -6) x 10
Ackerman 1993	Positive pelvic lymph nodes	Mean needle biopsy Gleason score higher in men with (mean = 6.4) vs without (mean = 5.3 - 5.4) node metastasis
Danella 1993	Positive pelvic lymph nodes	Needle biopsy Gleason score in men with positive nodes (mean = 7.1) higher than in men without positive nodes (mean = 5.8). PSA enhanced predictive value.
Narayan 1994	Positive pelvic lymph nodes	When needle biopsy Gleason score ≤6 and PSA ≤10 ng/ml, staging lymphadenectomy may not be needed since only 1% of lymph nodes positive
Bluestein 1994	Positive pelvic lymph nodes	Gleason grade, serum PSA and clinical stage used in nomogram to predict likelihood of positive nodes (like Partin tables)
Sands 1994	Positive pelvic lymph nodes	Gleason grade a significant predictor in univariate and multivariate analyses
Bishoff 1995	Positive pelvic lymph nodes	Trend (p = 0.08) toward Gleason score prediction of positive nodes. Used with clinical stage and PSA to determine probability of positive nodes
Weldon 1995	Positive pelvic lymph nodes	If Gleason score ≤6, PSA ≤11, and clinical stage ≤ T2b, then chance of a positive node = 1%
Rogers 1996	Positive pelvic lymph nodes	Needle biopsy Gleason score predictive in univariate and multivariate analyses but good model with PSA, and clinical stage could not be developed
Alagiri 1997	Positive pelvic lymph nodes	For Gleason score <8 and PSA <20, lymph node metastases were unlikely and avoidance of pelvic lymph node dissection was suggested in this setting
Hoenig 1997	Positive nodes by laparoscopic pelvic lymph node dissection (LPLND)	Gleason score predictive of lymph node metastasis in univariate and multivariate analysis; LPLND recommended when Gleason score ≥7, PSA > 20 and advanced clinical T stage
Haese 2002	Positive pelvic lymph nodes	High-grade Gleason pattern 4 used along with number of needle biopsy scores with pattern 4 to generate risk categories

specimens (Ackerman 1993, Arcangeli 1998, Huland 1996, Rabbani 1998, Watson 1996). Tumor size, location, stage, surgical technique, method of processing the radical prostatectomy specimen, and pathologist interpretation of margin status may be more important in determining margin positivity. The risk of metastasis to pelvic lymph nodes is closely related to needle biopsy Gleason score **t15.29, t15.30**.

Prediction of pathologic stage by needle biopsy Gleason grade alone is possible but is not absolutely accurate for the individual patient. Therefore, patients with lower-grade (Gleason score 2 to 6) carcinomas still are at risk for having cancer spread outside the prostate, and not all patients with a high-grade carcinoma component (Gleason score 7 to 10) will have carcinoma extension beyond the confines of the prostate gland **t15.30**. Clinically, needle biopsy Gleason grade usually is combined with other pretreatment factors, such as serum total PSA, percentage free PSA, local clinical T stage, and amount of tumor in needle biopsy, to predict pathologic stage. Perhaps the most commonly used data clinically are the so-called Partin tables (Partin 1993, 1997, Partin 2001), which combine needle biopsy Gleason grade, serum PSA, and clinical stage to provide estimates of risk of extraprostatic extension, seminal vesicle invasion, and lymph node metastasis. (These tables are available on the Web at http://urology.jhu.edu/Partin_tables/index.html). These nomograms, though useful, are also not absolutely accurate (Kattan 1997, Penson 2002, Vollmer 1998). Still, accurate needle biopsy Gleason grading and reporting is essential because patients are stratified into prognostic and therapeutic categories based in part on needle biopsy Gleason grade (O'Dowd 1997, Polascik 1998).

Needle biopsy Gleason grade has also been incorporated into models to predict potentially clinically "insignificant," "unimportant," or "harmless" prostate cancer (Arcangeli 1998, Cupp 1995, Epstein 1994A, 1998A, Humphrey 1998B, Irwin 1994, Noguchi 2001) **t15.31**. These models are not perfect, and even for the one with the best accuracy (highest positive predictive value) in predicting a small, lower-grade cancer (Epstein 1998A), the negative predictive value is only 77%. That is, when that model predicted a significant tumor, 23% were insignificant.

Gleason grade in larger tissue samples (TURP chips, open prostatectomy tissues, and radical prostatectomy tissues) is also related to pathologic endpoints. The relationships are not as strong for TURP chips and open prostatectomy tissues as for radical prostatectomy specimens because these former samples are selectively resected from the transition zone, where the grade often is lower and not as representative of the grade in the whole gland (Christensen 1990, Greene 1991, 1995) **t15.24**.

Gleason score in TURP chips is related to the amount of tumor in the chips, as previously noted (Christensen 1990, Fujita 1991, Gleason 1977, Greene 1991, Humphrey 1990). Well-differentiated Gleason score 2 to 4 carcinoma is most often focal, but these low-grade tumors can be extensive in chip tissue (Christensen 1990, Greene 1991). High-grade Gleason score 8 to 10 carcinomas tend to be of large size, with diffuse involvement of many chips (Humphrey 1988). TURP chip Gleason grade does not predict well Gleason grade or pathologic stage in whole gland. To reiterate, TURP chip Gleason grade typically is lower than the grade in the whole gland (Christensen 1990, Greene 1991, 1995) **t15.24** because the TURP procedure does not often sample the peripheral zone, where higher-grade carcinomatous

■ t15.30 Needle Biopsy Gleason Score in Prediction of Pathologic Stage[1]

Gleason Score	Extraprostatic Extension	Seminal Vesicle Invasion	Lymph Node Metastases
2-4	23%	3%	<1%
5	37%	4%	1%
6	40%	4%	3%
7	47%	14%	10%
8-10	39%	24%	20%

[1]In 4,133 men, with clinically localized prostate cancer, who underwent radical prostatectomy and pelvic lymph dissection (Partin 1997)

■ t15.31 Needle Biopsy Gleason Grade in Prediction of "Clinically Insignificant" Prostate Cancer in Whole Prostate

Study	Model[1]	Definition of "Insignificant Tumor"[2]	Accuracy[3]
Irwin 1994	PSA density ≤0.1 ng/mL/g and cancer ≤3mm of Gleason grade ≤2	Tumor volume ≤ 0.5cm³, organ- confined	82%
Epstein 1994	PSA density ≤0.1 ng/mL/g and good pathologic findings on needle biopsy (no Gleason pattern 4 or 5, fewer than 3 cores involved, no core with greater than 50% involvement)	Tumor volume < 0.2cm³, organ-confined, no Gleason grade 4 or 5 component	73%
Cupp 1995	Gleason score less than 7, 5% or less cancer or 3mm or less cancer in one core	Tumor volume < 0.5cm³	7-8%
Arcangeli 1998	Biopsy Gleason score alone	Tumor volume < 0.2cm³, organ-confined, Gleason score ≤ 6	Not significant; correlation coefficient = -0.02.
Epstein 1998	% free PSA ≥ 15, less than 3 cores involved, no core with greater than 50% involvement, Gleason score < 7	Tumor volume < 0.5cm³, organ-confined, Gleason score < 7	94%
Noguchi 2001	Best model was one positive core with cancer length less than 3mm that contained no Gleason grade 4/5	Tumor volume < 0.5cm³	75%

[1]Model based on pre-treatment parameters
[2]Definition based on characteristics of prostate cancer in whole gland (radical prostatectomy specimens)
[3]Accuracy = positive predictive value in determining how often a tumor predicted to be insignificant was insignificant

■ 15.32 Radical Prostatectomy Gleason Score in Relation to Pathologic Stage, Tumor Size, and Margin Status[1]

Gleason Score	Extraprostatic Extension[2]	Positive Margins	% Carcinoma[3]	Seminal Vesicle Invasion	Lymph Node Metastases
2-4	0%	0%	1%	0%	0%
5	16%	20%	9%	1%	1%
6	24%	29%	8%	4%	2%
7	62%	48%	13%	17%	12%
8-10	85%	59%	27%	48%	24%

[1]Data on Gleason scores 5-10 from Epstein 1998B; data on Gleason scores 2-4 and percentage carcinoma from Humphrey unpublished data on a series of 241 radical prostatectomies
[2]Established extraprostatic extension by carcinoma (more than a few malignant glands outside the capsule)
[3]Percentage carcinoma = mean percentage of prostate tissue involved by carcinoma as determined by a grid morphometric method (Humphrey 1990)

elements reside. For incidental T1a/b carcinomas, TURP chip Gleason grade, in combination with amount of tumor in the chips, is related to whole gland total tumor volume, extraprostatic extension, and seminal vesicle and lymph node spread. Although there is a correlation of TURP Gleason score with extension of carcinoma outside the whole gland, the relationship is sufficiently imprecise that definite prediction of pathologic stage based solely on Gleason grade in TURP chips is not possible. For example, a minority of patients with small, lower-grade, Gleason score 2 to 6, T1a carcinoma in TURP chips have carcinoma outside the gland. This is so because the greatest threat to patients with T1a/b transition zone disease usually is a separate, associated cancer in the peripheral zone that is not sampled by the TURP (Greene 1991). Furthermore, the presence of high-grade Gleason pattern 4 or 5 in TURP chips does not necessarily mean that carcinoma has already spread outside the prostate because 52% to 88% of patients with T1b disease have organ-confined prostate cancer t14.30. Gleason score is more predictive of radical prostatectomy pathologic T stage in T1b than in T1a disease: in one stage T1b (A2) series, the mean TURP Gleason score for men with organ-confined carcinoma was 4.6, compared with 6.6 for men with extraprostatic extension at radical prostatectomy (Christensen 1990).

Radical prostatectomy Gleason score is related to a number of pathologic findings, including vascular space invasion (De la Taille 2000, Herman 2000, Salomao 1995), tumor size, extraprostatic extension, positive margins, seminal vesicle invasion, and pelvic lymph node metastasis (Epstein 1994B, 1998B, Humphrey 1990, Iselin 1999, Ohori 1994B, 1995, Partin 1990, Stamey 1988, 1998) **t15.32**. The uncommon, pure well-differentiated Gleason score 2 to 4 adenocarcinomas usually are small, are located in the transition zone, and rarely extend outside the prostate gland (Chen 2000) **t15.32**. However, in some cases low-grade transition zone carcinomas are of high tumor volume (Chen 2000, Noguchi 2000). These are almost always associated with higher-grade peripheral zone carcinoma in the same gland (Chen 2000). At the other extreme, poorly differentiated Gleason score 8 to 10 carcinomas are commonly of large size, and most patients have carcinoma outside the prostate and positive margins. However, high-grade carcinomas of low tumor volume do exist (Epstein 1994B). There is a substantial risk of invasion of seminal vesicles and lymph node metastasis for patients with Gleason score 8 to 10 carcinomas **t15.32**. Moreover, there is a correlation between radical prostatectomy Gleason grade and cancer volume of metastatic deposits in the pelvic lymph nodes (Cheng 1998A). The percentage of the tumor that is high-grade Gleason pattern 4 or 5 seems to be related to tumor size, extraprostatic extension by carcinoma, and lymph node metastasis (Stamey 1988, 1998).

Relationship of Histologic Grade and Clinical Endpoints

Histologic grade of prostatic carcinoma is one of the most powerful, if not the dominant, predictor of clinical outcome for patients with this cancer. A number of clinical endpoints have been linked to histologic grade, including clinical stage, response to different therapies, PSA ("biochemical") failure, progression to metastatic disease, and survival, including prostate cancer–specific survival and overall survival **t15.33**.

Clinical stage is associated with histologic grade as increasing Gleason grade is related to increasing local, clinical T stage (Fowler 1985, Ohori 1994B, Ramos 1999) and increased incidence of metastatic spread to regional, pelvic lymph nodes. Gleason score is also related to the likelihood of the presence of distant metastasis in soft tissue or bone. The risk of detecting bony metastasis by radionuclide bone scan is highly related to histologic grade, including both WHO and Gleason grades (Bruwer 1999, Lin 1999, Rydh 1999, Shih 1991).

Clinical outcome measures have been linked to histologic grade in all types of prostatic tissue samples, including needle biopsy, TURP chips, and radical prostatectomy specimens. Many studies evaluating histologic grade as a prognostic indicator have used nonuniform patient populations, with mixtures of different clinical stages, tissue sampling methods, and treatments **t15.34**. Indeed, in a number of articles, the type of tissue sample used for grading was not even specified. Additionally, many studies were underpowered, with low numbers of patients followed for only a short period of time. It is therefore impressive that histologic grade, as assessed using different schemes **t15.1, t15.34** and applied to different patient populations, has been a dominant prognostic factor in determining patient outcome.

Needle core biopsy histologic grade, as determined by the Gleason method, has been shown in several contemporary studies that focused only on needle biopsies to be associated with therapy failure after radiation or radical prostatectomy treatment and progression to distant metastases (Anderson 1998, De la Taille 1999A, Eastham 1998, Lee 1996, Liebross 1998, Mohideen 1998, Narain 2001, Presti 1998, Sgrignoli 1994) **t15.34**. Any high-grade component, with a Gleason score of 7 to 10,

■ t15.33 Gleason Grade Linkage to Clinical Endpoints

Clinical stage: T stage and metastasis
Response to therapy
Cancer recurrence and progression
Survival

■ 15.34 Histologic Grade and Clinical Endpoints: Selected Studies

Study	Tissue Sample[1]	Clinical Stage	No. Patients	Findings
Muir 1934	NG	? to IV	24	Groups (grades) I & II survival 14-18 mos. vs 8 mos. for grade III
Evans 1942	NG	NG to IV	100	Average survival of grades I and II = 5.4 years vs 2.2 years for grade IV
Pool 1956	TURP chips (from 1926-1946 at Mayo-Clinic)	NG	1,534	At 5 years, grade 1: 50% survival; grade 2: 34%; grade 3: 16%; grade 4:5%
Shelley 1956	NG	NG	83	Average survival for class (grade I) = 3 years vs 1.9 years for grade II and 0.3 years for grade IV
Vickery 1963	Radical prostatectomy (at Massachusetts General Hospital, 1932-1956)	NG	148	% of patients surviving disease-free at 10 years = 40% for well-differentiated carcinoma vs 11% for poorly-differentiated carcinoma
Jewett 1968	Radical prostatectomy	II	92	35% survival for grades 1+2 vs 0% for grade 3, at 15 years after surgery
Mobley 1968	NG	IV	96	For patients with metastatic disease, grade 1 cases had better survival vs grade 2 and 3 at 1 and 2 years, but not 5 years
Gaeta 1982	Needle biopsies, TURP chips, prostatectomies	I-IV	169	16% cancer deaths for grade I, 64% for grade II, 89% for grade III, and 94% for grade IV, at 3.6 years of follow-up
Gleason 1977	60% on needle biopsy	I-IV	2,911	Cancer-specific mortality rate strongly linked to Gleason histologic pattern score at 3.3 years average follow-up
Brawn 1982	Needle biopsies and TURP chips	III	182	MD Anderson (MDAH) grade best in predicting 5-year survival vs Mostofi and Gleason systems
Böcking 1982	Punch biopsies, TURP chips, and open prostatectomy specimens	I-IV	108	Tumor-specific deaths at 25% for grade I, 47% for grade II, and 80% for grade III at 3-8 years
Schroeder 1985	Radical prostatectomy	T0-T3	257	98% survival for grade 1, 76% survival for grade 2, and 30% survival for grade 3, at 10 years follow-up
Sgrignoli 1994	Needle biopsy	T1-T3, N+	138	Biopsy Gleason score 8-10 associated with rapid progression to distant metastases in multivariate analysis
Lee 1996	Needle biopsy	T1-T3	224	Biopsy Gleason score not predictive of biochemical failure after radiation therapy at median follow-up of 2 years
D'Amico 1997	Needle biopsy	T1-T2	480	Biopsy Gleason score ≥8 placed patients at high risk for biochemical failure within 3 years after radical prostatectomy
Liebross 1998	Needle biopsy	T1-T3	133	Biopsy Gleason score not significant in predicting biochemical failure at 3 years after radiation therapy
Mohideen 1998	Needle biopsy	Tlc	75	Biopsy Gleason score > 6 predicted, in univariate and multivariate analyses, biochemical failure at 1.7 years after radiation therapy
Anderson 1998	Needle biopsy	T1-T3	226	Gleason score 2-6 vs 7-10 significant in univariate and multivariate analysis in predicting biochemical failure at 5 years after conformal external beam radiation therapy
Presti 1998	Needle biopsy	T1-T2	109	Biopsy Gleason score of 7-10 associated with biochemical failure after radical prostaectomy
Eastham 1998	Needle biopsy	T1-T2	782	Biopsy Gleason grade was prognostic for recurrence afer radical prostatectomy in univariate, but not multivariate analysis
De la Taille 1999	Needle biopsy	T1-T2	319	Biopsy Gleason score >7 significant in univariate but not multivariate analysis in linkage with biochemical failure at 2 years after radical prostatectomy
Khalifa 1976	TURP chips and enucleation	T1	48	Overall survival at 10 years was 39% for well-differentiated and 25% for poorly-differentiated carcinoma
Barnes 1976	TURP chips ("most"), needle biopsy ("some")	T1-T2	116	Survival at 15 years was 36% for grades I and II vs 19% for grades III and IV
Heaney 1977	TURP chips (n = 30), enucleation (n = 70)	T1	100	10-year survival for grade I = 57% vs 25% for grades II and III
Bauer 1960	enucleation	T1	55	10-year survival for well-differentiated carcinoma patients = 47%, vs 14% for moderate to poor differentiation
Cantrell 1981	63 TURPS, 54 enucleations	Tla/b	117	Gleason score predicted progression, but not as well as tumor extent
Epstein 1986	63 TURPs, 31 enucleations	Tla	94	Gleason grade did not predict progression
Humphrey 1988	TURP	I-IV	118	Gleason score significant in predicting risk of death in univariate, but not multivariate analysis
Foucar 1990	TURP	NG	79	Patients with Gleason score 8-10 had 13-fold increased risk of death compared to score of 2-4
Cheng 1999	TURP	Tla	102	Gleason grade did not predict progression

[1]NG = not given; TURP = transurethral resection of prostate

(continued on next page)

■ **15.34 Histologic Grade and Clinical Endpoints: Selected Studies (continued)**

Study	Tissue Sample[1]	Clinical Stage	No. Patients	Findings
Borre 2000	TURP	T1-T2	221	WHO grade was significant in univariate, but not multivariate analyses in predicting survival at median 15 years of follow-up
Gaeta 1980	Needle biopsies (78) TURPS (84) radical prostatectomies (16)	A-D	169	Mortality rates at 3.7 years: grade I: 16%, grade II: 64%, grade III: 89%, grade IV: 94%
Nemoto 1987	Needle biopsy (195) TURPs (24) enucleations (45) radical prostatectomy (3)	I-IV	287	In a Japanese series, Gleason grade was related to mortality, ranging from 0.09 deaths per patient-year of follow-up for pattern 1 vs 0.30 for pattern 5
Berner 1994	Needle biopsies (100) TURPs (75) enucleations (91)	A-D	266	WHO grading the most powerful prognosticator in survival analysis; Gleason system a poor prognosticator
El-Galley 1995	TURP (141) needle biopsies (39) enucleation (3)	T1-T4	191	Gleason score related to local progression and survival, in multivariate analysis, after radiotherapy
Aus 1995	FNA (67%) "surgical specimens" (24%) needle biopsy (4%)	T1-T4	514	WHO grade, applied to cytologic and histological specimens, was related to cause-specific survival after deferred treatment: Grade 1 mortality at 10 years = 30% vs 53% for grade 2 and 81% for grade 3
Zagars 1995	Needle biopsy (348) TURP (300)	T1-T4	648	Gleason score related to survival at 10 years after radiation therapy: score 2-3: 64%, 4-6: 60%, 7:46%, 8-10: 24%. Grade, in multivariate analysis, was the single most significant determinant of outcome
Albertsen 1998	TURP (60%) Needle biopsy (26%) enucleation (11%)	NG	767	Risk of death from prostate cancer within 15 years and after deferred treatment: Gleason score 2-4: 4%-7%; 5: 6%-11%; 6:18%-30%; 7:42%-70%; 8-10: 80%-87%
Johansson 1997	FNA (84%) TURP or enucleation (16%)	T0-T2	300	Death from prostate cancer in 6% of grade I patients, 17% of grade II, and 56% of grade III, but grading method not given
Ennis 1998	Needle biopsy TURP	T1-T4	238	Gleason score predictive of biochemical disease-free survival at 27 months after external beam radiotherapy
Sandblom 2000	FNA TURP	T0-T4	282	At 10 years, prostate cancer-specific survival rate for clinically localized tumors was 90% for WHO grade 1, 74% for grade 2, and 59% for grade 3
Egerad 2002	TURP	T1-T4	305	Gleason score, modified Gleason score (dominant + worst grade), and % Gleason 4/5 were all predictors of disease specific survival after deferred therapy
Myers 1983	Radical prostatectomy	B,C	562	Mayo grade correlated with local and systemic progression after surgery, but not survival
Gallee 1990	Radical prostatectomy	Localized	50	Mostofi-Schroeder and Broders grades best in predicting progression. MD Anderson and Mostofi methods also significant. Gleason grade not significant
Mukamel 1990	Radical prostatectomy	A2-B2	139	MD Anderson grade related to progression at 8 years after surgery: grade 1: 0%, 2: 19%, 3:31%, 4:40%
Paulson 1990	Radical prostatectomy	T1-T2	427	Biochemical failure at 10 years after surgery: 25% for Gleason score 2-7 vs 80% for score 8-10
Norberg 1994	Radical prostatectomy	A,B	51	At 5 years after surgery, rates of progression-free survival were 90% for Gleason scores 2-5, 84% for score of 6, and 44% for 7-10
Ravery 1994A	Radical prostatectomy	T1-T2	100	Rates of progression at 2 years after surgery were 40% for Gleason scores 2-7 and 52% for scores 8-10
D'Amico 1995	Radical prostatectomy	Localized	347	Gleason score, seminal vesicle invasion, and positive margins were significant indicators of PSA failure at 18 months after surgery
Ohori 1995	Radical prostatectomy	T1-T3	478	Gleason score, seminal vesicle invasion, and extracapsular extension were most significant in predicting progression. A unit increase in Gleason score doubles the risk of progression
Epstein 1996	Radical prostatectomy	Localized	721	Likelihood of progression at 10 years after surgery: Gleason score 2-4: 4%; 5-6: 18%; 7:48%; 8-10: 65%. In multivariate analysis, Gleason score, surgical margins, and capsular penetration were all significant
van den Ouden 1997	Radical prostatectomy	T1-T4	273	WHO grade significant in predicting biochemical progression and survival in univariate, but not multivariate analysis
Eastham 1998	Radical prostatectomy	Localized	728	For progression at 10 years, Gleason grade and pathologic stage were most significant in multivariate analysis
Catalona 1998	Radical prostatectomy	T1-T3	1,778	Moderately differentiated, and poorly-differentiated grades associated with 7-year cancer recurrence-free survival, with relative risks of 1.5 and 2.3, compared to well-differentiated tumor
D'Amico 1998	Radical prostatectomy	T1-T2	862	Gleason score, preop PSA, pathological stage and margin status were independent predictors of postop PSA failure at 42 months
Cheng 1998	Salvage radical prostatectomy after radiation therapy	T1-T3	86	In multivariate analysis, Gleason score and DNA ploidy were independent predictors of distant metastasis-free survival and cancer-specific survival
Tefilli 1998	Radical prostatectomy	T1-T2	93	In the presence of seminal vesicle invasion, Gleason score ≥7 was an adverse finding
Moul 1998	Radical prostatectomy	T1-T3	295	Combined WHO and Gleason grade was not significant in predicting recurrence after surgery

[1]NG = not given; TURP = transurethral resection of prostate

(continued on next page)

■ 15.34 Histologic Grade and Clinical Endpoints: Selected Studies (continued)

Study	Tissue Sample[1]	Clinical Stage	No. Patients	Findings
Tefilli 1999	Radical prostatectomy	Localized	652	Disease-free survival at 34 months was 91% for Gleason score 2-6, 75% for score of 7, and 35% for 8-10
Stamey 1999	Radical prostatectomy for peripheral zone cancer	Localized	379	Cancer progression after surgery was associated with % Gleason grade 4/5, tumor volume, positive lymph nodes and intraprostatic vascular invasion
Iselin 1999	Radical prostatectomy	Localized	1,242	Cancer-specific survival at 15 years after surgery: Gleason score 2-7: 78% vs median survival of 11 years for score 8-10
Jhaveri 1999	Radical prostatectomy	Localized	1,132	At 10 years overall survival was 93% for Gleason score ≤6 vs 86% for score ≥7
Cheng 1999A	Radical prostatectomy	Localized	298	Gleason score significant in univariate but not multivariate analysis in association with 5-year progression-free survival
Pound 1999	Radical prostatectomy	Localized	1,997	Gleason score, time to biochemical progression, and PSA doubling time were predictive of probability and time to development of metastasis
Pan 2000	Radical prostatectomy	Localized	114	Tertiary high-grade component had an adverse impact on progression
Epstein 2000A	Radical prostatectomy	Localized	60	In patients with seminal vesicle invasion, Gleason grade can be used along with margin status and vascular invasion to predict risk of postop progression
Carvalhal 2000	Radical prostatectomy	Localized	595	Gleason score, pathologic stage, and percentage carcinoma were independent predictors of biochemical failure
Koch 2000	Radical prostatectomy	Localized	165	Rapid PSA progression after surgery correlated with Gleason score and secondary grade
Zhou 2001	Radical prostatectomy	Localized	141	Gleason score, but not nuclear grade, in radical prostatectomy tissues predicted biochemical failure after surgery
Blute 2001	Radical prostatectomy	Localized	2,518	Gleason score, preop PSA, seminal vesicle status, and margin status used to predict postop failure
Vis 2001	Radical prostatectomy	Localized	218	Percentage Gleason 4/5 most strongly predicted PSA relapse in this screened population
Herman 2001	Radical prostatectomy	Localized	823	For Gleason score 7 carcinomas, primary Gleason pattern was predictive of disease progression in univariate, but not multivariate analysis.
Han 2001	Radical prostatectomy	Localized	2,404	Gleason grade groupings of 2-4 vs 5 vs 6 vs 7 vs 8-10 highly significant in predicting PSA recurrence at 15 years of follow-up.
Narain 2001	Needle biopsy Radical prostatectomy	Localized	1,031	Both needle biopsy and radical prostatectomy Gleason score correlated significantly with disease-free survival but there were differences in survival between biopsy and prostatectomy Gleason score categories
Sweat 2002	Radical prostatecromy	Localized	751	Risk of death from prostate cancer within 20 years: Gleason score 2-4: 6%-7%; 5: 10%-13%; 6: 15%-19%; 7: 29%-35%; 8-10: 36%-43%

[1]NG = not given; TURP = transurethral resection of prostate

was particularly ominous. Needle biopsy Gleason score has also been linked to patient survival, but most of these studies have added cases in which grade was assigned in TURP chips and open prostatectomy specimens **t15.34**. For example, 60% of Gleason's original large series of 2911 men were needle biopsy cases, but prognosis based on tissue specimen type was not analyzed (Gleason 1977). Not surprisingly, grade in the whole gland is more accurate than needle biopsy grade in predicting patient outcome. For example, in one large series needle biopsy Gleason grade was no longer significant in multivariate analysis in predicting failure after radical prostatectomy when Gleason grade and pathologic stage in the whole gland were known (Eastham 1998). Therefore, when needle biopsy and radical prostatectomy Gleason grades are both known for an individual patient, the radical prostatectomy grade should be used in stratifying patients for possible additional therapy and predicting the future.

Needle biopsy Gleason grade is routinely used to determine eligibility for clinical trials and plan treatment for patients. Men with lower Gleason scores are more likely to elect surveillance as initial management (Koppie 2000, Zietman 2001). Needle biopsy Gleason scores can be used in conjunction with serum PSA and clinical stage to plan for the type of radiation therapy and whether to administer hormonal therapy with radiation therapy (Nori 1997, Ragde 1997, Stock 1997). Needle biopsy Gleason score can also be used with serum PSA and clinical stage to predict response to radiotherapy (Kattan 2001, Movsas 1997, Ross 2001) or to radical prostatectomy (Kattan 1998, Ross 2001). Some nomograms are available as software programs for handheld computers (personal digital assistants), such that in a matter of seconds, by plugging in needle biopsy Gleason grade, serum PSA level, and clinical stage, one can find out the likelihood, for that individual patent, of disease-free survival 5 years after radical prostatectomy or radiation therapy.

Gleason grade in TURP chips and open prostatectomy tissues is also clearly associated with patient outcome. Again, only a few studies have focused solely on TURP chips or open prostatectomy tissues in linkage of clinical outcome with grade **t15.34**. For incidentally detected carcinoma in TURP chips and open prostatectomy (enucleation) specimens, histologic grade, as determined by several different grading schemes, has predicted response to therapy and patient survival. The one setting in these tissue samples in which histologic grade does not seem to impart prognostic information is for patients with T1a disease (≤5% of tissue involved by carcinoma), when the Gleason score range is 2 to 7 (Cheng 1999D, Epstein 1986). For all other clinical stages, high-grade carcinoma in any grading scheme is a threat to the patient's life. In multivariate analyses, the percentage of TURP tissue or chips involved by carcinoma harbors more prognostic information than Gleason grade (Cantrell 1981, Humphrey 1988).

Radical prostatectomy histologic grade, including Gleason grade, is one of the most powerful predictors of failure after surgery. Grade has been linked to postoperative progression and survival **t15.34**. Only uncommonly has grade been nonsignificant in univariate and multivariate analyses. Even in the face of seminal vesicle invasion, a highly adverse finding, Gleason score imparts additional prognostic information (Blute 2001, Herman 1999, Tefilli 1998) **t15.34**. Just as for other tissue samples, it is the presence of high-grade

■ **t15.35 Histologic Grade in Men with Metastatic Carcinoma**

Study	Tissue Sample	Site of Metastasis/Stage	No. Patients	Findings
Gleason 1977	Mixture	Clinical stage IV[1]	1,044	Gleason score strongly related to survival
Zincke 1984	Radical prostatectomy	Pelvic lymph nodes	100	Mayo grade not related to progression or survival
Mulders 1990	NG	Disseminated, hormone treated	175	Mostofi grade not related to survival
Schwartz 1991	TURP, needle biopsy	Bone	56	Gleason grade a predictor of response to orchiectomy
Ernst 1991	TURP, needle biopsy	Disseminated	162	Gleason grade not a prognostic factor
Kato 1993	NG	D2	138	Gleason primary pattern significant in multivariate analysis
Koutsilieris 1994	NG	D2	262	Aggressiveness score—using histological grade, serum PAP, serum alkaline phosphatase, and number of bone metastases—correlated with length of response and survival
Waaler 1994	NG	Bone(positive bone scan)	73	Grade not related to survival
Berner 1994	Needle biopsy (100) TURPs (75) enucleations (91)	Distant metastases	116	WHO grade added significant prognostic information in survival analysis
Sgrignoli 1994	Needle biopsy	Pelvic lymph nodes (D1)	113	High Gleason score correlated with rapid progression to distant metastases
Cipolla 1994	NG	D2	43	Gleason grade not significant in predicting progression or cancer-specific survival
Jøgensen 1995	NG	Bone	59	Neither Gleason grade nor WHO grade was of value in predicting progression or cancer-specific death
Fujikawa 1995	Needle biopsy (18) TURP (16) both (3)	D2	31	WHO and Gleason grade did not predict time to disease-specific death
Griebling 1997	NG	Positive pelvic lymph nodes	60	Gleason grade was strongest predictor of disease-specific survival in univariate and multivariate analyses
Cheng 1998	Radical prostatectomy	Positive pelvic lymph nodes	269	Gleason score significant in predicting systemic progression in univariate and multivariate analysis
Pound 1999	Radical prostatectomy	Distant metastasis	103	Gleason score and PSA level did not influence time until death

[1]Defined as an elevated serum prostatic acid phosphatase or distant metastasis by x-ray or biopsy

(Gleason pattern 4 or 5) disease that harbors the greatest risk for the patient. The presence of any high-grade carcinoma, even a tertiary component comprising just a small percentage of the total amount of tumor, has a deleterious impact on cure rates (Pan 2000). The amount or percentage of high-grade carcinoma may have an impact on the chance for cure (Herman 1999, Stamey 1999, Vis 2001). Therefore, patients with Gleason score 7 carcinoma have an outcome intermediate between patients with Gleason score 5 to 6 and 8 to 10 **t15.34**. Within the Gleason score 7 category, a 4 + 3 score, with more 4 pattern than 3, carries a worse prognosis than a 3 + 4 score, where pattern 3 dominates (Chan 2000, Han 2001, Herman 2001, Lau 2001, Sakr 2000, Skacel 2000). (However, this distinction between 4 + 3 and 3 + 4 does not appear to be significant in multivariate analysis when preoperative PSA, pathologic stage, and margin status are known [Han 2001, Herman 2001, Lau 2001].)

Radical prostatectomy Gleason grade can be used in models to predict high risk for recurrence after surgery. These models typically incorporate Gleason score, preoperative serum PSA, and pathologic stage, with or without tumor volume and margin status (Bauer 1998, D'Amico 1997C, Kattan 1999, Partin 1995, Roberts 2001, Stamey 1999). This information can be used to help stratify patients for consideration of closer surveillance or adjuvant therapy. One model predicts whether a rising PSA after surgery is caused by a local disease or distant metastasis. This program (called Partin II Calculation) is available on the Web (at http://www.prostatepointers.org/prostate/partin/partin2form.html) and is based on radical prostatectomy Gleason score and postoperative PSA velocity.

Gleason score of the primary tumor appears to be of prognostic value in the setting of pelvic lymph node metastasis (Cheng 1998A, McNeal 1990, Sgrignoli 1994) but is of uncertain value in the setting of distant and bony metastases **t15.35**. The data on use of histologic grade—including Mayo, Gleason, and WHO grades—as a prognostic factor in established distant metastatic disease are decidedly mixed, with a roughly equivalent number of studies showing significance and nonsignificance **t15.35**.

Experimental Approaches

Grade, as a measure of intrinsic biologic aggressiveness, may be assessed in the future by both structural (morphologic and morphometric) and functional means **t15.36**. One proposed morphologic approach is quantitation of the amount of high-grade (percentage Gleason pattern 4 or 5) carcinoma (Herman 1999, McNeal 1986B, 1990, Rubin 2001, Stamey 1995B, Stamey 1999). In transurethrally resected prostate chips, percentage Gleason grade 4 or 5 was a significant predictor of disease-specific survival and was a stronger predictor than standard Gleason score (Egevad 2002). The percentage of a tumor that is Gleason pattern 4 or 5 in the whole gland has been related to cancer volume, the presence of lymph node metastasis (McNeal 1986B,

■ **t15.36 Prostatic Carcinoma Experimental Grading Approaches**

% Gleason pattern 4/5
Quantitative nuclear features: size, shape, DNA content, chromatin texture
Structural alterations in carcinoma DNA, RNA, protein
Functional gene expression profiling (by gene chip microarrays)

1990), and progression after radical prostatectomy (Herman 1999, Stamey 1999). Indeed, in one study of peripheral zone cancers, percentage pattern 4 or 5 was a better predictor of biochemical (PSA) recurrence after surgery than pathologic stage or Gleason score (Stamey 1999), and in a second study (Vis 2001), the proportion of poorly differentiated cancer was the factor most strongly linked to the likelihood of biochemical failure. Therefore, this factor may be used in reporting grade in radical prostatectomy specimens in the future, but validation at other institutions and the question of reliability of the estimate (interobserver agreement) must be addressed. (Preliminary data suggest that a substantial level of interobserver reproducibility can be achieved [Glaessgen 2002].) Furthermore, it is not clear how to quantitate percentage pattern 4 or 5 cancer. In one study (Stamey 1999), 10% increments were used, whereas a different, 4-tiered categorization (<5%, 5% to 24%, 25% to 49%, and >50%) was applied in a second series (Vis 2001). Reporting of percentage Gleason grade 4 or 5 in cancer in needle biopsy has been advocated (Stamey 1995B), but only limited data have been published on the relationship of percentage Gleason pattern 4 or 5 in carcinoma in needle core tissue and pathologic and clinical endpoints. The percentage Gleason pattern 4 or 5 in needle cores is significantly related to percentage of that pattern in the whole gland (in radical prostatectomy specimens) (Bassily 2000, Bostwick 1994A, Rubin 2001, Stamey 1995B), but the correlation is variable (from a weak r^2 = .32 to a strong r^2 of .8 [Stamey 1995B]). Overall, use of the percentage Gleason pattern 4 or 5 parameter in needle biopsy seems to be limited by a high false-negative rate (Rubin 2001). The correlation of needle core percentage Gleason pattern 4 or 5 with other pathologic stage parameters, including extraprostatic extension, seminal vesicle involvement, and lymph node involvement has been weak (with r = .05 to .24) (Rubin 2001). Correlation of needle core percentage Gleason pattern 4 or 5 with failure after radical prostatectomy has been weak (Rubin 2001) or absent (Baschinsky 2002). Therefore, the amount of carcinoma of high-grade Gleason grade pattern 4 or 5 has potential for adding information to standard Gleason grade assignment in TURP chips and radical prostatectomy tissue, but its utility in needle core tissue is currently uncertain.

Quantitative measures of nuclear abnormalities have also been forwarded as grading tools (Bibbo 1993, Chiusa 1997, Diamond 1982, Eskelinen 1991, Fujikawa 1995A, 1998, Hurwitz 1999, Irinopoulou 1993, Lipponen 1996, Partin 1992, Robutti 1989, Tannenbaum 1982, Van der Poel 1992, 1997, Wenderoth 1994, Zhang 1999, 2000). These abnormal features can be divided into morphometric features, as in quantitation of DNA content and textural attributes related to chromatin patterns (Van der Poel 1992). Morphometric descriptors include nuclear area, nuclear diameter, nucleolar area, nuclear roundness, elongation factor, ellipticity, form factor, chain code, and percentage convex area fraction. These features have been used alone or in combination with other factors in linkage with pathologic and clinical endpoints. However, none of these features is an established and independent prognosticator. For example, the data on nuclear roundness and DNA content (ploidy) are conflicting (Van der Poel 1992). It has been suggested that DNA ploidy in needle biopsy could be used to predict Gleason grade shifting (Ross 1999) or when accuracy of Gleason grading is questioned (Brinker 1999), but in general DNA ploidy does not provide information that is independent of or supplemental to Gleason grade (Stamey 1995A). DNA ploidy of carcinoma in radical prostatectomy specimens is of little importance and is generally not used in models to predict cancer recurrence (Han 2001). Although quantitative, the methods used to measure nuclear abnormalities are time-consuming and expensive, typically necessitating a digital image analysis system. Moreover, multiple factors, such as method of tissue procurement, fixation, processing, and section preparation, could affect nuclear features (Van der Poel 1992). Additional potential problems with quantitative digital image analysis include reproducibility, subjectivity in field secretion, and lack of standardized methods (Bostwick 1999). For these reasons, quantitative measures of nuclear changes are unlikely to be used on a routine basis.

Structural alterations in carcinoma cell DNA, RNA, and protein have also been linked to pathologic and clinical endpoints in attempts to predict carcinoma aggressiveness (see Chapter 21), but these are currently experimental. Genotypic grading of DNA abnormalities might one day be used in conjunction with the current phenotypic grading.

Functional gene expression profiles of prostatic carcinoma might provide information on carcinoma aggressiveness or grade, but this is not of proven value. Historically, the expression of individual genes has been assessed one or a few at a time, but the simultaneous characterization of the expression of thousands of genes by gene chip microarray analysis holds more promise for the future in improving grading of prostate cancer (Singh 2002).

Reporting of Prostatic Carcinoma Histologic Grade

Histologic grade should be reported for carcinoma in every prostatic tissue sample (ADASP 1996, Algaba 1996, Bostwick 1999, 2000, Srigley 2000) **t15.37, t15.38**. The Gleason grade should be used (WHO 2003) and the "primary pattern plus secondary pattern equals" score should be recorded. Another scheme may be reported in addition to the Gleason grade, if desired, but the Gleason grade should always be included in the report.

t15.37 Reporting of Histologic Grade

Report Gleason grade of carcinoma for all prostate tissue samples[1]
Report primary Gleason pattern and secondary pattern = score
If only one pattern present, double to yield score
Provide Gleason grade for each separately submitted sample/container
For needle biopsy cases, provide composite Gleason score for the entire case based on Gleason score of all cores
For needle biopsy cases, note Gleason score of core with highest score
For needle biopsy cases in which more than two patterns are present and the worst grade is neither the predominant nor the secondary grade, the predominant and the highest grade should be added to arrive at a score
For radical prostatectomy cases in which more than two patterns are present and the worst grade is neither the predominant nor the secondary grade, mention the tertiary worst grade in a comment
Avoid lumping of Gleason scores
Provide Gleason grade for adenocarcinoma histologic variants - ductal, signet-ring, and mucinous
Provide Gleason grade for adenocarcinoma growth/cytologic variants, such as hypernephroid, atrophic, and pseudohyperplastic
If desired, additional grading scheme may be used, in addition to, but not replacing, Gleason scheme
Do not report Gleason grade in metastatic deposits of prostatic carcinoma
Do not report Gleason grade after hormonal therapy
Report Gleason grade after radiation therapy only if carcinoma shows no treatment effect

[1]That shows no radiation or hormonal therapy effect in the carcinoma

t15.38 Gleason Grade Reporting: Sample Format

NEEDLE BIOPSY

ONE GRADE (PATTERN) OF 3 PRESENT:
ADENOCARCINOMA, GLEASON GRADE 3+3 = SCORE OF 6

TWO GRADES (PATTERNS) PRESENT, WITH PRIMARY PATTERN OF 3 AND SECONDARY PATTERN OF 4:
ADENOCARCINOMA, GLEASON GRADE 3+4 = SCORE OF 7

THREE GRADES (PATTERNS) PRESENT, WITH PRIMARY = 3, SECONDARY = 4, AND TERTIARY = 5:
ADENOCARCINOMA, GLEASON GRADE 3+5 = SCORE OF 8

MULTIPLE CORES WITH DIFFERENT GLEASON SCORES:
PROVIDE SCORE FOR CORE(S) IN EACH SEPARATELY SUBMITTED CONTAINER
PROVIDE OVERALL, COMPOSITE SCORE FOR ALL CORES
INDICATE SCORE OF CORE WITH HIGHEST SCORE

RADICAL PROSTATECTOMY

ONE GRADE (PATTERN) OR TWO PATTERNS PRESENT:
REPORT IN STANDARD WAY (AS ABOVE FOR NEEDLE BIOPSY)

THREE GRADES (PATTERNS) PRESENT, WITH PRIMARY = 3, SECONDARY = 4, AND TERTIARY = 5:
ADENOCARCINOMA, GLEASON GRADE 3+4 = SCORE OF 7 (SEE COMMENT)
COMMENT: THERE IS A MINOR TERTIARY GLEASON GRADE 5 COMPONENT, OCCUPYING LESS THAN 5% OF THE TUMOR VOLUME

See **t14.22** and **t14.39** for reporting format for other pathologic features

For needle biopsy cores, histologic grade should be assigned to carcinoma in separately submitted tissues (containers), designated by site. The pertains mainly to needle biopsies specimens that are submitted separately. It has been recommended that for needle biopsies with different Gleason grades in different, separately submitted needle cores, a composite score be rendered (Bostwick 2000, Srigley 2000). In one study (Dunn 2002), the composite or global Gleason score for 6 needle core tissue samples from different locations had the strongest association with radical prostatectomy pT3 disease and margin status compared with the highest Gleason score for any single core or weighted Gleason score (the average Gleason score weighted by tumor amount on all cores). Further data are needed, but these data do support rendering a composite, overall, or global Gleason score for each case. Another recent study presented data that each core should also be given a separate grade (Epstein 2002). In needle biopsy tissue, if there is one Gleason pattern, it should be doubled to yield a score. Any high-grade pattern 4 or 5 should be incorporated into the score, no matter the amount in needle core tissue. In the uncommon event that there are more than 2 grades in needle core tissue, one should take the most common pattern as the primary Gleason grade and the higher grade of the next 2 most common patterns as the secondary Gleason grade (ADASP 1996, Bostwick 1999, Srigley 2000, WHO 2003). Gleason grade should be provided for all carcinomas in needle biopsy, even for minute, minimal, or limited carcinomas.

Gleason grade reporting in TURP chips and enucleation specimens should follow the standard Gleason method of reporting the predominant pattern as the primary grade and the second most common pattern as the secondary grade. How to handle a tertiary high-grade component is not clear because no data exist on this issue. In the circumstance that there is a small tertiary high-grade component, pattern 4 or 5, one should definitely describe its presence in a comment.

Radical prostatectomy Gleason grade should be assigned in standard fashion, with the most common and the secondary Gleason patterns in the whole gland used to determine the primary and secondary Gleason grades **t15.38**. There are published recommendations to grade only the "dominant nodule" (Allsbrook 1999) or to report separate grades for separate tumors in the whole gland (Srigley 2000), but many prostate glands lack a dominant nodule (Feng 2000), and no data exist to support reporting of separate tumors. A tertiary high-grade component, when present, should definitely be reported because this affects prognosis (Pan 2000). The evidence-based recommendation (Pan 2000) is to keep the original Gleason score (based on first most common and second most common patterns), with a notation on the presence of a tertiary high-grade component.

References

Abbas F, Kaplan M, Soloway MS, Induction androgen deprivation therapy before radical prostatectomy for prostate cancer-initial results. *Br J Urol* 77:423-428, 1996.

Ackerman DA, Barry JM, Wicklund RA, et al. Analysis of risk factors associated with prostate cancer extension to the surgical margin and pelvic lymph node metastasis at radical prostatectomy. *J Urol* 150:1845-1850, 1993.

ADASP (Association of Directors of Anatomical and Surgical Pathology). Recommendations for the reporting of resected prostate carcinomas. *Am J Clin Pathol* 105:667-670, 1996.

Ahlering TE, Lieskovsky G, Skinner DG, Salvage surgery plus androgen deprivation for radioresistant prostate adenocarcinoma. *J Urol* 147:900-902, 1992.

Aihara M, Wheeler TM, Ohori M, et al. Heterogeneity of prostate cancer in radical prostatectomy specimens. *Urology* 43:60-66, 1994.

Alagiri M, Colton MD, Seidmon EJ, et al. The staging pelvic lymphadenectomy: implications as an adjunctive procedure for clinically localized prostate cancer. *Br J Urol* 80:243-246, 1997.

Albertsen PC, Hanley JA, Gleason DF, et al. Competing risk analysis of men aged 55 to 74 years at diagnosis managed conservatively for clinically localized prostate cancer. *JAMA* 280:975-980, 1998.

Algaba F, Epstein JI, Aldape HC, et al. Assessment of prostate carcinoma in core needle biopsy: definition of minimal criteria for the diagnosis of cancer in biopsy material. *Cancer* 78:376-381, 1996.

Allsbrook WC Jr., Mangold KA, Yang X, et al. The Gleason grading system: an overview. *J Urol Pathol* 10:141-157, 1999.

Allsbrook WC Jr, Mangold KA, Johnson MH, et al. Interobserver reproducibility of Gleason grading of prostatic carcinoma. General pathologist. *Hum Pathol* 32:81-88, 2001A.

Allsbrook WC Jr, Mangold KA, Johnson MH, et al. Interobserver reproducibility of Gleason grading of prostatic carcinoma: urologic pathologists. *Hum Pathol* 32:74-80, 2001B.

Anderson PR, Hanlon AL, Patchefsky A, et al. Perineural invasion and Gleason 7-10 tumors predict increased failure in prostate cancer patients with pretreatment PSA <10 ng/ml treated with conformal external beam radiation therapy. *Int J Radiat Oncol Biol Phys* 41:1087-1092, 1998.

Arai Y, Yoshiki T, Yamabe H, et al. Value of prostate-specific antigen measurements in predicting lymph node involvement in prostatic cancer. *Urol Int* 45:356-360, 1990.

Arcangeli CG, Humphrey PA, Smith DS, et al. Percentage of free serum prostate-specific antigen as a predictor of pathologic features of prostate cancer in a screening population. *Urology* 51:558-565, 1998.

Arima K, Sugimura Y, Hioki T, et al. Stereologically estimated mean nuclear volume of prostatic cancer is a reliable prognostic parameter. *Br J Cancer* 76:234-237, 1997.

Armas OA, Aprikian AG, Melamed J, et al. Clinical and pathobiological effects of neoadjuvant total androgen ablation therapy on clinically localized prostatic adenocarcinoma. *Am J Surg Pathol* 18:979-991, 1994.

Aus G, Hugosson J, Norle L. Long-term survival and mortality in prostate cancer treated with noncurative intent. *J Urol* 154:460-465, 1995.

Babaian RJ, Grunow WA. Reliability of Gleason grading system in comparing prostate biopsies with total prostatectomy specimens. *Urology* 25:564-567, 1985.

Badalament RA, Miller MC, Peller PA, et al. An algorithm for predicting nonorgan-confined prostate cancer using the results obtained from sextant core biopsies with prostate specific antigen level. *J Urol* 156:1375-1380, 1996.

Bagshaw MA, Cox RS, Ramback JE. Radiation therapy for localized prostate cancer: justification by long-term follow-up. *Urol Clin North Am* 17:787-802, 1990.

Bain GO, Koch M, Hanson J. Feasibility of grading prostatic carcinomas. *Arch Pathol Lab Med* 106:265-267, 1982.

Barnes R, Hirst A, Rosenquist R. Early carcinoma of the prostate: comparison of stages A and B. *J Urol* 115:404-405, 1976.

Baschinsky D, Cheville JC, Riehle DL, et al. A comparison of Gleason scores and the percent Gleason patterns 4+5 of prostate carcinoma in needle biopsies to predict outcomes at radical retropubic prostatectomy (RRP) and cancer progression following RRP [abstract]. *Mod Pathol* 15:154-155A, 2002.

Bassily NH, Mucci NR, Rubin MA. Preoperative predictors of Gleason pattern 4/5 prostatic adenocarcinoma in radical prostatectomies [abstract]. *Mod Pathol* 13:93A, 2000.

Bauer JJ, Connelly RR, Sesterhenn IA, et al. Biostatistical modeling using traditional preoperative and pathological prognostic variables in the selection of men at high risk for disease recurrence after radical prostatectomy for prostate cancer. *J Urol* 159:929-933, 1998.

Bauer WC, McGavran MH, Carlin MR. Unsuspected carcinoma of prostate in suprapubic prostatectomy specimens; clinicopathological study of 55 consecutive cases. *Cancer* 13:370-378, 1960.

Bazinet M, Hamdy SM, Begin LR, et al. Prognostic significance of antigenic heterogeneity, Gleason grade, and ploidy of lymph node metastases in patients with prostate cancer. *Prostate* 20:311-326, 1992.

Berner A, Harvei S, Tretli S, et al. Prostatic carcinoma: a multivariate analysis of prognostic factors. *Br J Cancer* 69:924-930, 1994.

Bibbo M, Kim DH, Pfeifer T, et al. Histometric features for the grading of prostatic carcinoma. *Anal Quant Cytol Histol* 3:61-68, 1991.

Bibbo M, Bartels PH, Pfeifer T, et al. Belief network for grading prostate lesions. *Anal Quant Cytol Histol* 15:124-135, 1993.

Bishoff JT, Reyes A, Thompson IM, et al. Pelvic lymphadenectomy can be omitted in selected patients with carcinoma of the prostate: development of a system of patient selection. *Urology* 45:270-274, 1995.

Blackard CE, Mellinger GT, Gleason DF. Treatment of stage 1 carcinoma of the prostate: a preliminary report. *J Urol* 106:729-733, 1971.

Bluestein DL, Bostwick DG, Bergstralh EJ, et al. Eliminating the need for bilateral pelvic lymphadenectomy in select patients with prostate cancer. *J Urol* 151:1315-1320, 1994.

Blute MA, Bergstralh EJ, Iocca A, et al. Use of Gleason score, prostate specific antigen, seminal vesicle and margin status to predict biochemical failure after radical prostatectomy. *J Urol* 165:119-125, 2001.

Böcking A, Kiehn J, Heinzel-Wach M. Combined histologic grading of prostatic carcinoma. *Cancer* 50:288-294, 1982.

Böcking A, Sinagowitz E. Histologic grading of prostatic carcinoma. *Pathol Res Pract* 168:115-125, 1980.

Borre M, Stausbøl-Grøn B, Overgaard J. p53 accumulation associated with bcl-2, the proliferation marker MIB-1 and survival in patients with prostate cancer subjected to watchful waiting. *J Urol* 164:716-721, 2000.

Bostwick DG, Egbert BM, Fajardo LF. Radiation injury of the normal and neoplastic prostate. *Am J Surg Pathol* 6:541-551, 1982.

Bostwick DG. Gleason grading of prostatic needle biopsies. Correlation with grade in 316 matched prostatectomies. *Am J Surg Pathol* 18:796-803, 1994A.

Bostwick DG. Grading prostate cancer. *Am J Clin Pathol* 102(4 suppl 1):S38-S56, 1994B.

Bostwick DG, Qian J, Bergstralh E, et al. Prediction of capsular perforation and seminal vesicle invasion in prostate cancer. *J Urol* 155:1361-1367, 1995.

Bostwick DG, Aquilina JW. Finasteride shows modest pathologic changes in prostate cancer. *J Urol Pathol* 6:83-84, 1997A.

Bostwick DG, Dundore PA. Variants of prostatic adenocarcinomas. In: *Biopsy Pathology of the Prostate.* New York: Chapman & Hall Medical; 167, 1997B.

Bostwick DG, Foster CS. Predictive factors in prostate cancer: current concepts from the 1999 College of American Pathologists Conference on Solid Tumor Prognostic Factors and the 1999 World Health Organization Second International Consultation on Prostate Cancer. *Semin Urol Oncol* 17:222-272, 1999.

Bostwick DG, Grignon DJ, Hammond EH, et al. Prognostic factors in prostate cancer. College of American Pathologists Consensus Statement 1999. *Arch Pathol Lab Med* 124:995-1000, 2000.

Brawn P, Kuhl D, Johnson C III, et al. Stage D1 prostate carcinoma. The histological appearance of nodal metastases and its relationship to survival. *Cancer* 65:538-543, 1990.

Brawn PN, Ayala AG, von Eschenbach AC, et al. Histologic grading study of prostate adenocarcinoma: the development of a new system and comparison with other methods. A preliminary study. *Cancer* 49:525-532, 1982.

Brawn PN, Speights VO. The dedifferentiation of metastatic prostate carcinoma. *Br J Cancer* 59:85-88, 1989.

Brinker DA, Ross JS, Tran TA, et al. Can ploidy of prostate carcinoma diagnosed in needle biopsy predict radical prostatectomy stage and grade? *J Urol* 162:2036-2039, 1999.

Broders AC. Squamous cell epithelioma of the lip. *JAMA* 74:656-664, 1920.

Brown L, ed. In: *The New Shorter Oxford English Dictionary.* Oxford, UK: Clarendon Press; 1125, 1993.

Bruwer G, Heyns CF, Allen FJ. Influence of local tumour stage and grade on reliability of serum prostate-specific antigen in predicting skeletal metastasis in patients with adenocarcinoma of the prostate. *Eur Urol* 35:223-227, 1999.

Cantrell BB, DeKlerk DP, Eggleston JC, et al. Pathological factors that influence prognosis in stage A prostate cancer: the influence of extent versus grade. *J Urol* 125:516-520, 1981.

Carlson GD, Calvanese CB, Kahane H, et al. Accuracy of biopsy Gleason scores from a large uropathology laboratory: use of a diagnostic protocol to minimize observer variability. *Urology* 51:525-529, 1998.

Carvalhal G, Humphrey PA, Thorson P, et al. Visual estimate of percentage of cancer is an independent predictor of prostate cancer recurrence after radical prostatectomy. *Cancer* 89:1308-1314, 2000.

Catalona WJ, Stein AJ, Fair WR. Grading errors in prostatic needle biopsies: relation to the accuracy of tumor grade in predicting pelvic lymph node metastases. *J Urol* 127:919-922, 1982.

Catalona WJ, Smith DS. 5-year tumor recurrence rates after anatomical retropubic prostatectomy for prostate cancer. *J Urol* 152:1837-1842, 1994.

Catalona WJ, Smith DS. Cancer recurrence and survival rates after anatomic radical retropubic prostatectomy for prostate cancer: intermediate-term results. *J Urol* 160:2428-2434, 1998.

Cecchi M, Minervini R, Sepich CA, et al. Correlation between Gleason score of needle biopsy and radical prostatectomy tissue. *Int Urol Nephrol* 30:575-580, 1998.

Chan LW, Stamey TA. Calculating prostate cancer volume preoperatively: the D'Amico equation and some other observations. *J Urol* 159:1998-2003, 1998.

Chan TY, Partin AW, Walsh PC, et al. Prognostic significance of Gleason score 3+4 versus Gleason score 4+3 tumor at radical prostatectomy. *Urology* 56:823-827, 2000.

Chen ME, Johnston DA, Tang K, et al. Detailed mapping of prostate carcinoma foci. *Cancer* 89:1800-1809, 2000.

Cheng L, Bergstralh EJ, Cheville JC, et al. Cancer volume of lymph node metastasis predicts progression in prostate cancer. *Am J Surg Pathol* 22:1491-1520, 1998A.

Cheng L, Seho TJ, Slezak J, et al. Predictors of survival for prostate carcinoma patients treated with salvage radical prostatectomy after radiation therapy. *Cancer* 83:2164-2171, 1998B.

Cheng L, Darson MF, Bergstralh EJ, et al. Correlation of margin status and extraprostatic extension with progression of prostate carcinoma. *Cancer* 86:1775-1782, 1999A.

Cheng L, Slezak J, Bergstralh EJ, et al. Dedifferentiation in the metastatic progression of prostate carcinoma. *Cancer* 86:657-663, 1999B.

Cheng L, Cheville JC, Bostwick DG. Diagnosis of prostate cancer in needle biopsies after radiation therapy. *Am J Surg Pathol* 23:1173-1183, 1999C.

Cheng L, Bergstralh EJ, Scherer BG, et al. Predictors of cancer progression in T1a prostate adenocarcinoma. *Cancer* 85:1300-1304, 1999D.

Chibber PJ, McIntyre MA, Hindmarsh JR, et al. Transitional cell carcinoma involving the prostate. *Br J Urol* 53:605-609, 1981.

Chiusa L, Galliano D, Formiconi A, et al. High and low risk prostate carcinoma determined by histologic grade and proliferative activity. *Cancer* 79:1956-1963, 1997.

Christensen WN, Partin AW, Walsh PC, et al. Pathologic findings in clinical stage A2 prostate cancer. Relation of tumor volume, grade, and location to pathologic stage. *Cancer* 65:1021-1027, 1990.

Cintra ML, Billis A. Histologic grading of prostatic adenocarcinoma. Intraobserver reproducibility of the Mostofi, Gleason and Böcking grading systems. *Int Urol Nephrol* 23:449-454, 1991.

Cipolla B, Guille F, Moulinoux JP, et al. Erythrocyte polyamines and prognosis in stage D2 prostatic carcinoma patients. *J Urol* 151:629-633, 1994.

Civantos F, Marcial MA, Banks ER, et al. Pathology of androgen deprivation therapy in prostate carcinoma. A comparative study of 173 patients. *Cancer* 75:1634-1644, 1995.

Civantos F, Watson RB, Pinto JE, et al. Finasteride effect on prostatic hyperplasia and prostate cancer. A comparative clinicopathologic study of radical prostatectomies. *J Urol Pathol* 6:1-13, 1997.

Cookson MS, Fleshner NE, Soloway SM, et al. Correlation between Gleason score of needle biopsy and radical prostatectomy specimen: accuracy and clinical implications. *J Urol* 157:559-562, 1997.

Crook JM, Bahadur YA, Roberson SJ, et al. Evaluation of radiation effect, tumor differentiation, and prostate specific antigen staining in sequential prostate biopsies after external beam radiotherapy patients with prostate carcinoma. *Cancer* 79:81-89, 1997.

Cupp MR, Bostwick DG, Myers RP, et al. The volume of prostate cancer in the biopsy specimen cannot reliably predict the quantity of cancer in the radical prostatectomy specimen on an individual basis. *J Urol* 153:1543-1548, 1995.

D'Amico AV, Whittington R, Malkowicz SB, et al. A multivariate analysis of clinical and pathological factors that predict for prostate specific antigen failure after radical prostatectomy for prostate cancer. *J Urol* 154:131-138, 1995.

D'Amico AV, Chang H, Holupka E, et al. Calculated prostate cancer volume: the optimal predictor of actual cancer volume and pathologic stage. *Urology* 49:385-391, 1997A.

D'Amico AV, Whittington R, Malkowicz SB, et al. Combined modality staging of prostate carcinoma and its utility in predicting pathologic stage and postoperative prostate specific antigen failure. *Urology* 49(Suppl 3A):23-30, 1997B.

D'Amico AV, Whittington R, Schultz D, et al. Outcome based staging for clinically localized adenocarcinoma of the prostate. *J Urol* 158:1422-1426, 1997C.

D'Amico AV, Whittington R, Malkowicz SB, et al. The combination of preoperative prostate specific antigen and postoperative pathological findings to predict prostate specific antigen outcome in clinically localized prostate cancer. *J Urol* 160:2096-2101, 1998.

D'Amico AV, Renshaw AA, Arsenault L, et al. Clinical predictors of upgrading to Gleason grade 4 or 5 disease at radical prostatectomy: potential implications for patient selection for radiation and androgen suppression therapy. *Int J Radiat Oncol Biol Phys* 45:841-84, 1999.

Danella JF, deKernion JB, Smith RB, et al. The contemporary incidence of lymph node metastases in prostate cancer: implications for laparoscopic lymph node dissection. *J Urol* 149:1488-1491, 1993.

Danziger M, Shevchuk M, Antonescu C, et al. Predictive accuracy of transrectal ultrasound-guided prostate biopsy: correlations to matched prostatectomy specimens. *Urology* 49:863-867, 1997.

De la Taille A, Rubin MA, Bagiella E, et al. Can perineural invasion on prostate needle biopsy predict prostate specific antigen recurrence after radical prostatectomy? *J Urol* 162:103-106, 1999A.

De la Taille A, Katz A, Bagiella E, et al. Perineural invasion on prostate needle biopsy: an independent predictor of final pathologic stage. *Urology* 54:1039-1043, 1999B.

De la Taille A, Rubin MA, Buttyan R, et al. Is microvascular invasion on radical prostatectomy specimens a useful predictor of PSA recurrence for prostate cancer patients? *Eur Urol* 38:79-84, 2000.

De Las Morenas A, Siroky MB, Merriam J, et al. Prostatic adenocarcinoma: reproducibility and correlation with clinical stages of four grading systems. *Hum Pathol* 19:595-597, 1988.

DeMay RM. Prostate. In: *The Art and Science of Cytopathology. Aspiration Cytology.* Chicago: ASCP Press, 1996:1135-1155.

Deshmukh N, Foster CS. Grading prostate cancer. In: Foster CS, Bostwick DG, eds. *Pathology of the Prostate.* Philadelphia: WB Saunders; 191-227, 1998.

Devaney DM, Dorman A, Leader M. Adenosquamous carcinoma of the prostate: a case report. *Hum Pathol* 22:1046-1050, 1991.

Dhom G. Classification and grading of prostatic carcinoma. *Recent Results Cancer Res* 60:14-26, 1977.

Diamond DA, Berry SJ, Jewett HJ, et al. A new method to assess metastatic potential of human prostate cancer: relative nuclear roundness. *J Urol* 128:729-734, 1982.

di Loreto C, Fitzpatrick B, Underhill S, et al. Correlation between visual clues, objective architectural features, and interobserver agreement in prostate cancer. *Am J Clin Pathol* 96:70-75, 1991.

Djavan B, Kadesky K, Klopukh B, et al. Gleason scores from prostate biopsies obtained with 18-gauge biopsy needles poorly predict Gleason scores of radical prostatectomy specimens. *Eur Urol* 33:261-270, 1998.

Dunn RL, Shah R, Zhou M, et al. Global Gleason score, highest core Gleason score, or weighted Gleason score: what Gleason score should be reported in prostate needle biopsies? [abstract]. *Mod Pathol* 15: 161A, 2002.

Eastham JA, Scardino PT. Radical prostatectomy (Chapter 85). In: Walsh PC, Retik AB, Vaughan ED Jr, et al, eds. *Campbell's Urology.* Philadelphia: WB Saunders; 2547-2564, 1998.

Egawa S, Suyama K, Matsumoto K, et al. Improved predictability of extracapsular extension and seminal vesicle involvement based on clinical and biopsy findings in prostate cancer in Japanese men. *Urology* 52:443-440, 1998.

Egevad L, Norberg M, Mattson S, et al. Estimation of prostate cancer volume by multiple cores before radical prostatectomy. *Urology* 52:653-658, 1998.

Egevad L. Reproducibility of Gleason grading of prostate cancer can be improved by the use of reference images. *Urology* 57:291-295, 2001.

Egevad L, Granfors T, Karlberg L, et al. Percent Gleason grade 4/5 as prognostic factor in prostate cancer diagnosed at transurethral resection. *J Urol* 168:509-513, 2002.

El-Galley RE, Howard GC, Hawkyard S, et al. Radical radiotherapy for localized adenocarcinoma of the prostate. A report of 191 cases. *Br J Urol* 75:38-43, 1995.

Elder JS, Gibbons RP, Correa RJ Jr., et al. Efficacy of radical prostatectomy for stage A2 carcinoma of the prostate. *Cancer* 56:2151-2154, 1985.

Ennis RD, Malyszko BK, Rescigno J, et al. Biologic classification as an alternative to anatomic staging for clinically localized prostate cancer: a proposal based on patients treated with external beam radiotherapy. *Urology* 51:265-270, 1998.

Epstein JI, Paull G, Eggleston JC, et al. Prognosis of untreated stage A1 prostatic carcinoma: a study of 94 cases with extended follow-up. *J Urol* 136:837-839, 1986.

Epstein JI, Carmichael M, Partin AW, et al. Is tumor volume an independent predictor of progression following radical prostatectomy? A multivariate analysis of 185 clinical stage B adenocarcinomas of the prostate with 5 years of follow-up. *J Urol* 149:1478-1481, 1993.

Epstein JI, Walsh PC, Carmichael M, et al. Pathologic and clinical findings to predict tumor extent of nonpalpable (stage T1c) prostate cancer. *JAMA* 271:368-374, 1994A.

Epstein JI, Carmichael MJ, Partin AW, et al. Small high grade adenocarcinoma of the prostate in radical prostatectomy specimens performed for nonpalpable disease: pathogenetic and clinical implications. *J Urol* 151:1587-1592, 1994B.

Epstein JI. Diagnostic criteria of limited adenocarcinoma of the prostate on needle biopsy. *Hum Pathol* 26:223-229, 1995.

Epstein JI, Partin AW, Sauvageot J, et al. Prediction of progression following radical prostatectomy: a multivariate analysis of 721 men with long-term follow-up. *Am J Surg Pathol* 20:286-292, 1996.

Epstein JI, Chan DW, Sokoll LJ, et al. Nonpalpable stage T1c prostate cancer: prediction of insignificant disease using free/total prostate specific antigen levels and needle biopsy findings. *J Urol* 160:2407-2411, 1998A.

Epstein JI. The role of perineural invasion and other biopsy characteristics as prognostic markers for localized prostate cancer. *Semin Urol Oncol* 16(3):124-128, 1998B.

Epstein JI, Amin MB, Reuter VR, et al., and the Bladder Consensus Conference Committee. The World Health Organization/International Society of Urological Pathology Consensus classification of urothelial (transitional cell) neoplasms of the urinary bladder. *Am J Surg Pathol* 22:1435-1448, 1998C.

Epstein JI, Partin AW, Potter SR, et al. Adenocarcinoma of the prostate invading the seminal vesicle: prognostic stratification based on pathologic parameters. *Urology* 56:283-288, 2000A.

Epstein JI. Gleason score 2-4 adenocarcinoma of the prostate on needle biopsy. A diagnosis that should not be made. *Am J Surg Pathol* 24:477-478, 2000B.

Epstein JI, Walsh PC, Carter HB. Dedifferentiation of prostate cancer grade with time in men followed expectantly for stage T1c disease. *J Urol* 166:1688-1691, 2001.

Epstein JI, Kunz GM. Should each core with prostate cancer be assigned a separate Gleason score? (abstract) *J Urol* 167:226A, 2002.

Ernst DS, Hanson J, Venner PM. Analysis of prognostic factors in men with metastatic prostatic cancer. *J Urol* 146:372-376, 1991.

Eskelinen M, Lipponen P, Majapuro R, et al. Prognostic factors in prostatic adenocarcinoma assessed by means of quantitative histology. *Eur Urol* 19:274-278, 1991.

Evans N, Barnes RW, Brown AF. Carcinoma of the prostate. Correlation between the histologic observations and the clinical course. *Arch Pathol* 34:473-483, 1942.

Feng J, de Guia K, Gharibian A, et al. Changes in the frequency and volume of "index" tumors and HGPIN in radical prostatectomy specimens (RPS) in the 1990s [abstract]. *Mod Pathol* 13:99A, 2000.

Ferguson J, Zincke H, Ellison E, et al. Decrease of prostatic intraepithelial neoplasia following androgen deprivation therapy in patients with stage T3 carcinoma treated by radical prostatectomy. *Urology* 44:91-95, 1994.

Fergusson JD, Franks LM. The response of prostatic carcinoma to estrogen treatment. *Br J Surg* 40:422-428, 1953.

Fernandes ET, Sundaram CP, Long R, et al. Biopsy Gleason score: how does it correlate with the final pathological diagnosis in prostate cancer? *Br J Urol* 79:615-617, 1997.

Fleshner NE, Cookson MS, Soloway SM, et al. Repeat transrectal ultrasound-guided prostate biopsy: a strategy to improve the reliability of needle biopsy grading in patients with well-differentiated prostate cancer. *Urology* 52:659-662, 1998.

Foucar E, Haake G, Dalton L, et al. The area of cancer in transurethral resection specimens as a prognostic indicator in carcinoma of the prostate: a computer-assisted morphometric study. *Hum Pathol* 21:586-592, 1990.

Fowler JE Jr., Mills SE. Operable prostatic carcinoma: correlations among clinical stage, pathological stage, Gleason histological score and early disease-free survival. *J Urol* 133:49-52, 1985.

Franks LM. Estrogen-treated prostatic carcinoma. *Cancer* 13:490-501, 1960.

Freedland SJ, Sutter ME, Naitoh J, et al. Clinical characteristics in black and white men with prostate cancer in an equal access medical center. *Urology* 55:387-390, 2000.

Freeman VL, Coard K, Ogunbiyi O, et al. Gleason scoring system: high level of agreement between pathologists from three continents [abstract]. *Mod Pathol* 14:108A, 2001.

Fujikawa K, Sasaki M, Aoyama T, et al. Prognostic criteria in patients with prostate cancer: correlation with volume weighted mean nuclear volume. *J Urol* 154:2123-2127, 1995A.

Fujikawa K, Sasaki M, Aoyama T, et al. Prognostic criteria in patients with stage D2 prostate cancer. Correlation with mean nuclear volume. *Cancer* 76:91-95, 1995B.

Fujikawa K, Sasaki M, Itoh T, et al. Combining volume-weighted mean nuclear volume with Gleason score and clinical stage to predict more reliably disease outcome of patients with prostate cancer. *Prostate* 37:63-69, 1998.

Fujikawa K, Matsui Y, Kobayashi T, et al. Predicting pathological stage of localized prostate cancer using volume weighted mean nuclear volume. *J Urol* 164:1587-1590, 2000.

Fujita T, Kanimoto Y, Akino H, et al. (Study of incidental carcinoma of the prostate. Part 1. Pathological analysis related to the clinical features) [in Japanese] *Acta Urol Jpn* 37:695-703, 1991.

Gaeta JF, Asirwatham JE, Miller GJ, et al. Histologic grading of primary prostatic cancer: a new approach to an old problem. *J Urol* 123:689-693, 1980.

Gallee MP, ten Kate FJ, Mulder PG, et al. Histological grading of prostatic carcinoma in prostatectomy specimens. Comparison of prognostic accuracy of five grading systems. *Br J Urol* 65:308-375, 1990.

Garabedian EM, Humphrey PA, Gordon JI. A transgenic mouse model of metastatic prostate cancer originating from neuroendocrine cells. *Proc Natl Acad Sci* 95:15382-15387, 1998.

Gardner WA Jr. Histologic grading of prostate cancer: a retrospective and prospective overview. *Prostate* 3:555-561, 1982.

Garnett JE, Oyasu R, Grayhack JT. The accuracy of diagnostic biopsy specimens in predicting tumor grades by Gleason's classification of radical prostatectomy specimens. *J Urol* 131:690-693, 1984.

Gaudin PB, Zelefsky MJ, Leibel SA, et al. Histopathologic effects of three-dimensional conformal external beam radiation therapy on benign and malignant prostate tissues. *Am Surg Pathol* 23:1021-1031, 1999.

Glaessgen A, Hamberg H, Pihl CG, et al. Interobserver reproducibility of percent Gleason grade 4/5 in total prostatectomy specimens. *J Urol* 168:2006-2010, 2002.

Gleason DF. Classification of prostatic carcinoma. *Cancer Chemother Rep* 50:125-128, 1966.

Gleason DF, Mellinger GT, and The Veterans Administration Cooperative Urological Research Group. Prediction of prognosis for prostatic adenocarcinoma by combined histological grading and clinical staging. *J Urol* 111:58-64, 1974.

Gleason DF and The Veterans Administration Cooperative Urological Research Group. Histologic grading and clinical staging of prostatic carcinoma. (Chapter 9). In: Tannenbaum M, ed. *Urologic Pathology: The Prostate.* Philadelphia: Lea & Febiger; 171-197, 1977.

Gleason DF. Histologic grading of prostatic carcinoma. In: Bostwick DG, ed. *Pathology of the Prostate.* New York: Churchill Livingstone; 83-93, 1990.

Gleason DF. Histologic grading of prostate cancer: a perspective. *Hum Pathol* 23:273-279, 1992.

Goebbels R, Amberger L, Wernert N, et al. Urothelial carcinoma of the prostate. *Appl Pathol* 3:242-254, 1985.

Goldstein NS, Martinez A, Vicini F, et al. The histology of radiation therapy effect on prostate adenocarcinoma as assessed by needle biopsy after brachytherapy boost. Correlation with biochemical failure. *Am J Clin Pathol* 110:765-775, 1998.

Golimbu M, Schinella R, Morales P, et al. Differences in pathological characteristics and prognosis of clinical A2 prostatic cancer from A1 and B disease. *J Urol* 119:618-622, 1978.

Green GA, Hanlon AL, Al-Saleem T, et al. A Gleason score of 7 predicts a worse outcome for prostate carcinoma patients treated with radiotherapy. *Cancer* 83:971-976, 1998.

Greene DR, Egawa S, Neerhut G, et al. The distribution of residual cancer in radical prostatectomy specimens in stage A prostate cancer. *J Urol* 145:324-328, 1991.

Greene DR, Fitzpatrick JM, Scardino PT. Anatomy of the prostate and distribution of early prostate cancer. *Semin Surg Oncol* 11:9-22, 1995.

Greene LF, O'Dea MJ, Dockerty MB. Primary transitional cell carcinoma of the prostate. *J Urol* 116:761-763, 1976.

Griebling TL, Özkutlu D, See WA, et al. Prognostic implications of extracapsular extension of lymph node metastases in prostate cancer. *Mod Pathol* 10:804-809, 1997.

Grignon DJ, Sakr WA. Histologic effects of radiation therapy and total androgen blockade on prostate cancer. *Cancer* 75:1837-1841, 1995.

Guileyardo JM, Sarma DP, Johnson WD, et al. Incidental prostatic carcinoma: tissue extent versus histologic grade. *Urology* 20:40-42, 1982.

Haese A, Epstein JI, Nuland H, et al. Validation of a biopsy-based pathologic algorithm for predicting lymph node metastases in patients with clinically localized prostate carcinoma. *Cancer* 95:1016-1021, 2002.

Han M, Partin AW, Pound CR, et al. Long-term biochemical disease-free and cancer-specific survival following radical retropubic prostatectomy. The 15-year Johns Hopkins experience. *Urol Clin North Am* 28:555-565, 2001.

Hanks GE, Lee WR, Schultheiss TE. Clinical and biochemical evidence of control of prostate cancer at 5 years after external beam radiation. *J Urol* 154:456-459, 1995.

Harada M, Mostofi FK, Corle DK, et al. Preliminary studies of histologic prognosis in cancer of the prostate. *Cancer Treat Rep* 61:223-225, 1977.

Heaney JA, Chang HC, Daly JJ, et al. Prognosis of clinically undiagnosed prostatic carcinoma and the influence of endocrine therapy. *J Urol* 118:283-287, 1977.

Hellström M, Häggman M, Brändstedt S, et al. Histopathological changes in androgen-deprived localized prostatic cancer. *Eur Urol* 24:461-465, 1993.

Herman CM, Kattan MW, Scardino PT, et al. Quantification of high grade tumor is a predictive of disease progression in pT3NO prostate cancer [abstract]. *Mod Pathol* 12:97A, 1999.

Herman CM, Wilcox GE, Kattan MW, et al. Lymphovascular invasion as a predictor of disease progression in prostate cancer. *Am J Surg Pathol* 24:859-863, 2000.

Herman CM, Kattan MW, Ohori M, et al. Primary Gleason pattern as a predictor of disease progression in Gleason score 7 prostate cancer: a multivariate analysis of 823 men treated with radical prostatectomy. *Am J Surg Pathol* 25:657-660, 2001.

Hoenig DM, Chi S, Porter C, et al. Risk of nodal metastases at laparoscopic pelvic lymphadenectomy using PSA , Gleason score, and clinical stage in men with localized prostate cancer. *J Endourol* 11:263-265, 1997.

Hohbach M, Dhom G. Present problems in prostatic carcinoma [in German]. *Munch Med Wochenschr* 114:45-54, 1972.

Hugosson J, Abrahamsson PA, Ahlgren G, et al. The risk of malignancy in the surgical margin at radical prostatectomy reduced almost three-fold in patients given neo-adjuvant hormone treatment. *Eur Urol* 29:413-419, 1996.

Huland H, Hammerer P, Henke RP, et al. Preoperative prediction of tumor heterogeneity and recurrence after radical prostatectomy for localized prostatic carcinoma with digital rectal examination, prostate specific antigen and the results of 6 systematic biopsies. *J Urol* 155:1344-1347, 1996.

Humphrey P, Vollmer RT. The ratio of prostate chips with cancer. A new measure of tumor extent and its relationship to stage and prognosis. *Hum Pathol* 19:411-418, 1988.

Humphrey PA, Vollmer RT. Intraglandular tumor extent and prognosis in prostatic carcinoma: application of a grid method to prostatectomy specimens. *Hum Pathol* 21:799-804, 1990.

Humphrey PA, Baty J, Keetch DW. Relationship between serum prostate specific antigen, needle biopsy findings, and histopathologic features of prostatic carcinoma in radical prostatectomy tissues. *Cancer* 75:1842-1849, 1995.

Humphrey PA, Keetch DW, Smith DS, et al. Prospective characterization of pathological features of prostatic carcinomas detected via serum prostate specific antigen based screening. *J Urol* 155:816-820, 1996.

Humphrey PA, Kaleem Z, Swanson PE, et al. Pseudohyperplastic prostatic adenocarcinoma. *Am J Surg Pathol* 22:1239-1246, 1998A.

Humphrey PA, Vollmer RT. Relationships between serum prostate-specific antigen and histopathologic appearances of prostate carcinoma. In: Foster CS, Bostwick DG, eds. *Pathology of the Prostate.* Philadelphia: WB Saunders; 262, 1998B.

Hurwitz, MD, DeWee TL, Zinreich ES, et al. Nuclear morphometry predicts disease-free interval for clinically localized adenocarcinoma of the prostate treated with definitive radiation therapy. *Int J Cancer* 84:594-597, 1999.

Iczkowski KA, Bostwick DG. The pathologist as optimist. Cancer grade deflation in prostatic needle biopsies [editorial]. *Am J Surg Pathol* 22:1169-1170, 1998.

Irinopoulou T, Rigaut JP, Benson MC. Toward objective prognostic grading of prostatic carcinoma using image analysis. *Anal Quant Cytol Histol* 15:341-344, 1993.

Irwin MB, Trapasso JG. Identification of insignificant prostate cancers: analysis of preoperative parameters. *Urology* 44:862-868, 1994.

Iselin CE, Robertson JE, Paulson DF. Radical perineal prostatectomy: oncological outcome during a 20-year period. *J Urol* 161:163-168, 1999.

Jacobs DM, Vago JF, Weiss MA. Gleason grading of prostatic adenocarcinoma in fine-needle aspiration. *Diagn Cytopathol* 5:126-133, 1989.

Jewett HJ, Bridge RW, Gray GF Jr, et al. The palpable nodule of prostatic cancer: results 15 years after radical excision. *JAMA* 203:403-406, 1968.

Jhaveri FM, Zippe CD, Klein EA, et al. Biochemical failure does not predict overall survival after radical prostatectomy for localized prostate cancer: 10-year results. *Urology* 54:884-890, 1999.

Johansson JE, Holmberg L, Johansson S, et al. Fifteen-year survival in prostate cancer. A prospective, population-based study in Sweden. *JAMA* 277:467-471, 1997.

Johnson DE, Hogan JM, Ayala AG. Transitional cell carcinoma of the prostate. A clinical morphological study. *Cancer* 29:287-293, 1972.

Johnstone PA, Riffenburgh R, Saunders EL, et al. Grading inaccuracies in diagnostic biopsies revealing prostatic adenocarcinoma: implications for definitive radiation therapy. *Int J Radiat Oncol Biol Phys* 32:479-482, 1995.

Jørgensen T, Yogesan K, Skjørten F, et al. Histopathological grading and DNA ploidy as prognostic markers in metastatic prostatic cancer. Correlation with mean nuclear volume. *Br J Cancer* 71:1055-1060, 1995.

Jørgensen T, Yogesan K, Tveter KJ, et al. Nuclear texture analysis: a new prognostic tool in metastatic prostate cancer. *Cytometry* 24:277-283, 1996.

Kahler JE. Carcinoma of the prostate gland. *Mayo Clin Proc* 13:5809-592, 1938.

Kahler JE. Carcinoma of the prostate gland: a pathologic study. *J Urol* 41:557-574, 1939.

Kato M, Okada K, Yamashina M, et al. Clinical assessments on pre-treatment prognostic factors in 138 patients with advanced prostatic carcinoma (stage D2) [in Japanese]. *Acta Urol Jpn* 39:131-134, 1993.

Kattan MW, Stapleton AM, Wheeler TM, et al. Evaluation of a nomogram used to predict the pathologic stage of clinically localized prostate carcinoma. *Cancer* 79:528-537, 1997.

Kattan MW, Eastham JA, Stapleton AMF, et al. A preoperative nomogram for disease recurrence following radical prostatectomy for prostate cancer. *J Natl Cancer Inst* 90:766-771, 1998.

Kattan MW, Wheeler TM, Scardino PT. Postoperative nomogram for disease recurrence after radical prostatectomy for prostate cancer. *J Clin Oncol* 17:1499-1507, 1999.

Kattan MW, Potters L, Blasko JC, et al. Pretreatment nomogram for predicting freedom from recurrence after permanent prostate bradytherapy in prostate cancer. *Urology* 58:393-399, 2001.

Khalifa NM, Jarman WD. A study of 48 cases of incidental carcinoma of the prostate followed 10 years or longer. *J Urol* 116:329-331, 1976.

King CR, Long JP: Prostate biopsy grading errors: a sampling problem? *Int J Cancer* 90:326-330, 2000.

Koch MO, Foster RS, Bell S, et al. Characterization and predictors of prostates specific antigen progression rates after radical retropubic prostatectomy. *J Urol* 164:749-753, 2000.

Kojima M, Troncoso P, Babaian RJ. Use of prostate-specific antigen and tumor volume in predicting needle biopsy grade error. *Urology* 45:807-812, 1995.

Koppie TM, Grossfeld GD, Miller D, et al. Patterns of treatment of patients with prostate cancer initially managed with surveillance: results from the CaPSURE database. *J Urol* 164:81-88, 2000.

Koutsilieris M, Dupont A, Gomez J, et al. Stratification of stage D2 prostate cancer patients by a disease aggressiveness score and its use in evaluating disease response and outcome to combination hormonal treatment (GnRH-A plus flutamide). *Anticancer Res* 14:627-634, 1994.

Kramer SA, Spahr J, Bendler CB, et al. Experience with Gleason's histopathologic grading in prostatic cancer. *J Urol* 124:223-225, 1980.

Kramer SA, Farnham R, Glenn JF, et al. Comparative morphology of primary and secondary deposits of prostatic adenocarcinoma. *Cancer* 48:271-273, 1981.

Kronz JD, Silberman MA, Allsbrook WC Jr, et al. Pathology residents use of a web-based tutorial to improve Gleason grading of prostate carcinoma on needle biopsies. *Hum Pathol* 31:1044-1050, 2000.

Lange PH, Narayan P. Understaging and undergrading of prostate cancer. *Urology* 21:113-118, 1983.

Larsen MP, Carter HB, Epstein JI. Can stage A1 tumor extent be predicted by transurethral resection tumor volume, percent or grade? A study of 64 stage A1 radical prostatectomies with comparison to prostates removed for stages A2 and B disease. *J Urol* 146:1059-1063, 1991.

Lau WK, Blute ML, Bostwick DG, et al. Prognostic factors for survival of patients with pathological Gleason score 7 prostate cancer: differences in outcome between primary Gleason grades 3 and 4. *J Urol* 166:1692-1697, 2001.

Layfield LJ, Mukamel E, Hilborne LH, et al. Cytological grading of prostatic aspiration biopsy: a comparison with the Gleason grading system. *J Urol* 138:798-800, 1987.

Lee WR, Hanlon AL, Hanks GE. Systematic biopsies: do they add prognostic information in men with clinically localized prostate cancer treated with radiation therapy alone? *Radiology* 198:439-442, 1996.

Lehman TH, Kirchheim D, Braun E, et al. An evaluation of radical prostatectomy for incidentally diagnosed carcinoma of the prostate. *J Urol* 99:646-650, 1968.

Lessells AM, Burnett RA, Howatson SR, et al. Observer variability in the histopathologic reporting of needle biopsy specimens of the prostate. *Hum Pathol* 28:646-649, 1997.

Levi AW, Epstein JI. Pseudohyperplastic prostatic adenocarcinoma on needle biopsy and simple prostatectomy. *Am J Surg Pathol* 24:1039-1046, 2000.

Liebross RH, Pollack A, Lankford SP, et al. Relationship of ultrasound staging and bilateral biopsy positivity to outcome in stage T1c prostate cancer treated with radiotherapy. *Urology* 52:647-652, 1998.

Lilleby W, Torlakovic G, Torlakovic E, et al. Prognostic significance of histological grading for patients with prostate carcinoma who are assessed by the Gleason and World Health Organization grading systems in needle biopsies obtained prior to radiotherapy. *Cancer* 92:311-319, 2001.

Lin K, Szabo Z, Chin BB, et al. The value of a baseline bone scan in patients with newly diagnosed prostate cancer. *Clin Nucl Med* 24:579-582, 1999.

Lipponen P, Vesalainen S, Kasurinen J, et al. A prognostic score for prostatic adenocarcinoma based on clinical, histological, biochemical and cytometric data from the primary tumor. *Anticancer Res* 16:2095-2100, 1996.

Mai KT, Leahy CF. Squamous cell carcinoma occurring as a circumscribed nodule in the transition zone of the prostate. A case report and review of the literature. *J Urol Pathol* 5:85-92, 1996.

Makarov DV, Sanderson H, Partin AW, et al. Gleason score 7 prostate cancer on needle biopsy: is the prognostic difference between Gleason score 4+3 and 3+4 independent of the number of involved cores? *J Urol* 167:2440-2442, 2002.

Maksem JA, Resnick MI, Johenning PW. Can a cytological grading system be predictive of Gleason's scores in aspiration biopsy cytology specimens of prostate carcinoma. *World J Urol* 5:99-102, 1987.

Maksem JA, Johenning PW. Is cytology capable of adequately grading prostate carcinoma? Matched series of 50 cases comparing cytologic and histologic pattern diagnoses. *Urology* 31:437-444, 1988.

McCullough DL, Prout GR Jr, Daley JJ. Carcinoma of the prostate and lymphatic metastasis. *J Urol* 111:65-71, 1974.

McGowan DG, Bain GO, Hanson J. Evaluation of histological grading (Gleason) in carcinoma of the prostate: adverse influence of highest grade. *Prostate* 4:111-118, 1983.

McLean M, Srigley J, Banerjee D, et al. Interobserver variation in prostate cancer Gleason scoring: are there implications for the design of clinical trials and treatment strategies. *Clin Oncol* 9:222-225, 1997.

McNeal JE, Reese JH, Redwine EA, et al. Cribriform adenocarcinoma of the prostate. *Cancer* 58:1714-1719, 1986A.

McNeal JE, Bostwick DG, Kindrachuk RA, et al. Patterns of progression in prostate cancer. *Lancet* 1:60-63, 1986B.

McNeal JE, Villers AA, Redwine EA, et al. Histologic differentiation, cancer volume, and pelvic lymph node metastasis in adenocarcinoma of the prostate. *Cancer* 66:1225-1233, 1990.

McNeal JE. Prostatic microcarcinomas in relation to cancer origin and the evolution to clinical cancer. *Cancer* 71 (3 suppl):984-991, 1993.

McNeal JE, Yemoto CEM. Spread of adenocarcinoma within prostatic ducts and acini. *Am J Surg Pathol* 20:802-814, 1996.

McNeal JE, Cohen RJ, Brooks JD. Role of cytologic criteria in the histologic diagnosis of Gleason grade 1 prostatic adenocarcinoma. *Hum Pathol* 32:441-446, 2001.

Mellinger GT, Gleason D, Bailar J III. The histology and prognosis of prostatic cancer. *J Urol* 97:331-337, 1967.

Miller GJ. Pathologic aspects of prostate cancer: prediction of malignant potential. *Urology* 34(suppl):5-9, 1989.

Miller GJ. New developments in grading prostate cancer. *Semin Urol* 8:9-18, 1990.

Mills SE, Fowler JE Jr. Gleason histologic grading of prostatic carcinoma. Correlations between biopsy and prostatectomy specimens. *Cancer* 57:346-349, 1986.

Mobley TL, Frank IN. Influence of tumor grade on survival and on serum acid phosphatase levels in metastatic cancer of prostate. *J Urol* 99:321-323, 1968.

Mohideen MN, McCall AR, Feinstein J, et al. Factors that influence biochemical failure after radiation therapy for stage T1c prostate cancer. *Am J Clin Oncol* 21:6-11, 1998.

Montironi R, Magi-Galluzzi C, Muzzonigro G, et al. Effects of combination endocrine treatment on normal prostate, prostatic intraepithelial neoplasia, and prostatic adenocarcinomas. *J Clin Pathol* 47:906-913, 1994.

Montironi R, Schulman CC. Pathological changes in prostate lesions after androgen manipulation. *J Clin Pathol* 51:5-12, 1998.

Montironi R, Diamanti L, Santinelli A, et al. Effect of androgen ablation on pathologic stage and resection limit status of prostate cancer. Initial results of the Italian PROSIT study. *Pathol Res Pract* 195:201-208, 1999.

Mostofi FK. Grading of prostatic carcinoma. *Cancer Chemother Rep* 59:111-117, 1975.

Mostofi FK. Problems of grading carcinoma of prostate. *Semin Oncol* 3:161-169, 1976.

Mostofi FK, Sesterhenn I, Sobin LH. *Histological Typing of Prostate Tumours. International Histological Classification of Tumours,* No. 22. Geneva: World Health Organization, 1980.

Mott LJM. Squamous cell carcinoma of the prostate: report of 2 cases and review of the literature. *J Urol* 121:833-835, 1979.

Moul JW, Paulson DF. The role of radical surgery in the management of radiation recurrent and large volume prostate cancer. *Cancer* 68:1265-1271, 1991.

Moul JW, Connelly RR, Perahia B, et al. The contemporary value of pretreatment prostatic acid phosphatase to predict pathological stage and recurrence in radical prostatectomy cases. *J Urol* 159:935-940, 1998.

Movsas B, Hanlon AL, Teshima T, et al. Analyzing predictive models following definitive radiotherapy for prostate carcinoma. *Cancer* 80:1093-1102, 1997.

Muir EG. Carcinoma of the prostate. *Lancet* 1:667-672, 1934.

Mukamel E, deKernion JB, Dorey F, et al. Significance of histological prognostic indicators in patients with carcinoma of the prostate. *Br J Urol* 65:46-50, 1990.

Mulders PF, Dijkman GA, Fernandez del Moral PF, et al. Analysis of prognostic factors in disseminated prostatic cancer. An update. Dutch Southeastern Urological Cooperative Group. *Cancer* 65:2758-2761, 1990.

Müller H-A, Ackermann R, Frohmüller HGW. The value of perineal punch biopsy in estimating the histological grade of carcinoma of the prostate. *Prostate* 1:303-309, 1980.

Munsie WJ, Foster EA. Unsuspected very small foci of carcinoma of the prostate in transurethral resection specimens. *Cancer* 21:692-698, 1968.

Murphy WM, Soloway MS, Barrows GH. Pathologic changes associated with androgen deprivation therapy for prostate cancer. *Cancer* 68:821-828, 1991.

Myers RP, Neves RJ, Farrow GM, et al. Nucleolar grading of prostatic carcinoma. Light microscopic correlation with disease progression. *Prostate* 3:423-432, 1982.

Myers RP, Fleming TR. Course of localized adenocarcinoma of the prostate treated by radical prostatectomy. *Prostate* 4:461-472, 1983.

Narain V, Bianco FJ Jr, Grignon DJ, et al. How accurately does prostate biopsy Gleason score predict pathologic findings and disease-free survival? *Prostate* 49:185-190, 2001.

Narayan P, Fournier G, Gajendran V, et al. Utility of preoperative serum prostate-specific antigen concentration and biopsy Gleason score in predicting risk of pelvic lymph node metastases in prostate cancer. *Urology* 44:519-524, 1994.

Nemoto R, Uchida K, Harada M, et al. Experience with Gleason histopathologic grading of prostatic cancer in Japan. *Urology* 30:436-440, 1987.

Nielsen K, Berild GH, Bruun E, et al. The prognostic value of histological grading and mean nuclear volume in human prostatic cancer. *Prostate* 21:53-61, 1992.

Noguchi M, Stamey TA, McNeal JE, et al. An analysis of 148 consecutive transition zone cancers: clinical and histological characteristics. *J Urol* 163:1751-1755, 2000.

Noguchi M, Stamey TA, McNeal JE, et al. Relationship between systematic biopsies and histological features of 222 radical prostatectomy specimens: Lack of prediction of tumor significance for men with nonpalpable prostate cancer. *J Urol* 166:104-110, 2001.

Norberg M, Holmberg L, Wheeler T, et al. Five year follow-up after radical prostatectomy for localized prostate cancer: a study of the impact of different tumor variables on progression. *Scand J Urol Nephrol* 28:391-399, 1994.

Nori D, Moni J. Current issues in techniques of prostate brachytherapy. *Semin Surg Oncol* 13:444-453, 1997.

O'Dowd GJ, Veltri RW, Orozco R, et al. Update on the appropriate staging evaluation for newly diagnosed prostate cancer. *J Urol* 158:687-698, 1997.

Oesterling JE, Brendler CB, Epstein JI, et al. Correlation of clinical stage, serum prostatic acid phosphatase and preoperative Gleason grade with final pathological stage in 275 patients with clinically localized adenocarcinoma of the prostate. *J Urol* 138:92-98, 1987.

Ohki T, Akakura K, Uedu T, et al. Changes in histologic grade and argyrophilic nucleolar organizer regions during progression of prostate cancer. *Jpn J Clin Oncol* 26:82-87, 1996.

Ohori M, Goad JR, Wheeler TM, et al. Can radical prostatectomy alter the progression of poorly differentiated prostate cancer? *J Urol* 152:1843-1849, 1994A.

Ohori M, Wheeler TM, Scardino PT. The new American Joint Committee on Cancer and International Union Against Cancer TNM classification of prostate cancer. Clinicopathologic correlations. *Cancer* 74:104-114, 1994B.

Ohori M, Wheeler TM, Kattan MW, et al. Prognostic significance of positive surgical margins in radical prostatectomy specimens. *J Urol* 154:1818-1824, 1995.

Okamoto T, Ogiu K, Sato M, et al. Primary squamous cell carcinoma of the prostate: a case report [in Japanese]. *Acta Urol Jpn* 42:67-70, 1996.

Orozco R, O'Dowd G, Kunnel B, et al. Observations on pathology trends in 62,537 prostate biopsies obtained from urology private practices in the United States. *Urology* 51:186-195, 1998.

Özdamar SO, Sarikaya S, Yildiz L, et al. Intraobserver and interobserver reproducibility of WHO and Gleason histologic grading systems in prostatic adenocarcinomas. *Int Urol Nephrol* 28:73-77, 1996.

Pan CC, Potter SR, Partin AW, et al. The prognostic significance of tertiary Gleason patterns of higher grade in radical prostatectomy specimens: a proposal to modify the Gleason grading system. *Am J Surg Pathol* 24: 563-569, 2000.

Partin AW, Carter HB, Chan DW, et al. Prostate specific antigen in the staging of localized prostate cancer: influence of tumor differentiation, tumor volume and benign hyperplasia. *J Urol* 143:747-752, 1990.

Partin AW, Steinberg GD, Pitcock RV, et al. Use of nuclear morphometry, Gleason histologic scoring, clinical stage, and age to predict disease-free survival among patients with prostate cancer. *Cancer* 70:161-168, 1992.

Partin AW, Yoo J, Carter HB, et al. The use of prostate specific antigen, clinical stage, and Gleason score to predict pathological stage in men with localized prostate cancer. *J Urol* 150:110-114, 1993.

Partin AW, Piantadosi S, Sanda MG, et al. Selection of men at high risk for disease recurrence for experimental adjuvant therapy following radical prostatectomy. *Urology* 45:831-838, 1995.

Partin AW, Kattan MW, Subong ENP, et al. Combination of prostate-specific antigen, clinical stage, and Gleason score to predict pathological stage of localized prostate cancer. A multi-institutional update. *JAMA* 277:1445-1451, 1997.

Partin AW, Mangold LA, Lamm DM, et al. Contemporary update of prostate cancer staging nomograms (Partin Tables) for the new millenium. *Urology* 58:843-848, 2001.

Paulson DF, Piserchia PV, Gardner W. Predictors of lymphatic spread in prostatic adenocarcinoma: uro-oncology research group study. *J Urol* 123:697-699, 1980.

Paulson DF, Moul JW, Walther PJ. Radical prostatectomy for clinical stage T1-2N0M0 prostatic adenocarcinoma: long-term results. *J Urol* 144:1180-1184, 1990.

Paulson DF. Impact of radical prostatectomy in the management of clinically localized disease. *J Urol* 152:1826-1830, 1994.

Peller PA, Young DC, Marmaduke DP, et al. Sextant prostate biopsies. A histopathologic correlation with radical prostatectomy specimens. *Cancer* 75:530-538, 1995.

Penson DF, Grossfeld GD, Li YP, et al. How well does the Partin nomogram predict pathological stage after radical prostatectomy in a community based population? *J Urol* 167:1653-1657, 2002.

Pilepich MV, Krall JM, Sause WT, et al. Prognostic factors in carcinoma of the prostate: analysis of RTOG 75-06. *Int J Radiat Oncol Biol Phys* 13:339-349, 1987.

Polascik TJ, Pearson JD, Partin AW. Multivariate models as predictors of pathological stage using Gleason score, clinical stage, and serum prostate-specific antigen. *Semin Urol Oncol* 16:160-171, 1998.

Pontes JE, Montie J, Klein E, et al. Salvage surgery for radiation failure in prostate cancer. *Cancer* 71(3 suppl):976-980, 1993.

Pool TL, Thompson GJ. Conservative treatment of carcinoma of the prostate. *JAMA* 160:833-837, 1956.

Pound CR, Partin AW, Epstein JI, et al. Prostate-specific antigen after anatomic radical retropubic prostatectomy. Patterns of recurrence and cancer control. *Urol Clin North Am* 24:395-406, 1997.

Presti JC Jr., Shinohara K, Bacchetti P, et al. Positive fraction of systematic biopsies predicts risk of relapse after radical prostatectomy. *Urology* 52:1079-1084, 1998.

Prestidge BR, Hoak DC, Grimm PD, et al. Post-treatment biopsy results following interstitial brachytherapy in early-stage prostate cancer. *Int J Radiat Oncol Biol Phys* 37:31-39, 1997.

Prout GR Jr, Heaney JA, Griffin PP, et al. Nodal involvement as a prognostic indicator in patients with prostatic carcinoma. *J Urol* 124:226-231, 1980.

Puppo P, Perachino M. Clinical stage, prostate-specific antigen and Gleason grade to predict extracapsular disease or nodal metastasis in men with newly diagnosed, previously untreated prostate cancer. A multicenter study. *Eur Urol* 32:273-279, 1997.

Rabbani F, Bastar A, Fair WR. Site specific predictors of positive margins at radical prostatectomy: an argument for risk based modification of technique. *J Urol* 160:1727-1733, 1998.

Ragde H, Blasko JC, Grimm PD, et al. Brachytherapy for clinically localized prostate cancer: results at 7- and 8-year follow-up. *Semin Surg Oncol* 13:438-443, 1997.

Ramos CG, Carvalhal GF, Smith DS, et al. Clinical and pathological characteristics, and recurrence rates of stage T1c versus T2a or T2b prostate cancer. *J Urol* 161:1525-1529, 1999.

Ravery V, Boccon-Gibod LA, Meulemans A, et al. Predictive value of pathological features for progression after radical prostatectomy. *Eur Urol* 26:197-201, 1994A.

Ravery V, Boccon-Gibod LA, Dauge-Geffroy MC, et al. Systematic biopsies accurately predict extracapsular extension of prostate cancer and persistent recurrent detectable PSA after radical prostatectomy. *Urology* 44:371-376, 1994B.

Reuter VE. Pathological changes in benign and malignant prostatic tissue following androgen deprivation therapy. *Urology* 49(3A suppl):16-22, 1997.

Roach M III, Marquez C, Yuo HS, et al. Predicting the risk of lymph node involvement using the pre-treatment prostate specific antigen and Gleason score in men with clinically localized prostate cancer. *Int J Radiat Oncol Biol Phys* 28:33-37, 1994.

Roberts WW, Bergstralh EJ, Blute ML, et al. Contemporary identification of patients at high risk of early prostate cancer recurrence after radical retropubic prostatectomy. *Urology* 57:1033-1037, 2001.

Robutti F, Pilato FP, Betta PG. A new method of grading malignancy of prostate carcinoma using quantitative microscopic nuclear features. *Pathol Res Pract* 185:701-703, 1989.

Rogers E, Ohori M, Kassabian VS, et al. Salvage radical prostatectomy: outcome measured by serum prostate specific antigen levels. *J Urol* 153:104-110, 1995.

Rogers E, Gurnipar T, Dillioglugil O, et al. The role of digital rectal examination, biopsy Gleason sum and prostate-specific antigen in selected patients who require lymph node dissections for prostate cancer. *Br J Urol* 78:419-425, 1996.

Ross JS, Sheehan CE, Ambros RA, et al. Needle biopsy DNA ploidy status predicts grade shifting in prostate cancer. *Am J Surg Pathol* 23:296-301, 1999.

Ross PL, Scardino PT, Kattan MW. A catalog of prostate cancer nomograms. *J Urol* 165:1562-1568, 2001.

Rubin MA, de La Taille A, Bagiella E, et al. Cribriform carcinoma of the prostate and cribriform prostatic intraepithelial neoplasia: Incidence and clinical implications. *Am J Surg Pathol* 22:840-848, 1998.

Rubin MA, Dunn R, Kambham N, et al. Should a Gleason score be assigned to a minute focus of carcinoma on prostate biopsy? *Am J Surg Pathol* 24:1634-1640, 2000.

Rubin MA, Mucci NR, Manley S, et al. Predictors of Gleason pattern 4/5 prostate cancer on prostatectomy specimens. Can high grade tumor be predicted preoperatively? *J Urol* 165:114-118, 2001.

Ruijter ET, van de Kaa CA, Schalken JA, et al. Histological grade heterogeneity in multifocal prostate cancer. Biological and clinical implications. *J Pathol* 180:295-299, 1996.

Russell KJ, Dunatov C, Hafermann MD, et al. Prostate specific antigen in the management of patients with localized adenocarcinoma of the prostate treated with primary radiation therapy. *J Urol* 146:1046-1052, 1991.

Rydh A, Tomic R, Tavelin B, et al. Predictive value of prostate-specific antigen, tumor stage, and tumor grade for the outcome of bone scintigraphy in patients with newly diagnosed prostate cancer. *Scand J Urol Nephrol* 33:89-93, 1999.

Sagalowsky AI, Milam H, Reveley LR, et al. Prediction of lymphatic metastases by Gleason histologic grading in prostatic cancer. *J Urol* 128:951-952, 1982.

Sakr WA, Tefilli MV, Grignon DJ, et al. Gleason score 7 prostate cancer: a heterogeneous entity? Correlation with pathologic parameters and disease-free survival. *Urology* 56:730-734, 2000.

Salomao DR, Graham SD, Bostwick DG. Microvascular invasion in prostate cancer correlates with pathologic stage. *Arch Pathol Lab Med* 119:1050-1054, 1995.

Sandblom G, Dufmats M, Varenhorst E. Long-term survival in a Swedish population-based cohort of men with prostate cancer. *Urology* 56:442-447, 2000.

Sands ME, Zagars GK, Pollack A, et al. Serum prostate-specific antigen, clinical stage, pathological grade, and the incidence of nodal metastases in prostate cancer. *Urology* 44:215-220, 1994.

San Francisco IF, DeWolf WC, Rosen S, et al. Extended prostate needle biopsy improves concordance of Gleason grading between prostate needle biopsy and radical prostatectomy. *J Urol* 169:136-140, 2003.

Schroeder FH, Blom JH, Hop WC, et al. Grading of prostatic cancer (1): an analysis of the prognostic significance of single characteristics. *Prostate* 6:81-100, 1985A.

Schroeder FH, Blom JHM, Hop WCJ, et al. Grading of prostatic cancer: II. The prognostic significance of the presence of multiple architectural patterns. *Prostate* 6:403-415, 1985B.

Schroeder FH, Hop WCJ, Blom JHM, et al. Grading of prostatic cancer. III. Multivariate analysis of prognostic parameters. *Prostate* 7:13-20, 1985C.

Schwartz CB, Bekirov H, Melman A. Gleason's histologic grading as clinical prognostic marker in patients with advanced prostatic carcinoma. *Urology* 37:198-201, 1991.

Scott R Jr., Mutchnik DL, Laskowski TZ, et al. Carcinoma of the prostate in elderly men: incidence, growth characteristics and clinical significance. *J Urol* 101:602-607, 1969.

Sgrignoli AR, Walsh PC, Steinberg GD, et al. Prognostic factors in men with stage D1 prostate cancer: identification of patients less likely to have prolonged survival after radical prostatectomy. *J Urol* 152:1077-1081, 1994.

Sheldon CA, Williams RD, Fraley EE. Incidental carcinoma of the prostate: a review of the literature and critical reappraisal of classification. *J Urol* 124:626-631, 1980.

Shelley HS, Auerbach SH, Classen HL, et al. Carcinoma of the prostate. A new system of classification. *Arch Surg* 77:751-756, 1958.

Shih WJ, Mitchell B, Wierzbinski B, et al. Prediction of radionuclide bone imaging findings by Gleason histologic grading of prostate carcinoma. *Clin Nucl Med* 16:763-766, 1991.

Siders DB, Lee F. Histologic changes of irradiated prostatic carcinoma diagnosed by transrectal ultrasound. *Hum Pathol* 23:344-351, 1992.

Siders DB, Lee F, Mayman DM. Diagnosis of prostate cancer altered by ionizing radiation with and without neoadjuvant antiandrogen hormonal ablation. In: Foster CS, Bostwick DG, eds. *Pathology of the Prostate.* Philadelphia: WB Saunders; 315-326, 1998.

Singh D, Febbo PG, Ross K, et al. Gene expression correlates of clinical prostate cancer behavior. *Cancer Cell* 1:203-209, 2002.

Skacel M, Ormsby AH, Abrahams N, et al. The relative amount of Gleason pattern (GP) 4 tumor and surgical margin status are independent prognostic factors in Gleason score (GS)7 prostate carcinoma (PCa) treated by radical prostatectomy (abstract). *Mod Pathol* 13:108A, 2000.

Southwick PC, Catalona WJ, Partin AW, et al. Prediction of post-radical prostatectomy outcome for stage T1c prostate cancer with percent free prostate specific antigen: a prospective multicenter clinical trial. *J Urol* 162:1346-1351, 1999.

Spires SE, Cibull ML, Wood DP Jr., et al. Gleason histologic grading in prostatic carcinoma. Correlation of 18-gauge core biopsy with prostatectomy. *Arch Pathol Lab Med* 118:705-708, 1994.

Srigley JR, Amin MB, Bostwick DG, et al., for Members of the Cancer Committee, College of American Pathologists. Updated protocol for the examination of specimens from patients with carcinoma of the prostate gland. *Arch Pathol Lab Med* 124:1034-1039, 2000.

Stamey TA, McNeal JE, Freiha FS, et al. Morphometric and clinical studies on 68 consecutive radical prostatectomies. *J Urol* 139:1235-1241, 1988.

Stamey TA. DNA ploidy status. *Urology* 45:563-565, 1995A.

Stamey TA. Making the most out of six systematic sextant biopsies. *Urology* 45:2-12, 1995B.

Stamey TA, Sözen TS, Yemoto CM, et al. Classification of localized untreated prostate cancer based on 791 men treated only with radical prostatectomy: common ground for therapeutic trials and TNM subgroups. *J Urol* 159:2009-2012, 1998.

Stamey TA, McNeal JE, Yemoto CM, et al. Biological determinants of cancer progression in men with prostate cancer. *JAMA* 281:1395-1400, 1999.

Stamey TA, Yemoto CM, McNeal JE, et al. Prostate cancer is highly predictable: a prognostic equation based on all morphological variables in radical prostatectomy specimens. *J Urol* 163:1155-1160, 2000.

Steinberg DM, Sauvageot J, Piantadosi S, et al. Correlation of prostate needle biopsy and radical prostatectomy Gleason grade in academic and community settings. *Am J Surg Pathol* 21:566-576, 1997.

Stock RG, Stone NN. The effect of prognostic factors on therapeutic outcome following transperineal prostate brachytherapy. *Semin Surg Oncol* 13:454-460, 1997.

Svanholm H, Mygind H. Prostatic carcinoma. Reproducibility of histologic grading. *Acta Pathol Microbiol Immunol Scand* 93:67-71, 1985.

Sweat SD, Bergstralh EJ, Slezak J, et al. Competing risk analysis after radical prostatectomy for clinically nonmetastatic prostate adenocarcinoma according to clinical Gleason score and patient age. *J Urol* 168:525-529, 2002.

Tannenbaum M, Tannenbaum S, DeSanctis PN, et al. Prognostic significance of nucleolar surface area in prostate cancer. *Urology* 19:546-551, 1982.

Tefilli MV, Gheiler EL, Tiguert R, et al. Prognostic indicators in patients with seminal vesicle involvement following radical prostatectomy for clinically localized prostate cancer. *J Urol* 160:802-806, 1998.

Tefilli MV, Gheiler EL, Tiguert R, et al. Should Gleason score 7 prostate cancer be considered a unique grade category? *Urology* 53:372-377, 1999.

Ten Kate FJN, Gallee MPW, Schmitz PIM, et al. Problems in the grading of prostatic carcinoma: interobserver reproducibility of five different grading systems. *World J Urol* 4:147-152, 1986.

Tetu B, Srigley JR, Boivin JC, et al. Effect of combination endocrine therapy (LHRH agonist and flutamide) on normal prostate and prostatic adenocarcinoma. *Am J Surg Pathol* 15:111-120, 1991.

Thickman D, Speers WC, Philpott PJ, et al. Effect of the number of core biopsies of the prostate on predicting Gleason score of prostate cancer. *J Urol* 156:110-113, 1996.

Thompson IM, Zeidman EJ. Extended follow-up of stage A1 carcinoma of prostate. *Urology* 33:455-458, 1989.

Thorson P, Vollmer RT, Arcangeli C, et al. Minimal carcinoma in prostate needle biopsy specimens: diagnostic features and radical prostatectomy follow-up. *Mod Pathol* 11:543-551, 1998.

Tran TA, Jennings TA, Ross JS, et al. Pseudomyxoma ovariilike post-therapeutic alteration in prostatic adenocarcinoma. A distinctive pattern in patients receiving neoadjuvant androgen ablation therapy. *Am J Surg Pathol* 22:347-354, 1998.

True LD. Surgical pathology examination of the prostate gland. Practice survey by American Society of Clinical Pathologists. *Am J Clin Pathol* 102:572-579, 1994.

Uchida T, Go M, Nakajo H, et al. Correlation between histological grading and the prognosis of prostatic carcinoma — a comparative study of the Japanese General Rules of Prostatic Cancer (JGRPC) and Gleason's classification [in Japanese]. *Acta Urol Jpn* 34:116-122, 1988.

Utz DC, Farrow GM. Pathologic differentiation and prognosis of prostatic carcinoma. Results 15 years after radical excision. *JAMA* 209:1701-1703, 1969.

Vaillancourt L, Tetu B, Fradet Y, et al. Effect of neoadjuvant endocrine therapy (combined androgen blockade) on normal prostate and prostatic carcinoma. A randomized study. *Am J Surg Pathol* 20:86-93, 1996.

Van de Voorde WM, Elgamal AA, Van Poppel HP, et al. Morphologic and immunohistochemical changes in prostate cancer after preoperative hormonal therapy. A comparative study of radical prostatectomies. *Cancer* 74:3164-3175, 1994.

Van den Ouden D, Hop WCJ, Kranse R, et al. Tumour control according to pathological variables in patients treated by radical prostatectomy for clinically localized carcinoma of the prostate. *Br J Urol* 79:203-211, 1997.

Van der Poel HG, Schaafsma HE, Vooijs GP, et al. Quantitative light microscopy in urological oncology. *J Urol* 148:1-13, 1992.

Van der Poel HG, Oosterhof GON, Schaafsma HE, et al. Intratumoral nuclear morphologic heterogeneity in prostate cancer. *Urology* 49:652-657, 1997.

Vargas SO, Jiroutek M, Welch WR, et al. Perineural invasion in prostate needle biopsy specimens. Correlation with extraprostatic extension at resection. *Am J Clin Pathol* 111:223-228, 1999.

Vickery AL Jr, Kerr WS Jr. Carcinoma of the prostate treated by radical prostatectomy. A clinicopathological survey of 187 cases followed for 5 years and 148 cases followed for 10 years. *Cancer* 16:1598-1608, 1963.

Vis AN, Hoedemaeker RF, van der Kwast TH, et al. Defining the window of opportunity in screening for prostate cancer: validation of a predictive tumor classification model. *Prostate* 46:154-162, 2001.

Voges GE, Mottrie AM, Stöckle M, et al. Hormone therapy prior to radical prostatectomy in patients with clinical stage C prostate cancer. Prostate 5(suppl):4-8, 1994.

Vollmer RT, Keetch DW, Humphrey PA. Predicting the pathology results of radical prostatectomy from preoperative information. A validation study. *Cancer* 83:1567-1580, 1998.

Waaler G, Nilssen MO. Prognostic factors in disseminated prostatic cancer, with special emphasis on extent of disease. *Urol Int* 53:130-134, 1994.

Wang Q, Lin CS, Unger PD. Squamous cell carcinoma arising in hormonally treated adenocarcinoma of the prostate. *Int J Surg Pathol* 4:13-16, 1996.

Watson RB, Civantos F, Soloway MS. Positive surgical margins with radical prostatectomy: detailed pathological analysis and prognosis. *Urology* 48:80-90, 1996.

Weldon VE, Tavel FR, Neuwirth H, et al. Patterns of positive specimen margins and detectable prostate specific antigen after radical perineal prostatectomy. *J Urol* 153:1565-1569, 1995.

Wenderoth UK, Gerlach B, Köppen A, et al. Computerized nuclear morphometry: prognostic value for carcinoma of the prostate and renal cell carcinoma. *Investig Urol* 5:16-19, 1994.

Wheeler JA, Zagars GK, Ayala AG. Dedifferentiation of locally recurrent prostate cancer after radiation therapy. Evidence for tumor progression. *Cancer* 71:3783-3787, 1993.

WHO (World Health Organization). *International Histological Classification of Tumours No. 10. Histological Typing of Urinary Bladder Tumours.* Geneva: World Health Organization, 1973.

WHO: *World Health Organization Classification of Tumours: Tumours of the Urinary System and Male Genital Organs.* Lyon, France: IARC Press; in press, 2003.

Wills ML, Sauvageot J, Partin AW, et al. Ability of sextant biopsies to predict radical prostatectomy stage. *Urology* 51:759-764, 1998.

Wolf JS Jr, Shinohara K, Carroll PR, et al. Combined role of transrectal ultrasonography, Gleason score, and prostate-specific antigen in predicting organ-confined prostate cancer. *Urology* 42:131-137 1993.

Yang XJ, Lecksell K, Short K, et al. Does long-term finasteride therapy affect the histologic features of benign prostatic tissue and prostate cancer on needle biopsy? PLESS Study Group. Proscar long-term efficacy and safety study. *Urology* 53:696-700, 1999.

Young HH, Davis DM. *Young's Practice of Urology.* Philadelphia: Saunders, 1926.

Zagars GK, Ayala AG, von Eschenbach AC, et al. The prognostic importance of Gleason grade in prostatic adenocarcinoma: a long-term follow-up study of 648 patients treated with radiation therapy. *Int J Radiat Oncol Biol Phys* 31:237-245, 1995.

Zhang YH, Kanamaru H, Oyama N, et al. Comparison of nuclear morphometric results between needle biopsy and surgical specimens from patients with prostate cancer. *Urology* 54:763-766, 1999.

Zhang YH, Kanamaru H, Oyama N, et al. Prognostic value of nuclear morphometry on needle biopsy from patients with prostate cancer: is volume-weighted mean nuclear volume superior to other morphometric parameters? *Urology* 55:377-381, 2000.

Zhou M, Hayasaka S, Taylor JMG, et al. Lack of association of prostate carcinoma nuclear grade with prostate specific antigen recurrence after radical prostatectomy. *J Urol* 166:2193-2197, 2001.

Zietman AL, Edelstein RA, Coen JJ, et al. Radical prostatectomy for adenocarcinoma of the prostate: the influence of preoperative and pathologic findings on biochemical disease-free outcome. *Urology* 43:828-833, 1994.

Zietman AL, Thakral H, Wilson L, et al. Conservative management of prostate cancer in the prostate specific antigen era: the incidence and time course of subsequent therapy. *J Urol* 166:1702-1706, 2001.

Zincke H, Utz DC. Observations in surgical management of carcinoma of prostate with limited nodal metastases. *Urology* 24:137-145, 1984.

Staging of Prostatic Carcinoma

[16.1] TNM AJCC/UICC Staging Classification **377**

[16.2] Clinical Staging **378**

[16.3] Pathologic TNM Staging **379**

[16.4] Pretreatment Models of Pathologic Stage **381**

[16.5] Stage Relationships with Pathologic Findings **382**

[16.6] Stage and Patient Outcome **382**

[16.7] Experimental Staging Procedures **384**

[16.8] Reporting of Pathologic Stage **385**

CHAPTER 16

S*tage* has been defined as "a definite period in the development of a disease, marked by specific symptoms" (Stage 1993). For prostatic carcinoma, symptoms are not used to determine the stage of the cancer; rather, it is anatomic extent of prostate cancer that determines its stage. Determination of extent of prostate cancer stage is important for evaluating prognosis and selecting therapy **t16.1** (Carter 2002, Montie 2000).

In 1956, the first clinical staging scheme for prostatic carcinoma was devised by Whitmore **t16.2** (Whitmore 1956). This 4-tiered staging design formed the foundation for currently used stage groups. In 1975 a modification, the Whitmore-Jewett system, was introduced (Jewett 1975). This 4-tiered A to D stage grouping was widely used for the next several decades **t16.3**. During that time, there was a movement to adopt a TNM (T = primary tumor, N = regional lymph nodes, M = distant metastases) form of anatomic staging. In 2002, the sixth and most recent TNM staging system was adopted by the American Joint Committee on Cancer (AJCC) and the International Union Against Cancer (UICC) (Greene 2002). This latest 2002 TNM staging system is the one most widely used in clinical practice, clinical trials, and the medical literature.

■ t16.1 Staging of Prostate Cancer

Stage = anatomic extent of cancer
Stage is related to prognosis and treatment selection
2002 TNM system most widely used
Distinguish between clinical and pathologic staging

■ t16.2 1956 Whitmore Clinical Staging Scheme for Prostate Cancer

I. Clinically latent prostate cancer
II. Clinically manifest early prostate cancer
III. Clinically manifest locally advanced prostate cancer
IV. Clinically manifest advanced prostate cancer with evidence of distant metastases

From Whitmore 1956

■ t16.3 Whitmore-Jewett 1975 Staging Scheme

Stage	A	Tumor not clinically manifest but found microscopically within surgically removed obstructing tissue
	A1	Focal
	A2	Diffuse
Stage	B	Clinically manifest tumor without metastasis but palpably localized to the prostate
	B1	Less than one lobe involved
	B2	One lobe or more involved
Stage	C	Locally extensive beyond the prostate but without metastasis
Stage	D	Metastases

From Jewett 1975

[16.1] TNM AJCC/UICC Staging Classification

The 2002 TNM clinical and pathologic staging schemes are given in **t16.4**. This staging scheme applies only to adenocarcinomas of the prostate, not to sarcomas and prostatic carcinoma variants.

■ t16.4 2002 TNM Staging Scheme

Primary Tumor, Clinical (T)

TX	Primary tumor cannot be assessed
T0	No evidence of primary tumor
T1	Clinically inapparent tumor not palpable nor visible by imaging
T1a	Tumor incidental histologic finding in 5% or less of tissue resected
T1b	Tumor incidental histologic finding in more than 5% tissue resected
T1c	Tumor identified by needle biopsy (eg, because of elevated PSA)
T2	Tumor confined within prostate[1]
T2a	Tumor involves one half of one lobe or less
T2b	Tumor involves more than one half of one lobe but not both lobes
T2c	Tumor involves both lobes
T3	Tumor extends through the prostate capsule[2]
T3a	Extracapsular extension (unilateral or bilateral)
T3b	Tumor invades seminal vesicle(s)
T4	Tumor is fixed or invades adjacent structures other than seminal vesicles: bladder neck, external sphincter, rectum, levator muscles, and/or pelvic wall
[1]Note:	Tumor found in one or both lobes by needle biopsy, but not palpable or reliably visible by imaging, is classified as T1c
[2]Note:	Invasion into the prostatic apex or into (but not beyond) the prostatic capsule is not classified as T3, but as T2

Primary Tumor, Pathologic (pT)

pT2[3]	Organ confined
pT2a	Unilateral, involving one half of one lobe or less
pT2b	Unilateral, involving more than one half of one lobe but not both lobes
pT2c	Bilateral
pT3	Extraprostatic extension
pT3a	Extraprostatic extension
pT3b	Seminal vesicle invasion
pT4	Invasion of bladder, rectum
[3]Note:	There is no pathologic T1 classification
[4]Note:	Positive surgical margin should be indicated by an R1 descriptor (residual microscopic disease)

Regional Lymph Nodes (N)

NX	Regional lymph nodes cannot be assessed
N0	No regional lymph node metastasis
N1	Metastasis in regional lymph node or nodes

Distant Metastasis[5] (M)

MX	Distant metastasis cannot be assessed
M0	No distant metastasis
M1	Distant metastasis
M1a	Nonregional lymph node(s)
M1b	Bone(s)
M1c	Other site(s)
[5]Note:	When more than one site of metastasis is present, the most advanced category is used. pM1c is most advanced

Stage Grouping

Stage I	T1a	N0	M0	G1 (Gleason score 2-4)
Stage II	T1a	N0	M0	G2,3-4 (Gleason score 5-10)
	T1b	N0	M0	Any G
	T1c	N0	M0	Any G
	T1	N0	M0	Any G
	T2	N0	M0	Any G
Stage III	T3	N0	M0	Any G
Stage IV	T4	N0	M0	Any G
	Any T	N1	M0	Any G
	Any T	Any N	M1	Any G

From Greene 2002

The 2002 TNM scheme (Greene 2002) differs from the 1997 TNM scheme (Fleming 1997) in that the 2002 scheme once again (as in the 1992 scheme) divides T2 disease into T2a, T2b, and T2c subcategories. The 1997 TNM scheme had been criticized for changing the T2 subclassification into T2a and T2b, compared with the 1992 TNM subgroupings of T2a, T2b, and T2c. Evidence does exist that, based on the 1992 TNM definitions, T2a cancer is pathologically and clinically different from T2b cancer (Han 2000, Iyer 1999, Stamey 1998).

[16.2] Clinical Staging

Clinical staging commences after a histologic diagnosis of prostatic carcinoma is established. The modalities most commonly used to assess prostate carcinoma extent include digital rectal examination (DRE), radiologic imaging, serum tumor markers (usually serum total prostate-specific antigen [PSA] and sometimes serum prostatic acid phosphatase [PAP]), histologic grading, and surgical lymphadenectomy (Carter 1998, Gee 1998, Montie 2000, O'Dowd 1997) **t16.5**.

DRE is routinely used to evaluate local extent or clinical T stage of prostate cancer, particularly in determining whether the cancer is organ confined (T2) or not (T3 or T4). However, the DRE is subjective and is fraught with high interexaminer variability (Philips 1991, Varenhorst 1993, Smith 1995). Moreover, clinical staging by DRE is inaccurate in defining true pathologic stage. Although both understaging and overstaging occur, the most common difficulty is the inability of the DRE to detect pathologic stage T3 disease. Indeed, in a recent review of 17 studies of 12 984 prostate cancers that were deemed clinically organ confined, 48% were pathologically not organ confined, based on examination of radical prostatectomy slides (O'Dowd 1997). Even when the prostatic carcinoma is not palpable (in T1c disease), carcinoma extends outside the gland in 30% to 49% of cases (Humphrey 1996). DRE is more accurate when the carcinoma is judged to be outside the prostate gland (T3) by palpation. When the carcinoma was felt to be clinically extraprostatic, it was extraprostatic in 70% to 93% of cases by histopathologic assessment of radical prostatectomy specimens (O'Dowd 1997, Ohori 1994B, Partin 1993, Schroeder 1975).

Radiologic imaging approaches, including intravenous urography, transrectal ultrasound (TRUS), computed tomography (CT), magnetic resonance imaging (MRI), and bone scintigraphy (radionuclide bone scan) have all been used in attempts at clinical staging (Carter 1998, Montie 2000, O'Dowd 1997). Bone scan is the most commonly ordered imaging test in staging of newly diagnosed prostate cancer, being requested by urologists in 48% of cases of newly diagnosed prostate cancer (Gee 1998). In comparison, CT scans were ordered in 21% of cases and MRI scans in 1% to 3% of cases (Gee 1998). Intravenous urography, TRUS, CT, and MRI do not demonstrate sufficient accuracy for routinely predicting pathologic stage (O'Dowd 1997), particularly local T stage. In prediction of organ-confined carcinoma, TRUS exhibited 58% accuracy (Rifkin 1990), body coil MRI was 69% accurate (Rifkin 1990), and endorectal coil MRI was 52% accurate (Tempany 1994). CT was of similar sensitivity and specificity in this prediction (Hricak 1987, Platt 1987). CT and MRI also are not routinely used for staging pelvic lymph nodes because they have a low sensitivity (on the order of 35%) in detecting pathologically proven lymph node metastases (O'Dowd 1997). CT assessment of pelvic lymph node status may be warranted in select cases, where the patient is at high risk for nodal metastases (locally advanced cancer by DRE, PSA greater than 20 ng/mL, or Gleason score 8 to 10 on needle biopsy) (Carter 1998, Montie 2000). In such cases, fine needle aspiration biopsy or laparoscopic lymphadenectomy can be used to confirm metastatic disease in nodes that appear positive by CT scan (Carter 1998, Van Poppel 1993). Bone scintigraphy (radionuclide bone scan) is commonly used to evaluate for metastatic spread to bone (stage M1b) **i13.10**, p 241. The likelihood of a positive scan is directly related to the serum PSA level, with a positive scan in asymptomatic patients being rare when the PSA is less than 10 ng/mL (Chybowski 1991, Lee 1997). Still, some urologists obtain a bone scan in all newly diagnosed patients as part of the initial staging workup in order to have a baseline scan.

Tumor marker levels—that is, serum PSA and PAP levels—are directly related to clinical stage (Hudson 1989, Polascik 1999), but there is overlap in levels between stages such that total serum PSA levels do not provide accurate clinical staging information for the individual patient (Hudson 1989, Polascik 1999). Serum PSA contributes to only 1 formal staging category: clinical stage T1c. This is defined as clinically inapparent tumor not palpable by DRE or visible by imaging and detected by needle biopsy performed solely because of an elevated serum PSA level **t16.4.**

Histologic grade of carcinoma has been used to distinguish between clinical stage T1a and T1b carcinoma but is only used in the 2002 TNM staging scheme to separate Stage I T1a from Stage II T1a **t16.4**. The formal distinction between T1a and T1b tumor, which is carcinoma incidentally detected in transurethral resection chips or open (enucleation) prostatectomy specimens, is tumor in 5% or less of tissue (T1a) or in more than 5% of tissue resected (T1b). Most studies allow only low-grade carcinoma in clinical stage T1a disease (Humphrey 1993A), but the Gleason grade in T1a disease has varied, with use of Gleason score 2 to 4 (Zhang 1991), 2 to 6 (Voges 1992), 2 to 7 (Epstein 1986, Cheng 1999), or 2 to 10 (Partin 1997). Given the deleterious prognostic effect of high-grade elements, any high-grade carcinoma with Gleason pattern 4 or 5 (or score 7 to 10) of any extent should be considered T1b disease.

Extraprostatic tissue sampling, including seminal vesicle biopsy, pelvic lymph node biopsy or excision, and biopsy or excision of distant metastatic deposits, can be used for clinical staging. Local T staging by periprostatic soft tissue (Lee 1998, Okihara 2002) or seminal vesicle biopsy (Allepuz Losa 1995, O'Dowd 1997, Okihara 2002, Pandey 1995, Stone 1998, Terris 1993, 1997, Vallancien 1994), has been attempted

t16.5 Staging of Prostate Cancer

- Methods: DRE, radiologic imaging, serum PSA and PSAP, histologic grade, and extraprostatic tissue sampling
- DRE used to determine local primary T stage but is often inaccurate, with understaging common, being seen in about ½ of all cases
- Radiologic staging tools most often used include bone scan (in about one-half of cases) and CT scan (in about 20% of cases). Radiologic modalities of TRUS, MRI, CT, are too inaccurate for routine use in T and N staging
- Serum PSA elevation used to define clinical stage T1c
- Histologic grade not formally included in clinical TNM staging definitions, but it is used to separate T1a stage I vs stage II, and by many to distinguish stage T1a vs T1b cancer
- Extraprostatic tissue sampling such as seminal vesicle biopsy, pelvic lymph node biopsy/excision, and biopsy of distant metastatic deposit can be used for clinical staging

■ **t16.6 Seminal Vesicle Biopsy in Clinical Staging**

Not routinely done since it is low yield, with low sensitivity
A caution: Microscopically, seminal vesicle tissue my be difficult to distinguish from ejaculatory duct tissue in small needle biopsies
May be indicated in high-risk patients (T2b or higher, PSA greater than 10-15 ng/mL) if this biopsy result will change therapy

t16.6. However, the usefulness of seminal vesicle biopsy in clinical staging is limited by the low percentage of patients with seminal vesicle invasion in clinically localized disease. In this current era, only about 4% of patients who undergo radical prostatectomy have positive seminal vesicles (stage T3b disease) (Partin 2001). The incidence of directed, positive seminal vesicle biopsies in 161 men with a median PSA of 17 was 3.7% (Terris 1997); it is likely that the true incidence is even lower because most men who undergo biopsy have a PSA between 4 and 10 ng/mL. In the presence of already-diagnosed prostatic carcinoma, the incidence of directed, positive seminal vesicle biopsies in 5 recent series with a total of 517 men was 19% (Allepuz Losa 1995, Stone 1998, Terris 1993, 1997, Vallancien 1994). Another important mitigating factor is the high false-negative biopsy rate due to sampling error. That is, in a high percentage of cases (40%), a needle biopsy of seminal vesicle is negative when the patient actually has carcinoma in the seminal vesicle (Vallancien 1994). A final problem is that in small biopsies seminal vesicle tissue can be difficult to distinguish from ejaculatory duct tissue, which is intraprostatic and has an epithelial lining identical to that of the seminal vesicle. Seminal vesicle biopsy therefore should not typically be a part of routine pretreatment staging of patients with newly diagnosed prostatic carcinoma (Pandey 1995, Terris 1997). Seminal vesicle biopsies have been recommended when detection of seminal vesicle invasion would change clinical treatment (Terris 1997), particularly for high-risk patients with PSAs more than 10 ng/mL, DRE stage of T2b or greater, and palpably or sonographically abnormal seminal vesicles (O'Dowd 1997, Terris 1997). Prostatic carcinoma can be uncommonly seen in inadvertently sampled periprostatic adipose tissue in prostate needle biopsy, but needle biopsy directed specifically at periprostatic soft tissue is rarely done. Needle biopsy sampling of periprostatic soft tissue, like seminal vesicle sampling, usually is not done intentionally as a clinical staging maneuver.

Pelvic lymph node sampling to clinically stage newly diagnosed prostate cancer is performed in a minority of patients, with one third of patients undergoing an open lymph node dissection and only 2% of patients undergoing a laparoscopic pelvic lymph node dissection (Gee 1998) **t16.7**. A third option for detecting nodal metastases is imaging-guided fine needle aspiration biopsy (O'Dowd 1997). A limitation of this last approach is the 70% sensitivity (O'Dowd 1997).

■ **t16.7 Pelvic Lymph Node Sampling in Clinical Staging**

Can be done by open dissection, laparoscopic sampling, and imaging-guided fine needle aspiration biopsy.
Current incidence of positive nodes in clinically localized prostatic carcinoma: 2%
Routinely done as part of radical prostatectomy operation
Pretreatment decision to sample laparoscopically, at frozen section or at all, may be driven by T stage, PSA level, and needle biopsy Gleason grade of carcinoma

The current incidence of histologically diagnosed prostatic carcinoma in pelvic lymph nodes is only about 2% (Partin 2002). Therefore, it has been recommended that the indication for laparoscopic lymph node dissection or open pelvic lymph node dissection with frozen section should be high-risk disease, defined as a serum PSA greater than 20 ng/mL, Gleason score 8 to 10 carcinoma in needle biopsy, 5 or more positive cores, clinical T stage T3 or T4, positive seminal vesicle biopsy, or enlarged pelvic lymph nodes by imaging (Carter 1998, O'Dowd 1997). Indeed, because of the low yield rate, some urologists have stopped requesting frozen section of the pelvic lymph nodes before performing the radical prostatectomy and instead submit the lymph nodes in formalin for routine sections. Some have suggested that pelvic lymph node dissection at the time of radical prostatectomy is unnecessary for men at low risk of harboring nodal metastatic carcinoma, based on preoperative T stage, serum PSA, and tumor grade (Bluestein 1994, Kerbl 1993, Narayan 1994). A number of models have been generated in attempts to predict lymph node metastasis **t2.11**, p 45, and these can help the physician decide whether to sample pelvic lymph nodes before treatment or intraoperatively for frozen section or for routine sections. The most widely used model is the Partin tables (Partin 1997). (These tables are available on the Web at http://urology.jhu.edu/Partin_tables/index.html (as of January 2003) and are also available on handheld computers, in which one can enter pretreatment serum PSA level, biopsy Gleason grade, and clinical T stage and generate risk of lymph node metastasis, with 95% confidence intervals.) None of these models is 100% accurate, and histologic detection of nodal metastases remains the gold standard for the "N" category of clinical staging.

Limitations of clinical staging by the TNM system do exist. They relate mainly to the inaccuracy of clinical staging relative to pathologic staging. They include clinical understaging with transurethral resection and by DRE, the limited ability of radiologic imaging studies to define the extent of prostatic carcinoma, and heterogeneity of clinical stage T1c adenocarcinoma (Bostwick 1997). Transurethrally detected incidental prostatic carcinoma is deemed low-stage T1a or T1b, yet when radical prostatectomy is done after the transurethral resection, pathologic T3 or even N disease is found in a substantial minority of patients **t14.30.** Because pathologic T3 disease often is microscopic, it is not surprising that DRE and radiologic imaging studies are inaccurate. Finally, within the clinical staging subgroups, pathologic and clinical outcome heterogeneity exists. For example, the homogenous clinical stage T1c cancers are pathologically heterogeneous, ranging from minute organ-confined pathologic T2a (pT2a) cancers to large, bulky, high-grade carcinoma, with extraprostatic extension of cancer (pT3) (Humphrey 1998). Also, clinical outcome for patients within clinical stage T2 is variable. In a study of 1314 men clinically staged as T2c, 71% experienced biochemical progression-free survival at 10 years after surgery (Han 2000). It is preferable that clinical stages predict a uniform response to specific therapies. Nevertheless, clinical TNM staging is still critically important for predicting patient prognosis and selecting appropriate therapy.

[16.3] Pathologic TNM Staging

Pathologic T staging generally entails histologic examination of radical prostatectomy tissues, including the prostate gland and

■ **t16.8 Pathologic TNM Staging of Prostatic Carcinoma**

Requires examination of radical prostatectomy specimens[1]
Primary tumor pathologic "T" stage: pT2-4 categories
No pathologic stage pT1 exists
pT4 rarely utilized
Regional node pathologic "N" stage: NX, N0, N1
Distant metastasis pathologic "M" stage: Often MX (cannot be assessed) or assume M0 (since patient undergoing radical prostatectomy should have been clinically staged as M0)

[1]Except for a biopsy with prostatic carcinoma in rectal tissue = pT4

seminal vesicles (Greene 2002, Grignon 1996) **t16.8**. Pathologic N staging is based on histologic examination of resected regional lymph nodes (Greene 2002). Pathologic M staging occurs with histologic diagnosis of prostatic carcinoma in nonregional lymph nodes, bone, or other distant metastatic sites. (Recommendations on reporting pathologic stage are provided in Chapter 14.)

Pathologic staging of the primary tumor, designated pT, differs from the clinical staging scheme in that there is no pT1 category corresponding to clinical T1 cancer, and pT4 carcinoma is defined as bladder or rectal invasion, compared with the broader clinical T4 definition of fixation or invasion of bladder neck, external sphincter, rectum, levator muscles, or pelvic wall (Greene 2002). Pathologic T2 and T3 definitions are identical to clinical definitions of anatomic extent **f16.1**.

Pathologic stage T2 disease (pT2) is organ-confined carcinoma, which is subdivided into pT2a (unilateral, involving one half of one lobe or less), pT2b (unilateral, involving more than one half of one lobe but not both lobes), and pT2c (bilateral) carcinoma. Needle biopsy findings may be incorporated into the final pathologic stage determination based on a radical prostatectomy specimen. For example, if carcinoma is identified only in radical prostatectomy sections from the right side, and needle biopsies from both the right and left sides were positive for carcinoma, then the final pT stage assignment would be pT2c rather than pT2a or pT2b.

A significant problem with the current T classification scheme is that there is no guidance for stage designation when there is surgical incision into the gland, with carcinoma at the margin, such that it is not possible to determine whether the tumor is pT2 or pT3 **f16.2**. These cases, which have been characterized as capsule incision positive and margin positive, iatrogenic, equivocal, and indeterminate (Wiedner 1998), should be distinguished from cases in which there is clear extraprostatic extension, with a positive margin. One proposal has been to consider such cases T2+ (Sakr 1996), although this is not part of the current TNM staging system. In these cases, one could describe the findings in the report and comment that the pT stage is indeterminate and could be either pT2 or pT3.

Pathologic stage T3 disease (pT3) is the histologically detected presence of carcinoma outside the prostate gland, in any tissue sample. This can be extraprostatic carcinoma in periprostatic soft tissue (pT3a) or seminal vesicle wall involvement by carcinoma (pT3b). (Diagnosis of this extraprostatic extension [EPE] by carcinoma is discussed in Chapter 14.) The current TNM scheme does not include a quantitative assessment of amount of extraprostatic disease, but it seems worthwhile to report anatomic sites of EPE **t14.39, t14.44, pp 306-307**, and whether the tumor is focal or

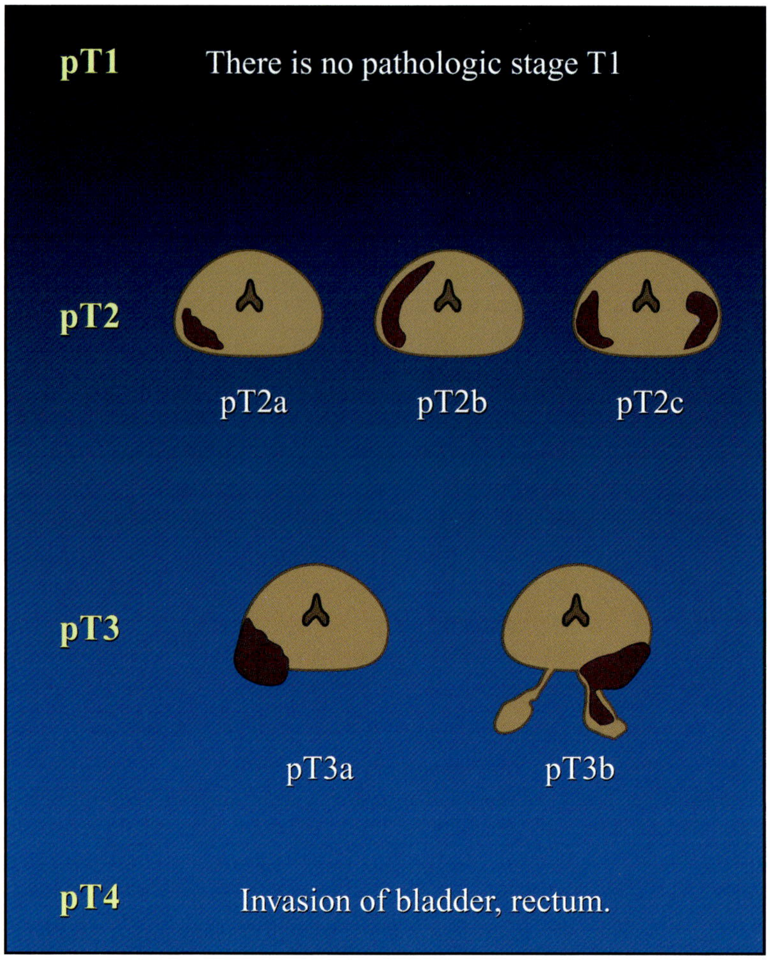

■ **f16.1** *Pathologic T stages in radical prostatectomy tissues:*
pT2a : Unilateral organ-confined carcinoma, involving one-half of one lobe or less
pT2b : Unilateral involving more than one-half of one lobe but not both lobes
pT2c : Bilateral organ-confined carcinoma
pT3a : Unilateral or bilateral extraprostatic extension
pT3b : Seminal vesicle wall invasion (unilateral or bilateral)

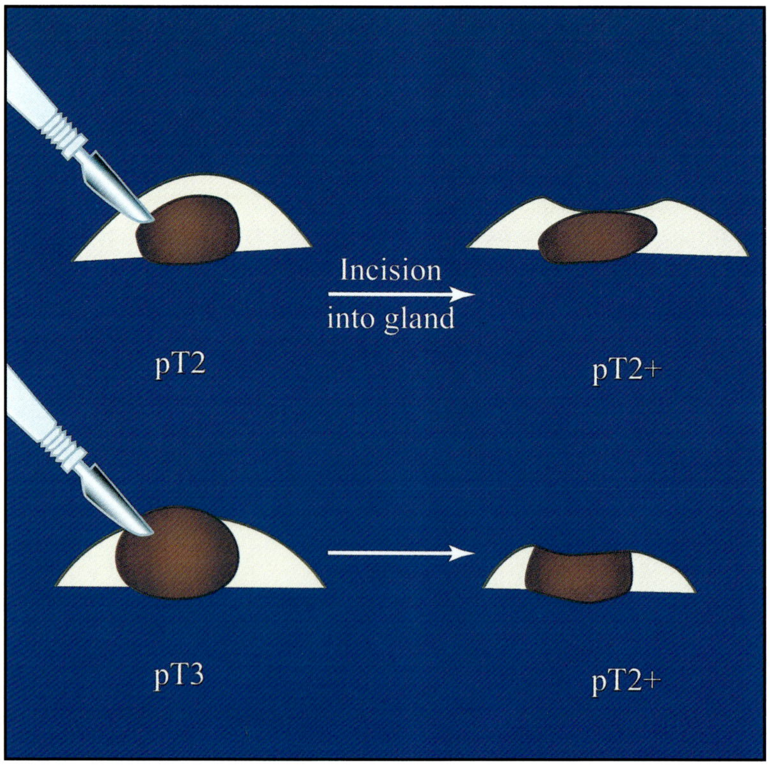

■ **f16.2** *Surgical incision can create stage pT2+ from either pT2 or pT3 disease. pT2+ is a proposed stage category where there is margin positivity, but no definitive histologic evidence of extraprostatic extension by carcinoma.*

nonfocal, extensive, or established (Bostwick 1999, Epstein 1993, Wheeler 1998). Focal EPE by carcinoma has been defined as a few neoplastic glands exterior to the prostate (Epstein 1993) or tumor outside the prostate that is equal to or less than 2 high-power (40×) microscopic fields (Bostwick 1999, Wheeler 1998). For T3b cancer, carcinoma should be identified in the smooth muscle wall of the one or both seminal vesicles. Carcinoma in soft tissue surrounding the seminal vesicle does not count as T3b carcinoma but rather is T3a carcinoma. Although it does not affect staging, seminal vesicle invasion should be specified or unilateral or bilateral. Beyond this, it is not necessary to quantitate the amount of tumor in the seminal vesicle or the pathway of spread into the seminal vesicle (Sakr 1996).

Pathologic pT4 stage should rarely, if ever, be an assignment in radical prostatectomy specimens. This is so because patients with gross clinical stage T4 lesions are not candidates for surgery (Sakr 1996). In certain radical prostatectomy cases it is possible to detect prostatic carcinoma infiltrating into the thick smooth muscle bundles of the bladder neck and carcinoma in the bladder neck margin. This latter finding was present in 2% to 19% of radical prostatectomy cases (Ackerman 1993, Blute 1997, Obek 1999, Ohori 1995, Shelfo 1998, Stamey 1990, Watson 1996). It is not established that microscopic bladder neck involvement by carcinoma warrants such a high stage appointment. Indeed, in a radical prostatectomy study in which 3% of cases had bladder neck involvement, the failure rate after surgery for this apparent pT4 disease was significantly less than that for pT3b carcinoma (Yossepowitch 2002). In another recent investigation, bladder neck involvement was associated with a risk of recurrence after surgery that was less than that of pT3b disease and not substantially different from that of pT3a cancer (Dash 2002). Clarification of pT4 carcinoma in radical prostatectomy tissue should be attempted in future TNM schemes. According to the *AJCC Cancer Staging Manual* (Greene 2002), it is clear that pT4 carcinoma can be diagnosed without radical prostatectomy in the case of a positive rectal biopsy.

Surgical margin status, tumor size (beyond unilateral or bilateral), and histologic grade do not affect the pathologic TNM stage designation. In the 2002 TNM scheme, it was recommended that a positive surgical margin be indicated by an R1 descriptor (residual microscopic disease) (Greene 2002). (However, it should be recognized that a positive margin does not always mean there is residual carcinoma left behind in the patient.) Some doctors and studies have equated a positive surgical margin with pT3 carcinoma (Lerner 1996, Ramos 1999), but this is not appropriate; surgical margin status should be reported independently of stage. Other factors that do not influence pathologic stage assignment include serum PSA level, presence of perineural invasion, presence of lymphvascular space invasion, multifocality of carcinoma, carcinoma location (transition vs peripheral zone), and histologic type of carcinoma.

Pathologic stage category is affected by the degree of sampling of the radical prostatectomy specimen. Partial embedding of prostatic tissue from radical prostatectomy specimens has been reported to miss 7% to 20% of cases of extraprostatic extension by carcinoma compared with complete embedding (Cohen 1994, Donohue 1991, Haggman 1993, Hall 1992, Sehdev 2001). A key question here is whether these cases of missed EPE translate into prognostic and therapeutic differences (Grossfeld 2000). This is not known with certainty. The most accurate and thorough pathologic pT staging would be complete embedding of the prostate gland and seminal vesicles, with serial sectioning through the blocks. Yet this takes thousands of slides per case (2678 for one prostate gland, to be precise [Humphrey 1993B]). Even complete embedding of all prostatic tissue, with a single hematoxylin and eosin section from each block, is not typical practice, being done in only 12% of hospitals nationwide (True 1994). Whole mount sections do not provide any advantage over partially sampled glands in detecting EPE or seminal invasion by carcinoma (Hollenbeck 2000). As for selecting a sampling protocol for radical prostatectomy specimens, each laboratory should make a decision based on cost-benefit considerations. (See Chapter 2 for a summary of available sampling protocols.)

In overview, current limitations of pathologic TNM staging include lack of incorporation of the prognostic indicators of tumor size, margin status, and amount of EPE by carcinoma into stage groups. The current pathologic TNM system is also limited by failure to account for T2+ tumors, lack of clarity on significance and severity for pT4 classification of bladder neck involvement by carcinoma, and the impact of variable radical prostatectomy sampling protocols on pT staging accuracy. Despite these difficulties, pathologic stage, as currently defined, is still one of the most powerful predictors of patient prognosis and response to therapy.

[16.4] Pretreatment Models of Pathologic Stage

Preoperative clinical and pathologic findings have been used in models to predict pathologic stage **t16.9**. The most popular of these, the so-called Partin tables uses clinical stage, preoperative serum PSA level, and needle biopsy or transurethral resection chip Gleason score to stratify patients in prediction of organ-confined (pT2) carcinoma, established capsular penetration (pT3a), seminal vesicle involvement (pT3b), and lymph node metastasis (pN1) in radical prostatectomy and pelvic lymph node tissues (Partin 1997, Partin 2001). Other models have used various combinations of clinical stage, histologic grade, serum PSA, serum prostatic acid phosphatase, amount of tumor in biopsy tissue, nuclear grade, DNA ploidy, transrectal ultrasound, PSA density, and percentage free PSA **t16.9.**

The power of the Partin tables resides in the large numbers of patients (4133 men), the multi-institutional nature of the study, the use of confidence intervals, and attempts to validate the model by the original group (Partin 1997) and others, using independent data sets (Blute 2000, Kattan 1997, Naitoh 1997, Vollmer 1998). Also, the tables are easy to use and are widely available in journal publications (Partin 1997, Partin 2001, Polascik 1998), in textbooks (Carter 2002), on handheld computers, and on the Web. Weaknesses of the Partin tables include the rather broad confidence intervals in some categories and difficulty in validation in some but not all independent data sets (Blute 2000, Kattan 1997, Naitoh 1997, Penson 2002, Vollmer 1998). Even in their own validation analysis, the nomograms did not predict the probability of pathologic stage to within 10% in a substantial minority (28%) of patients. Clearly, further refinement of the model (possibly with new serum markers or additional parameters such as amount of tumor in needle biopsy tissue) is desirable. Even so, the Partin tables are of substantial clinical value in counseling patients regarding the probability of their tumor being a specific pathologic stage and in rationally selecting patients for specific therapies based on their predicted pathologic stage.

■ t16.9 Pretreatment Models to Predict Pathologic T Stage

Study	Model	Comment
Oesterling 1987	Gleason grade and serum prostatic acid phosphatase or clinical stage used	Probability plots constructed to predict capsular penetration and seminal vesicle invasion
Partin 1993	Initial publication of probability plots in Partin Tables, using serum PSA, Gleason score, and clinical stage	Data used to generate nomograms for predicting final pathologic stage. A combination of all three variables was more accurate than any single variable alone
Wolf 1993	Algorithm for staging clinically localized prostate cancer using (in sequence) needle biopsy Gleason score, serum PSA, and transrectal ultrasound	Staging accuracy of 77% in predicting organ-confined disease
Kleer 1993	Probability plots generated from local clinical stage (determined by DRE), Mayo histologic grade, and serum PSA	Predicted probability curves for organ confined and extracapsular disease generated, but Gleason grading not used
Nishiya 1994	PSA density> 0.3 ng/mL/mL and Gleason score > 6	These patients had a high probability of having extraprostatic carcinoma
Narayan 1995	Biopsy-based stage (T2a vs T2b vs T3), serum PSA and Gleason score used	Probability plots made for 813 men; biopsy T3 stage not very useful: 3% of men were T3 on biopsy but 32% of men T3 in radical prostatectomy tissues
Badalament 1996	Quantitative nuclear grade, preop PSA, % tumor in needle cases, needle biopsy Gleason score, base and/or apex tumor involvement more than 5%, DNA ploidy all used	Actual model not published
Bostwick 1996	PSA and % cancer in needle biopsy tissue best for predicting capsular perforation and seminal vesicle invasion	PSA and Gleason score only slightly less predictive
Puppo 1997	Clinical stage, PSA, and Gleason grade used in probability plots	Useful in this population of 1,738 patients form 34 Italian urology departments
Partin 1997	Clinical stage, needle biopsy or TURP chip Gleason grade, and preop PSA	Most widely used model; based on 4,133 patients from 3 hospitals
Egawa 1998	Number of positive cores, maximum cancer length, PSA, clinical stage and biopsy Gleason score	Amount of tumor in needle biopsy significantly improved prediction of pT3 disease
Wills 1998	Biopsy Gleason score, number of involved cores, and bilaterality of positive cores	Best model to predict pathologic stage
Southwick 1999	% free PSA and biopsy Gleason score	% free PSA > 15 and Gleason score < 7: 87% of patients had pT2 disease
Fujikawa 2000	Mean nuclear volume, PSA, estimated tumor volume	Each independently predicted stage but how to predict probability of risk not given

■ t16.10 Clinical and Pathological Stage: Histopathologic Findings with Increasing Stage

Increasing histological grade of primary tumor
Increasing tumor size (volume, % cancer) of primary tumor
Increasing incidence of lymphvascular space invasion by carcinoma
Peripheral rather than transition zone origin of carcinoma

[16.5] Stage Relationships with Pathologic Findings

Increasing clinical and pathologic stages are related to unfavorable pathologic findings **t16.10**. With increasing clinical and pathologic stage of prostatic carcinoma, there tends to be increasing histologic grade (see Chapter 15), tumor size, and lymphovascular space invasion by carcinoma (Bahnson 1989, Herman 2000, Salomao 1995). Exceptions do exist such that, uncommonly, low-volume primary tumors can exhibit extraprostatic spread, for example (Donohue 1991, Humphrey 1996, McNeal 1986, Miller 1994), or high-grade tumors can be organ-confined (Epstein 1994, Peeroti 1998, Tefilli 1999). In general, though, in higher-stage tumors the primary tumor in the prostate often is of higher grade and larger size.

[16.6] Stage and Patient Outcome

Clinical and pathologic stage are strongly related to response to specific therapies and patient outcome. Responses to the commonly applied local therapies of radiation **t16.11** and radical prostatectomy **t16.12** clearly correspond to clinical T stage (Amling 1996, Bagshaw 1993,

■ 16.11 Survival for Patients Treated with External-Beam Radiation Therapy: Relationship with Clinical T Stage

	Overall suvival[1]	
Clinical T Stage	**10 Years**	**15 Years**
T1	54%-64%	41%
T2	43%-46%	22%
T3	35%-45%	18%-31%
T4	15%	15%

Data from Hanks 1993, Perez 1993, Bagshaw 1993, and Zagars 1993
[1]Note that this is overall survival. There is no difference after 15 years between expected survival and overall survival of treated T1 patients (Kuban 2000), but T2-T4 patients clearly fare worse than men without prostate cancer

■ t16.12 Prostatic Carcinoma Recurrence after Radical Prostatectomy: Relationship with Clinical T Stage

	% of patients free of recurrence	
Clinical T Stage	**5 Years**	**10 Years**
T1a	100%[1]	100%[1]
T1b	89%[1]	89%[1]
T1c	85-89%[1-4]	86%[1]
T2a	69-85%[1-4]	57-68%[1]
T2b	63-74%[1,3,4]	53%[1]
T3a	61%[1]	52%[1,5]

[1]Data from a series of 1,579 patients (Pound 1997)
[2]Data from a series of 1,337 patients (Eastham 2000)
[3]Data from a series of 4,774 patients (Amling 1996)
[4]Data from a series of 1,620 patients (Ramos 1999)
[5]8-year rather than 10-year follow-up

■ **t16.13 Prostatic Carcinoma Recurrence and Metastases-free Survival after Radical Prostatectomy: Relationship with Pathologic Stage**

	% of patients free of recurrence[1]		Metastasis-free survival[2]	
Pathologic stage	**5 years**	**10 years**	**5 years**	**10 years**
T2	94%	92%	99%	99%
T3a	74%	68%	99%	91%-99%
T3b	40%	33%	92%	77%
N+[3]	16%	—	78%[4]-96%	47%[4]-68%

[1]Data from Eastham 2000 (1,337 patients)
[2]Data from Pound 1997 (1,579 patients)
[3]Microscopically detected pelvic lymph node metastases
[4]Data from Iselin 1999

Eastham 2000, Han 2000, Hanks 1993, Iyer 1999, Kuban 2000, Perez 1993, Pound 1997, Ramos 1999, Stamey 1998, Zagars 1993). Local clinical stage was an independent predictor of survival in 1 large, multi-institution study (Gerber 1996) but not in 2 single-institution series (Pound 1999, Zincke 1994). In the former study, patients with cT1 carcinoma treated by radical prostatectomy had a 10-year disease-specific survival rate of 90%, compared with 82% of cT2 patients. Pathologic T stage is also closely tied to response to radical prostatectomy **t16.13** and indeed is more predictive of survival than clinical stage (Pound 1997).

Cure is much more likely to be achieved when prostatic carcinoma is confined to the prostate **t13.25, p 245; t16.13**. It is striking that the 5-year relative survival for prostate cancer diagnosed in the United States from 1989 through 1996 was 98% to 100% for localized or regional disease and 30% to 32% for patients with distant metastasis (Greenlee 2001).

Pretreatment Models Using Clinical T Stage to Predict Response to Local Therapy

Initial clinical T stage can be used with pretreatment serum PSA level and biopsy Gleason score to predict the likelihood of response to radical prostatectomy (D'Amico 1998A, 1999B, 2000, Kattan 1998, Ross 2001) and radiation therapy **t16.14**. A model that is in widespread use is a nomogram that predicts 5-year probability of recurrence-free survival among men with clinically localized prostate cancer treated with radical prostatectomy (Kattan 1998). Using clinical T stage, PSA level, and Gleason score, the model yields an estimate, with 95% confidence of the percentage of men who would be free of tumor at 5 years. Similar models for predicting outcome after 3-dimensional conformal radiotherapy and brachytherapy are available (D'Amico 1999B, Kattan 2001). Risk stratification prediction systems that condense risk spectra into discrete groups have also been developed **t16.15**. These prediction models can assist in treatment selection (both initial and adjuvant) and design of clinical trials. Limitations of these current models include the high level of uncertainty in prediction, the short follow-up (short for prostate cancer, that is, at 5 years), use of PSA failure rather than survival as an endpoint, and lack of prospective validation. The high level of uncertainty is expressed in the rather broad 95% confidence intervals. In the future, reduction of uncertainty and refinement of the models may be possible with use of additional biologic, pathologic (such as amount of tumor in needle biopsy), and clinical markers.

Postoperative Models Using Pathologic Stage to Predict Response to Surgery

After radical prostatectomy, pathologic T or N stage can be used in postoperative models to predict the patient's chance of being cured **t16.16**. The power of the information in histopathologic, rather than clinical, definition of disease extent is highlighted by the greater accuracy (judged by area under receiver-operating characteristic curve) of postoperative rather than preoperative models that predict patient outcome (Kattan 1999). The limitations of these models are similar to those of the pretreatment models discussed earlier; increased accuracy, longer follow-up, use of survival as an endpoint, and validation are desirable goals for the future.

■ **t16.14 Models Using Clinical Stage to Predict Response to Radical Prostatectomy and Radiation Therapy**

Use initial clinical T stage, pre-treatment serum PSA and biopsy Gleason score
Can be used in continuous risk scale or in risk stratification systems that use discrete groups (low-risk vs intermediate-risk vs high-risk)
Currently related to PSA failure at 5 years after therapy
Need longer follow-up and use of survival as end-point

■ **t16.15 Combined Modality Risk Stratification System Using Clinical T Stage to Predict Response to Radical Prostatectomy and Radiation Therapy**

Low risk	= Greater than 85% 5-year freedom from PSA failure = 1992 AJCC clinical stage T1c or T2a and PSA of 10 ng/mL or less and biopsy Gleason score of 6 or less
Intermediate risk	= 50% 5-year freedom from PSA failure = 1992 AJCC clinical stage T2b or PSA of 10-20 ng/mL or biopsy Gleason score of 7
High risk	= 33% 5-year freedom from PSA failure = 1992 AJCC clinical stage T2c or PSA > 20 ng/mL or biopsy Gleason score of 8 or higher

Definitions from D'Amico 2000

■ **t16.16 Postoperative Models Using Pathologic Stage to Predict Response to Surgery**

Study	Model	Comments
Partin 1995	RW = (0.061 × PSAST) + (0.54 × postop Gleason score) + (1.87 × pathologic stage)	Log relative risk, RW of recurrence for 212 patients included stage definition as "specimen-confined"
Bauer 1997	Rr = exp [(0.70 × race) + (0.79 × PSA [4.1-10)] + (1.34 × PSA [> 10]) + (0.91 × organ confinement) + [(0.65 × p53 [1,2+]) + (1.45× p53 [3,4+]) + (0.70 × bcl-2)]	Relative risk of recurrence (PSA failure) for 132 patients followed for 5 years
Bauer 1998	Rr = exp [0.51 × race] + (0.12 x PSAST) + (0.25 × post Gleason sum) + (0.89 × organ confined)	Relative risk of recurrence (PSA failure) based in part on pT stage
D'Amico 1998B	Nomogram uses preop PSA, pathological stage, margin status and prostatectomy Gleason score	pT stage incorporated into PSA failure model based on 862 men, but only 2 year follow-up
Kattan 1999	Nomogram uses preop PSA, and radical prostatectomy Gleason sum, EPE, seminal vesicle invasion, and lymph node status	7-year recurrence free probability predicted, based on 996 men
Blute 2001	Prognostic score = Gleason +1 (PSA 4-10), +2 (PSA 10.1-20), +3 (PSA > 20), +2 (positive seminal vesicle) and + 2 (positive margin)	T3b disease (positive seminal vesicle) used in this large study of 2,518 patients, with validation performed

[16.7] Experimental Staging Procedures

Experimental staging methods include a huge number of clinical, radiologic, pathologic, and molecular biologic approaches **t16.17**. Indeed, of the hundreds of identified putative predictive and prognostic factors for prostatic carcinoma, all could be considered potentially useful in staging (Bostwick 1999). This list would be even longer if one were to add all the molecules that are of biologic importance in prostatic carcinoma (Chapter 21) but that were not tested for linkage with pathologic or clinical endpoints. Incorporation of any new methods or definition into the formal TNM staging scheme will require compelling and overwhelming evidence of staging utility, based on extensive experience gathered over a long period of time.

Promising clinical staging tools include serum markers such as percentage of free PSA (Arcangeli 1998, Catalona 2000, Pannek 1998, Southwick 1999), the PSA cousin, human glandular kallikrein 2 (Haese 2000), and serum polypeptide growth factors (Duque 1999, Naughton 2001).

■ **t16.17 Experimental Staging: Selected Approaches[1]**

Total serum PSA, PSA density, percentage of free PSA, human glandular kallikrein 2
Use of new non-PSA serum markers (such as polypeptide growth factors)
Imaging: Radioimmunoimaging (eg, ProstaScint scans), transrectal ultrasound, endorectal coil magnetic resonance imaging, PET scans
Calculated prostate cancer volume (pretreatment)
Needle biopsy characteristics: Gleason score, amount of tumor in needle biopsy tissue, perineural invasion, tumor in fat or seminal vesicle tissue
Biomarkers in needle biopsy tissue: "Quantitative nuclear grade," DNA ploidy, mean nuclear volume, p53, bcl-2, proliferation index (Ki-67), microvessel density
Radical prostatectomy tumor size (% carcinoma, tumor volume), predominant tumor location, multifocality, Gleason grade, level of "capsular" invasion, amount of extraprostatic tumor, margin status, amount of margin positivity
Radical prostatectomy biomarkers: morphometric, immunophenotypic, and genotypic markers
Use of immunohistochemistry and/or PCR to detect prostatic cells in lymph nodes, blood, bone marrow
Neural networks

[1]Not currently used in TNM clinical or pathological staging

Functional imaging using antibodies against prostate-specific membrane antigen in radioimmunoimaging (indium-111 capromab pendetide [ProstaScint] scan) (Lang 2001, Sartor 2001), functional MRI, and PET scans (DeGrado 2001) are new avenues for radiologic attempts at staging. A combination of serum PSA, biopsy Gleason score, and prostate ultrasound volume was used to generate so-called calculated prostate cancer volume, which was reported to be the only significant predictor of pathologic T3 disease in patients with clinically localized disease (D'Amico 2001), but this technique was not reproduced by others (Chan 1998). Histopathologic staging information in needle biopsy tissue is limited by the small tissue sample size, but Gleason grade and amount of tumor contribute to stage prediction. Needle biopsy tumor extent may be useful in future refinement of pretreatment models of stage prediction. Biomarker assessment in needle biopsy tissue for staging purposes is similarly likely to be compromised by small sample size and marker heterogeneity. Histopathologic information is radical prostatectomy specimens could readily contribute to new pathologic substage groupings. In particular, a tumor volume (or percentage carcinoma)–based prognostic index could be generated (Bostwick 1993), and stage subgroupings could also be formulated based on margin status, extent of margin positivity, and extent of extraprostatic carcinoma. A plethora of new biomarkers based on gene expression (gene chip) profiling of prostatic carcinoma from radical prostatectomy tissues will emerge soon; however, it will take some time to determine whether any of these will be clinically significant for staging. Ever more sensitive techniques such as polymerase chain reaction to detect circulating and metastatic prostatic carcinoma also must be judged for clinical applicability based on clinical outcome studies. Computerized neural networks (Batuello 2001, D'Amico 2000) may help with refinement of current TNM staging, which only roughly predicts prognosis and response to therapy.

Finally, one could ask whether the current TNM system is sufficient to characterize the dynamic state of prostate cancer. TNM staging is static in that a stage is assigned at the time of initial diagnosis. One proposal to capture the evolving natural history and treated history of disease is use of a clinical states model that would provide a framework to assess and reassess prognosis over time **f16.3** (Scher 2000).

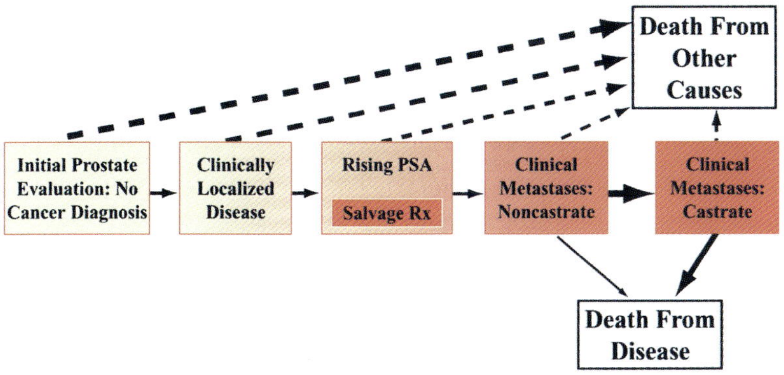

■ **f16.3** *Clinical states model of prostatic carcinoma evolution over time, with possible outcomes. In contrast, the TNM system assigns one stage — that at initial diagnosis (Scher 2000, with permission from Elsevier Science).*

[16.8] Reporting of Pathologic Stage

Pathologic stage information from the radical prostatectomy specimen and dissected pelvic lymph nodes may be provided in the diagnostic field (ADASP 1998, Greene 2002) or checklist field (examples are given in **t14.39, t14.40**, pp 306-307). Diagrams illustrating extent of disease (Greene 2002) are optional.

References

Ackerman DA, Barry JM, Wicklund RA, et al. Analysis of risk factors associated with prostate cancer extension to the surgical margin and pelvic node metastasis at radical prostatectomy. *J Urol* 150:1845-1850, 1993.

ADASP (Association of Directors of Anatomic and Surgical Pathology). Recommendations for reporting of resected prostatic carcinomas. *Am J Clin Pathol* 105:667-670, 1998.

Alagiri M, Colton MD, Seidmon EJ, et al. The staging pelvic lymphadenectomy: implications as an adjunctive procedure for clinically localized prostate cancer. *Br J Urol* 80:243-246, 1997.

Allepuz Losa CA, Sanz Velez JI, Gil Sanz MJ, et al. Seminal vesicle biopsy in prostate cancer staging. *J Urol* 154:1407-1411, 1995.

Amling CL, Blute ML, Lerner SE, et al. Influence of prostate-specific antigen testing on the spectrum of patients with prostate cancer undergoing radical prostatectomy at a large referral practice. *Mayo Clin Proc* 73:401-406, 1996.

Arai Y, Yoshiki T, Yamabe H, et al. Value of prostate-specific antigen measurements in predicting lymph node involvement in prostatic cancer. *Urol Int* 45:356-360, 1990.

Arcangeli CG, Humphrey PA, Smith DS, et al. Percentage of free serum prostate-specific antigen as a predictor of pathological features of prostate cancer in a screening population. *Urology* 51:558-564, 1998.

Badalament RA, Miller MC, Peller PA, et al. An algorithm for predicting non–organ-confined prostate cancer using the results obtained from sextant core biopsies with prostate-specific antigen level. *J Urol* 156:1375-1380, 1996.

Bagshaw MA, Kaplan ID, Cox RC. Prostate cancer: radiation therapy for localized disease. *Cancer* 71 (3 suppl):939-952, 1993.

Bahnson RR, Dresner SM, Gooding W, et al. Incidence and prognostic significance of lymphatic and vascular invasion in radical prostatectomy specimens. *Prostate* 15:149-155, 1989.

Bangma CH, Hop WC, Schroder FH. Eliminating the need for pre-operative frozen section analysis of pelvic lymph nodes during radical prostatectomy. *Br J Urol* 76:595-599, 1995.

Batuello JT, Gamito EJ, Crawford ED, et al. Artificial neural network model for the assessment of lymph node spread in patients with clinically localized prostate cancer. *Urology* 57:481-485, 2001.

Bauer JJ, Connelly RR, Sesterhenn IA, et al. Biostatistical modeling using traditional variables and genetic biomarkers for predicting the risk of prostate carcinoma recurrence after radical prostatectomy. *Cancer* 79:952-962, 1997.

Bauer JJ, Connelly RR, Sesterhenn IA, et al. Biostatistical modeling using traditional preoperative and pathological prognostic variables in the selection of men at high risk for disease recurrence after radical prostatectomy for prostate cancer. *J Urol* 159:929-933, 1998.

Bishoff JT, Reyes A, Thompson IM, et al. Pelvic lymphadenectomy can be omitted in selected patients with carcinoma of the prostate: development of a system of patient selection. *Urology* 45:270-274, 1995.

Bluestein DL, Bostwick DG, Bergstralh EJ, et al. Eliminating the need for bilateral pelvic lymphadenectomy in select patients with prostate cancer. *J Urol* 151:1315-1320, 1994.

Blute ML, Bostwick DG, Bergstralh EJ, et al. Anatomic site-specific positive margins in organ confined prostate cancer and its impact on outcome after radical prostatectomy. *Urology* 50:733-739, 1997.

Blute ML, Bergstralh EJ, Partin AW, et al. Validation of Partin tables for predicting pathological stage of clinically localized prostate cancer. *J Urol* 164:1591-1595, 2000.

Blute ML, Bergstralh EJ, Iocca A, et al. Use of Gleason score, prostate specific antigen, seminal vesicle and margin status to predict biochemical failure after radical prostatectomy. *J Urol* 165:119-125, 2001.

Bostwick DG, Graham SD Jr, Napalkov P, et al. Staging of early prostate cancer: a proposed tumor volume-based prognostic index. *Urology* 41:403-411, 1993.

Bostwick DG, Qian J, Bergstralh E, et al. Prediction of capsular perforation and seminal vesicle invasion in prostate cancer. *J Urol* 155:1361-1367, 1996.

Bostwick DG, Montironi R. Evaluating radical prostatectomy specimens: therapeutic and prognostic importance. *Virchows Arch* 430:1-16, 1997.

Bostwick DG, Foster CS. Predictive factors in prostate cancer: current concepts from the 1999 College of American Pathologists Conference on Solid Tumor Prognostic Factors and the 1999 World Health Organization Second International Consultation on Prostate Cancer. *Semin Urol Oncol* 17:222-272, 1999.

Carter HB, Partin AW. Diagnosis and staging of prostate cancer. In: Walsh PC, Retik AB, Vaughan ED Jr, et al, eds. *Campbell's Urology.* 8th ed. Philadelphia: Saunders; 3070-3071, 2002.

Catalona WJ, Partin AW, Slawin KM, et al. Percentage of free PSA in black versus white men for detection and staging of prostate cancer: a prospective multicenter clinical trial. *Urology* 55:372-376, 2000.

Chan LW, Stamey TA. Calculating prostate cancer volume preoperatively: the D'Amico equation and some other observations. *J Urol* 159:1998-2003, 1998.

Cheng L, Bergstralh EJ, Scherer BG, et al. Predictors of cancer progression in T1a prostate adenocarcinoma. *Cancer* 85:1300-1304, 1999.

Chybowski FM, Larson-Keller JJ, Bergstralh EJ, et al. Predicting radionuclide bone scan findings in patients with newly diagnosed untreated prostate cancer: prostate specific antigen is superior to all other clinical parameters. *J Urol* 145:313-318, 1991.

Cohen MB, Soloway MS, Murphy WM. Sampling of radical prostatectomy specimens. How much is adequate? *Am J Clin Pathol* 101:250-252, 1994.

D'Amico AV, Chang H, Holupka E, et al. Calculated prostate cancer volume: the optimal predictor of actual cancer volume and pathologic stage. *Urology* 49:385-391, 1997.

D'Amico AV, Whittington R, Malkowicz SB, et al. Biochemical outcome after radical prostatectomy, external beam radiation therapy, or interstitial radiation therapy for clinically localized prostate cancer. *JAMA* 280:969-974, 1998A.

D'Amico AV, Whittington R, Malkowicz SB, et al. The combination of preoperative prostate specific antigen and postoperative pathological findings to predict prostate specific antigen outcome in clinically localized prostate cancer. *J Urol* 160:2096-2101, 1998B.

D'Amico AV, Whittington R, Malkowicz SB, et al. Optimizing patient selection for dose escalation techniques using the prostate-specific antigen level, biopsy Gleason score, and clinical T stage. *Int J Radiat Oncol Biol Phys* 45:1227-1233, 1999A.

D'Amico AV, Whittington RS, Malkowicz SB, et al. Pretreatment nomogram for prostate specific antigen recurrence after radical prostatectomy or external-beam radiation therapy for clinically localized prostate cancer. *J Clin Oncol* 17:168-172, 1999B.

D'Amico AV, Moul JW, Kattan MW. Emerging prognostic factors for outcome prediction in clinically localized prostate cancer: prostate-specific antigen level, race, molecular markers, and neural networks. In: Vogelzang NJ, Scarcino PT, Shipley WU, et al, eds. *Genitourinary Oncology.* 2nd ed. Philadelphia: Lippincott Williams & Wilkins; 680-700, 2000.

Danella JF, deKernion JB, Smith RB, et al. The contemporary incidence of lymph node metastases in prostate cancer: implications for laparoscopic lymph node dissection. *J Urol* 149:1488-1491, 1993.

Dash A, Sanda MG, Yu M, et al. Prostate cancer involving the bladder neck: recurrence-free survival and implications for AJCC staging modification. *Urology* 60: 276-280, 2002.

De GradoTR, Coleman RE, Wang S, et al. Synthesis and evaluation of 18F-labeled choline as an oncologic tracer for position emission tomography: initial findings in prostate cancer. *Cancer Res* 61:110-117, 2001.

Donohue RE, Miller GJ. Adenocarcinoma of the prostate: biopsy to whole mount. Denver VA experience. *Urol Clin North Am* 18:449-452, 1991.

Duque JL, Loughlin KR, Adam RM, et al. Plasma levels of vascular endothelial growth factor are increased in patients with metastatic prostate cancer. *Urology* 54:523-527, 1999.

Eastham JA, Scardino PT. Radical prostatectomy for clinical stage T1 and T2 prostate cancer. In: Vogelzang NJ, Scardino PT, Shipley WU, et al, eds. *Genitourinary Oncology.* 2nd ed. Philadelphia: Lippincott Williams & Wilkins; 722-738, 2000.

Egawa S, Suyama K, Matsumoto K, et al. Improved predictability of extracapsular extension and seminal vesicle involvement based on clinical and biopsy findings in prostate cancer in Japanese men. *Urology* 52:433-440, 1998.

Epstein JI, Paull G, Eggleston JC, et al. Prognosis of untreated stage A1 prostatic carcinoma: a study of 94 cases with extended follow-up. *J Urol* 136:837-839, 1986.

Epstein JI, Carmichael MJ, Pizov G, et al. Influence of capsular penetration on progression following radical prostatectomy: a study of 196 cases with long-term follow-up. *J Urol* 150:135-141, 1993.

Epstein JI, Carmichael MJ, Partin AW, et al. Small high grade adenocarcinoma of the prostate in radical prostatectomy specimens performed for nonpalpable disease: pathogenetic and clinical implications. *J Urol* 151:1587-1592, 1994.

Fleming ID, Cooper JS, Henson DE, et al. Prostate. *AJCC Cancer Staging Manual.* 5th ed. Philadelphia: Lippincott-Raven; 1997.

Fujikawa K, Matsui Y, Kobayashi T, et al. Predicting pathological stage of localized prostate cancer using volume weighted mean nuclear volume. *J Urol* 164:1587-1590, 2000.

Gee WF, Holtgrewe L, Blute ML, et al. 1997 American Urological Association Gallup survey: changes in diagnosis and management of prostatic cancer and benign prostatic hyperplasia, and other practice trends from 1994 to 1997. *J Urol* 160:1804-1807, 1998.

Gerber GS, Thisted RA, Scardino PT, et al. Results of radical prostatectomy in men with clinically localized prostate cancer. Multi-institutional pooled analysis. *JAMA* 276:615-619, 1996.

Greene FL, Page DL, Fleming ID, et al. Prostate. *AJCC Cancer Staging Manual.* 6th ed. New York: Springer Verlag; 309-316, 2002.

Greenlee RT, Hill-Harmon MB, Murray T, et al. Cancer statistics, 2001. *CA Cancer J Clin* 51:15-36, 2001.

Grignon DJ, Sakr WA. Pathologic staging of prostate carcinoma. What are the issues? *Cancer* 78:337-340, 1996.

Grossfeld GD, Chang JJ, Broering JM, et al. Does the completeness of prostate sampling predict outcome for patients undergoing radical prostatectomy? Data from the CaPSURE database. *Urology* 56:430-435, 2000.

Haese A, Becker C, Noldus J, et al. Human glandular kallikrein 2: a potential serum marker for predicting the organ confined versus nonorgan-confined growth of prostate cancer. *J Urol* 163:1491-1497, 2000.

Haese A, Epstein JI, Huland K, et al. Validation of a biopsy-based pathologic algorithm for predicting lymph node metastases in patients with clinically localized prostate carcinoma. *Cancer* 95:1016-1021, 2002.

Haggman M, Norberg M, de la Torre M, et al. Characterization of localized prostatic cancer: distribution, grading and pT-staging in radical prostatectomy specimens. *Scand J Urol Nephrol* 27:7-13, 1993.

Hall GS, Kramer CE, Epstein JI. Evaluation of radical prostatectomy specimens: a comparative analysis of sampling methods. *Am J Surg Pathol* 16:315-324, 1992.

Han M, Walsh PC, Partin AW, et al. Ability of the 1992 and 1997 American Joint Committee on Cancer staging systems for prostate cancer to predict progression-free survival after radical prostatectomy for stage T2 disease. *J Urol* 164:89-92, 2000.

Hanks GE, Krall JM, Hanlon AL, et al. Patterns of care and RTOG studies in prostate cancer: long-term survival, hazard rate observations, and possibilities of cure. *Int J Radiat Oncol Biol Phys* 28:39-45, 1993.

Herman CM, Wilcox GE, Kattan MW, et al. Lymphovascular invasion as a predictor of disease progression in prostate cancer. *Am J Surg Pathol* 24:859-863, 2000.

Hoenig DM, Chi S, Porter C, et al. Risk of nodal metastases at laparoscopic pelvic lymphadenectomy using PSA, Gleason score, and clinical stage in men with localized prostate cancer. *J Endourol* 11:263-265, 1997.

Hollenbeck BK, Bassily N, Wei JT, et al. Whole mounted radical prostatectomy specimens do not increase detection of adverse pathological features. *J Urol* 164:1583-1586, 2000.

Hricak H, Dooms GC, Jeffrey RB, et al. Prostatic carcinoma: staging by clinical assessment, CT, and MRI. *Radiology* 162:331-336, 1987.

Hudson MA, Bahnson RR, Catalona WJ. Clinical use of prostate specific antigen in patients with prostate cancer. *J Urol* 142:1011-1017, 1989.

Humphrey PA, Walther PJ. Adenocarcinoma of the prostate. Part II: Tissue prognosticators. *Am J Clin Pathol* 100:256-269, 1993A.

Humphrey PA. Complete histologic serial sectioning of a prostate gland with adenocarcinoma. *Am J Surg Pathol* 17:468-472, 1993B.

Humphrey PA, Keetch DW, Smith DS, et al. Prospective characterization of pathological features of prostatic carcinomas detected via serum prostate specific antigen based screening. *J Urol* 155:816-820, 1996.

Humphrey PA, Vollmer RT. Relationships between serum prostate-specific antigen and histopathologic appearances of prostate carcinoma. In: Foster CS, Bostwick DG, eds. *Pathology of the Prostate.* Philadelphia: WB Saunders; 264, 1998.

Iselin CE, Robertson JE, Paulson DF. Radical perineal prostatectomy: oncological outcome during a 20-year period. *J Urol* 161:163-168, 1999.

Iyer RV, Hanlon AL, Pinover WH, et al. Outcome evaluation of the 1997 American Joint Committee on Cancer Staging System for Prostate Carcinoma treated by radiation therapy. *Cancer* 85:1816-1821, 1999.

Jewett HJ. The present status of radical prostatectomy for stages A and B prostatic cancer. *Urol Clin North Am* 2:105-124, 1975.

Kattan MW, Stapleton AMF, Wheeler TM, et al. Evaluation of a nomogram used to predict the pathologic stage of clinically localized prostate carcinoma. *Cancer* 79:528-537, 1997.

Kattan MW, Eastham JA, Stapleton AMF, et al. A preoperative nomogram for disease recurrence following radical prostatectomy for prostate cancer. *J Natl Cancer Inst* 90:766-771, 1998.

Kattan MW, Wheeler TM, Scardino PT. Postoperative nomogram for disease recurrence after radical prostatectomy for prostate cancer. *J Clin Oncol* 17:1499-1507, 1999.

Kattan MW, Zelefsky MJ, Kupelian PA, et al. Pretreatment nomogram for predicting the outcome of three-dimensional conformal radiotherapy in prostate cancer. *J Clin Oncol* 18:3352-3359, 2000.

Kattan MW, Potters L, Blasko JC, et al. Pretreatment nomogram for predicting freedom from recurrence after permanent prostate brachytherapy in prostate cancer. *Urology* 58:393-399, 2001.

Kerbl K, Clayman RV, Petros JA, et al. Staging pelvic lymphadenectomy for prostate cancer: a comparison of laparoscopic and open techniques. *Urology* 150:396-398, 1993.

Kleer E, Larson-Keller JJ, Zincke H, et al Ability of preoperative serum prostate-specific antigen value to predict pathologic stage and DNA ploidy. Influence of clinical stage and tumor grade. *Urology* 41:207-216, 1993.

Kuban DA, Schellhammer PF, El-Mahdi AM. External-beam radiation therapy for stage T1 and T2 prostate cancer. In: Vogelzang NJ, Scardino PT, Shipley WU, et al, eds. *Genitourinary Oncology.* 2nd ed. Philadelphia: Lippincott Williams & Wilkins; 739-754, 2000.

Lange PH. ProstaScint Scan for staging prostate cancer (editorial). *Urology* 57:402-406, 2001.

Lee CT, Oesterling JE. Using prostate-specific antigen to eliminate the staging bone scan. *Urol Clin North Am* 24:389-394, 1997.

Lee F, Bahn DK, Siders DB, et al. The role of TRUS-guided biopsies for determination of internal and external spread of prostate cancer. *Semin Urol Oncol* 16:129-136, 1998.

Lerner SE, Seay TM, Blute ML, et al. Prostate specific antigen detected prostate cancer (clinical stage T1c): an interim analysis. *J Urol* 155:821-826, 1996.

McNeal JE, Bostwick DG, Kindrachuk RA, et al. Patterns of progression in prostate cancer. *Lancet* 1:60-63, 1986.

Miller GJ, Cygan JM. Morphology of prostate cancer: the effects of multifocality on histological grade, tumor volume and capsule penetration. *J Urol* 152:1709-1713, 1994.

Montie JE. Staging systems for prostate cancer. In: Vogelzang NJ, Scardino PT, Shipley WU, et al, eds. *Genitourinary Oncology.* 2nd ed. Philadelphia: Lippincott Williams & Wilkins; 673-679, 2000.

Naitoh J, Dorey F, deKernion J. Predicting pathological stage of localized prostate cancer [letter]. *JAMA* 278:980-982, 1997.

Narayan P, Fournier G, Gajendran V, et al. Utility of preoperative serum prostate-specific antigen concentration and biopsy Gleason score in predicting risk of pelvic lymph node metastases in prostate cancer. *Urology* 44:519-524, 1994.

Narayan P, Gajendran V, Taylor SP, et al. The role of transrectal ultrasound-guided biopsy-based staging, preoperative serum prostate-specific antigen, and biopsy Gleason score in prediction of final pathologic diagnosis in prostate cancer. *Urology* 46:205-212, 1995

Narayan P, Tewari A. Systematic biopsy-based staging of prostate cancer: scientific background, individual variables, combination of parameters, and current integrative models. *Semin Urol Oncol* 16:172-181, 1998.

Naughton M, Picus J, Zhu X, et al. Scatter factor–hepatocyte growth factor elevation in the serum of patients with prostate cancer. *J Urol* 165:1325-1328, 2001.

Nishiya M, Miller GJ, Lookner DH, et al. Prostate specific antigen density in patients with histologically proven prostate carcinoma. *Cancer* 74:3002-3009, 1994.

O'Dowd GJ, Veltri RW, Orozco R, et al. Update on the appropriate staging evaluation for newly diagnosed prostate cancer. *J Urol* 158:687-698, 1997.

Obek S. Sadek S, Lai S, et al. Positive surgical margins with radical retropubic prostatectomy: anatomic site-specific pathologic analysis and impact on prognosis. *Urology* 54:682-688, 1999.

Oesterling JE, Brendler CB, Epstein JI, et al. Correlation of clinical stage, serum prostatic acid phosphatase, and preoperative Gleason grade with final pathological stage in 275 patients with clinically localized adenocarcinoma of the prostate. *J Urol* 138:92-98, 1987.

Ohori M, Goad JR, Wheeler TM, et al. Can radical prostatectomy alter the progression of poorly differentiated prostate cancer? *J Urol* 152:1843-1859, 1994A.

Ohori M, Wheeler TM, Scardino PT. The new American Joint Committee on Cancer and International Union Against Cancer TNM Classification of Prostate Cancer. Clinicopathologic correlations. *Cancer* 74:104-114, 1994B.

Ohori M, Wheeler TM, Kattan MW, et al. Prognostic significance of positive surgical margins in radical prostatectomy specimens. *J Urol* 154:1818-1824, 1995.

Okihara K, Kamoi K, Lane RB, et al. Role of systematic ultrasound-guided staging biopsies in predicting extraprostatic extension and seminal vesicle invasion in men with prostate cancer. *J Clin Ultr* 30:123-131, 2002.

Pandey P, Fowler JE, Seaver LE, et al. Ultrasound guided seminal vesicle biopsies in men with suspected prostate cancer. *J Urol* 154:1798-1801, 1995.

Pannek J, Rittenhouse HG, Chan DW, et al. The use of percent free prostate specific antigen for staging clinically localized prostate cancer. *J Urol* 159:1238-1242, 1998.

Partin AW, Yoo J, Carter HB, et al. The use of prostate specific antigen, clinical stage and Gleason score to predict pathological stage in men with localized prostate cancer. *J Urol* 150:110-114, 1993.

Partin AW, Piantadosi S, Sanda MG, et al. Selection of men at high risk for disease recurrence for experimental adjuvant therapy following radical prostatectomy. *Urology* 45:831-838, 1995.

Partin AW, Subong ENP, Walsh PC, et al. Combination of prostate-specific antigen, clinical stage, and Gleason score to predict pathological stage of localized prostate cancer: a multi-institutional update. *JAMA* 277:1445-1451, 1997.

Partin AW, Mangold LA, Lamm DM, et al. Contemporary update of prostate cancer staging nomograms (Partin Tables) for the new millenium. *Urology* 58:843-848, 2001.

Penson DF, Grossfeld GD, Li YP, et al. How well does the Partin nomogram predict pathological stage after radical prostatectomy in a community based population. *J Urol* 167:1653-1657, 2002.

Perez CA, Lee HK, Georgiou A, et al. Technical and tumor related factors affecting outcome of definitive irradiation for localized carcinoma of the prostate. *Int J Radiat Oncol Biol Phys* 26:581-591, 1993.

Perrotti M, Rabbani F, Russo P, et al. Early prostate cancer detection and potential for surgical cure in men with poorly differentiated tumors. *Urology* 52:106-110, 1998.

Philips TH, Thompson IM. Digital rectal examination and cancer of the prostate. *Urol Clin North Am* 18:459-465, 1991.

Pisansky TM, Kahn MJ, Bostwick DG. An enhanced prognostic system for clinically localized carcinoma of the prostate. *Cancer* 79:2154-2161, 1997.

Platt JF, Bree RL, Schwab RE. The accuracy of CT in the staging of carcinoma of the prostate. *AJR Am J Roentgenol* 149:315-318, 1987.

Polascik TJ, Pearson JD, Partin AW. Multivariate models as predictors of pathological stage using Gleason score, clinical stage, and serum prostate-specific antigen. *Semin Urol Oncol* 16:160-171, 1998.

Polascik TJ, Oesterling JI, Partin AW. Prostate specific antigen: a decade of discovery—what have we learned and where are we going. *J Urol* 162:293-306, 1999.

Pound CR, Partin AW, Epstein JI, et al. Prostate-specific antigen after anatomic radical retropubic prostatectomy. Patterns of recurrence and cancer control. *Urol Clin North Am* 24:395-406, 1997.

Pound CR, Partin AW, Eisenberger MA, et al. Natural history of progression after PSA elevation following radical prostatectomy. *JAMA* 281:1591-1597, 1999.

Puppo P, Perachino M. Clinical stage, prostate-specific antigen and Gleason grade to predict extracapsular disease or nodal metastasis in men with newly diagnosed, previously untreated prostate cancer. A multicenter study. *Eur Urol* 32:293-279, 1997.

Ramos CG, Carvalhal GF, Smith DS, et al. Clinical and pathological characteristics, and recurrence rates of stage T1c versus T2a or T2b prostate cancer. *J Urol* 161:1525-1529, 1999.

Rifkin MD, Zerhouni EA, Gatsonis CA, et al. Comparison of magnetic resonance imaging and ultrasonography in staging early prostate cancer. Results of a multi-institutional cooperative trial. *N Engl J Med* 323:621-626, 1990.

Roach M III, Marquez C, Yuo HS, et al. Predicting the risk of lymph node involvement using the pre-treatment prostate specific antigen and Gleason score in men with clinically localized prostate cancer. *Int J Radiat Oncol Biol Phys* 28:33-37, 1993.

Rogers E, Gurpinar T, Dillioglugil O, et al. The role of digital rectal examination, biopsy Gleason sum and prostate-specific antigen in selecting patients who require pelvic lymph node dissections for prostate cancer. *Br J Urol* 78:419-425, 1996.

Ross PL, Scardino PT, Kattan MW. A catalog of prostate cancer nomograms. *J Urol* 165:1562-1568, 2001.

Sakr WA, Wheeler TM, Blute M, et al. Staging and reporting of prostate cancer-sampling the radical prostatectomy specimen. *Cancer* 78:366-368, 1996.

Salomao DR, Graham SD, Bostwick DG. Microvascular invasion in prostate cancer correlates with pathologic stage. *Arch Pathol Lab Med* 119:1050-1054, 1995.

Sands ME, Zagars GK, Pollack A, et al. Serum prostate-specific antigen, clinical stage, pathologic grade, and the incidence of nodal metastases in prostate cancer. *Urology* 44:215-220, 1994.

Sartor O, McLeod D. Indium-111-Capromab pendetide scans: an important test relevant to clinical decision making. *Urology* 57:399-401, 2001.

Scher HI, Heller G. Clinical states in prostate cancer: toward a dynamic model of disease progression. *Urology* 55:323-327, 2000.

Schroeder FH, Belt E. Carcinoma of the prostate: a study of 213 patients with stage c tumors treated by total perineal prostatectomy. *J Urol* 114:257-260, 1975.

Sehdev AE, Pan CC, Epstein JI. Comparative analysis of sampling methods for grossing radical prostatectomy specimens performed for nonpalpable (stage T1c) prostatic adenocarcinoma. *Hum Pathol* 32:494-499, 2001.

Shelfo SW, Obek C, Soloway MS. Update on bladder neck preservation during radical retropubic prostatectomy: impact on pathologic outcome, anastomotic strictures, and continence. *Urology* 51:73-78, 1998.

Southwick PC, Catalona WJ, Partin AW, et al. Prediction of post–radical prostatectomy pathological outcome for stage T1c prostate cancer with percent free prostate specific antigen: a prospective multicenter clinical trial. *J Urol* 162:1346-1351, 1999.

Smith DS, Catalona WJ. Interexaminer variability of digital rectal examination detecting prostate cancer. *Urology* 45:70-74, 1995.

Spevack L, Killion KT, West JC Jr, et al. Predicting the patient at low risk for lymph node metastasis with localized prostate cancer: an analysis of four statistical models. *Int J Radiat Oncol Biol Phys* 34:543-547, 1996.

Stage (a) *Med.* In: Brown L, ed. *The New Shorter Oxford English Dictionary.* Oxford, England: Clarendon Press; 3020, 1993.

Stamey TA, Villers AA, McNeal JE, et al. Positive surgical margins at radical prostatectomy: importance of the apical dissection. *J Urol* 143:1166-1173, 1990.

Stamey TA, Sözen TS, Yemoto CM, et al. Classification of localized untreated prostate cancer based on 791 men treated only with radical prostatectomy: common ground for therapeutic trials and TNM subgroups. *J Urol* 159:2009-2012, 1998.

Stone NN, Stock RG, Parikh D, et al. Perineural invasion and seminal vesicle involvement predict pelvic lymph node metastasis in men with localized carcinoma of the prostate. *J Urol* 160:1722-1726, 1998.

Tefilli MV, Gheiler EL, Tiguert R, et al. Role of radical prostatectomy in patients with prostate cancer of high Gleason score. *Prostate* 39:60-66, 1999.

Tempany CM, Zhou X, Zerhouni EA, et al. Staging of prostate cancer: results of radiology diagnostic oncology group project comparison of three different MR imaging techniques. *Radiology* 192:47-54, 1994.

Terris MK, McNeal JE, Freiha FS, et al. Efficacy of transrectal ultrasound–guided seminal vesicle biopsies in the detection of seminal vesicle invasion by prostate cancer. *J Urol* 149:1035-1039, 1993.

Terris MK, Pham TQ, Issa MM, et al. Routine transition zone and seminal vesicle biopsies in all patients undergoing transrectal ultrasound guided prostate biopsies are not indicated. *J Urol* 157:204-206, 1997.

True LD. Surgical pathology examination of the prostate gland. Practice survey by American Society of Clinical Pathologists. *Am J Clin Pathol* 102:572-579, 1994.

Vallancien G, Bochereau G, Wetzel O, et al. Influence of preoperative positive seminal vesicle biopsy on the staging of prostate cancer. *J Urol* 152:1152-1156, 1994.

Van Poppel H, Ameye F, Oyen R, et al. Accuracy of combined computerized tomography and fine needle aspiration cytology in lymph node staging of localized prostate carcinoma. *J Urol* 151:1310-1314, 1994.

Varenhorst E, Berglund K, Lofman O, et al. Inter-observer variation in assessment of the prostate by digital rectal examination. *Br J Urol* 72:173-176, 1993.

Voges GE, McNeal JE, Redwine EA, et al. The predictive significance of substaging stage A prostate cancer (A1 vs A2) for volume and grade of total cancer in the prostate. *J Urol* 147:858-863, 1992.

Vollmer RT, Keetch DW, Humphrey PA. Predicting the pathology results of radical prostatectomy from preoperative information. *Cancer* 83:1567-1580, 1998.

Watson RB, Civantos F, Soloway MS. Positive surgical margins with radical prostatectomy: detailed pathological analysis and prognosis. *Urology* 48:80-90, 1996.

Wiedner JA, Soloway MS. Incidence, etiology, location, prevention, and treatment of positive surgical margins after radical prostatectomy for prostate cancer. *J Urol* 160:299-315, 1998.

Weldon VE, Tavel FR, Neuwirth H, et al. Patterns of positive specimen margins and detectable prostate specific antigen after radical perineal prostatectomy. *J Urol* 153:1565-1569, 1995.

Wheeler TM, Dillioglugil O, Kattan MW, et al. Clinical and pathological significance of the level and extent of capsular invasion in clinical stage T1-2 prostate cancer. *Hum Pathol* 29:856-862, 1998.

Whitmore WF Jr. Hormone therapy in prostatic cancer. *Am J Med* 697:613, 1956.

Wills ML, Sauvageot J, Partin AW, et al. Ability of sextant biopsies to predict radical prostatectomy stage. *Urology* 51:759-764, 1998.

Wolf JS Jr, Shinohara K, Carroll PR, et al. Combined role of transrectal ultrasonography, Gleason score, and prostate-specific antigen in predicting organ-confined prostate cancer. *Urology* 42:131-137, 1993.

Yossepowitch O, Engelstein D, Konichezky M, et al. Bladder neck involvement in pathological stage pT4 radical prostatectomy specimens is not an independent prognostic factor. *J Urol* 168:2011-2015, 2002.

Zagars GK, von Eschenbach AC, Ayala AG. Prognostic factors in prostate cancer. Analysis of 874 patients treated with radiation therapy. *Cancer* 72:1709-1725, 1993.

Zelefsky MJ, Leibel SA, Gaudin PB, et al. Dose escalation with three-dimensional conformal radiation therapy affects the outcome in prostate cancer. *Int J Radiat Oncol Biol Phys* 41:491-500, 1998.

Zhang G, Wasserman NF, Sidi AA, et al. Long-term follow-up after expectant management of stage A1 prostatic cancer. *J Urol* 146:99-103, 1991.

Zincke H, Oesterling JE, Blute ML, et al. Long term (15 years) results after radical prostatectomy for clinically localized (stage T2c or lower) prostate cancer. *J Urol* 152:1850-1857, 1994.

Variants of Prostatic Carcinoma

[17.1] Prostatic Ductal Adenocarcinoma **391**
[17.2] Mucinous (Colloid) Adenocarcinoma **400**
[17.3] Signet-Ring Carcinoma **403**
[17.4] Adenosquamous and Squamous Carcinomas **406**
[17.5] Basaloid and Adenoid Cystic "Carcinomas" **408**
[17.6] Transitional Cell (Urothelial) Carcinoma **410**
[17.7] Small Cell Carcinoma **414**
[17.8] Sarcomatoid Carcinoma (Carcinosarcoma) **419**
[17.9] Others **422**

CHAPTER 17

t17.1 Ductal Adenocarcinoma of the Prostate

Known previously as endometrioid or endometrial, or papillary or papillary ductal adenocarcinoma
Incidence = 1.3% of all prostatic carcinomas (range: 0.4%-7.5% in 6 large series)
Men same age as those with acinar adenocarcinoma, but present with obstruction and hematuria
DRE usually abnormal and serum PSA usually elevated
Cystoscopically: Can project into urethra as papillary fronds
Microscopically: A papillary, cribriform, and glandular adenocarcinoma
Comedocarcinoma can be seen
Cytologically: Tall columnar cells, basally situated nuclei, amphophilic or clear cytoplasm
Clinical outcome worse than for acinar adenocarcinoma

Most primary carcinomas of the prostate are conventional or usual acinar adenocarcinomas. Unusual histologic variants, or types, account for about 5% to 10% of all carcinomas that originate in the prostate gland (Young 2000). The word *variant* is defined as "a form or version of something differing in some respect from other forms of the same thing" (Brown 1993). For prostatic carcinoma these unusual forms differ in histologic appearance from usual acinar adenocarcinoma and from other variants. These variants often differ from usual prostatic adenocarcinomas in many other ways, including different clinical, immunophenotypic, ultrastructural, and genetic features. These variants frequently display divergent differentiation compared with usual acinar carcinomas, yet epithelial differentiation is the common binding attribute of these carcinomas. Other patterns or cell appearances that are sometimes included in variant lists (Bostwick 1997, Delahunt 1998) include atrophic pattern adenocarcinoma (Cina 1997, Egan 1997, Kaleem 1998), pseudohyperplastic pattern adenocarcinoma (Humphrey 1998, Levi 2000), foamy gland carcinoma (Nelson 1996, Tran 2001), and carcinoma with oncocytic change (Ordóñez 1992, Pinto 1994). These are discussed and illustrated in Chapter 14. In this chapter, 9 histologic variants or types of primary prostatic carcinoma are discussed. The classification of these variants follows a recently tabulated arrangement (Young 2000). These variants are important to diagnose because many differ in prognosis from acinar adenocarcinoma, they may prompt a different therapeutic approach, and they are important in differential diagnosis of both benign and malignant conditions in the prostate.

[17.1] Prostatic Ductal Adenocarcinoma

Ductal adenocarcinoma of the prostate, which has also been called endometrioid, endometrial, papillary, or papillary ductal adenocarcinoma, has historically been a controversial entity **t17.1**. In 1950, the designation of "duct-celled type" was applied to prostatic carcinomas originating in the "ductile zone" (Foot 1950), but the first description of ductal adenocarcinoma was made in 1967 by Melicow and Pachter (Melicow 1967). In this article on a single case and a follow-up 1971 article with 5 additional cases (Melicow 1971), the argument was made that this carcinoma was an endometrial carcinoma arising in the prostatic utricle, which is a müllerian remnant present in normal male subjects. Accordingly, it was felt that standard hormonal treatments with estrogen and orchiectomy would be contraindicated because they might fuel the growth of this müllerian neoplasm. Since that time, however, data from multiple lines of inquiry, including data on immunohistochemical features, ultrastructural features, and response to therapy, indicate that these so-called endometrial or endometrioid carcinomas of the prostate, are, in fact, of prostate origin and should be treated like standard prostatic adenocarcinoma. Specifically, these carcinomas are almost always immunoreactive with antibodies directed against prostate-specific antigen (PSA) and prostate-specific acid phosphatase (Armonis 1993, Aydin 1993, Fujino 1998, Ishizu 1992, Küllü 1991, Lee 1994, Ma 1998, Millar 1996, Oxley 1998A, Samaratunga 1997, Vale 1992), the ultrastructural features are more consistent with a prostatic rather than an endometrial carcinoma (Bostwick 1985, Ro 1988B, Tannenbaum 1975B, Walther 1985, Zaloudek 1976), and there is hormonal dependence similar to that of prostatic acinar adenocarcinoma (Epstein 1986, Fukuoka 1984, Lemberger 1984, Ro 1988B, Scott 1976, Witters 1986). Recently, the very existence of prostatic ductal adenocarcinoma as a discrete clinicopathologic entity has been questioned (Bock 1999). Here, the authors concluded that the only specific feature of ductal adenocarcinoma is the characteristic growth location, that being large periurethral ducts (Bock 1999). Given that most (but not all) series indicate a more aggressive clinical course for ductal adenocarcinomas **t17.2**, it seems reasonable to diagnostically separate this morphologic variant from pure acinar adenocarcinoma.

Ductal adenocarcinoma is the most common histologic variant of prostatic carcinoma **t17.1, t17.2**. The incidence of ductal adenocarcinoma, including both pure ductal and mixed ductal-acinar adenocarcinomas, is 3.2% of all prostatic carcinomas. (This is based on summed figures from 6 large series, with 347 of 10 951 patients with prostatic carcinoma diagnosed with ductal adenocarcinoma [Bostwick 1985, Brinker 1999, Dube 1973, Epstein 1986, Lemberger 1984].) Mixed ductal-acinar carcinoma is more common than pure ductal carcinoma. In the largest series (by far) of ductal carcinomas in the literature (262 patients), the incidence of pure ductal carcinoma was 1.3%, whereas the incidence of mixed ductal-acinar adenocarcinoma was 4.8% (Dube 1973).

Men with prostatic ductal adenocarcinoma typically are aged 63 to 72 years, with a range of 41 to 89 years **t17.2**. Obstruction and hematuria are common clinical manifestations. The digital rectal examination (DRE) usually is abnormal and often suspicious for malignancy. Most patients (56% to 100%) have a serum PSA above 4 ng/mL (Armonis 1993, Brinker 1999, Christensen 1991, Millar 1996, Vale 1992), with medians of 7.9 ng/mL (Brinker 1999) to 13.8 ng/mL (Millar 1996). A substantial minority of men with ductal prostatic adenocarcinoma can present with "metastatic" levels of serum PSA in the hundreds to thousands of nanograms per milliliter, bone pain, and skeletal metastases **t17.2**. Indeed, clinical stage is more often advanced compared with standard acinar carcinomas, with a higher percentage of men with non–organ-confined disease (Lemberger 1984, Ro 1988B, Tannenbaum 1977).

Few radiologic studies of localized ductal adenocarcinoma have been reported (Egawa 1992, Rubinowicz 2000, Vale 1992). Computed tomography (CT) scans have been used in several cases to demonstrate extent of a bulky tumor (Vale 1992, Witters 1986), and based

■ t17.2 Ductal Adenocarcinoma of the Prostate: Clinical Features in Series with Ten or More Patients

Author	No.[1]	Incidence[2]	Mean Age[3]	Presentation	Sample[4]	Outcome
Dube 1973	55	6.1%	69 (41-81)	Obstruction: 93% Gross hematuria: 18% DRE Suspicious: 85% Cystoscopy: Villous/polypoid intraurethral tumor or infiltrative tumor Bony mets: 24%	TUR	5-year survival: 24%-43%
Lemberger 1984	39	7.5%	72 (57-89)	Prostatism: 38% Retention: 33% Hematuria: 10% Bony mets: 10%	TUR: 62% Needle bx: 23% Both: 15%	40% 5-year survival without bony mets; 0% with mets
Bostwick 1985	13	0.8%	65 (49-81)	Hematuria Obstruction DRE: Enlargement, hardness (39%), nodularity (23%) Cystoscopy: Friable, exophytic white fronds of tumor protruding into urethra at verumontanum	TUR: 100%	15% crude 5-year survival
Epstein 1986	10	0.4%	63 (46-76)	Obstruction: 50% Gross hematuria: 40% DRE: Suspicious: 43% Cystoscopy: 60% with papillary lesions in and around verumontanum	TUR: 70% Needle bx: 40%	5 patients had mets; two patients died at 3.5- 4 years
Wernert 1987	50	NG	71 (51-86)	DRE: 80% suspicious Urethroscopy: 20% villous	TUR, needle bx, open prostatectomy	24% with mets; 6% died
Ro 1988B	35	NG	65 (51-86)	Obstruction: 45% Hematuria: 23% Bone pain: 9%; Bony mets: 36% DRE: Hard, enlarged prostate in 82% 41% with clinical stage C or D		30% 5-year survival; survival stage dependent
Christensen 1991	15	NG	63 (52-73)	Obstruction: 60% Hematuria: 20% DRE: 80% with palpable abnormality Elevated serum PSA: 100% Cystoscopy: 50% with papillary urethral lesions	11 needle bx 2 TUR 2 aspirate	All treated by radical prostatectomy; 47% recurred after 3-18 months
Millar 1996	16	NG	72 (65-87)	Hematuria: 75% Obstruction: 19% Cystoscopy: Papillary urethral lesion: 25%, nodular urethra: 6%, normal urethra: 25% Elevated serum PSA: 56%, where median = 13.8 ng/mL (range 0 - 200)	TUR, prostatic urethral biopsy, radical prostatectomy	"Good prognosis" —one cancer-caused death at mean 3.4 year follow-up
Oxley 1998A	12	NG	76 (67-84)	Obstruction: 66% Hematuria: 33% Cystoscopy: Urethral "fronded appearance": (33%) or narrowing (66%) Skeletal mets: 33%	11 TURP 1 retropubic prostatectomy	58% dead of disease at mean of 2.4 years (range 1- 4)
Bock 1999	17	5%	64 (52-77)	NG	Radical prostatectomy and corresponding needle biopsies	NG
Brinker 1999	55	NG	69 (50-89)	Abnormal DRE: 76% Elevated PSA (median 7.9 ng/mL; range 1.5 -2719) Clinical stage T1: 23% T2a: 37% T2b: 10% T3a: 14% T3b: 2% T4: 2% M⊕: 12%	Needle biopsy series; 20 men treated by radical prostatectomy	Risk of progression at 2 years: 42%

[1]Number of cases
[2]Incidence out of all prostatic carcinomas
[3]Mean age (range)
[4]Tissue sample used for diagnosis
NG = not given

only on 2 cases it was written that a predominantly hyperechoic look, rather than the hypoechoic look of acinar adenocarcinoma, suggests the presence of a high-grade ductal adenocarcinoma (Egawa 1992).

The clinical macroscopic appearance of ductal adenocarcinoma by cystoscopy (urethroscopy) is in many cases that of an exophytic, villous or polypoid growth, with white fronds of wormlike tumor

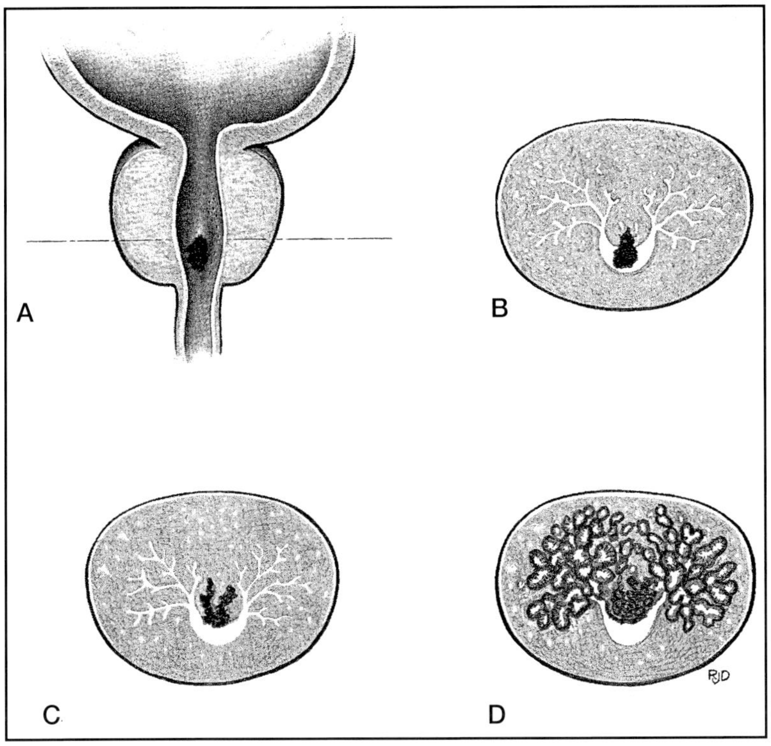

■ **f17.1** *Spread of ductal adenocarcinoma. A,B: Exophytic, "wormy", papillary projections into prostatic urethra at area of verumontanum. C: Predominantly intraductal spread at verumontanum. D: Extensive central ductal and peripheral duct-acinar growth. (Melicow 1971, with permission from Lippincott Williams and Wilkins).*

protruding into the urethra at or near the verumontanum **f17.1; t17.2**. The prostatic urethra can also appear narrowed, nodular, or normal.

The gross characteristics of ductal adenocarcinoma in resected prostatic tissue have not been defined. Many cases of ductal adenocarcinoma are diagnosed in transurethral resection of the prostate (TURP) chips (because of their central location; **t17.2**), but no gross features of ductal adenocarcinoma in this tissue sample type have been reported. Similarly, in the few reported radical prostatectomy cases (Bock 1999, Bostwick 1985, Brinker 1999, Christensen 1991, Dube 1973, Rubinowicz 2000), no mention and illustrations of the gross findings are provided, save for a single case report that shows a dilated peripheral prostatic duct filled with a nodular and papillary tumor (Rubinowicz 2000). Possible patterns of growth are illustrated in **f17.1**. Ductal adenocarcinomas often are exophytic **f17.1A, B** but can be intraductal **f17.1C** and can spread throughout the entire prostate gland **f17.1D**. This latter mode of permeation accounts for the high frequency of DREs that are suspicious for malignancy. Although ductal adenocarcinomas are classically centrally located, they can be central and peripheral or even isolated in the peripheral zone (Bock 1999, Brinker 1999).

Microscopically, 2 forms of ductal adenocarcinoma growth have been noted (Dube 1973, Melicow 1971, Millar 1996, Ro 1988B). These have been defined as adenocarcinoma of the primary prostatic ducts (or type A) and adenocarcinoma of the secondary prostatic ducts (or type B) (Dube 1973, Ro 1988B) **t17.3**). The relative frequency of occurrence of the 2 patterns is not definitively established because in one large study, type B was predominant (Dube 1973), but in another they were found with equal frequency (Ro 1988B). These 2 growth patterns are not mutually exclusive and can be mixed. Their main importance is in diagnostic recognition of ductal adenocarcinoma. The data are mixed as to whether these two patterns are associated with a different prognosis (Dube 1973, Ro 1988B). Moreover, the dividing line between them often is blurred because the patterns merge. Therefore, it does not appear necessary to distinguish between these 2 patterns (Ro 1988B).

Adenocarcinoma of the so-called primary ducts is an exuberant, complex, and branching papillary adenocarcinoma that expands and projects into or fills large, central, periurethral prostatic ducts (Dube 1973, Ro 1988B) **i17.1**. A papillary ductal adenocarcinoma should be suspected if numerous cleftlike spaces or complex branching architectural patterns are visualized **i17.2-i17.4**. The papillary nature of adenocarcinoma can easily be overlooked when frond fusion occurs **i17.5**, where only the thin, numerous fibrovascular cores and columnar shape of the tumor cells provide evidence of ductal differentiation **i17.6**. The neoplastic cells are high columnar and may be

■ **t17.3 Adenocarcinoma of Primary vs Secondary Ducts vs Mixed Ductal-Acinar Adenocarcinoma[1]**

Feature	1° Ducts (Type A)[2]	2° Ducts (Type B)[2]	Mixed Ductal-Acinar
Incidence	0.002%[3]	1.1%	4.8%
Age	Average = 69 years	Average = 69 years	NG
Symptoms	Obstruction in most patients	Obstruction in most patients	
DRE	Suspicious: 50%	Suspicious: 91%	NG
Cystoscopy	71% with villous or polypoid intraurethral tumor	6% with villous intraurethral projection; 60% with infiltrative growth suspicious for cancer	NG
Microscopic	Exuberant papillary adenocarcinoma in large central periurethral ducts. Single layer tall columnar epithelium with uniform, elongated, basal nuclei	Growth in intermediate to small ducts. Single layer to multilayered, with small papillary projections. Intraluminal eosinophilic debris present. Some cribriform areas	NG
Metastasis at presentation	50%	19%	18%
Five-year survival	43%[4,5]	24%[5]	46%[4]

[1]Data from a large, single institutional 20 year review of 4,286 cases of prostatic adenocarcinoma (Dube 1973)
Note that the cases were diagnosed from 1950-1970
[2]1° duct growth pattern has also been classified as type A, and the 2° duct pattern as type B (Ro 1988B)
[3]Data are mixed as to which pattern predominates. A second study (Werneet 1987) also found 2° duct/type B to be much more common, while a third study (Ro 1988B) reported type A = type B in frequency
[4]Survival rates similar to that of patients with acinar adenocarcinoma at that time
[5]No difference in survival rate between types A and B in a more recent study (Ro 1988B)
NG = not given

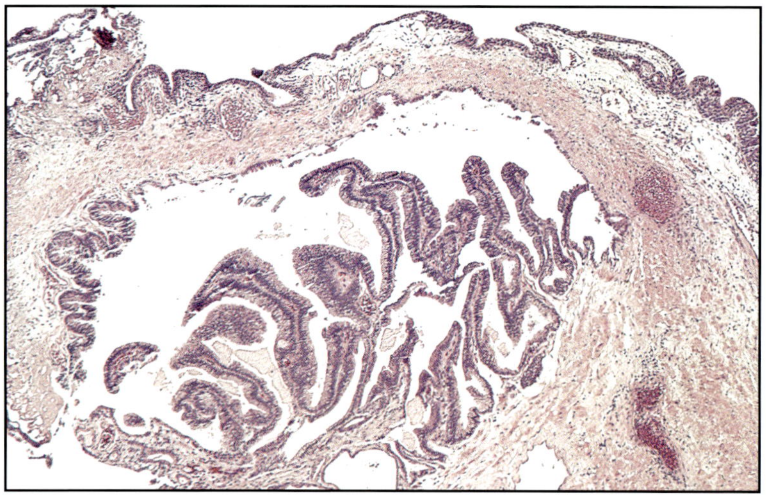

■ **i17.1** *Ductal adenocarcinoma of the prostate. Expansion of a prostatic duct by papillary adenocarcinoma. Prostatic urethral urothelium is on top.*

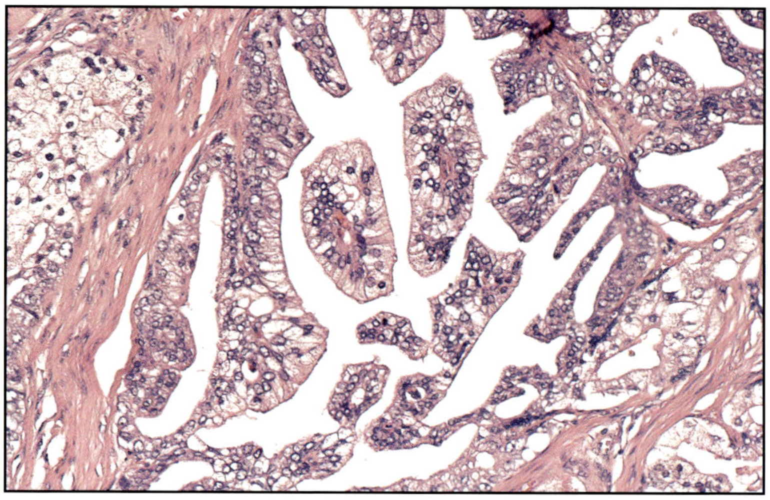

■ **i17.2** *Tall columnar neoplastic cells cover fibrovascular cores in ductal adenocarcinoma.*

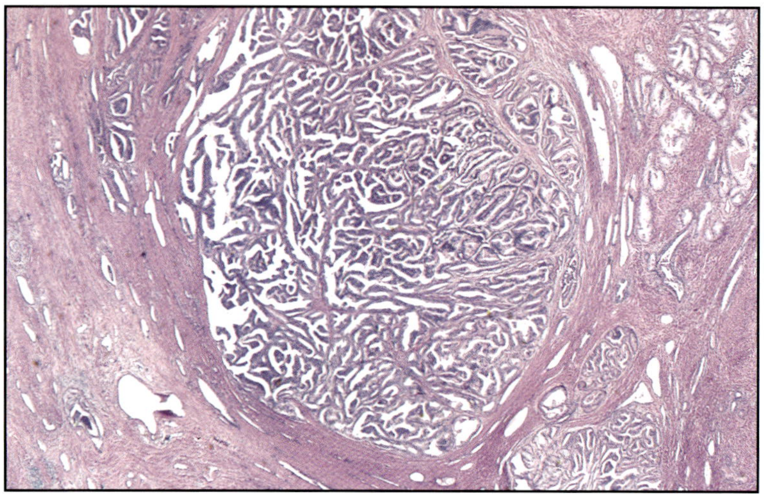

■ **i17.3** *Nodule of prostatic ductal adenocaricnoma with clefted or slit-like glandular spaces.*

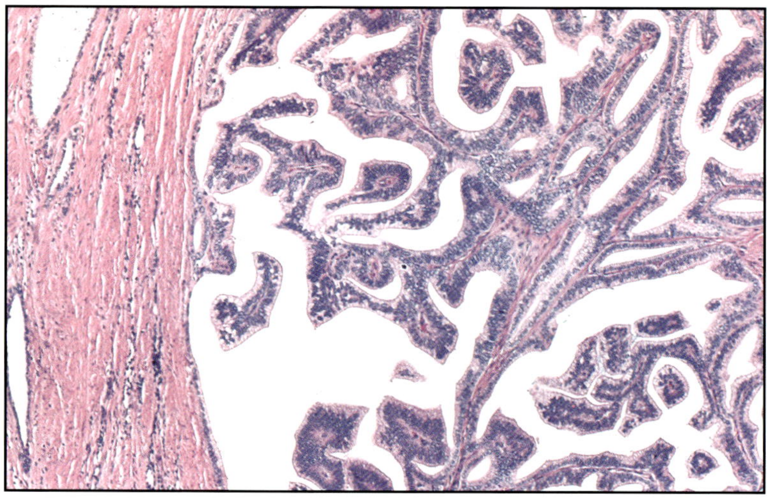

■ **i17.4** *Prostatic ductal adenocarcinoma: nodular, intracystic, complex branching growth.*

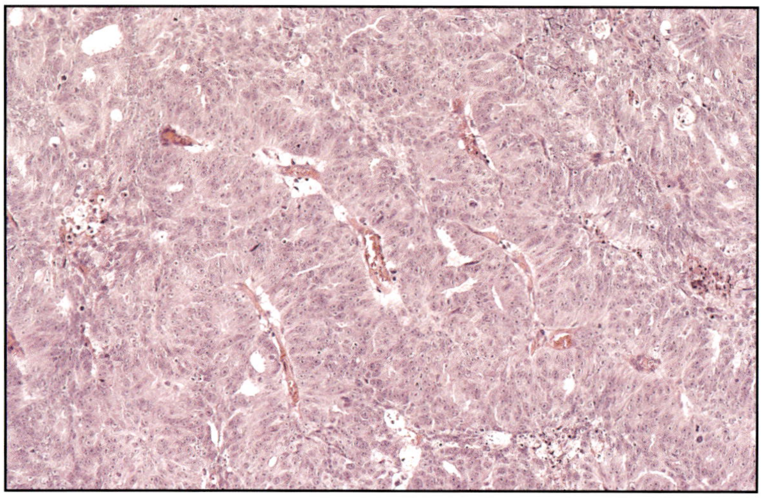

■ **i17.5** *Fused papillary prostatic duct adenocarcinoma. A few scattered glandular lumina and thin fibrovascular cores.*

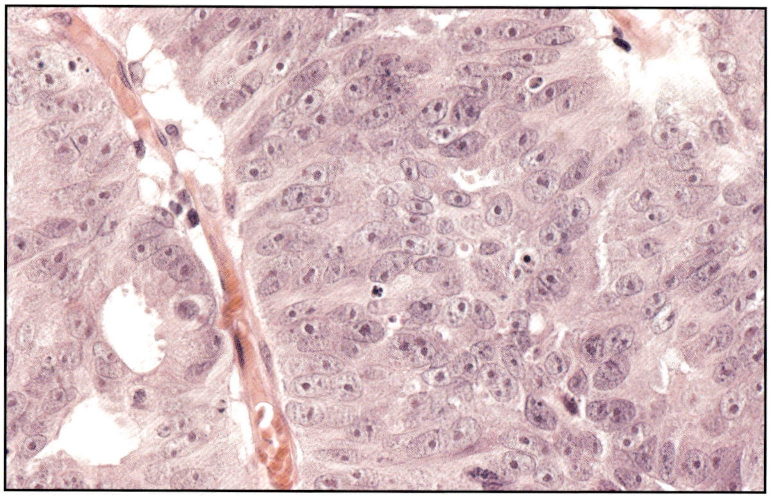

■ **i17.6** *Ductal adenocarcinoma: Cytologic features of nucleomegaly and true macronucleoli.*

single layered or multilayered. The nuclei often are basally situated and elongated, with a fairly uniform degree of nucleomegaly and true macronucleoli **i17.6, i17.7**. Cytoplasm is abundant and usually eosinophilic to amphophilic but can be vacuolated. Apocrine-like snouts may be common (Millar 1996), and subnuclear vacuoles can be seen in a few cases (Epstein 1986, Ro 1988B). Significant mucin production is not evident, and psammoma bodies, which are often detected in papillary adenocarcinomas elsewhere, are uncommon (Ro 1988B).

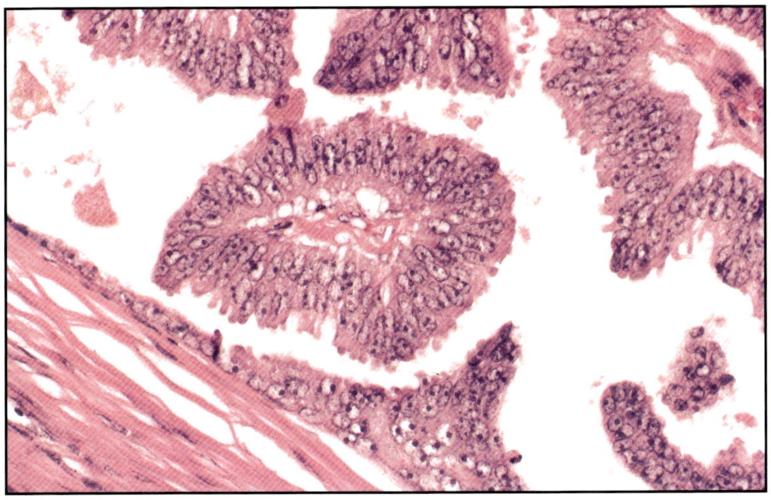

■ **i17.7** *Prostatic ductal adenocarcinoma. A papillary adenocarcinoma with mainly columnar cells and elongated nuclei.*

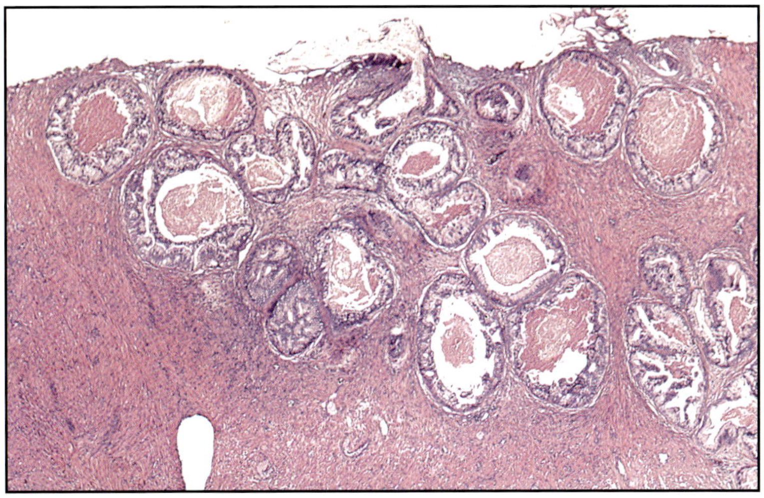

■ **i17.8** *Prostatic ductal adenocarcinoma in TURP chip.*

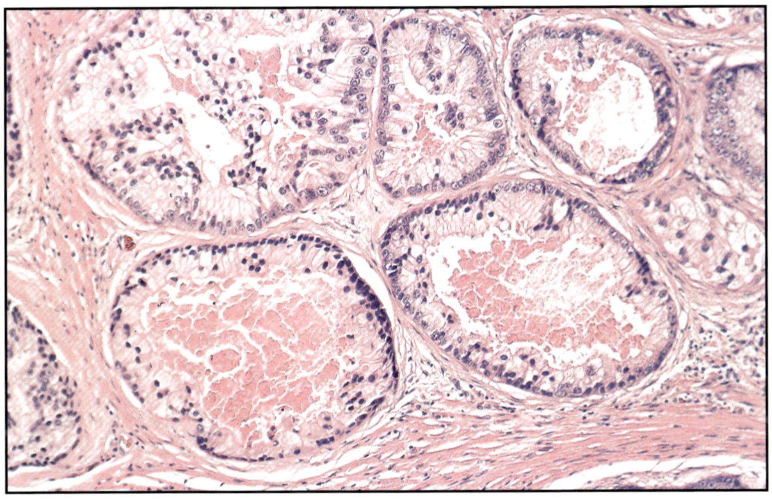

■ **i17.9** *Prostatic ductal adenocarcinoma: Eosinophilic intraluminal debris and cleared cytoplasm.*

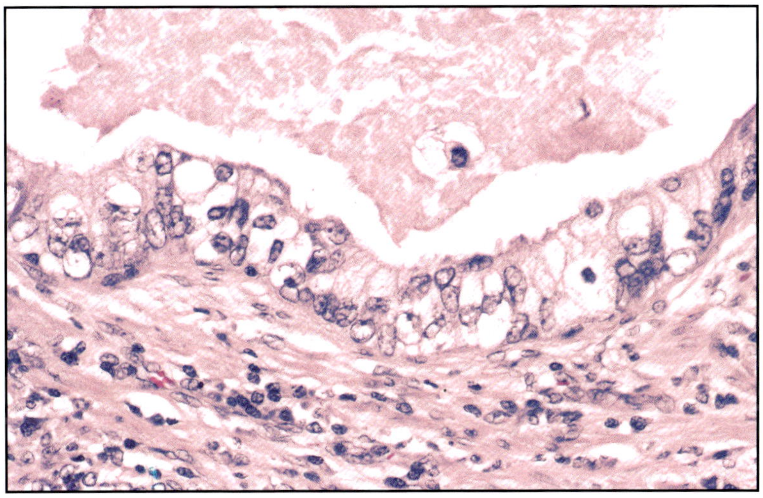

■ **i17.10** *Prostatic ductal adenocarcinoma: Flat lining layer composed of neoplastic cells with cleared cytoplasm.*

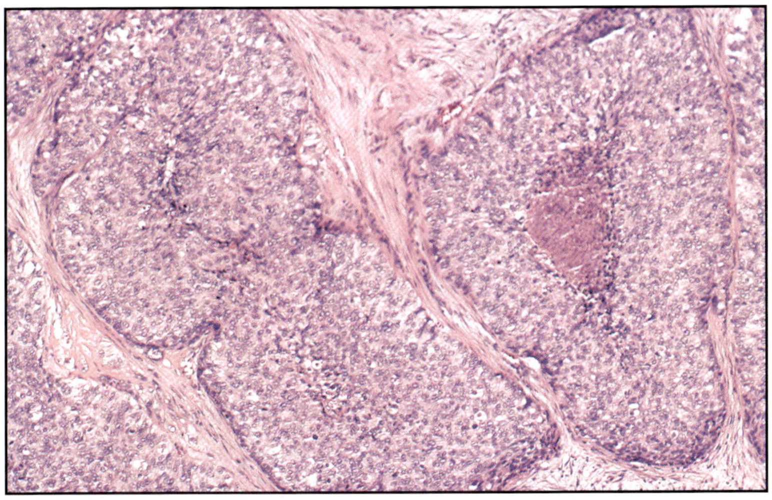

■ **i17.11** *Solid carcinoma and comedocarcinoma, with central necrosis, in prostatic ductal adenocarcinoma.*

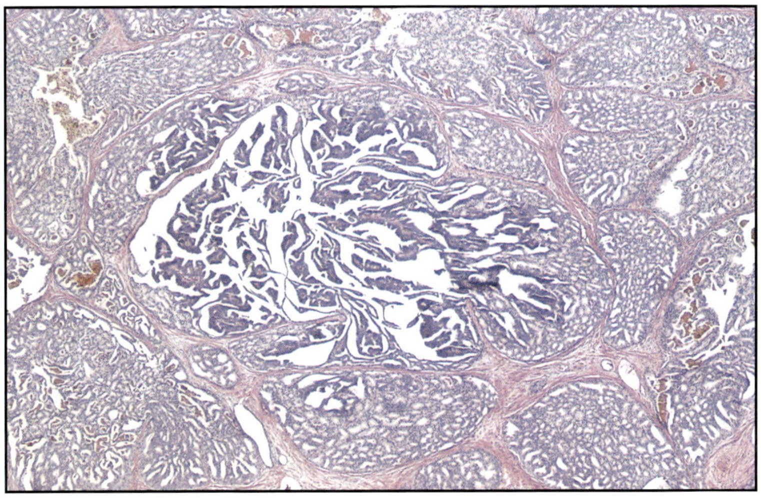

■ **i17.12** *Prostatic ductal adenocarcinoma with central papillary region, with surrounding confluent cribriform growth.*

Contrary to early reports (Melicow 1967, 1971, Tannenbaum 1975B), cilia (as found in müllerian differentiation) are not present.

Adenocarcinoma of so-called secondary prostatic ducts (type B) display an intraductal proliferation with multicentric, complex glandular, solid, and comedo patterns, often with intermediate to small-sized glandular spaces (called ducts in Dube 1973, but they could be ducts or acini) (Dube 1973, Ro 1988B) **i17.8-i17.15**. A particularly distinctive finding is cylinders of tumor with eosinophilic luminal

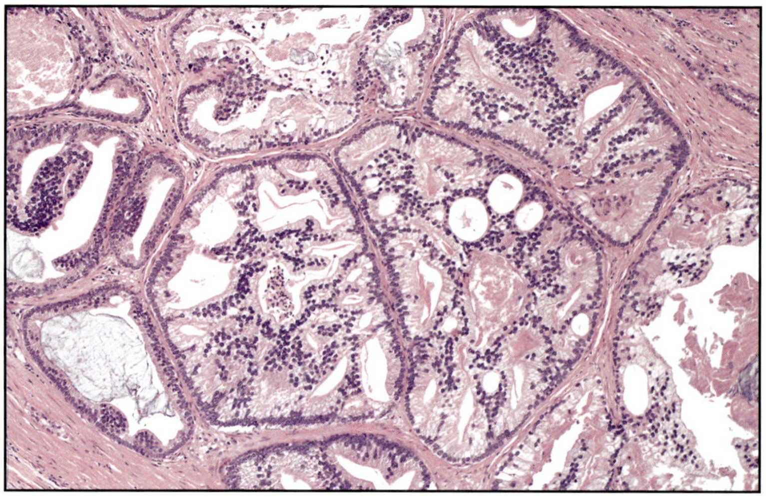

■ **i17.13** *Prostatic ductal adenocarcinoma, with cribriform arrangement of neoplastic cells.*

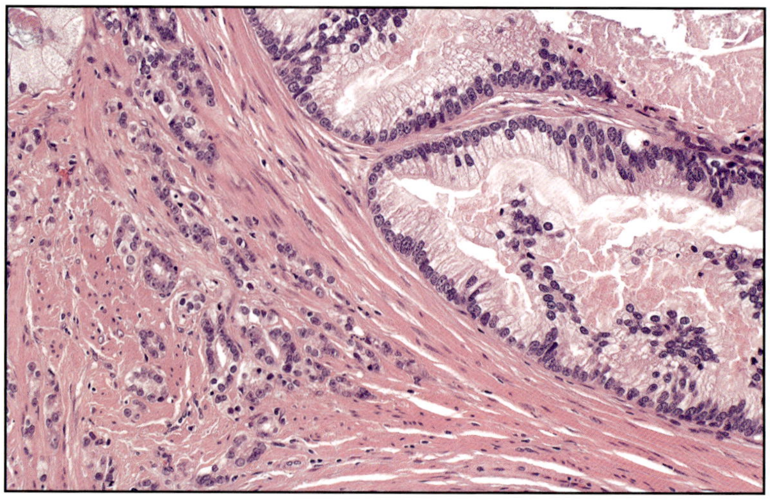

■ **i17.14** *Prostatic ductal adenocarcinoma (right) adjacent to acinar adenocarcinoma (left). The ductal component is characterized by larger glands composed of tall columnar cells with cleared cytoplasm and basal nuclei.*

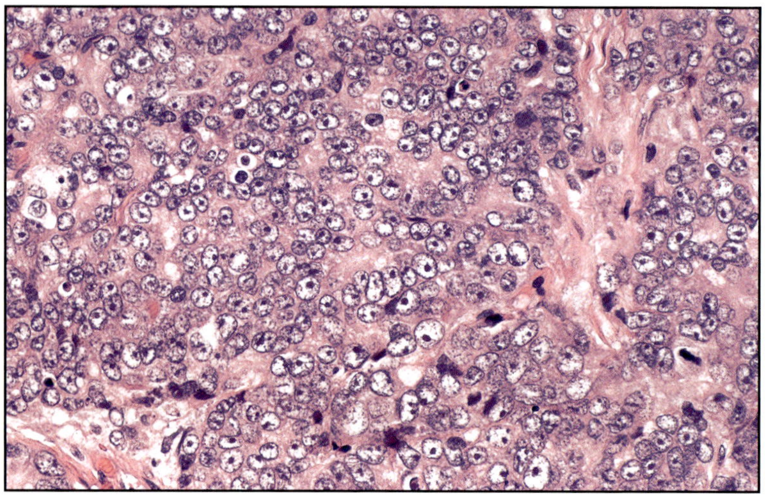

■ **i17.15** *Nuclear atypia in solid pattern ductal adenocarcinoma.*

debris **i17.8, i17.9**. This is not comedo necrosis since necrotic tumor cells are not present in the eosinophilic debris. True comedo carcinoma can be a component of ductal adenocarcinoma **i17.11**. Cribriform-papillary growth arrangements also typify this second form of prostatic ductal adenocarcinoma **i17.12, i17.13**. An additional clue that one might be dealing with a prostatic ductal adenocarcinoma is the presence of high columnar or cuboidal cells with basal nuclei and abundant, clear cytoplasm **i17.14**. Another diagnostic hint is that the glands of ductal adenocarcinoma often are embedded within a fibrotic stroma (Brinker 1999), which is unusual for small acinar adenocarcinoma. Cytologically, the nuclear atypia in this adenocarcinoma of secondary ducts can be substantial, with large, pleomorphic, and hyperchromatic nuclei (Dube 1973).

Overall, for both patterns, the carcinoma cell nuclei are moderately to severely atypical, with pleomorphism, hyperchromasia, chromatin clumping, and occasional large prominent nucleoli (Bostwick 1985, Ro 1988B). In a few cases, the nuclei may be quite uniform and bland (Brinker 1999, Millar 1996). In needle biopsy tissue, nuclear atypia may be more difficult to appreciate, as it was reported that only a minority of ductal adenocarcinoma cases exhibited hyperchromasia (41%) and nucleomegaly (12%) (Brinker 1999). Prominent nucleoli were observed in 71% of needle biopsy cases (Brinker 1999).

Mitotic activity in ductal carcinoma is variable but is higher than in most acinar adenocarcinomas, where it can be difficult to find any mitoses at all. Mitotic figures averaged about 6 per 10 high-power fields (range 2 to 10) in one series (Bostwick 1985), and in a second series (Ro 1988B), 10 of 35 cases had 10 or more mitoses per 10 high-power fields. Another quantitative study (Oxley 1998A) yielded a high mitotic count of more than 4/mm^2 in 8 of 12 cases, but the range was 0.5 to 5.5. In needle biopsy tissue, 41% of cases had mitotic figures (Brinker 1999). Atypical mitoses were common in 1 series (Bostwick 1985).

Prostatic ductal adenocarcinoma has a significant in situ component, with extension of the carcinoma inside preexisting ducts and acini, with a discontinuous to continuous layer of basal cells (Bostwick 1985, Millar 1996, Samaratunga 1997). This is true for all growth configurations: cribriform, papillary, comedo, and solid (Samaratunga 1997). Additionally, the neoplastic epithelium can merge with the pseudostratified transitional epithelium of the adjacent urethra (Dube 1973) or, uncommonly, exhibit pagetoid spread of tumor cells in benign periurethral ductal epithelium (Bostwick 1985). "Telescoping" or projections of solid masses of adenocarcinoma into benign luminal spaces can be found.

Prostatic ductal adenocarcinoma may be diagnosed in prostatic tissue in transrectal prostate needle biopsies **i17.16-i17.19**, transurethral prostatic biopsies, TURP chips **i17.8**, simple (open or suprapubic) prostatectomies (enucleations) and radical prostatectomy specimens **t17.2**. In needle biopsy tissue of prostate, papillary or cribriform structures are predominant (Brinker 1999) **t17.4**. Sometimes this proliferation is discovered at the tip of the needle core tissue **i17.17**. Stromal fibrosis and individual glands with tall columnar cells are also helpful findings **i17.18**. The columnar cells can also assume a colonic-like arrangement **i17.19**, with nuclear elongation. Usually 1 or 2 cores have cancer, with a substantial amount of tumor, with a mean, for positive cores, of 47% (range 10% to 100%) of needle core tissue involved (Brinker 1999). In one half of the cases, there is a minor coexisting acinar component, which was most often of a Gleason score of 6 or 7 (Brinker 1999). The percentage of adenocarcinoma that is ductal in needle biopsy tissue correlates with the percentage of ductal cancer in radical prostatectomy tissues: when more than 50% of the adenocarcinoma is ductal in needle core tissue, 80% of the corresponding radical prostatectomies have more than 50% ductal adenocarcinoma (Brinker 1999).

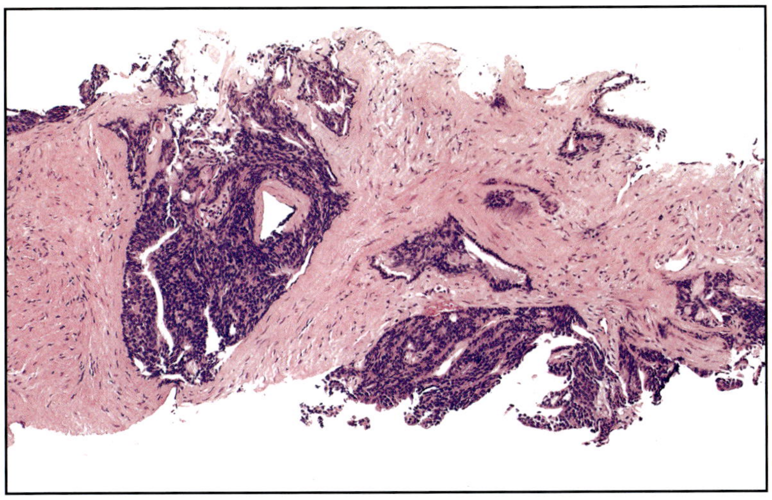

■ **i17.16** *Ductal adenocarcinoma in needle biopsy tissue.*

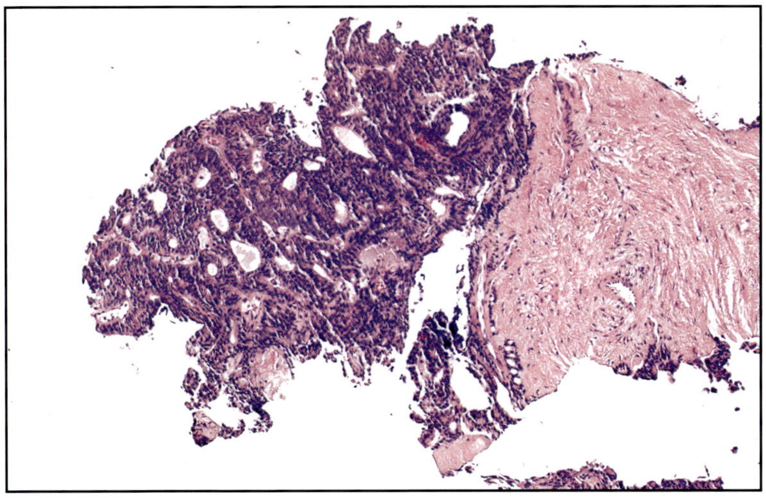

■ **i17.17** *Cribriform ductal adenocarcinoma at tip of needle core.*

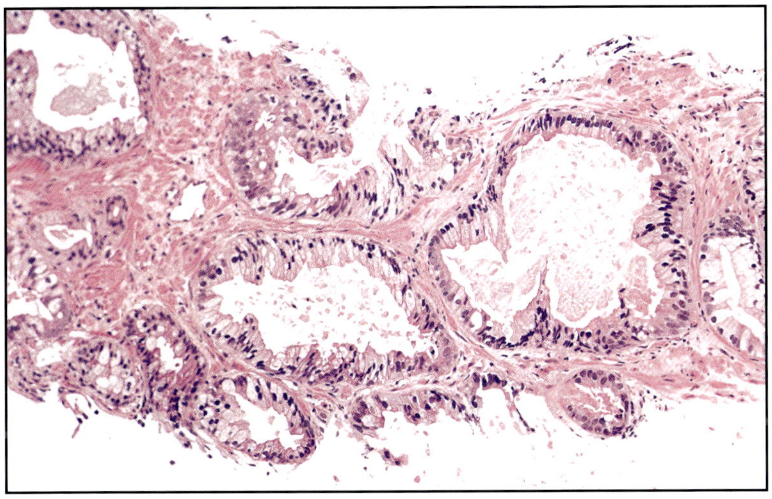

■ **i17.18** *Ductal adenocarcinoma that appears deceptively benign at lower magnification. The high columnar cells had nuclear atypia at higher power views. A few small malignant acini are also present.*

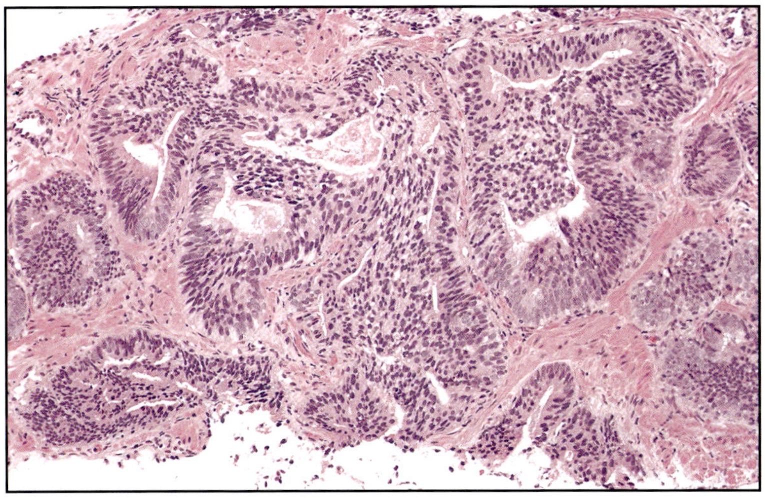

■ **i17.19** *Prostatic ductal adenocarcinoma with some resemblance to a colonic neoplasm. Prostatic origin was substantiated by strong, diffuse tumor cell immunoreactivity for PSA and PSAP.*

In radical prostatectomy specimens, the ductal adenocarcinoma consists of confluent masses of papillary or cribriform adenocarcinoma **i17.3, i17.12**, (Carney 1973) that are admixed with usual acinar adenocarcinoma **i17.14**. The ductal adenocarcinoma is almost always intimately admixed with acinar adenocarcinoma, with the proportion of the tumor showing ductal differentiation ranging from 5% to 100%. In one series (Bock 1999), the mean percentage of the tumor occupied by ductal adenocarcinoma was 29%. It is striking that in radical prostatectomy specimens ductal adenocarcinoma is predominantly located in the peripheral zone **i17.20**, with focal extension into the transition zone in only a minority of cases (Bock 1999, Brinker 1999). The intraurethral and periurethral duct extension that is characteristic of primary duct or type A tumors **t17.3** is not seen in radical prostatectomy specimens. This is undoubtedly due to selection bias, where these patients were selected for this surgery based on peripheral carcinomas diagnosed by transrectal needle biopsy. Ductal adenocarcinoma in radical prostatectomy specimens tends to be of higher stage and larger tumor size **t17.5** than pure acinar adenocarcinoma. Most ductal adenocarcinomas exhibit extraprostatic extension, whereas most pure acinar adenocarcinomas do not, and the size of ductal adenocarcinoma is about twice that of acinar adenocarcinomas (Christensen 1991). The majority of cases are high grade in the ductal and acinar components, although in almost one half of cases the acinar component is intermediate, at Gleason score 6 (Brinker 1999).

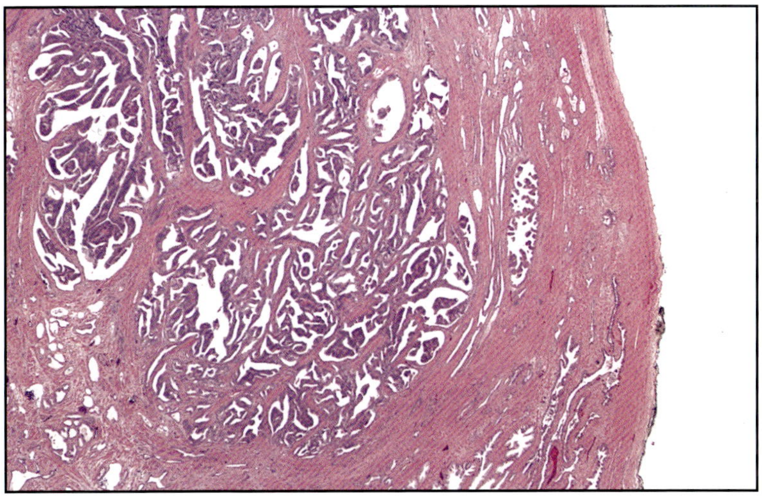

■ **i17.20** *Prostatic ductal adenocarcinoma of papillary pattern with peripheral extension. Inked peripheral surgical margin is at right.*

■ **t17.4 Ductal Adenocarcinoma in Prostate Needle Biopsy Tissue[1]**

Cribriform and/or papillary architecture most common
A minority pattern: Individual glands with tall columnar cells and elongated nuclei, resembling colonic carcinoma
Stromal fibrosis and mitoses can be found, unlike most usual acinar adenocarcinomas
Nuclear atypia: Prominent nucleoli in 71%, hyperchromasia in 41%, nucleomegaly in 12%
Perineural invasion: 22%
Coexistent acinar component in one-half of cases

[1]Brinker 1999

■ **t17.5 Ductal Adenocarcinoma in Radical Prostatectomy Tissues**

Limited number of cases studied [n = 59 in 5 reports (Dube 1973, Christensen 1991, Egawa 1992, Bock 1999, Brinker 1999)]
Cribriform and papillary structures mainly in peripheral zone
Mixed with acinar component in vast majority of cases
Most have high grade element: mean Gleason score of ductal adenocarcinoma = 7 (range 5-9); acinar component usually Gleason score 6-7
Large size: Mean volume 5.2 cc (range 0.1cc-35cc) and mean % carcinoma = 23% (range 3%-73%)
Most (65%-93%) exhibit extraprostatic extension, with seminal vesicle involvement in 10%-40% and positive margins in 20%-47%

Ductal adenocarcinoma spreads outside the prostate gland in the same fashion as pure acinar adenocarcinoma (Bostwick 1985, Brinker 1999, Christensen 1991, Dube 1973, Lemberger 1984, Oxley 1998A, Ro 1988B). The papillary and cribriform growths can involve periprostatic soft tissue, seminal vesicles, pelvic lymph nodes **i17.21,** and distant sites **i17.22, i17.23**, including lung (Copeland 2002) and bone. Ductal adenocarcinomas appear to have a propensity to metastasize to testis, penis and lung (Copeland 2002, Tu 2002). Mixed ductal-acinar adenocarcinomas can penetrate outside the prostate gland and metastasize as pure ductal adenocarcinoma, pure acinar adenocarcinoma, or mixed ductal-acinar adenocarcinoma (Christensen 1991, Ro 1988B).

Ductal adenocarcinoma is admixed with usual acinar adenocarcinoma in a majority of cases. This does not represent dual carcinomas of the prostate in the same gland (Rotterdam 1975) but rather probably reflects the variability in growth of a single prostatic neoplasm. Although it has been written that ductal adenocarcinoma should be diagnosed when it is predominant, occupying more than 50% (Samaratunga 1997) or 80% (Ro 2000) of the tumor, and that adenocarcinoma with ductal differentiation or features should be diagnosed when less than 50% of the tumor is ductal (Samaratunga 1997), there is no evidence linking percentage ductal component to patient outcome. In one series, patients with 100% secondary duct or type B adenocarcinoma had a worse prognosis than those with mixed ductal-acinar and pure primary duct adenocarcinoma (Dube 1973), but in a second series, patients with type A and type B adenocarcinoma had a similar survival (Ro 1988B). An approach this author favors would be to diagnose ductal adenocarcinoma if the neoplasm is pure ductal and mixed ductal-acinar if both components are present, with a comment describing the percentage of the tumor that is ductal. Rare reported admixtures of ductal adenocarcinoma with other histologic types of carcinomas include ductal adenocarcinoma with sarcomatoid carcinoma (Ma 1998, Millar 1996), mucinous pools (Ro 1988B) and mucinous carcinoma (Nishimura 1995), and transitional cell carcinoma (Kopelson 1978).

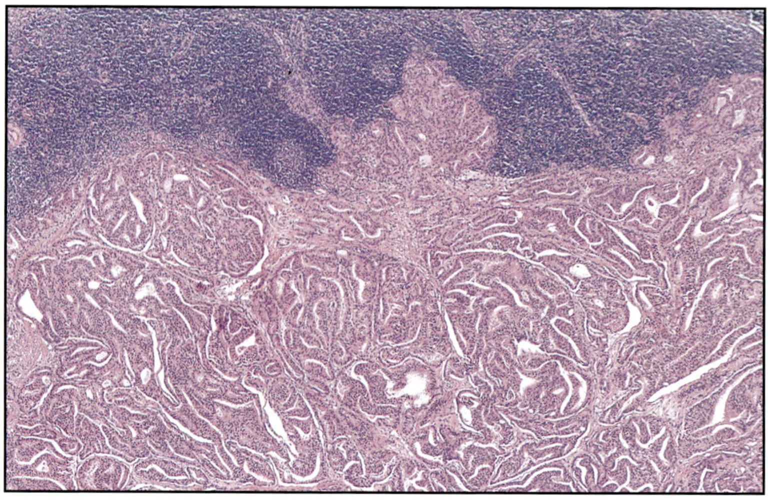

■ **i17.21** *Prostatic ductal adenocarcinoma of papillary pattern in pelvic lymph node.*

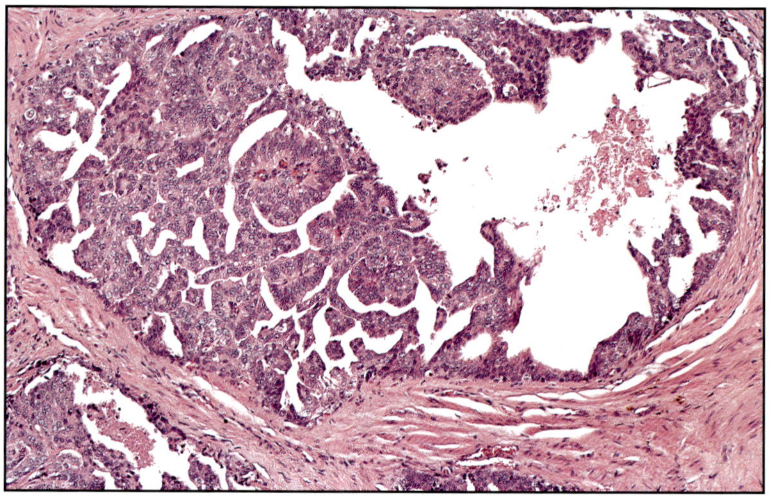

■ **i17.22** *Ductal prostatic adenocarcinoma metastatic to penis. The patient presented with a penile mass of unknown primary origin. A papillary growth configuration is evident.*

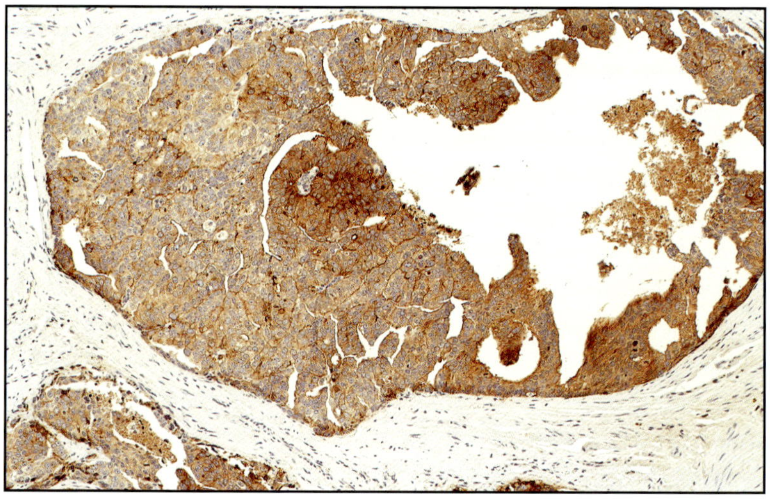

■ **i17.23** *PSA immunoreactivity in the metastatic deposit of prostatic ductal adenocarcinoma depicted in* **i17.22**.

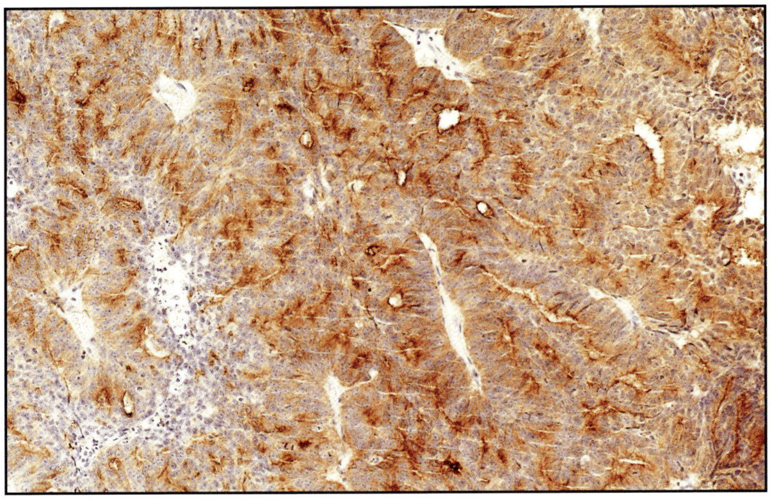

■ **i17.24** *PSA immunolabeling of this prostatic ductal adenocaricnoma exhibits luminal accentuation.*

Histologic grading of ductal adenocarcinoma has been inconsistently performed, including lack of any grading and use of unspecified grading systems, using such terms such as grade 1 or well- or moderately differentiated adenocarcinoma. Authors of the largest series used their own 4-tiered grading scheme (Dube 1973). In some studies, only the acinar and not the ductal component was graded. Gleason grading of ductal adenocarcinoma has been performed in only a few studies (Bircan 1991, Bock 1999, Egawa 1992, Lemberger 1984, Rubinowicz 2000). The assigned grade is moderately to poorly differentiated adenocarcinoma of Gleason scores 5 to 10. In the largest series (with $n = 17$) with specific data on individual patients, the mean Gleason score was 7, with a range of 5 to 9 (Bock 1999). Gleason wrote that ductal adenocarcinomas ("intraductal carcinoma and endometrial carcinoma") should be graded using the Gleason system, with application of the same guidelines as other prostatic adenocarcinomas (Gleason 1990). It has been recommended that cribriform ductal adenocarcinoma be graded as pattern 3, and the comedocarcinoma ductal pattern should be graded as pattern 5 (Bostwick 1994). Gleason pattern 4 ductal adenocarcinoma with fused microacini in a cribriform arrangement and solid Gleason pattern 5 also clearly exist. So the range of Gleason patterns that should be applied to a ductal adenocarcinoma component is 3 to 5 (and score of 6 to 10). For mixed ductal-acinar adenocarcinomas, separate grades should not be given but rather a combined score, just as for pure acinar adenocarcinomas. The ductal component usually is of higher grade than the acinar proliferation (Ro 1988B).

Special studies used to characterize ductal adenocarcinoma include histochemistry (Bostwick 1985, Dube 1973, Küllü 1991, Ro 1988B, Zaloudek 1976), immunohistochemistry, electron microscopy (Bostwick 1985, Ro 1988B, Tannenbaum 1975B, Walther 1985, Zaloudek 1976), and DNA quantitation by image cytometry (Christensen 1991). Histochemical studies have documented the presence of acid phosphatase (Dube 1973, Zaloudek 1976) in ductal carcinoma cells, but only minimal to faint neutral and acidic mucin staining using periodic acid-Schiff (PAS) with diastase and Alcian blue, respectively (Bostwick 1985, Dube 1973, Küllü 1991, Ro 1988B), along the apical border and inside lumina. Intracytoplasmic mucin was not evident. This mucin staining profile is different from acinar adenocarcinomas, which are apt to be mucin-positive by histochemistry. However, associated extracellular mucinous pools, seen in 3 cases, stained positively for PAS with diastase and mucicarmine. The immunophenotype of prostatic ductal adenocarcinoma is similar to that of acinar adenocarcinoma. Although they are heterogenous in stain distribution and intensity, immunostains for PSA and prostate-specific acid phosphatase (PSAP) are almost always positive **i17.23, i17.24** in both primary and metastatic sites (Copeland 2002, Fujino 1998). As in acinar adenocarcinomas, estrogen receptor immunostaining is negative (Oxley 1998A), and a low percentage of ductal adenocarcinoma cases stain for carcinoembryonic antigen (CEA) (Bostwick 1985, Lee 1994, Ro 1988B) and p53 (Oxley 1998A). Androgen receptor immunoreactivity has been detected in a high percentage of ductal adenocarcinomas (Oxley 1998A). There are differences between ductal and acinar adenocarcinomas in the Ki67 and 34βE12 immunoprofiles. In accord with mitotic counting on hematoxylin and eosin (H&E)-stained sections, the Ki67 labeling index appears to be higher in ductal adenocarcinomas (Ali-Fehmi 2001, Oxley 1998A), but it is not clear whether this is a statistically significant difference. The 34βE12 immunohistochemical reaction with basal cells is different because basal cells are, by definition, absent in acinar adenocarcinoma, but some allow basal cells in the intraductal component of ductal adenocarcinoma (Brinker 1999, Samaratunga 1997). Despite the presence of basal cells, certain authors would still diagnose ductal adenocarcinoma (Brinker 1999), whereas for acinar carcinomas the in situ proliferation phase is designated high-grade prostatic intraepithelial neoplasia (PIN). Electron microscopy of ductal adenocarcinoma substantiates prostatic rather than müllerian differentiation. Light cells, with secretory droplets, lipid-laden vacuoles, and pinocytic vesicles, and dark cells with membrane-bound organelles are seen. No ciliated cells are visualized. Finally, the DNA ploidy profiles of ductal adenocarcinoma do not differ substantially from those of acinar adenocarcinoma (Christensen 1991).

The differential diagnosis of prostatic ductal adenocarcinoma includes benign prostatic urethral polyps, nephrogenic adenoma, urethral villous adenoma, prostatic acinar adenocarcinoma, high-grade PIN, transitional cell carcinoma, and colonic adenocarcinoma. Benign prostatic urethral polyps can exhibit intraurethral polypoid growth, just as for some ductal adenocarcinomas, but the lining prostatic epithelium is cytologically bland, with both secretory columnar cells and basal cells identified (Chapter 23). Papillary and fused cribriform masses, with high columnar cells, suggest ductal over acinar differentiation. However, cribriform growth and tall columnar cells with basally located nuclei, are not specific for ductal differentiation (Humphrey 1998, McNeal 1996, Rubin 1998). Tall columnar cells with cleared cytoplasm can be present in pseudohyperplastic (Humphrey 1998) and well-differentiated adenocarcinomas, and cribriform adenocarcinomas can be acinar. This overlap may account for some of the difficulties in interobserver agreement on the diagnosis of ductal adenocarcinoma. Papillary adenocarcinoma, with or without exophytic intraurethral extension, is the central finding in the diagnosis of ductal adenocarcinoma. The in situ or intraductal component of ductal adenocarcinoma differs from high-grade PIN in that it may exhibit necrosis and solid areas of growth. Cribriform high-grade PIN may be difficult, and occasionally impossible, to separate from ductal adenocarcinoma with cribriform intraductal spread. Features that would favor ductal adenocarcinoma in needle biopsy include associated papillary tumor, stromal fibrosis, and large, confluent back-to-back cribriform glands (Brinker 1999). Transitional cell (urothelial) carcinoma can be confused with prostatic ductal adenocarcinoma because of its capacity to grow as papillary carcinoma in the urethra and prostatic ducts and because of comedocarcinoma patterns generated by in situ spread in prostatic ducts and acini. However, cells of transitional cell carcinoma do not appear secretory, do not form cribriform structures, and are only rarely associated with an intimately admixed prostatic acinar adenocarcinoma. In cases that are not clearly diagnostic by examination of H&E-stained sections, immunostains for PSA and PSAP, which are positive in almost all cases of prostatic ductal adenocarcinoma but not transitional cell carcinoma should be helpful. (A thrombomodulin immunostain tentatively appears to be helpful; in preliminary reports it stains transitional cell carcinoma [in 91% of cases] but not prostatic ductal adenocarcinoma (Ordóñez 1998, Oxley 1998B]. Further validation of the sensitivity and specificity of this immunoreaction is needed.) Finally, prostatic ductal adenocarcinoma with crowded individual glands lined by pseudostratified columnar epithelium may simulate enteric epithelium **i17.19**. However, colonic adenocarcinoma rarely involves the prostate in the absence of clinically known disease. PSA and PSAP immunostains are of aid here. A diagnosis of metastatic prostatic ductal adenocarcinoma in a man may be missed if one does not think of a metastatic papillary adenocarcinoma of unknown primary origin as potentially emanating from the prostate. We have seen cases of metastatic prostatic ductal adenocarcinoma in lung (Copeland 2002) and mediastinal lymph nodes that mimicked primary lung adenocarcinoma. Prostatic ductal papillary adenocarcinoma involving the bladder by metastasis through lymphovascular channels or direct extension could easily be confused with a primary transitional cell carcinoma of the bladder. In cases such as these, one should inquire about the clinical findings (such as history of prostate cancer, serum PSA level, and cystoscopic appearance of the bladder). Also, PSA and PSAP immunostains should always be included in an immunohistochemical nuclear panel as part of the workup of metastatic adenocarcinoma of unknown primary in a man.

In most studies, the outcome for men with prostatic ductal adenocarcinoma is worse than the outcome for men with prostatic acinar adenocarcinoma **t17.2**. Survival and response to therapy appear to be related to stage. Many patients with prostatic ductal adenocarcinoma present with large tumors and advanced stage, including bony metastasis; this may account for the poor prognosis. Some patients respond to radical prostatectomy, hormonal therapy, and radiotherapy (Brinker 1999, Ro 1988B). Factors other than stage that predict outcome have not been well characterized. In needle biopsy tissue only the extent of tumor correlated with time to biochemical failure (Brinker 1999). It is not known whether the combination of Gleason grade (including the ductal component), pretreatment serum PSA, and clinical stage are helpful in determining response to treatment, as is the case for acinar adenocarcinoma.

The origin of prostatic ductal adenocarcinoma remains unsettled. The name *ductal* may not be a completely accurate label because this adenocarcinoma can arise peripherally and could originate within acinar units. It is now well established that prostatic ductal adenocarcinoma does not spring from the prostatic utricle. Ductal adenocarcinoma has been reported to arise in a single case of villous polyp (Walker 1982). A few (n = 3) cases of prostatic papillary hyperplasia near the urethra have been described (Ito 1995, Sogbein 1989), but it is not known whether there is a relationship of this proliferation with prostatic ductal adenocarcinoma. Similarly, there is no evidence implicating PIN as a precursor for prostatic ductal adenocarcinoma. In an animal model of ductal prostatic adenocarcinoma (induced in rats treated with testosterone and estradiol-17ß or diethylstilbestrol), atypical hyperplasia in the periurethral prostatic ducts appears to be the precursor proliferation (Bosland 1995).

[17.2] Mucinous (Colloid) Adenocarcinoma

Mucinous prostatic adenocarcinoma is defined as adenocarcinoma with at least 25% of tumor consisting of lakes of extracellular mucin, with exclusion of a nonprostatic origin **t17.6**. When it was so defined, the incidence in 3 large series was 0.2% (or 27 cases of mucinous adenocarcinoma out of 11 100 cases of prostatic carcinoma) (Dhom 1990, Epstein 1985, Ro 1990). The incidence figure of 1.9% (Brooks 1986) must be an overestimate because only about 60 well-documented cases have been reported (Saito 1999). Since the initial description by Boyd in 1881 (Boyd 1881), most published reports have been on single case reports, with only a few series available for analysis **t17.7**. When rigorously defined, mucinous adenocarcinoma is one of the rarer variants of prostatic adenocarcinoma.

Clinically, the average age for men diagnosed with mucinous adenocarcinoma is similar to that of acinar adenocarcinoma at 66, with a range of 32 to 93 (Saito 1999). Most patients present with obstructive symptoms and, less commonly, irritative symptoms and hematuria (Saito 1999). The DRE often is abnormal, with a palpable mass. Substantially elevated serum PSA levels (mean = 271 ng/mL) have been detected in several patients at presentation (Lopez 1995, Outwater 1992, Ro 1990, Teichman 1994). In only a few cases (n = 3) has the primary tumor been studied by CT (Dunnick 1982) or magnetic resonance imaging (Outwater 1992) scanning; in the latter procedure, the T2-weighted signal intensity of primary prostatic mucinous adenocarcinoma was higher than that of typical acinar adenocarcinoma. The clinical stage at presentation often is advanced: in one series (Ro 1990), all patients presented with locally advanced (stage C) or metastatic (stage D) disease.

Mucinous adenocarcinoma has been diagnosed in needle aspirates, needle biopsy tissue, transurethrally resected chips, open (enucleation) prostatectomy tissue, and a few radical prostatectomy specimens. It is not feasible to establish a definitive diagnosis of mucinous adenocarcinoma in prostate needle biopsy because it is not possible to determine whether at least 25% of the entire neoplasm is mucinous, based solely on needle biopsy sampling. However, one should certainly note whether mucinous features (mucin lakes) are present in adenocarcinoma in needle biopsy.

The gross findings of mucinous prostatic adenocarcinoma are limited to a few communications (Elbadawi 1979,Proia 1981, Franks 1964, Lopez 1995, Odom 1986) **t17.8**. Open or radical prostatectomy tissues were described as having opalescent, sticky, and gelatinous cut surfaces. Grossly evident tumor measured 5.5 and 2 cm in greatest dimension in 2 cases, and an ulcerated, necrotic mass replaced the prostate in a third (Franks 1964, Lopez 1995, Odom 1986). The tumor was multinodular (Lopez 1995) and cystic (Proia 1981) in single examples.

Microscopically, the prototypical mucinous adenocarcinoma exhibits tumor cells floating or embedded in prominent lakes or

■ t17.6 Mucinous Adenocarcinoma of Prostate

Also previously called mucus-forming, mucogenic, mucoid, gelatinous or colloid adenocarcinoma
At least 25% of tumor with lakes of extracellular tumor = mucinous adenocarcinoma
Less than 25% mucinous component = adenocarcinoma with mucinous features
Intraluminal mucin without lakes of mucin ≠ mucinous adenocarcinoma
Nonprostatic mucinous adenocarcinoma primary should be excluded

■ **t17.7 Mucinous Adenocarcinoma of Prostate: Clinical Features in Largest Series**

Study	No.[1]	Incidence[2]	Age[3]	Presentation	Sample	Outcome
Sika 1964	7	NG	68 (55-72)	Prostatism (4) Back pain (2)	PP (3)[4] TURP (2) RPP (1) autopsy (1)	Survival 1-4 years
Epstein 1985	6	0.4%	62 (46-82)	Obstruction (5) Hematuria (2) Lymphadenopathy (1)	TURP (5) autopsy (1)	Survival 1 month to 8 years
Ro 1990	12	0.4%	66 (57-81)	Obstruction Hematuria Irritative symptoms Stage C (3) Stage D (5) Serum PSA mean = 369 ng/mL for 3 patients tested	TURP	58% died of disease at 56 months

[1]Number of cases
[2]Incidence out of total number of prostatic carcinomas
[3]Mean age (range)
[4]Abbreviations: PP = perineal prostatectomy; TURP = transurethral resection of prostate, RPP = retropubic prostatectomy

■ **t17.8 Mucinous Adenocarcinoma of Prostate: Pathologic Features**

Grossly: Gelatinous cut surface
Microscopically: Cribriform nests or cords, strands, papillae, tubules or acini of tumor cells floating in mucin lakes
Cytologically bland nuclei, occasional nucleoli, rare mitoses
Gleason grade most commonly high-grade pattern 4
Immunophenotype: PSA+, PSAP+, CEA-

pools of extracellular mucin that represents at least 25% of the tumor **i17.25-i17.31**. (This 25% cutoff is strictly a visual inspection ["eyeball"] estimate and does not entail morphometric or computer-assisted image analysis quantitation.) The proportion of mucinous carcinoma varies from 25% to 90%, with an average of 59% in one series (Ro 1990). Fibrous, stromal strands **i17.26** may separate areas of mucin, and collagenous micronodules can also be seen in about one third of mucin lakes. The mucin-stromal interface can be sharp and rounded **i17.25, i17.28, i17.29**, or the mucinous component can merge into an infiltrative small acinar component **i17.30**. Cribriform or gyriform arrangements are the dominant architectural patterns of tumor cells in the mucinous lakes (Epstein 1985, Ro 1990), although nests (McNeal 1991), cords or strands (Epstein 1985, Sika 1964), papillae (Elbadawi 1979), acini or tubules (Alfthan 1970, Elbadawi 1979, Epstein 1985) **i17.27**, and signet-ring cells (Alfthan 1970, Manne 1989, Uyama 1979) have also been identified. (The presence of signet-ring adenocarcinoma cells should be considered diagnostic of the signet-ring carcinoma variant, even if these cells are found in mucinous areas.) Cytologically, the tumor cell nuclei appear bland with finely dispersed chromatin, occasional prominent nucleoli, and rare mitoses (Elbadawi 1979, Epstein 1985, Ro 1990). The nonmucinous component can show a variety of patterns, including acinar, cribriform, comedo, solid, and hypernephroid patterns (Epstein 1985, Ro 1990). The mean Gleason score of the nonmucinous carcinoma was 7 in one series (Ro 1990), with a range of 5 to 9. The Gleason grade of mucinous adenocarcinoma typically is high-grade, pattern 4 (Bostwick 1994, McNeal 1991), although patterns 3 and 5 have also been detected (Epstein 1985, Lopez 1995, Manne 1989, Outwater 1992, Teichman 1994). The histologic appearance of metastatic deposits of mucinous prostatic adenocarcinoma can be identical to the mucinous or acinar component of the primary tumor (Ro 1990).

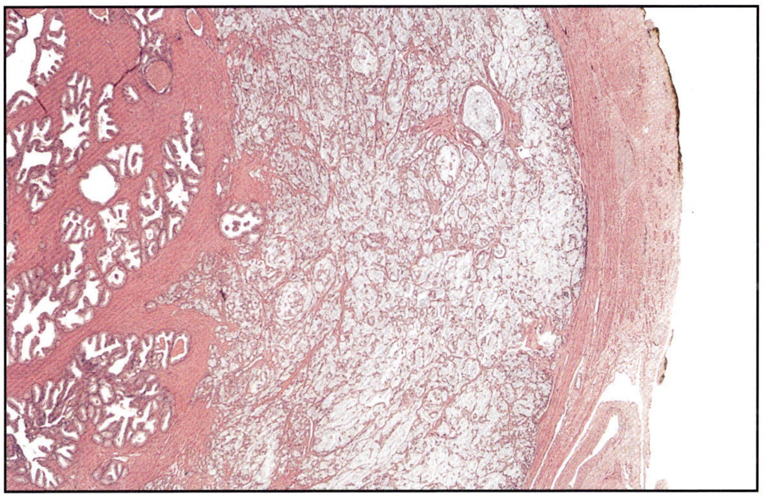

■ **i17.25** *Mucinous adenocarcinoma with large pools of blue mucin in peripheral zone. A minor acinar component was evident elsewhere in this radical prostatectomy case.*

The most important special study is immunohistochemical staining for PSA and PSAP to substantiate that the mucinous adenocarcinoma is prostatic. Mucinous prostatic adenocarcinoma is positive for these 2 markers (Epstein 1985, Ishibashi 1992, Lee 1990, Lopez 1995, Manne 1989, Nagakura 1986, Odom 1986, Proia 1981, Rodriguez Fernandez 1992, Saez 1998, Saito 1999, Watarai1994) and is negative for CEA (Lee 1990, Lopez 1995, Odom 1986, Ro 1990), which is often expressed in nonprostatic adenocarcinomas. Other special studies have included histochemical characterization of the mucin and electron microscopic examination of a single case (Proia 1981). By histochemical staining, the mucin lakes and intraluminal spaces in mucinous prostatic adenocarcinoma are positive with Alcian blue (at pH 2.7), mucicarmine, and PAS with and without diastase (Alfthan 1970, Proia 1981, Franks 1964, Hsueh 1984, Joshi 1967, Lee 1990, McNeal 1991, Odom 1986, Ro 1990, Saez 1998, Uyama 1979) and negative with Alcian blue at pH 0.9, indicating the presence of neutral and nonsulfated acidic mucins. Acidic mucins that are 0-acylated are the major secretory

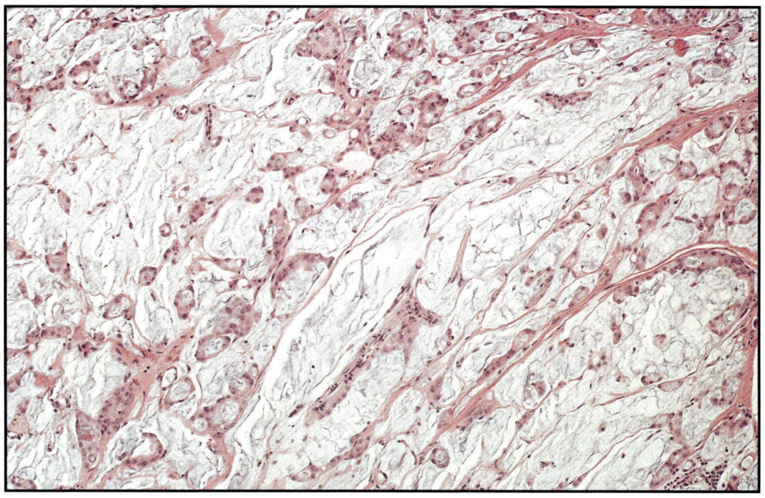

■ **i17.26** *Thin, fibrous strands in mucinous adenocarcinoma.*

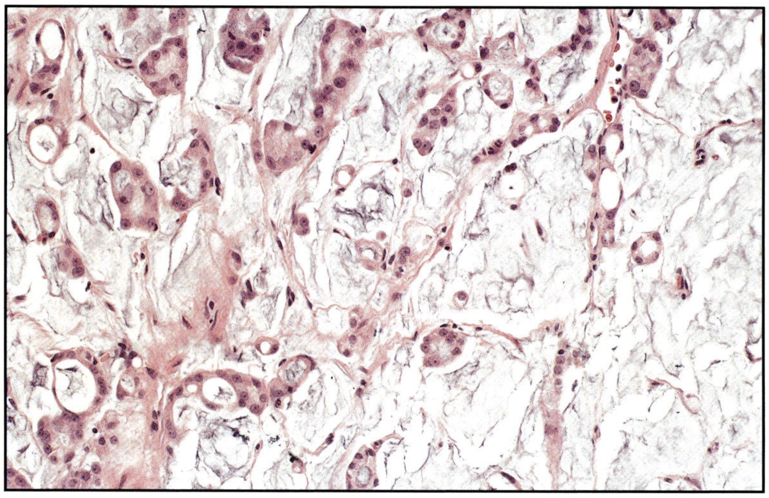

■ **i17.27** *Malignant tubules "floating" in mucin in mucinous adenocarcinoma.*

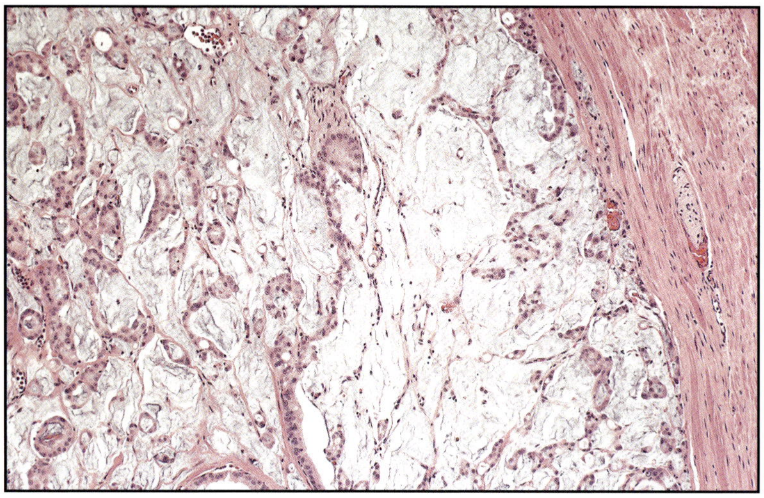

■ **i17.28** *Mucinous adenocarcinoma with sharp tumor-stromal interface.*

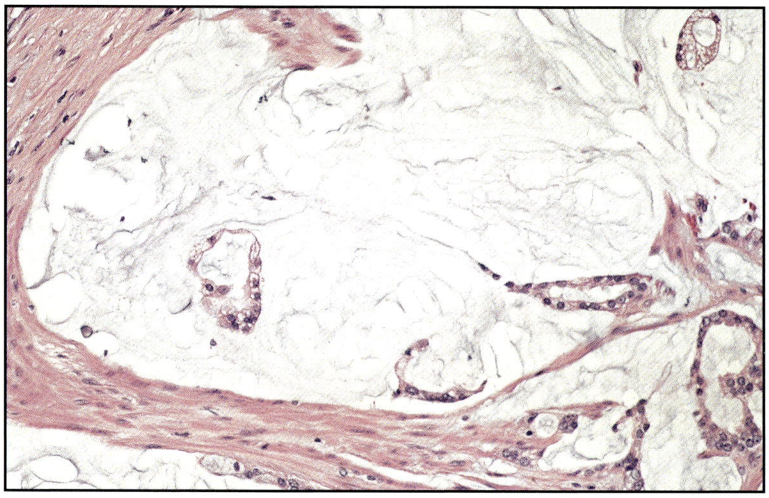

■ **i17.29** *Mucinous adenocarcinoma exhibiting rounded mucin-stromal junction, without epithelial lining.*

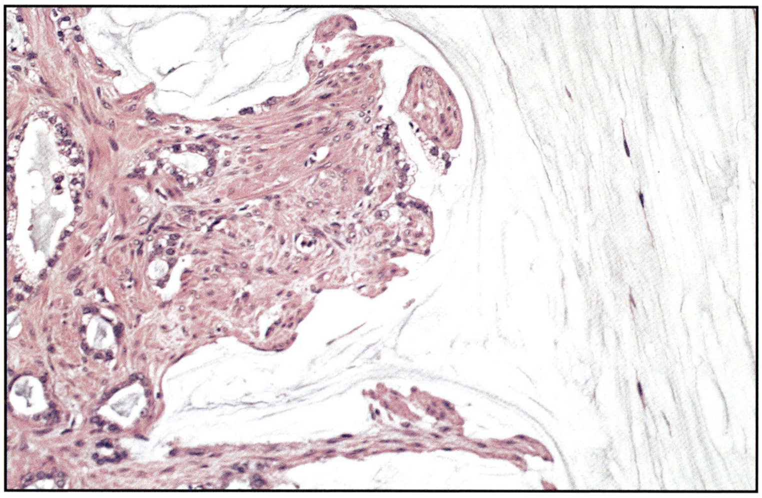

■ **i17.30** *Mucinous adenocarcinoma, with large collection of mucin adjacent to small acinar adenocarcinoma.*

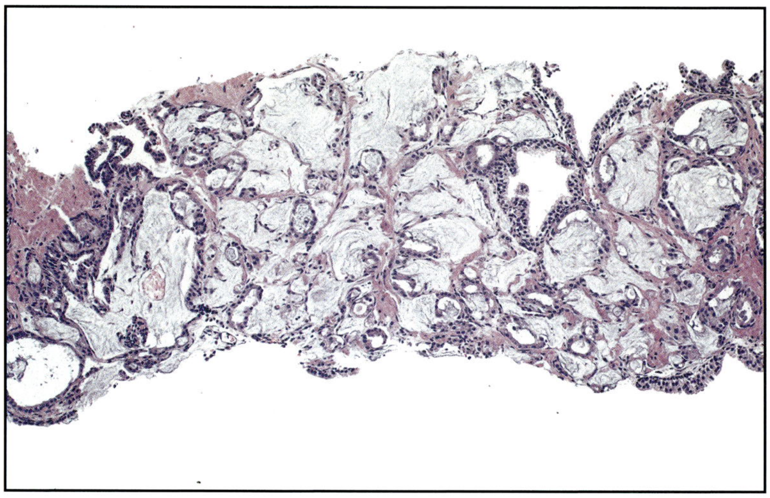

■ **i17.31** *Mucinous adenocarcinoma in needle biopsy tissue. It is not known if amount of mucinous carcinoma in needle biopsy predicts amount of mucinous carcinoma in the whole gland.*

product (Saez 1998). The mucin staining profile of mucinous adenocarcinoma is in general similar to acinar adenocarcinomas. Furthermore, the 0-acylation in mucinous prostatic adenocarcinoma is associated with high-grade acinar adenocarcinomas of Gleason score 8 to 10 (Saez 1998). Ultrastructurally, mucinous carcinoma cells contain mucigen granules (Proia 1981), but mucin histochemical stains do not typically highlight intracellular mucin (Ro 1990). It is not known whether there is a genotypic difference between mucinous and nonmucinous adenocarcinomas of the prostate; in a single case of mucinous adenocarcinoma (Wullich 2001), there was high-frequency microsatellite instability, which is rare in nonmucinous prostatic adenocarcinoma.

The differential diagnosis of mucinous prostatic adenocarcinoma in the prostate focuses on nonprostatic mucinous adenocarcinomas, including direct extension of a mucinous carcinoma of the bladder, urethra (Tran 1996), colon (Yamaguchi 1993), or Cowper's gland. An admixture of usual acinar adenocarcinoma is one hint that the mucinous adenocarcinoma is of prostatic origin. Also, goblet cells should be absent in mucinous adenocarcinomas of the prostate. Clinical and radiologic correlations as to the location of a dominant mass can be most helpful in the differential diagnosis. Immunopositivity for PSA and PSAP, with a negative immunoreaction for CEA, will help confirm the source of the mucinous adenocarcinoma as prostatic, with the caveat that rare cases of periurethral gland adenocarcinoma and bladder adenocarcinoma have been reported to be immunoreactive with PSA and PSAP antibodies (mainly polyclonal antibodies) **t14.17, t14.18, pp 205-206**. Additional differential diagnostic considerations in the prostate consist of hormonal therapy effect and adenocarcinoma with mucinous features. Androgen deprivation therapy effect can generate pools of mucin, which lack tumor cells; this alteration has been called pseudomyxoma ovariilike post-therapeutic alteration (Tran 1998). Adenocarcinomas with focal mucin lakes representing less than 25% of the tumor volume should be designated as adenocarcinoma with mucinous features or adenocarcinoma with a focal mucinous component (Epstein 1985, Ro 1990). The incidence and biological behavior of those neoplasms compared with those of mucinous adenocarcinoma and nonmucinous acinar adenocarcinomas are not well defined. In one series (McNeal 1991), the incidence of focal colloid carcinoma was 11% (11 of 100 cases). Finally, mucinous adenocarcinoma with its abundant extracellular mucin should be distinguished from standard acinar adenocarcinoma with intraluminal mucin. Such mucin can be seen in 18% to 52% (in needle biopsy) to 72% (in radical prostatectomy) of usual acinar adenocarcinomas on H&E-stained sections **t14.11, p 280**, and intraluminal mucin can be identified in 60% to 90% of standard acinar prostatic adenocarcinomas by histochemical stains (Allsbrook 1998). One should not equate detection of any mucin with the specific diagnosis of mucinous adenocarcinoma. In metastatic sites, mucinous prostatic adenocarcinoma can potentially simulate mucinous adenocarcinoma in many other organ systems. Mucinous adenocarcinoma of the prostate spreads in the same manner as acinar adenocarcinoma, with local infiltration into periprostatic soft tissue and seminal vesicles and distant metastases to lymph nodes, lungs, and bone (Epstein 1985, Ro 1990), where the metastases are osteoblastic. Rarely, patients may present with metastatic mucinous prostatic adenocarcinoma (Epstein 1985, Lee 1990), such that prostate cancer should be in the differential diagnosis for any man with a mucinous adenocarcinoma of unknown or uncertain origin.

More than 30 years ago, it was believed that mucinous prostatic adenocarcinoma was indolent and uncommonly metastasized to the skeleton (Cricco 1979, Joshi 1967). Actually, the opposite is true: mucinous prostatic adenocarcinoma often presents with advanced stage, including bony metastasis (Epstein 1985, Ro 1990), and appears to be quite aggressive **t17.7**. For cases reported from 1960 through 1986, the survival rate appeared to be slightly worse than that for acinar adenocarcinoma (Nagakura 1986). Recently calculated 3- and 5-year survival rates were 50% and 25%, respectively (Saito 1999). The treatment approach for mucinous prostatic adenocarcinoma should be the same as for nonmucinous adenocarcinoma. However, response to androgen deprivation therapy appears to be modest (Epstein 1985, Ishizu 1991, Ro 1990, Saito 1999, Teichman 1994). Stage appears to be the best predictor of outcome; histopathologic indicators such as grade of the nonmucinous element and proportion of the mucinous component were not significantly associated with patient outcome (Ro 1990).

[17.3] Signet-Ring Carcinoma

Signet-ring carcinoma is a rare prostatic carcinoma variant, with about 48 cases reported in the literature **t17.9**. Most published reports are of single cases, with only a few small series available for evaluation **t17.10**. The true incidence is not known because the definition of a primary signet-ring prostatic carcinoma based on percentage of signet-ring cells in the tumor is not set. Some authors

■ t17.9 Signet-Ring Carcinoma of the Prostate

Rare and clinically aggressive
Various cutoffs of % signet-ring calls used for definition. Most use 25%
Clinical presentation: Prostatism, abnormal DRE and/or quite high serum PSA
Microscopically: Signet-ring cells = nuclear displacement and indentation by cytoplasmic vacuole
Differential diagnosis vs other signet-ring carcinomas: Prostatic signet-ring cells often mucin-negative, and usually PSA and PSAP-positive

■ t17.10 Signet-Ring Carcinoma: Clinical Features of Largest Series

Author	N[1]	Incidence[2]	Age[3]	Presentation	Sample[4]	Outcome
Ro 1988C	8	NG	68(50-80)	Five: Stage C Three: Stage D	TURP: 6 Needle biopsy: 2	5 died of disease at 32-60 months
Guerin 1993	5	2.5%	79(70-84)	NG	TURP	3 died of disease at 1-50 months
Torbenson 1998	12	NG	69(54-82)	Mean serum PSA = 23.7 (range 4.4-92.6)	RP: 7 Needle biopsy: 4 TURP: 1	1 died of disease at 18 months; 4 alive with disease at 21-34 months

[1]Number of cases
[2]Incidence out of total number of prostatic carcinomas
[3]Mean age (range)
[4]Abbreviations: NG = not given; TURP = transurethral resection of prostate; RP = radical prostatectomy

have suggested that at least 25% of the neoplasm should consist of signet-ring cells to establish a diagnosis of signet-ring carcinoma (Bostwick 1997, Young 2000), but other investigators have classified cases as signet-ring cell carcinoma when more than 50% (Ro 1988C) or as little as 5% of the tumor was composed of signet-ring cells (Guerin 1993, Torbenson 1998). When the 5% threshold was used, the incidence of signet-ring cell carcinoma was 2.5% in a series of 200 primary prostate carcinomas (Guerin 1993). The presence of *any* signet-ring cell differentiation raises this incidence substantially: in a consecutive series of 308 primary prostatic carcinomas, fully 22% had signet-ring cells, but only 0.6% of cases had 30% signet-ring cells and none had 50% or more (Bostwick 1995). The key issue here is whether different cutoffs of signet-ring cell percentages relate to patient outcome. Because this is not known, use of any cutoff is arbitrary. Use of the 25% mark is currently recommended.

Clinically, a man with signet-ring prostatic carcinoma presents at an average age of 71 with prostatism, an abnormal DRE, or an elevated serum PSA. Urinary retention and hematuria are less common (Picurelli 1994, Saito 1999). The serum PSA elevation can be pronounced, with the majority of men having a level above 15 ng/mL (Torbenson 1998). Only a few men had modest increases in the range of 4 to 10 ng/mL (Alline 1992, Attaran 1987, Torbenson 1998,), the typical level for men with usual acinar adenocarcinoma. A normal serum PSA at presentation has been reported (Skodras 1993). Many men present with advanced clinical stage, including metastatic carcinoma (see reviews in Leong 1996, Saito 1999).

Gross observations can only be gathered from a few cases with large tumors. In one autopsy case (Giltman 1981), the prostate was described as diffusely rock hard and yellowish. In a second case, the prostate was not enlarged, and cut surfaces were yellowish-white, firm, and homogenous (Hejka 1984). Local gross extension of tumor into periprostatic soft tissue (Giltman 1981, Remmele 1988), seminal vesicles (Remmele 1988), and bladder (Smith 1994) was macroscopically evident at autopsy (Giltman 1981, Remmele 1988) and in a radical prostatectomy specimen (Smith 1994).

Microscopically, signet-ring cells with nuclear displacement and indentation by clear cytoplasmic vacuoles should be identified by visual inspection in at least 25% of the tumor **i17.32-i17.36**. The signet-ring cells can grow in sheets **i17.32**, small clusters **i17.33**, and as single cells **i17.33, i17.36** (Guerin 1993, Ro 1988C, Torbenson 1998). As for all signet-ring carcinomas, this single-cell infiltrate can be insidiously infiltrative and occasionally difficult to recognize. A transition with high-grade acinar adenocarcinoma is commonly seen (Guerin 1993, Ro 1988C, Torbenson 1998). Although a pure signet-ring cell population may rarely be noted in smaller samples such as needle biopsy tissue, in the whole gland the signet-ring cells are invariably mixed with acinar adenocarcinoma. The average proportion of signet-ring cells in the largest series in the literature (with $n = 12$ patients [Torbenson 1998]) was 39%, with up to 75% of the tumor composed of signet-ring cells in the whole gland. The admixed acinar carcinoma component can exhibit solid, comedo, cribriform, and raggedly infiltrative patterns (Ro 1988C). Rarely, signet-ring cells have been found within mucin lakes (Alfthan 1970, Manne 1989, Uyama 1979). Other rare morphologic structures include glomerulations with signet-ring cells **i17.34** and signet-ring cells in preexisting glands (Reyes 1997, Ro 1988C), which could represent high-grade signet-ring cell PIN or in situ spread of signet-ring cells (Reyes 1997).

The histologic grade assigned to signet-ring prostatic carcinoma should be high grade. Although grading of this variant was not addressed in the Gleason scheme, the recommended Gleason pattern is 5 (Bostwick 1994). The few Gleason scores assigned to signet-ring prostatic carcinoma in the literature have ranged from 6 to 10, with a mean of 9 (Leong 1996, Reyes 1997, Ro 1988C, Torbenson 1998).

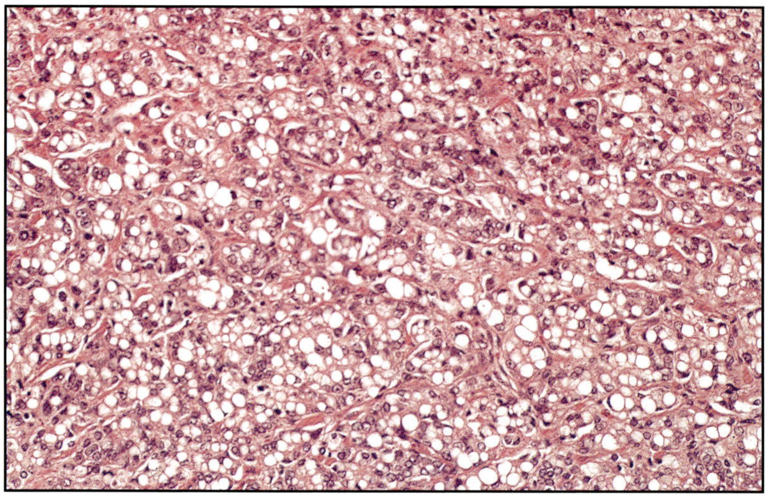

■ **i17.32** *Signet-ring prostatic carcinoma: Sheet-like growth*

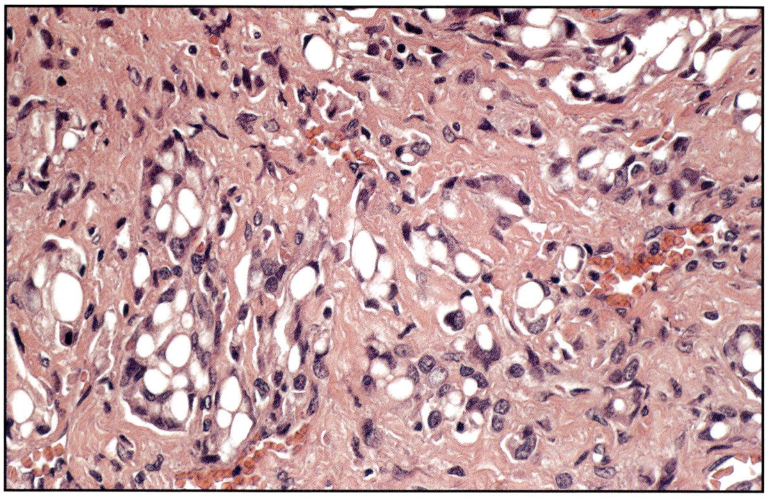

■ **i17.33** *Signet-ring prostatic carcinoma growing as small clusters and single cells.*

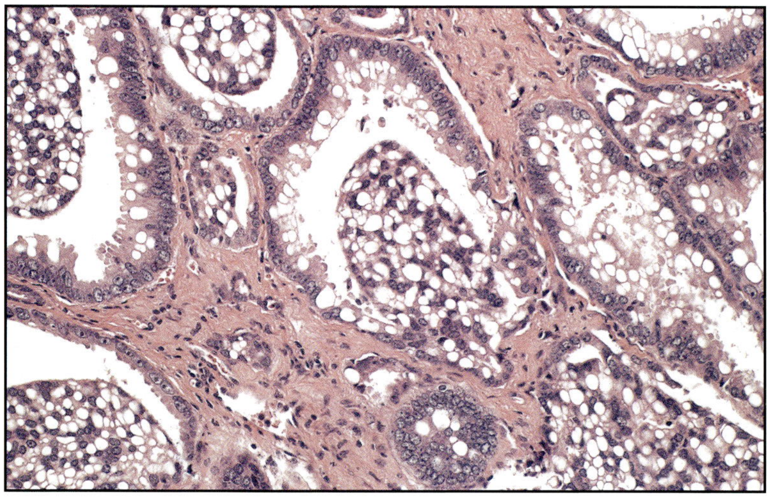

■ **i17.34** *An unusual pattern of prostatic signet-ring carcinoma: glomeruloid signet-ring cell architecture.*

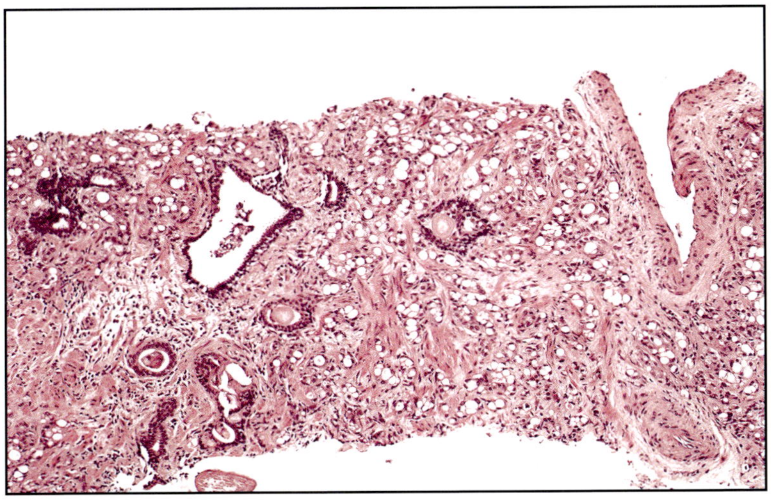

■ **i17.35** *Signet-ring cell prostatic carcinoma in needle biopsy tissue.*

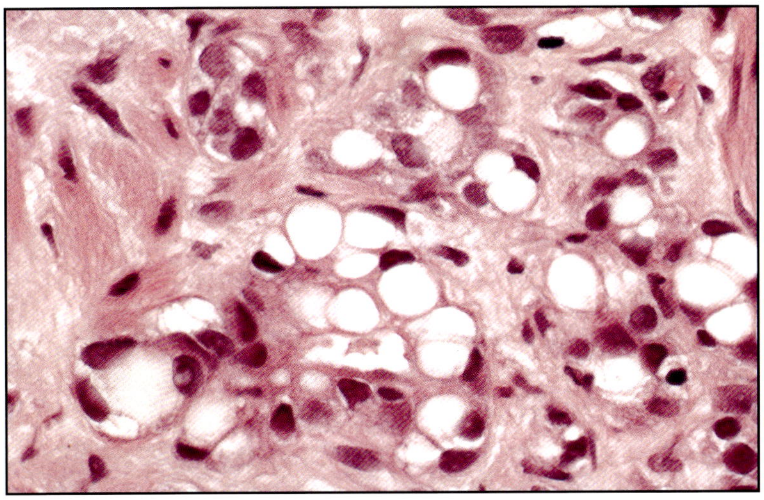

■ **i17.36** *Signet-ring cell prostatic carcinoma: Higher power view of* **i17.35**.

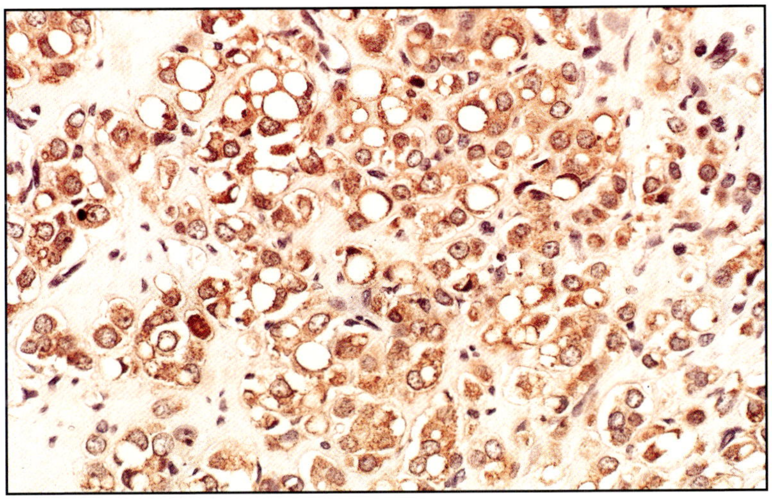

■ **i17.37** *PSA immunoreactivity in prostatic signet-ring carcinoma is a consistent finding.*

The basis for the vacuole formation in prostatic signet-ring carcinoma, as demonstrated by histochemical stains and electron microscopy (Alline 1992, Ben-Izhak 1992, Catton 1992, Guerin 1993, Hejka 1984, Leong 1996, Ro 1988C, Tran 2000), is heterogenous, with mucin-negative intracytoplasmic lumina and vacuoles with lipid predominating. An important characteristic of prostatic carcinoma signet-ring cells is that in many cases intracellular mucin may not be detected (by PAS-diastase, mucicarmine, and Alcian blue stains) (Ben-Izhak 1992, Guerin 1993, Ro 1988C) and when detected tends to be weak and focal (Guerin 1993, Torbenson 1998) and concentrated on the rims of the vacuoles (Guerin 1993).

Immunostains for PSA and PSAP, pan-cytokeratin (AE1/AE3 and CAM5.2), are positive in most cases of signet-ring carcinoma of the prostate **i17.37** (Ben-Izhak 1992, Catton 1992, Guerin 1993, Hejka 1984, Kanematsu 1997, Kuroda 1999, Reyes 1997, Ro 1988C, Skodras 1993, Smith 1994, Torbenson 1998, Uchijma 1990). Immunoreaction for CEA, EMA, bcl-2, c-MET, CD44v6, and CD44v7 may be noted in some but not all cases (Alline 1992, Catton 1992, Guerin 1993, Hejka 1984, Kanematsu 1997, Remmele 1988, Ro 1988C, Skodras 1993, Smith 1994), whereas stains for chromogranin (Guerin 1993) and CK7 and CK20 (Kuroda 1999, Leong 1996), are negative. High-molecular-weight cytokeratins labeled by 34βE12 binding are also not detected (Torbenson 1998), as expected for an invasive carcinoma. Curiously, despite its aggressive nature, the proliferation index of prostatic signet-ring carcinoma, as calculated based on MIB1-immunostains, is low at about 8% (range 1% to 10%) (Torbenson 1998).

The differential diagnosis for prostatic signet-ring carcinoma includes both benign and malignant entities. Benign signet-ring cells can be seen in the prostate. Both benign stromal cells and lymphocytes can undergo artifactual signet-ring cell change as a function of trauma or diathermy during TURP (Alguacil-Garcia 1986, Schned 1987). We have also seen a case of a benign stromal nodule with extensive signet-ring cell change, without associated trauma or cautery artifact as an inducing factor (Wang 2002). Haphazardly distributed lymphocytes with signet-ring cell change may appear infiltrative and thereby mimic infiltrative signet-ring cell carcinoma. The lymphocytic nuclei usually are smaller, but in cases where doubt persists, pan-cytokeratin, PSA and PSAP immunostains, in conjunction with a positive CD45 (leukocyte common antigen) or smooth muscle actin immunostain, will provide reassurance as to the lymphocytic or smooth muscle cell nature, respectively, of the signet-ring cells. The main diagnostic problem for signet-ring carcinoma is determining the anatomic site of origin. Even in prostate tissue samples, not all signet-ring carcinomas originate in the prostate. There are rare examples of metastatic signet-ring carcinoma of the stomach that were diagnosed in prostate needle biopsy tissue and TURP chips (Ehara 1991, Plancke 1994). In nonprostatic anatomic sites, one should always rule out prostatic carcinoma when confronted with a signet-ring cell carcinoma of unknown primary. Like usual acinar adenocarcinoma, signet-ring carcinoma spreads to lymph nodes and bone; additional, less common documented sites of metastasis include lung, liver, pleura, peritoneum, gastrointestinal tract, adrenal, pancreas, kidney, and ascites fluid (Leong 1996). A mucin-negative signet-ring carcinoma in one of these locations suggests a prostatic primary. In contrast, bladder and gastric signet-ring carcinomas usually are diffuse and strongly mucin positive (Torbenson 1998). Further support for a prostatic primary would be positive PSA and PSAP immunostains, although these are not absolutely specific for prostatic carcinoma. It is particularly alarming that in one recent study PSA and PSAP polyclonal antibodies bound to several bladder and gastric signet-ring carcinomas in immunohistochemical reactions (Torbenson 1998). Three of 6 bladder and 2 of 7 gastric signet-ring carcinomas were PSAP-positive (Torbenson 1998). Greater specificity was realized with a PSA monoclonal antibody, but still a case of signet-ring carcinoma of the bladder was PSA positive. Just as

PSA immunoreactivity does not definitely rule in prostatic signet-ring carcinoma, so does negativity fail to exclude prostatic signet-ring carcinoma (Alline 1992, Remmele 1988, Smith 1994). PSA and PSAP are best used in a panel of immunohistochemical markers to point to a possible primary anatomic site of origin of carcinomas of unknown origin (DeYoung 2000), including signet-ring carcinomas. Radiologic and clinical correlations, especially with the serum PSA level, should be suggested. Finally, hormonal therapy can potentially induce signet-ring cell change (Fergusson 1953), although the cytoplasm of the single, treated neoplastic cells is more often vacuolated with nuclear pyknosis, imparting a histiocytoid rather than a signet-ring cell appearance (Reuter 1997).

The outcome for patients with signet-ring carcinoma of the prostate generally is poor (Guerin 1993, Ro 1988C, Saito 1999). Response to androgen-deprivation therapy is minimal (Ro 1988C, Saito 1999), and the 3-year survival rate was 27% and 5-year survival 0% (Saito 1999).

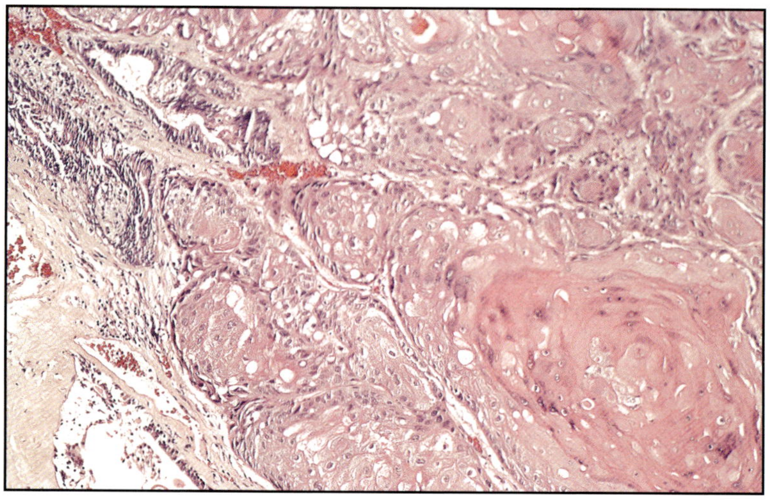

■ **i17.38** *Keratinizing squamous cell carcinoma of the prostate.*

[17.4] Adenosquamous and Squamous Carcinomas

Squamous cell carcinoma and adenosquamous carcinomas that originate in the prostate are so rare that no series of more than 6 cases has been described in detail from any one hospital **t17.11**. Rather, almost all reports in the literature are of 1 or 2 cases. The incidence of prostatic squamous cell carcinoma in earlier articles (Arnheim 1948, Franks 1954, Kahler 1939) and 1 later publication (Samsonov 1984) was 1.4% to 3%, whereas other investigators place the incidence at closer to 0.2% (Dhom 1980, Sarma 1991). The incidence depends on how the patient population was treated because many carcinomas in the prostate with squamous differentiation arise after radiation or hormonal therapy. The incidence of adenosquamous carcinoma is lower than that of pure squamous cell carcinoma, with only about 20 cases of adenosquamous carcinoma reported (Bainborough 1952, Bassler 1999, Bennett 1973, Devaney 1991, Fergusson 1953, Gattuso 1995, Kim 1999, Moyana 1987, Orhan 1996, Saito 1984). In addition to admixture with adenocarcinoma, a few patients have had prostatic squamous cell carcinoma mixed with transitional cell carcinoma and adenocarcinoma (Bennett 1973) and transitional cell carcinoma (Ishigooka 1994, Wernert 1990).

Clinically, patients with primary prostatic squamous cell carcinoma or adenosquamous carcinoma are 52 to 79 years of age, with an average of 64 years (Little 1993). These men present with findings and symptoms closely resembling those of advanced prostatic adenocarcinoma, with urinary obstructive symptoms, hematuria, and bone pain (Kim 1999, Little 1993). The DRE often is remarkable for stony hard induration. Serum acid phosphatase is normal in all patients, and serum PSA usually is normal. Serum PSA has been elevated in 2 cases of adenosquamous carcinoma (Gattuso 1995, Orhan 1996) and in 1 patient with squamous cell carcinoma (Miller 1995). In a couple of patients radiologic studies of the primary tumor disclosed extraprostatic extension, seminal vesicle and pelvic floor invasion by pelvic CT (Ishigooka 1994), and irregular, anterior and hyperechoic intraprostatic lesions by transrectal ultrasound (Terris 1999B).

■ **t17.11 Squamous Cell Carcinoma and Adenosquamous Carcinoma of Prostate**

Rare; incidence = 0.2%-3% (probably closest to 0.2%)
Predisposition: Treatment of prior pure adenocarcinoma with hormonal therapy or radiotherapy
Men 64 years of age (mean) present with advanced prostate cancer
Serum PAP, PSA usually normal
Grossly: Large, solid, white-gray
Microscopically: Polygonal cells with variable nuclear atypia and degrees of keratinization
Outcome: Generally poor and much worse than acinar adenocarcinoma

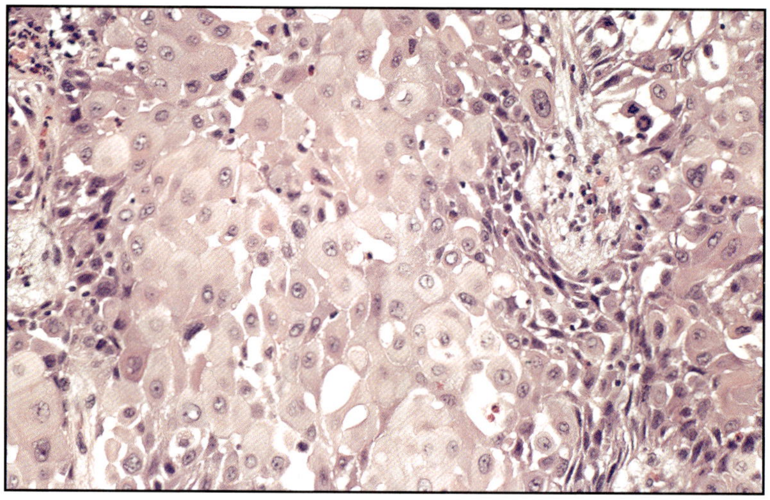

■ **i17.39** *Well to moderately differentiated prostatic squamous cell carcinoma, with abundant eosinophilic cytoplasm.*

Grossly, the tumors usually are large, measuring up to 6.5 cm in the greatest dimension and often replacing a substantial portion of the prostate (Corder 1976, Gattuso 1995, Gray 1975, Kastendieck 1974, Mai 1996, Sarma 1991, Wang 1996). Cut surfaces reveal a solid, firm, whitish-yellow, white-gray, or gray-tan mass. Central extension, with compression of prostatic urethra, and local invasion into the bladder, rectum, and seminal vesicle were macroscopically apparent in several cases (Bainborough 1952, Gray 1975, Sarma 1991, Wang 1996). Microscopically, pure squamous cell carcinoma was typified by infiltrating nests, strands, and sheets of polygonal cells with nuclear atypia, with squamous differentiation manifested as individual cell keratinization, intercellular bridges, or keratin pearl formation **i17.38-i17.42**. In examples of

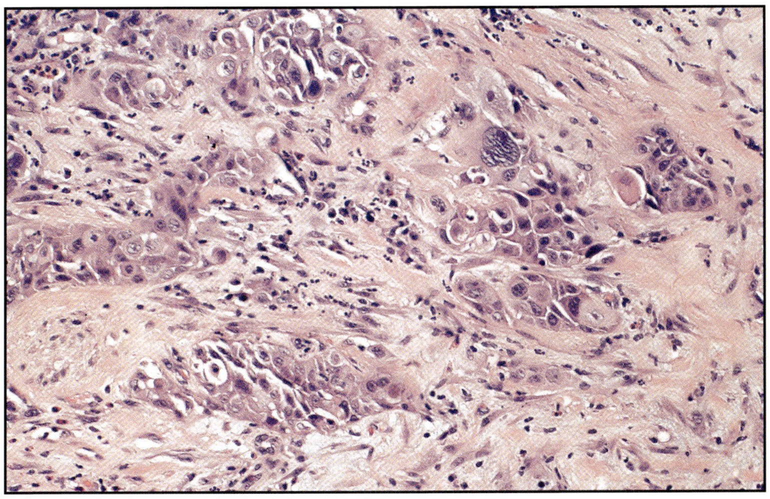

■ **i17.40** *Infiltrative moderately to poorly differentiated prostatic squamous cell carcinoma.*

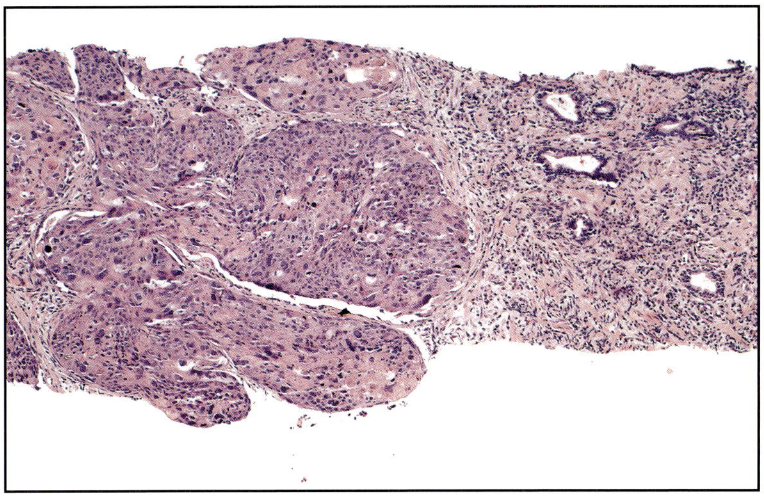

■ **i17.41** *Squamous cell carcinoma in prostate needle biopsy tissue (left), with adjacent benign atrophy (right).*

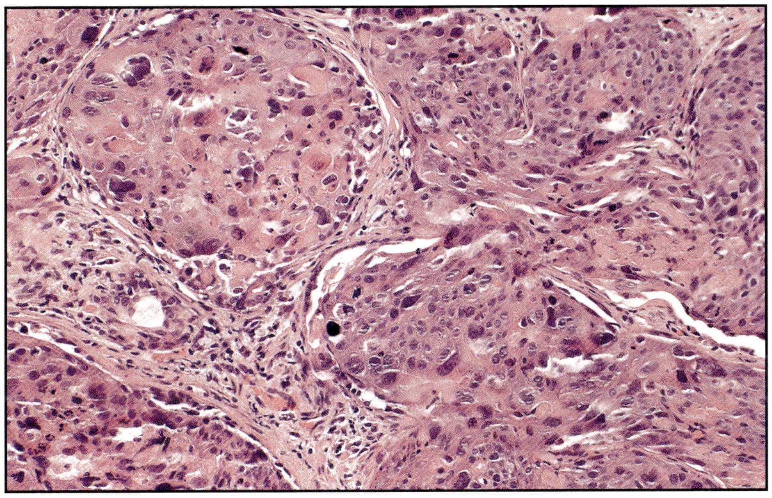

■ **i17.42** *Squamous cell carcinoma with eosinophilic cytoplasm and nuclear atypia (Higher magnification of* **i17.41***).*

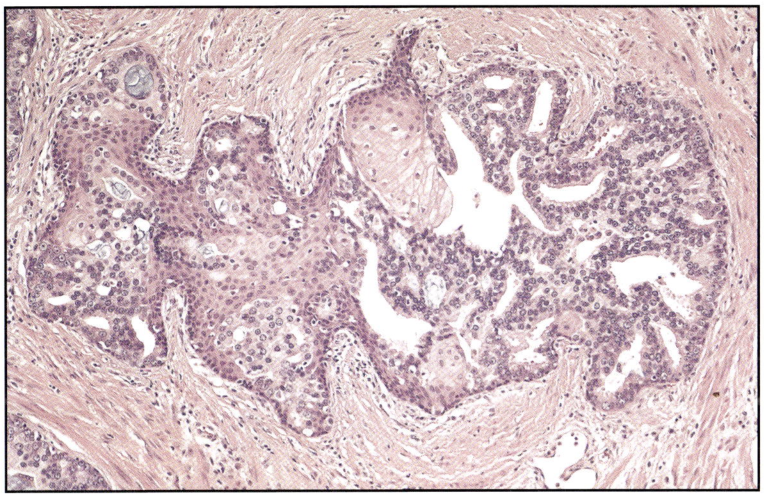

■ **i17.43** *Adenosquamous carcinoma of the prostate, with continuity between squamous and glandular epithelium.*

adenosquamous carcinoma, glandular and squamous components could be distinct or could exhibit direct transitions **i17.43, i17.44**. The grade of the adenocarcinoma ranges from moderately to poorly differentiated. The histologic grade of the squamous element is also variable, with reports of well-, moderately, and poorly differentiated growths. The application of a 3-tiered grading scheme to squamous cell carcinomas of the prostate seems reasonable. The Gleason grading scheme can be used for the glandular component but not the squamous component.

Special studies are of limited use in diagnosis. The malignant squamous cells are most often negative for PSA and PSAP immunostains (Accetta 1983, Devaney 1991, Gattuso 1995, Lager 1988, Mai 1996, Miller 1995, Orhan 1996, Uchibayashi 1996, Wang 1996), and this correlates with the normal serum PSA and PSAP levels found in most patients with prostatic squamous cell carcinoma. A few reports (Al Adnani 1985, Moyana 1987, Saito 1984, Turhan 1999) did describe PSA or PSAP immunoreactivity in the squamous carcinoma cells. Ultrastructurally, the neoplastic cells show desmosomes, tonofibrils, and tight junctions as well as microvilli (Devaney 1991, Moyana 1987). Almost nothing is known of molecular genetic abnormalities in these neoplasms. DNA content can be diploid or aneuploid (Bassler 1999, Mai 1996, Tran 2001). Accumulation of p53 protein was observed in both the squamous and glandular components in one case of adenosquamous carcinoma (Orhan 1996).

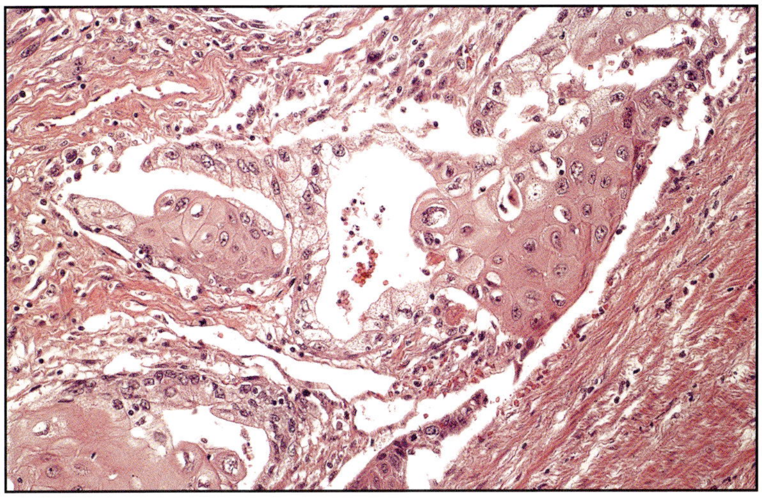

■ **i17.44** *Adenosquamous carcinoma of the prostate with admixed malignant squamous and glandular elements. The patient had been treated with radiation and hormonal therapy.*

Prostatic squamous cell carcinoma and adenosquamous carcinoma, like glandular adenocarcinomas, can spread along

■ t17.12 **Differential Diagnosis of Squamous Carcinoma in the Prostate**

Squamous metaplasia secondary to hormonal or radiation therapy
Squamous metaplasia adjacent to infarcts or secondary to inflammation
Urothelial carcinoma with squamous features extending into prostate
Squamous cell carcinoma from bladder
Squamous cell carcinoma metastasis from distant site (such as lung)

nerves, extend locally into periprostatic soft tissue, bladder and seminal vesicles, and metastasize to lymph nodes and bone. In bone, however, the metastases are routinely osteolytic rather than osteoblastic (Little 1993). In widely disseminated disease, metastatic deposits have been detected in glans penis, peritoneum, diaphragm, liver, and lung (Little 1993, Wang 1996).

The differential diagnosis of squamous carcinoma in prostatic tissue includes squamous metaplasia, urethral or vesical transitional cell carcinoma with squamous features, direct extension of nonprostatic squamous cell carcinoma into the prostate, and metastasis of a squamous cell carcinoma from a distant site into the prostate **t17.12**. Squamous metaplasia is common in benign glands after radiation therapy and hormonal therapy of prostatic adenocarcinoma and so shares the clinical setting in which prostatic squamous cell carcinoma and adenosquamous carcinoma occur. Squamous metaplasia has been misdiagnosed as carcinoma (Samsonov 1984), although this mistake can be avoided by diagnosing squamous cell carcinoma only in the setting of significant architectural disarray and nuclear atypia. More problematic is squamous metaplasia with dysplasia (Wernert 1990). However, this is not a well-defined entity in the prostate. Reactive nuclear atypia certainly can be seen in squamous metaplasia adjacent to infarcts and inflammation, so one should be cautious in diagnosing carcinoma in this context. If squamous cell carcinoma is detected in the prostate, one should clinically rule out spread from another site, particularly urothelial carcinoma with squamous features and primary squamous cell carcinoma of the bladder growing into the prostate (Wernert 1990). In metastatic sites, the possibility that a metastatic deposit of squamous cell carcinoma or adenosquamous carcinoma of unknown primary might be of prostatic origin should be contemplated, particularly in an older man with a history of radiation or androgen deprivation treatment of prostatic adenocarcinoma. Squamous cell carcinoma or adenosquamous carcinoma of the prostate can be found as metastatic deposits after treatment of a pure adenocarcinoma in the prostate (Accetta 1982, 1983).

Prostatic squamous cell carcinoma and adenosquamous carcinoma are extremely aggressive neoplasms that are consistently nonresponsive to androgen deprivation and radiation therapies. This should not be so surprising, given that many of these tumors arise from treated tumors and therefore probably represent therapy-resistant clones. The mean survival is only 6 months to a year. There have been a few responses to chemotherapy (Imamura 2000, Okada 2000) and a few patients surviving 5 to 9 years (Imamura 2000, Little 1993, Sieracki 1955), but the outlook is generally dismal.

The mechanism underlying the development of squamous cell carcinoma or adenosquamous carcinoma after radiation or androgen deprivation therapy is not known. Clearly, this pathway is generated in only very small minority of patients with adenocarcinoma of the prostate treated with hormonal therapy or radiotherapy. The pathway can develop after different forms of androgen deprivation and radiation therapy. These treatment forms included diethylstilbestrol, orchiectomy, luteinizing hormone–releasing hormone analogs, androgen receptor blockers, external beam radiation, and radioactive seed implantation. The time course for the appearance of squamous differentiation in the carcinoma varies from 3 months (Orhan 1996, Wang 1996) to many (up to 9) years after therapy (Miller 1995). Squamous metaplasia and human papillomavirus infection do not appear to predispose to this development (Little 1993, Mai 1996). It is not possible to completely exclude a second squamous malignancy in these cases, although a more plausible explanation would be clonal evolution and divergence of persistent carcinoma, secondary to the selective pressure of therapy. Finally, other pathways for squamous prostatic carcinogenesis must exist because in some cases no therapy was administered before the diagnosis of squamous carcinoma (Accetta 1983, Bassler 1999, Corder 1976, Gray 1975, Little 1993, Mai 1996, Okamoto 1996, Orhan 1996, Sarma 1991, Uchibayashi 1996), and prostatic squamous cell carcinoma has been shown to occur in association with prostatic schistosomiasis (Al Adnani 1985). In rats, squamous carcinoma of the prostate can be induced by intraprostatic placement of the chemical carcinogen methylcholanthrene (Segaloff 1963). No chemical carcinogen has been associated with prostatic squamous cell carcinoma in men.

[17.5] Basaloid and Adenoid Cystic "Carcinomas"

This is a poorly defined diagnostic category that includes malignant basaloid proliferations (basaloid carcinomas) and also neoplasms that resemble, to a certain degree, adenoid cystic carcinomas of the salivary glands **t17.13**. A large number of terms have been used for these neoplasms and related growths such as *adenoid basal cell tumor* (Devaraj 1993, Grignon 1988, Reed 1984), *adenoid cystic tumor, adenoid cystic-like tumor* (Young 1988), *basal cell carcinoma* (Sesterhenn 1987), and *adenoid basal proliferation of uncertain significance* (McKenney 2001). Some of these cases probably represent adenoid cystic-like hyperplasia (McKenney 2001). The difficulty in classifying these proliferations resides in the facts that they are rare, there is no agreement on histologic criteria, and follow-up of the few reported cases is of minimal duration.

Basaloid and adenoid cystic carcinomas are extraordinarily rare, with only about 30 reported cases (Ahn 1991, Cecchi 2000, Cohen 1993, Denholm 1992, Grignon 1988, McKenney 2001, Nkanza 1988, Osorio Acosta 1997, Shindo 1998, Terris 1999A, Van Renterghem 1994, Yang 1998). It is unclear how many of these might be adenoid cystic-like hyperplasia. The term *basaloid carcinoma* has been used to include tumors with islands or cords of basaloid epithelial cells with peripheral palisading, which is morphologically similar to basal cell carcinoma of the skin, and adenoid

■ 17.13 **Basaloid/Adenoid Cystic "Carcinomas" of Prostate**

Rare — about 30 reported cases
Histologic criteria for diagnosis not set
Some cases may represent hyperplasia
Two patterns: Basaloid and adenoid cystic-like
A neoplasm of low malignant potential

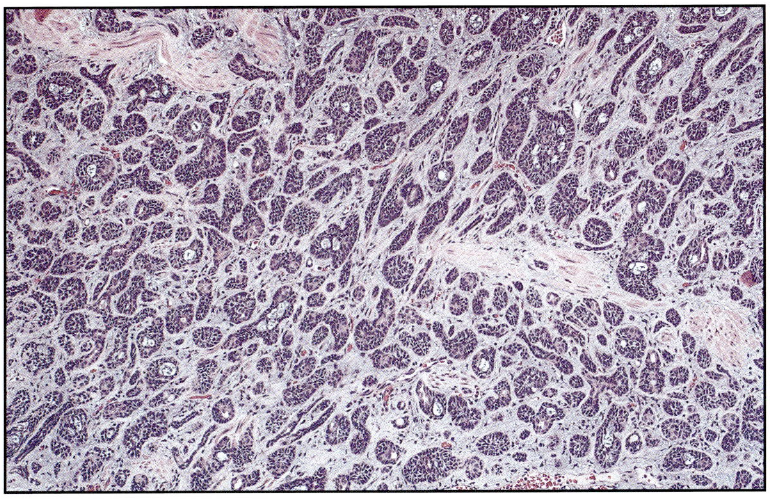

■ **i17.45** *Basaloid/adenoid cystic tumor with haphazardly dispersed nests and tubules of basaloid cells.*

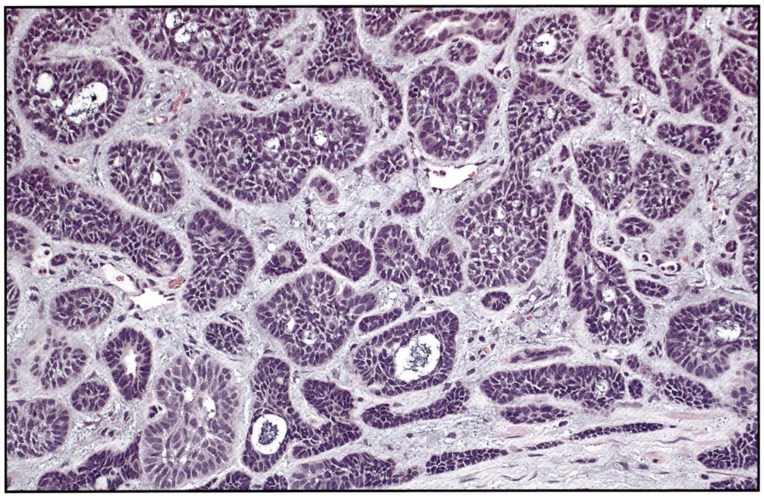

■ **i17.46** *Basaloid/adenoid cystic tumor: Nested and glandular pattern of growth.*

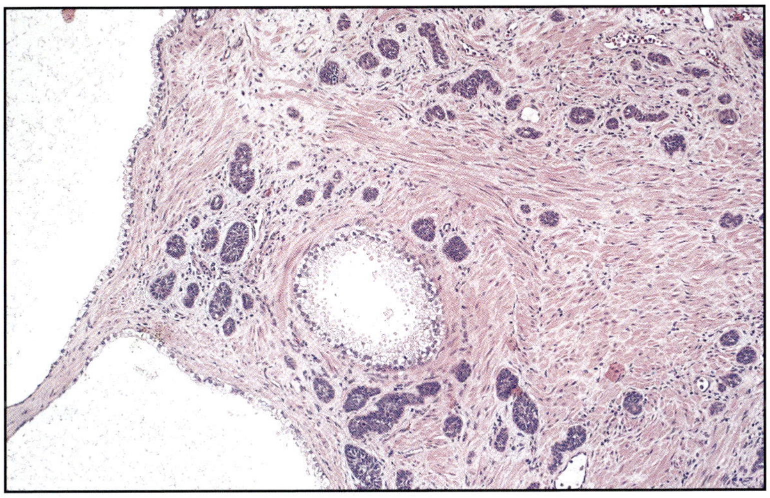

■ **i17.47** *Infiltrative permeation of basaloid nests around benign glands in basaloid/adenoid cystic tumor.*

cystic carcinomas (Yang 1998). Only a few ($n = 5$) of the former type have been described (Denholm 1992, Yang 1998). Clinical features were not given for 4 of these; the fifth patient was a 28-year-old man with a history of increasing urinary outflow obstruction (Denholm 1992). Microscopically, basaloid carcinomas exhibit extraprostatic extension, perineural invasion, or necrosis. There is often an associated desmoplastic stromal response to invasive tumor. Immunohistochemical stains show strong staining for bcl-2 (Yang 1998) and cytokeratins, including those bound by antibody 34βE12 (Denholm 1992), and negative immunostains for PSA, vimentin, desmin, and neuron-specific enolase (Denholm 1992). No evidence of metastatic disease was reportedly present in these cases, but clinical follow up was not available (except in 1 case). Therefore, the clinical behavior of basaloid carcinoma of the prostate remains unknown.

Patients with the reported adenoid cystic type of growth pattern were of a mean age of 61 (range 38 to 74). These men present with obstructive and irritative symptoms. The DRE often is notable for an enlarged prostate that is not typically hard and irregular. The serum PSA was slightly elevated in 2 cases (to 4.5 and 4.6 ng/mL [Terris 1999A]). Transrectal ultrasound yields an unusual appearance of a monotonous pattern of multiple small cysts of similar size (Terris 1999A). TURP or open prostatectomy usually was performed. The gross features were related in only 2 cases: a well-defined pinkish-gray, firm mass with discrete areas of hemorrhage, necrosis, and microcystic change was illustrated (Ahn 1991), and numerous whitish-yellow nodules were described (Manrique 1978). Microscopically, the basaloid cell proliferation should be infiltrative **i17.45-i17.47**, with a prominent cribriform architecture. Cordlike, glandular, and nested basaloid patterns can also be present. The cribriform spaces often contain hyalinized, basement membrane–like material or basophilic mucinous secretions. Cytologically, small ovoid basaloid cells with a scant amount of cytoplasm and finely stippled chromatin are present. Cells lining glandular spaces have more conspicuous eosinophilic cytoplasm. Necrosis, perineural invasion, lymphvascular space invasion, and extraprostatic extension may be present but are not present in all cases (Young 2000). Apoptotic bodies are commonly present, and nuclear atypia and mitotic activity are variable (Young 2000). Unlike in salivary gland adenoid cystic carcinomas, sebaceous and squamous differentiation can be seen (Young 2000). Histochemical stains show the material in the glandular lumina to be PAS-positive, diastase-resistant, Alcian blue-positive, and mucicarmine-positive (Frankel 1974, Kuhajda 1984, Nkanza 1988, Tannenbaum 1975D, Young 1988). Electron microscopic examination shows basal lamina material in the lumina, admixed with amorphous material that includes collagen fibers (Cohen 1993). Basal lamina also surrounds tumor cell nests (Cohen 1993, Young 1988). Intercellular true glandular lumina with microvilli are also identified (Young 1988).

Ultrastructural and immunophenotypic analysis demonstrates that prostatic adenoid cystic carcinoma, in contrast to salivary gland adenoid cystic carcinomas, lacks myoepithelial cells (Cohen 1993, Denholm 1992, Grignon 1988, Young 1988). Specifically, immunoreactive muscle-specific actin (MSA) is not detectable, S-100 protein is only focally present or absent, cytokeratin labeling with antibody CAM 5.2 is focal, and CEA is present (Cohen 1993, Grignon 1988, Young 1988). In contrast, salivary gland adenoid cystic carcinomas are MSA positive, CAM5.2 positive, and CEA negative (Cohen 1993, Ellis 1996). Variable reactivity with PSA and PSAP antibodies has been reported, although many cases are negative (Cohen 1993, Kuhajda 1984, Young 1988). High-molecular-weight cytokeratins, highlighted in normal and hyperplastic basal cells by antibody 34βE12, are also expressed in adenoid cystic carcinoma cells (Grignon 1988).

Admixed usual acinar adenocarcinoma should not be overlooked because focal well- to moderately differentiated adenocarcinoma was

■ **t17.14 Comparison of Prostatic Adenoid Cystic "Carcinoma" and Salivary Gland Adenoid Cystic Carcinoma**

Feature	Prostatic Adenoid Cystic "Carcinoma"	Salivary Gland Adenoid Cystic Carcinoma[1]
Cribriform, tubular, and solid growth patterns	+	+
Myoepithelial cells	–	Most cells
Squamous metaplasia	Can be present	–
Perineural invasion	Variable	Characteristic
S-100	±	+
Muscle specific actin	–	+
CEA	–	+
Metastasis	Uncommon (3 cases)[2]	Distant metastasis in 50% of patients
Outcome	Uncertain; most patients free of disease with short follow-up	Good 5-year survival; low 10-20 year survival rates

[1]Cohen 1993 and Ellis 1996
[2]Manrique 1978, Shindo 1948, Cecchi 2000

found in a few cases (Young 1988). In 2 other cases, prostatic adenoid cystic carcinoma was admixed with anaplastic carcinoma (Nkanza 1988) and squamous cell carcinoma with myxoid and chondroid areas, which was interpreted as a malignant mixed tumor of salivary gland type (Manrique 1978).

Grading generally is not done, although there is one recommendation to apply Gleason patterns of 3 to 5 (Bostwick 1994).

The differential diagnosis of prostatic basaloid or adenoid cystic "carcinomas" includes other basal cell proliferations, such as usual basal cell hyperplasia and basal cell hyperplasia with prominent nucleoli (also known as atypical basal cell hyperplasia), and cribriform proliferations in the prostate, including normal central zone epithelium, cribriform hyperplasia, cribriform PIN, and cribriform adenocarcinoma. Neuroendocrine carcinoma and carcinomas from other sites should also be contemplated. In contrast to basal cell hyperplasias, including the proposed adenoid cystic-like hyperplasia, basaloid and adenoid cystic carcinomas appear infiltrative rather than lobulated, with invasion around nerves, into vessels, or into soft tissues. Necrosis, bcl-2 expression, and proliferation index (assessed by Ki-67 immunostaining) may also be helpful in distinguishing basaloid carcinoma from benign basal cell proliferations, where basaloid carcinoma had strongly positive bcl-2 immunoreaction and a higher Ki-67 index (Yang 1998). Mitotic activity may also be useful for separating adenoid cystic carcinoma from adenoid cystic-like hyperplasia (Young 2000), but an appropriate cutoff has not been established. In regard to glandular cribriform proliferations, the N:C rations of the basaloid cells in basaloid and adenoid cystic carcinoma are higher than in glandular cells of cribriform hyperplasia, PIN, and adenocarcinoma. These basaloid cells might elicit a consideration of neuroendocrine carcinoma; neuroendocrine immunomarkers should be helpful here. Extension of an anal basaloid (cloacogenic) carcinoma or adenoid cystic carcinoma of Cowper's gland (Carpenter 1971) into the prostate is also a possibility. Clinical and radiologic correlations as to the location of the bulk of the mass would be of value in this circumstance.

The outcome for patients diagnosed with basaloid or adenoid cystic "carcinoma" of the prostate is uncertain. Prostatic adenoid cystic carcinoma is different from salivary gland adenoid cystic carcinoma in many ways **t17.14**, so one should not assume that they will behave in a similar fashion. In some cases of prostatic basaloid or adenoid cystic carcinoma, local invasion into surrounding tissue has been documented, but there have been only 3 cases of metastasis (Cecchi 2000, Manrique 1978, Shindo 1998) and 3 deaths (Manrique 1978, Shindo 1998, Young 2000). Overall, basaloid or adenoid cystic carcinoma of the prostate should be provisionally viewed as a neoplasm of low malignant potential.

[17.6] Transitional Cell (Urothelial) Carcinoma

Most (76% to 100%) transitional cell (urothelial) carcinomas involving the prostate are associated with bladder or urethral transitional cell carcinoma (Chapter 23). This association may result from intraprostatic extension from the bladder or urethra, implantation from one of these sites, or multifocal disease as a result of a field effect of urothelial carcinogenesis (Cheville 1998B, Johnson 1972), where urothelium normally lining the intraprostatic ducts might be affected. Therefore, it has been argued that the terms *primary* and *secondary* should not be used for prostatic urothelial carcinoma (Cheville 1998B). Indeed, it is often difficult to know with certainty the primary site of origin, so prostatic urethral and periurethral prostatic ductal sites often are lumped together.

Prostatic transitional cell carcinomas diagnosed in the absence of a bladder transitional cell carcinoma are rare **t17.15**. The mean incidence in 9 series of 11 678 patients was 1.1% (range 0.2% to 3.5%) of all prostatic carcinomas (Busto Castanon 1990, Ende 1963, Goebbels 1985, Kopelson 1978, Losi 1994B, Rhamy 1973, Rubenstein 1969, Zincke 1985). Men of an average age of 66 years (range 45 to 91) present with obstructive symptoms of short duration and rapid progression (Goebbels 1985, Greene 1973, Kopelson 1978, Nicolaisen 1984, Rhamy 1973, Sawczuk 1985) **t17.16.** Hematuria and irritative symptoms are also common. On DRE, the prostate is felt to be enlarged, and in about one half of cases it is

■ **t17.15 Transitional Cell Carcinoma Primary in Prostate**

Most transitional cell carcinomas (TCC) in prostate are associated with bladder carcinoma
By definition, primary prostatic TCC occurs in the absence of bladder carcinoma
Men of average age of 66 present in same fashion as men with prostatic adenocarcinoma
Microscopically, TCC in-situ is common, with solid plugs of cytologically pleomorphic tumor cells, often with comedo necrosis, mitoses, and stromal inflammation
Immunophenotype of PSA–, PSAP–, CK7+,34βE12+, helpful in differential diagnosis with prostatic adenocarcinoma
Outcome excellent for CIS alone and unfavorable for stromal invasion

■ **t17.16 Transitional Cell Carcinoma of Prostate: Clinical Features in Largest Series**

Author	No.[1]	Incidence[2]	Age[3]	Presentation	Sample	Outcome
Rhamy 1973	20	2.5%	64 (52-76)	Obstruction Prostatism Hematuria DRE: Suspicious in 50% Bony metastasis: 15%	Needle bx TURP	Average survival 18 months (range 1-59)
Greene 1976	39	NG	67 (45-91)	Obstruction Hematuria Stage A: 16% Stage B: 16% Stage C: 50% Stage D: 18%	NG[4]	Average survival 17 months (range 1-60)
Goebbels 1985	46	1.7%	NG	Stage A: 8% Stage B: 33% Stage C: 33% Stage D: 25%	Needle bx, TURP, Prostatectomy Cystoprostatectomy	Average survival 24-29 months (range 1-93)

[1]Number of patients
[2]% of all prostatic carcinomas
[3]Mean age (range)
[4]Not given

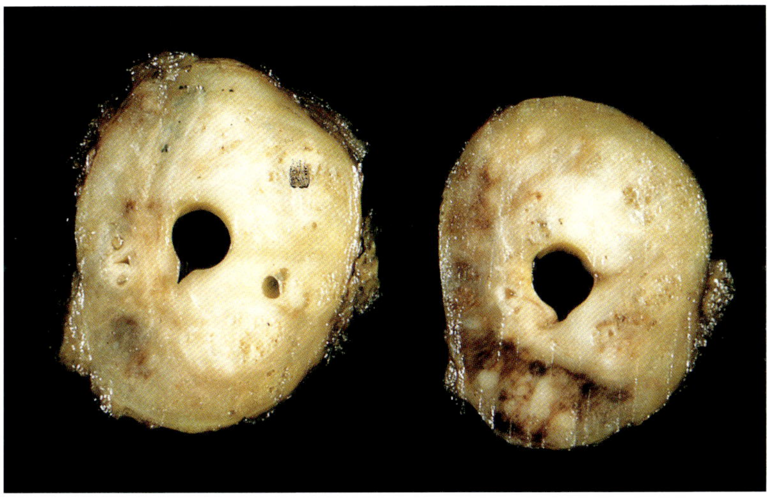

■ **i17.48** *Transitional cell carcinoma primary in the prostate. Extensive, solid white tumor in cut sections of a prostate gland from a cystoprostatectomy specimen. This 63-year-old man did not have disease in the bladder or urethra.*

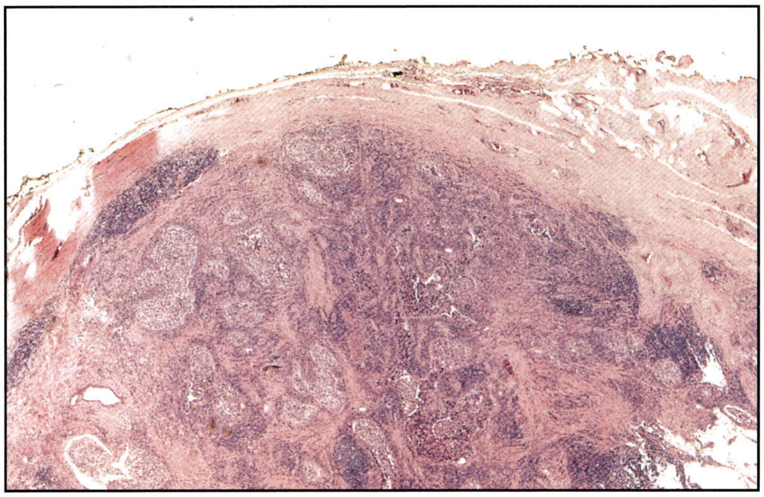

■ **i17.49** *Extensive transitional cell carcinoma in prostate, with spread into peripheral zone, and lymphoid response.*

stony-hard and suspicious for malignancy. Insufficient data are available on whether the serum PSA is elevated, but apparently this can occur with prostatic involvement by transitional cell carcinoma in general (Oliai 2001). Why this is so is not clear, but the basis may be analogous to that for serum acid phosphatase, which can be elevated (Cheville 1998A, Nicolaisen 1984), apparently because of coexisting usual adenocarcinoma. Alternatively, the characteristic marked prostatic inflammatory infiltrate associated with transitional cell carcinoma in the prostate might elevate the serum PSA. By cystoscopy, the tumors are shaggy, obstructive, and infiltrating (Sawczuk 1985). Fourteen percent are polypoid-papillary. It is unclear whether this represents urethral involvement or intraurethral protrusion of papillary transitional cell carcinoma from the periurethral prostatic ducts. Many patients in the 1970s and 1980s presented with advanced stage disease (Goebbels 1985, Greene 1973) **t17.16**. On the whole, the clinical presentation of prostatic transitional cell carcinoma is not different from that of usual prostatic adenocarcinoma. The main exception is in the setting of bony metastasis, which tends to be osteolytic for prostatic transitional cell carcinoma (Greene 1973, Nicolaisen 1984, Sawczuk 1985), compared with the typical osteoblastic metastasis of prostatic acinar adenocarcinoma. Also, urine cytology can be positive in prostatic transitional cell carcinoma (Kopelson 1978, Sawczuk 1985), whereas prostatic adenocarcinoma is hardly ever first diagnosed in a urine specimen (DeMay 1996).

No reliable gross features of prostatic transitional cell carcinoma have been reported (Greene 1973, Rubenstein 1969) **i17.48**. Microscopically, prostatic transitional cell carcinoma has a striking propensity for growth within prostatic ducts and acini **i17.49-i17.57**. Rounded or elongated cylinders and plugs of solid tumor within ducts are characteristic profiles **i17.50, i17.51**. Comedo necrosis can also commonly be found **i17.55** (Goebbels 1985) and may undergo dystrophic calcification (Greene 1973). Partial involvement of benign prostatic glands is typical (Goebbels 1985) and includes nodular or tonguelike tumoral protuberances **i17.52** and an undermining growth pattern in which the transitional carcinoma cells insinuate themselves underneath benign luminal prostatic epithelium **i17.53** (Cheville 1998B, Goebbels 1985). Pagetoid

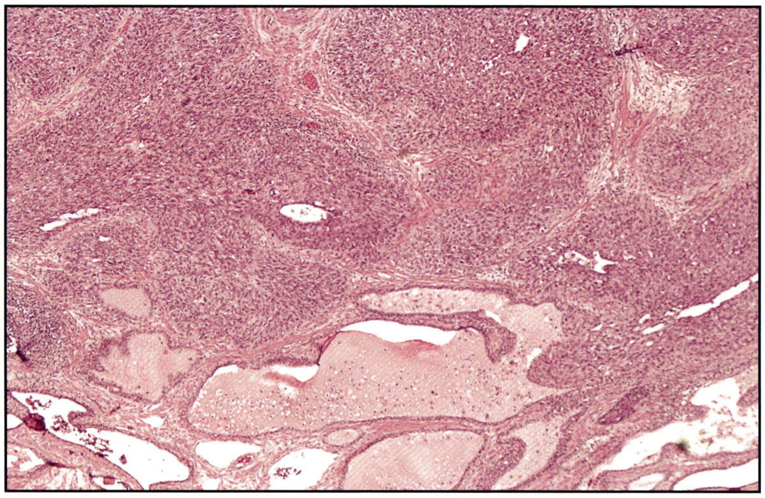

■ **i17.50** *Transitional cell carcinoma in prostate with solid intraductal spread. Benign prostate glands with open lumina are below.*

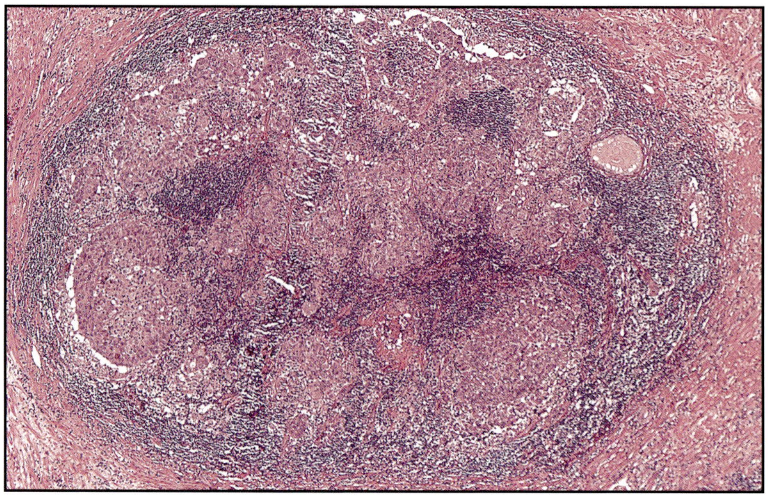

■ **i17.51** *Transitional cell carcinoma in the prostate: Rounded, solid masses with a lymphoid response.*

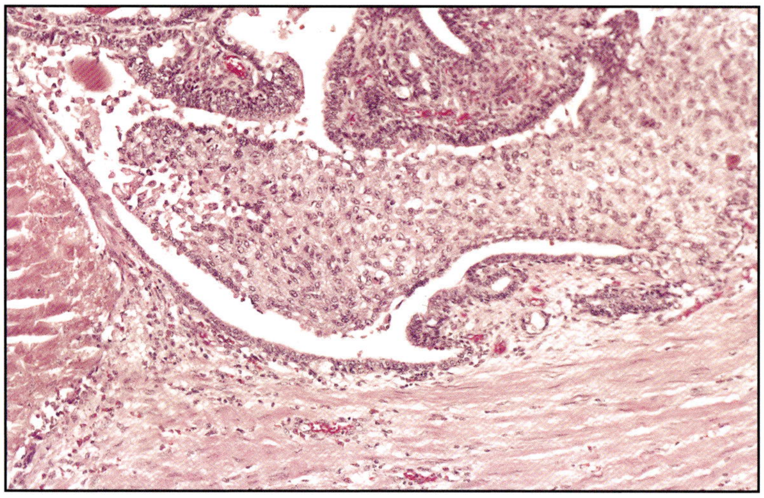

■ **i17.52** *Transitional cell carcinoma in prostate showing band-like protrusion into prostatic gland.*

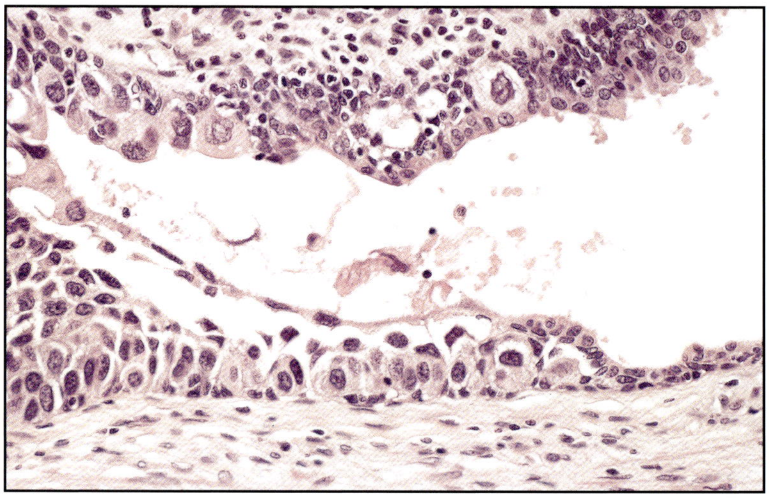

■ **i17.53** *Transitional cell carcinoma spread within benign prostatic epithelium: Undermining growth with splitting of epithelium (below) and pagetoid spread (above).*

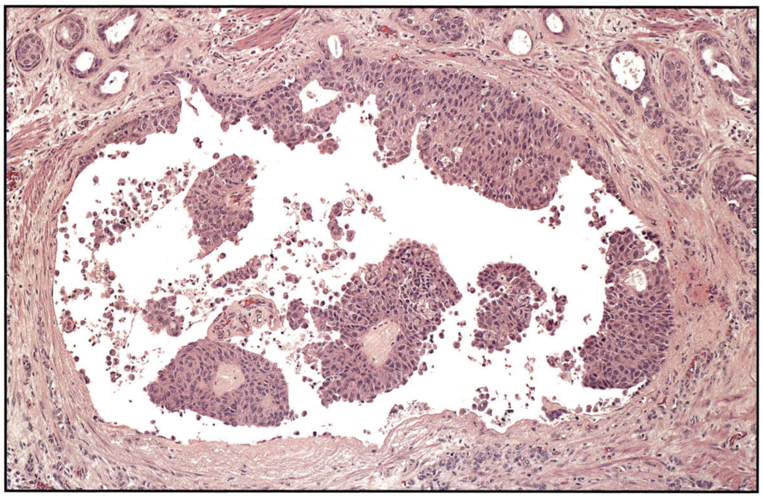

■ **i17.54** *Intraductal papillary transitional cell carcinoma in the prostate: A rare architectural configuration.*

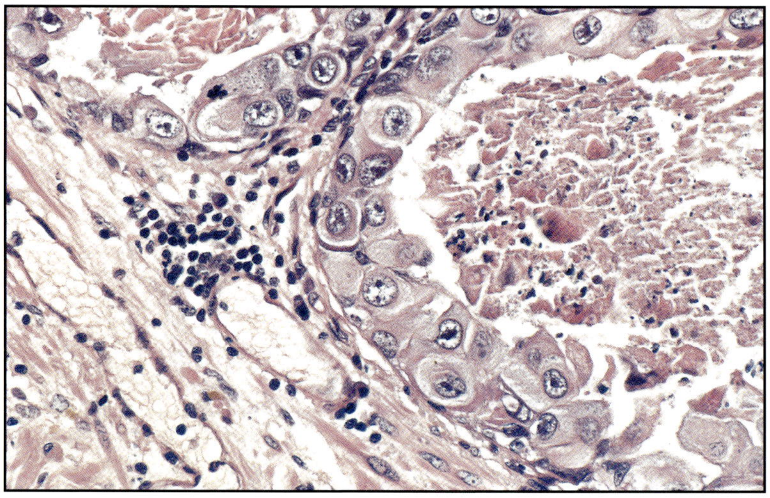

■ **i17.55** *Transitional cell carcinoma in prostate with comedo necrosis and pronounced cytologic atypia.*

spread can also be found **i17.53**. Intraductal papillary transitional cell carcinoma is rarely detected **i17.54** (Ende 1963, Goebbels 1985, Rhamy 1973). Why this is so is unknown, but there is a definite preference for in situ spread in the prostate by higher-grade transitional carcinoma cells. Another explanation is that the limited intraluminal volume of prostatic ducts and acini might only rarely permit formation of papillary structures (Ende 1963, Goebbels 1985). The presence of prostatic basal cells attests to the in situ nature of these transitional cell

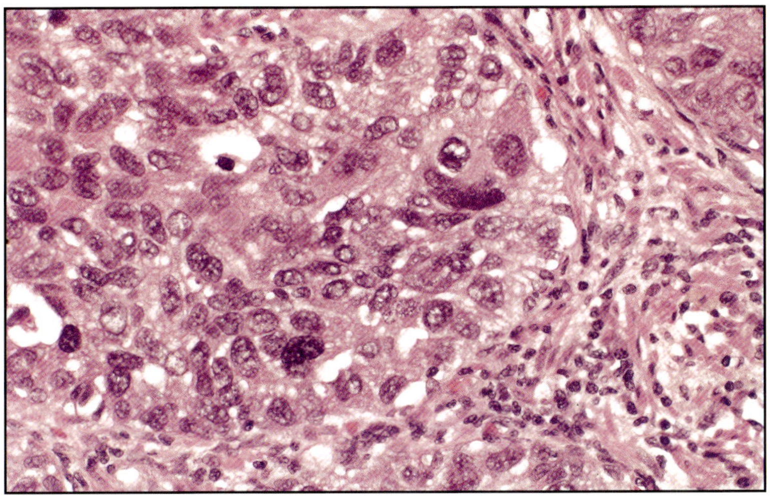

■ **i17.56** *Nuclear atypia in transitional cell carcinoma in the prostate is more pronounced than prostatic adenocarcinoma.*

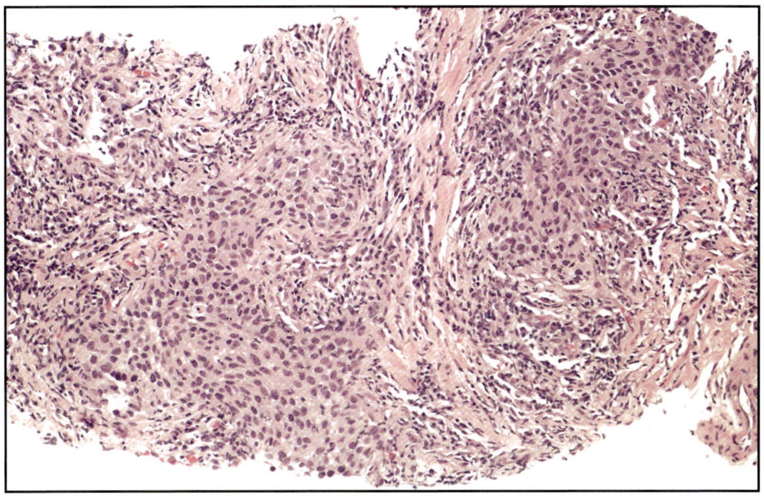

■ **i17.57** *Transitional cell carcinoma in prostate needle biopsy tissue: Irregular nodules of poorly differentiated carcinoma.*

carcinoma proliferations. Prostatic stromal invasion by transitional cell carcinoma is typified by irregular solid nests and cords (Johnson 1972, Kopelson 1978) that extend beyond the rounded, smooth outer profile of the transitional cell carcinoma in situ (CIS). Cytologically, transitional cell carcinoma in the prostate has a high nuclear grade with substantial nucleomegaly, nuclear pleomorphism, and nuclear hyperchromasia **i17.55, i17.56**. Prominent nucleoli often are evident. The cytoplasm often has an eosinophilic squamoid appearance. Glandular differentiation in the transitional cell carcinoma is absent (Greene 1973). Stromal sclerosis and inflammation often are pronounced **i17.49, i17.51** (Goebbels 1985, Greene 1976, Rhamy 1973); the inflammation can consist of acute and chronic inflammatory cells and can be associated with both in situ and invasive phases of growth.

The immunophenotypic profile of prostatic transitional cell carcinoma is the same as for urothelial carcinomas elsewhere (**t14.16, p 284**). They are PSA and PSAP negative and often are positive for the cytokeratins CK7, CK20, and high molecular weight cytokeratins bound by antibody 34βE12 (CK903) (Cheville 1998B, Oliai 2001). CEA staining is variable (Cheville 1998B).

Prostatic transitional cell carcinoma is thought to arise centrally in the large periurethral ducts via a pathway of urothelial dysplasia, with progression to carcinoma in situ (Ende 1963, Franks 1956, Karpas 1969, Ullman 1967). Because the neoplasm is more centrally located, in the past tissue diagnosis was mainly achieved by examination of TURP chips. However, transitional cell carcinoma in the prostate can be extensive, and both transitional cell CIS and invasive carcinoma can extend into the peripheral zone, such that transrectal needle biopsy sampling of transitional cell carcinoma is possible **i17.57** (Oliai 2001). In the past, it was stated that needle biopsy would miss more than 90% of cases (Rhamy 1973). It is not known how often prostatic transitional cell carcinoma would be missed using the current 6- to 12-core sampling of the prostate gland.

Spread of prostatic transitional cell carcinoma within ducts and acini can be extensive, without stromal invasion. Prostatic stromal infiltration is associated with lymphvascular space invasion in a substantial percentage (44%) of cases, but perineural invasion is much less common (at 14% of cases) (Goebbels 1985). Many cases exhibit locally aggressive growth, with extension into the bladder and pelvis (Nicolaisen 1984). Lymph node, lung, and osteolytic (with a few osteoblastic) bone metastases have been identified (Nicolaisen 1984). Rare sites of metastasis include kidney, pancreas, gallbladder, thymus, penis, skin, and testis (Han 2000, Rodrigues Netto 1990, Rodriguez Martinez 1999, Takashi 1990).

Grading and staging have been inconsistently performed. Three-tiered (Johnson 1972) and 4-tiered (Greene 1976) grading systems have been used. Most cases (89%) were high grade. The Gleason system should not be applied. It is not clear how to stage primary prostatic transitional cell carcinoma. In the past, the Whitmore-Jewett A-D staging scheme for adenocarcinoma was used (Greene 1973, Kopelson 1978) **t17.16**. The current primary tumor, regional lymph nodes, distant metastases (TNM) staging manual of the American Joint Committee on Cancer (AJCC) (Greene 2002) presents TNM definitions **t17.17**, but the T1 category is confusing because the prostate lacks a well-defined subepithelial connective tissue compartment. What is definitive is that the distinction between prostatic transitional cell CIS and stromal invasion, with or without associated bladder carcinoma, is critical for prognosis (Cheville 1998A).

The differential diagnosis of prostatic transitional cell carcinoma focuses on poorly differentiated prostatic adenocarcinoma, especially because they can present clinically in the same manner. Another potentially confounding factor is that in up to 30% of cases of primary prostatic transitional cell carcinoma, there is an associated prostatic acinar adenocarcinoma (Nicolaisen 1984). This applies to larger tissue specimens and not needle biopsy tissue samples. Histologically, a clue that one may be dealing with an unusual carcinoma is the presence of abundant inflammation in combination with rounded, solid nests of pleomorphic cells. Indeed, in one needle biopsy series, a majority of cases harbored only intraductal transitional cell CIS (Oliai 2001). Another diagnostic clue arguing for transitional cell carcinoma rather than prostatic adenocarcinoma is the greater degree of nuclear atypia in the former cancer. Mitoses and a squamoid cytoplasm also favor transitional cell carcinoma, whereas intraductal comedo-type necrosis may be seen in either ductal adenocarcinoma in situ or transitional cell CIS. In doubtful cases, immunostains for PSA, PSAP, high molecular weight cytokeratins (using 34βE12), and CK7 (and perhaps thrombomodulin [Ordóñez 1998]) can be extremely helpful (**t14.16**, p 284). Whenever one diagnoses transitional cell carcinoma in the prostate, one should raise the possibility of spread from the urethra or bladder. However, in prostatic tissue samples it is not morphologically possible to distinguish primary from secondary prostatic transitional cell carcinoma. Finally, transitional cell

t17.17 2002 AJCC TNM Staging Scheme for Primary Urothelial (Transitional Cell) Carcinoma of the Prostate

Primary Tumor (T)

Tis pu	Carcinoma in situ, with involvement of the prostatic urethra
Tis pd	Carcinoma in situ, with involvement of the prostatic ducts
T1	Tumor invades subepithelial connective tissue
T2	Tumor invades any of the following: prostatic stroma, corpus spongiosum, periurethral muscle
T3	Tumor invades any of the following: corpus cavernosum, beyond prostatic capsule, bladder neck (extraprostatic extension)
T4	Tumor invades other adjacent organs (invasion of the bladder)

Regional Lymph Nodes (N)

NX	Regional lymph nodes cannot be assessed
N0	No regional lymph node metastasis
N1	Metastasis in a single lymph node 2 cm or less in greatest dimension
N2	Metastasis in a single node more than 2 cm in greatest dimension, or in multiple nodes

Distant Metastasis (M)

MX	Distant metastasis cannot be assessed
M0	No distant metastasis
M1	Distant metastasis

Stage Grouping

Stage 0a	Ta	N0	M0
Stage 0is	Tis	N0	M0
Tis pu	N0	M0	
Tis pd	N0	M0	
Stage I	T1	N0	M0
Stage II	T2	N0	M0
Stage III	T1	N1	M0
	T2	N1	M0
	T3	N0	M0
	T3	N1	M0
Stage IV	T4	N0	M0
	T4	N1	M0
	Any T	N2	M0
	Any T	Any N	M1

Greene 2002

metaplasia is readily distinguished from transitional cell carcinoma based on the bland nuclei of the metaplastic cells.

The outcome for patients diagnosed with primary transitional cell carcinoma in the 1970s and 1980s was dismal, with an average survival of 17 to 29 months in the largest series **t17.16**. However, it is now abundantly clear that the prognosis for pure transitional cell CIS in the prostate is excellent, with or without bladder CIS, with 100% 5-year survival, compared with 45% of patients with prostatic stromal invasion (Cheville 1998A, 1998B). This early detection before the development of invasion is vital. Accurate diagnosis of prostatic transitional cell carcinoma is also essential because these neoplasms do not respond to androgen deprivation therapy used to treat some patients with high-grade prostatic adenocarcinoma (Nicolaisen 1984, Sawczuk 1985). The best therapeutic management for primary prostatic transitional cell carcinoma has not been defined (Sawczuk 1985).

[17.7] Small Cell Carcinoma

Small cell carcinoma primary in the prostate is a rare, extremely aggressive tumor that often presents with disseminated disease **t17.18**. Incidence estimates range from 0.3% (Losi 1994B) to 1% (Têtu 1987) of all prostatic carcinomas. In about one half of cases the carcinoma is pure small cell carcinoma, and in the other half there is a mixture with prostatic acinar adenocarcinoma. An intriguing and important aspect of prostatic small cell carcinoma diagnosis is that in one third of patients there was an initial diagnosis of adenocarcinoma, followed by therapy, usually hormonal, in turn followed (at median of 18 to 49 months, range 7 months to 8 years [Amato 1992, Hindson 1985, Têtu 1987]) by a subsequent diagnosis of small cell carcinoma. This could relate to tissue sampling error or emergence or progression of an aggressive androgen-insensitive neuroendocrine clone related to therapeutic selection pressure.

There are significant differences in the clinical features of prostatic small cell carcinoma and prostatic acinar adenocarcinoma. Distinctive clinical features include a lower percentage of men who present with an elevated serum PSA despite presentation at advanced stages, marked clinical symptomatology, large prostatic/pelvic mass, bulky lymphadenopathy, the propensity for rapid and widespread metastasis with visceral involvement, lack of hormonal responsiveness, and a short survival (Abbas 1995, Amato 1992, Hindson 1985, Papandreou 2002, Schwartz 1998, Têtu 1987) **t17.19**. This aggressive clinical behavior is similar to that of small cell carcinomas arising at other anatomic sites.

Most patients are men aged 65 to 72 years of age (range 24 [Okada 1996, Taylor 1983] to 89). The most common presenting symptoms are related to bladder outlet obstruction and disseminated disease (Abbas 1995). In a few cases paraneoplastic syndromes have been reported; these include Cushing syndrome (most common, caused by tumoral adrenocorticotropic hormone production), hypercalcemia, syndrome of inappropriate secretion of antidiuretic hormone, hyperparathyroidism, thyrotoxicosis, hyperglucagonemia, Eaton-Lambert syndrome, and limbic encephalitis (Abbas 1995, Stern 1999). The presence of such paraneoplastic syndromes in a patient with prostatic carcinoma should prompt a search, at the histologic level, for a small cell carcinoma element, but these syndromes are not specific for the small cell histologic type. One third to two thirds of patients with prostatic small cell carcinoma present with an elevated serum PSA; this elevation could be caused by an admixed adenocarcinomatous component. The DRE often is suspicious for malignancy, with an enlarged, irregular, and stony-hard prostate. Another dramatic difference compared with prostatic acinar adenocarcinoma is that 92% of patients with prostatic small cell carcinoma have advanced disease at presentation, and three quarters of patients have metastatic disease (Abbas 1995). The sites of clinically evident metastasis are also different, with spread to viscera, including liver and lung, being much more common in prostatic small cell carcinomas (Abbas 1995, Amato 1992, Hindson 1985, Têtu 1987). Also, widespread dissemination and metastatic deposits in unusual locations (such as omentum, vocal cord, temporal bone, axillary lymph node, epididymis, pericardium, and soft tissue [Hindson 1985, Smith 1992, Têtu 1987]) are more often seen with prostatic small cell

t17.18 Small Cell Carcinoma of Prostate

Rare: 0.3%-1% of all prostatic carcinomas
50% pure and 50% mixed with adenocarcinoma
Clinical presentation: advanced stage and widespread metastases
Microscopically identical to pulmonary small cell carcinoma (except for high rate of admixture with acinar adenocarcinoma)
Outcome poor

t17.19 Small Cell Carcinoma of Prostate: Clinical Features in Largest Series

Author	No.[1]	Incidence[2]	Age[3]	Presentation	Outcome
Têtu 1987	20	1%	67(30-89)	Rapid onset of urinary tract obstruction with dysuria, nocturia, urgency	55% died of disease at 10 months
Oesterling 1992	27	NG	72(48-87)	Stage A: 0% Stage B: 0% Stage C: 59% Stage D: 41% Serum PSA elevated in 66% of patients	Median survival 17.5 months (average 2-90)
Amato 1992	21	NG	65(55-77)	All had metastatic disease. Serum PSA increased in 1/14 (7%) Metastatic sites: Bone: 76% Lymph nodes: 57% Liver: 43% Lung: 33%	Median survival 9.4 months (range 1-25)
Schwartz 1998	12	NG	NG	One-third with elevated serum PSA; median = 1.7 ng/mL (range 0-110)	NG
Papandreou 2002	38	NG	65(40-80)	89% had metastases, 69% had bone pain and urinary symptoms	Overall survival 10.5 months. 22 patients had partial response to chemotherapy

[1]Number of patients
[2]Percentage of all prostatic carcinomas
[3]Median age (range)
[4]NG = not given

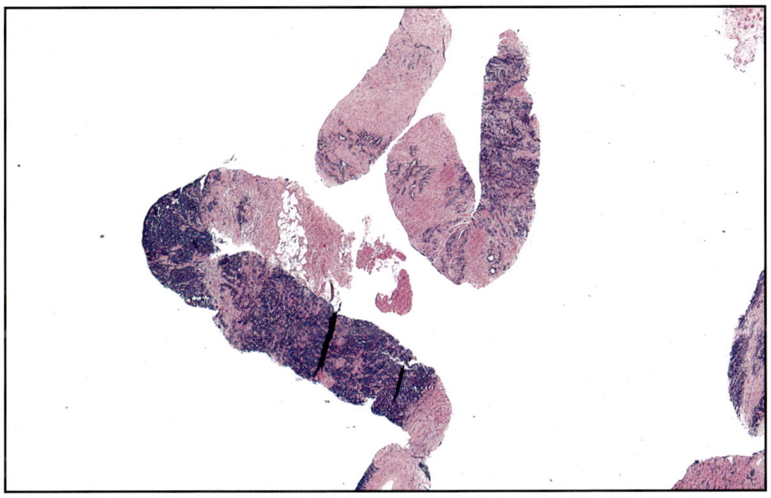

i17.58 *Small cell carcinoma in prostate needle biopsy tissue: Blue biopsy tissue at low-power magnification.*

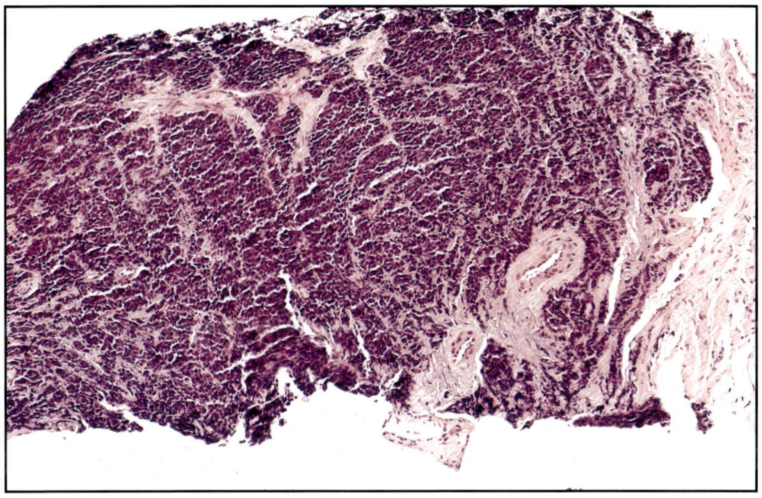

i17.59 *Small cell carcinoma in prostate needle core biopsy tissue: Sheet-like arrangement of small blue tumor cells. (High-power magnification of* **i17.58***).*

carcinomas than with prostatic acinar adenocarcinoma. Additionally, there is a high prevalence of lytic bone metastases (Papandreaou 2002). Finally, the low volume of osseous disease in the presence of visceral metastases should lead one to suspect small cell carcinoma (Amato 1992). Radiologically, CT and magnetic resonance imaging are useful in defining the extent of bulky, local disease and presence of metastases (Blunt 1996, Munechika 1995, Schwartz 1998).

Grossly, there is usually extensive involvement of the prostate, sometimes with replacement of the entire prostate by tumor (Amato 1992, Ghandur-Mnaymneh 1986, Patel 1993, Sarma 1989). At autopsy, cut surfaces are gray-whitish and nodular (Ghandur-Mnaymneh 1986, Hagood 1991), and extraprostatic extension into seminal vesicles, periprostatic soft tissue, and bladder can be visualized. In rare cases, prostatic small cell carcinoma is not clinically, radiologically, or grossly evident but is an incidental finding in patients with known prostatic carcinoma, discovered by examination of prostate sections from a radical prostatectomy specimen (Bolton 1994) or at autopsy (Turbat-Herrera 1988). Microscopically, prostatic small cell carcinoma is identical to its more common counterpart in the lung **i17.58-i17.64**, except that admixture with adenocarcinoma is much more common in the prostate. Histologically, prostatic small cell carcinoma grows as sheets, with ribbons, nesting, palisading along fibrous bands, and rosette-like structures occasionally noted. The polygonal, round, or spindled tumor cells exhibit only scanty cytoplasm, with hyperchromatic nuclei, salt-and-pepper stippled chromatin, and inconspicuous nucleoli. Nuclear molding can be evident. Both individual cell necrosis, manifested by karyorrhectic debris, and large areas of geographic necrosis can be seen. Encrustation of vessels with DNA (the Azzopardi phenomenon) can also be appreciated. Crush artifact is present in most cases **i17.61**. Mitoses are readily found. In one study (Christopher 1991), an average of 1 to 2 mitotic figures were detected per high-power field. Cytologically, prostatic small cell carcinoma has been diagnosed in pleural fluid (Renshaw 1996) and urine specimens (Nguyen-Ho 1994).

The acinar adenocarcinoma component in mixed small cell carcinoma–adenocarcinoma in the prostate is variable in grade and extent. The glandular component varies from focal to 70% (Têtu 1987) of the tumor volume. In most cases, particularly those in which adenocarcinoma preceded a diagnosis of small cell carcinoma (Hindson 1985), the histologic grade of the adenocarcinoma portion was

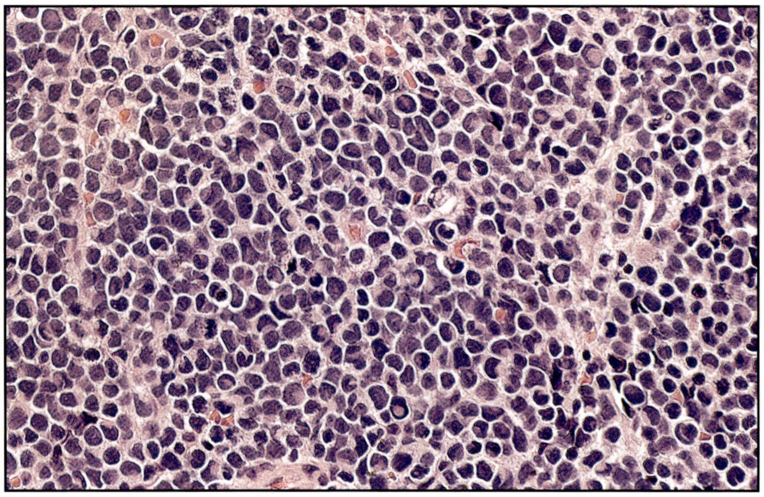

■ **i17.60** *Small cell carcinoma in the prostate. Sheet of neoplastic cells with scanty cytoplasm. Abundant nuclear debris and mitotic figures are typically appreciated.*

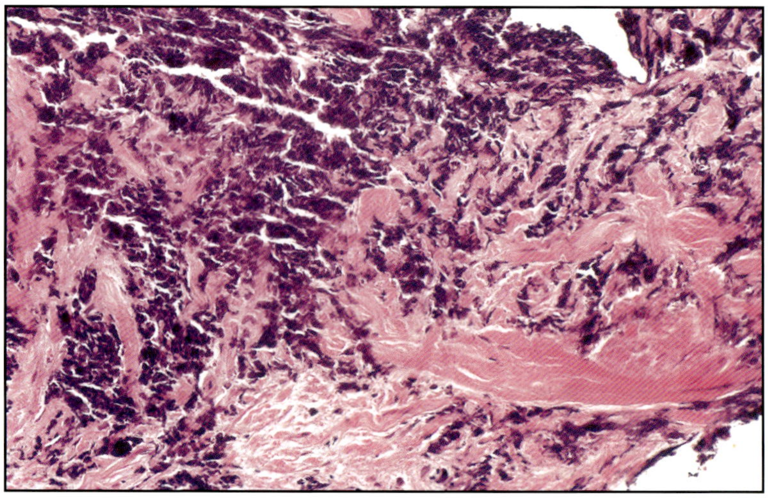

■ **i17.61** *"Crush" artifact in prostatic small cell carcinoma.*

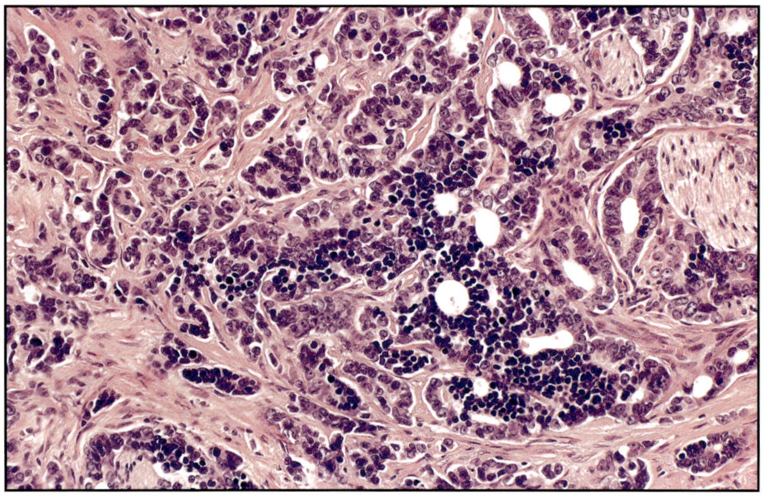

■ **i17.62** *Mixed small cell carcinoma-adenocarcinoma*

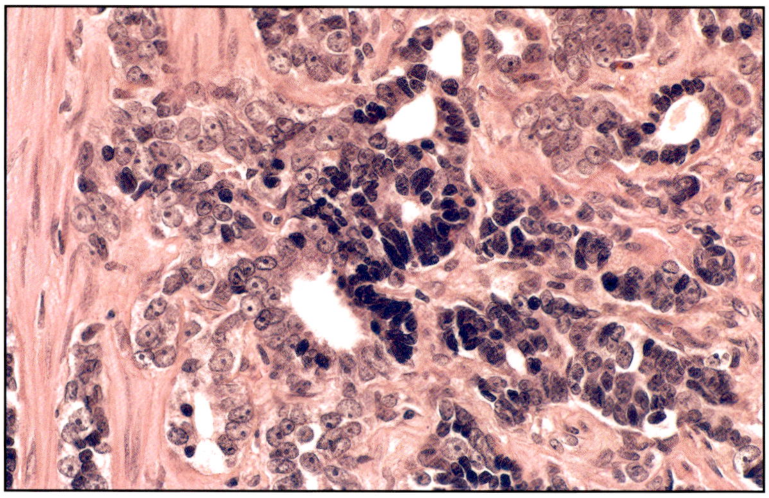

■ **i17.63** *Mixed small cell carcinoma-adenocarcinoma: The malignant glandular and neuroendocrine cells are admixed. (High-power magnification of* **i17.62***).*

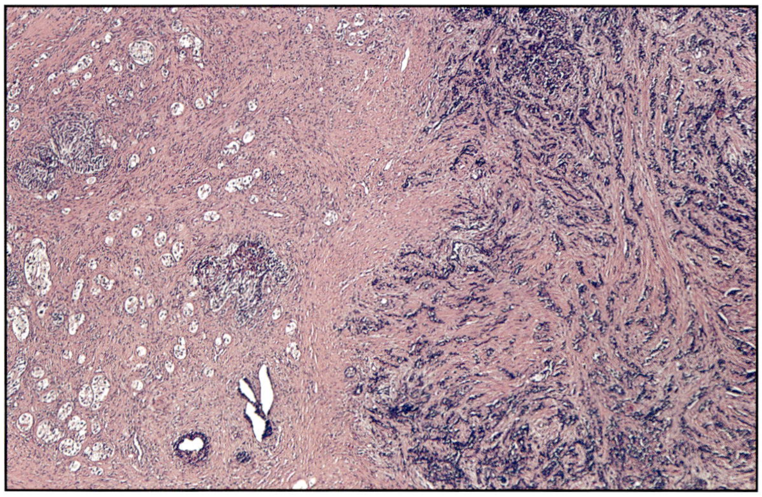

■ **i17.64** *Mixed small cell carcinoma-adenocarcinoma in hormone-refractory disease. The patient was treated with androgen-deprivation therapy and suffered progression. The small cell carcinoma component (left) was unaffected by the treatment, while the adenocarcinoma (right) exhibited cytoplasmic vacuolization and nuclear pyknosis.*

low grade (Gleason grade 2 or 3 [Hindson 1985] and M.D. Anderson grade I and II [Têtu 1987]), but high-grade Gleason pattern 4 and M.D. Anderson grades III and IV were reported in about one third of cases. In two thirds of cases the malignant epithelium of the adenocarcinoma and small cell carcinoma merge directly into each other **i17.62**. In one third of cases, there is physical separation of these components **i17.64**. In metastatic deposits derived from primary mixed small cell carcinoma–adenocarcinoma, the small cell carcinoma element often is found, although both components can be seen (Schron 1984). Rare examples of admixture of small cell carcinoma with malignant cells other than adenocarcinoma include coexistence with Paneth cell–like change (Weaver 1992), squamous cell carcinoma (Mahadevia 1983, Têtu 1987), and a spindle cell sarcomatoid component.

The immunophenotypic profile of prostatic small cell carcinoma can be valuable in confirming the diagnosis **t17.20**. Epithelial and neuroendocrine differentiation **i17.65** is best demonstrated by applying a panel of antibodies because no single marker is 100% sensitive **t17.20**. The prostatic markers PSA and PSAP are identified in only a small percentage of small cell carcinoma cases **t17.20**, so these immunostains are most often noncontributory in establishing a prostatic origin for a rare metastatic small cell carcinoma of unknown primary origin. The adenocarcinomatous component of mixed small cell carcinoma–adenocarcinoma is positive for PSA and PSAP in almost all cases. Immunohistochemical evidence of biosynthesis of a variety of

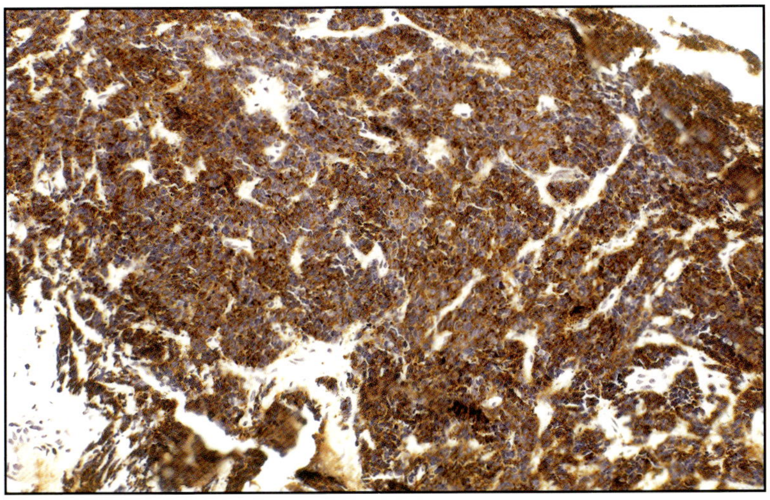

■ **i17.65** *Strong and diffuse chromogranin immunoreactivity in small cell carcinoma of prostate.*

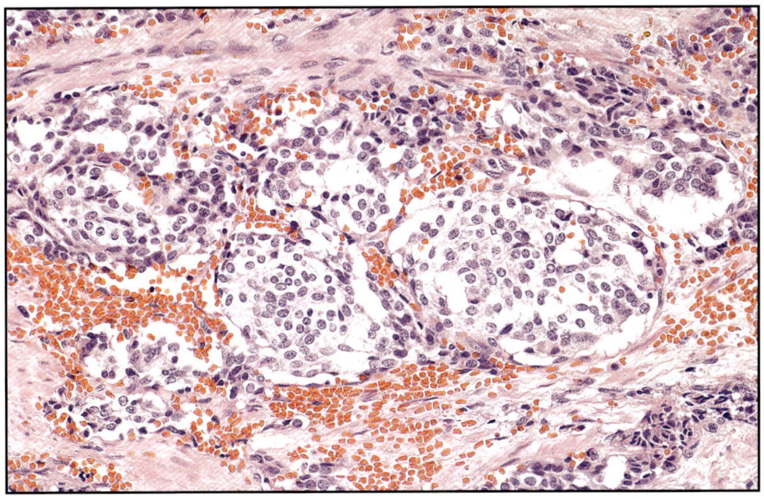

■ **i17.66** *The rare prostatic carcinoid tumor, with nested growth pattern (Case courtesy of Dr John Srigley).*

hormones can be obtained, including adrenocorticotropic hormone, calcitonin, serotonin, parathormone, antidiuretic hormone, gastrin, vasoactive intestinal peptide, bombesin, somatostatin, and thyrotropin (Abbas 1995). Expression of these bioactive molecules by prostatic small cell carcinoma can result in elevated serum levels in some cases and production of a paraneoplastic syndrome in a few cases.

Histochemical silver stains and electron microscopy have also been used to verify neuroendocrine differentiation in prostatic small cell carcinoma but are not routinely used because of their lower sensitivity (histochemical stains) and time and expense (electron microscopy). Histochemical argyrophil (Grimelius) and argentaffin (Fontana-Masson) stains are positive in only 35% and 5% of prostatic small cell carcinoma cases, respectively (Abbas 1995). Ultrastructural examination shows 75nm to 350nm intracytoplasmic dense core granules in 39% of prostatic small cell carcinoma cases (Abbas 1995, Bolton 1994, Christopher 1991, Nguyen-Ho 1994, Ro 1987, Sarma 1989, Turbat-Herrera 1988).

The differential diagnosis of prostatic small cell carcinoma encompasses small blue round cell tumors, poorly differentiated prostatic adenocarcinoma, usual prostatic adenocarcinoma with neuroendocrine differentiation, prostatic carcinoid tumor, prostatic large cell neuroendocrine carcinoma, and small cell carcinoma from

■ **t17.20 Small Cell Carcinoma of Prostate: Immunophenotype[1]**

Marker	% Cases Positive[2]
Cytokeratin	47%
Epithelial membrane antigen (EMA)	75%
Carcinoembryonic antigen (CEA)	47%
Neuron-specific enolase (NSE)	74%
Chromogranin A	60%
Synaptophysin	31%
Prostate specific antigen	12%
Prostate specific acid phosphatase	6%
ACTH	29%
Calcitonin	21%
Androgen receptor	Rare
Leukocyte common antigen (CD45)	0%

[1]Data compiled from Ro 1987, Krijnen 1993, Abbas 1995, Aqel 1995, Okada 1996, Sandhu 1997, Stern 1999, Helpap 1999, Lee 2001.
[2]The percentages refer to small cell carcinoma cells, either in pure or mixed form. The adenocarcinoma immunophenotype in mixed small cell-adenocarcinoma is the same as for pure adenocarcinoma.

other anatomic sites. The small blue round cell tumors to be considered include lymphoma, neuroblastoma, Ewing's sarcoma/primitive neuroectodermal tumor (PNET), and rhabdomyosarcoma. Lymphoma is the main consideration and can be excluded with negative CD45 and positive epithelial immunostains. Neuroblastoma and Ewing's sarcoma/PNET are hardly ever seen in the prostate, and prostatic rhabdomyosarcoma is found predominantly in children. Poorly differentiated prostatic adenocarcinomas lack the classic architectural and cytologic characteristics of small cell carcinoma and are more likely to exhibit diffuse and strong PSA and PSAP immunostaining. Neuroendocrine markers are not of benefit here because conventional prostatic adenocarcinomas can express these proteins (Di Sant'Agnese 2000). Indeed, the most common type of neuroendocrine differentiation in prostatic carcinoma is neuroendocrine differentiation detected by chromogranin A and serotonin immunostaining of acinar adenocarcinoma cells (Di Sant'Agnese 2000). Such neuroendocrine marker expression can be seen in almost all garden-variety prostatic acinar adenocarcinomas, although it is usually focal and minimal, with only about 10% of conventional adenocarcinomas harboring large numbers of neoplastic neuroendocrine cells (Di Sant'Agnese 2000). Prostatic carcinoid tumors (well-differentiated neuroendocrine carcinomas) and large cell neuroendocrine carcinomas are part of the neuroendocrine carcinoma spectrum in the prostate. As in the lung, prostatic carcinoids lack necrosis, and the tumor cells have more cytoplasm than small cell carcinoma **i17.66**. Large cell neuroendocrine carcinoma is not currently a defined entity in the prostate (Wynn 2000), but this author has seen several cases with features of large cell neuroendocrine carcinoma, where, as in the lung, the tumor cells are larger, with more vesicular nuclei and occasionally prominent nucleoli **i17.67-i17.71**. In the prostate, one should also clinically exclude small cell carcinoma spread from the bladder, lung, or other anatomic site. Exceptionally rare cases ($n = 2$) of small cell carcinoma of the lung presenting as a prostatic tumor have been reported (Madersbacher 1994, Smedley 1983). For men with metastatic deposits of small cell carcinoma, one should always consider the possibility of prostatic small cell carcinoma, particularly in men with a history of treated prostatic adenocarcinoma who have advanced or progressive disease in the absence of an elevated serum PSA. Distinction of prostatic small cell carcinoma from other small cell carcinomas in men with an unknown primary can be addressed with PSA and PSAP immunostains, although this is a low-yield procedure. Clinical and

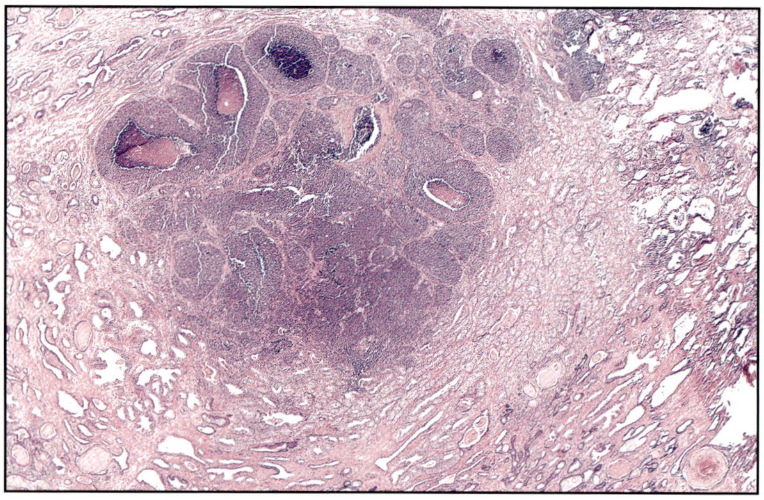

■ **i17.67** *Mixed large cell neuroendocrine carcinoma-adenocarcinoma: Nodule of neuroendocrine carcinoma, with adjacent peripheral adenocarcinoma.*

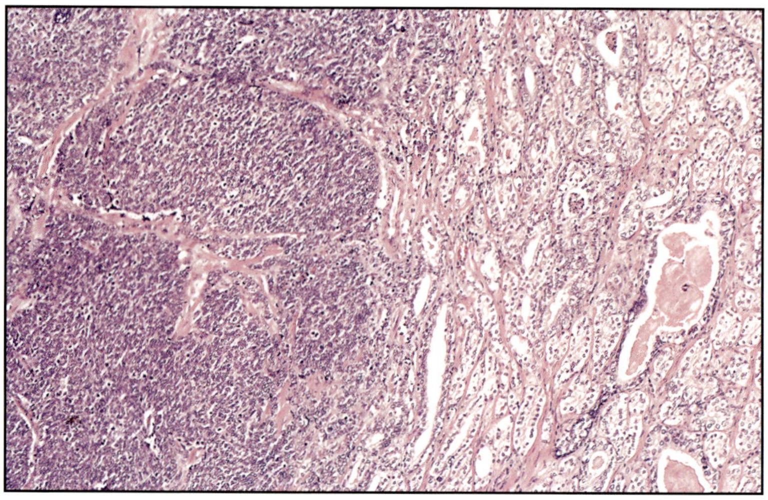

■ **i17.68** *Prostatic large cell neuroendocrine carcinoma, with adjacent adenocarcinoma.*

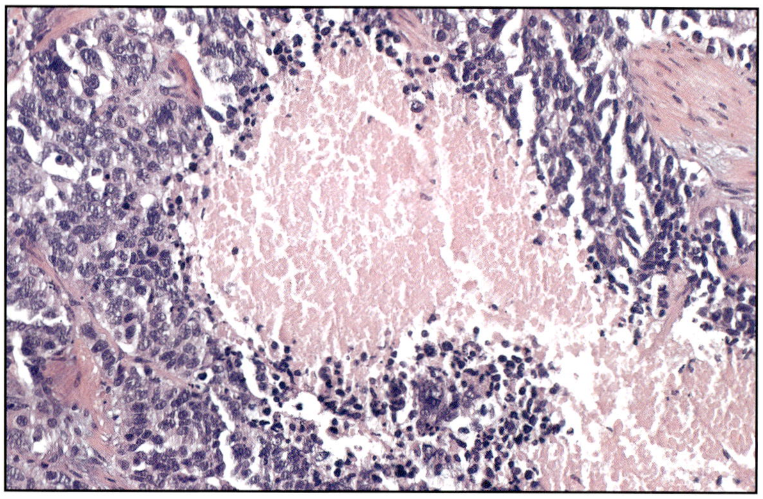

■ **i17.69** *Prostatic large cell neuroendocrine carcinoma, with abundant necrosis.*

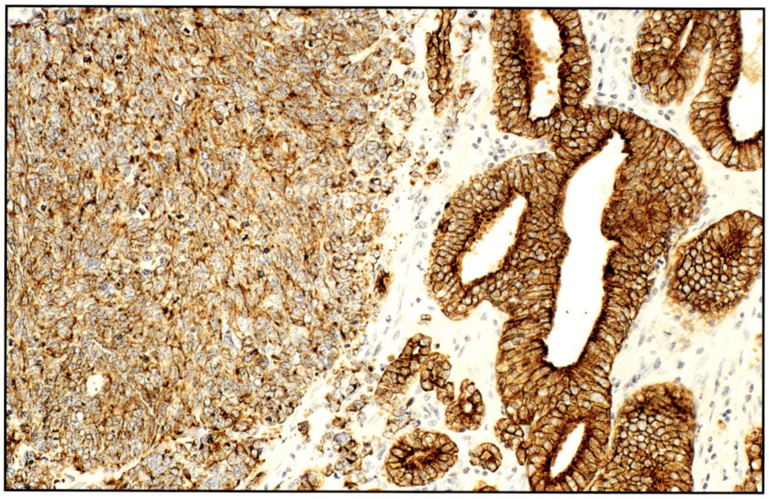

■ **i17.70** *Prostatic large cell neuroendocrine carcinoma: Cytokeratin positivity, with dot-like accentuation (left). The adenocarcinoma displays a different labeling pattern (right).*

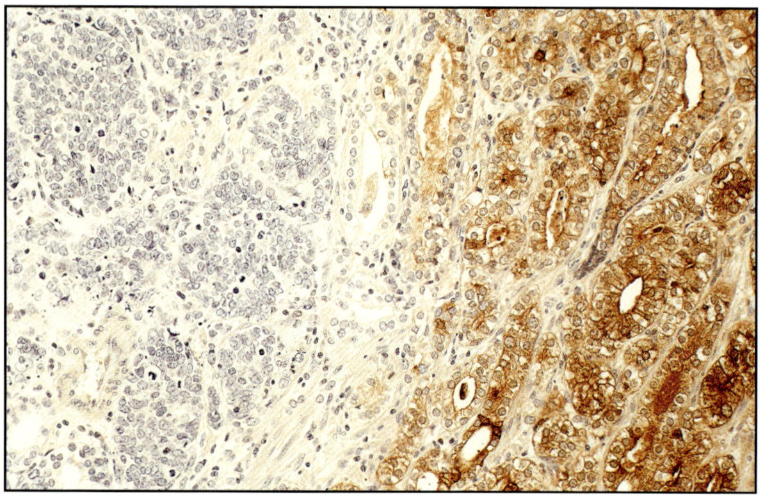

■ **i17.71** *Prostatic large cell neuroendorine carcinoma: PSA negative, with adjacent adenocarcinoma (right) being positive.*

radiologic correlations as to the location of a dominant mass are likely to be more fruitful.

The outcome for patients with small cell carcinoma of the prostate is dismal, with median average survival of 9 to 17 months. These are highly proliferative tumors (with a mean MIB-1 proliferation labeling index of 83% [Helpap 1999]) that generate early, widespread metastases. The neoplasms are not responsive to hormonal therapy, and although there may be an initial response to chemotherapy, in one study only primary surgery predicted survival (Mackey 1998, Papandreou 2002). However, because almost all patients present with advanced stage disease, few patients are treated with surgery. In one study, performance status, serum albumin level, and number of organs involved by metastases were predictors of survival time in multivariate analysis (Papandreou 2002). Patient age, sex, primary tumor size, stage, and serum PSA and neuroendocrine markers were not determinants of survival (Mackey 1998).

Diagnostic reporting of prostatic small cell carcinoma should include typing as pure small cell carcinoma or mixed small cell carcinoma–adenocarcinoma. Of critical importance, the presence of any amount of small cell carcinoma in mixed small cell carcinoma–adenocarcinoma should be diagnosed because the amount of small cell cancer does not affect survival (Têtu 1987). That is, patients with pure small cell carcinoma and mixed small cell carcinoma–adenocarcinoma have the same prognosis (Hindson 1985, Têtu 1987). If mixed, a Gleason grade should be given to the adenocarcinoma (if the patient has not been treated with hormones). Prostatic small cell carcinoma is not graded, and it is not necessary to distinguish oat cell from intermediate cell size because this is not a prognostic factor (Têtu 1987).

The cellular and clinical origins of prostatic neuroendocrine carcinoma are not clearly established. Many authors hold the view that prostatic small cell carcinoma originates from a common stem cell or a multipotential cell with the capacity to differentiate along both glandular and neuroendocrine lines (Abbas 1995). However, in a recently described transgenic animal model of high-grade prostatic neuroendocrine carcinoma, the carcinoma was shown to derive from the extremely small resident normal neuroendocrine cell population (Garabedian 1998). Both of these carcinogenesis models could be in operation. The initial progression pathway in this mouse model always proceeded through high-grade PIN. In humans, small cell neuroendocrine high-grade PIN and small cell carcinoma have been described in only a few cases (Bostwick 1997, Di Sant'Agnese 2000, Reyes 1997, Sarma 1989). Because of the typically bulky, extensive invasive carcinoma in the prostate, it is possible that in other cases, the invasive disease effaced the previously existing in situ neuroendocrine disease. In later clinical stages, it has been hypothesized that prostatic neuroendocrine and small cell carcinoma represents a progression pathway in the emergence of hormone-resistant cancer (Di Sant'Agnese 2000, Logothetis 1996). Prostatic small cell carcinomas lack the androgen receptor, are resistant to hormonal therapy, and can emerge or progress from hormonally treated usual acinar adenocarcinoma. Such emergence seems to be uncommon **i17.64**. Another proposed neuroendocrine pathway of prostate cancer progression is expansion of chromogranin-positive neuroendocrine cells in usual acinar adenocarcinomas, but this is controversial (Di Sant'Agnese 2000).

[17.8] Sarcomatoid Carcinoma (Carcinosarcoma)

Sarcomatoid carcinoma is a rare biphasic malignancy in the prostate **t17.21**. Fewer than 60 cases have been reported in the literature (Berney 1999, Delahunt 1999, Dundore 1995, Kaneko 1992, Kubosawa 1993, Lauwers 1993, Lindboe 1992, Luque Barona 2000, Poblet 2000, Reuter 1993, Sak 1997, Shannon 1992). More than one half of the cases are found in the 2 largest series (Dundore 1995, Shannon 1992) **t17.22**. The 2 elements of sarcomatoid carcinoma are a malignant epithelial (carcinomatous) component and a malignant mesenchymal or mesenchymal-like (sarcomatous) component. Sarcomatoid carcinoma may be either homologous, where the mesenchymal-like areas have the appearance of an undifferentiated sarcoma, or heterologous, where the sarcoma exhibits differentiation along the lines of specific mesenchymal cells such as bone and cartilage. *Carcinosarcoma* is a term that is synonymous with *heterologous sarcomatoid carcinoma.* Other terms that are equivalent to *sarcomatoid carcinoma* include *metaplastic carcinoma, spindle cell carcinoma,* and *malignant mixed mesodermal tumor.*

Clinically, most patients are around 70 years of age (range 50 to 89) and present with urinary tract obstruction and symptoms of frequency, urgency, and nocturia. On DRE, the palpable prostate is enlarged, nodular, and hard. An equal number of men have normal and elevated serum PSA levels (Berney 1999, Dundore 1995, Poblet 2000). Of note, in about half of all cases the initial diagnosis is a usual acinar adenocarcinoma, followed by hormonal or radiation therapy, with a subsequent diagnosis of sarcomatoid carcinoma **t17.22** (Berney 1999, Dundore 1995, Shannon 1992). There are several descriptions of the appearance of these tumors at TURP. In one a large, white glistening tumor was found (Meeter 1960), and in a second the tumor was characterized as rock-hard, gritty, and difficult to resect (Locke 1986).

Grossly, prostatic sarcomatoid carcinomas at pelvic exenteration, prostatectomy, and autopsy are large (5.5cm to 18cm), gray-white to pink masses with hemorrhage, necrosis, and local extension into surrounding structures such as seminal vesicle and rectal wall

t17.21 Sarcomatoid Carcinoma of the Prostate

- Rare: less than 60 reported cases
- Also known as carcinosarcoma (when heterologous mesenchymal elements are present), spindle cell carcinoma, metaplastic carcinoma
- Clinically, in men 70 years of age; one-half had prior diagnosis of pure adenocarcinoma followed by hormonal and/or radiation therapy
- A biphasic malignant neoplasm comprised of carcinomatous (usually adenocarcinoma) and spindled, pleomorphic sarcomatous (usually MFH-like, osteosarcoma and/or chondrosarcoma) elements
- Outcome poor

t17.22 Sarcomatoid Carcinoma of Prostate: Clinical Features in Largest Series

Author	No.[1]	Incidence[2]	Age[3]	Presentation	Sample[4]	Outcome
Shannon 1992	12	NG	71 (58-85)	Urinary tract obstruction; in 9/12 patients, sarcomatoid carcinoma appeared at a mean of 36 months (range 2-89) after initial diagnosis of adenocarcinoma	TURP Needle bx	Median survival 37 months (range 8-100) after initial diagnosis and median of 12 months (range 5-48) after appearance of sarcomatoid component
Dundore 1995	21	NG	68 (50-89)	Obstructive voiding symptoms; in 10/21 patients, sarcomatoid carcinoma appeared at a mean of 33 months (range 2-73) after initial diagnosis of adenocarcinoma. Eight of these 10 received hormonal and/or radiation therapy after the initial diagnosis. Metastatic disease present at initial diagnosis in 11 patients.	TURP	5-year survival: 41% 7-year survival: 14%

[1]Number of patients
[2]Not given
[3]Mean age (range)
[4]Tissue sample used to make diagnosis

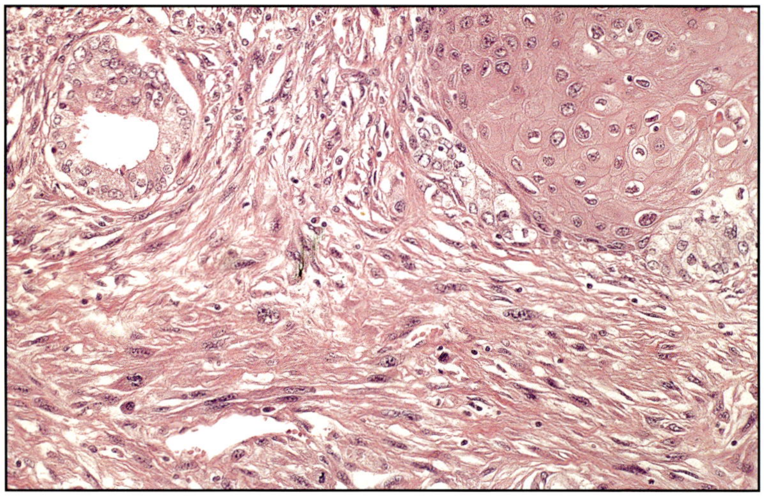

■ **i17.72** *Sarcomatoid carcinoma of the prostate with glandular (upper left), squamous (upper right), and homologous spindled elements.*

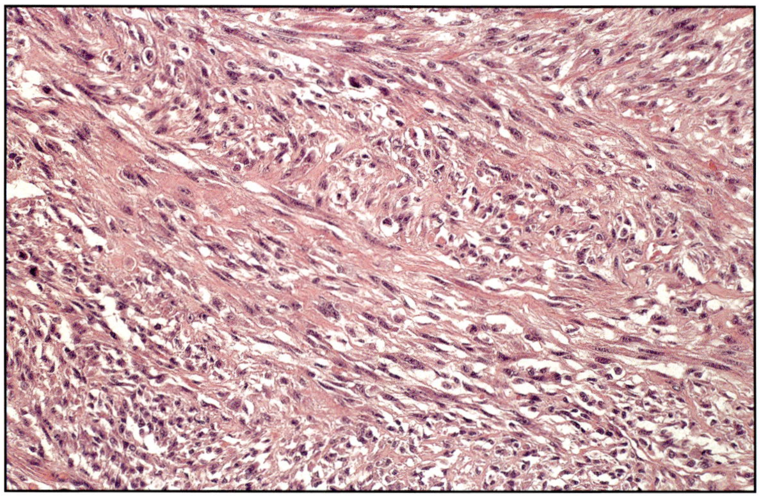

■ **i17.73** *Sarcomatoid carcinoma of the prostate : Homologous malignant cell population with fascicular growth.*

(Martin 1979, Meeter 1960, Nazeer 1991, Wick 1989, Zenklusen 1990). Translucent areas indicative of cartilage were present in one case (Martin 1979). In one autopsy case, extensive osteosarcoma led to "bony enlargement of the prostate," where the tumorous prostate had to be "chiseled loose" (Meeter 1960).

Microscopically, the carcinomatous and sarcomatous components are admixed, with blending in some areas **i17.72**. The carcinomatous element is almost always glandular and acinar. Two cases were ductal adenocarcinoma (Ma 1998, Poblet 2000), and 3 cases demonstrated squamous differentiation or adenosquamous carcinoma (Berney 1999, Martin 1979). I have seen a case of mixed acinar, ductal, and squamous differentiation in a sarcomatoid carcinoma. The adenocarcinoma typically is high grade, with a mean Gleason score of 9 (range 7 to 10) in the 2 largest series (Dundore 1995, Shannon 1992). In most cases, the adenocarcinoma component was a minor component, but it was dominant in one third of cases (Dundore 1995). The sarcomatoid component often exhibits large areas of undifferentiated spindled and pleomorphic cells arranged in sheets, pinwheels, or fascicles **i17.73, i17.74**. These patterns often resemble those of malignant fibrous histiocytoma (Shannon 1992). Cellularity is variable, from higher degrees to lower degrees in more hyalinized areas **i17.75**. Osteosarcoma **i17.76** and chondrosarcoma were by far the most frequently identified heterologous elements **t17.23**. Areas of fibrosarcoma, leiomyosarcoma, angiosarcoma, and rhabdomyosarcoma are rarely found. Different types of sarcoma can be found together in the same case. Cytologically, nuclear

■ **t17.23 Differentiation in Prostatic Sarcomatoid Carcinoma**

Carcinomatous Element[1]	Sarcomatous Element[1]
Adenocarcinoma: 95%	Osteosarcoma: 40%
Squamous cell and adenosquamous: 12%	MFH-like: 23%
	Chondrosarcoma: 21%
	Fibrosarcoma: 4%
	Rhabdomyosarcoma: 4%
	Leiomyosarcoma: 4%
	Angiosarcoma: 1%
	Liposarcoma: 0%

[1]Does not add up to 100% since specific pattern was not reported in some cases. In some cases more than one sarcomatous pattern can be seen

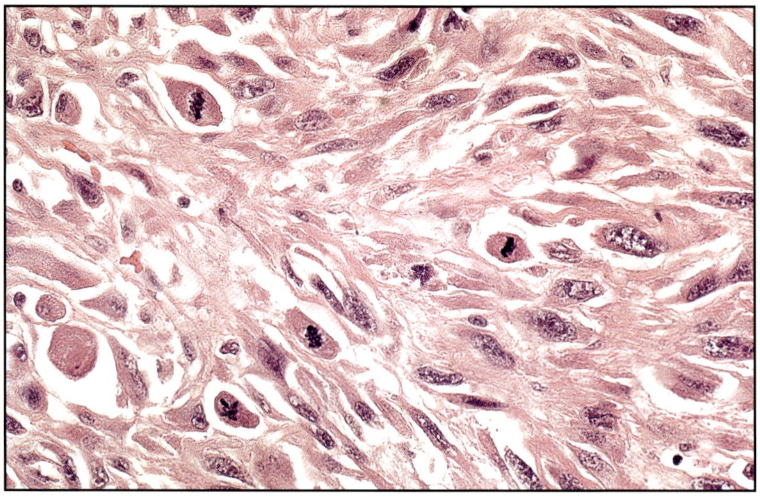

■ **i17.74** *Sarcomatoid carcinoma displaying nuclear atypia and a high mitotic rate.*

pleomorphism is moderate to marked (Shannon 1992), with numerous mitotic figures, including atypical ones, readily identified **i17.74**. In one study, an average of 14.8 mitoses were recognized per 10 high-power fields, with a range of 6 to 36 (Shannon 1992). Tumor giant cells, including osteoclast-like giant cells (Delahunt 1999), can be seen. Overall, the recommended Gleason grade for sarcomatoid carcinoma is pattern 5 (Bostwick 1994).

Immunohistochemical stains and electron microscopy have demonstrated mesenchymal or epithelial differentiation in the sarcomatoid component (Dundore 1995, Hokamura 1985, Kaneko 1992, Lauwers 1993, Locke 1986, Nazeer 1991, Ordóñez 1982, Poblet 2000, Reuter 1993, Shannon 1992, Tannenbaum 1975A, Wick 1989, Zenklusen 1990). Epithelial markers (cytokeratin, PSA, PSAP) and muscle markers can be detected by immunohistochemistry in the malignant spindle cells **t17.24**. Vimentin immunostains are uniformly positive, and S-100 protein is consistently found in chondrosarcomatous regions. In one case, skeletal muscle and vascular differentiation was substantiated by positivity for myoglobin and ulex europaeus I agglutinin, respectively (Wick 1989). Ultrastructural examination of the spindle cells has shown epithelial differentiation manifested as well-developed desmosomes, microvillus projections, intracytoplasmic keratin bundles (Shannon 1992), smooth muscle differentiation in the form of

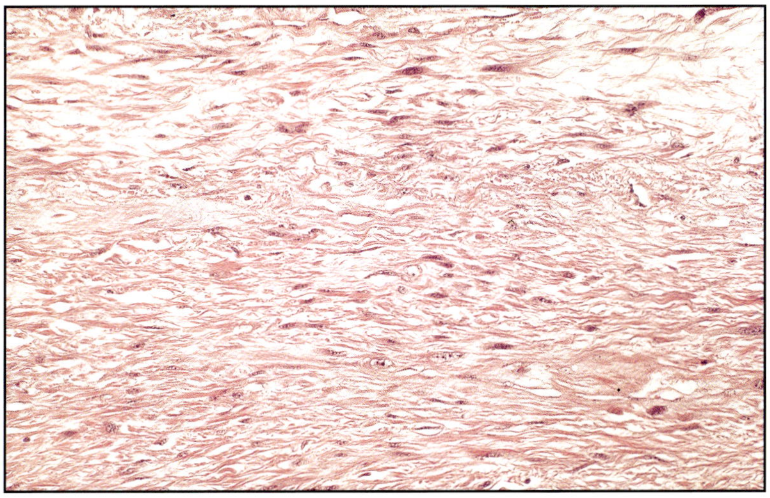

■ **i17.75** *Hypocellular area of sarcomatoid carcinoma of prostate.*

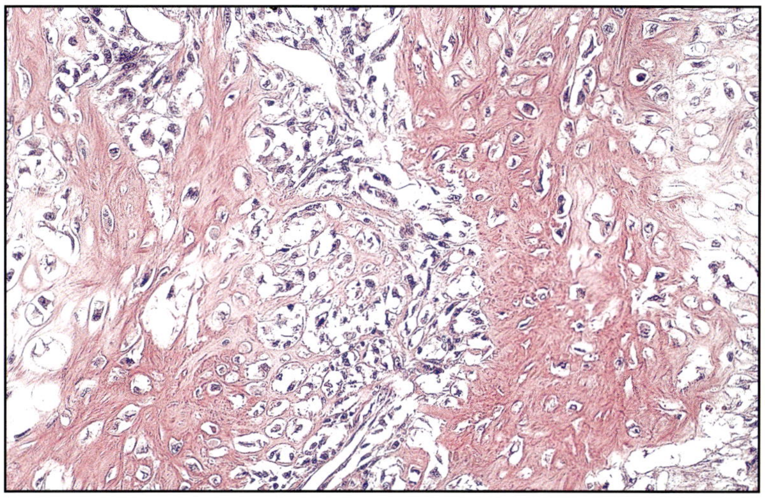

■ **i17.76** *Sarcomatoid carcinoma of prostate with heterologous osteosarcoma component.*

intracytoplasmic dense bodies or myofilaments (Martin 1979, Nazeer 1991), or no specific differentiation (Shannon 1992).

The differential diagnosis includes postoperative spindle cell nodule, inflammatory myofibroblastic tumor (also known as pseudosarcomatous fibromyxoid tumor and inflammatory pseudotumor), and stromal hyperplasia. These benign spindle cell proliferations enter into consideration if only a spindle cell proliferation is sampled. Certainly, it is possible to sample, in needle biopsy or TURP specimens, only the sarcomatoid component of a sarcomatoid carcinoma (Shannon 1992). In such cases, a clinical history of previous surgery should be sought, which might contribute to a stronger consideration of postoperative spindle cell nodule. Overall, significant nuclear atypia, with mitotic figures, especially atypical ones, with or without necrosis, would favor a malignant spindle cell proliferation, including sarcomatoid carcinoma. PSA and PSAP immunoreactivity in the spindle cells would argue for sarcomatoid carcinoma, whereas cytokeratin immunopositivity is not useful because it can be present in both sarcomatoid carcinoma cells and myofibroblasts in the benign entities. Other tumors to exclude before diagnosing sarcomatoid carcinoma include prostatic stromal proliferation of uncertain malignant potential (PSPUMP), primary prostatic sarcomas, and prostatic carcinoma with a pseudosarcomatous, fibrogenic stroma. Unlike in sarcomatoid carcinoma, mitoses are absent to rare in PSPUMP (Gaudin 1998). Primary prostatic sarcomas in older adults are rare and include mainly prostatic stromal sarcoma (Gaudin 1998) and leiomyosarcoma. These can be difficult or impossible to separate from sarcomatoid carcinoma if only the malignant spindle cell component is sampled. The detection of muscle markers should exclude prostatic stromal sarcoma (Gaudin 1998) but obviously not leiomyosarcoma. Because leiomyosarcoma can be seen in sarcomatoid carcinoma, it is usually not feasible, in a limited tissue sample (ie, not the whole prostate) and in the absence of a malignant epithelial component, to distinguish between primary prostatic leiomyosarcoma and sarcomatoid carcinoma. Cytokeratins can be found in both leiomyosarcoma (Iwata 2000) and the sarcomatoid element of sarcomatoid carcinoma. Only immunoreactive PSA or PSAP in the spindle cells would favor a diagnosis toward sarcomatoid carcinoma. "Collision tumors" of separate primary prostatic sarcomas and adenocarcinoma in the same prostate gland could potentially occur (Dundore 1995, Palma 1983), but criteria for what constitutes physically separate tumors is not set. These could also be viewed as sarcomatoid carcinoma because proof of separate origin would be difficult or impossible to procure. Finally, one should not confuse prostatic adenocarcinoma in a reactive, fibrogenic stroma with sarcomatoid carcinoma. This distinction is readily made if one pays attention to absence of nuclear atypia, lack of stromal overgrowth, and paucity of mitoses in the reactive stroma.

■ **t17.24 Immunophenotype of Sarcomatoid Component in Sarcomatoid Carcinoma of Prostate[1]**

Marker	% Cases Positive
PSAP	33%
Cytokeratin	11%
PSA	7%
Vimentin	100%
S-100	100%[2]
Muscle specific (common) actin	55%
Smooth muscle actin	43%
Desmin	10%

[1]Adenocarcinoma in sarcomatoid carcinoma exhibits same immunoprofile as pure adenocarcinoma
[2]In chondrosarcoma areas

The prognosis of patients with prostatic sarcomatoid carcinoma is poor, with a median survival of 3 years and 7-year survival of 14% (Haddad 1970, Reuter 1993). The disease can be locally aggressive, with local recurrences and formation of large pelvic masses. Sites of metastasis include, in order of frequency, lung, bone, lymph nodes, and brain, with rare cases of metastatic spread to skin, liver, peritoneum, adrenal, pleura, and kidney. Both epithelial and mesenchymal components can be seen in metastatic deposits (Haddad 1970, Hamlin 1967, Martin 1979, Shannon 1992). Treatment has varied (Dundore 1995, Shannon 1992); nonsurgical therapy was ineffective (Dundore 1995). The histologic pattern did not predict progression and survival (Dundore 1995).

The development of sarcomatoid carcinoma after treatment of an acinar adenocarcinoma with androgen deprivation therapy or radiotherapy is provocative. In some of these cases, particularly those in which the sarcomatoid carcinoma was diagnosed shortly (less than 1 year) after the pure adenocarcinoma, it is possible that the sarcomatoid part was just not sampled initially. However, there are at least 25 cases in which sarcomatoid carcinoma was diagnosed 1 year or more after acinar adenocarcinoma, and during the time interval there was hormonal treatment or radiotherapy. Indeed, the average time for developing sarcomatoid carcinoma after acinar adenocarcinoma is about 3 years (Dundore 1995, Shannon 1992) **t17.22**. One could then argue that this might be treatment selection pressure, where evolution and progression of an aggressive sarcomatoid clone from the adenocarcinoma occurred. In support of this notion are the findings of morphologic transitions between the adenocarcinoma and sarcomatoid elements and the mixed epithelial and mesenchymal phenotype in the spindle cell population. The molecular mechanisms underlying such selection have not been elucidated, although a role of abnormal p53 protein accumulation has been suggested (Delahunt 1999). Certainly, treatment is not the sole trigger because sarcomatoid carcinomas can occur de novo. Moreover, it appears to be a rare stimulus because sarcomatoid carcinoma itself is so rare.

[17.9] Others

There are single case reports of lymphoepithelioma-like carcinoma (Adlakha 1994) and tubulocystic clear cell adenocarcinoma of the prostate (Pan 2000). The patient with lymphoepithelioma-like carcinoma was a 66-year-old man who underwent transrectal needle biopsy because of an elevated serum PSA of 5.5 and bilateral palpable nodularity of the prostate. Although the needle biopsy tissue had only a typical Gleason score 7 acinar adenocarcinoma, the radical prostatectomy sections revealed, in one half of the tumor, cohesive sheets and syncytial nests of undifferentiated carcinoma accompanied by a dense lymphocytic inflammatory cell infiltrate. Unlike in histologically similar head and neck carcinomas, no Epstein-Barr virus presence was detected. The Gleason grade was considered high-grade pattern 5 because of the solid sheets of tumor. It was proposed that at least 25% of tumor be lymphoepithelioma-like to qualify for this diagnosis, but this was admittedly arbitrary. One of the main entities in the differential diagnosis is transitional cell carcinoma with a prominent lymphoid response, but unlike transitional cell carcinoma, lymphoepithelioma-like carcinoma is positive for PSA and PSAP immunohistochemical reactivity. Lymphoma may be a passing thought, but in lymphoepithelioma-like carcinoma, malignant epithelium was clearly present, and the lymphoid infiltrate is a mixture of T and polyclonal B cells (Adlakha 1994).

Tubulocystic clear cell adenocarcinoma of the prostate was reported in a 47 year-old man who had a 1-year history of painful gross hematuria (Pan 2000). Histologically, this intraprostatic neoplasm was indistinguishable from classic clear cell adenocarcinoma of the ovary, with tubulocystic and papillary structures lined by clear or hobnail cells. The patient developed testicular and pulmonary metastases. The differential diagnosis includes nephrogenic adenoma of the prostatic urethra and prostatic adenocarcinoma with cleared cytoplasm, direct extension from clear cell adenocarcinoma of the urethra or bladder, direct extension of transitional cell carcinoma with clear cells, and metastatic renal cell carcinoma of clear cell type.

References

Abbas F, Civantos F, Benedetto P, et al. Small cell carcinoma of the bladder and prostate. *Urology* 46:617-630, 1995.

Abe K, Ohishi Y, Onodera S, et al. A case of primary transitional cell carcinoma of the prostate responsive to combination chemotherapy with methotrexate, epirubicin and cisplatin [in Japanese]. *Acta Urol Jpn* 44:415-417, 1998.

Accetta PA, Gardner WA. Squamous metastases from prostatic adenocarcinoma. *Prostate* 3:515-521, 1982.

Accetta PA, Gardner WA Jr. Adenosquamous carcinoma of prostate. *Urology* 32:73-75, 1983.

Adlakha K, Bostwick DG. Lymphoepithelioma-like carcinoma of the prostate. A new histologic variant of prostatic adenocarcinoma. *J Urol Pathol* 2:319-325, 1994.

Ahn SK, Kim K, Choi IJ, et al. Adenoid cystic carcinoma of the prostate gland. Pathological review with a case report. *Yonsei Med J* 32:74-78, 1991.

Al Adnani MS. Schistosomiasis, metaplasia and squamous cell carcinoma of the prostate: histogenesis of the squamous cancer cells determined by localization of specific markers. *Neoplasma* 32:613-622, 1985.

Alfthan O, Koivuniemi A. Mucinous carcinoma of the prostate. Case report. *Scand J Urol Nephrol* 4:78-80, 1970.

Alguacil-Garcia A. Artifactual changes mimicking signet ring cell carcinoma of transurethral prostatectomy specimens. *Am J Surg Pathol* 10:795-800, 1986.

Ali-Fehmi R, Merati K, Grignon D, et al. Proliferative index and cell cycle regulators expression in high grade prostatic intraepithelial neoplasia (HGPIN) and ductal "endometrioid" prostatic carcinoma [abstract]. *Mod Pathol* 14:100A, 2001.

Alline KM, Cohen MB. Signet-ring cell carcinoma of the prostate. *Arch Pathol Lab Med* 116:99-102, 1992.

Allsbrook WC Jr, Pfeifer EA. Histochemistry of the prostate. In: Foster CS, Bostwick DG, eds. *Pathology of the Prostate.* Philadelphia: WB Saunders; 296-298, 1998.

Amato RJ, Logothetis CJ, Hallinan R, et al. Chemotherapy for small cell carcinoma of prostate origin. *J Urol* 147:935-937, 1992.

Aqel NM, El-Hady S, Henry K, et al. Small cell carcinoma of the prostate. A case report and discussion of histogenesis. *Int J Surg Pathol* 2:237-244, 1995.

Armonis BN, Harland SJ, Milroy EJG, et al. Misdiagnosis of prostatic primary duct carcinoma. *Br J Urol* 72: 978-979, 1993.

Arnheim FK. Carcinoma of the prostate: a study of the postmortem findings in one hundred and seventy-six cases. *J Urol* 60:599-603, 1948.

Aseuro Mantero M, Gomez Velazquez M, Leal Arenas J. A case of epidermoid carcinoma of the prostate [in Spanish]. *Arch Esp Urol* 40:681-684, 1987.

Attaran SY, Daneshbod K. Primary signet-ring cell adenocarcinoma of the prostate (a case report). *Ind J Pathol Microbiol* 30:379-382, 1987.

Aydin F. Endometrioid adenocarcinoma of prostatic urethra presenting with anterior urethral implantation. *Urology* 41:91-95, 1993.

Aygun C. Small cell carcinoma of the prostate: a case report and review of the literature. *Md Med J* 46:353-356, 1997.

Bainborough AR. Squamous metaplasia of prostate following estrogen therapy. *J Urol* 68:324-336, 1952.

Bassler TJ Jr, Orozco R, Bassler IC, et al. Adenosquamous carcinoma of the prostate: case report with DNA analysis, immunohistochemistry and literature review. *Urology* 53:832-834, 1999.

Bates HR, Thornton JL. Carcinoma of the prostate ducts. *Am J Clin Pathol* 45:96-98, 1966.

Bates HR. Transitional cell carcinoma of the prostate. *J Urol* 101:206-207, 1969.

Ben-Izhak O, Lichtig C. Signet-ring cell carcinoma of the prostate mimicking primary gastric carcinoma. *J Clin Pathol* 45:452-454, 1992.

Bennett RS, Edgerton EO. Mixed prostatic carcinoma. *J Urol* 110:561-563, 1973.

Berney DM, Ravi R, Baithun SI. Prostatic carcinosarcoma with squamous cell differentiation: a consequence of hormonal therapy: report of two cases and review of the literature. *J Urol Pathol* 11:123-132, 1999.

Bircan K, Usar I, Ergen A, et al. Histopathological pattern in prostatic adenocarcinoma: is it a prognostic criterion? *Int Urol Nephrol* 23:57-64, 1991.

Bleichner JC, Chun B, Klappenbach RS. Pure small-cell carcinoma of the prostate with fatal liver metastasis. *Arch Pathol Lab Med* 110:1041-1044, 1986.

Blunt DM, Sansom HE, King DM. Imaging of small cell carcinoma of the male urogenital tract. *Clin Radiol* 51:724-727, 1996.

Bock BJ, Bostwick DG. Does prostatic ductal adenocarcinoma exist? *Am J Surg Pathol* 23:781-785, 1999.

Bodner DR, Cohen JK, Resnick MI. Primary transitional cell carcinoma of the prostate. *J Urol* 92:121-122, 1986.

Bolton DM, Chiu ST, Clarke S, et al. Primary small cell carcinoma of the prostate: unusual modes of presentation. *Aust N Z J Surg* 64:91-94, 1994.

Bosland MC, Ford H, Horton L. Induction at high incidence of ductal prostate adenocarcinomas in NBL/Cr and Sprague-Dawley Hsd: SD rats treated with a combination of testosterone and estradiol-17β or diethylstilbestrol. *Carcinogenesis* 16:1311-1317, 1995.

Bostwick DG, Kindrachuk RW, Rouse RV. Prostatic adenocarcinoma with endometrioid features. Clinical, pathologic, and ultrastructural findings. *Am J Surg Pathol* 9:595-609, 1985.

Bostwick DG. Grading prostate cancer. *Am J Clin Pathol* 102(suppl):S38-S56, 1994.

Bostwick DG, Wollan P, Adlakha K. Collagenous micronodules in prostate cancer. A specific but infrequent diagnostic finding. *Arch Pathol Lab Med* 119:444-447, 1995.

Bostwick DG, Dundore PA. Variants of prostatic adenocarcinoma. In: *Biopsy Pathology of the Prostate.* London: Chapman & Hall Medical; 167-189, 1997.

Boyd S. Case of colloid scirrhus of prostate. *Trans Pathol Soc London* 33:200-203, 1881.

Braslis KG, Davi RC, Nelson E, et al. Squamous cell carcinoma of the prostate: a transformation from adenocarcinoma after the use of a luteinizing hormone-releasing hormone agonist and flutamide. *Urology* 45:329-331, 1995.

Brinker DA, Potter SR, Epstein JI. Ductal adenocarcinoma of the prostate diagnosed on needle biopsy. Correlation with clinical and radical prostatectomy findings and progression. *Am J Surg Pathol* 23:1471-1479, 1999.

Brooks B, Miller GJ. Evaluation of prostatic cancer histology and grade distribution: experience with the Colorado Central Cancer Registry. *Prostate* 8:139-150, 1986.

Brown L, ed. *The New Shorter Oxford English Dictionary.* Oxford, England: Clarendon Press; 3547, 1993.

Busto Castanon L, Sousa Escandon A, Rodriguez Garcia J, et al. Transitional cell carcinoma of the prostate [in Spanish]. *Acta Urol Esp* 14:365-367, 1990.

Carney JA, Kelalis PP. Endometrial carcinoma of the prostatic utricle. *Am J Clin Pathol* 60:565-573, 1973.

Carpenter AA, Bernardo JR Jr. Adenoid cystic carcinoma of Cowper's gland: case report. *J Urol* 106:701-703, 1971.

Catton PA, Hartwick RWJ, Srigley JR. Prostate cancer presenting with malignant ascites: signet ring cell variant of prostate adenocarcinoma. *Urology* 39:495-497, 1992.

Cecchi M, Sepich CA, Bertolini L, et al. Adenoid cystic carcinoma of the prostate. Clinical case [in Italian]. *Minerva Urol Nefrol* 52:73-75, 2000.

Cheville JC, Dundore PA, Bostwick DG, et al. Transitional cell carcinoma of the prostate. Clinicopathologic study of 50 cases. *Cancer* 82:703-707, 1998A.

Cheville JC. Urothelial carcinoma of the prostate. An immunohistochemical comparison with high grade prostatic adenocarcinoma and review of the literature. *J Urol Pathol* 9:141-154, 1998B.

Chica G, Johnson DE, Ayala AG. Mucinous adenocarcinoma of the prostate. *J Urol* 118:124-125, 1977.

Chikazawa H, Uchihayashi T, Ohtaki M. Mucus-forming adenocarcinoma of the prostate: report of a case. *Jpn J Clin Urol* 28:743, 1974.

Christensen WN, Steinberg G, Walsh PC, et al. Prostatic duct adenocarcinoma. Findings at radical prostatectomy. *Cancer* 67:2118-2124, 1991.

Christopher ME, Seftel AD, Sorenson K, et al. Small cell carcinoma of the genitourinary tract: an immunohistochemical, electron microscopic and clinicopathological study. *J Urol* 146:382-388, 1991.

Cia EMM, Moriyama H, Billis A, et al. Metastases in epididymides from papillary adenocarcinoma of prostate. *Urology* 18:607-608, 1981.

Cina SJ, Epstein JI. Adenocarcinoma of the prostate with atrophic features. *Am J Surg Pathol* 21:289-295, 1997.

Cohen RJ, Goldberg RD, Verhaart MJS, et al. Adenoid cyst-like carcinoma of the prostate gland. Arch Pathol Lab Med 117:799-801, 1993.

Colpaert C, Gentens P, Van Marck E. Ductal ("endometrioid") adenocarcinoma of the prostate. *Acta Urol Belg* 66:29-32, 1998.

Copeland JN, Amin MB, Humphrey PA, et al. The morphologic spectrum of metastatic prostatic adenocarcinoma to the lung: special emphasis on histologic features overlapping with other pulmonary neoplasms. *Am J Clin Pathol* 117:552-557, 2002.

Corder MP, Cicmil GA. Effective treatment of metastatic squamous cell carcinoma of the prostate with adriamycin. *J Urol* 115:222, 1976.

Cricco RP, Kassis J. Mucinous adenocarcinoma of prostate. *Urology* 14:276-278, 1979.

Das S. Endometrial carcinoma of the prostate. *Urology* 27:543-545, 1986.

Daugherty RL, Cos LR, Keller JW, et al. Nondetectable prostate specific antigen in moderately differentiated adenocarcinoma of the prostate. *Urology* 39:552-555, 1992.

Delahunt B, Nacey JN. Broadsheet number 45: thin core biopsy of prostate. *Pathology* 30:247-256, 1998.

Delahunt B, Eble JN, Nacey JN, et al. Sarcomatoid carcinoma of the prostate: progression from adenocarcinoma associated with p53 over-expression. *Anticancer Res* 19:4279-4283, 1999.

DeMay RM. Urine. In: *The Art and Science of Cytopathology.* Chicago: ASCP Press; 409, 1996.

Denholm SW, Webb JN, Howard GCW, et al. Basaloid carcinoma of the prostate gland: histogenesis and review of the literature. *Histopathology* 20:151-155, 1992.

Devaney DM, Dorman A, Leader M. Adenosquamous carcinoma of the prostate: a case report. *Hum Pathol* 22:1046-1050, 1991.

Devaraj LT, Bostwick DG. Atypical basal cell hyperplasia of the prostate. Immunophenotypic profile and proposed classification of basal cell proliferations. *Am J Surg Pathol* 17:645-659, 1993.

DeYoung BR, Wick MR. Immunohistologic evaluation of metastatic carcinomas of unknown origin: an algorithmic approach. *Semin Diagn Pathol* 17:184-193, 2000.

Dhom G. Pathologie des Prostata-Carcinoms. *Verh Dtsch Ges Urol* 32:9-16, 1980.

Dhom G. Unusual prostatic carcinomas. *Pathol Res Pract* 186:28-36, 1990.

Di Sant'Agnese PA. Divergent neuroendocrine differentiation in prostatic carcinoma. *Semin Diagn Pathol* 17:149-161, 2000.

Dube VE, Farrow GM, Greene LF. Prostatic adenocarcinoma of ductal origin. *Cancer* 32:402-409, 1973.

Dundore PA, Cheville CJ, Nascimento AG, et al. Carcinosarcoma of the prostate. Report of 21 cases. *Cancer* 76:1035-1042, 1995.

Dunnick NR, Walther PJ, Ford KK, et al. Mucinous adenocarcinoma of the prostate. *J Comput Assist Tomogr* 6:1198-1199, 1982.

Efros MD, Choudhury M, Fischer J, et al. Unusual primary prostatic malignancies. *Urology* 39:407-410, 1992.

Egan AJM, Lopez-Beltan A, Bostwick DG. Prostatic adenocarcinoma with atrophic features: malignancy mimicking a benign process. *Am J Surg Pathol* 21:931-935, 1997.

Egawa S, Wheeler TM, Greene DR, et al. Unusual hyperechoic appearance of prostate cancer on transrectal ultrasonography. *Br J Urol* 69:169-174, 1992.

Ehara H, Ito M, Yamaha M, et al. Secondary tumor of the prostate: a case report [in Japanese]. *Acta Urol Jpn* 37:923-925, 1991.

Elbadawi A, Craig W, Linke CA, et al. Prostatic mucinous carcinoma. *Urology* 13:658-666, 1979.

Ellis GL, Auclair PL. Malignant epithelial tumors. In: *Tumors of the Salivary Glands.* Washington, DC: Armed Forces Institute of Pathology; 1996.

Ende N, Woods LP, Shelley HS. Carcinoma originating in ducts surrounding the prostatic urethra. *Am J Clin Pathol* 40:183-189, 1963.

Epstein JI, Lieberman PH. Mucinous adenocarcinoma of the prostate gland. *Am J Surg Pathol* 9:299-308, 1985.

Epstein JI, Woodruff JM. Adenocarcinoma of the prostate with endometrioid features. A light microscopic and immunohistochemical study of ten cases. *Cancer* 57:111-119, 1986.

Ezura M, Kimura N, Nagura H. A case of mucinous adenocarcinoma of the prostate [in Japanese]. *Jpn J Cancer Clin* 36:563-566, 1990.

Fergusson JD, Franks LM. The response of prostatic carcinoma to oestrogen treatment. *Br J Surg* 40:422-428, 1953.

Ferrero G, Mastroberardino E, Del Vino A, et al. Mucinous adenocarcinoma of the prostate: description of a case [in Italian]. *Pathologica* 92:86-88, 2000.

Foot NC, Humphreys GA, Coats EC. Carcinoma of the prostate. A review of 162 cases with a pathologic classification. *N Y State J Med* 50:84-88, 1950.

Frankel K, Craig JR. Adenoid cystic carcinoma of the prostate. Report of a case. *Am J Clin Pathol* 62:639-645, 1974.

Franks LM. Latent carcinoma of prostate. *J Pathol Bacteriol* 68:603-616, 1954.

Franks LM, Chesterman FC. Intraepithelial carcinoma of the prostatic urethra, periurethral glands and prostatic ducts (Bowen's disease of urinary epithelium). *Br J Cancer* 10:223-225, 1956.

Franks LM, O'Shea JD, Thomson AER. Mucin in the prostate: a histochemical study in normal glands, latent, clinical, and colloid cancers. *Cancer* 17:983-991, 1964.

Freedy RM, Miller KD Jr. Small cell carcinoma of the prostate: metastases to the brain as shown by CT and MR with pathologic correlation. *AJNR Am J Neuroradiol* 11:947-948, 1990.

Frkovic-Grazio S, Kraljic I, Trnski D, et al. Immunohistochemical staining and serotest markers during development of a sarcomatoid and small cell prostate tumor. *Anticancer Res* 14:2151-2156, 1996.

Fujino A. A case of prostatic ductal adenocarcinoma with endometrioid features, associated with rectal invasion and multiple liver metastases [in Japanese]. *Jpn J Urol* 89:792-795, 1998.

Fukuoka H, Yamazaki A, Kitamura H. A case of papillary adenocarcinoma of the prostate [in Japanese]. *Acta Urol Jpn* 30:663-669, 1984.

Garabedian EM, Humphrey PA, Gordon JI. A transgenic mouse model of metastatic prostatic cancer from neuroendocrine cells. *Proc Natl Acad Sci* 95:15382-15387, 1998.

Gattuso P, Carson HJ, Candel A, et al. Adenosquamous carcinoma of the prostate. *Hum Pathol* 26:123-126, 1995.

Gaudin PB, Rosai J, Epstein JI. Sarcomas and related proliferative lesions of specialized prostatic stroma. A clinicopathologic study of 22 cases. *Am J Surg Pathol* 22:148-162, 1998.

Ghandur-Mnaymneh L, Satterfield S, Block NL. Small cell carcinoma of the prostate gland with inappropriate antidiuretic hormone secretion: morphological, immunohistochemical and clinical expressions. *J Urol* 135:1263-1266, 1986.

Gillatt DA, O'Reilly PH, Reeve NL. Endometrioid carcinoma of the prostatic utricle. *Br J Urol* 58:559-560, 1986.

Gilmour AM, Bell TJ. Adenoid cystic carcinoma of the prostate. *Br J Urol* 58:105-106, 1986.

Giltman LI. Signet ring adenocarcinoma of the prostate. *J Urol* 126:134-135, 1981.

Ginesin Y, Bolkier M, Moskovitz B, et al. Carcinosarcoma of the prostate. *Eur Urol* 12:441-442, 1986.

Gleason DF. Atypical hyperplasia, benign hyperplasia, and well-differentiated adenocarcinoma of the prostate. *Am J Surg Pathol* 9:53-67, 1985.

Gleason DF. Histologic grading of prostatic carcinomas. In: Bostwick DG, ed. *Pathology of the Prostate.* New York: Churchill Livingstone; 89, 1990.

Goebbels R, Amberger L, Wernert N, et al. Urothelial carcinoma of the prostate. *Appl Pathol* 3:242-254, 1985.

Gray GF Jr, Marshall VF. Squamous carcinoma of the prostate. *J Urol* 113:736-738, 1975.

Greene FL, Page DL, Fleming ID, et al. Urethra. *AJCC Cancer Staging Manual.* 6th ed. New York: Springer Verlag; 341-343, 2002.

Greene LF, Mulchay JJ, Warren MM, et al. Primary transitional cell carcinoma of the prostate. *J Urol* 110:235-237, 1973.

Greene LF, O'Dea MJ, Dockerty MB. Primary transitional cell carcinoma of the prostate. *J Urol* 116:761-763, 1976.

Grignon DJ, Ro JY, Ordóñez NG, et al. Basal cell hyperplasia, adenoid basal cell tumor, and adenoid cystic carcinoma of the prostate gland: an immunohistochemical study. *Hum Pathol* 19:1425-1433, 1988.

Guerin D, Hosan N, Keen CE. Signet ring cell differentiation in adenocarcinoma of the prostate: a study of five cases. *Histopathology* 22:367-371, 1993.

Haddad JR, Reyes EC. Carcinosarcoma of the prostate with metastasis of both elements: case report. *J Urol* 103:80-83, 1970.

Hagood PG, Johnson FE, Bedrossian CWM, et al. Small cell carcinoma of the prostate. *Cancer* 67:1046-1050, 1991.

Hamlin WB, Lund PK. Carcinosarcoma of the prostate: a case report. *J Urol* 97:518-522, 1967.

Han M, Kronz JD, Schoenberg MP. Testicular metastasis of transitional cell carcinoma of the prostate. *J Urol* 164:2026, 2000.

Hashimoto Y, Kimura G, Tsuboi N, et al. A case of prostatic small cell carcinoma [in Japanese]. *Acta Urol Jpn* 46:425-427, 2000.

Hashine K, Nakatsuji H, Karashima T, et al. Small cell carcinoma of the prostate: a case report [in Japanese]. *Acta Urol Jpn* 44:607-610, 1998.

Haukaas SA, Halvorsen OJ, Nygaard SJ, et al. Cushing's syndrome in prostate cancer. An aggressive course of prostatic malignancy. *Urol Int* 63:126-129, 1999.

Hejka AG, England PM. Signet-ring cell carcinoma of prostate: immunohistochemical and ultrastructural study of a case. *Urology* 34:155-158, 1989.

Helpap B, Kollermann J. Undifferentiated carcinoma of the prostate with small cell features: immunohistochemical subtyping and reflections on histogenesis. *Virchows Arch* 434:385-391, 1999.

Hindson DA, Knight LL, Ocker JM. Small-cell carcinoma of prostate. Transient complete remission with chemotherapy. *Urology* 26:182-184, 1985.

Hokamura K, Kurozumi T, Tanaka K, et al. Carcinosarcoma of the prostate. *Acta Pathol Jpn* 35:481-487, 1985.

Howell LP, Teplitz RL. Papillary carcinoma of prostatic ductal origin: a cytologic case report with immunohistochemical and quantitative DNA correlation. *Diagn Cytopathol* 5:211-216, 1989.

Hsueh Y, Tsung SH. Prostatic mucinous adenocarcinoma. *Urology* 24:626-627, 1984.

Humphrey PA, Kaleem Z, Swanson PE, et al. Pseudohyperplastic prostatic adenocarcinoma. *Am J Surg Pathol* 22:1239-1246, 1998.

Ichijo S, Date T, Imamura J. A case of papillary adenocarcinoma of the prostate. *Jpn J Urol* 67:201-204, 1976.

Imamura M, Nishiyama H, Ohmori K, et al. Squamous cell carcinoma of the prostate without evidence of recurrence 5 years after operation. *Urol Int* 65:122-124, 2000.

Ishibashi Y, Kishida T, Yamaguchi T, et al. Two cases of mucinous adenocarcinoma of the prostate [in Japanese]. *Acta Urol Jpn* 38:463-467, 1992.

Ishigooka M, Yaguchi H, Tomaru M, et al. Mixed prostatic carcinoma containing malignant squamous element. Reports of two cases. *Scand J Urol Nephrol* 28:425-427, 1994.

Ishizu K, Yoshihiro S, Joko K, et al. Mucinous adenocarcinoma of the prostate with good response to hormonal therapy: a case report. *Acta Urol Jpn* 37:1057-1060, 1991.

Ishizu K, Konishi M, Joko K, et al. Papillary adenocarcinoma of the prostate with good response to antiandrogen therapy and delayed radiotherapy: a case report [in Japanese]. *Acta Urol Jpn* 38:343-346, 1992.

Ito T, Furusato M, Akiyama A, et al. A clinical and immunohistochemical study of papillary adenocarcinoma of the prostate. *Prostate* 26:23-27, 1995.

Iwata J, Fletcher CD. Immunohistochemical detection of cytokeratin and epithelial membrane antigen in leiomyosarcoma: a systematic study of 100 cases. *Pathol Int* 50:7-14, 2000.

Johnson DE, Hogan JM, Ayala AG. Transitional cell carcinoma of the prostate. A clinical morphological study. *Cancer* 29:287-293, 1972.

Joshi DP, Seery WH, Neier CR. Mucogenic adenocarcinoma of the prostate. *J Urol* 98:241-243, 1967.

Kahler JE. Carcinoma of the prostate gland: a pathologic study. *J Urol* 41:557-574, 1939.

Kaleem Z, Swanson PE, Vollmer RT, et al. Prostatic adenocarcinoma with atrophic features: a study of 202 consecutive, completely-embedded radical prostatectomy specimens. *Am J Clin Pathol* 109:695-703, 1998.

Kaneko Y, Yoshiki T, Fukumoto M, et al. Carcinosarcoma of the prostate. *Urol Int* 49:105-107, 1992.

Kanematsu A, Hiura M. Primary signet ring cell adenocarcinoma of the prostate treated by radical prostatectomy after preoperative androgen deprivation. *Int J Urol* 4:522-523, 1997.

Kanetsuna Y. An autopsy case of prostatic neuroendocrine cell carcinoma and adenocarcinoma initially found by brain and abdominal wall metastasis [in Japanese]. *Jpn J Urol* 91:530-533, 2000.

Karpas CM, Moumgis B. Primary transitional cell carcinoma of prostate gland: possible pathogenesis and relationship to reserve cell hyperplasia of prostatic periurethral ducts. *J Urol* 101:201-205, 1969.

Kastendieck H, Altenahr E. The squamous-cell carcinoma of the prostate as an example of metaplasia in a tumor [in German]. *Cancer Res Clin Oncol* 82:355-340, 1974.

Kim YW, Park YK, Park JH, et al. Adenosquamous carcinoma of the prostate. *Yonsei Med J* 40:396-399, 1999.

Kin T, Tsukamto T, Yonese J, et al. Adenosquamous carcinoma of the prostate with elevated serum parathyroid hormone-related protein and squamous cell carcinoma antigen. *BJU Int* 86:562, 2000.

Konya E, Nose K, Kiwamoto H, et al. A case of primary transitional cell carcinoma of the prostate [in Japanese]. *Acta Urol Jpn* 45:439-442, 1999.

Kopelson G, Harisiadis L, Romas NA, et al. Periurethral prostatic duct carcinoma. Clinical features and treatment results. *Cancer* 42:2894-2902, 1978.

Kramer SA, Bredael JJ, Krueger RP. Adenoid cystic carcinoma of the prostate: report of a case. *J Urol* 120:383-384, 1978.

Krastanova LJ, Addonizio JC. Carcinosarcoma of prostate. *Urology* 18:85-88, 1981.

Krijnen JLM, Janssen PJA, Ruizeveld de Winter JA, et al. Do neuroendocrine cells express androgen receptor? *Histochemistry* 100:393-398, 1993.

Kubo T, Kato T, Wantanabe H, et al. Two cases of gluey cancer of prostate. *Clin Dermatol Urol* 18:655-658, 1964.

Kubosawa H, Matsuzaki O, Kondo Y, et al. Carcinosarcoma of the prostate. *Acta Pathol Jpn* 43:209-214, 1993.

Kuhajda FP, Mann RB. Adenoid cystic carcinoma of the prostate. A case report with immunoperoxidase staining for prostate-specific acid phosphatase and prostate-specific antigen. *Am J Clin Pathol* 81:257-260, 1984.

Küllü S, Ersev A, Simsek F, et al. Adenocarcinoma of the prostate with endometrioid features. *Int Urol Nephrol* 23:577-580, 1991.

Kums JJM, Helsdingen PJRO. Signet-ring cell carcinoma of the bladder and prostate. Report of 4 cases. *Urol Int* 40:116-119, 1985.

Kuroda N, Yamasaki I, Nakayama H, et al. Prostatic signet-ring cell carcinoma: case report and literature review. *Pathol Int* 49:457-461, 1999.

Kuwahara M, Matsushita K, Yoshinaga H, et al. Primary squamous cell carcinoma of the prostate: a case report [in Japanese]. *Acta Urol Jpn* 39:77-80, 1993.

Lager DJ, Goeken JA, Kemp JD, et al. Squamous metaplasia of the prostate. An immunohistochemical study. *Am J Clin Pathol* 90:597-601, 1988.

Lauwers GY, Schevchuk M, Armenakas N, et al. Carcinosarcoma of the prostate. *Am J Surg Pathol* 17:342-349, 1993.

Lee DW, Ro JY, Sahin AA, et al. Mucinous adenocarcinoma of the prostate with endobronchial metastasis. *Am J Clin Pathol* 94:641-645, 1990.

Lee M, de Peralta Venturina M, Lim S, et al. Small cell carcinoma of prostate gland: immunohistochemical assessment of relationship to adenocarcinoma of prostate [abstract]. *Mod Pathol* 14:115A, 2001.

Lee SS. Endometrioid adenocarcinoma of the prostate: a clinicopathologic and immunohistochemical study. *J Surg Oncol* 55:235-238, 1994.

Lemberger RJ, Bishop MC, Bates CP, et al. Carcinoma of the prostate of ductal origin. *Br J Urol* 56:706-709, 1984.

Leong FJ, Leong AS, Swift J. Signet-ring carcinoma of the prostate. *Pathol Res Pract* 192:1232-1241, 1996.

Levi AW, Epstein JI. Pseudohyperplastic prostatic adenocarcinoma on needle biopsy and simple prostatectomy. *Am J Surg Pathol* 24:1039-1046, 2000.

Lightbourn GA, Abrams M, Seymour L. Primary mucoid adenocarcinoma of the prostate with bladder invasion. *J Urol* 101:78-80, 1969.

Lindboe CF, Mjones J. Carcinosarcoma of the prostate: immunohistochemical and ultrastructural observations. *Urology* 40:376-380, 1992.

Little NA, Wiener JS, Walther PJ, et al. Squamous cell carcinoma of the prostate: 2 cases of a rare malignancy and review of the literature. *J Urol* 149:137-139, 1993.

Lo Re G, Canzonieri V, Veronesi A, et al. Extrapulmonary small cell carcinoma: a single-institution experience and review of the literature. *Ann Oncol* 5:909-913, 1994.

Locke JR, Soloway MS, Evans J, et al. Osteogenic differentiation associated with x-ray therapy for adenocarcinoma of the prostate gland. *Am J Clin Pathol* 85:375-378, 1986.

Logothetis CJ, Hoosein NH, Ro J. Neuroendocrine progression. In: Vogelzang NJ, Scardino PT, Shipley WU, et al, eds. *Comprehensive Textbook of Genitourinary Oncology.* Baltimore: Williams & Wilkins; 914-919, 1996.

Lopez JI, Laforga JB. Mucinous (colloid) adenocarcinoma of the prostate. *Br J Urol* 76:805-806, 1995.

Losi L, Di Gregori C, Brausi M, et al. Expression of p53 protein in prostate cancers of different histologic types. *Pathol Res Pract* 190:384-388, 1994A.

Losi L, Brausi M, Di Gregorio C. Rare prostatic carcinomas: histogenesis and morphologic pattern. *Pathologia* 86:366-370, 1994B.

Luque Barona RJ, Gonzalez Campora R, Vicioso Recio L, et al. Synchronous prostatic carcinosarcoma: report of 2 cases and review of the literature [in Spanish]. *Acta Urol Esp* 24:173-178, 2000.

Lyster MT, Kies MS, Kuzel TM. Neurologic complications of patients with small cell prostate carcinoma. Report of two cases. *Cancer* 74:3159-3163, 1994.

Ma TKF, Chapman WB, McLean M, et al. Prostatic carcinosarcoma consisting of the unusual combination of ductal adenocarcinoma with osteogenic sarcoma: a report of a case and review of the literature. *J Urol Pathol* 8:111-120, 1998.

Mackey JR, Au HJ, Hugh J, et al. Genitourinary small cell carcinoma: determination of clinical and therapeutic factors associated with survival. *J Urol* 159:1624-1629, 1998.

Madersbacher S, Schatzl G, Susani M, et al. Prostatic metastasis of a small cell lung cancer in a young male. *Eur Urol* 26:267-269, 1994.

Mahadevia PS, Ramaswamy A, Greenwald ES, et al. Hypercalcemia in prostatic carcinoma. A report of eight cases. *Arch Intern Med* 143:1339-1342, 1983.

Mai KT, Leahy CF. Squamous cell carcinoma occurring as a circumscribed nodule in the transition zone of the prostate. *J Urol Pathol* 5:85-96, 1996.

Manne RK, Haddad FS. Mucinous adenocarcinoma of prostate. *Urology* 33:247-249, 1989.

Manrique JJ, Albores-Saavedra J, Orantes A, et al. Malignant mixed tumor of the salivary gland type, primary in the prostate. *Am J Clin Pathol* 70:932-937, 1978.

Manson AL, Terhune D, MacDonald G. Small cell carcinoma of the prostate. *Urology* 33:78-79, 1989.

Marchal Escalona C, Caballero Alcantara J, Padilla Leon M, et al. Primary transitional cell carcinoma of the prostate. An infrequent tumor [in Spanish]. *Acta Urol Esp* 21:926-930, 1997.

Martin SA, Fowler M, Catalona WJ, et al. Carcinosarcoma of the prostate: report of a case with ultrastructural observations. *J Urol* 122:709-711, 1979.

Matzkin H, Soloway MS, Hardeman S. Transitional cell carcinoma of the prostate. *J Urol* 146:1207-1212, 1991.

McKenney JK, Amin MB, Srigley JR, et al. Adenoid basal proliferations of the prostate other than usual basal cell hyperplasia: A study of 23 cases with a proposed classification [abstract]. *Mod Pathol* 14:117A, 2001.

McNeal JE, Alroy J, Villers A, et al. Mucinous differentiation in prostatic adenocarcinoma. *Hum Pathol* 22:979-988, 1991.

McNeal JE, Yemoto CEM. Spread of adenocarcinoma of the prostate within prostatic ducts and acini: morphologic and clinical correlations. *Am J Surg Pathol* 20:802-814, 1996.

Meeter UL, Richards JN. Osteogenic sarcoma of the prostate. *J Urol* 84:654-657, 1960.

Melicow MM, Pachter MR. Endometrial carcinoma of prostatic utricle (uterus masculinus). *Cancer* 20:1715-1722, 1967.

Melicow MM, Tannenbaum M. Endometrial carcinoma of uterus musculinus (prostatic utricle). Report of 6 cases. *J Urol* 106:892-902, 1971.

Millar EKA, Sharma NK, Lessels AM. Ductal (endometrioid) adenocarcinoma of the prostate: a clinicopathological study of 16 cases. *Histopathology* 29:11-19, 1996.

Miller VA, Reuter V, Scher HI. Primary squamous cell carcinoma of the prostate after radiation seed implantation for adenocarcinoma. *Urology* 46:111-113, 1995.

Monsalve Rodriguez M, Parra Muntaner LE, Kilani S, et al. Colloid carcinoma of the prostate [in Spanish]. *Arch Esp Urol* 45:369-371, 1992.

Moore SR, Reinberg Y, Zhang G. Small cell carcinoma of prostate: effectiveness of hormonal versus chemotherapy. *Urology* 39:411-416, 1992.

Morikawa T, Kobayashi S, Yamadori I, et al. Three cases of extrapulmonary small cell carcinoma occurring in the prostate, stomach, and pancreas. *Indian J Cancer* 31:268-273, 1994.

Moskovitz B, Munichor M, Bolkier M, et al. Squamous cell carcinoma of the prostate. *Urol Int* 51:181-183, 1993.

Mostofi FK, Price EB Jr. Endometrial carcinoma. In: *Tumors of the Male Genital System.* Washington, DC: Armed Forces Institute of Pathology; 241-244, 1973.

Mott LJ. Squamous cell carcinoma of the prostate: report of 2 cases and review of the literature. *J Urol* 121:833-835, 1979.

Moyana TN. Adenosquamous carcinoma of the prostate. *Am J Surg Pathol* 11:403-407, 1987.

Munechika H, Kitanosono T, Gokan T, et al. Small cell carcinoma of the prostate: CT and MRI findings. *Radiat Med* 13:137-142, 1995.

Murao T, Tanahashi T. A case of small cell carcinoma of the prostate. *Jpn J Cancer Clin* 34:1624-1628, 1988.

Nabi G, Ansari MS, Singh I, et al. Primary squamous cell carcinoma of the prostate. A rare clinicopathological entity. Report of 2 cases and review of literature. *Urol Int* 66:216-219, 2001.

Nagakura K, Hayakawa M, Mukai K, et al. Mucinous adenocarcinoma of prostate: a case report and review of the literature. *J Urol* 135:1025-1028, 1986.

Nazeer T, Barada JH, Fisher HAG, et al. Prostatic carcinosarcoma: case report and review of literature. *J Urol* 146:1370-1373, 1991.

Nelson RS, Epstein JI. Prostatic carcinoma with abundant xanthomatous cytoplasm. Foamy gland carcinoma. *Am J Surg Pathol* 20:419-426, 1996.

Nguyen-Ho P, Nguyen GK, Villanueva RR. Small cell anaplastic carcinoma of the prostate: report of a case with positive urine cytology. *Diagn Cytopathol* 10:159-161, 1994.

Nicolaisen GS, Williams RD. Primary transitional cell carcinoma of prostate. *Urology* 24:544-549, 1984.

Nishimura K, Higashino M, Hara T, et al. Prostatic adenocarcinoma showing features of endometrioid and mucinous carcinomas: a case report [in Japanese]. *Acta Urol Jpn* 41:805-807, 1995.

Nkanza N. Adenoid cystic carcinoma of the prostate. *Cent Afr J Med* 34:166-168, 1988.

Novak J, Hanus T, Dvoracek J. Small-cell carcinoma of the prostate [in Czech]. *Cas Lek Cesk* 137:522-524, 1998.

Nyi KM, Rangwala AF. Small cell carcinoma of the prostate with adenocarcinoma of the rectum. *N J Med* 88:733-735, 1991.

Odom DG, Donatucci CF, Deshon GE. Mucinous adenocarcinoma of the prostate. *Hum Pathol* 17:863-865, 1986.

Oesterling JE, Hauzeur CG, Farrow GM. Small cell anaplastic carcinoma in clinical, pathological and immunological study of 27 patients. *J Urol* 147:804-807, 1992.

Okada E, Kamizaki H. Primary squamous cell carcinoma of the prostate. *Int J Urol* 7:347-350, 2000.

Okada H, Tatsumi N, Nakano Y, et al. Small cell carcinoma of the prostate [in Japanese]. *Jpn J Urol* 85:1002-1005, 1994.

Okada H, Gotoh A, Ogawa T, et al. Two cases of small cell carcinoma of the prostate. *Scand J Urol Nephrol* 30:503-508, 1996.

Okamoto T, Ogiu K, Sato M, et al. Primary squamous cell carcinoma of the prostate: a case report. *Acta Urol Jpn* 42:67-70, 1996.

Okamura K, Ito K, Sahashi M, et al. Primary squamous cell carcinoma of the prostate: a case report [in Japanese]. *Jpn J Urol* 75:979-983, 1984.

Oliai BR, Kahane H, Epstein JI. A clinicopathologic analysis of urothelial carcinomas diagnosed in prostate needle biopsy. *Am J Surg Pathol* 25:794-801, 2001.

Olivas TP, Brady TW. Mucinous adenocarcinoma of the prostate: a report of a case of long-term survival. *Urology* 47:256-258, 1996.

Ordóñez NG, Ayala AG, von Eschenbach AC, et al. Immunoperoxidase localization of prostatic acid phosphatase in prostatic carcinoma with sarcomatoid changes. *Urology* 19:210-214, 1982.

Ordóñez NG, Ro JY, Ayala AG. Metastatic prostatic carcinoma presenting as an oncocytic tumor. *Am J Surg Pathol* 16:1007-1012, 1992.

Ordóñez NG. Thrombomodulin expression in transitional cell carcinoma. *Am J Clin Pathol* 110:385-390, 1998.

Orhan D, Sak SD, Yaman Ö, et al. Adenosquamous carcinoma of the prostate. *Br J Urol* 78:646-647, 1996.

Osorio Acosta V, Borrajero Martinez I. Cystic adenoid carcinoma of the prostate. Report of a case [in Spanish]. *Arch Esp Urol* 50:67-71, 1997.

Outwater E, Schiebler ML, Tomaszewski JE, et al. Mucinous carcinomas involving the prostate: atypical findings at MR imaging. *J Magn Reson Imaging* 2:597-600, 1992.

Oxley JD, Abbott CD, Gillatt DA, et al. Ductal carcinomas of the prostate: a clinicopathological and immunohistochemical study. *Br J Urol* 81:109-115, 1998A.

Oxley J, Abbott C. Thrombomodulin immunostaining and ductal carcinoma of the prostate [letter]. *Histopathology* 33:391-392, 1998B.

Palma PGR, Rodriguez NJN, Ikari O, et al. Leiomyosarcoma in association with incidental adenocarcinoma of the prostate. *J Urol* 129:156-157, 1983.

Pan CC, Chiang H, Chang YH, et al. Tubulocystic clear cell adenocarcinoma arising within the prostate. *Am J Surg Pathol* 24:1433-1436, 2000.

Papandreou CN, Daliani DD, Thall PF, et al. Results of a phase II study with doxorubicin, etoposide, and cisplatin in patients with fully characterized small cell carcinoma of the prostate. *J Clin Oncol* 20:3072-3080, 2002.

Parker DC, Folpe AL, Bell J, et al. Potential utility of uroplakin III, thrombomodulin, high molecular weight cytokeratin, and cytokeratin 20 in noninvasive, invasive, and metastatic urothelial (transitional cell) carcinomas. *Am J Surg Pathol* 27:1-10, 2003.

Parra Muntaner L, Verdu Martinez M, Kilani Elmasri S, et al. Transitional cell carcinoma of the prostate. Report of a case treated with chemotherapy [in Spanish]. *Arch Esp Urol* 46:909-912, 1993.

Patel A, Ball AJ, Chappell M. Pure primary small cell carcinoma of the prostate. *Br J Urol* 72:380-381, 1993.

Perez Garcia FJ, Veiga Gonzalez M, Rodriguez Martinez JJ, et al. Squamous cell carcinoma of the prostate. Presentation of a case and review of the literature [in Spanish]. *Acta Urol Esp* 21:931-935, 1997.

Picurelli L, Sendra A, Fernandez A, et al. Prostatic signet ring cell carcinoma [in Spanish]. *Acta Urol Esp* 18:903-905, 1994.

Pinder SE, McMahon RFT. Mucins in prostatic carcinoma. *Histopathology* 16:43-46, 1990.

Pinto JA, Gonzalez JE, Granadillo MA. Primary carcinoma of the prostate with diffuse oncocytic changes. *Histopathology* 25:286-288, 1994.

Plancke HR, Delaere KP, Theunissen P. Secondary signet ring cell tumour of the prostate. *Urol Int* 52:223-224, 1994.

Poblet E, Gomez-Tierno A, Alfaro L. Prostatic carcinosarcoma: a case originating in a previous ductal adenocarcinoma of the prostate. *Pathol Res Pract* 196:569-572, 2000.

Proia AD, McCarty KS Jr, Woodard BH. Prostatic mucinous adenocarcinoma. A Cowper gland carcinoma mimicker. *Am J Surg Pathol* 5:701-706, 1981.

Quay SC, Proppe KH. Carcinosarcoma of the prostate: case report and review of the literature. *J Urol* 125:436-438, 1981.

Queipo Zaragoza JA, Budia Alba A, Perez Ebri M, et al. Mucinous prostate adenocarcinoma initially presented as an intestinal subocclusive picture [in Spanish]. *Acta Urol Esp* 23:712-716, 1999.

Rahmanou F, Koo J, Marinbakh AY, et al. Squamous cell carcinoma at the prostatectomy site: squamous differentiation of recurrent prostate carcinoma. *Urology* 54:744, 1999.

Raica M. Pathology and histochemistry of small cell carcinoma of the prostate. *Rom J Morphol Embryol* 41:107-110, 1995.

Reed RJ. Consultation case. *Am J Surg Pathol* 8:699-704, 1984.

Remmele W, Weber A, Harding P. Primary signet-ring cell carcinoma of the prostate. *Hum Pathol* 19:478-480, 1988.

Renshaw AA, Nappi D, Cibas ES. Cytology of metastatic adenocarcinoma of the prostate in pleural effusions. *Diagn Cytopathol* 15:103-107, 1996.

Reuter VE. Sarcomatoid lesions of the urogenital tract. *Semin Diagn Pathol* 10:188-201, 1993.

Reuter VE. Pathological changes in benign and malignant prostatic tissue following androgen deprivation therapy. *Urology* 49(suppl 3A):16-22, 1997.

Reyes AO, Swanson PE, Carbone JM, et al. Unusual histologic types of high-grade prostatic intraepithelial neoplasia. *Am J Surg Pathol* 21:1215-1222, 1997.

Rhamy RK, Buchanan RD, Spalding MJ. Intraductal carcinoma of the prostate gland. *J Urol* 109:457-460, 1973.

Ro JY, Têtu B, Ayala AG, et al. Small cell carcinoma of the prostate. II. Immunohistochemical and electron microscopic studies of 18 cases. *Cancer* 59:977-982, 1987.

Ro JY, Grignon DJ, Troncoso P, et al. Mucin in prostatic adenocarcinoma. *Semin Diagn Pathol* 5:273-283, 1988A.

Ro JY, Ayala AG, Wishnow KI, et al. Prostatic duct adenocarcinoma with endometrioid features: immunohistochemical and electron microscopic study. *Semin Diagn Pathol* 5:301-311, 1988B.

Ro JY, El-Naggar A, Ayala AG, et al. Signet ring cell carcinoma of the prostate. Electron-microscopic and immunohistochemical studies of eight cases. *Am J Surg Pathol* 12:453-460, 1988C.

Ro JY, Grignon DJ, Ayala AG, et al. Mucinous adenocarcinoma of the prostate: histochemical and immunohistochemical studies. *Hum Pathol* 21:593-600, 1990.

Ro JY, Amin MB, Sahin AA, et al. Tumors and tumours conditions of the male genital tract. In: Fletcher CDM, ed. *Diagnostic Histopathology of Tumors.* London: Churchill Livingstone; 764-765, 2000.

Rodrigues Netto N Jr, de Almeida Claro JF, Balthazar Saldanha L. Transitional cell carcinoma of the prostate metastatic to penis as cause of priapism. *Arch Esp Urol* 43:321-322, 1990.

Rodriguez Fernandez A, Garcia Gonzalez A, Bengoechea Miranda O, et al. Mucinous adenocarcinoma of the prostatic gland. Histochemical and immunohistochemical studies [in Spanish]. *Arch Esp Urol* 45:572-575, 1992.

Rodriguez Martinez JJ, Madrigal Rubiales B, Perez Garcia FJ, et al. Mucinous adenocarcinoma of the prostate. Report of 3 cases and review of the literature [in Spanish]. *Arch Esp Urol* 50:952-958, 1997.

Rodriguez Martinez JJ, Cerrato Rodriquez ME, Garica Perez FJ, et al. Skin metastases of primary transitional cell carcinoma of the prostate [in Spanish]. *Arch Esp Urol* 52:885-887, 1999.

Rotterdam HZ, Melicow MM. Double primary prostatic adenocarcinoma. *Urology* 6:245-248, 1975.

Rubenstein AB, Rubnitz ME. Transitional cell carcinoma of the prostate. *Cancer* 24:543-546, 1969.

Rubin MA, de La Taille A, Bagiella E, et al. Cribriform carcinoma of the prostate and prostatic intraepithelial neoplasia: incidence and clinical implications. *Am J Surg Pathol* 22:840-848, 1998.

Rubinowicz DM, Soloway MS, Lief M, et al. Hemospermia and expressed tumor in the urethra: an unusual presentation of ductal carcinoma of the prostate. *J Urol* 163:915, 2000.

Saez C, Japon MA, Conde AF, et al. Sialomucins are characteristically O-acylated in poorly differentiated and colloid prostatic adenocarcinomas. *Mod Pathol* 11:1193-1197, 1998.

Saito R, Davis BK, Ollapally EP. Adenosquamous carcinoma of the prostate. *Hum Pathol* 15:87-89, 1984.

Saito S, Iwaki H. Mucin-producing carcinoma of the prostate: review of 88 cases. *Urology* 54:141-144, 1999.

Sak SD, Orhan D, Yaman O, et al. Carcinosarcoma of the prostate. A case report and possible evidence on the role of hormonal therapy. *Urol Int* 59:50-52, 1997.

Samaratunga H, Singh M. Distribution pattern of basal cells detected by cytokeratin 34βE12 in primary prostatic duct adenocarcinoma. *Am J Surg Pathol* 21:435-440, 1997.

Samsonov VA, Kolomoitsev SV. Association of prostatic adenocarcinoma with transitional cell and squamous cell carcinomas of the same origin [in Russian]. *Arkh Patol* 45:28-34, 1983.

Samsonov VA. Prostatic squamous cell cancer and its differential diagnostic contrast with squamous cell metaplasia [in Russian]. *Arkh Patol* 46:23-29, 1984.

Sandhu SS, Denton A, Jarmulowicz M, et al. Pure small cell carcinoma of the prostate. *Clin Oncol* 9:412-414, 1997.

Sano K, Miyai K, Yoshida S. Small cell carcinoma of the prostate: a case report. *Int J Urol* 4:321-323, 1997.

Saphir O, Vass A. Carcinosarcoma. *Am J Cancer* 33:331-361, 1938.

Sarma DP, Weilbaecher TG. Small-cell carcinoma of prostate. *Urology* 33:332-335, 1989.

Sarma DP, Weilbaecher TG, Moon TD. Squamous cell carcinoma of prostate. *Urology* 37:260-262, 1991.

Sawczuk I, Tannenbaum M, Olsson CA, et al. Primary transitional cell carcinoma of prostatic periurethral ducts. *Urology* 25:339-343, 1985.

Schned AR. Artifactual signet-ring cells [letter]. *Am J Surg Pathol* 11:736-737, 1987.

Schron DS, Gipson T, Mendelsohn G. The histogenesis of small cell carcinoma of the prostate. An immunohistochemical study. *Cancer* 53:2478-2480, 1984.

Schwartz LH, Latrenta LR, Bonaccio E, et al. Small cell and anaplastic prostate cancer-correlation between CT findings and prostate-specific antigen level. *Radiology* 208:735-738, 1998.

Scott MB, Goldstein AMB, Onofrio RC, et al. Papillary adenocarcinoma of prostate. *Urology* 8:227-230, 1976.

Segaloff A. Discussion on experimental tumors: observations of a squamous cell carcinoma. *J Natl Cancer Inst Monogr* 12:407-408, 1963.

Sesterhenn I, Mostofi FK, Davis CJ. Basal cell hyperplasia and basal cell carcinoma [abstract]. *Lab Invest* 56:71A, 1987.

Shannon RL, Ro JY, Grignon DJ, et al. Sarcomatoid carcinoma of the prostate. A clinicopathologic study of 12 patients. *Cancer* 69:2676-2682, 1992.

Sharma SK, Malik AK, Bapna BC. Squamous cell carcinoma of prostate. *Indian J Cancer* 17:134-135, 1980.

Shindo M, Aoki S, Ikeda E. Adenoid cystic carcinoma of the prostate. A case report [in Japanese]. *Jpn J Urol* 89:670-673, 1998.

Sieracki JC. Epidermoid carcinoma of the human prostate; report of 3 cases. *Lab Invest* 4:232-240, 1955.

Sika JV, Buckley JJ. Mucus-forming adenocarcinoma of prostate. *Cancer* 17:949-952, 1964.

Sim SJ, Glassman AB, Ro JY, et al. Serum calcitonin in small cell carcinoma of the prostate. *Ann Clin Lab Sci* 26:487-495, 1996.

Skodras G, Wang J, Kragel PJ. Primary prostatic signet-ring cell carcinoma. *Urology* 42:338-342, 1993.

Smedley HM, Brown C, Turner A. Ectopic ACTH-producing lung cancer presenting with prostatic metastasis. *Postgrad Med J* 59:371-372, 1983.

Smith BD, Flegel G. Primary transitional cell carcinoma of the prostate: report of two cases. *J Am Osteopath Assoc* 82:547-548, 1983.

Smith C, Feddersen RM, Dressler L, et al. Signet ring cell adenocarcinoma of prostate. *Urology* 43:397-400, 1994.

Smith DC, Tucker JA, Trump DL. Hypercalcemia and neuroendocrine carcinoma of the prostate: A report of three cases and a review of the literature. *J Clin Oncol* 10:499-505, 1992.

Sogbein SK, Steele AA. Papillary prostatic epithelial hyperplasia of the urethra: a cause of hematuria in young men. *J Urol* 142:1218-1220, 1989.

Stavropoulos NE, Ioackim-Velogianni E, Sidoni K, et al. Endometrioid carcinoma of the prostate. The diagnostic value of Leu 7 and prostate specific antigen. *Br J Urol* 71:309-312, 1993.

Stern RC, Hulette CM. Paraneoplastic limbic encephalitis associated with small cell carcinoma of the prostate. *Mod Pathol* 12:814-818, 1999.

Sule-Suso J, Brunt AM. Small cell carcinoma of the prostate. *Br J Radiol* 65:726-728, 1992.

Svanholm H, Starklint H, Barlebo H, et al. Histological evaluation of prostatic cancer. 1. Reproducibility of tumour type. *APMIS* 97:699-704, 1989.

Takashi M, Sahashi M, Sakata T, et al. Primary transitional cell carcinoma of prostate: case with lymph node metastasis eradicated by neoadjuvant methotrexate, vinblastine, doxorubicin, and cisplatin (M-VAC) therapy. *Urology* 36:96-98, 1990.

Tannenbaum M. Carcinoma with sarcomatoid changes or carcinosarcoma of prostate. *Urology* 6:91-97, 1975A.

Tannenbaum M. Endometrial tumors and/or associated carcinomas of prostate. *Urology* 6:372-375, 1975B.

Tannenbaum M. Mucin-secreting carcinoma of the prostate. *Urology* 5:543-544, 1975C.

Tannenbaum M. Adenoid cystic or "salivary gland" carcinomas of prostate. *Urology* 6:238-239, 1975D.

Tannenbaum M. Histopathology of the prostate gland. In: Tannenbaum M, ed. *Urologic Pathology: The Prostate.* Philadelphia: Lea & Febiger; 312-315, 1977.

Taylor HG, Blom J. Transitional cell carcinoma of the prostate. Response to treatment with adriamycin and cis-platinum. *Cancer* 51:1800-1802, 1983.

Teichman JMH, Shabaik A, Demby AM. Mucinous adenocarcinoma of the prostate and hormone sensitivity. *J Urol* 151:701-702, 1994.

Terris MK. The appearance of adenoid cystic carcinoma of the prostate on transrectal ultrasonography. *BJU Int* 83:875-876, 1999A.

Terris MK. Transrectal ultrasound appearance of squamous cell carcinoma involving the prostate. *Urol Int* 63:133-135, 1999B.

Têtu B, Ro JY, Ayala AG, et al. Small cell carcinoma of the prostate. Part 1. A clinicopathologic study of 20 cases. *Cancer* 59:1803-1809, 1987.

Têtu B, Ro JY, Ayala AG, et al. Small cell carcinoma of the prostate associated with myasthenic (Eaton-Lambert) syndrome. *Urology* 33:148-152, 1989.

Thompson GJ, Albers DD, Broders AC. Unusual carcinomas involving the prostate gland. *J Urol* 69:416-425, 1953.

Torbenson M, Dhir R, Nangia A, et al. Prostatic carcinoma with signet ring cells: a clinicopathologic and immunohistochemical analysis of 12 cases, with review of the literature. *Mod Pathol* 11:552-559, 1998.

Tran KP, Epstein JJ. Mucinous adenocarcinoma of urinary bladder type arising from the prostatic urethra: distinction from mucinous adenocarcinoma of the prostate. *Am J Surg Pathol* 20:1346-1350, 1996.

Tran TA, Jennings TA, Ross JS, et al. Pseudomyxoma ovariilike posttherapeutic alteration in prostatic adenocarcinoma. A distinctive pattern in patients receiving neoadjuvant androgen ablation therapy. *Am J Surg Pathol* 22:347-354, 1998.

Tran TT, Sengupta E, Yang XJ. Signet ring cell carcinoma (SRCC) of the prostate: resulted from intracytoplasmic lumina and lipid [abstract]. *Mod Pathol* 13:117A, 2000.

Tran TT, Sengupta E, Yang XY. Prostatic foamy gland carcinoma with aggressive behavior. Histologic, immunohistochemical, and ultrastructural analysis. *Am J Surg Pathol* 25:618-623, 2001.

Tu SM, Reyes A, Maa A, et al. Prostate carcinoma with testicular or penile metastases. Clinical, pathologic, and immunohistochemical features. *Cancer* 94:2610-2617, 2002.

Turbat-Herrera EA, Herrera GA, Gore I, et al. Neuroendocrine differentiation in prostatic carcinomas. A retrospective autopsy study. *Arch Pathol Lab Med* 112:1100-1105, 1988.

Turhan OI, Aydin NE, Sariyuce O. Adenosquamous carcinoma of the prostate. *Int Urol Nephrol* 31:89-93, 1999.

Uchibayashi T, Hisazumi H, Hasegawa M, et al. Squamous cell carcinoma of the prostate. *Scand J Urol Nephrol* 31:223-224, 1996.

Uchijma Y, Ito H, Takahashi M, et al. Prostate mucinous adenocarcinoma with signet ring cell. *Urology* 36:267-268, 1990.

Uemura M, Imamura R, Inoue H, et al. Primary transitional cell carcinoma of the prostate: a case report [in Japanese]. *Acta Urol Jpn* 46:495-498, 2000.

Ullman AS, Ross OA. Hyperplasia, atypism and carcinoma in situ in prostatic periurethral glands. *Am J Clin Pathol* 47:497-504, 1967.

Ulloa SA, Iturregui JR, Amezquita M, et al. Squamous cell carcinoma of the prostate: case report and review of the literature. *Bol Asoc Med P R* 89:192-194, 1997.

Uyama T, Moriwaki S. Papillary and mucus-forming adenocarcinomas of prostate. *Urology* 13:432-434, 1979.

Vale JA, Patel A, Ball AJ, et al. Endometrioid carcinoma of the prostate: a misnomer? *J R Soc Med* 85:394-396, 1992.

Valle J, von Boguslawsky K, Stenborg M, et al. Progression from adenocarcinoma to small cell carcinoma of the prostate with normalization of prostate-specific antigen (PSA) levels. *Scand J Urol Nephrol* 30:509-512, 1996.

Van Renterghem K, Mattelaer J, Billiet I. Adenoid cystic carcinoma of the prostate. *Acta Urol Belg* 62:69-70, 1994.

Vandersteen DP, Wiemerslage SJ, Cohen MB. Prostatic duct adenocarcinoma: a cytologic and histologic case report with review of the literature. *Diagn Cytopathol* 17:480-483, 1997.

Vera-Donoso CD, Vidal J, Gómez S, et al. Carcinoma of prostatic ducts. *Eur Urol* 19:8-11, 1991.

Virseda Rodriguez JA, Martin de Francisco J. Colloid or mucinous adenocarcinoma of the prostate. *Arch Esp Urol* 44:827-829, 1991.

Vuitch MF, Mendelsohn G. Relationship of ectopic ACTH production to tumor differentiation: a morphologic and immunohistochemical study of prostatic carcinoma with Cushing's syndrome. *Cancer* 47:296-299, 1981.

Walker AN, Mills SE, Fechner RE, et al. Endometrial adenocarcinoma of the prostatic urethra arising in a villous polyp. *Arch Pathol Lab Med* 106:624-627, 1982.

Walther MM, Nassar V, Harruff RC, et al. Endometrial carcinoma of the prostatic utricle: a tumor of prostatic origin. *J Urol* 134:769-773, 1985.

Wang HL, Humphrey PA. Exaggerated signet-ring cell change in stromal module of prostate: a pseudoneoplastic proliferation. *Am J Surg Pathol* 26:1066-1070, 2002.

Wang Q, Lin CS, Unger PP. Squamous cell carcinoma arising in hormonally treated adenocarcinoma of the prostate. *Int J Surg Pathol* 4:13-16, 1996.

Watarai Y, Demura T, Togashi M, et al. Mucinous adenocarcinoma of the prostate. A case report and analysis of the literature [in Japanese]. *Jpn J Urol* 85:1276-1279, 1994.

Weaver MG, Abdul-Karim FW, Srigley JR. Paneth cell–like change and small cell carcinoma of the prostate. Two divergent forms of prostatic neuroendocrine differentiation. *Am J Surg Pathol* 16:1013-1016, 1992.

Wendelken JR, Schellhammer PF, Ladaga LE, et al. Transitional cell carcinoma: cause of refractory cancer of prostate. *Urology* 13:557-560, 1979.

Wenk RE, Bhagavan BS, Levy R, et al. Ectopic ACTH, prostatic oat cell carcinoma, and marked hypernatremia. *Cancer* 40:773-778, 1977.

Wernert N, Lüchtrath H, Seeliger H, et al. Papillary carcinoma of the prostate, location, morphology, and immunohistochemistry: the histogenesis and entity of so-called endometrioid carcinoma. *Prostate* 10:123-131, 1987.

Wernert N, Goebbels R, Bonkhoff H, et al. Squamous cell carcinoma of the prostate. *Histopathology* 17:339-344, 1990.

Wick MR, Young RH, Malvesta R, et al. Prostatic carcinosarcomas. Clinical, histologic, and immunohistochemical data on two cases, with a review of the literature. *Am J Clin Pathol* 92:131-139, 1989.

Witters S, Moerman P, Vanden Bussche L, et al. Papillary adenocarcinoma of the prostatic urethra. *Eur Urol* 12:143-144, 1986.

Wullich B, Rohde V, Moll V, et al. High frequency microsatellite instability in mucinous adenocarcinoma of the prostate. *J Urol* 165:912-913, 2001.

Wynn SS, Nagabundi S, Koo J, et al. Recurrent prostate carcinoma presenting as omental large cell carcinoma with neuroendocrine differentiation and resulting in bowel obstruction. *Arch Pathol Lab Med* 124:1074-1076, 2000.

Yamaguchi S, Hashimoto H, Kaneko S, et al. Secondary mucinous adenocarcinoma of the prostate in a patient with ulcerative colitis. *Urol Int* 50:231-233, 1993.

Yang XJ, McEntee M, Epstein JI. Distinction of basaloid carcinoma of the prostate from benign basal cell lesions by using immunohistochemistry for bcl-2 and Ki-67. *Hum Pathol* 29:1447-1450, 1998.

Yashi M, Suzuki K, Tokue A. A case of giant small cell carcinoma of the prostate. *Acta Urol Jpn* 47:55-57, 2001.

Yoshikawa H, Ikeuchi T, Onodera Y, et al. A case of transitional cell carcinoma of the prostate [in Japanese]. *Acta Urol Jpn* 40:257-260, 1954.

Yoshimura K, Fukui I, Ishikawa Y, et al. Locally-confined signet-ring cell carcinoma of the prostate: a case report of a long-term survivor. *Int J Urol* 3:406-407, 1996.

Young BW, Lagios MD. Endometrial (papillary) carcinoma of the prostatic utricle-response to orchiectomy. *Cancer* 32:1293-1300, 1973.

Young RH, Frierson HF Jr, Mills SE, et al. Adenoid cystic-like tumor of the prostate gland. A report of two cases and review of the literature on "adenoid cystic carcinoma" of the prostate. *Am J Clin Pathol* 89:49-56, 1988.

Young RH, Srigley JR, Amin MB, et al. Variants of prostatic adenocarcinoma, other primary carcinomas of prostate, and secondary carcinomas. In: *Tumors of the Prostate Gland, Seminal Vesicles, Male Urethra, and Penis.* Washington, DC: Armed Forces Institute of Pathology; 217-255, 2000.

Zaloudek C, Williams JW, Kempson RL. "Endometrial" adenocarcinoma of the prostate. A distinctive tumor of probably prostatic duct origin. *Cancer* 37:2255-2262, 1976.

Zenklusen HR, Weymuth G, Rist M, et al. Carcinosarcoma of the prostate in combination with adenocarcinoma of the prostate and adenocarcinoma of the seminal vesicles. A case report with immunocytochemical analysis and review of the literature. *Cancer* 66:998-1001, 1990.

Zincke H, Utz DC, Farrow GM. Review of Mayo Clinic experience with carcinoma in situ. *Urology* 26(suppl 4):39-46, 1985.

Zrara I, al Bouzidi A, Rimani M, et al. Small cell cancer of the prostate: 1 case [in French]. *J d Urol* 102:188-190, 1996.

Unusual Prostatic Neoplasms

[18.1] Adenomas **431**

[18.2] Soft Tissue (Stromal) Tumors **432**

[18.3] Hematolymphoid Neoplasms **441**

[18.4] Miscellaneous Neoplasms **446**

[18.5] Secondary Neoplasms **446**

CHAPTER 18

The dominant proliferations in the prostate are epithelial-stromal hyperplasia and prostatic carcinoma; the latter disease is by far the most common neoplastic process. Other neoplasms are distinctly uncommon in the prostate. These include adenomas; mixed epithelial stromal tumor (phyllodes tumor); soft tissue neoplasms such as leiomyoma, leiomyosarcoma, rhabdomyosarcoma, and stromal sarcoma; hematolymphoid neoplasms such as lymphoma and leukemia; endocrine and neuroendocrine neoplasms such as paraganglioma and carcinoid tumors; secondary neoplasms; and miscellaneous neoplasms such as malignant melanoma and germ cell tumors. This chapter presents these primary and secondary neoplasms that are uncommon in the prostate gland.

[18.1] Adenomas

Given that epithelial hyperplasia and malignant epithelial neoplasms are so common in the prostate, it is striking and curious that benign epithelial neoplasms, adenomas, are so rare in the prostate. In the past, nodular hyperplasia of usual type has been called adenoma, and nodules of basal cell hyperplasia have sometimes been called basal cell adenoma. Also, fibroadenoma-like foci can be found in usual hyperplasia. However, the prevailing view is that all these nodules are hyperplastic rather than neoplastic. There is a single case report of a prostatic oncocytoma (or oncocytic adenoma) (Beer 1990), and about 20 cases of cystadenoma, also called giant multilocular cystadenoma, have been diagnosed (Blum 1960, Choi 2000, Douille 1963, Kanomata 1996, Kirkland 1967, Kirsch 1996, Levy 1993, Lim 1993, Maluf 1991, Melen 1932, Seong 1998, Watanabe 1990) **t18.1**.

The oncocytoma occurred in an 87-year-old man who presented with urinary retention (Beer 1990). The patient underwent transurethral resection of the prostate (TURP), and histologic examination of the chips showed nodules of tubules and acini lined by polygonal tumor cells with abundant eosinophilic cytoplasm. No nuclear atypia, mitotic activity, and necrosis were apparent. The differential diagnosis includes prostatic carcinoma with oncocytic features (Ordóñez 1992), where the diagnosis was made based on a metastatic deposit from an inguinal lymph node. This malignant oncocytic tumor appeared to have a greater degree of nuclear atypia than the oncocytoma. However, no follow-up was provided (Beer 1990), so it is not firmly established that this was a benign tumor.

Cystadenoma of the prostate is found in men of an average age of 56 years (range 28 to 80) who present with symptoms of urinary obstruction with or without a palpable abdominal mass. Clinically and radiologically, the origin of the mass is not always clear, and the anatomic location often is just generally pelvic. The mass usually is palpable on digital rectal examination (DRE). Computed tomography (CT) and magnetic resonance imaging (MRI) typically show a large, complex mass displacing but not invading the bladder and rectum (Choi 2000, Levy 1993, Lim 1993). In a few cases needle biopsies were done and were nondiagnostic. Fine needle aspiration was performed in one case and yielded bloody fluid (Levy 1993), and biopsies in a second case were interpreted as fragments of prostatic tissue with hyalinized and fibroblastic stroma (Maluf 1991). Intraoperatively, some of the masses were physically separate from the prostate gland, whereas others were attached to the prostate via a thin pedicle. In one case, the tumor arose in the bladder (Goudale 1928), presumably from ectopic prostatic tissue. Complete excision of the mass in 7 cases entailed pelvic exenteration. The masses have a bosselated, smooth external surface, and cut surfaces are remarkable for multiple cysts varying in size from 0.1cm to 2cm, with separation by white fibrous septae **i18.1**. The cystic contents are brown to yellowish brown fluid, with or without gray inspissated material and brown semisolid material (Choi 2000, Levy 1993, Lim 1993, Maluf 1991). Microscopically, the cysts are lined by benign 2-cell-layered prostatic epithelium **i18.2**, which is flattened in some larger cysts by intraluminal pressure. Epithelial denudation with replacement

■ t18.1 Giant Multilocular Cystadenoma of Prostate

- Rare: Around 20 cases reported in adult men
- Men at mean age of 56 present with obstruction and/or palpable abdominal mass
- Mass can be pelvic without attachment to prostate, can be attached via pedicle, or intraprostatic
- Gross: Very large (average = 18cm), multiloculated, cystic mass
- Microscopically: Benign prostatic epithelial cysts surrounded by hypocellular stroma
- Completely benign

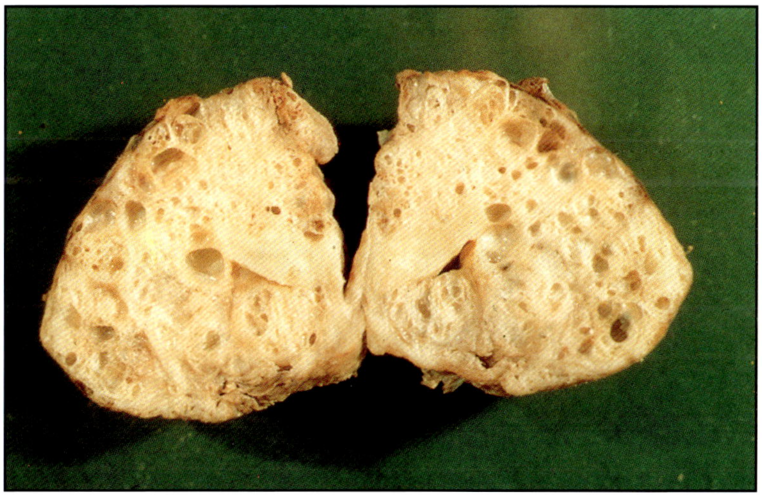

■ i18.1 *Giant multilocular cystadenoma: multiple cysts are evident. (Courtesy of Dr Horacio Maluf).*

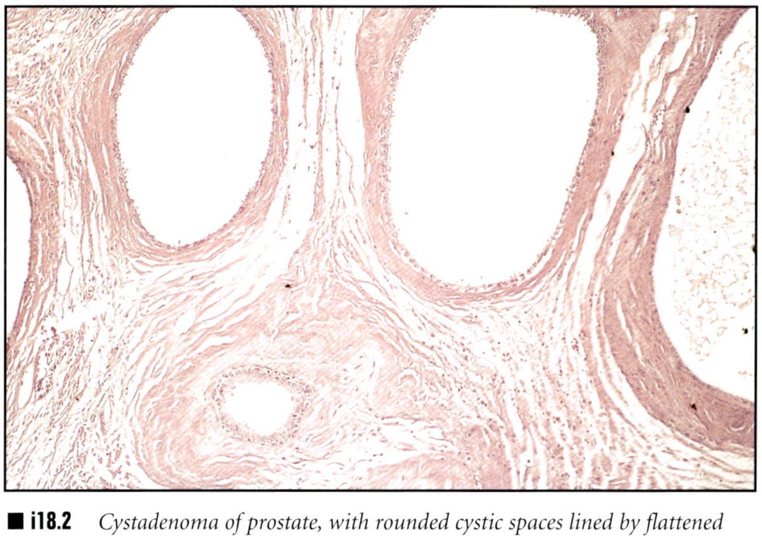

■ i18.2 *Cystadenoma of prostate, with rounded cystic spaces lined by flattened layer of benign prostatic epithelial cells.*

by granulation tissue can also be seen (Levy 1993). Focally, intraluminal small papillary projections or cribriform glands can be seen. There is no evidence of cytologic atypia or mitotic figures. The epithelium is prostatic in nature, as substantiated by positive immunohistochemical stains for prostate-specific antigen (PSA). The stroma is hypercellular to hyalinized, with a few chronic inflammatory cells. In one case (Lim 1993), the seminal vesicle was entrapped within the cystic mass, but in no case was there infiltration into adjacent bladder or rectum. The differential diagnosis includes usual hyperplasia, prostatic phyllodes tumors, and retrovesical and retroperitoneal multilocular tumors such as multilocular peritoneal inclusion cysts, lymphangiomas, müllerian duct cysts, and seminal vesicle cysts (Maluf 1991). Cystadenomas lack the leaflike projections and hypercellular stroma of phyllodes tumors, and the other tumors can be excluded based on the prostatic epithelial lining of the cysts in the cystadenoma. Usual prostatic hyperplasia can be cystic, but in contrast to cystadenoma, it is classically a multinodular stromal and epithelial cell proliferation. Prostatic cystadenomas are completely benign, based on clinical follow-up of 4 months to 8 years (Levy 1993, Maluf 1991). Recurrence was seen in one case (Maluf 1991). However, no report exists of association with or progression to malignancy.

[18.2] Soft Tissue (Stromal) Tumors

A wide variety of mesenchymal neoplasms can originate in the prostate gland **t18.2**. These are all infrequently encountered. The most common benign mesenchymal neoplasm is the leiomyoma, and the most common malignant mesenchymal neoplasms are rhabdomyosarcoma in children and leiomyosarcoma in adults.

Leiomyoma

The incidence of leiomyoma in the prostate is uncertain because leiomyomatous stromal nodules in usual hyperplasia have been diagnosed as leiomyoma. Prostatic leiomyoma may be defined as a solitary, well-circumscribed smooth muscle mass measuring >1cm in diameter (Ayala 1999, Kaufman 1951) **t18.3**. (This size cutoff is admittedly arbitrary, and the existence of the prostatic leiomyoma has been questioned [Têtu 1990]. It could very well be that prostate "leiomyomas" are examples of solitary, nodular, leiomyomatous stromal hyperplasia.) Recent reviews (Ayala 1999, Têtu 1988) compiled about 50 to 60 cases of prostatic leiomyoma (Belis 1979, Károlyi 1988, Leader 1998, Leonard 1988, Muzafer 1987, Persaud 1982, Prabhu 1995, Regan 1987, Rosen 1980, Schumacher 1996, Têtu 1988, 1990). The average age at diagnosis is 60 years (range 24 to 80) (Kaufman 1951). Most patients present with urinary difficulties. Grossly, the mean diameter was 4.7cm (range 1.2cm to 13.5cm) (Kaufman 1951). Microscopically, prostatic leiomyoma is a bland spindle cell proliferation without an epithelial component. Sheetlike, whorled, or fascicular growth patterns can be identified **i18.3, i18.4**. Cellularity is variable. Of significance, necrosis and more than rare mitotic figures should not be evident. Specifically, there should be fewer than 2 mitoses per 10 high-power fields. Nuclear pleomorphism is also absent, except in rare cases of "bizarre" or "atypical" leiomyomas (Károlyi 1988, Persaud 1982, Rosen 1980), where degenerative-type nuclear atypia with smudged chromatin can be visualized. Such degenerative nuclear alterations are similar to those seen in "ancient" schwannomas or "symplastic" uterine leiomyomas and are found in the absence of mitotic activity. Histologic variants of prostatic leiomyoma include these atypical (bizarre or symplastic) leiomyomas (Károlyi 1988, Persaud 1982, Rosen 1980) and also cellular leiomyomas, epithelioid leiomyoma (Schumacher 1996), and leiomyoblastoma (Benassayag 1975). There is no evidence to suggest malignant behavior of these variants. The principal entities in the differential diagnosis are leiomyomatous stromal nodules and leiomyosarcoma. Size is the main distinguishing feature between leiomyomatous stromal nodule and leiomyoma. Also, the stromal nodules tend to occur with a background of usual hyperplasia. Criteria for separating benign from malignant smooth muscle tumors in the prostate are not fully defined, but necrosis, nondegenerative nuclear atypia, a high mitotic rate, and atypical mitotic figures should not be detected in leiomyomas.

Other benign mesenchymal neoplasms in the prostate recognized in isolated case reports include solitary fibrous tumor (Mentzel 1997, Takeshima 1997, Westra 2000), hemangiomas (Fiorelli 1991, Holtl 1982, Sundarasivarao 1973), chondroma (Sloan 1985), granular cell tumor (Furihata 1996), ganglioneuroma (Nassiri 1994), and neurofibroma (Chung 1996, Elbadawi 1979, Niku 1995) found in the setting of neurofibromatosis. Fibromatosis can also involve the prostate (Scholtmeijer 1988). Tumors described as prostatic fibromas probably are part of the spectrum of usual hyperplasia (Kafandaris 1983).

Stromal Proliferations of Uncertain Malignant Potential

Prostatic stromal proliferations of uncertain malignant potential include atypical stromal hyperplasia, inflammatory

t18.2 Soft Tissue (Stromal) Tumors of the Prostate

Benign
Leiomyoma
Others: solitary fibrous tumor, hemangioma, chondroma, granular cell tumor, neurofibroma, ganglioneuroma

Stromal Proliferations of Uncertain Malignant Potential
Atypical stromal hyperplasia [prostatic stromal proliferation of uncertain malignant potential, pattern 1; atypical (bizarre or symplastic) leiomyoma]
Inflammatory myofibroblastic tumor (pseudosarcomatous fibromyxoid tumor, atypical fibromyxoid tumor)
Phyllodes tumor
Hemangiopericytoma

Malignant
Rhabdomyosarcoma
Leiomyosarcoma
Prostatic stromal sarcoma
Others: Angiosarcoma, malignant peripheral nerve sheath tumor, malignant fibrous histiocytoma, synovial sarcoma, chondrosarcoma, Ewing's sarcoma, malignant rhabdoid tumor, malignant mesenchymoma, ectomesenchymoma, undifferentiated sarcoma.

t18.3 Leiomyoma of Prostate

Most common benign mesenchymal neoplasm but only 50-60 cases reported
Men 60 years of age (range 20-80) present with urinary difficulties
Grossly: 4.7cm average size (range 1cm-13.5cm)
Microscopically: Similar to leiomyomas elsewhere.
Not allowable: Necrosis, > 2 mitoses/10 HPF, nondegenerative nuclear atypia

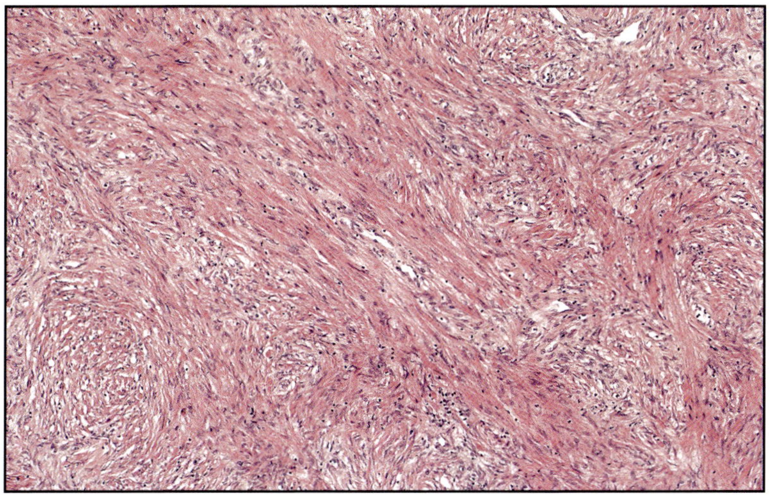

■ **i18.3** *Leiomyoma of prostate. Bundles of smooth muscle cells typify this proliferation.*

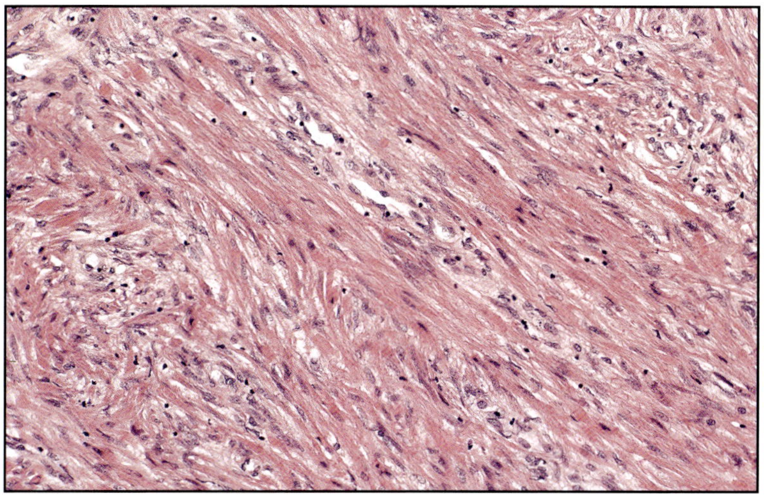

■ **i18.4** *Leiomyoma of prostate: Higher power view of* **i18.3** *revealing cytologically bland smooth muscle cells.*

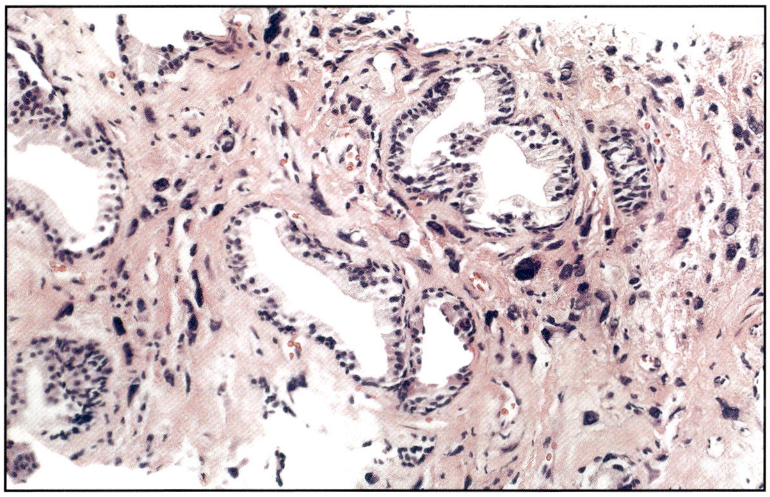

■ **i18.5** *Atypical stromal hyperplasia in prostate needle biopsy tissue: Atypical stromal cells course around benign glands.*

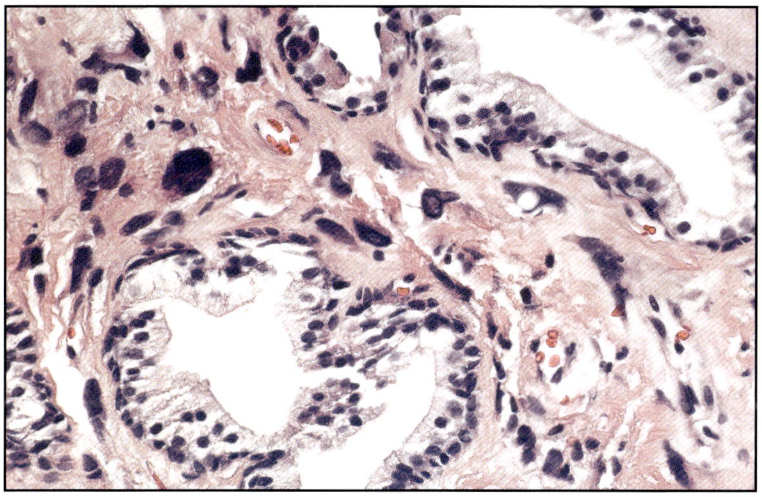

■ **i18.6** *Atypical stromal hyperplasia. Stromal cells with nuclear atypia are evident, but no mitoses are seen.*

myofibroblastic tumor, certain phyllodes tumors, and certain hemangiopericytomas **t18.2**.

Atypical Stromal Hyperplasia

Atypical stromal hyperplasia has been considered both a variant of prostatic hyperplasia (Young 2000) and a prostatic stromal proliferation of uncertain malignant potential (PSPUMP) (Gaudin 1998) **t18.4**. Some also include atypical (bizarre or symplastic) leiomyomas in this category (Attah 1977, Ayala 1999, Wang 1997). The incidence is unknown,

■ **t18.4 Atypical Stromal Hyperplasia of Prostate**

aka prostatic stromal proliferation of uncertain malignant potential, pattern 1, and atypical (bizarre or symplastic) leiomyomas
Less than 32 reported cases
Men 62 years old (range 27-80) present with obstruction or abnormal DRE
Two patterns: leiomyoma-like and infiltrative
Microscopically, both patterns have scattered large, atypical, cells with smudged chromation and sporadic multinucleation
Differential diagnosis vs sarcoma: No stromal overgrowth, no necrosis, no mitoses

but <30 cases have been reported (Attah 1977, Eble 1991, Gaudin 1998, Károlyi 1988, Leong 1988, Medina Perez 2000, Persaud 1982, Rosen 1980, Têtu 1988, Wang 1997, Young 1987). The average age at presentation is 62 (range 27 to 80), and most men present urinary obstruction or abnormal DRE (Attah 1977, Wang 1997). A few men had an elevated serum PSA level (Wang 1997). The diagnostic procedure was either TURP or needle biopsy, with a few cases diagnosed in suprapubic (open) prostatectomy tissues (Gaudin 1998, Wang 1997). Histologically, the process may exhibit growth as a solid, circumscribed stromal nodule (called leiomyoma-like [Wang 1997]) or as an infiltrative process (the latter being equivalent to PSPUMP, pattern 1 [Gaudin 1998]). The lesional cells are scattered within the smooth muscle nodules or between benign glands **i18.5**. Nuclei are enlarged, pleomorphic, and hyperchromatic **i18.6**, with occasional multinucleation, bubbly or vacuolated appearances and nuclear pseudoinclusions. Mitotic figures are rare or, most commonly, are absent. Immunohistochemically, the atypical stromal cells in the leiomyoma-like pattern exhibit intense desmin and actin immunoreactivity, with weak to moderate vimentin staining, whereas the atypical cells in the infiltrative pattern show intense vimentin immunopositivity but weak or no staining for desmin and actin (Wang 1997). The main diagnostic problem is that these atypical cells may cause concern for a sarcoma. (At least one case was misdiagnosed as a leiomyosarcoma [Têtu 1988]). However, features of sarcoma such as stromal overgrowth, necrosis, and mitotic activity are generally absent.

Difficulty may arise in limited sampling such as needle biopsy, where distinction between atypical stromal hyperplasia, phyllodes tumor, and sarcoma may be difficult or impossible. In these cases a descriptive diagnosis of atypical spindle cell proliferation, with a comment on the differential diagnosis, might be appropriate. The nature of the atypical cells in prostatic atypical stromal hyperplasia is not known with certainty, with different camps favoring reactive (Wang 1997), hyperplastic (Young 2000), and neoplastic (Gaudin 1998) processes. Local recurrence of atypical stromal hyperplasia can occur with incomplete excision, but thus far no metastases have developed (Ayala 1999, Gaudin 1998, Wang 1997).

Inflammatory Myofibroblastic Tumor

Inflammatory myofibroblastic tumor is a distinctive, spindle cell proliferation with fibroinflammatory and pseudosarcomatous appearances (Coffin 1995, 1998). It is also known as pseudosarcomatous fibromyxoid tumor, inflammatory pseudotumor, pseudosarcoma, plasma cell granuloma, plasma cell pseudotumor, xanthomatous pseudotumor, pseudosarcomatous myofibroblastic proliferation, inflammatory myofibrohistiocytic proliferation, and atypical fibromyxoid tumor (Cespedes 1996, Coffin 1995, 1998, Griffin 1999, Hafiz 1984, Lawrence 2000, Nochomovitz 1985, Sahin 1991). One proposal is that it is a visceral form of nodular fasciitis (Nochomovitz 1985). Recent evidence suggests that these proliferations are true neoplasms, with findings of clonal genetic abnormalities, especially at 2p22-24 (Griffin 1999, Lawrence 2000, Weiss 2001A). Anaplastic lymphoma kinase (ALK) is a valuable immunohistochemical marker for diagnosis (Cook 2001). In the prostate, the terms "pseudosarcomatous fibromyxoid tumor" (Cespedes 1996, Sahin 1991) and "atypical fibromyxoid tumor" (Hafiz 1984) have been applied. Only a few cases have involved the prostate (Cespedes 1996, Hafiz 1984, Sahin 1991). The patients were 22, 42, and 56 years of age. These men presented with complaints related to urinary obstruction. Cystoscopy revealed protrusion of a mass into the urethra (Sahin 1991) or bladder (Hafiz 1984). TURP (Cespedes 1996, Sahin 1991) and radical cystoprostatectomy (Hafiz 1984) were the surgical modes of treatment. Microscopically, these inflammatory myofibroblastic tumors were characterized by a spindle cell proliferation within an edematous and myxoid stroma. Effacement of benign prostatic ducts and acini, with extension into the bladder wall, was present in one case (Sahin 1991). The spindle cell nuclei were large, hyperchromatic, and pleomorphic. Mitotic figures were uncommon (at 1 per 10 high-power fields [Sahin 1991]) or nonexistent (Hafiz 1984), and no atypical mitoses were found. Immunohistochemical stains were positive for vimentin, with scattered cells positive for smooth muscle actin, with no immunopositivity for desmin, myoglobin, S-100 protein, or cytokeratin (Sahin 1991). Ultrastructural analysis revealed peripheral condensations of microfilaments with dense bodies, indicative of myofibroblastic differentiation (Sahin 1991). The differential diagnosis includes a postoperative spindle cell nodule and sarcoma. For postoperative spindle cell nodule there is a history of previous surgery, whereas it is more difficult to rule out a myxoid sarcoma. Indeed, in these 3 cases, initial biopsies were interpreted as "possible low-grade sarcoma" (Sahin 1991), "low-grade leiomyosarcoma or rhabdomyosarcoma" (Hafiz 1984), and suspicious for possible sarcoma (Cespedes 1996). Abundant mitoses, with or without atypical forms, should raise the suspicion of sarcoma. Clinical follow-up of 1 to 3.5 years has revealed an uneventful course for the 3 patients with prostatic inflammatory myofibroblastic tumor. In general, these tumors should be viewed as having an indeterminate or low malignant potential (Coffin 1998).

Phyllodes Tumor

Prostatic stromal proliferations that resemble phyllodes tumor of the breast have been categorized as phyllodes-like hyperplasia, phyllodes type of atypical prostatic hyperplasia, cystadeno-leiomyofibroma, phyllodes tumor, high-grade phyllodes tumor, malignant phyllodes tumor, cystosarcoma phyllodes, malignant cystosarcoma phyllodes, prostatic stromal proliferation of uncertain malignant potential (pattern 3), epithelial-stromal tumor, malignant cystic epithelial-stromal tumor, and mixed epithelial-stromal tumor (Chatelain 2000, De Siati 1999, Gaudin 1998, Jackson 1999, Kim 1999, Schapmans 2000, Têtu 1988, Tijare 1999, Yamamoto 2000, Young 2000) **t18.5**. Given the similarities with phyllodes tumor of the breast, the term *phyllodes tumor* seems preferable for this prostatic lesion. The true incidence is unknown, but the condition is rare, with around 35 reported cases. Almost all reports are of single cases; the largest "series" is of 6 patients (Halling 1993). For 34 patients, the average age was 50 years (range 22 to 74) (De Siati 1999, Gaudin 1998; reviews: Chatelain 2000, Schapmans 2000). The clinical presentation can mimic that of benign prostatic hyperplasia (BPH), with obstruction, dysuria, hematuria, and urinary retention. Additionally, because the tumor often is large, many patients present with a palpable abdominal mass (Kevwitch 1993). Initial treatment often is suprapubic prostatectomy or TURP, which provides diagnostic tissue. Only 1 tumor was an incidental finding (at radical prostatectomy) (Gaudin 1998). Needle biopsy diagnosis has been reported (Gaudin 1998), but recognition of phyllodes tumor in needle biopsy must be arduous. CT and MRI scans show a solid and cystic heterogeneous mass (Hessel 1993, Kerley 1992, Kevwitch 1993, Mai 1994, Young 1992). The serum PSA may or may not be elevated; the few reported elevations were 13 (De Siati 1999) and 17 ng/mL (Kevwitch 1993). Initial treatment often is suprapubic prostatectomy or TURP. Radical prostatectomy, cystoprostatectomy, and pelvic exenteration were performed in a few ($n = 8$) cases (Gaudin 1998, Schapmans 2000). These masses selected for complete resection were quite large, with a mean diameter of 20cm (range 6cm to 58cm) (Chatelain 2000, De Siati 1999, Hessel 1993, Kerley 1992, Kevwitch 1993, Schapmans 2000, Young 1992). Macroscopically, these excised tumors have smooth, lobulated outer surfaces and white-gray, solid to multiloculated cut surfaces. The cystic spaces contain yellowish brown, serous fluid. In one case, polypoid projections were noted grossly (Schapmans 2000). In single cases, hemorrhage and necrosis (Hessel 1993) and invasion through the bladder wall (Young 1992) were detected

■ t18.5 Phyllodes Tumor of Prostate

Also known as epithelial-stromal tumor and cystosarcoma phyllodes
About 35 reported cases
Clinical: Men 50 years of age (range 22-74), who present with BPH-like symptoms
Resected masses can be massive: 20cm average diameter (range 6cm-58cm)
Microscopically leaf-like fronds with variable stromal cellularity; nuclear atypia, and mitotic count. High-grade tumors = sarcomatous areas
Variable outcome

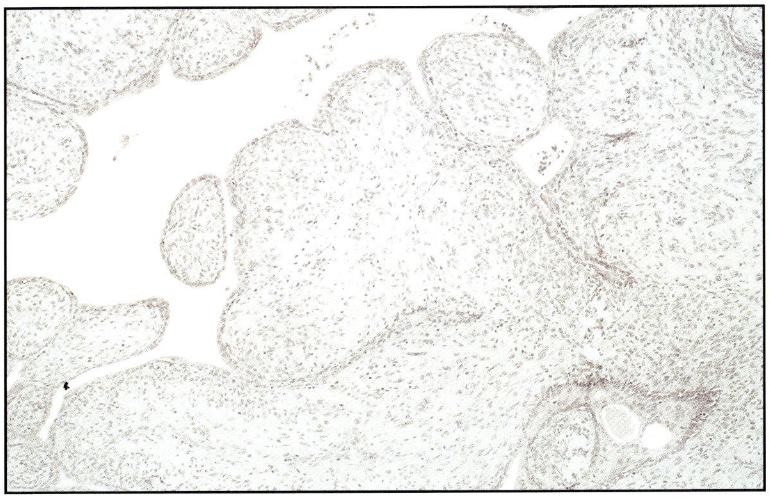

■ **i18.7** *Phyllodes tumor of prostate, with broad leaflike protrusions into a cystic space.*

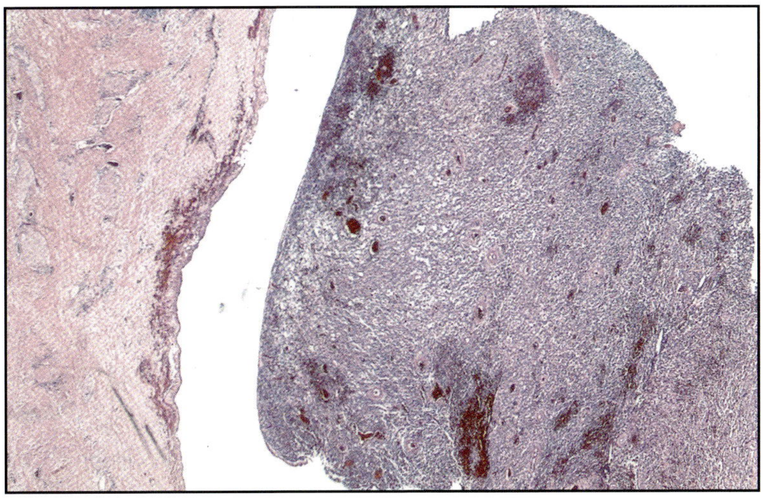

■ **i18.8** *Malignant phyllodes tumor of prostate: Cellular mass protruding into cystic cavity. (Courtesy of Dr Robert Young, Boston, MA.)*

grossly. Microscopically, prostatic phyllodes tumors display broad leaflike growths that are reminiscent of phyllodes tumors of the mammary gland **i18.7**. Like breast tumors, phyllodes tumors are essentially stromal cell proliferations with benign glandular elements. The stromal proliferation can result in intracystic protrusions of the fronds or polypoid nodules. Compression of glandular elements results in elongated clefts (Gaudin 1998). There is wide variability in stromal to epithelial ratio, stromal cellularity, cytologic atypia, and mitotic activity. Low-grade or benign prostatic phyllodes tumors, like those in the breast, exhibit uniform stromal expansion, few if any mitoses (usually less than 1 per 10 high-power fields), modest cellularity, and minimal nuclear pleomorphism. At the other end of the spectrum, clearly malignant or high-grade phyllodes tumors **i18.8–i18.9** are typified by sarcomatoid overgrowth and prominent cellularity **i18.9**, with necrosis, easily recognized mitotic figures, and nuclear pleomorphism. The sarcomatous component most often appears homologous, comprising malignant spindle cells arranged in bundles and fascicles, without obvious cell lineage–specific differentiation on hematoxylin and eosin (H&E)-stained sections. Fibrosarcoma-like and leiomyosarcoma-like areas may be seen. In 3 cases, poorly differentiated leiomyosarcoma was found in recurrent tumor (De Siati 1999, Young 1992, Yum 1991). Isolated examples of heterologous differentiation in the sarcomatous element include rhabdomyomatous (De Raeve 2001, Yokota 1984), angiosarcoma **i18.9**, and osteosarcoma. The epithelium in prostatic phyllodes tumors is nonneoplastic but can exhibit metaplastic or proliferative alterations, such as basal cell hyperplasia, adenosis, sclerosing adenosis, and squamous metaplasia (Gaudin 1998). Three cases have had an associated incidental adenocarcinoma (Kerley 1992, Kevwitch 1993, Lukl 1987). Immunohistochemical stains show cytokeratin, epithelial membrane antigen (EMA), and prostate-specific acid phosphatase (PSAP) in the epithelium, and the presence of basal cells is substantiated by 34βE12 binding and immunolabeling. The stromal cells are vimentin and actin positive, with variable or focal staining for desmin and CD34; immunostains for S-100 are negative (Chatelain 2000, Gaudin 1998, Gueft 1975, Ito 1989, Jackson 1999, Kerley 1992, Kevwitch 1993, Manivel 1986, Schapmans 2000, Young 1992). Features of both fibroblasts and smooth muscle cells are detected by electron microscopy of the stromal compartment (Hessel 1993, Ito 1989, Mishina 1990, Young 1992).

The differential diagnosis for phyllodes tumor includes usual hyperplasia and fibroadenomatoid change in usual hyperplasia, but

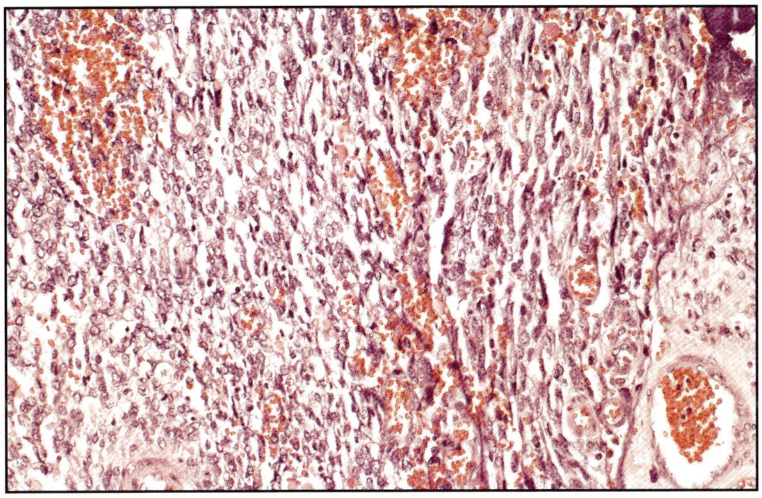

■ **i18.9** *Malignant phyllodes tumor of prostate: Angiosarcomatous heterologous component, with red blood cells in slit-like spaces. (Courtesy of Dr Robert Young).*

these lack the leaflike architecture, stromal cellularity, and cytologic atypia of phyllodes tumor. For higher-grade tumors, sarcomatoid carcinoma or a pure sarcoma are possibilities, but recognizing the benign epithelium in phyllodes tumor as a intrinsic part of the neoplasm aids in establishing correct diagnosis.

Local recurrence is common in patients with prostatic phyllodes tumor (Schapmans 2000). This results in part from use of transurethral or suprapubic prostatectomy (Kevwitch 1993), with apparently incomplete resection. Grade appears to be related to outcome in that patients with an overtly malignant, sarcomatoid component are at risk for extensive local pelvic invasion, distant metastasis, and death (Lopez-Beltran 1990, Lukl 1987, Yamamoto 2000, Yokota 1984, Young 1992, Yum 1991). Metastatic spread is to lungs, bone, and liver (Lopez-Beltran 1990, Lukl 1987, Yamamoto 2000, Yum 1991). Lymph node metastases have not been seen. It is difficult to predict the clinical behavior of prostatic phyllodes tumor because there are so few cases in the literature. One proposal is to grade these tumors as low, intermediate, and high grade (Halling 1993), but this approach has not been validated. Stratification into low-grade and high-grade neoplasms, as defined here, could also be performed. The best treatment for prostatic phyllodes tumor is not defined, but complete excision appears desirable.

Hemangiopericytoma

Seven cases of hemangiopericytoma in the prostate have been published (Chen 1987, Ishiguro 1984, Reyes 1977, Stout 1956, Velasco 1993, Wunsch 1982). These men had an average age of 61 (range 47 to 82) and presented with obstructive symptoms or hematuria. Diagnosis usually was made on sections of TURP chips and in one case (Wunsch 1982) on punch biopsy tissue. Gross observations of one case at autopsy disclosed a 7cm tumor that invaded the posterior wall of the urinary bladder (Chen 1987). The light microscopic appearance is identical to that of hemangiopericytomas of soft tissue, with uniform oval to spindle cells with little pleomorphism, a prominent, branding vasculature, and few mitotic figures. In one case with aggressive local infiltration, up to 4 mitoses per 10 high-power fields were found in certain areas (Chen 1987). Incidental adenocarcinoma was also found in one case (Ishiguro 1984). Lack of diagnostic awareness of the existence of prostatic hemangiopericytoma contributed to diagnosis of cellular leiomyoma and undifferentiated carcinoma in one case (Reyes 1977). Recurrence and locally aggressive behavior have been noted in 2 cases (Chen 1987, Reyes 1977), but it is not feasible to predict such behavior based on clinical or histologic attributes.

Malignant Soft Tissue Tumors

Sarcomas of the prostate are rare, accounting for 0.1% of all prostatic malignancies (Mackenzie 1968). The most common malignant mesenchymal neoplasms in the prostate are rhabdomyosarcoma and leiomyosarcoma (Smith 1972) **t18.6**. Overall, rhabdomyosarcoma is more common: 60% to 70% of all prostatic sarcomas are rhabdomyosarcomas (Smith 1972). These muscular sarcomas have a distinctive age predilection, with rhabdomyosarcoma striking mainly children and adolescents and leiomyosarcoma occurring most often in adults. Other sarcomas primary in the prostate are decidedly rare.

Rhabdomyosarcoma

Rhabdomyosarcoma is the most common prostate cancer in children and adolescents (Coffin 1992, 1997B, Crist 1995, El-Sherbiny 2000, Husain 2001, Maurer 1995, Newton 1995, O'Shea 1997, Parham 2001, Smith 1972, Weiss 2001B, Wijnaendts 1994) **t18.7**. The rarity of prostate cancer in this age group is underscored by the fact that the incidence is <0.1% of all primary prostatic cancers (Mackenzie 1968). The median age at diagnosis is 3.5 to 6.5 years, with a range of a few months to 68 years (Hays 1982A, Lemmon 1960, Shapiro 1992, Timmons 1975). Less than a dozen prostatic rhabdomyosarcomas have been reported in adults of 18 to 68 years (Waring 1992). Both boys and men present with symptoms related to urinary obstruction and with suprapubic pain (Rogers 1976, Shapiro 1992, Smith 1972, Tefft 1973, Timmons 1975, Waring 1992). Rectal wall compression or invasion can lead to constipation. On physical examination a palpable suprapubic mass can be detected. In adults with prostatic rhabdomyosarcoma, the DRE is remarkable for an enlarged, firm, smooth prostate compared with the nodular, hard palpable prostatic carcinoma (Waring 1992). Another difference is that serum PSAP levels are normal in patients with prostatic rhabdomyosarcoma (Waring 1992). Also unlike prostatic carcinoma, which is classically hypoechoic, prostatic rhabdomyosarcoma is isoechoic by transrectal ultrasound (Terris 1994).

Grossly (and clinically), determination that a rhabdomyosarcoma is primary in the prostate rather than the bladder can be difficult or impossible, primarily because of the large size of these neoplasms and concurrent involvement of the bladder and prostate. Therefore, many series have lumped prostatic rhabdomyosarcomas as bladder-prostate rhabdomyosarcoma, lower urinary tract rhabdomyosarcoma, genitourinary rhabdomyosarcoma, or pelvic rhabdomyosarcoma (Crist 1995, El-Sherbiny 2000, Enzinger 1995, Exelby 1978, Hays 1982B, Maurer 1995, O'Shea 1997). For tumors of definite prostatic origin, the average size was 9cm (range 6cm to 20cm) (Hays 1982A, Smith 1972). They tend to be solid masses with a gelatinous appearance (Shapiro 1992, Smith 1972). Microscopically, most are embryonal nonbotryoid rhabdomyosarcomas, with a small percentage of cases being of the alveolar subtype, according to the International Classification of Rhabdomyosarcoma (ICR) (Newton 1995, Parham 2001). The embryonal subtype is composed of diffuse sheets or nests of small rounded or elongated hyperchromatic cells with a moderate amount of eosinophilic cytoplasm (Coffin 1992, Smith 1972). Cellularity is variable, ranging from compact areas to loose myxoid regions (O'Shea 1997, Smith 1972). This can create an alternating light and dark pattern. Condensation of cells along protrusions into adjacent cavities can create the compact "cambium layer" (Smith 1972). Cytologically, there is a range of differentiation, from primitive stellate or fusiform cells **i18.10** to "tadpole" and ribbon-like "strap" cells that have cross-striations indicative of skeletal muscle lineage (O'Shea 1997). Mitotic activity is variable, usually moderate in degree, and more often seen in the more primitive zones **i18.11** (O'Shea 1997, Smith 1972). The alveolar subtype, as defined by the ICR scheme, need not always have the classic alveolar structure of delicate anastomosing fibrous septa with tumor cells floating in the alveolar space; rather, solid patterns are also allowable (Newton 1995, O'Shea 1997, Parham 2001) **i18.12A**. It is critical that cytologically, these alveolar rhabdomyosarcomas be of high grade, with pleomorphic, hyperchromatic nuclei, coarse chromatin, and numerous mitotic figures (O'Shea 1997). When the histologic subtypes are mixed, any amount of alveolar subtype defines the tumor as alveolar rhabdomyosarcoma. Treatment can lead to necrosis, fibrosis, and "maturation," in which the tumor cells appear well differentiated (Coffin 1997B). Immunohistochemical stains are of immense utility in confirming muscular differentiation, especially in neoplasms that are poorly differentiated in H&E-stained sections.

t18.6 Sarcomas of the Prostate

Rare: 0.1% or less of all prostate cancer
Most common types (by far): rhabdomyosarcoma and leiomyosarcoma
Rhabdomyosarcomas usually occur in children and adolescents
Leiomyosarcoma usually found in adults
Other 1^0 sarcomas: Many types but only a few reported cases for each one

t18.7 Rhabdomyosarcoma of the Prostate

Most common prostatic neoplasm in children and adolescents but still very rare overall
Most cases in young boys but exceptional cases in adults reported
Grossly large (average 9 cm); sometimes so bulky it is difficult to tell if bladder or prostate is primary site
Microscopically, most embryonal subtype (intermediate prognosis), with a few alveolar subtype (poor prognosis)
Prognosis related to histologic subtype and TNM stage

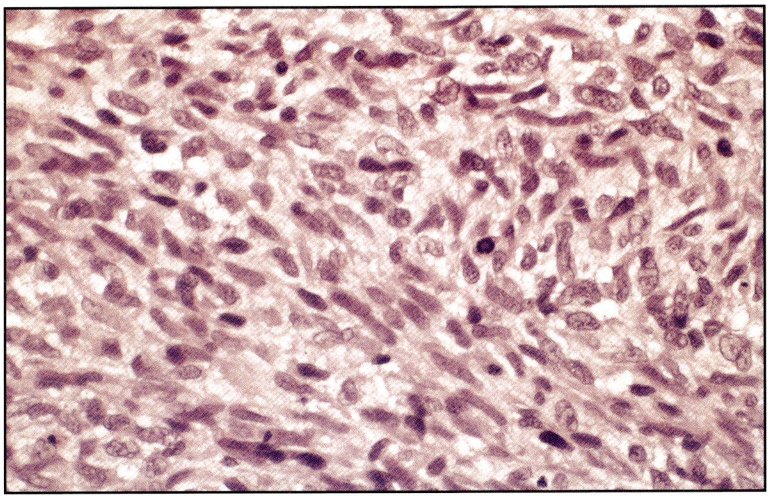

■ **i18.10** *Embryonal rhabdomyosarcoma with spindled neoplastic cells that do not exhibit differentiation in H&E-stained sections.*

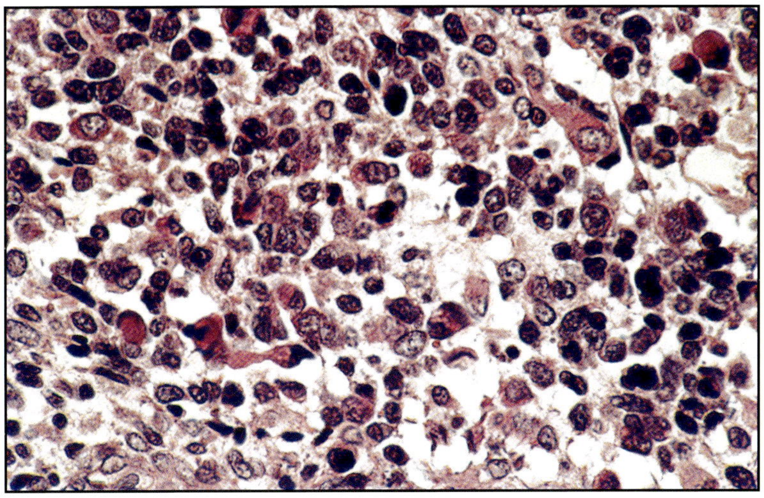

■ **i18.11** *Embryonal rhabdomyosarcoma with scattered elongated cells with eosinophilic cytoplasm (rhabdomyoblasts).*

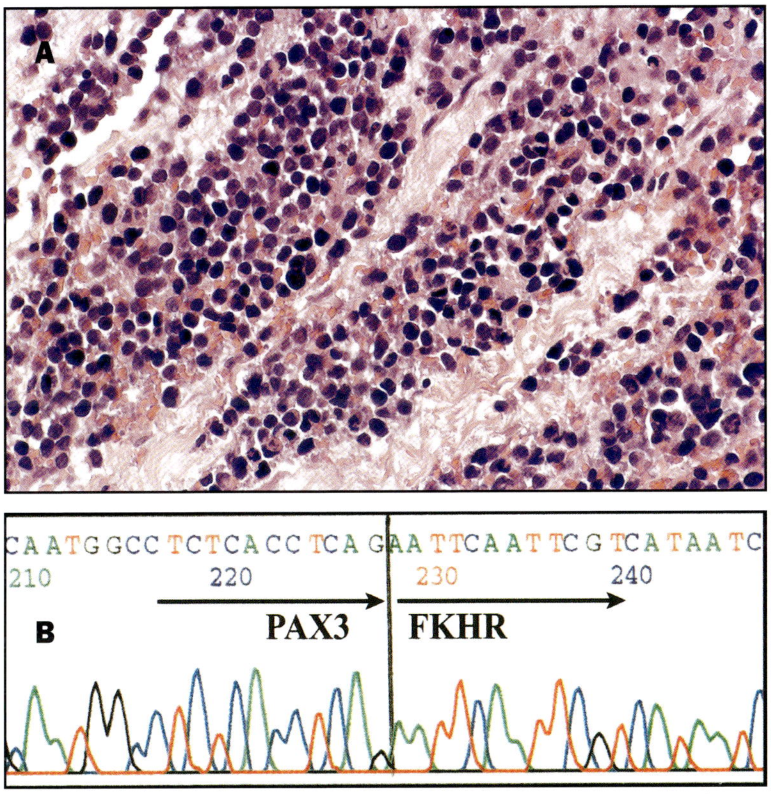

■ **i18.12** *A: Alveolar rhabdomyosarcoma of prostate, solid pattern. B: Gene fusion sequence of PAX3-FKHR, characteristic of alveolar rhabdomyosarcoma. RT-PCR of RNA extracted from formalin-fixed, paraffin-embedded tissue from block corresponding to section shown in (A) was performed, followed by cloning of PCR products, and automated sequencing. (Courtesy of Dr Xiaopei Zhu and Dr John Pfeifer).*

Positivity for vimentin, muscle-specific actin, and desmin is the rule, whereas antibodies to p30/32 (MIC2 protein), synaptophysin, S-100, cytokeratin, CD45, L26, and MT1 generally are nonreactive (Coffin 1997A, Parham 2001). Rare examples of p30/32 MIC2 glycoprotein and B-cell lymphoid marker expression have been reported (O'Shea 1997, Pinto 1997). Specific useful markers of skeletal muscle differentiation include myoglobin, MyoD, and myogenin (Parham 2001). Myoglobin is less useful because of its low sensitivity; antibodies to it react only with the better-differentiated cells (O'Shea 1997, Parham 2001). In most cases, light microscopy and immunostains are sufficient to establish the diagnosis of prostatic rhabdomyosarcoma (O'Shea 1997). Genetic studies and electron microscopy can be helpful when histologic features are not consistent with the immunohistochemical stain results (Parham 2001). An extremely useful diagnostic genetic alteration is the characteristic t(2:13) and t(1:13) translocations found in about two thirds of alveolar rhabdomyosarcoma cases (O'Shea 1997, Parham 2001). These translations, which fuse genes PAX3 or PAX7 and FKHR, can be detected by cytogenetics or reverse transcriptase polymerase chain reaction (Barr 1995, Kelly 1996). The latter technique can be performed using formalin-fixed, paraffin-embedded tissue **i18.12B**. A diagnostic genetic alteration has not been discovered in embryonal rhabdomyosarcomas (Parham 2001). Electron microscopy of rhabdomyosarcoma reveals cells that are somewhat similar to those of embryonal muscle, with 12- to 15-mm myosin filaments and parallel bundles of thick and thin filaments that can have Z-band–like arrays (O'Shea 1997).

The differential diagnosis of prostatic rhabdomyosarcoma includes other small round cell tumors of childhood, including leukemia, lymphoma, neuroblastoma, and primitive neuroectodermal tumor (PNET)/Ewing sarcoma (Bale 1983, O'Shea 1997). An immunohistochemical marker panel allows one to distinguish most of these childhood entities. Ectomesenchymoma and malignant rhabdoid tumor should also enter into the deliberation in childhood; ectomesenchymoma has admixed muscle and neural elements (Govender 1999), whereas epithelial markers (cytokeratin, EMA, and carcinoembryonic antigen) are positive in the rhabdoid tumor (Ekfors 1985) but not rhabdomyosarcoma (Coffin 1997A, O'Shea 1997). Before diagnosing embryonal rhabdomyosarcoma, one should consider spindle cell and myxoid lesions such as leiomyosarcoma, inflammatory myofibroblastic tumor, malignant peripheral nerve sheath tumor, malignant fibrous histiocytoma, fibrosarcoma, and stromal sarcoma and sarcomatoid carcinoma with a rhabdomyosarcomatous component. The tumors in this differential diagnosis occur mainly in adults, so adult rhabdomyosarcoma is the principal consideration. Again, immunohistochemical stains, including those targeting skeletal muscle antigens, are valuable for diagnosis.

Prostatic rhabdomyosarcoma is an aggressive neoplasm that exhibits direct, local extension into the bladder neck, posterior portion of the urethra, and perirectal and rectal tissues (Shapiro 1992, Tefft 1973). Lymph node metastases are fairly common for a sarcoma, being seen in 20% to 40% of patients (Lawrence 1987, Tefft 1973). Distant metastasis is mainly to lungs, liver, and bone. In adults, the bony

■ **t18.8 TNM Staging of Prostatic Rhabdomyosarcoma**

Stage	T Invasiveness	T Size	N	M
II	T_1 or T_2	a	N_0 or N_x	M_0
III	T_1 or T_2	a	N_1	M_0
IV	All	a or b	N_0 or N_1	M_1

From Wexler 1994: pretreatment staging classification for Intergroup Rhabdomyosarcoma Study - IV, T_1 = confined to anatomic site of origin; T_2, extension, a = ≤ 5cm in diameter; b, > 5cm in diameter, N = regional nodes; N_0, not clinically involved; N_1, clinically involved; Nx, clinical status unknown, M = metastases; M_0, no distant metastases; M_1, distant metastases present

metastases often are osteolytic and generalized, compared with the osteoblastic metastasis of prostatic carcinoma, which often is localized to pelvic and vertebral bones.

Multimodal therapy, including chemotherapy, surgery, and radiation therapy, has dramatically improved survival for patients with childhood prostatic rhabdomyosarcoma. Currently, survival at 5 years is 83% (Crist 1995), whereas in 1973 survival was 20% (Tefft 1973). However, the disease in adults is lethal, with all patients dying of disseminated cancer at a mean of 8 months after diagnosis (Waring 1992). Prognosis for rhabdomyosarcoma is related to histologic subtype, where embryonal rhabdomyosarcoma has an intermediate prognosis and alveolar rhabdomyosarcoma a poor prognosis (Newton 1995, Wijnaendts 1994). TNM (T = primary tumor, N = regional lymph nodes, M = distant metastases) staging of childhood and prostatic rhabdomyosarcoma is also linked to prognosis (Wijnaendts 1994). The Intergroup Rhabdomyosarcoma Study uses a modified TNM staining system in which primary anatomic site of origin plays a role in stage assignment (Wexler 1994). Bladder and prostate rhabdomyosarcomas are automatically stage II or III, reflecting their worse prognosis compared with that of orbital, head and neck, and non–bladder or prostate genitourinary primaries **t18.8**. It has not been established that DNA content, p53 protein accumulation, or transcriptional expression profiles are of prognostic value (O'Shea 1997).

Leiomyosarcoma

Leiomyosarcoma is the most common sarcoma originating the adult prostate, accounting for 30% of all prostatic sarcomas (Smith 1972) but is rare, with about 100 reported cases (Aragona 1985, Cheville 1995, Christoffersen 1973, Cordonnier 1996, Danckers 1960, Mackenzie 1971, Mottola 1985, Narayana 1978A, Romero Perez 1990, Russo 1993, Sexton 2001, Tadera 1986) **t18.9, t18.10**. The mean age at diagnosis is about 57, with a range of 19 to 78 (Cheville 1995, Mackenzie 1968, Narayana 1978A, Smith 1972, Tadera 1986). Several cases have been reported in children below age 10 (Christoffersen 1973, Danckers 1960, Mackenzie 1971), but these may have been rhabdomyosarcomas. Patients typically present with urinary frequency, dysuria, urgency, retention, and nocturia (Cheville 1995, Smith 1972). For the few patients tested, the serum PSA level was normal (Sexton 2001). In one case, MRI was used to gauge the local extent of tumor, but otherwise little is known of the radiologic appearance. Grossly, mean and median sizes of 9cm and 5cm, respectively, were reported (Cheville 1995, Smith 1972), with a size range of 2cm to 24cm. The tumors are nodular and firm (Smith 1972) and are often necrotic and cystic (Cheville 1995). Microscopically, interlacing fascicles, handles, and whorls of neoplastic spindle cells are found, with effacement of the normal prostatic tissue **i18.13-i18.14**. In a minority of cases, the neoplastic smooth muscle cells are epithelioid **i18.15** (Cheville 1995). Histologic grade is variable, with about one third being low grade (Broder's grade 1 of 4) **i18.16**, with the remainder high grade (grade 3 to 4 of 4) (Cheville 1995). Higher-grade tumors are cellular, with marked nuclear pleomorphism, hyperchromasia, and macronucleoli. Of substantial importance, mitotic figures are present, with a mean approaching 1 per high-power field (mean 8.4 in 10 high-power fields [Cheville 1995] and a range of 2 to 24). Also, abnormal mitoses are readily found. Necrosis is evident in one half of cases, and on average, one half of the tumor is necrotic (range 10% to 90%).

Prostatic leiomyosarcoma has been reported to arise in a phyllodes tumor (Yum 1991), in sarcomatoid carcinoma **t17.23, p 420**, and 10 years after radiation therapy for prostatic adenocarcinoma (Cheville 1995). By immunohistochemical staining, all tumor cells are vimentin positive, two thirds are actin positive, and weak desmin staining is seen in 20% of cases (Cheville 1995). Keratin was identified (using AE1/AE3) in 27% of cases, in both epithelioid and nonepithelioid cells. S-100 immunostains were negative.

■ **t18.9 Leiomyosarcoma of the Prostate**

Most common sarcoma of prostate in adults
Men at average age of 57 (range 19-78) present with obstruction
Grossly large (5cm-9cm) with frequent necrosis and cysts
Microscopically, most appear like high-grade leiomyosarcomas found elsewhere, with hypercellularity, high mitotic counts, and nuclear atypia
Outcome poor: Almost all tumors recur after surgery and average survival is 2-4 years

■ **t18.10 Leiomyosarcoma of the Prostate: Clinical Features in Largest Series**

Author	Year	No.[1]	Age	Presentation	Outcome
Smith and Dehner	1972	14	58[2] (42-71)	Urinary frequency and urgency	median survival = 49 months
Cheville et al.	1995	23	61[3] (41-78)	Urinary obstruction: nocturia, frequency and urgency Perineal pain: 25% Serum PSA: normal	71% died of disease at a mean of 22 months (range 3-72) after diagnosis
Sexton et al.	2001	12	53[3] (40-79)	Not given	75% died of disease at a mean of 13 months (range 3-41) after diagnosis

[1]Number of cases
[2]Median age (range)
[3]Mean age (range)

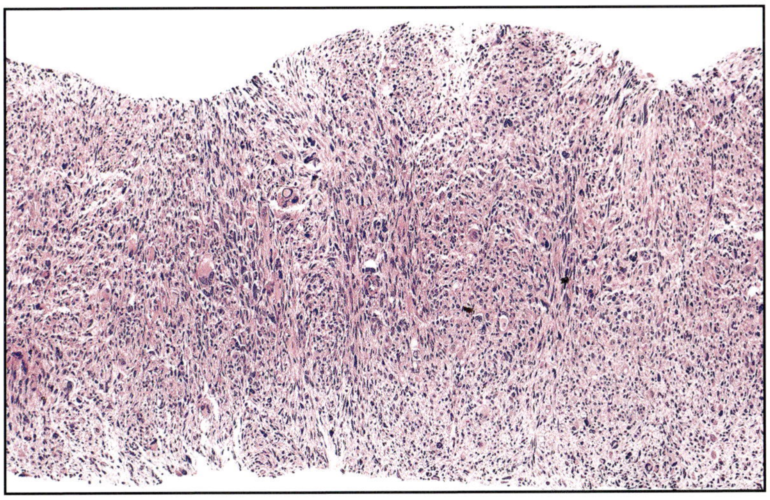

■ **i18.13** *Leiomyosarcoma of prostate in needle biopsy, with destructive, fascicular growth pattern.*

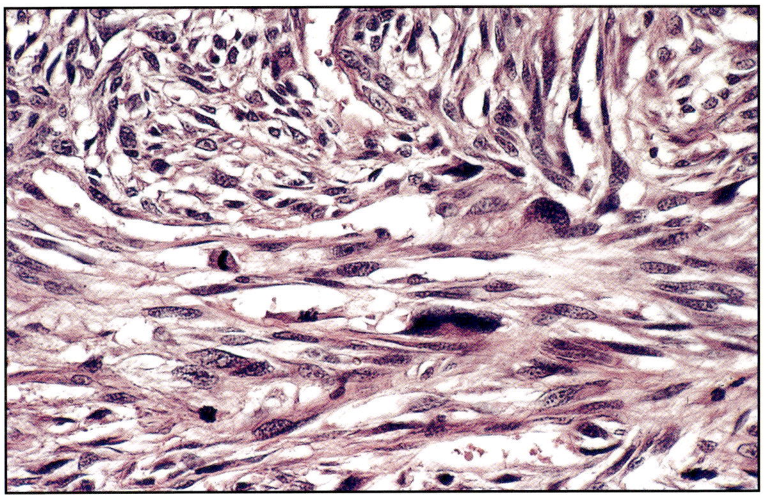

■ **i18.14** *Prostatic leiomyosarcoma: cytologic atypia.*

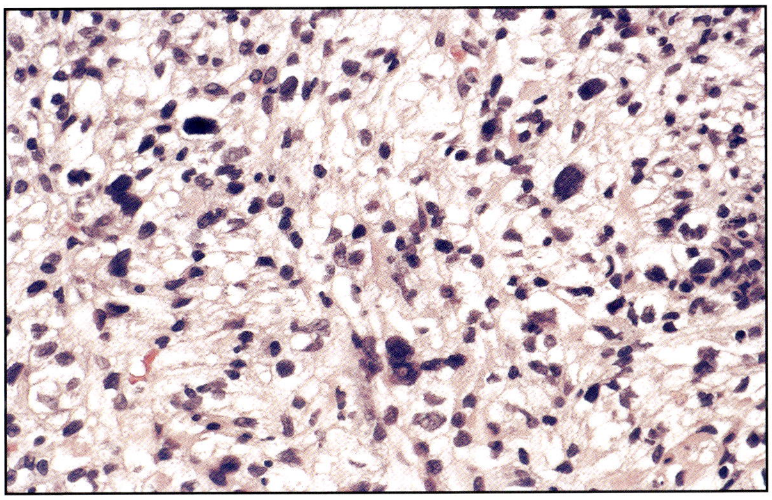

■ **i18.15** *Area of epithelioid cells with clear cell cytoplasmic change in leiomyosarcoma of prostate. Smooth muscle markers were strongly positive (muscle specific actin, smooth muscle actin) and epithelial markers (immunostains for cytokeratin and PSA) were negative.*

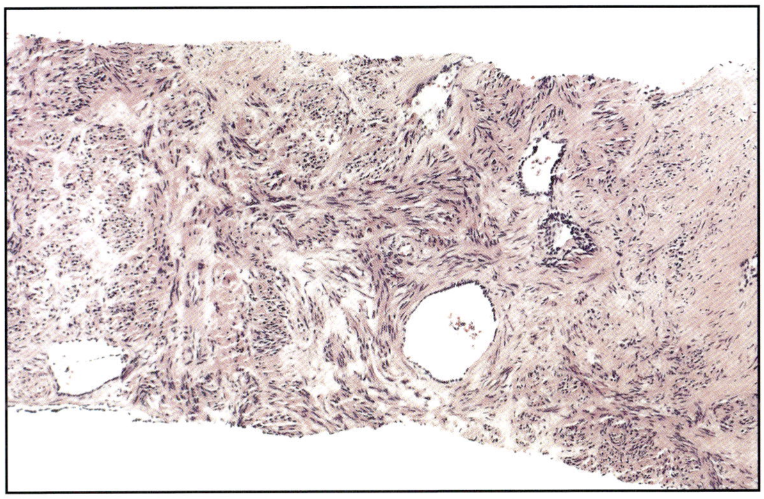

■ **i18.16** *Low-grade leiomyosarcoma in prostate needle biopsy. Distinction from leiomyoma may be difficult to impossible in needle biopsy.*

The differential diagnosis includes both benign and malignant spindle cell proliferations. One should exclude stromal hyperplasia, with or without atypia, inflammatory myofibroblastic tumor, postoperative spindle cell nodule, and leiomyoma, before diagnosing a malignant smooth muscle neoplasm. The key histologic indicators of malignancy are infiltrative growth with destruction of benign prostatic tissue, high cellularity, and mitotic activity (Cheville 1995). In needle biopsy, infiltrative growth of the smooth muscle cells can be difficult to assess, and high cellularity, necrosis, nuclear atypia, and mitoses, particularly atypical ones, are important. Yet because nuclear grade can be low and mitotic counts low, it may not be feasible in some cases to diagnose leiomyosarcoma in limited tissue samples, such as needle biopsy. Here, a descriptive diagnosis such as atypical smooth muscle cell proliferation seems appropriate, with a note in the report that clinical follow-up and additional biopsies or TURP are recommended. Other spindle cell malignancies of adulthood should be excluded, particularly sarcomatoid carcinoma and prostatic stromal sarcoma. Sarcomatoid carcinoma harbors a leiomyosarcomatous component in only a small percentage of cases **t17.23**, so in a limited tissue sample, it is not possible to definitively distinguish between a sampled leiomyosarcomatous component of a sarcomatoid carcinoma and a pure leiomyosarcoma. One should not misconstrue keratin immunoreactivity or epithelioid areas as being diagnostic of carcinoma because leiomyosarcoma can have one or both. Prostatic stromal sarcomas lack the actin and desmin immunopositivity seen in leiomyosarcoma (Gaudin 1998). Poorly differentiated prostatic carcinoma could be confused with epithelioid leiomyosarcoma; in this situation, PSA, PSAP, actin, and desmin immunostains usually identify cell type.

Leiomyosarcomas of the prostate are aggressive neoplasms, with most (10/11) patients suffering recurrence after surgical resection (Cheville 1995). One half of the men developed distant metastases, with lung being the most common site for metastatic spread (Cheville 1995). Additional metastatic deposits were detected in abdominal wall, brain, axillary lymph nodes, liver, kidney, and bone (Cheville 1995). Average survival was 2 to 4 years after diagnosis (Cheville 1995, Smith 1972). Radical surgery appears to offer the best chance for cure (Cheville 1995, Sexton 2001), although there may also be a role for multimodality therapy with radiotherapy and chemotherapy (Sexton 2001). There are no established prognostic factors (including grade, tumor size, and stage [Sexton 2001]), although it has been suggested that low mitotic activity and ability to achieve complete surgical resection with negative margins may predict survival (Cheville 1995, Sexton 2001). Cytogenetic abnormalities involving chromosomes 2, 3, 9, 11, and 19 have been described in a single case (Limon 1986), but so far there is no role for genetic abnormalities in the management of prostatic leiomyosarcoma.

Prostatic Stromal Sarcoma

Only 4 cases of prostatic stromal sarcoma have been reported (Gaudin 1998, Probert 2000). An additional 5 cases of malignant phyllodes tumor were reclassified as prostatic stromal sarcoma (Gaudin 1998). All but 1 of these 10 cases resembled malignant phyllodes tumor of the mammary gland. It is not clear whether this new classification is justified because clinical outcome for the original 4 cases of prostatic stromal sarcoma (Gaudin 1998) has not been proven to be different from prostatic stromal proliferation of uncertain malignant potential (Colby 1999). Further research should attempt to clarify the behavior of various stromal proliferations, including prostatic stromal sarcoma, to determine which classification scheme will improve therapeutic patient stratification.

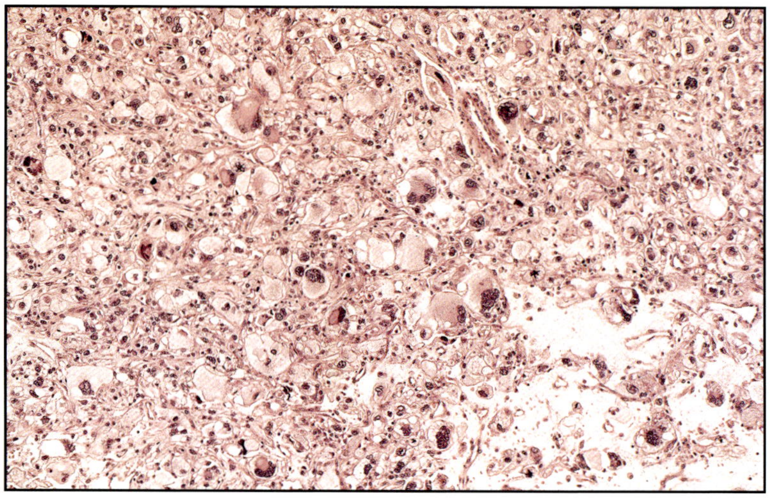

■ **i18.17** *Malignant fibrous histiocytoma with xanthomatous cells and giant cells.*

Other Sarcomas

Additional sarcomas primary in the prostate have been the subject of case reports **t18.11**. These include angiosarcoma (Boucher 2000, K Chan 1990, Lowsley 1934, Oliva Encina 2001, Smith 1986), malignant peripheral nerve sheath tumors (Rames 1999, Rober 1991, Schuppler 1971, Smith 1972, Tefft 1973), malignant fibrous histiocytoma **i18.17** (Bain 1985, Chin 1986, Heising 1985, Sexton 2001), synovial sarcoma (Fritsch 2000, Iwasaki 1999), chondrosarcoma (Dogra 1999), Ewing sarcoma (Szakacs 1974), malignant rhabdoid tumor (Ekfors 1985), malignant mesenchymoma (Ohta 1996), and ectomesenchymoma (Govender 1999). A few cases of osteogenic sarcoma have been described as originating in the prostate (Lerut 1967, Locke 1976, McKenzie 1999, Meeter 1960, Nishiyama 2001), but most appeared after treatment for adenocarcinoma, so it is uncertain whether these cases should be deemed sarcomatoid carcinoma with an osteosarcomatous element or pure osteosarcoma. *Fibrosarcoma* (Kumanov 1981, Tannenbaum 1975), *fibromyxosarcoma* (Derdoy 1967, Tannenbaum 1975), *myosarcoma,* and *spindle cell sarcoma* are diagnostic terms applied to a few prostatic sarcomas in the older literature (Tefft 1973), when immunohistochemistry and electron microscopy were not available for more precise characterization of tumor cell differentiation. *Undifferentiated sarcoma* or *unclassified sarcoma* remains a viable diagnostic category for prostatic sarcomas not exhibiting any specific mesenchymal cell type differentiation after morphologic, immunophenotypic, and genotypic evaluations. Liposarcoma has been reported as a secondary neoplasm in the prostate (Smith 1972) but not as a primary sarcoma.

Prostatic sarcomas of various histologic types have been reported to occur after radiation therapy to the prostate or pelvis. These are extremely rare, with only a few documented cases. These postradiation or radiation-induced sarcomas are mainly osteogenic

■ **t18.11 Exceptionally Rare Sarcomas of the Prostate**

Sarcoma	References	No.[1]	Comments
Angiosarcoma	*	7	Median age 37 (range 2-60). Factor VIII-related antigen positive in three cases. Metastases to lymph nodes, lung, spleen, liver reported. Most men died of disease 1-6 months after diagnosis.
MPNST[2]	**	6	Median age 25 years (range 1-67). Two cases in setting of neurofibromatosis type 1. Two patients died of disease in less than 1 year.
Malignant fibrous histiocytoma[3]	***	4	Patients 54,63,74, and 80 years of age. Rapid growth in two cases, pulmonary metastasis in one case. Two men died of disease in less than six months. One man died of disease at 94 months.
Synovial sarcoma	****	2	Men aged 34 and 37 years. t(X;18) detected in both cases. Metastases to lungs in both cases, liver in one. Both men died of disease in 32-35 months.
Chondrosarcoma	Dogra 1999	1	54-year-old man with bony, hard nodular mass by DRE. 6.5cm tumor at radical prostatectomy. No evidence of recurrence at 6 months.
Ewing's sarcoma	Szakacs 1974	1	15-year-old boy with tumor in posterior bladder wall and prostate.
Malignant rhabdoid tumor	Ekfors 1985	1	14-year-old boy with tumor in prostatic region. Widespread metastases and death 5 months after presentation.
Malignant mesenchymoma	Ohta 1996	1	40-year-old man with tumor with MFH, chondrosarcoma and rhabdomyosarcoma areas. Metastases to abdominal wall and lung, with death 6 months after presentation.
Ectomesenchymoma	Govender 1999	1	5-month-)old infant with prostatic embryonal rhabdomysosarcoma-ganglioneuroma. Patient died 8 months after presentation.

[1]N = number of cases
[2]MPNST = malignant peripheral nerve sheath tumor (neurofibrosarcoma, malignant schwannoma and malignant neurilemmoma in older literature)
*(Lowsley 1934, Smith 1986, K Chan 1990, Boucher 2000, Oliva Encina 2001)
**(Smith 1972, Tefft 1973, Rober 1991, Rames 1999, Schuppler 1991)
***(Sexton 2001, Bain 1985, Heising 1985, Chin 1986)
****(Iwasaki 1999, Fritsch 2000)

(Locke 1976, McKenzie 1999, Meeter 1960, Nishiyam 2001) but can also be leiomyosarcoma (Cheville 1995) and undifferentiated sarcoma (Nghiem 1995). In several cases, histologic typing of the sarcoma was not performed (Scully 1990, Terris 1998B). They are usually discovered years (range 2 to 25 years) after radiation therapy for prostatic adenocarcinoma. As noted earlier, it is unknown whether these sarcomatous neoplasms result from divergent differentiation in an adenocarcinoma and are therefore sarcomatoid carcinoma or are pure sarcomas. There are at least 2 true postradiation prostatic sarcomas that arose in men without a history of prostate cancer. Both of these patients were diagnosed with prostatic sarcoma 18 years after pelvic irradiation for testicular cancer (Nghiem 1995, Terris 1998B).

[18.3] Hematolymphoid Neoplasms

Hematolymphoid neoplasms may involve the prostate, including leukemia, lymphoma, Hodgkin disease, and multiple myeloma **t18.12**. For many decades it has been known that leukemia and lymphoma can infiltrate the prostate. Lymphomatous infiltration of the prostate was first described in 1877 (Coupland 1877), and leukemia infiltration was first reported in 1933 (Ascoli 1933). Leukemia and lymphoma commonly involve the prostate gland at postmortem examination, but clinical manifestations of such infiltrates are rare, occurring in <1% of patients with lymphoma or leukemia (Blank 1980, Fishman 1963, Freeman 1972, Melchior 1974, Rosenberg 1961, Zein 1985). However, there are cases in which the initial clinical presentation of the leukemia or lymphoma was symptoms referable to the prostate. However, with or without a previous history of leukemia or lymphoma, prostatic involvement usually is clinically attributed to prostatitis, BPH, or prostatic carcinoma (Bell 1995, Boe 1981, Bostwick 1998, Cos 1984, Doll 1978, Ferry 1997, Lewi 1984, Sridhar 1983, Waddington 1973). Therefore, diagnostic awareness of potential involvement of the prostate gland by leukemia or lymphoma is vital. Hematolymphoid neoplasms that rarely involve the prostate include Hodgkin disease and multiple myeloma.

■ t18.12 Hematolymphoid Neoplasms of the Prostate

Leukemia (including rare cases of granulocytic sarcoma)
Lymphoma, non-Hodgkin's: Primary and secondary
Hodgkin's disease (lymphoma) :11 reported cases
Multiple myeloma: 6 reported cases

Leukemia

Leukemic infiltrates in the prostate almost always indicate secondary spread, except for 1 reported case of primary extramedullary leukemia of the prostate (Quien 1996). The incidence of histologic detection of leukemic infiltrates in the prostate depends on the clinical setting **t18.13**. For 4863 men who underwent prostatectomy for BPH, only 6, or 0.1%, had leukemic infiltrates in TURP chips (Butler 1973). The incidence is much higher, at 10% to 36%, in prostatectomy or autopsy tissue from patients with known leukemia (Melchior 1974, Viadana 1978, Watson 1949, Zein 1985,). Such infiltrates apparently only rarely produce clinical symptoms (Blank 1980, Fishman 1963, Freeman 1972, Melchior 1974, Rosenberg 1961, Zein 1985). In several patients with leukemia, urinary obstruction, with or without retention, was the initial presentation (Dajani 1976, Flaherty 1940, Johnson 1953, Lubin 1947, Mitch 1970, Sridhar 1983). Additionally, some patients with known leukemia can develop obstruction necessitating surgery. In such cases, leukemic infiltrates (all of which were chronic lymphocytic leukemia [CLL]) were detected in 36% of prostatectomy tissues (Lewi 1984, Melchior 1974, Wilbur 1981). Although it is difficult to know for certain to what extent the leukemic infiltrates contribute to symptoms, it is felt that prostatic leukemic infiltrates may be a significant factor in precipitating acute retention of urine but only in the presence of other factors such as BPH (Dajani 1976).

There is little knowledge of the gross appearance of leukemic infiltrates in the prostate. A few reports of diffuse white parenchyma (Flaherty 1940) and white to yellow prostatic nodules (Dajani 1976, Jacobi 1937) exist. In one case (Jacobi 1937), the prostate was described as resembling a lymph gland (node), much as the extrinsic lymphoid infiltrates in Hashimoto thyroiditis can cause the thyroid to look like lymph node tissue. Most cases of prostatic leukemic infiltrates detected in living patients have been diagnosed in TURP chips or open enucleation prostatectomy tissue removed to treat obstruction. Several cases of CLL in these prostatic tissues were incidental diagnoses in older patients without a known history of leukemia (Butler 1973, Dajani 1976). In only a few cases has a prostatic leukemic infiltrate been diagnosed in needle biopsy tissue (Fishman 1963, Lewi 1984, Merimsky 1981). Microscopically, the most

■ t18.13 Leukemia and Lymphoma of the Prostate: Incidence

Neoplasm	Histologic incidence in all prostatectomies	Clinical incidence of urinary symptoms in L/L[1] patients	Histologic incidence in prostatectomies from L/L patients	Histologic incidence at autopsy of L/L patients
Leukemia	0.1%[2]	< 1%[3]	36%[4]	14%[5]
Lymphoma[6]	Unknown	< 1%[3]	Unknown	8%[7]

[1]L/L = leukemia or lymphoma patients
[2]Data from Butter 1973 on 4,863 prostatectomies for obstruction
[3]Data from Zein 1985, Fishman 1963, Melchior 1974, Blank 1980, Rosenberg 1961, Freeman 1972
[4]Combined data from Melchior 1974, Lewi 19842, Wilbur 1981
[5]Combined data from Zein 1985, Lucia 1952, Watson 1949, Melchior 1974, Viadana 1978,on 1,170 cases
[6]Non-Hodgkin's lymphoma data. Hodgkin's disease rarely involves the prostate, even at autopsy (Zein 1985)
[7]Combined data from Zein 1985, Watson 1949

■ **t18.14 Prostatic Leukemia: Type of Leukemias**

Leukemia Type	Prostates Involved at Autopsy
Chronic lymphocytic (CLL)	20%-22%
Acute lymphoblastic (ALL)	12%-13%*
Acute myelogenous (AML)	9%
Chronic myelogenous (CML)	4-5%

Data from Zein 1985, Barcos 1987
*In one series (Viadana 1978), 39% involvement was detected

common type of prostatic leukemic infiltrate is CLL, followed in order by acute lymphocytic leukemia, acute myelogenous leukemia, and chronic myelogenous leukemia (Barcos 1987, Zein 1985) **t18.14**. The leukemic cells are variable in number and distribution (Dajani 1976). Growth in a diffuse sheetlike fashion, with replacement of benign prostatic parenchyma, can be observed. The proliferation is predominantly stromal based **i18.18, i18.19**, with dispersion around prostatic glands, which can be compressed and destroyed by the infiltrate. The splitting of fibromuscular bundles can be seen (Fishman 1963, Melchior 1974), with linear arrays or rows (Melchior 1974) of leukemic cells that can simulate the appearance of carcinoma cells **i18.18**. Individual CLL cells can insinuate themselves into benign prostatic epithelium (Dajani 1976). In one case (Guerrier 1969) leukemic infiltrate and prostatic carcinoma were found together.

Rare ($n = 5$) cases of granulocytic sarcoma (chloroma) of the prostate, related to myelogenous leukemia or myeloproliferative disorder of the marrow, have been published (Y Chan 1990, Frame 1987, Muss 1973, Thalhammer 1994). Granulocytic sarcoma infrequently involves the prostate. Out of 58 cases, only 1 case (2%) was found in the prostate (Liu 1973, Muss 1973). Men with prostatic chloroma are of an average age of 68 (range 59 to 72) and present with hematoma, gross hematuria, and anemia. The prostate is enlarged by DRE. One patient had known myelodysplastic syndrome, and 2 patients had known active or remote acute myelogenous leukemia, but in 2 other cases a diagnosis of acute myeloid leukemia was established only after the diagnosis of granulocytic sarcoma was rendered in TURP chips. In another case (Quien 1996), acute nonlymphocytic leukemia, M2 by French-American-British classification, developed several months after an initial diagnosis of extramedullary leukemia (chloroma) in TURP chips. In this case, positive immunostains for myeloperoxidase, CD68, and lysozyme, with negative T cell (CD3, CD45RO) and B cell (CD20) immunostains, were instrumental in confirming the diagnosis. Microscopically, prostatic chloromas are characterized by confluent collections to patchy infiltrates of blasts, usually with immature granulocytes, including eosinophilic metamyelocytes or myelocytes. Naphthyl-ASD-chloroacetate esterase stain (Leder stain) and immunostains for myeloperoxidase and lysozyme are critical in substantiating the diagnosis of granulocytic sarcoma (chloroma); CD117 may also be helpful.

The differential diagnosis of leukemic infiltrates in the prostate should include inflammation, poorly differentiated and neuroendocrine carcinoma, and lymphoma. Inflammatory cell infiltrates in the prostate often are of a mixed cell population, unlike CLL, for example, and generally do not efface benign prostatic tissue. Immunostains demonstrating a mixed T- (CD3) and B- (CD20) cell population argue against CLL when there is a dense lymphoid infiltrate. The nuclear atypia in myeloid leukemias and granulocytic

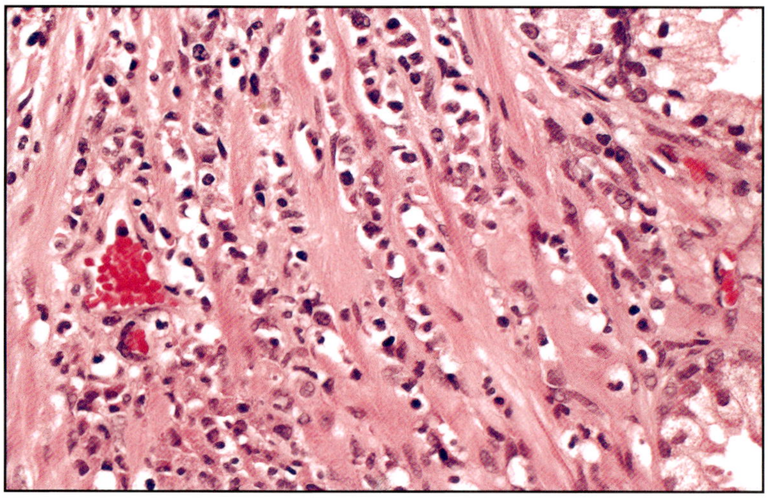

■ **i18.18** *Leukemic infiltrate in the prostate. Acute myeloblastic cells infiltrating as cords, resembling carcinoma.*

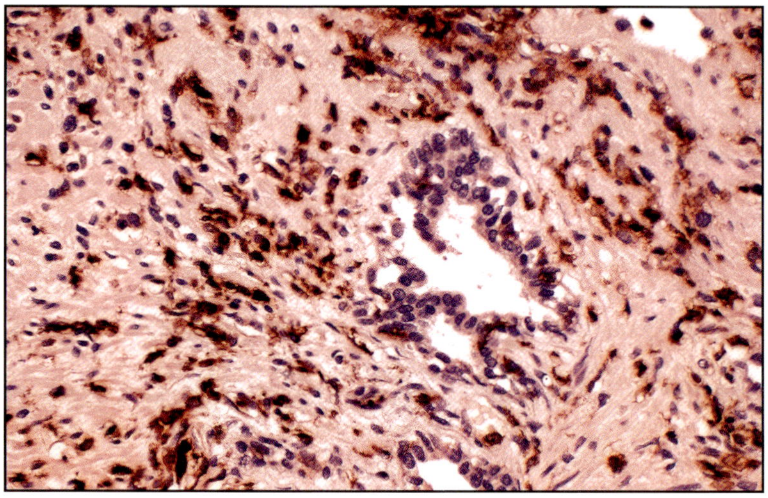

■ **i18.19** *Myeloperoxidase immunostain highlights the extent and infiltration of leukemic cells shown in* **i18.18**.

sarcoma would not be seen in inflammatory infiltrates in the prostate. A leukemic infiltrate was misdiagnosed as "undifferentiated carcinoma" in needle biopsy in the pre-immunohistochemistry era (Flaherty 1940), but immunostains for cytokeratin, PSA, and PSAP in a panel will prevent this pitfall. Leukemic infiltrates are distinguished from lymphoma based on hematologic studies. Chloromas, which often are initially misdiagnosed as lymphoma (Quien 1996), can be distinguished from lymphoma using Leder stain and an immunohistochemical marker panel.

Lymphoma

Both primary and secondary lymphomas of the prostate have been recognized **t18.15, t18.16**. These are rare diseases in prostate, with <200 reported cases. It is difficult to gauge the precise number of cases and incidence because lymphoma classification has varied over time (and no doubt will continue to change), and older reports refer to lymphosarcoma, lymphoblastoma, reticulum and round cell sarcoma, malignant lymphocytoma, with classification under the broad heading of *sarcoma* (Cartagena 1975, Ferguson 1932, Hampel 1977, Kaufmann 1941, King 1951, Kirshbaum 1943, Lucia 1952, Smith 1972, Symmers 1923, Waller 1949,

■ t18.15 Lymphoma of Prostate

Primary and secondary lymphomas exist; both rare
Incidence of primary lymphomas: 0.09% of all prostatic neoplasms
Men aged 57 (range 5-89) present with obstruction
Microscopically, suspect lymphoma is there is a dense monomorphous stromal infiltrate of atypical lymphoid cells
Most common types: diffuse large cell lymphoma and small lymphocytic B cell lymphoma, but many histologic types described
Outcome: Unfavorable. Median survival about 2 years

Watson 1949, West 1962). Clinically, the mean age at presentation is around 57 years, with a wide age range of 5 to 89 years (Bostwick 1998, Ferry 1997). Patients present with obstructive symptoms, including urgency and frequency, sometimes with hematuria and retention (Bostwick 1998, Ferry 1997). Systemic symptoms (fever, chills, night sweats, weight loss) are rare (Bostwick 1998). On DRE, the prostate is felt to be enlarged, smooth, rubbery, and firm. Serum PSA and PSAP levels usually are within normal limits but are elevated above 4 ng/mL in about 20% of patients (Bostwick 1998, Ferry 1997). The PSA serum level was substantially elevated (to 69 and 903 ng/mL) in 2 cases (Drinis 2001, Tomura 1999). Transrectal ultrasound can show a hypoechoic mass (Rainwater 1990, Swierz 1996) but is generally noninformative (Terris 1998A). Cystoscopically, the appearance of the prostate is identical to that in BPH (Bostwick 1998).

Clinically, the main difference between patients with primary and secondary lymphoma of the prostate is that, by definition, patients with secondary lymphoma had their disease diagnosed in an extraprostatic site first (usually lymph nodes), or extraprostatic site involvement was discovered within 1 month of diagnosis of prostatic involvement (Bostwick 1985, 1998). Secondary prostatic lymphoma has been diagnosed from 2 to 3 months after presentation at extraprostatic sites (Bostwick 1998). The criteria for a diagnosis of primary prostatic lymphoma are given in **t18.16**. Patients with primary prostatic lymphoma are slightly younger (60 years, on average) than patients with secondary prostatic lymphoma (whose average age is 66) (Bostwick 1998).

Little is written of the gross appearance of prostatic lymphoma, probably because most cases are diagnosed on needle biopsy or TURP chip tissue and because radical excision (prostatectomy) is

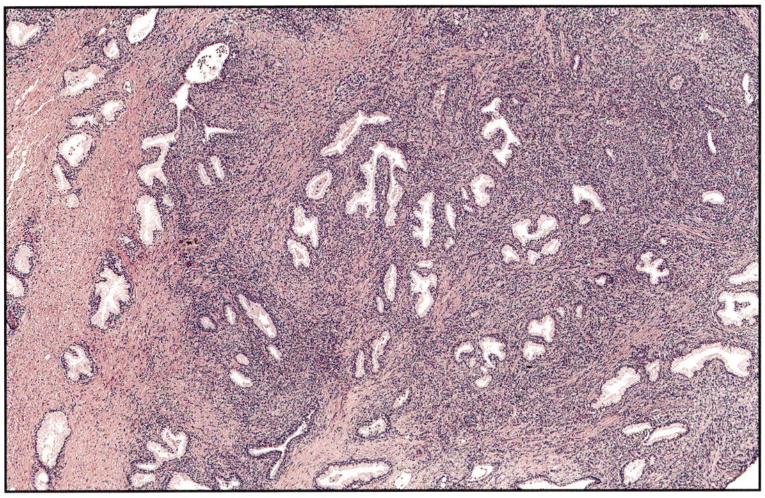

■ i18.20 *Malignant lymphoma in TURP chip, with stromal infiltration, without glandular destruction.*

not indicated as treatment. The few cases diagnosed as incidental findings in radical prostatectomy tissues (Bostwick 1998, Terris 1997, 1998A) were unlikely to be mass-formative. The few macroscopic descriptions that do exist are from autopsy observations of advanced cases published in the older literature (Ferguson 1932, Kaufmann 1941, King 1951, Kirshbaum 1943, Mason 1933, Rathbun 1937-1938, Smith 1937, Waller 1949). These prostatic lymphomas from more than one half century ago were large masses 6.5cm to 22cm in greatest dimension that often completely replaced the prostate and filled the entire pelvis. The palpable character was described as exhibiting "rubbery elasticity" (Ferguson 1932), or being firm, or even hard (Kaufmann 1941). Cut surfaces are homogenous, "perfectly smooth" and variable in coloration, ranging from yellow-brown to white to yellowish-white to grayish-pink or grayish yellow. Necrosis was mentioned in several reports (Kaufmann 1941, Kirshbaum 1943). Gross extension into local, adjacent structures, especially the bladder, often was noted. Microscopically, there is usually a patchy, stromal, atypical lymphoid infiltrate **i18.20-i18.22**, although the neoplasm can be extensive **i18.23, i18.24**, obliterative **i18.25**, perivascular, or focal **i18.26-i18.28** (Bostwick 1998, Doll 1978). For angiotropic or intravascular lymphomas (of which there are 6 reported cases (Banerjee 1988, Ben-Ezra 1986, Chim 2002, DeGiuseppe 1994, Stroup 1990)), the tumor cells are confined to vascular lumens. The

■ 18.16 Primary Lymphoma of Prostate[1]

Rare: 0.1% of all non-Hodgkin's lymphomas and 0.09% of all neoplasms of the prostate[2]
35% of lymphomas in the prostate are primary
Criteria:
1. Symptoms due to prostatic enlargement
2. Predominant involvement of prostate with or without involvement of adjacent tissue
3. Absence of involvement of liver, spleen, lymph nodes, or peripheral blood within 1 month of diagnosis of prostatic involvement

Mean age at presentation: 60 years (range 5-86)
Clinical presentation: lower urinary tract obstruction
Diagnosis established in needle biopsy in one-third of cases, in TURP chips in two-thirds
Extraprostatic involvement (usually in lymph nodes) diagnosed in 73% of patients 1-59 months after diagnosis of prostatic lymphoma
All B-cell lymphomas
Histologic subtypes: diffuse large B-cell (55%); small lymphocytic (18%); Burkitt-lymphoma (9%); follicular lymphoma, grade 1 of 3, (9%), follicular lymphoma, grade 2 of 3 (5%)
Six cases of MALToma of prostate reported[3]
Median survival: 23 months (same as secondary lymphoma)

[1]Data from Bostwick 1998
[2]Sarris 1995
[3]Pelstring 1991, Araki 1998, Tomikawa 1998, Tomaru 1999, Jhavar 2001, Tissier 2002

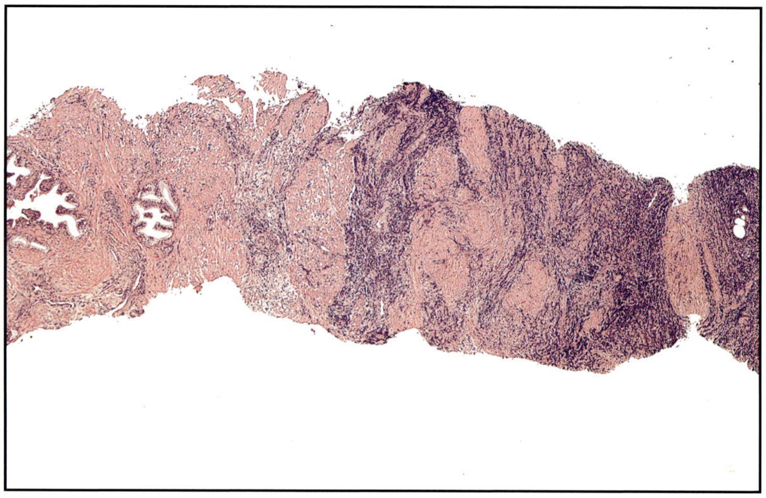

■ **i18.21** *Malignant lymphoma in prostate needle biopsy tissue . Patchy infiltrates in prostatic stroma.*

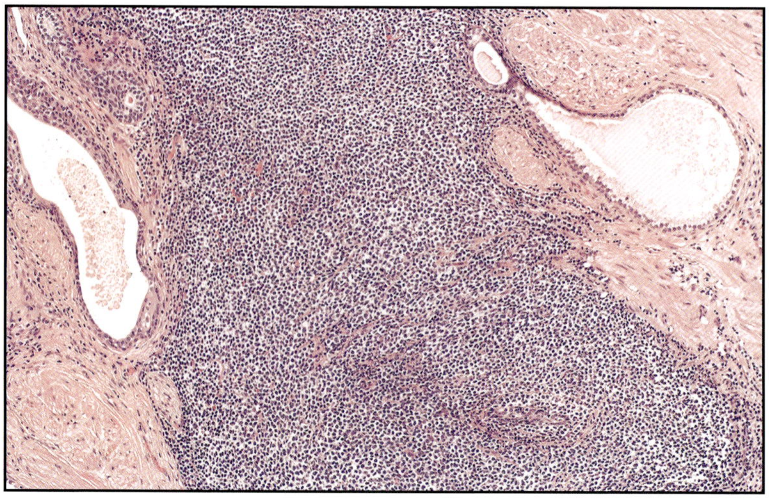

■ **i18.22** *Malignant lymphoma in prostate, with solid growth and spread between benign prostatic glands.*

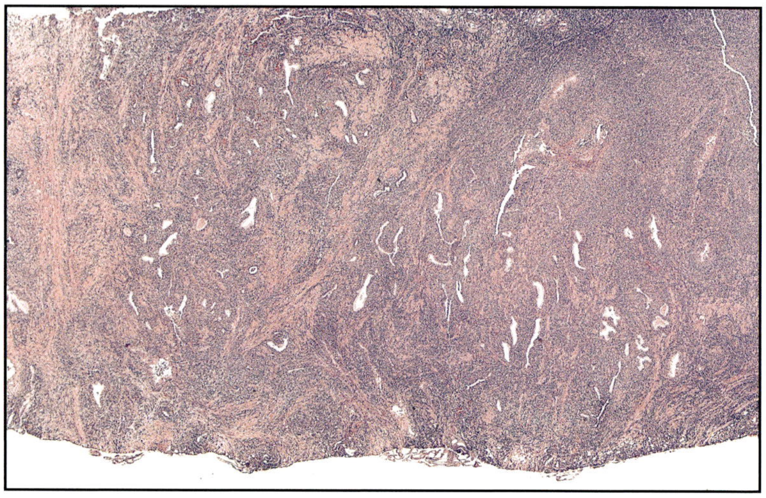

■ **i18.23** *Extensive malignant lymphoma in TURP chip. This was a non-Hodgkin's lymphoma, large cell, B cell type.*

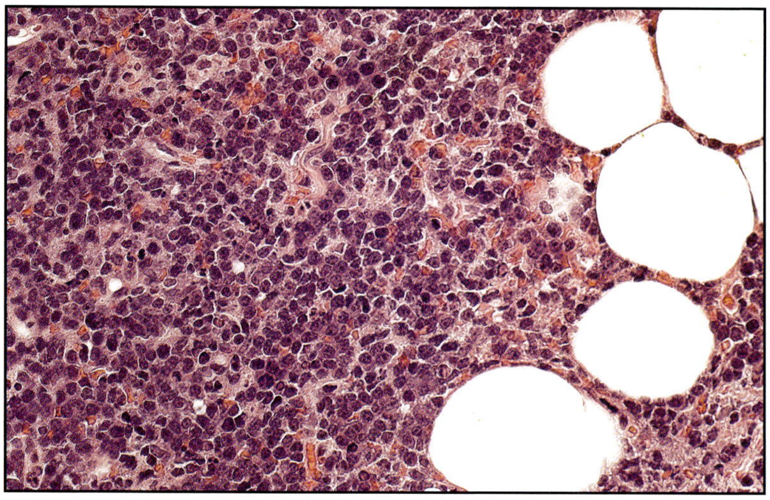

■ **i18.24** *Extension of malignant lymphoma of prostate into periprostatic adipose tissue.*

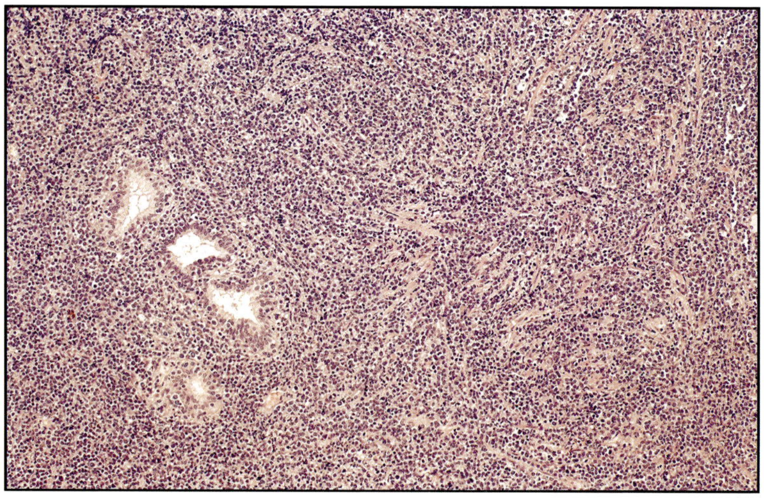

■ **i18.25** *Destructive growth pattern of malignant lymphoma in prostate, with only a few residual prostatic glands in this field.*

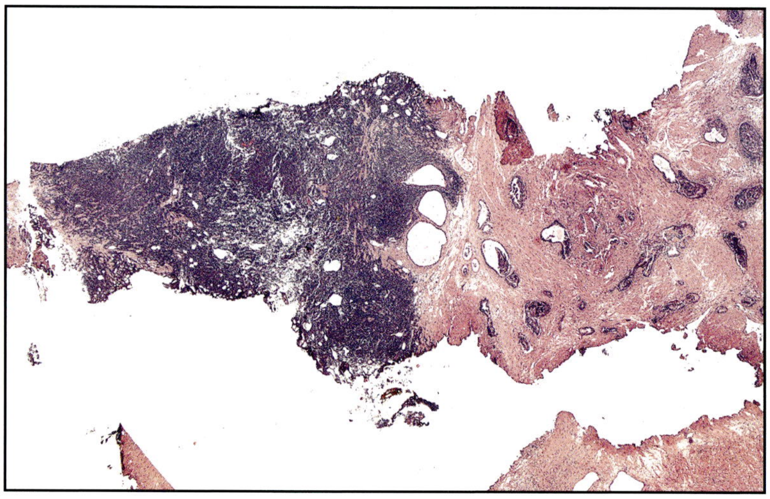

■ **i18.26** *Malignant lymphoma involving end of a TURP chip.*

neoplastic lymphoid cells can extend into prostatic epithelium in some cases **i18.29, i18.30** (Bostwick 1985, 1998, Ferry 1997), and for the reported cases of prostatic B-cell lymphoma of mucosa-associated lymphoid tissue (MALToma), lymphoepithelial lesions were formed (Araki 1998, Jhavar 2001, Pelstring 1991, Tissier 2002, Tomikawa 1998, Tomaru 1999). A wide variety of lymphoma types have been diagnosed in the prostate. Ninety percent are B-cell lymphomas (Bostwick 1998), and the most common types are diffuse large lymphoma in 40% of all cases

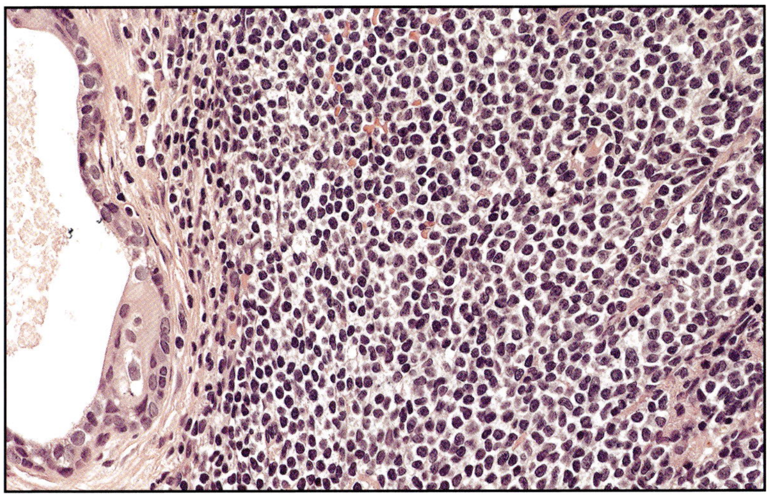

■ **i18.27** *Malignant lymphoma in the prostate: A monomorphous lymphoid infiltrate. Higher power view of* **i18.27**.

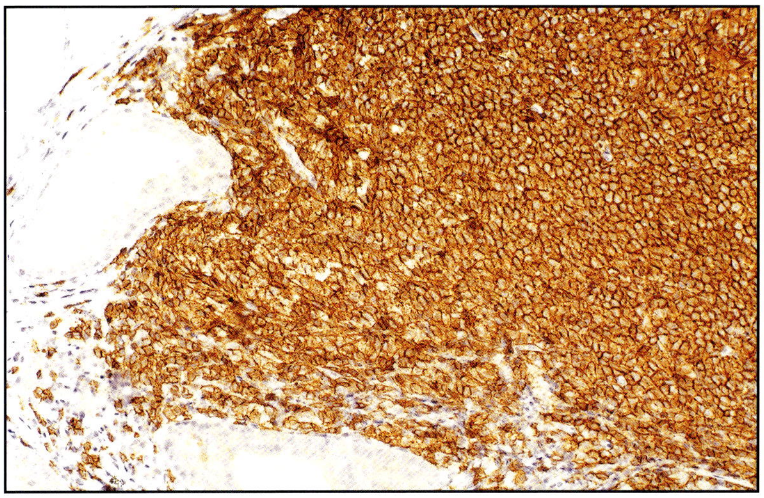

■ **i18.28** *Malignant lymphoma (depicted in* **i18.27** *and* **i18.28***) marked as a B-cell, mantle cell lymphoma [CD20 positive(shown here) and cyclin D1 positive].*

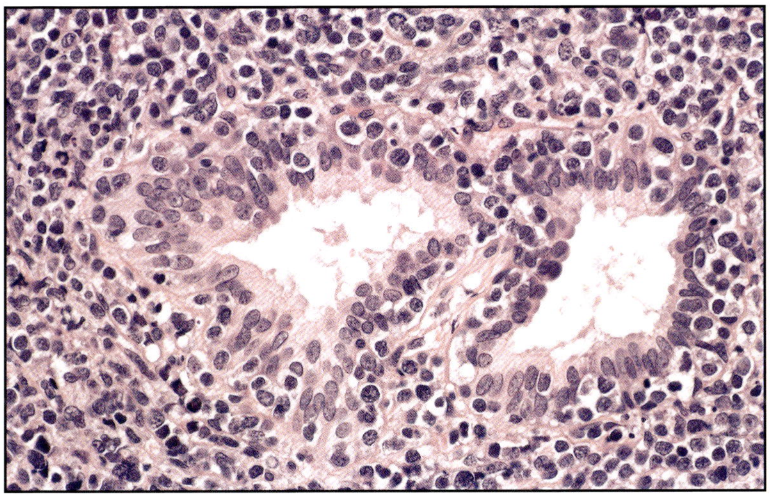

■ **i18.29** *Malignant lymphoma of prostate with intraepithelial extension: Focal, single cell intraepithelial involvement.*

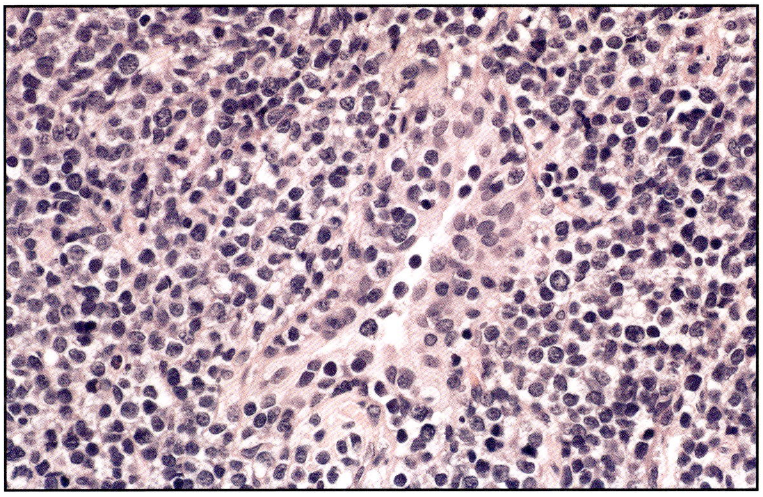

■ **i18.30** *Malignant lymphoma of prostate with extensive intraepithelial involvement and compression of gland lumen into slit-like space.*

and small lymphocytic lymphoma in 27% of cases. Other types include lymphoblastic lymphoma, Burkitt lymphoma, monocytoid B-cell lymphoma, lymphomas of follicular center cell origin, and lymphomatoid granulomatosis (Bostwick 1998, Ferry 1997). We have seen a single example of mantle cell lymphoma in the prostate **i18.26-i18.28**. Small lymphocytic lymphomas tended to be secondary, but otherwise no difference in histologic type could be discerned between primary and secondary lymphomas (Bostwick 1998). Admixed prostatic adenocarcinoma has been found in a few cases (Ben-Ezra 1986, Bostwick 1998, Ferry 1997, Gros 1984, Lopez 2000). "Collision" between the lymphoma and adenocarcinoma has been depicted (Bostwick 1998, Lopez 2000).

The differential diagnosis of malignant lymphoma in the prostate includes inflammation and poorly differentiated carcinoma, as noted earlier for leukemic infiltrates. A dense, monomorphous atypical lymphoid infiltrate in H&E-stained sections of prostatic tissue should prompt an immunohistochemical and clinical workup to evaluate for lymphoma. Pseudolymphoma has been reported in the prostate (Peison 1977) and should be considered in the differential diagnosis, but it is important in these cases to exclude MALToma by immunohistochemical marker panels. In the older literature some cases diagnosed as prostatic lymphoma before the use of immunohistochemistry probably represented poorly differentiated carcinoma or sarcoma (Bostwick 1985). The same diagnostic difficulty can be encountered today, as highlighted by a fairly recent case in which biopsy misdiagnosis of a prostatic lymphoma as "anaplastic carcinoma" led to an unnecessary radical cystoprostatectomy (Kerbl 1988). The outcome for patients with prostatic lymphoma is generally unfavorable, with a median survival of 23 to 28 months. Outcome did not differ according to histologic type (Bostwick 1998), except for prostatic angiotropic (intravascular) lymphoma, which has an extremely poor prognosis (Ferry 1997). Survival also did not differ based on whether the prostatic lymphoma was primary or secondary.

Hodgkin Disease (Lymphoma)

Only a few cases (about 10) of Hodgkin disease involving the prostate have been reported (Bostwick 1998, Klotz 1986, Lucia 1952, Smith 1972, Sridhar 1983, Terris 1998A, West 1962, Zein 1985). Few details have been provided, except in one case report (Klotz 1986). The incidence of prostatic involvement in patients with known Hodgkin disease is extremely low at 0.5% (Zein 1985). The median patient age in 4 cases was 49 (range 30 to 71). Histologically, both nodular sclerosis and mixed cellularity subtypes have been seen in prostatic tissue (Bostwick 1998).

Multiple Myeloma

Multiple myeloma has been found in the prostate in about 6 cases (Batts 1939, Estrada 1971, Franklin 1982, Hollenberg 1978, Yasuda 1994). The median age at presentation was 51, with a range of 43 to 77. For one patient with urinary retention, microscopic examination of TURP chip sections established the diagnosis of multiple myeloma (Hollenberg 1978). Sheets of anaplastic plasma cells were seen. In another patient with a subcutaneous mass, a prostate biopsy revealed diffuse infiltration by IgD (λ)-positive myeloma cells (Yasuda 1994). In 2 additional cases, prostatic involvement was diagnosed 9 months (Estrada 1971) and 2 years (Franklin 1982) after the initial diagnosis of myeloma; in the other 2 cases, prostatic involvement was detected at postmortem examination (Batts 1939, Yasuda 1994). Of the 4 cases tested, 2 were IgA myeloma (Franklin 1982, Hollenberg 1978) and 2 were IgD(λ) myeloma (Yasuda 1994).

[18.4] **Miscellaneous Neoplasms**

Paraganglioma

Fewer than 10 cases of paraganglioma (pheochromocytoma) of the prostate have been described (Dennis 1989, Hasselager 1997, Jimemez 1999, Nielsen 1987, Shapiro 1997, Voges 1990). Most patients are boys or young adults (mean age 23 years, range 8 to 37). Clinical presentations have included hypertension (with headaches, sweating, and blurred vision), perineal pain, and hematuria. ^{123}I-metaiodobenzylguanidine, CT, MRI, and ultrasound scans have been useful in defining extent of disease. In one case there was a synchronous adrenal pheochromocytoma (Voges 1990) and in another, multiple paragangliomas were present (Nielsen 1987). Tissue diagnoses have been made on needle biopsy (Jimemez 1999, Shapiro 1997), lumpectomy (Voges 1990), and radical prostatectomy (Dennis 1989, Jimemez 1999). Microscopically, the characteristic nested (Zellballen) arrangement of tumor cells with rounded nuclei and abundant cytoplasm is evident. Immunohistochemical stains confirm the neuroendocrine nature of the tumor cells, with positive staining for chromogranin and neuron-specific enolase (NSE) and negative immunostains for S-100 and desmin. Clinical correlation with urinary catecholamine and catecholamine metabolite levels is essential. These prostatic-based paragangliomas should be distinguished from urethral paragangliomas, which can occur in the prostatic urethra and tend to occur in older men, without metastatic spread (Boyle 1996). Metastatic spread to pelvic lymph nodes has been detected in several cases of prostatic paraganglioma (Jimemez 1999, Shapiro 1997), but no distant metastasis has been reported. No histologic features of the primary are predictive of metastatic nodal spread. Long-term follow-up data are not available for patients with prostatic paraganglioma.

Melanocytic Neoplasms

Malignant melanoma is rarely found in the prostate (Abeshouse 1958, Bamberger 1990, Berry 1953, Das Gupta 1965, Grignon 1989, Hubler 1980, Spasic 1980, Stein 1984, Wang 1995). Most cases represent metastatic spread from a cutaneous primary. Moreover, it is felt that most cases considered to be of prostatic origin are actually of prostatic urethral origin (Stein 1984). Only a few cases of primary malignant melanoma of the prostate have been published (Berry 1953, Hubler 1980, Wang 1995). This malignancy should be distinguished from prostatic melanosis and blue nevus (Chapter 9), which lack the destructive growth and cytologic atypia of melanoma. Metastatic spread to the prostate is also rare (Abeshouse 1958, Bamberger 1990, Das Gupta 1965, Grignon 1989, Johnson 1974, Spasic 1980, Zein 1985), even in patients dying of melanoma (Das Gupta 1965). Overall, at autopsy 1% (24/2083) of patients with melanoma had metastases to the prostate (Das Gupta 1965, Johnson 1974, Zein 1985). Two cases of malignant melanoma metastatic to prostatic adenocarcinoma in the prostate (tumor-to-tumor metastasis) have been reported (Grignon 1989, Spasic 1980).

Germ Cell Tumors

Rare primary and secondary germ cell tumors have been described in the prostate (Aria 1988, Benson 1978, Dalla Palma 1988, Dvoracek 1949, Hayman 1995, Khandekar 1993, Kimura 1995, Michel 1986, Prym 1927, Tay 1995, Zein 1985). The primaries were 3 cases of endodermal sinus (yolk sac tumors) (Benson 1978, Dalla Palma 1988, Tay 1995), 2 choriocarcinomous (Dvoracek 1949, Prym 1927), 2 seminomas (Hayman 1995, Khandekar 1993), and 1 mixed malignant germ cell tumor composed of embryonal carcinoma, teratoma, and a neuroectodermal element (Michel 1986). The basis for extragonadal occurrence of germ cell tumors is uncertain; one explanation is sequestration of germ cells during embryonic migration from the yolk sac to the gonadal ridge. A rigorous search for testicular or extragonadal, nonprostatic primary is mandated before assignment of the germ cell tumor to prostate as a primary. Synchronous (Aria 1988) or metachronous (Kimura 1995) prostate and testicular germ cell tumors interpreted as separate primaries could easily represent a testicular primary, with prostatic metastasis. Germ cell tumor metastatic to the prostate was found in 2.3% of germ cell tumor autopsy cases (Zein 1985). Of these 3 cases, 2 were from a testicular primary and the third was an extragonadal primary (Zein 1985).

Others

A few prostatic carcinoids have been reported (Azumi 1984, Tash 2002, Wasserstein 1979, 1981, Whelan 1995) **i17.66**, p 417. These should be distinguished from the equally rare prostatic adenocarcinomas that assume a carcinoid-like appearance (Almagro 1985, Ansari 1981, Ghali 1984). A single case report of primary prostatic Wilms tumor exists (Casiraghi 1991). This tumor occurred in a 32-year-old man and had the classic triphasic appearance (Casiraghi 1991). The initial needle biopsy was misinterpreted as rhabdomyosarcoma. Pulmonary metastases were detected on chest radiograph. The patient was alive with active disease at 3 years after chemotherapy.

[18.5] **Secondary Neoplasms**

Malignancies from other anatomic sites can involve the prostate by direct extension or by metastatic spread **t18.17**. Overall, both are uncommon events. In 2 series of a total of 7436 autopsies, 346 (5%)

■ **t18.17 Secondary Neoplasms of the Prostate: Incidence**

Primary Malignancy	% Prostates Involved
Direct Extension	
Bladder urothelial carcinoma	23%[1]
Colonic adenocarcinoma	Rare
Pelvic lymphoma	Rare
Metastatic Spread	
Primary Malignancy	**% Prostates Involved[2]**
Leukemia	14%
Lymphoma, non-Hodgkin's	8%
Germ cell tumor	2.3%
Thyroid papillary carcinoma	1.5%
Stomach adenocarcinoma	1.2%
Malignant melanoma	1%
Pancreatic carcinoma	1%
Renal cell carcinoma	0.9%
Lung carcinoma	0.6%
Hodgkin's disease	0.5%
Laryngeal adenocarcinoma	0.1%

[1]Combined data from 1,001 radical cystoprostatectomy specimens (Sakamoto 1993, Esrig 1990, Farrow 1976, Kardeman 1990, Mahaderia 1986, Tobisu 1991, Wood 1989)
[2]Autopsy data. Leukemia data: Zein 1985, Lucia 1952, Watson 1949, Melchior 1974, Viadana 1978. Lymphoma data: Zein 1985 and Watson 1949.
Others: Zein 1985 and Johnson 1974

had a secondary tumor in the prostate (Johnson 1974, Zein 1985). However, secondary spread can be detected in a substantial minority of patients with bladder carcinoma, leukemia, and non-Hodgkin lymphoma **t18.17**. Direct contiguous invasion accounted for 44% of secondary tumors in the prostate at autopsy, with carcinoma of bladder or urethra and colon being most common (Zein 1985). Secondary metastatic spread was seen most often in patients with leukemia and lymphoma (Zein 1985). The most common neoplasm to secondarily involve the prostate is transitional cell carcinoma of the bladder **t18.18**. The reported frequency of prostatic involvement by transitional cell carcinoma of the bladder is highly variable, ranging from 5% to 58%. This incidence variability results largely from tissue sampling differences. Therefore, in general, detection rates are lower with biopsy than with examination of cystoprostatectomy specimens (**t23.12, p 535**). Multi-institutional data on 1001 radical

■ **t18.18 Secondary Transitional Cell (Urothelial) Carcinoma of Prostate**

Incidence: 23% of cases of urinary bladder carcinoma involve prostate	
Pathways of spread	Intraepithelial into prostatic urethra and/or prostatic ducts/acini
	implantation
	multifocal disease
	direct extension via perivesical/periprostatic soft tissue
	direct extension via bladder neck
	lymphovascular space invasion
Microscopically	CIS of urethra
	Pagetoid, undermining, and expansile in-situ growth in prostatic ducts/acini
	Prostatic stromal invasion
Outcome	Dependent on whether stromal invasion is present or not

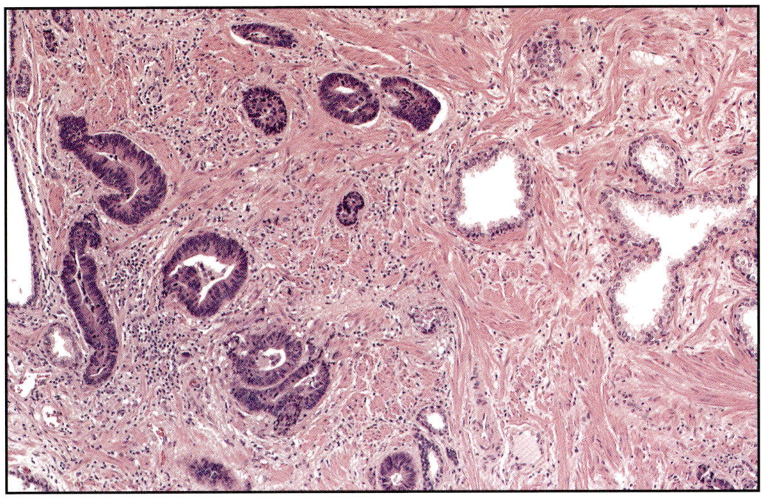

■ **i18.31** *Colonic adenocarcinoma with direct extension into prostate.*

cystoprostatectomies done for urinary bladder transitional cell carcinoma indicate an overall incidence of 23% (Esrig 1990, Farrow 1976, Hardeman 1990, Mahadevia 1986, Sakamoto 1993, Tobisu 1991, Wood 1989). This so-called secondary involvement could represent direct extension, multifocal disease, implantation (seeding), or lymphvascular space invasion by carcinoma. The direct extension pathway can be through the bladder neck (Donat 2001) or via soft tissue around the bladder and prostate. Anatomic sites of involvement include the prostatic urethra, prostatic ducts and acini, and prostatic stroma. Microscopically, patterns of urinary bladder transitional cell (urothelial) carcinoma growth into the urethra and prostate are identical to primary transitional cell carcinomas at these sites (see Chapters 17 and 23). Secondary transitional cell carcinomas can be seen in urethral biopsies, transrectal prostatic needle biopsies (Oliai 2001), TURP chips, and radical cystoprostatectomy specimens. In one series of transrectal prostatic needle biopsies with urothelial carcinoma, one half of the cases were associated with a previous, current, or subsequent bladder carcinoma primary (Oliai 2001). The distinction between in situ transitional cell carcinoma in the prostate and bladder carcinoma with prostatic stromal invasion is important because this affects treatment and survival (Esrig 1990, Herr 1999, Pagano 1996, Schellhammer 1977). Noninvasive spread into the urethra or the prostatic duct and acinar system may be treated conservatively with aggressive TURP and intravesical bacille Calmette-Guérin, whereas prostatic stromal invasion is best managed by radical cystoprostatectomy (Donat 2001, Herr 1998). The 5-year survival for patients with transitional cell carcinoma with prostatic stromal invasion is 36% to 48%, compared with 71% to 82% for patients without prostatic stromal invasion (Esrig 1990, Herr 1998). Direct extension into the prostate has also been observed for colonic carcinoma **i18.31** and pelvic lymphoma, although most of these are advanced stage cases, seen at autopsy (Zein 1985).

Metastatic spread to the prostate gland by lymphatic or blood vessels is most often seen with leukemia and lymphoma **t18.13, t18.17**. Solid tumors, even those that are well known for their capacity for widespread dissemination, such as melanoma and renal cell carcinoma, rarely metastasize to the prostate **t18.17**. It is also rare for metastatic solid tumor deposits in the prostate to produce clinical symptoms **t18.13** (Rub 1999, Thompson 1953), where biopsy or TURP chips resected to relieve obstruction disclosed clinically unsuspected metastatic tumor (Chihak 1980, Madersbacher 1994, Rub 1999, Smedley 1983).

References

Abeshouse BS. Primary and secondary melanoma of the genitourinary tract. *South Med J* 51:994-1006, 1958.

Almagro UA. Argyrophilic prostatic carcinoma. Case report with literature review on prostatic carcinoid and "carcinoid-like" prostatic carcinoma. *Cancer* 55:608-614, 1985.

Ansari MA, Pintozzi RL, Choi YS, et al. Diagnosis of carcinoid-like prostatic carcinoma by an immunoperoxidase method. *Am J Clin Pathol* 76:94-98, 1981.

Aragona F, Serretta V, Marconi A, et al. Leiomyosarcoma of the prostate in adults. *Ann Chir Gynaecol* 74:191-194, 1985.

Araki K, Kubota Y, Iijima Y, et al. Indolent behaviour of low-grade B-cell lymphoma of mucosa-associated lymphoid tissue involved in salivary glands, renal sinus and prostate. *Scand J Urol Nephrol* 32:234-236, 1998.

Aria Y, Watanabe J, Kounami T, et al. Retroperitoneal seminoma with simultaneous occurrence in the prostate. *J Urol* 139:382-383, 1988.

Ascoli R. La leucemia della prostata. *Arch Ital Chir* 35:849, 1933.

Attah EB, Powell MEA. Atypical stromal hyperplasia of the prostate gland. *Am J Clin Pathol* 67:324-327, 1977.

Attah EB, Nkposong EO. Phyllodes type of atypical prostatic hyperplasia. *J Urol* 115:762-764, 1976.

Ayala AG. Stromal lesions of the prostate. Presentation at International Society of Urologic Pathology, United States and Canadian Academy of Pathology Annual Meeting, 1999.

Azumi N, Shibuya H, Ishikura M. Primary prostatic carcinoid tumor with intracytoplasmic prostatic acid phosphatase and prostate-specific antigen. *Am J Surg Pathol* 8:545-550, 1984.

Bain GO, Danyluk JM, Shnitka TK, et al. Malignant fibrous histiocytoma of prostate gland. *Urology* 26:89-91, 1985.

Bale PM, Parsons RE, Stevens MM. Diagnosis and behavior of juvenile rhabdomyosarcoma. *Hum Pathol* 14:596-611, 1983.

Bamberger MH, Romas NA. Clinically significant metastatic melanoma to prostate. *Urology* 35:445-447, 1990.

Banavali SD, Mohandas KM, Iyer R, et al. Non-Hodgkin's lymphoma of prostate: a rare site of primary extranodal presentation (a report of two cases). *Indian J Cancer* 28:70-74, 1991.

Banerjee SS, Harris M. Angiotropic lymphoma presenting in the prostate. *Histopathology* 12:667-670, 1988.

Barcos M, Lane W, Gomez GA, et al. An autopsy study of 1206 acute and chronic leukemias (1958 to 1982). *Cancer* 60:827-837, 1987.

Barone AM, Joelson JJ. Leiomyosarcomas of the prostate: report of a case. *J Urol* 63:533-538, 1950.

Barr FG, Chatten J, D'Cruz CM, et al. Molecular assays for chromosomal translocations in the diagnosis of pediatric soft tissue sarcomas. *JAMA* 273:553-557, 1995.

Batts M Jr. Multiple myeloma: review of 40 cases. *Arch Surg* 39:807-823, 1939.

Beer M, Occhionero F, Welsch U. Oncocytoma of the prostate: a case report with ultrastructural and immunohistochemical evaluation. *Histopathology* 17:370-372, 1990.

Belis JA, Post GJ, Rochman SC, et al. Genitourinary leiomyomas. *Urology* 13:424-429, 1979.

Bell CRW, Napier MP, Morgan RJ, et al. Primary non-Hodgkin's lymphoma of the prostate gland: case report and review of the literature. Clin Oncol 7:409-410, 1995.

Bell R, Stinson RF Jr. Leiomyosarcoma of the prostate. *J Urol* 73:716-717, 1955.

Ben-Ezra J, Sheibani K, Kendrick FE, et al. Angiotropic large cell lymphoma of the prostate gland: an immunohistochemical study. *Hum Pathol* 17:964-966, 1986.

Benassayag EV, Galian P. Leiomyoblastoma of the prostate in a young man [in French]. *J Urol Nephrol* 81:831-833, 1975.

Benson RC Jr, Segura JW, Carney JA. Primary yolk-sac (endodermal sinus) tumor of the prostate. *Cancer* 41:1395-1398, 1978.

Berry NE, Reese L. Malignant melanoma which had its first clinical manifestations in the prostate gland. *J Urol* 69:286-290, 1953.

Blank B, Hodges CV. Leukemic infiltration of the prostate: a case report. *J Urol* 123:789-790, 1980.

Blum E, Batzenschlager A, Le Gal Y. Adenoma prostatique cystico-papillaire a evolution polykystique. *J Urol* 66:411-414, 1960.

Boe S, Nielsen H, Ryttov N. Burkitt's lymphoma mimicking prostatitis. *J Urol* 125:891-892, 1981.

Bostwick DG, Mann RB. Malignant lymphomas involving the prostate. A study of 13 cases. *Cancer* 56:2932-2938, 1985.

Bostwick DG, Iczkowski KA, Amin MB, et al. Malignant lymphoma involving the prostate. Report of 62 cases. *Cancer* 83:732-738, 1998.

Boucher LD, Swanson PE, Stanley MW, et al. Cytology of angiosarcoma. Findings in fourteen fine-needle aspiration biopsy specimens and one pleural fluid specimen. *Am J Clin Pathol* 114:210-219, 2000.

Boyle ET Jr, Reiman HM, Kramer SA, et al. Embryonal rhabdomyosarcoma of bladder and prostate: nuclear DNA patterns studied by flow cytometry. *J Urol* 140:1119-1121, 1988.

Boyle M, Gaffney EF, Thurston A. Paraganglioma of the prostatic urethra. A report of three cases and review of the literature. *Br J Urol* 77:445-448, 1996.

Bretton PR, Herr HW, Whitmore WF Jr, et al. Intravesical bacillus Calmette-Guérin therapy for in situ transitional cell carcinoma involving the prostatic urethra. *J Urol* 141:853-856, 1989.

Butler MR, O'Flynn JD. Prostatic disease in leukemic patient, with particular reference to leukemic infiltration of the prostate. *Br J Urol* 45:179-183, 1973.

Cachia PG, McIntyre MA, Dewar AE, et al. Prostatic infiltration in chronic lymphatic leukaemia. *J Clin Pathol* 40:342-345, 1987.

Cacic M, Petrovic D, Tentor D, et al. Cystosarcoma phyllodes of prostate. *Scand J Urol Nephrol* 30:501-502, 1996.

Cartagena R, Baumgartner G, Wajsman Z, et al. Preliminary reticulum cell sarcoma of prostate gland. *Urology* 5:815-816, 1975.

Casiraghi O, Martinez-Madrigal F, Mostofi FK, et al. Primary prostatic Wilms tumor. *Am J Surg Pathol* 15:885-890, 1991.

Cespedes RD, Lynch SC, Grider DJ. Pseudosarcomatous fibromyxoid tumor of the prostate. A case report with review of the literature. *Urol Int* 57:249-251, 1996.

Chan KW. Angiosarcoma of the prostate. An immunohistochemical study of a case. *Pathology* 22:108-110, 1990.

Chan YF. Granulocytic sarcoma (chloroma) of the kidney and prostate. *Br J Urol* 65:655-656, 1990.

Chatelain D, Coppola S, De Pinieux G, et al. Prostatic phyllodes tumor, a rare entity. Anatomo-clinical and immunohistochemical study of 1 case [in French]. *Ann Pathol* 20:629-632, 2000.

Chen KTK. Hemangiopericytoma of the prostate. *J Surg Oncol* 35:42-43, 1987.

Cheville JC, Dundore PA, Nascimento AG, et al. Leiomyosarcoma of the prostate. Report of 23 cases. *Cancer* 76:1422-1427, 1995.

Chihak RW, Haas R Jr, Koenen CT, et al. Metastatic renal cell carcinoma to the prostate gland: presentation as prostatic hypertrophy. *J Urol* 123:791-792, 1980.

Chim CS, Loong F. Intravascular lymphomatosis of the prostate gland. *Br J Haematol* 119:2, 2002.

Chin W, Fay R, Ortega P. Malignant fibrous histiocytoma of prostate. *Urology* 27:363-365, 1986.

Choi YH, Namkung S, Ryu BY, et la. Giant multilocular prostatic cystadenoma. *J Urol* 163:246-247, 2000.

Christoffersen J. Leiomyosarcoma of the prostate. *Acta Chir Scand* 433(suppl):75-84, 1973.

Chung AK, Michels V, Poland GA, et al. Neurofibromatosis with involvement of the prostate gland. *Urology* 47:448-451, 1996.

Coffin CM, Watterson J, Preist JR, et al. Extrapulmonary inflammatory myofibroblastic tumor (inflammatory pseudotumor). A clinicopathologic and immunohistochemical study of 84 cases. *Am J Surg Pathol* 19:859-872, 1995.

Coffin CM, Dehner LP. Neurogenic tumors of soft tissue. In: Coffin CM, Dehner LP, O'Shea PA, eds. *Pediatric Soft Tissue Tumors.* Baltimore: Williams & Wilkins; 113, 1997A.

Coffin CM, Rulon J, Smith L, et al. Pathologic features of rhabdomyosarcoma before and after treatment: a clinicopathologic and immunohistochemical analysis. *Mod Pathol* 10:1175-1187, 1997B.

Coffin CM, Humphrey PA, Dehner LP. Extrapulmonary inflammatory myofibroblastic tumor: a clinical and pathological survey. *Semin Diagn Pathol* 15:75-101, 1998.

Colby TV, Bostwick DG. Sarcomas and related proliferative lesions of specialized prostatic stroma [letter]. *Am J Surg Pathol* 23:243, 1999.

Cook JR, Dehner LP, Collins MH, et al. Anaplastic lymphoma kinase (ALK) expression in inflammatory myofibroblastic tumor. A comparative immunohistochemical study. *Am J Surg Pathol* 25:1364-1371, 2001.

Cordonnier C, Sevestre H, Petit J, et al. Rare tumors of the prostate or seminal vesicle. Report of a case of leiomyosarcoma [in French]. *Ann Pathol* 16:37-40, 1996.

Cos LR, Rashid HA. Primary non-Hodgkin lymphoma of the prostate presenting as benign prostate hyperplasia. *Urology* 23:176-179, 1984.

Coupland S. Lymphoma (lymphosarcoma) of the prostate, secondary nodules in the pancreas and the suprarenal capsule. *Trans Pathol Soc London* 28:179-185, 1877.

Cox R, Dawson IMP. A curious prostatic tumor: probably a true mixed tumour (cystadeno-leiomyofibroma). *Br J Urol* 32:306-311, 1960.

Crist W, Gehan EA, Ragab AH, et al. The third intergroup rhabdomyosarcoma study. *J Clin Oncol* 13:610-630, 1995.

Cummine HG, Johnson AS. Report of a retrovesical polycystic tumor of probably prostatic origin. *Aust NZ J Surg* 19:91-92, 1950.

Dajani YF, Burke M. Leukemic infiltration of the prostate. A case study and clinicopathologic review. *Cancer* 38:2442-2446, 1976.

Dalla Palma PA, Dante S, Guazzieri S, et al. Primary endodermal sinus tumor of the prostate: report of a case. *Prostate* 12:255-261, 1988.

Danckers VF, Philipsborn HF, Baylor JE, et al. Sarcomas of the prostate, periprostatic tissue and bladder neck in children. *Am J Roentgenol* 84:555-561, 1960.

Das Gupta T, Grabstald H. Melanoma of the genitourinary tract. *J Urol* 93:607-614, 1965.

De Raeve H, Jeuris W, Wyndaele JJ, et al. Cystosarcoma phyllodes of the prostate with rhabdomyoblastic differentiation. *Pathol Res Pract* 197:657-662, 2001.

De Siati M, Busolo A, Contin F, et al. High grade phyllodes tumor of the prostate. *Arch Ital Urol Androl* 71:225-227, 1999.

DeGiuseppe JA, Nelson WG, Seifter EJ, et al. Intravascular lymphomatosis: a clinicopathologic study of 10 cases and assessment of response to chemotherapy. *J Clin Oncol* 12:2573-2579, 1994.

Dennis PJ, Lewandowski AE, Rohner TJ Jr, et al. Pheochromocytoma of the prostate: an unusual location. *J Urol* 141:130-132, 1989.

Derdoy JB, Garimaldi JE. Fibromyxosarcoma of the prostate [in Spanish]. *Rev Argent Microbiol* 36:262-268, 1967.

Dogra PN, Aron M, Rajeev TP, et al. Primary chondrosarcoma of the prostate. *BJU Int* 83:150-151, 1999.

Doll DC, Weiss RB, Shah S. Lymphoma of the prostate presenting as benign prostatic hypertrophy. *South Med J* 71:1170-1171, 1978.

Donat SM, Genega EM, Herr HW, et al. Mechanisms of prostatic stromal invasion in patients with bladder cancer: clinical significance. *J Urol* 165:1117-1120, 2001.

Douille MC, Couderc P, Coste M. Cystadenoma papillaire de la prostate. *J Urol Nephrol* 69:339-643, 1963.

Drinis S, Finkelstein MP, Tortorelis DG, et al. Five-year prognosis after radical prostatectomy in a patient with localized prostate cancer and incidental non-Hodgkin's lymphoma. *Urol Int* 66:105-107, 2001.

Dupree WC, Fisher C. Rhabdomyosarcoma of prostate in adult. Long-term survival and problem of histologic diagnosis. *Urology* 19:80-82, 1982.

Dvoracek C. Primarni chorionepitheliom prostaty s gynekomastii. *Cas Lek Cesk* 88:198, 1949.

Eble JN, Tejada E. Prostatic stromal hyperplasia with bizarre nuclei. *Arch Pathol Lab Med* 115:87-89, 1991.

Ekfors TO, Aho HJ, Kekomaki M. Malignant rhabdoid tumor of the prostatic region. Immunohistochemical and ultrastructural evidence of epithelial origin. *Virchows Arch* [A] *Pathol Anat Histopathol* 406:381-388, 1985.

El-Sherbiny MT, El-Mekresh MH, El-Baz MA, et al. Paediatric lower urinary tract rhabdomyosarcoma: a single-centre experience of 30 patients. *BJU Int* 86:260-267, 2000.

Elbadawi A. Pathology of male accessory genital glands. II. Proliferative lesions and neoplasms. In: Spring-Mills E, Hafez ESE, eds. *Perspectives of Human Reproduction.* Vol 6. Ann Arbor: Ann Arbor Science; 205, 1979.

Esrig D, Freeman JA, Elmajian DA, et al. Transitional cell carcinoma involving the prostate with a proposed staging classification for stromal invasion. *J Urol* 156:1071-1076, 1996.

Estrada PC, Scardino PL. Myeloma of the prostate: a case report. *J Urol* 106:586-587, 1971.

Exelby PR, Ghavimi F, Jereb B. Genitourinary rhabdomyosarcoma in children. *J Pediatr Surg* 13:746-752, 1978.

Franco V, Florena AM, Quintini G, et al. Monocytoid B-cell lymphoma of the prostate. *Pathologica* 84:411-417, 1992.

Farrow GM, Utz DC, Rife CC. Morphological and clinical observations of patients with early bladder cancer treated with total cystectomy. *Cancer Res* 36:2495-2501, 1976.

Feinberg SM, Leslie KO, Colby TV. Bladder outlet obstruction by so-called lymphomatoid granulomatosis (angiocentric lymphoma). *J Urol* 137:989-990, 1987.

Fell P, O'Connor M, Smith JM. Primary lymphoma of the prostate presenting as bladder outflow obstruction. *Urology* 29:555 556, 1987.

Ferguson RS, Stewart FW. Lymphosarcoma of the prostate. *J Urol* 28:93-104, 1932.

Ferry JA, Young RH. Malignant lymphoma of the genitourinary tract. *Curr Diagn Pathol* 4:145-169, 1997.

Fiorelli RL, Koolpe HA, Klaus RL. Use of polyvinyl alcohol in treatment of bladder and prostatic hemangioma. *Urology* 38:480-482, 1991.

Fishman A, Taylor WN. Leukemic infiltration of the prostate. *J Urol* 89:65-72, 1963.

Fitzpatrick TJ, Stump G. Leiomyosarcoma of the prostate: case report and review of the literature. *J Urol* 83:80-83, 1960.

Flaherty SA, Cope HE, Shecket HA. Prostatic obstruction as the presenting symptom of acute monocytic leukemia. *J Urol* 44:488-497, 1940.

Frame R, Head D, Lee R, et al. Granulocytic sarcoma of the prostate. Two cases causing urinary obstruction. *Cancer* 59:142-146, 1987.

Franklin RM, Kenyon KR, Green WR, et al. Epibulbar IgA plasmacytoma occurring in multiple myeloma. *Arch Ophthalmol* 100:451-456, 1982.

Freeman C, Berg JW, Cutler SJ. Occurrence and prognosis of extranodal lymphoma. *Cancer* 29:252-260, 1972.

Fritsch M, Epstein JI, Perlman EJ, et al. Molecularly confirmed primary prostatic synovial sarcoma. *Hum Pathol* 31:246-250, 2000.

Fujita K, Matsushima H, Munakata A. Phyllodes type of atypical prostatic hyperplasia. *Int J Urol* 3:158-160, 1996.

Furihata M, Sonobe H, Iwata J, et al. Granular cell tumor expressing myogenic markers in the prostate. *Pathol Int* 46:298-300, 1996.

Gaudin PB, Rosai J, Epstein JI. Sarcomas and related proliferative lesions of specialized prostatic stroma. A clinicopathologic study of 22 cases. *Am J Surg Pathol* 22:148-162, 1998.

Ghali VS, Garcia RL. Prostatic adenocarcinoma with carcinoidal features producing adrenocorticotropic syndrome. Immunohistochemical study and review of the literature. *Cancer* 54:1043-1048, 1984.

Goudale RH. Cystadenoma of the bladder from aberrant prostatic gland. *Arch Pathol* 6:210-214, 1928.

Govender D, Hadley GP. Ectomesenchymoma of the prostate: histological diagnostic criteria. *Pediatr Surg Int* 15:68-70, 1999.

Grier EA, Phillips FL. Rhabdomyosarcoma of the prostate. *J Urol* 69:695-702, 1953.

Griffin CA, Hawkins AL, Dvorak C, et al. Recurrent involvement of 2p23 in inflammatory myofibroblastic tumors. *Cancer Res* 59:2776-2780, 1999.

Grignon DJ, Ro JY, Ayala AG. Malignant melanoma with metastasis to adenocarcinoma of the prostate. *Cancer* 63:196-198, 1989.

Gros R, Richter S, Bechar L. Prostatic carcinoma with concomitant non-Hodgkin lymphoma: report of 2 cases. *Urol Int* 39:121-122, 1984.

Gueft B, Walsh MA. Malignant prostatic cystosarcoma phyllodes. *NY State J Med* 75:2226-2228, 1975.

Guerrier KR, Persky L. Combined leukemia, carcinoma, and hyperplasia of the prostate. *Arch Surg* 98:365-366, 1969.

Hafiz MA, Toker C, Sutula M. An atypical fibromyxoid tumor of the prostate. *Cancer* 54:2500-2504, 1984.

Halling AC, Farrow GM, Bostwick DG. Prostatic phyllodes tumor [abstract]. A report of 6 cases. *Am J Clin Pathol* 100:320, 1993.

Hampel N, Richter-Levin D, Gersh I. Primary lymphosarcoma of prostate. *Urology* 9:461-463, 1977.

Hardeman SW, Soloway MS. Urethral recurrence following radical cystectomy. *J Urol* 144:666-669, 1990.

Hasselager T, Horn T, Rasmussen F. Paraganglioma of the prostate. A case report and review of the literature. *Scand J Urol Nephrol* 31:501-503, 1997.

Hayman R, Patel A, Fisher C, et al. Primary seminoma of the prostate. *Br J Urol* 76:273-274, 1995.

Hays DM, Raney RB Jr, Lawrence W Jr, et al. Bladder and prostatic tumors in the Intergroup Rhabdomyosarcoma Study (IRS-1). Results of therapy. *Cancer* 50:1472-1482, 1982A.

Hays DM, Raney RB Jr, Lawrence W Jr, et al. Primary chemotherapy in the treatment of children with bladder-prostate tumors in the Intergroup Rhabdomyosarcoma Study (IRS-II). *J Pediatr Surg* 17:812-820, 1982B.

Hays DM. Bladder/prostate rhabdomyosarcoma: results of multi-institutional trials of the Intergroup Rhabdomyosarcoma Study. *Semin Surg Oncol* 9:520-523, 1993.

Heising J, Cremer H, Davidts H. Malignant fibrous histiocytoma of the prostate capsule [in German]. *Urologe* A 24:118-121, 1985.

Herr HW, Donat SM. Prostatic tumor relapse in patients with superficial bladder tumors: 15-year outcome. *J Urol* 161:1854-1857, 1999.

Herr HW. Extravesicular tumor relapse in patients with superficial bladder tumors. *J Clin Oncol* 16:1099-1102, 1998.

Hessel RG, Reyes CV, Jensen J, et al. Malignant cystic epithelial-stromal tumor of the prostate. *Diagn Cytopathol* 9:314-317, 1993.

Hollenberg GM. Extraosseous multiple myeloma simulating primary prostatic neoplasm. *J Urol* 119:292-294, 1978.

Holtl W, Hruby W, Redtenbacher M. Cavernous hemangioma originating from prostatic plexus. *Urology* 20:184-185, 1982.

Hubler J, Pajor L, Kincses I. Primary malignant melanoma of the prostate [in German]. *Acta Chir Acad Sci Hung* 21:239-243, 1980.

Husain AN, Selby DM, Dehner LP. The male reproductive system including intersex disorders. In: Stocker JT, Dehner LP, eds. *Pediatric Pathology, 2nd ed.* Philadelphia: Lippincott, Williams & Wilkins; 973-974, 2001.

Ishiguro K, Yamakoshi T, Okishio N, et al. Hemangiopericytoma of the prostate [in Japanese]. *Acta Urol Jpn* 30:931-934, 1984.

Ito H, Ito M, Mitsuhata N, et al. Phyllodes tumor of the prostate: a case report. *Jpn J Clin Oncol* 19:299-304, 1989.

Iwasaki H, Ishiguro M, Ohjimi Y, et al. Synovial sarcoma of the prostate with t(X:18) (p11.2; q11.2). *Am J Surg Pathol* 23:220-226, 1999.

Jackson D, Clements R. Sonographic and radiological features of cystosarcoma phyllodes of the prostate. *Clin Radiol* 54:473-475, 1999.

Jacobi M, Panoff CE, Herzlich J. Leukemic infiltration of the prostate. *J Urol* 68:494-499, 1937.

Jhavar S, Agarwal JP, Naresh KN, et al. Primary extranodal mucosa associated lymphoid tissue (malt) lymphoma of the prostate. *Leuk Lymphoma* 41:445-449, 2001.

Jimenez RE, Tiguert R, Harb JF, et al. Prostatic paraganglioma: 5-year follow-up. *J Urol* 161:1909-1910, 1999.

Johnson DE, Chalbaud R, Ayala AG. Secondary tumors of the prostate. *J Urol* 112:507-508, 1974.

Johnson MA, Gunderson AH. Infiltration of the prostate gland by chronic lymphatic leukaemia. *J Urol* 69:681-685, 1953.

Kafandaris PM, Polyzonis MB. Fibroadenoma-like foci in human prostatic nodular hyperplasia. *Prostate* 4:33-36, 1983.

Kamat MR, Kulkarni JN, Tongaonkar HB, et al. Rhabdomyosarcoma of the bladder and prostate in children. *J Surg Oncol* 48:180-182, 1991.

Kanomata N, Eble JN, Ohbayashi C, et al. Ectopic prostate in the retrovesical space. *J Urol Pathol* 7:121-126, 1996.

Károlyi P, Endes P, Krasznai G, et al. Bizarre leiomyoma of the prostate. *Virchows Arch* [A] *Pathol Anat Histopathol* 412:383-386, 1988.

Kaufman JJ, Berneike RR. Leiomyoma of the prostate. *J Urol* 65:297-310, 1951.

Kaufmann W, Wright AW. Lymphosarcoma of the prostate. With report of a case. *Arch Surg* 43:1061-1075, 1941.

Kelly KM, Womer RB, Barr FG. Minimal disease detection in patients with alveolar rhabdomyosarcoma using a reverse transcriptase-polymerase chain reaction method. *Cancer* 78:1320-1326, 1996.

Kerbl K, Pauer W. Primary non-Hodgkin lymphoma of the prostate. *Urology* 32:347-349, 1988.

Kerley SW, Pierce P, Thomas J. Giant cystosarcoma phyllodes of the prostate associated with adenocarcinoma. *Arch Pathol Lab Med* 116:195-197, 1992.

Kevwitch MK, Walloch JL, Waters WB, et al. Prostatic cystic epithelial-stromal tumors: a report of 2 new cases. *J Urol* 149:860-864, 1993.

Khandekar JD, Holland JM, Rochester D, et al. Extragonadal seminoma involving urinary bladder and arising in the prostate. *Cancer* 71:3972-3974, 1993.

Kim HS, Lee JH, Nam JH, et al. Malignant phyllodes tumor of the prostate. *Pathol Int* 49:1105-1108, 1999.

Kimura F, Watanabe S, Shimizu S, et al. Primary seminoma of the prostate and embryonal cell carcinoma of the left testis in one patient: a case report [in Japanese]. *Jpn J Urol* 86:1497-1500, 1995.

King LS, Cox TR. Lymphosarcoma of the prostate. *Am J Pathol* 27:801-820, 1951.

Kirkland KL, Bale PM. A cystic adenoma of the prostate. *J Urol* 97:324-327, 1967.

Kirsch AJ, Newhouse J, Hibshoosh H, et al. Giant multilocular cystadenoma of the prostate. *Urology* 48:303-305, 1996.

Kirshbaum JD, Larkin HS, Culver H. Retothel sarcoma of the prostate gland: report of a case. *J Urol* 50:597-607, 1943.

Klotz LH, Herr HW. Hodgkin's disease of the prostate: a detailed case report. *J Urol* 135:1261-1262, 1986.

Kumanov K, Sivchev S, Tsvetkov M, et al. Fibrosarcoma of the prostate [in Bulgarian]. *Khirurgiia* 34:190-194, 1981.

Lawrence B, Perez-Atayde A, Hibbard MK, et al. TPM3-ALK and TPM4-ALK oncogenes in inflammatory myofibroblastic tumors. *Am J Pathol* 157:377-384, 2000.

Lawrence W Jr, Hays DM, Heyn R, et al. Lymphatic metastases with childhood rhabdomyosarcoma. A report from the Intergroup Rhabdomyosarcoma Study. *Cancer* 60:910-915, 1987.

Leader M, Kay E, Walsh CB. Soft tissue neoplasms and other unusual tumors of prostate, including uncommon carcinomas. In: Foster CS, Bostwick DG, eds. *Pathology of the Prostate.* Philadelphia: WB Saunders; 364-383, 1998.

Lemmon WT Jr, Holland JM, Ketcham AS. Rhabdomyosarcoma of the prostate. *Surgery* 59:736-740, 1960.

Leonard A, Baert L, Van Praet F, et al. Solitary leiomyoma of the prostate. *Br J Urol* 62:184-185, 1988.

Leong SS, Vogt PJ, Yu GS. Atypical stromal smooth muscle hyperplasia of prostate. *Urology* 31:163-167, 1988.

Lerut R, Lerut H. Osteogenic sarcoma of the prostate [in French]. *Acta Urol Belg* 35:401-407, 1967.

Leung TW, Tung SY, Sze WK, et al. Primary non-Hodgkin's lymphoma of the prostate. *Clin Oncol* 9:264-266, 1997.

Levy DA, Gogate PA, Hampel N. Giant multilocular prostatic cystadenoma: a rare clinical entity and review of the literature. *J Urol* 150:1920-1922, 1993.

Lewi HJ, White A, Cassidy M, et al. Lymphocytic infiltration of the prostate. *Br J Urol* 56:301-303, 1984.

Li CK, Yeung CK, Chow J, et al. Prostatic non-Hodgkin's lymphoma causing urinary retention in childhood. *Med Pediatr Oncol* 25:420-422, 1995.

Lim DJ, Hayden RT, Murad T, et al. Multilocular prostatic cystadenoma presenting as a large complex pelvic cystic mass. *J Urol* 149:856-859, 1993.

Limon J, Dal Cin P, Sandberg AA. Cytogenetic findings in a primary leiomyosarcoma of the prostate. *Cancer Genet Cytogenet* 22:159-167, 1986.

Liu PI, Ishimaru T, McGregor DH, et al. Autopsy study of granulocytic sarcoma (chloroma) in patients with myelogenous leukemia, Hiroshima-Nagasaki, 1949-1969. *Cancer* 31:948-955, 1973.

Locke JR, Soloway MS, Evans J, et al. Osteogenic differentiation associated with x-ray therapy for adenocarcinoma of the prostate gland. *Am J Clin Pathol* 85:375-378, 1976.

Lopez JI, Elorriaga K, Irizar E, et al. Adenocarcinoma and non-Hodgkin's lymphoma involving the prostate [letter]. *Histopathology* 36:373-374, 2000.

Lopez-Beltran A, Gaeta JF, Huben R, et al. Malignant phyllodes tumor of prostate. *Urology* 35:164-167, 1990.

Loughlin KR, Retik AB, Weinstein HJ, et al. Genitourinary rhabdomyosarcoma in children. *Cancer* 63:1600-1606, 1989.

Lowsley OS, Kimball FN. Sarcoma of the prostate: with a review of the literature. *Br J Urol* 8:328-348, 1934.

Lubin EN, Fetter TR, Erf LA. Subacute monocytic leukemia presenting symptoms of prostatism: a case report. *J Urol* 58:272-276, 1947.

Lucia SP, Mills H, Lowenhaupt E, et al. Visceral involvement in primary neoplastic diseases of the reticulo-endothelial system. *Cancer* 5:1193-1200, 1952.

Lukl P, Bacon JA, Gherardi G, et al. Cystosarcoma phyllodes of the prostate with widespread hematogenous metastases [abstract]. *Pathol Res Pract* 182:520, 1987.

Mackenzie AR, Whitmore WF Jr, Melamed MR. Myosarcomas of the bladder and prostate. *Cancer* 22:833-844, 1968.

Mackenzie AR, Sharma TC, Whitmore WF Jr, et al. Non-extirpative treatment of myosarcomas of the bladder and prostate. *Cancer* 28:329-334, 1971.

Madersbacher S, Schatzl G, Susani M, et al. Prostatic metastasis of a small cell lung cancer in a young male. *Eur Urol* 26:267-269, 1994.

Mahadevia PS, Koss LG, Tar IJ. Prostatic involvement in bladder cancer. Prostate mapping in 20 cystoprostatectomy specimens. *Cancer* 58:2096-2102, 1986.

Mai KT, Walley VM. Adenofibroma of the ejaculatory duct. *J Urol Pathol* 301-305, 1994.

Maluf HM, King ME, DeLuca FR, et al. Giant multilocular prostatic cystadenoma: a distinctive lesion of the retroperitoneum in men. A report of two cases. *Am J Surg Pathol* 15:131-135, 1991.

Manivel C, Shenoy BV, Wick MR, et al. Cystosarcoma phyllodes of the prostate. A pathologic and immunohistochemical study. *Arch Pathol Lab Med* 110:534-538, 1986.

Martin Plata C, Rojo Todo FG, Tremps Velazquez D, et al. Primary lymphoma of the prostate: report of a clinico-pathological case and review of the literature [in Spanish]. *Acta Urol Esp* 24:437-441, 2000.

Masih K, Bhalla S. Primary non-Hodgkin's lymphoma of the prostate gland: a case report. *Ind J Pathol Microbiol* 37(suppl):S56-57, 1994.

Mason DG. Primary malignant lymphocytoma of the prostate gland. *Arch Pathol* 16:803-808, 1933.

Maurer HM, Gehan E, Beltaugady M, et al. The Intergroup Rhabdomyosarcoma Study. *J Clin Oncol* 13:610-630, 1995.

McDougal WS, Persky L. Rhabdomyosarcoma of the bladder and prostate in children. *J Urol* 124:882-885, 1980.

McKenzie M, MacLennan I, Kostashuk E, et al. Postradiation sarcoma after external beam radiation therapy for localized adenocarcinoma of the prostate: report of three cases. *Urology* 53:1228, 1999.

McLorie GA, Abara OE, Churchill BM, et al. Rhabdomyosarcoma of the prostate in childhood: current challenges. *J Pediatr Surg* 24:977-981, 1989.

Medina Perez M, Valero Puerta JA, Perez Martin D. Atypical stromal hyperplasia of the prostate (stromal proliferation of uncertain malignant potential) [in Spanish]. *Arch Esp Urol* 53:722-723, 2000.

Meeter UI, Richards JN. Osteogenic sarcoma of the prostate. *J Urol* 84:654-657, 1960.

Melchior J, Valk WL, Foret JD, et al. The prostate in leukemia: evaluation and review of the literature. *J Urol* 111:647-651, 1974.

Melen DR. Multilocular cyst of the prostate. *J Urol* 27:343-349, 1932.

Mentzel T, Bainbridge TC, Katenkamp D. Solitary fibrous tumor: clinicopathological, immunohistochemical, and ultrastructural analysis of 12 cases arising in soft tissues, nasal cavity and nasopharynx, urinary bladder and prostate. *Virchows Arch* 430:445-453, 1997.

Merguerian PA, Agarwal S, Greenberg M, et al. Outcome analysis of rhabdomyosarcoma of the lower urinary tract. *J Urol* 160:1191-1194, 1998.

Merimsky E, Baratz M, Kahn Y. Leukaemic infiltration of the prostate. *Br J Urol* 53:150-151, 1981.

Meyer LM. Pathology of the urinary tract in leukemia. *Urol Cut Rev* 45:693-695, 1941.

Michaels MM, Brown HE, Favino CJ. Leiomyoma of the prostate. *Urology* 3:617-620, 1974.

Michel F, Gattegno B, Roland J, et al. Primary nonseminomatous germ cell tumor of the prostate. *J Urol* 135:597-599, 1986.

Mincione GP, Grechi G. Urinary cytology of rhabdomyosarcoma in children. Report of two cases located in the urinary bladder and in the prostate. *Pathologica* 75:797-801, 1983.

Mishina T, Shimada N, Toki J, et al. A case report of phyllodes tumor of the prostate: review of the literature and analysis of bizarre giant cell origin. *Acta Urol Jpn* 36:1185-1188, 1990.

Mitch WE Jr, Serpick AA. Leukemic infiltration of the prostate: a reversible form of urinary obstruction. *Cancer* 26:1361-1365, 1970.

Mottola A, Selli C, Carini M, et al. Leiomyosarcoma of the prostate. *Eur Urol* 11:131-133, 1985.

Muss HB, Moloney WC. Chloroma and other myeloblastic tumors. *Blood* 42:721-728, 1973.

Muzafer MH. Large leiomyoma of prostate. *Br J Urol* 59:192-193, 1987.

Narayana AS, Leoning S, Weimar GW, et al. Sarcoma of the bladder and prostate. *J Urol* 119:72-76, 1978A.

Narayana AS, Leoning S, Leoning V, et al. Sarcoma of the urinary bladder and prostate in children. *Eur Urol* 4:401-404, 1978B.

Nassiri M, Ghazi C, Stivers JR, et al. Ganglioneuroma of the prostate. A novel finding in neurofibromatosis. *Arch Pathol Lab Med* 118:938-939, 1994.

Newton WA, Gehan EA, Webber BL, et al. Classification of rhabdomyosarcomas and related sarcomas. *Cancer* 76:1073-1085, 1995.

Nghiem HV, Sommer FG, Moretto JC. MRI of radiation-induced prostate sarcoma. *Clin Imaging* 19:54-56, 1995.

Nielsen VM, Skovgaard N, Krist N. Phaeochromocytoma of the prostate. *Br J Urol* 59:478-479, 1987.

Niku SD, Mattrey RF, Kalota SJ, et al. MRI of pelvic neurofibromatosis. *Abdom Imaging* 20:176-178, 1995.

Nishiyama T, Ikarashi T, Terunuma M, et al. Osteogenic sarcoma of the prostate. *Int J Urol* 8:199-201, 2001.

Nochomovitz LE, Orenstein JM. Inflammatory pseudotumor of the urinary bladder: possible relationship to nodular fasciitis. *Am J Surg Pathol* 9:366-373, 1985.

Ohta S, Takaki R, Ishizawa S. Malignant mesenchymoma arising from the prostate in Gardner's syndrome. *Urol Int* 56:256-258, 1996.

Oliai BR, Kahane H, Epstein JI. A clinicopathologic analysis of urothelial carcinomas diagnosed on prostate needle biopsy. *Am J Surg Pathol* 25:794-801, 2001.

Oliva Encina J, Gil Martinez P, Allepuz Losa C, et al. Prostatic angiosarcoma: report of a new case [in Spanish]. *Acta Urol Esp* 25:78-80, 2001.

Olson EM, Trambert MA, Mattrey RF. Cystosarcoma phyllodes of the prostate: MRI findings. *Abdom Imaging* 19:180-181, 1994.

Ordóñez NG, Ro JY, Ayala AG. Metastatic prostatic carcinoma presenting as an oncocytic tumor. *Am J Surg Pathol* 16:1007-1012, 1992.

Orihuela E, Herr HW, Whitmore WF Jr. Conservative treatment of superficial transitional cell carcinoma of prostatic urethra with intravesical BCG. *Urology* 34:231-237, 1989.

O'Shea PA. Myogenic tumors of soft tissue. In: Coffin CM, Dehner LP, O'Shea PA, eds. *Pediatric Soft Tissue Tumors. A Clinical, Pathological, and Therapeutic Approach.* Baltimore: Williams & Wilkins; 214-253, 1997.

Pagano F, Bassi P, Ferrante GL, et al. Is stage pT4a (D1) reliable in assessing transitional cell carcinoma involvement of the prostate in patients with a concurrent bladder cancer? A necessary distinction for contiguous or noncontiguous involvement. *J Urol* 155:244-247, 1996.

Palou J, Xavier B, Laguna P, et al. In situ transitional cell carcinoma involvement of prostatic urethra: bacillus Calmette-Guérin therapy without previous transurethral resection of the prostate. *Urology* 47:482-484, 1996.

Parham DM. Pathologic classification of rhabdomyosarcomas and correlations with molecular studies. *Mod Pathol* 14:506-514, 2001.

Parks RW, Henry PG, Abram WP, et al. Primary non-Hodgkin's lymphoma of the prostate mimicking acute prostatitis. *Br J Urol* 76:409, 1995.

Patel DR, Gomez GA, Henderson ES, et al. Primary prostatic involvement in non-Hodgkin's lymphoma. *Urology* 32:96-98, 1988.

Peison B, Benisch B, Nicora B, et al. Acute urinary obstruction secondary to pseudolymphoma of prostate. *Urology* 10:478-479, 1977.

Pelstring RJ, Essell JH, Kurtin PJ, et al. Diversity of organ site involvement among malignant lymphomas of mucosa-associated tissues. *Am J Clin Pathol* 96:738-745, 1991.

Pereira Arias JG, Prieto Ugidos N, Larrinaga Simon J, et al. Primary prostatic infiltration by Burkitt's lymphoma [in Spanish]. *Arch Esp Urol* 50:906-908, 1997.

Persaud V, Douglas LL. Bizarre (atypical) leiomyoma of the prostate gland. *West Indian Med J* 31:217-220, 1982.

Pinto A, Tallini G, Novak RW, et al. Undifferentiated rhabdomyosarcoma with lymphoid phenotype expression. *Med Pediatr Oncol* 28:165-170, 1997.

Prabhu GGL, Rao MS, Venugopal N. Conservatively managed symptomatic leiomyoma of the prostate. *J Indian Med Assoc* 93:209, 1995.

Prince CL, Vest SA. Leiomyosarcoma of the prostate. *J Urol* 46:1129-1143, 1941.

Probert JL, O'Rourke JS, Farrow R, et al. Stromal sarcoma of the prostate. *Eur J Surg Oncol* 26:100-101, 2000.

Prym P. Spontanheilung eines bosortigen, wahrscheinlich Chorionepitheliiomatosen gewachses im Hoden. *Virchows Arch* [A] 265:239, 1927.

Pyrah LN. Retrovesical tumours. A report of three cases. *Br J Urol* 26:75-83, 1954.

Quien ET, Wallach B, Sandhaus L, et al. Primary extramedullary leukemia of the prostate: case report and review of the literature. *Am J Hematol* 53:267-271, 1996.

Rader ES. Leukemic infiltration of prostate. *Urology* 3:779-781, 1974.

Rainwater LM, Barrett DM. Primary lymphoma of the prostate: transrectal ultrasonic appearance. *Urology* 36:522-525, 1990.

Rames RA, Smith MT. Malignant peripheral nerve sheath tumor of the prostate: a rare manifestation of neurofibromatosis type 1. *J Urol* 162:165-166, 1999.

Rathbun ND, de Veer JA. Lymphosarcoma of the prostate. With report of a case. *Mt Sinai Hosp* 4:771-780, 1937-1938.

Reese JH, Lombard CM, Krone K, et al. Phyllodes type of atypical prostatic hyperplasia: a report of 3 new cases. *J Urol* 138:623-626, 1987.

Regan JB, Barrett DM, Wold LE. Giant leiomyoma of the prostate. *Arch Pathol Lab Med* 111:381-382, 1987.

Reyes JW, Shinozuka H, Garry P, et al. A light and electron microscopic study of a hemangiopericytoma of the prostate with local extension. *Cancer* 40:1122-1126, 1977.

Rober PE, Smith JB, Sakr W, et al. Malignant peripheral nerve sheath tumor (malignant schwannoma) of the urinary bladder in von Recklinghausen neurofibromatosis. *Urology* 38:473-476, 1991.

Rodary C, Rey A, Olive D, et al. Prognostic factors in 281 children with nonmetastatic rhabdomyosarcoma (RMS) at diagnosis. *Med Pediatr Oncol* 16:71-77, 1988.

Rodriguez-Calvillo M, Panizo C, Rifon J, et al. Prostatic infiltration by non-Hodgkin's lymphoma: report of a case [in Spanish]. *Rev Clin Esp* 200:640, 2000.

Rogers PC, Howards SS, Komp DM. Urogenital rhabdomyosarcoma in childhood. *J Urol* 115:738-739, 1976.

Romero Perez P, Lobato Encinas JJ, Megias Garrigos J, et al. Leiomyosarcoma of the prostate. Report of a case [in Spanish]. *Arch Esp Urol* 43:1019-1023, 1990.

Rosen Y, Ambiavagar PC, Vuletin JC, et al. Atypical leiomyoma of prostate. *Urology* 15:183-185, 1980.

Rosenberg EM, Diamond HL, Jaslowitz B, et al. Lymphosarcoma: a review of 1269 cases. *Medicine* 40:31-84, 1961.

Rub R, Jossiphov J, Avidor Y. Macroscopic hematuria as an initial manifestation of carcinoma of the colon. *J Urol* 161:922, 1999.

Russo P, Demas B, Reuter V. Adult prostatic sarcoma. *Abdom Imaging* 18:399-401, 1993.

Sahin AA, Ro JY, El-Naggar AK, et al. Pseudosarcomatous fibromyxoid tumor of the prostate. A case report with immunohistochemical, electron-microscopic, and DNA flow cytometric analysis. *Am J Clin Pathol* 96:253-258, 1991.

Sakamoto N, Tsuneyoshi M, Naito S, et al. An adequate sampling of the prostate to identify prostatic involvement by urothelial carcinoma in bladder cancer patients. *J Urol* 149:318-321, 1993.

Samsonov VA. Nodular hyperplasia of the prostate with focal changes of phyllode type [in Russian]. *Arkh Patol* 46:66-69, 1984.

Sarkar K, Tolnai G, McKay DE. Embryonal rhabdomyosarcoma of the prostate. An ultrastructural study. *Cancer* 31:442-448, 1973.

Sarris A, Dimopoulos M, Pugh W, et al. Primary lymphoma of the prostate: good outcome with doxorubicin-based combination chemotherapy. *J Urol* 153:1852-1854, 1995.

Schapmans S, Van Leuven L, Cortvriend J, et al. Phyllodes tumor of the prostate. *Eur Urol* 38:649-653, 2000.

Schellhammer PF, Bean MA, Whitmore WF Jr. Prostatic involvement by transitional cell carcinoma: pathogenesis, patterns and prognosis. *J Urol* 118:399-403, 1977.

Scholtmeijer RJ, van Unnik AM, ten Kate FW. Acute urine retention in a child due to fibromatosis of the prostate. *Eur Urol* 14:412-413, 1988.

Schumacher S, Moll R, Muller SC, et al. Epithelioid leiomyoma of the prostate. *Eur Urol* 30:125-126, 1996.

Schuppler J. Malignant neurilemmoma of prostate gland. *J Urol* 106:903-905, 1971.

Scully JM, Uno JM, McIntyre M, et al. Radiation-induced prostatic sarcoma: a case report. *J Urol* 144:746-748, 1990.

Seong BM, Cheon J, Lee JG, et al. A case of multilocular prostatic cystadenoma. *J Korean Med Sci* 13:554-558, 1998.

Sexton WJ, Lance RE, Reyes AO, et al. Adult prostatic sarcoma. The M.D. Anderson Cancer Center Experience. *J Urol* 166:521-525, 2001.

Shapiro B, Gonzalez E, Weissman A, et al. Malignant paraganglioma of the prostate: case report, depiction by meta-iodobenzylguanidine scintigraphy and review of the literature. *Q J Nucl Med* 41:36-41, 1997.

Shapiro E, Strother D. Pediatric genitourinary rhabdomyosarcoma. *J Urol* 148:1761-1768, 1992.

Sloan SE, Rapoport JM. Prostatic chondroma. *Urology* 25:319-321, 1985.

Smedley HM, Brown C, Turner A. Ectopic ACTH-producing lung cancer presenting with prostatic metastasis. *Postgrad Med J* 59:371-372, 1983.

Smith BH, Dehner LP. Sarcoma of the prostate gland. *Am J Clin Pathol* 58:43-50, 1972.

Smith DM, Manivel C, Kapps D, et al. Angiosarcoma of the prostate: report of 2 cases and review of the literature. *J Urol* 135:382-384, 1986.

Smith LD. Lymphosarcoma of the prostate. A case report. *J Urol* 38:375-382, 1937.

Spasic P, Brankovan K, Petrov B. Malignant melanoma metastasis into prostate carcinoma and adrenal adenoma [in Serbo-Croatian]. *Vojnosanit Pregl* 37:115-116, 1980.

Sridhar KN, Woodhouse CRJ. Prostatic infiltration in leukaemia and lymphoma. *Eur Urol* 9:153-156, 1983.

Stein BS, Kendall AR. Malignant melanoma of the genitourinary tract. *J Urol* 132:859-868, 1984.

Stout AP. Tumors featuring pericytes. *Lab Invest* 5:217-233, 1956.

Stroup RM, Sheibani K, Moncada A, et al. Angiotropic (intravascular) large cell lymphoma. A clinicopathologic study of seven cases with unique clinical presentations. *Cancer* 66:1781-1788, 1990.

Sundarasivarao D, Banerjea S, Nageswararao A, et al. Hemangioma of the prostate: a case report. *J Urol* 110:708-709, 1973.

Suzuki H, Nakada T, Iijima Y, et al. Malignant lymphoma of the prostate. Report of a case. *Urol Int* 47:172-175, 1991.

Swierz J, Zielinski H, Dabek A. Primary non-Hodgkin's lymphoma of the prostate [in Polish]. *Pol Merkuriusz Lek* 1:278-279, 1996.

Symmers D. Primary lymphosarcoma of the prostate. *Arch Surg* 6:755-763, 1923.

Szakacs JE, Carta M, Szakacs MR. Ewing's sarcoma, extraskeletal and of bone. Case report with ultrastructural analysis. *Ann Clin Lab Sci* 4:306-322, 1974.

Tadera S, Oka N, Sako M, et al. A case of prostatic leiomyosarcoma [in Japanese]. *Acta Urol Jpn* 32:462-467, 1986.

Takeshima Y, Yoneda K, Sanda N, et al. Solitary fibrous tumor of the prostate. *Pathol Int* 47:713-717, 1997.

Tannenbaum M. Sarcomas of the prostate gland. *Urology* 5:810-814, 1975.

Tash JA, Reuter V, Russo P. Metastatic carcinoid tumor of the prostate. *J Urol* 167:2526-2527, 2002.

Tay HP, Bidair M, Shabaik A, et al. Primary yolk sac tumor of the prostate in a patient with Kleinefelter's syndrome. *J Urol* 153:1066-1069, 1995.

Tefft M, Jaffe N. Sarcoma of the bladder and prostate in children. *Cancer* 32:1161-1177, 1973.

Terris MK, Eigner EB, Briggs EM, et al. Transrectal ultrasound in the evaluation of rhabdomyosarcoma involving the prostate. *Br J Urol* 74:341-344, 1994.

Terris MK, Hausdorff J, Freiha FS. Hematolymphoid malignancies diagnosed at the time of radical prostatectomy. *J Urol* 158:1457-1459, 1997.

Terris MK, Freiha FS. Transrectal ultrasound appearance of hematolymphoid malignancies involving the prostate. *Urology* 51:339-341, 1998A.

Terris MK. Transrectal ultrasound appearance of radiation-induced prostatic sarcoma. *Prostate* 37:182-186, 1998B.

Têtu B, Ro JY, Ayala AG, et al. Atypical spindle cell lesions of the prostate. *Semin Diagn Pathol* 5:284-293, 1988.

Têtu B, Srigley JR, Bostwick DG. Soft tissues tumors. In: Bostwick DG, ed. *Pathology of the Prostate.* New York: Churchill Livingstone; 117-135, 1990.

Thalhammer F, Gisslinger H, Chott A, et al. Granulocytic sarcoma of the prostate as the first manifestation of a late relapse of acute myelogenous leukemia. *Ann Hematol* 68:97-99, 1994.

Thompson GJ, Albers DD, Broders AC. Unusual carcinomas involving the prostate gland. *J Urol* 89:416-425, 1953.

Tijare JR, Shrikhande AV, Shrikhande VV. Phyllodes type of atypical prostatic hyperplasia. *J Urol* 162:803-804, 1999.

Timmons JW Jr, Burgert EU Jr, Soule EH, et al. Embryonal rhabdomyosarcoma of the bladder and prostate in children. *J Urol* 113:694-697, 1975.

Tissier F, Badoual C, Saporta F, et al. Prostatic lymphoma of mucosa-associated lymphoid tissue: an uncommon location [letter]. *Histopathology* 40:103-113, 2002.

Tobisu KI, Tanaka Y, Mizutani T, et al. Transitional cell carcinoma of the urethra in men following cystectomy for bladder cancer: multivariate analysis for risk factors. *J Urol* 146:1551-1553, 1991.

Tobisu K, Kanai Y, Sakamoto M, et al. Involvement of the anterior urethra in male patients with transitional cell carcinoma of the bladder undergoing radical cystectomy with simultaneous urethrectomy. *Jpn J Clin Oncol* 27:406-409, 1997.

Tomikawa S, Okumura H, Yoshida T, et al. Primary prostatic lymphoma of mucosa-associated lymphoid tissue. *Intern Med* 37:628-630, 1998.

Tomaru U, Ishikura H, Kon S-I, et al. Primary lymphoma of the prostate with features of low grade B-cell lymphoma of mucosa associated lymphoid tissue: a rare cause of urinary obstruction. *J Urol* 162:496-497, 1999.

Vassilakis GB. Pure leiomyoma of prostate. *Urology* 11:93-94, 1978.

Velasco A, Mora X, Baeza R, et al. Hemangiopericytoma: report of 4 cases [in Spanish]. *Rev Med Chil* 121:1305-1308, 1993.

Viadana E, Bross ID, Pickren JW. An autopsy study of the metastatic patterns of human leukemias. *Oncology* 35: 87-96, 1978.

Viskens D, Van Hove C, Fransen G, et al. Phyllodes type of atypical prostatic hyperplasia [in Dutch]. *Acta Chir Belg* 91:22-26, 1991.

Voges GE, Wippermann F, Düber C, et al. Pheochromocytoma in the pediatric age group: the prostate—an unusual location. *J Urol* 144:1219-1221, 1990.

Waddington RT. Leukemic infiltration of the prostate in a patient with chronic lymphatic leukemia: a case report. *Br J Urol* 45:184-186, 1973.

Waller JI, Shullenberger WA. Lymphosarcoma of the prostate. *J Urol* 62:480-487, 1949.

Wang CJ, Chen YT, Shun CT, et al. Primary malignant melanoma of the prostate. *J Urol* 154:1865, 1995.

Wang X, Bostwick DG. Prostatic stromal hyperplasia with atypia: a study of 11 cases. *J Urol Pathol* 6:15-26, 1997.

Waring PM, Newland RC. Prostatic embryonal rhabdomyosarcoma in adults. A clinicopathologic review. *Cancer* 69:755-762, 1992.

Wasserstein PW, Goldman RL. Primary carcinoid of prostate. *Urology* 13:318-320, 1979.

Wasserstein PW, Goldman RL. Diffuse carcinoid of the prostate. *Urology* 18:407-409, 1981.

Watanabe J, Konishi T, Takeuchi H, et al. A case of giant prostatic cystadenoma. *Acta Urol Jpn* 36:1077-1079, 1990.

Watson EM, Sauer HR, Sadugor MG. Manifestations of the lymphoblastomas in the genito-urinary tract. *J Urol* 61:626-642, 1949.

Weiss SW, Goldblum JR. Fibrous tumors of infancy and childhood. In: *Enzinger and Weiss' Soft Tissue Tumors*, 4th ed. St Louis: Mosby; 383-388, 2001A.

Weiss SW, Goldblum JR. Rhabdomyosarcoma. In: *Enzinger and Weiss' Soft Tissue Tumors*, 4th ed. St Louis: Mosby; 785-835, 2001B.

West WO. Primary lymphosarcoma of the prostate gland. *Arch Intern Med* 109:469-472, 1962.

Westra WH, Grenko RT, Epstein JI. Solitary fibrous tumor of the lower urogenital tract: a report of five cases involving the seminal vesicles, urinary bladder, and prostate. *Hum Pathol* 31:63-68, 2000.

Wexler LH, Helman LJ. Pediatric soft tissue sarcoma. *CA Cancer J Clin* 44:211-247, 1994.

Whelan T, Gatfield CT, Robertson S, et al. Primary carcinoid of the prostate in conjunction with multiple endocrine neoplasia IIb in a child. *J Urol* 153:1080-1082, 1995.

Wijnaendts LC, van der Linden JC, van Unnick AJ, et al. Histopathological classification of childhood rhabdomyosarcoma: relationship with clinical parameters and prognosis. *Hum Pathol* 25:900-907, 1994.

Wilbur H, Taylor RJ. Prostatectomy in patients with leukemia. *Urology* 18:580-581, 1981.

Williams E, Hanchard B, Brooks SE, et al. Immunohistochemistry of lymphocyte B-cell lymphoma of the prostate gland. *West Indian Med J* 41:126-129, 1992.

Wood DP Jr, Montie JE, Pontes JE, et al. Transitional cell carcinoma of the prostate in cystoprostatectomy specimens removed for bladder cancer. *J Urol* 141:346-349, 1989.

Wunsch PH, Muller HA. Hemangiopericytoma of the prostate, a light microscopic study of an unusual tumor. *Pathol Res Pract* 173:334-338, 1982.

Yamamoto S, Ito T, Miki M, et al. Malignant phyllodes tumor of the prostate. *Int J Urol* 7:378-381, 2000.

Yasuda N, Ohmori SI, Usui T. IgD myelomas involving the prostate. *Am J Hematol* 47:65-66, 1994.

Yokota T, Yamashita Y, Okuzono Y, et al. Malignant cystosarcoma phyllodes of prostate. *Acta Pathol Jpn* 34:663-668, 1984.

Young JF, Jensen PE, Wiley CA. Malignant phyllodes tumor of the prostate. A case report with immunohistochemical and ultrastructural studies. *Arch Pathol Lab Med* 116:296-299, 1992.

Young RH, Scully RE. Pseudosarcomatous lesions of the urinary bladder, prostate gland, and urethra. *Arch Pathol Lab Med* 111:354-358, 1987.

Young RH, Srigley JR, Amin MB, et al. Miscellaneous tumors of the prostate. In: *Tumors of the Prostate Gland, Seminal Vesicles, Male Urethra, and Penis.* Washington, DC: Armed Forces Institute of Pathology; 257, 2000.

Yum M, Miller JC, Agrawal BL. Leiomyosarcoma arising in atypical fibromuscular hyperplasia (phyllodes tumor) of the prostate with distant metastasis. *Cancer* 68:910-915, 1991.

Zein TA, Huben R, Lane W, et al. Secondary tumors of the prostate. *J Urol* 133:615-616, 1985.

Treatment Effects

[19.1] Surgery **457**
[19.2] Hormonal Therapy **457**
[19.3] Radiation Therapy **464**
[19.4] Chemotherapy **468**
[19.5] Miscellaneous Therapies **469**
[19.6] Medical Therapy for BPH **469**
[19.7] Minimally Invasive Therapy for BPH **469**
[19.8] Experimental Prostate Cancer Therapy **470**

CHAPTER 19

Treatments for disease of the prostate, mainly benign prostatic hyperplasia (BPH) and cancer, can have a profound effect on the histopathologic appearance of prostatic tissues, benign and malignant. Knowledge of these alterations is critical so that treatment-induced alterations in benign tissues are not misdiagnosed as malignancy and, conversely, so that treatment effects on persistent or recurrent malignant proliferations are not misinterpreted as benign conditions. Additionally, histologic grading and pathologic staging after treatment merit special consideration. Forms of therapy documented to have a histologic effect are discussed in this chapter.

[19.1] Surgery

Transurethral resection of the prostate (TURP) or biopsy can generate postbiopsy or postresection granulomatous prostatitis. These distinctive fibrinoid granulomas bear a passing resemblance to rheumatoid nodules and have also been misdiagnosed as tuberculous granulomas. (A full discussion of these granulomas is found in Chapter 4.) TURP can also lead to fibrosis and reactive epithelial changes, such as squamous metaplasia. However, the relative amount of glandular and stromal tissue is not different in TURP chips from repeat transurethral resection for BPH in comparison with chips from the initial resection (Jonler 1995).

[19.2] Hormonal Therapy

Endocrine or androgen deprivation therapy has been a common treatment modality for patients with locally advanced or metastatic prostate cancer (Furr 1999, Khoury 1999, Lytton 2001, McLeod 2000, Schröeder 2002, Stenner 1999) **t19.1**. More recently, preoperative neoadjuvant hormonal therapy has been used in patients with clinically localized prostate cancer in efforts to downstage the tumor before radical prostatectomy.Clinically, in this neoadjuvant setting, this androgen suppression leads to a decrease in the size of the prostate (by transrectal ultrasound), a drop in the serum prostate-specific antigen (PSA, often to normal or undetectable levels), and regression in palpable induration by digital rectal examination (DRE) (Armas 1994). Hormonal therapy in the form of a 5α-reductase inhibitor (finasteride) has also been used to treat patients with BPH. It follows that one may encounter androgen deprivation–induced effects in needle biopsy, TURP chips, open prostatectomy, or radical prostatectomy tissues. Needle biopsy tissue can be procured from patients with BPH previously treated with androgen deprivation agents who undergo transrectal needle biopsy to rule out prostate cancer in the setting of an elevated serum PSA or abnormal DRE. TURP tissue or open prostatectomy samples can be submitted from patients in whom finasteride medical therapy failed or from patients with hormone-treated advanced prostate cancer who underwent a channel TURP to relieve obstruction. One can also be confronted with androgen deprivation therapy effects in radical prostatectomy tissues from patients treated with neoadjuvant hormonal therapy. Finally, hormone-induced changes can be seen in biopsies of locally recurrent or metastatic tumor deposits.

The major initial studies on the effects of androgen deprivation on prostate tissue were performed in the 1940s through 1960s, based on the seminal and Nobel prize–winning work of Huggins and Hodges on the androgen dependence of prostate cancer (Huggins 1941A, 1941B, Lytton 2001). These first studies characterized the effect of estrogen (usually diethylstilbestrol) on benign and malignant prostatic tissues (Bainborough 1952, Fergusson 1953, Franks 1960, Heckel 1942, Moore 1938, Rezek 1951, Schenken 1942) **t19.2**. In this earlier literature, squamous metaplasia of benign glands was emphasized **t19.2**. Since that time, additional changes in benign cells and tissues have been defined **t19.3**.As early as 1942, the classic cytologic changes induced by hormones on responsive prostatic carcinoma cells were described (Schenken 1942). These include both nuclear and cytoplasmic alterations. Nuclei were noted to be pyknotic, with reduction in size, loss of nucleoli, and chromatin condensation. Cytoplasmic vacuolization was also a regressive feature in treated carcinoma cells, as well as rupture of cell membranes with coalescence of vacuoles of neighboring cells, whereby free-floating or naked nuclei were generated (Schenken 1942). Nuclear pyknosis and cytoplasmic vacuolization are now recognized as hallmarks of all forms of androgen deprivation therapy. Since the mid-20th century, the only major additional feature of hormone-induced histologic change that has been added is the "mucinous degeneration" (Reuter 1997) or pseudomyxomatous stromal changes (De Voot 1987).

Even in the 1940s it was evident that there was heterogeneity of hormone responsiveness of prostate cancer cells because variability

t19.1 Major Methods of Androgen Deprivation

Orchiectomy
Estrogen therapy (such as diethylstilbestrol)
Luteinizing hormone-releasing hormone agonists (such as leuprolide and goserelin)
Antiandrogens
- Steroidal (such as cyproterone and megestrol)
- Nonsteroidal (such as flutamide, nilutamide, and bicalutamide)
- Nonclassical (such as ketoconazole; aminoglutethimide, and finasteride[1])

Combined androgen blockade (antiandrogen and LHRH analog or orchiectomy)

Classification from McLeod 2000
[1]Finasteride (Proscar) is used for treatment of BPH

t19.2 Effect of Estrogen on Prostatic Tissues: 1940-1960 Studies

Benign prostatic tissue
Squamous metaplasia (glycogenated, nonkeratinizing)

Adenocarcinoma
Decrease in size and number of cells
Nuclear pyknosis
Cytoplasmic vacuolization, including swollen balloon or signet cells
Cell rupture with dissolution of sharp epithelial-stromal margin and release of discohesive cells into glandular lumina
Stroma pale-staining and vacuolated to fibrotic

Descriptions from Schenken 1942, Heckel 1942, Moore 1938, Rezek 1951, Bainborough 1952, and Fergusson 1953

■ **t19.3 Effect of Androgen Deprivation Therapy on Prostatic Tissue**

Benign prostatic tissue
Atrophy, with loss of undulating hyperplastic architecture
Basal cell prominence and hyperplasia
Squamous metaplasia, both glycogenated and immature types
Secretory epithelium with nuclear pyknosis and cytoplasmic clearing
Stromal dominance, with focal stromal hypercellularity
Stromal lymphocytic/histiocytic infiltrative, focal

Prostatic intraepithelial neoplasia (PIN)
Lower prevalence and extent
Flattening of luminal epithelium
Shed cells in lumen
Less nuclear crowding
Nuclear pyknosis and hyperchromasia
Inconspicuous nucleoli
Cytoplasmic clearing

Adenocarcinoma
Decrease in gland number, with increased stroma
Glands tend to be small and atrophic, with compressed or absent lumina
Single tumor cells, often histiocyte-like, can be present
Nuclear pyknosis and hyperchromasia
Inconspicuous nucleoli ("nucleolus-poor")
Cytoplasmic clearing and vacuolization
Occasionally: branching clefts, mucinous stromal pools (pseudomyxoma), large tumor cells in inflammatory background

in the degree of nuclear pyknosis was quantitated and "foci of unaltered neoplastic cells" were detected (Schenken 1942). There was variation in morphologic alterations from patient to patient and also from "part to part of the same tumor" (Franks 1960).

Grossly, prostates treated with neoadjuvant hormonal therapy (luteinizing hormone–releasing hormone [LHRH] analog or antiandrogens) are small, and hyperplasia and carcinoma are more difficult to macroscopically identify, compared with untreated glands. Treated glands are shrunken and have a rubbery to soft consistency (Armas 1994, Reuter 1997). The treated prostate weights are an average of 33% (down to a mean of 33 g) lower than those of untreated controls (Armas 1994, Civantos 1996). This difference in gross size correlates with the prostate volume reduction that can be clinically quantitated by transrectal ultrasound (Armas 1994, Soloway 1994, Voges 1994) On cut sections, fewer nodules of hyperplasia are seen in treated prostates (Armas 1994). Grossly visible prostatic carcinoma was evident in only 15% of treated prostate glands, compared with 60% of untreated glands (Armas 1994).

Microscopically, the first clue, captured at scanning magnification, of androgen deprivation therapy effect is stromal dominance **i19.1**. That is, the prostate tissue often is made up predominantly of stroma, with the identified epithelium being atrophic **t19.3**. In hormonally treated benign prostatic tissue there is "global senescence or involution" (Gaudin 1998), with a decrease in number and size of glands **i19.1**. Normal (De Voot 1987) and hyperplastic glands are simplified in that they lose their branching complexity and intraluminal undulations and appear small, ovoid, round, or comma-shaped **i19.2** (Armas 1994, Civantos 1996, De Voot 1987, Grignon 1995, Montironi 1998, Murphy 1991, Reuter 1997, Tetu 1991). The secretory, luminal epithelium often is atrophic, with loss of cytoplasmic volume **i19.2, i19.3**, and displays nuclear pyknosis and cytoplasmic clearing. Basal cell prominence and hyperplasia are also stereotypical responses of benign prostatic glands to withdrawal of androgens **i19.4, i19.5**. Glycogenated squamous

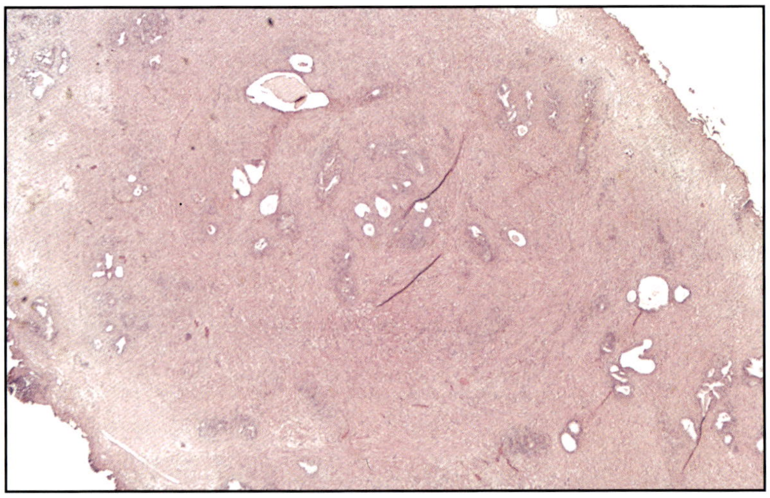

■ **i19.1** *Androgen deprivation therapy effect on benign prostatic tissue: Stromal dominance with abundant fibromuscular stroma, and few atrophic prostatic glands.*

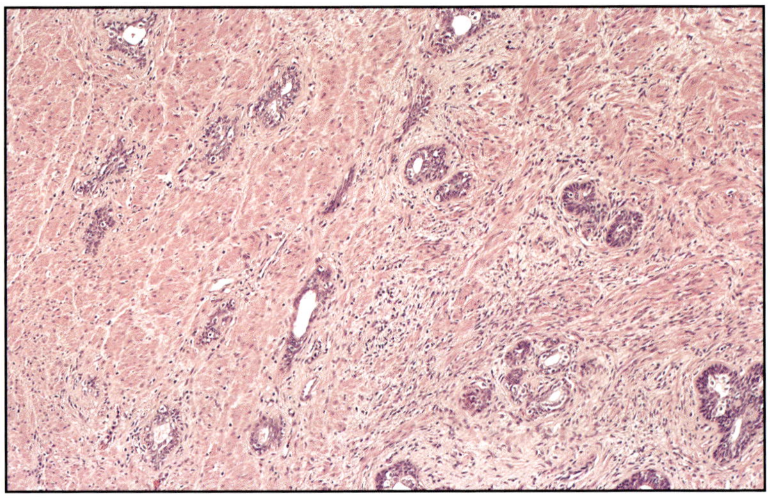

■ **i19.2** *Androgen deprivation therapy effect on benign glands: Small, rounded to elongated glands.*

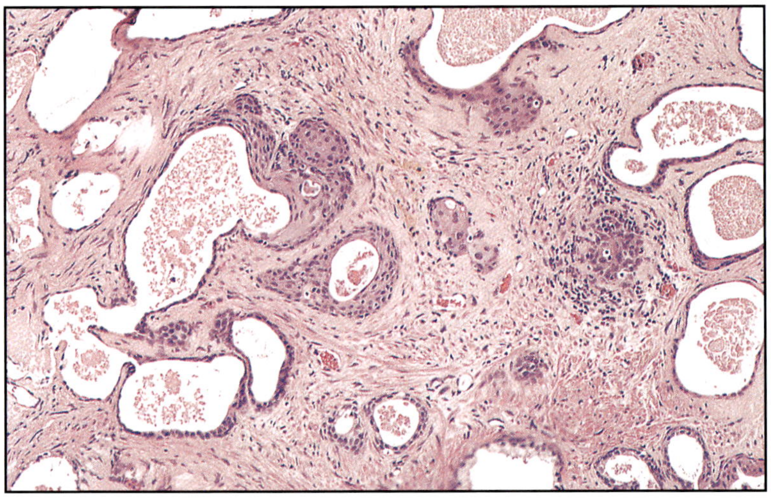

■ **i19.3** *Androgen deprivation therapy effect: Atrophic glands with flattened epithelial lining. There is focal squamous metaplasia.*

metaplasia **i19.6** is much less common in nonestrogenic hormonal treatments than in estrogen- or diethylstilbestrol-treated glands. Immature squamous metaplasia can be seen. The frequency of squamous metaplasia is debated, with the incidence being reported as

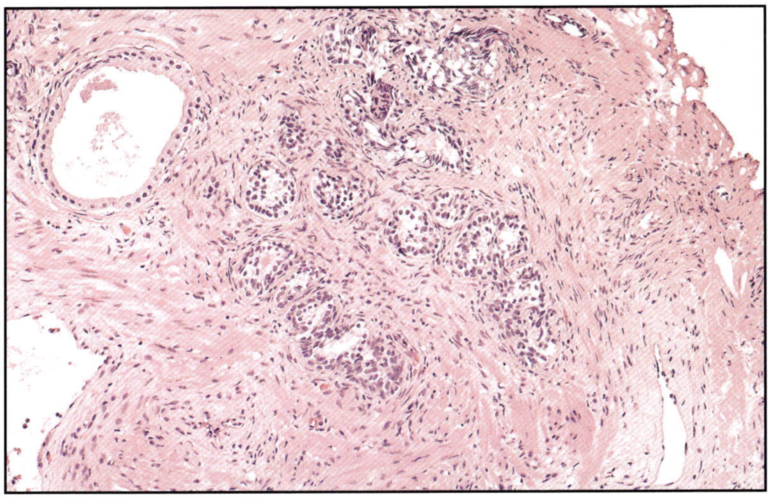

■ **i19.4** *Basal cell prominence is a common finding in benign prostatic glands after androgen deprivation. This pseudoinfiltrative appearance of these treated glands should not be mistaken for infiltrating adenocarcinoma.*

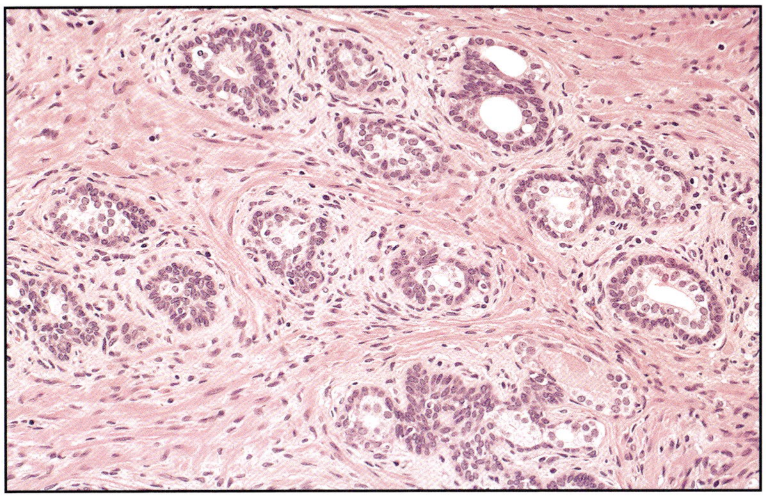

■ **i19.5** *Androgen deprivation therapy effect on benign glands: Basal cell prominence.*

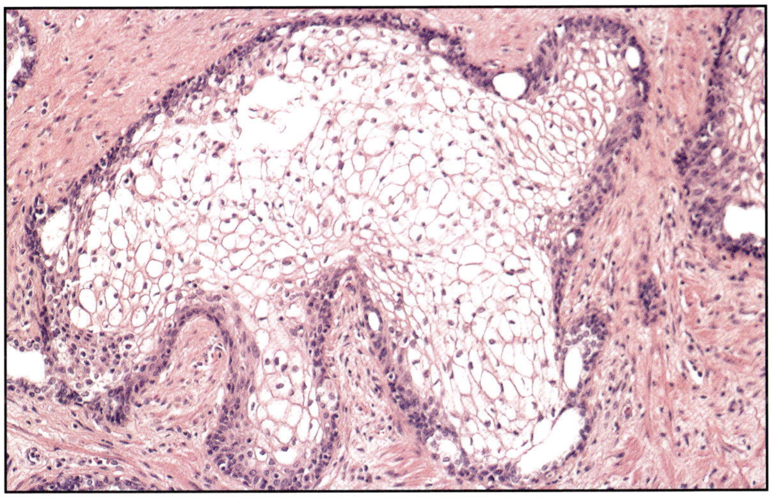

■ **i19.6** *Androgen deprivation therapy (estrogen treatment) on benign glands: Glycogenated squamous metaplasia.*

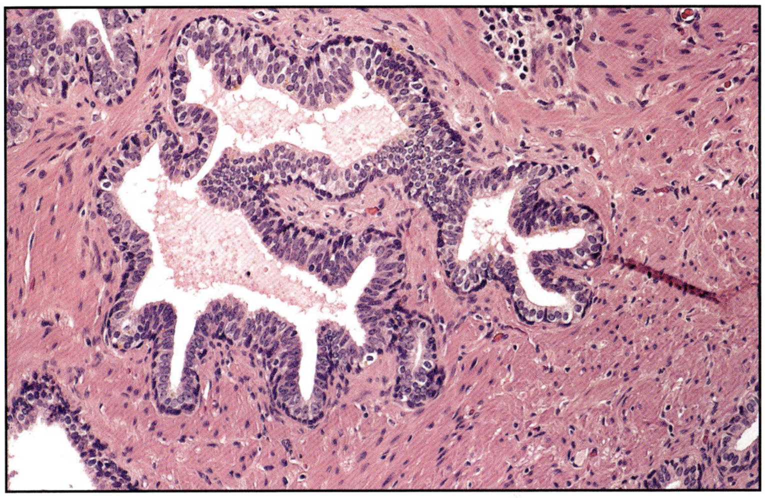

■ **i19.7** *Prostatic intraepithelial neoplasia after androgen deprivation: Flattening of luminal cell lining.*

0% (Murphy 1991), to rare and focal (Armas 1994, Tetu 1991), to common at 53% (Civantos 1995). Transitional cell metaplasia is not usually associated with androgen deprivation therapy. (However, one study [Civantos 1995] found an incidence of 59% in androgen-deprived glands and 3% of control glands). The reason for the differences in reported frequency of squamous metaplasia and transitional metaplasia in androgen deprivation therapy probably is related to different definitions of squamous metaplasia and transitional cell metaplasia. Also, immature squamous metaplasia, transitional cell metaplasia, and basal cell hyperplasia can display a degree of morphologic overlap. Androgen deprivation does not result in an increase in neuroendocrine Paneth-like cells (Civantos 1995). Stromal changes, aside from an apparent increase in area, are less conspicuous than the epithelial alterations. The apparent increase in amount of stroma appears to result from a reduction in glandular elements. Stromal hyperplasia may be found and may result from a true increase in the number of stromal cells or shrinkage of stromal cell cytoplasm (Armas 1994). Scattered lymphocytes may be present in the benign stroma (Armas 1994). Androgen blockade treatment of prostatic hyperplasia induces epithelial involution by a combined reduction in proliferative activity and enhancement of apoptosis (Montironi 1994A). Androgen deprivation therapy morphologic effects can persist for years.

Prostatic intraepithelial neoplasia (PIN) is reduced in prevalence and extent after androgen deprivation therapy (Armas 1994, Civantos 1995, Ferguson 1994, Tetu 1991, Vaillancourt 1996, Wheeler 1996). Microscopically, treated PIN glands show diminished luminal architectural complexity **i19.7**, with flat and low tufted patterns predominating, rather than high tufted and micropapillary patterns (Bullock 2002). Basal cells are usually prominent (Bullock 2002). The glands exhibit less nuclear crowding and can reveal luminal cell detachment and shedding . Apoptotic bodies can be seen easily (Montironi 1994B). The cytologic alterations in the luminal cells are the same as for adenocarcinoma, with nuclear pyknosis, inconspicuous nucleoli, and cytoplasmic shedding. Luminal cell cytoplasm may also be diminished (Bullock 2002). Because of these changes, it is often not feasible to grade PIN after hormonal treatment. The decrease in PIN volume after androgen deprivation has important implications for prostate cancer chemoprevention. That is, if one can cause regression of a putative prostate cancer precursor by androgen blockade, then perhaps one can thereby prevent prostate cancer development with such treatment. This concept has not been tested in a clinical trial of LHRH agonists or antiandrogens.

The histomorphologic effects of neoadjuvant androgen deprivation therapy on adenocarcinoma include a decrease in

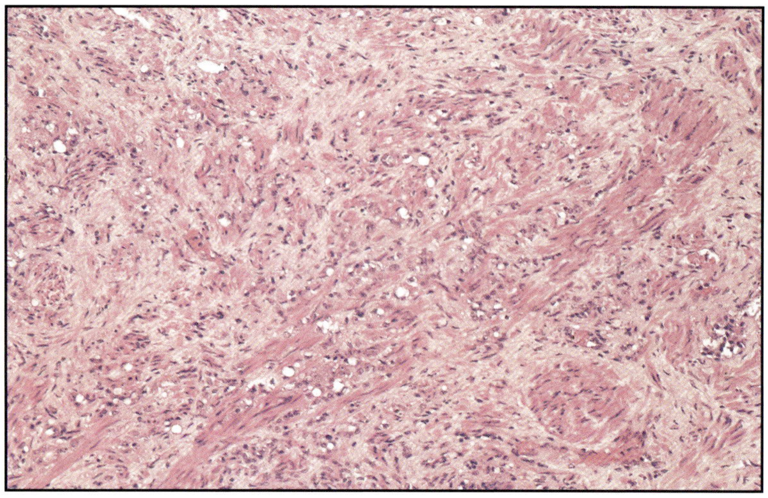

■ **i19.8** *Androgen deprivation therapy effect on carcinoma: Small, scattered, atrophic prostatic adenocaricnoma glands with treatment effect are often difficult to identify at low magnification.*

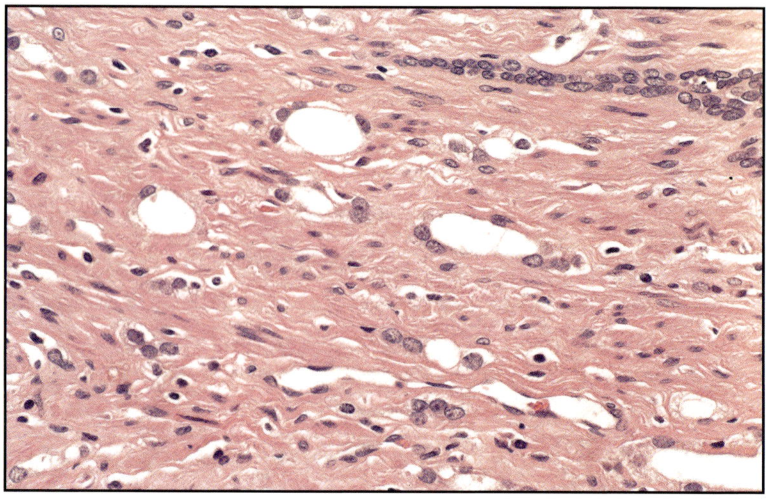

■ **i19.9** *Atrophic pattern of prostatic adenocarcinoma induced by hormonal therapy.*

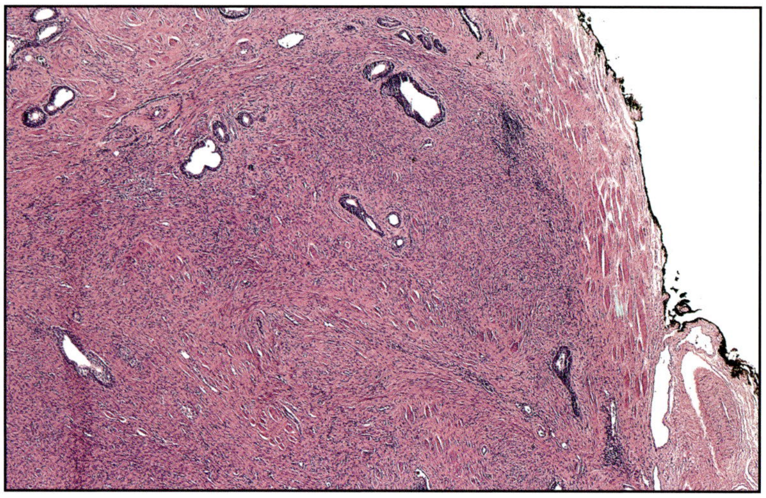

■ **i19.10** *Androgen-deprivation therapy effect on nodule of carcinoma. Here, it is impossible to recognize malignancy at scanning magnification.*

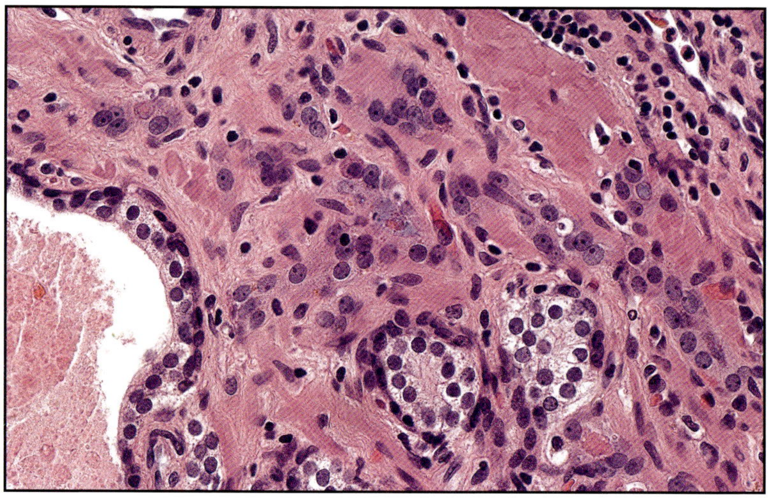

■ **i19.11** *Androgen-deprivation therapy effect on nodule of carcinoma. Even at high-power views of* **i19.10**, *the carcinoma infiltrate is subtle; here it is visualized as basophilic nests and cords.*

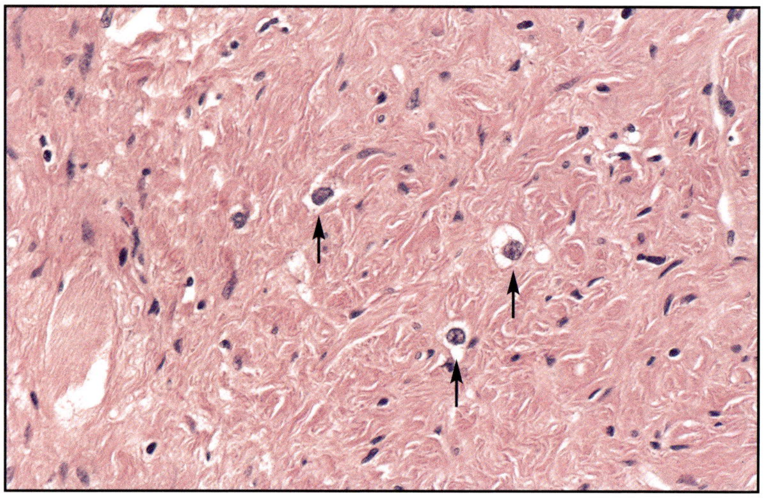

■ **i19.12** *Androgen-deprivation treatment effect on prostatic carcinoma: Widely dispersed single malignant cells (arrows).*

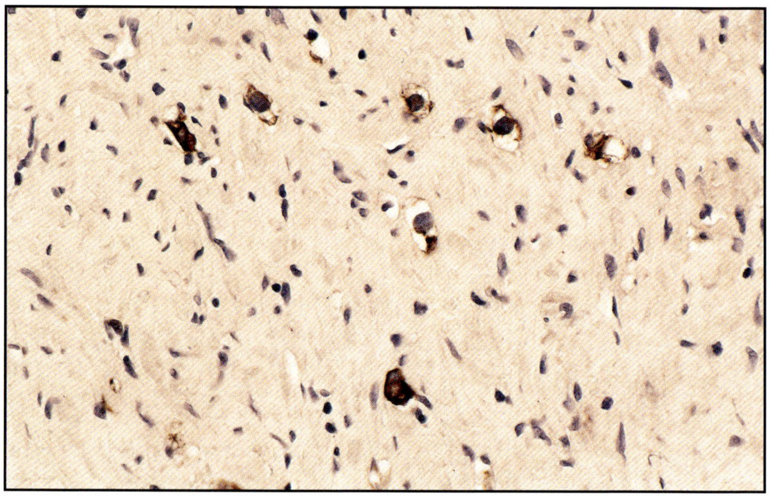

■ **i19.13** *Androgen-deprivation treatment effect on prostatic carcinoma. Immunostains for PSA (shown here) and/or pan-cytokeratin can aid in detection of subtle single carcinoma cell infiltrates depicted in* **i19.12**.

tumor amount and number of malignant glands, with loss of luminal glandular spaces (luminal collapse), increased stroma, nuclear pyknosis, and cytoplasmic vacuolization **t19.3**. A decrease in tumor size in radical prostatectomy specimens from treated patients is observed in comparison with control, untreated cases. A 44% reduction in tumor volume (Vaillancourt 1996), a decrease in number of quadrants with tumor (Armas 1994), and an increase in cases with focal tumor (Armas 1994, Tetu 1991) were reported. A small

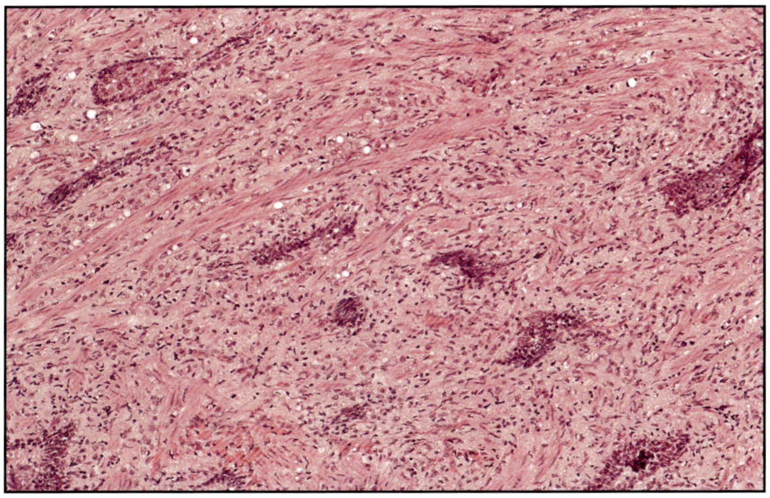

■ **i19.14** *Androgen deprivation therapy effect on prostatic carcinoma. The treated carcinoma cells invade between and around benign, atrophic glands with basal cell prominence.*

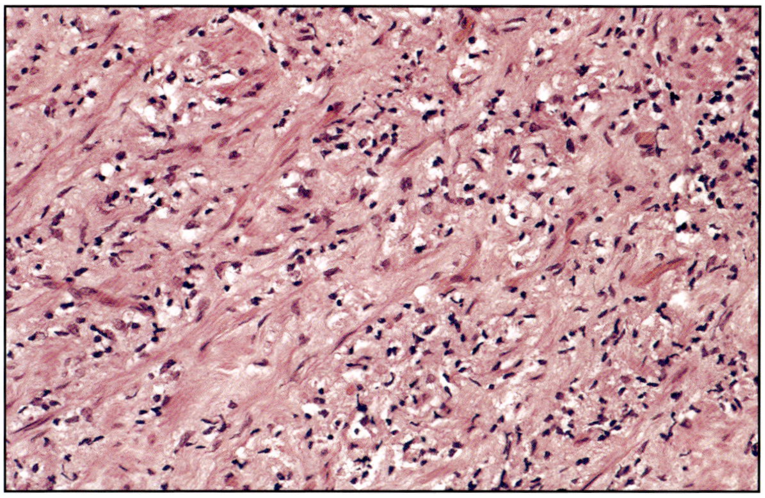

■ **i19.15** *Androgen deprivation therapy effect on prostatic carcinoma. At higher magnification, this is the prototypical image of treated prostatic carcinoma cells with loss of glandular lumina, nuclear pyknosis, and cytoplasmic vacuolization.*

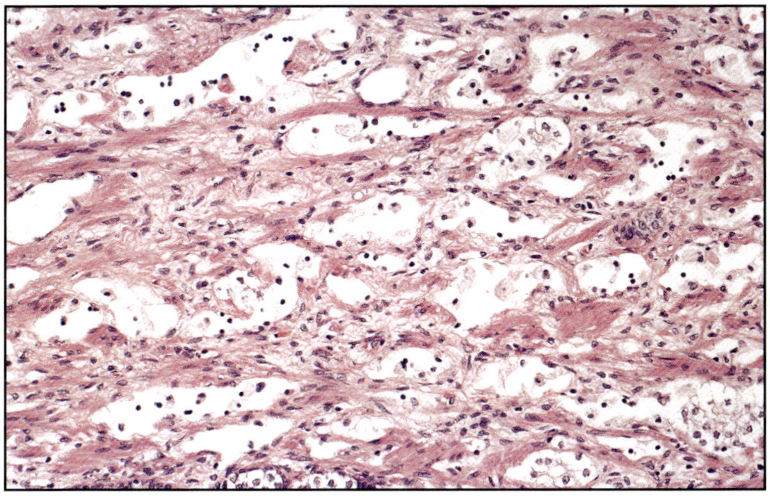

■ **i19.16** *Androgen deprivation therapy effect on prostatic carcinoma: Pyknotic tumor cells shed into clefted spaces.*

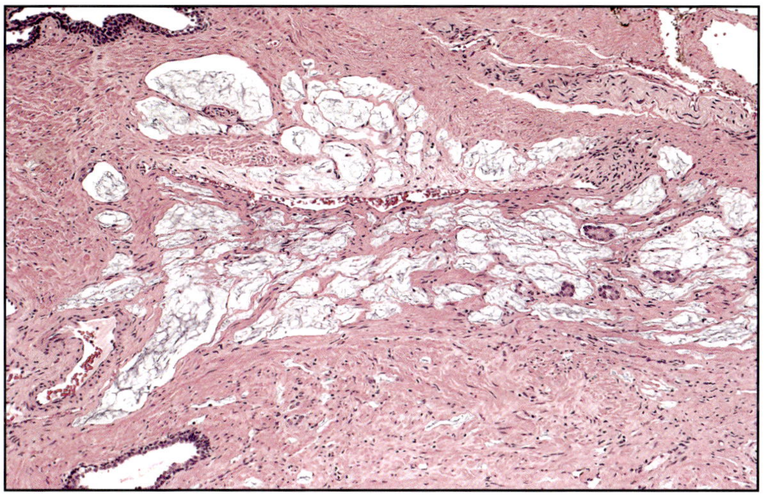

■ **i19.17** *Androgen deprivation therapy effect on prostatic carcinoma: "pseudomyxoma"-like appearance, with clefts and pools of mucin, which contained only a few residual malignant glands.*

percentage of cases with no residual tumor after hormonal treatment have been reported (Gleave 2000, Kollerman 2000, Schulman 1994, Tetu 1991, Tunn 1996, Vaillancourt 1996, Van der Kwast 1997), but in some of these cases complete embedding of the prostate gland was not performed (Tetu 1991, Vaillancourt 1996). In many other studies of completely embedded glands, residual carcinoma was found in every case (Armas 1994, Civantos 1995, Hellström 1993, Van de Voorde 1994, Voges 1994). Microscopically, there is a decrease in malignant glandular density, with abundant stroma often separating small groups of dispersed glands **i19.8, i19.9** or cords of cells **i19.10, i19.11**. A decrease in size of the adenocarcinoma glands is also characteristic (Murphy 1991), where the glands often are small and atrophic, with compressed or absent lumina **i19.9, i19.11**. A particularly insidious pattern of growth that can be difficult to detect on hematoxylin and eosin (H&E)-stained sections is the presence of widely scattered single tumor cells embedding in a wide expanse of stroma **i19.12**. Hormonally treated carcinoma cells can resemble vague lymphohistiocytic infiltrates **i19.14, i19.15**. Another distinctive effect of hormonal therapy is the formation of branching clefts, which may or may not contain degenerated tumor cells **i19.16** or wispy-blue mucin **i19.17, i19.18**. The branched architecture with scattered tumor cells with pyknotic nuclei and foamy vacuolated cytoplasm has been deemed "hemangiopericytoma-like" (Tetu 1991), and the mucinous clefts and spaces without tumor cells have been designated "pseudomyxoma ovarii-like" (Tran 1998) and "mucinous breakdown" (Bullock 2002). The wispy blue mucin and crystalloids associated with adenocarcinoma can

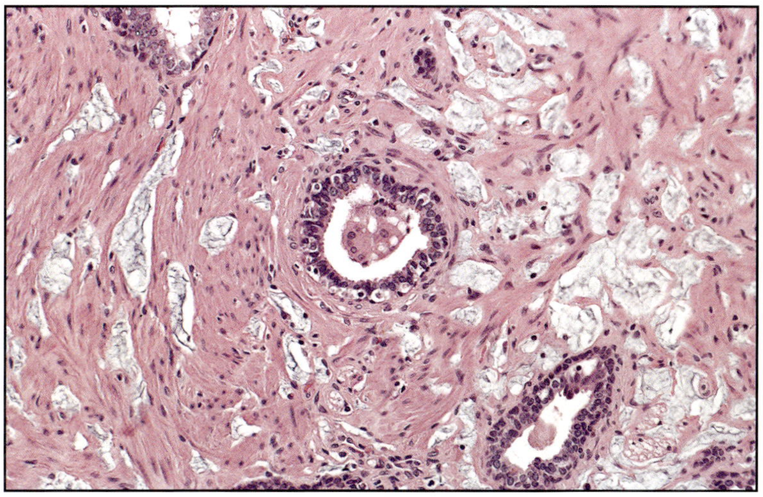

■ **i19.18** *Androgen deprivation therapy effect on prostatic carcinoma. The infiltrative nature of the treated carcinoma is indicated by the dissecting pattern of the residual clefts and aggregates of mucin.*

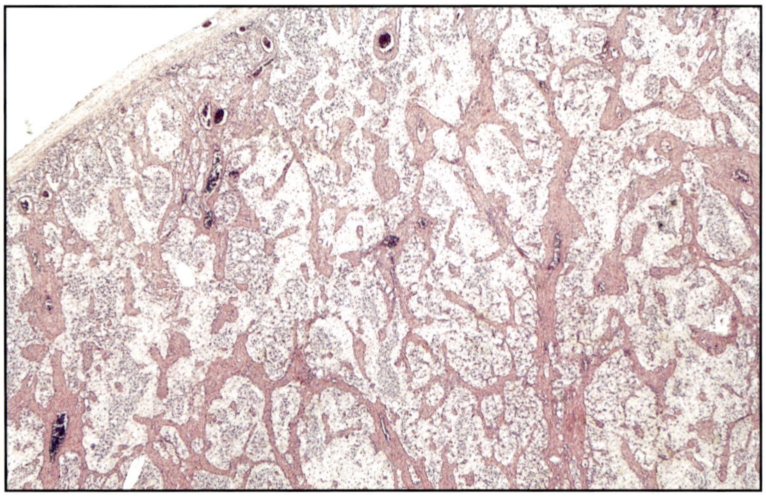

■ **i19.19** *Androgen deprivation therapy effect on prostatic carcinoma metastatic to a pelvic lymph node: masses of pale cells.*

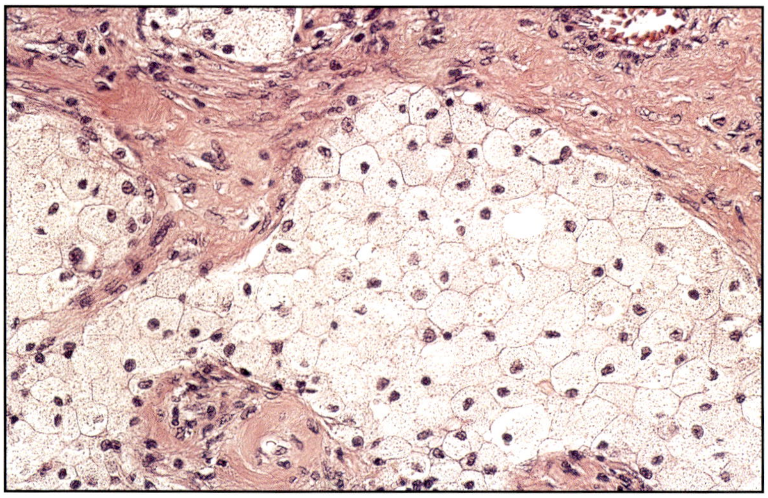

■ **i19.20** *Androgen deprivation therapy effect on prostate carcinoma metastatic to a pelvic lymph node: histiocytoid appearance of the carcinoma cells. (Higher power magnification of a field from* **i19.19***.)*

still be seen after hormonal therapy (Civantos 1996, Grignon 1995, Montironi 1998), although a lower frequency of intraluminal crystalloids has been noted (Montironi 1998, Vaillancourt 1996). Perineural invasion is also less common (Vaillancourt 1996). A pattern seen in a small minority (10%) of cases is one of large tumor cells with cleared cytoplasm within an exuberant lymphohistiocytic response (Civantos 1996). Such a marked lymphohistiocytic response can also be found in pelvic lymph nodes with treated carcinoma (Armas 1994, Schned 1996). Higher numbers of lymphocytic, eosinophilic, and granulomatous inflammatory cell infiltrates in the prostate are found in the treated than in the untreated patients. The prostatic stroma is sometimes edematous, fibrotic, or hyalinized and sclerotic (Civantos 1995, Helpap 1985, Van de Voorde 1994). Cytologically, carcinoma cells classically show nuclear pyknosis, hyperchromasia, and inconspicuous nucleoli **i19.15**. These features, in conjunction with cytoplasmic clearing and vacuolization, can impart a histiocytoid appearance to the treated tumor cells **i19.19, i19.20**.

The type of androgen deprivation **t19.1**, drug dosage, and treatment duration can all affect the observed histologic changes. Most earlier studies assessed the effect of estrogen treatment (with or without orchiectomy) **t19.2**, whereas more recent studies have focused on combined (also called total or complete) androgen blockade using LHRH analogs and nonsteroidal antiandrogens **t19.3**. Various studies have also evaluated single-agent therapies for histologic effects (Aus 1994, Eri 2001, Hellström 1993, Murphy 1991, Tetu 1991, Van Poppel 1993). Another confounding factor in comparative assessment of histologic alterations induced by various treatments is variable dosing and duration of treatment in different studies. Heterogeneity of tissue responsiveness (Murphy 1991, Tetu 1991) or minimal morphologic effects can result from variable duration (Reuter 1997) or low dosage (Eri 2001) and intrinsically variable androgen responsiveness of tumor cells. A morphologic response to androgen deprivation can occur after 1 week of therapy (Cosar 2001, Stattin 1998). Most studies have documented pathologic changes after several months of androgen deprivation therapy. Limited data exist on morphologic effects of treatment beyond 3 months, but a few studies suggest that increasing combined androgen blockade from 3 to 6 months further reduces tumor volume (Van der Kwast 1997), extraprostatic extension in clinical stage C disease (Bono 2001), and positive margins (Montironi 1999). With 8 months of neoadjuvant androgen withdrawal therapy before radical prostatectomy, the positive margin rate in one study was very low (at 4%) (Van der Kwast 1997). Tumor cell proliferation, as gauged by proliferating cell nuclear antigen and Ki-67 immunostains, was not increased in carcinoma cells exposed to 8 months of neoadjuvant therapy (Paterson 1999, Van der Kwast 1997). This finding was forwarded as an argument against one concern of prolonged androgen deprivation therapy: that it would select for highly proliferative androgen-independent clones, with progression during the prolonged therapy. Such a selection process may still have occurred, and the continuing concern is that after cessation of the androgen suppression, outgrowth of these androgen-independent, more lethal clones might ensue.

Hormonal therapy has been associated, in rare cases, with the emergence (or selection and progression) of prostatic carcinoma variants, including small cell carcinoma, sarcomatoid carcinoma, and squamous cell carcinoma (see Chapter 17). A few cases of these variants have been diagnosed after treatment of a typical acinar adenocarcinoma with hormonal therapy. The mechanistic basis for this is unknown.

Finasteride, a 4-aza analog of testosterone, is an androgen deprivation agent via its inhibition of 5α-reductase and the conversion of testosterone to dihydrotestosterone. It is clinically indicated for treating BPH, where it results in increased urine flow, decreased voiding symptoms, decreased serum PSA, and decreased prostate size, especially in men with larger prostates (Gormley 1992, McConnell 1998). Finasteride is also being tested as a chemopreventive agent in the placebo-controlled Prostate Cancer Prevention Trial, which enrolled 18 000 men with PSA levels = 3 ng/mL and a normal DRE. After 7 years, biopsy will be done to assess for the prevalence of carcinoma. The results of this clinical trial should be available sometime between 2004 and 2006 (McLeod 2000). Finasteride exhibits some of the same morphologic alterations as combined androgen blockage, but the effects are more prominent in benign epithelium (Andriole 1994, Bostwick 1997, Civantos 1997, Cote 1998, Epstein 1999, Marks 1997, 1999, McConnell 1998, Montironi 1996A, 1996B, Rittmaster 1996, Yang 1999). Most of the work on finasteride relates to its effects on benign and hyperplastic prostate tissue. Finasteride induces prostatic involution in benign tissues via atrophy and cell death of benign prostatic epithelium (Rittmaster 1996). There is a corresponding increase in the stromal-epithelial ratio (Marks 1997, Montironi 1996A). Apoptotic cell death, as indicated by increased TUNEL staining, is

■ **t19.4 Handling and Reporting Prostatic Tissues Hormonal Therapy**[1]

Confirm clinical history of hormonal therapy (if not provided)[2]
Submit all tissue
Histologic grading (Gleason or WHO) not recommended[3]
Grading of degree of treatment effect not recommended[4]
Routine pan-cytokeratin immunostaining not recommended[5]

[1]Modified from Grignon 1999
[2]Hormonal therapy effect can usually be recognized in histologic sections (Murphy 1991, Smith 1994, Drew 1997)
[3,4]Except for research purposes
[5]Pan-cytokeratin, 34βE12, PSA, and PSAP immunostains can be of value in selected cases

seen at 6 to 18 days (Rittmaster 1996), and long-term treatment of 24 to 40 months leads to progressive contraction of both transition zone and peripheral zone epithelium (Marks 1999). Basal cell prominence, cytoplasmic clearing, and squamous metaplasia have been described in a few patients (Andriole 1994, Civantos 1997, Montironi 1996B), but the precise finasteride-induced incidence of these changes is not clear. The effects of finasteride on PIN and carcinoma appear to be modest or nonexistent. The incidence and morphologic characteristics of PIN seem to be unaltered in finasteride-treated patients (Civantos 1997, Cote 1998, Yang 1999). In carcinoma, changes including apoptosis, cleared cytoplasm, less prominent nucleoli, small tumor glands separated by stroma, empty or mucin-filled gland spaces, and inflammation were described in a few cases (Civantos 1997), whereas no effect was observed in another series (Yang 1999).

Histologic grading of prostatic carcinoma after androgen deprivation therapy generally is not recommended (Grignon 1999) because the architectural changes of luminal collapse simulate high-grade carcinoma **t19.4**. That is, hormonal treatment (with the possible exception of finasteride) causes an upgrading of carcinoma such that after androgen deprivation, most prostatic carcinomas appear to be of high World Health Organization or Gleason grade (Armas 1994, Civantos 1995, Ferguson 1994, Hugosson 1996, Murphy 1991, Vaillancourt 1996). The argument may be made that this posttreatment appearance results from persistence of high-grade androgen-resistant clones. Arguing against this idea is the finding of a predominance of diploid tumors with low proliferation index in treated patients (Armas 1994).

Grading of hormonal therapy treatment effect has been attempted, with variable success (Ahlgren 1999, Bentley 2000, Dhom 1982, Helpap 1985, Stattin 1998, Van de Voorde 1994). Such regression grading systems are not generally recommended (Grignon 1999), although providing an estimate of the amount of tumor with treatment effect is an option. Development of posttherapy histologic grading and regression grading schemes that predict clinical outcome is a desirable goal for the future.

Pathologic staging is affected by androgen deprivation therapy in several ways. First, neoadjuvant androgen deprivation therapy is associated with a lower prevalence of extraprostatic extension (lower pT stage) and a lower frequency of positive margins. A recent meta-analysis of 7 randomized clinical trials comparing neoadjuvant androgen ablation and radical prostatectomy with radical prostatectomy alone for clinically localized prostatic cancer indicated that neoadjuvant treatment was associated with lower pathologic stage and negative surgical margins to a highly significant degree (Bonney 1998). Thus far, however, these favorable pathologic endpoints have not correlated with improved recurrence rates after surgery (Aus 1998, Klotz 1999, Schulman 2000). Second, pathologic staging and evaluation of surgical margins in radical prostatectomy specimens from patients treated with neoadjuvant hormonal therapy can be difficult. Specifically, if one is not aware of the architectural and cytologic alterations caused by androgen deprivation, carcinoma cells with treatment effect may not be recognized. A particular pattern that can be exceedingly challenging to appreciate as neoplastic is the scattered single cell arrangement **i19.12**. Here, pan-cytokeratin, PSA, and prostate-specific acid phosphatase (PSAP) immunostains can facilitate detection of a few scattered carcinoma cells outside the prostate glands or at the surgical margin. Routine use of these immunostains to assess stage and margins is not recommended (Grignon 1999); rather, they should be applied when uncertainty exists in interpretation of H&E-stained sections. In one study, use of AE1/AE3 anticytokeratin antibodies in immunohistochemistry increased detection of extraprostatic extension by carcinoma and positive surgical margins (Bazinet 1997). A related staging problem is the diagnosis of minimal residual carcinoma in radical prostatectomy tissues after neoadjuvant hormonal therapy. Complete embedding of prostate glands from patients treated with hormonal therapy probably is desirable but not absolutely necessary (Grignon 1999). Up-front, initial complete embedding of all prostatic tissue from radical prostatectomy specimens from these patients probably is the most efficient approach, given the often focal nature of the carcinoma. Certainly, before designating a case as no residual carcinoma (pT0), one should completely embed all prostatic tissue. If no carcinoma is seen in the initial sections of the completely blocked prostate, one should obtain deep H&E recuts or flip the blocks to obtain recuts. Only then should one resort to cytokeratin, PSA, and PSAP immunostains to aid in the search for histologically insidious carcinoma. In the literature, there are a few cases of residual carcinoma diagnosed with the aid of immunostains after an initial histologic pT0 assignment (Bazinet 1997, Gleave 1996). Immunostains for CD68 and high-molecular-weight cytokeratin (using antibody 34βE12) can be also helpful if there is a question of focal, residual, or treated carcinoma versus histiocytes or benign atrophic glands as mimics of treated carcinoma.

Immunoreactive PSA and PSAP in prostatic tissue sections can be reduced after hormonal therapy, in terms of both intensity of cellular staining and number of cells staining (Grignon 1985, Helpap 1985, Murphy 1991, Paterson 1999, Tetu 1991, Van de Voorde 1994). Cytokeratin expression is unaltered by hormonal therapy, so cytokeratin immunostains reactive with treated carcinoma (AE1/AE3 or CAM5.2) and benign glands (34βE12) are more helpful in difficult cases, although I usually run a panel of pan-cytokeratin, 34βE12, PSA, and PSAP immunostains, recognizing that PSA and PSAP may be less informative than in untreated cases.

Special studies other than immunohistochemistry are not currently of diagnostic usefulness in assessing hormonally treated prostatic carcinoma. Electron microscopic examination of treated prostatic carcinoma cells has been performed in a few cases (Armas 1994). The cleared epithelial cell cytoplasm contained few organelles and large liposomes. Apoptotic neoplastic cells were characterized by small nuclei with clumped chromatin. DNA ploidy did not distinguish treated from untreated carcinomas (Armas 1994).

In the differential diagnosis of hormonally treated prostatic tissues, one should note that benign prostatic tissue can mimic malignancy and, conversely, treated carcinoma can simulate benign proliferations. The changes induced in benign glands by hormonal treatment are among the most common pseudoneoplastic lesions in the prostate: atrophy and basal cell hyperplasia. Architectural order, lack of significant nuclear atypia, and presence of benign basal cells in a background of stromal dominance should direct one toward a benign diagnosis. Treated carcinoma cells can be mistaken for histiocytes and lymphocytes, particularly in tumor cells with marked treatment effect in the form of cytoplasmic vacuolization and nuclear shrinkage. Distinguishing treated carcinoma from inflammatory cells can be facilitated by paracytokeratin, PSA, PSAP, CD68, and CD45 immunohistochemical stains. Another pitfall is that a nodular and cellular stroma can be written off at low-power magnification as benign stromal nodule **i19.10**, whereas at higher magnification, clandestine growth of single cells **i19.12** or small nests or cords of tumor cells **i19.11** might be appreciated. The point here is that although untreated prostatic carcinoma often is suspected at low magnification because of architectural disturbances, higher-power views often are necessary to detect subtle infiltrates of hormonally treated carcinoma.

Experimental factors that predict, in preliminary studies, response to hormonal therapy include p53 and bcl-2 immunoreactivity (Apakama 1996) and DNA ploidy (Pollack 1997) in prostatic carcinoma tissues before institution of hormonal therapy. Patients with long CAG repeats also responded better to endocrine therapy (Bratt 1999). After androgen deprivation therapy, patients with androgen receptor gene amplification (Palmberg 2000) and lower proliferation index (Ahlgren 1999) in treated carcinoma tissue had a favorable response to second-line combined androgen blockade and longer progression-free survival, respectively. Unlike immunostains for hormone (estrogen and progesterone) receptors in breast carcinoma, immunostains for the androgen receptor in prostate carcinoma do not reliably predict response to androgen deprivation therapy (Noordzij 1997, Pertschuk 1994, 1995, Prins 1998, Ruizeveld de Winter 1994, Sadi 1991, Takeda 1996,). Expression of large numbers (hundreds) of genes and proteins is clearly modulated in prostatic carcinoma by androgens and androgen deprivation (Bostwick 2000, Xu 2001). Cell cycle and apoptotic pathways are clearly perturbed by androgen deprivation (Chapter 21) and are attractive avenues for further study. A more pressing objective for future research is discovery of markers that predict response to specific forms of androgen deprivation.

[19.3] Radiation Therapy

Radiation therapy can be used to treat clinically localized and locally advanced prostate cancer (Blasko 2000, D'Amico 2002, Porter 1999). The radiation can be delivered from an external source (external beam therapy), by implantation of radioactive sources ("seeds") into the gland (interstitial brachytherapy) (Horwitz 2000), or both. Radiation therapy can also be combined with hormonal therapy for patients advanced disease (Horwitz 2000). The most common tissue sample submitted after radiation therapy is a prostate needle biopsy specimen, in the setting of a rising serum PSA after therapy. Even though prostate rebiopsy after radiation therapy is not deemed necessary as standard follow-up care (ASTROCP 1999), rebiopsy remains an important research tool and is an independent predictor of clinical outcome (Crook 2000, Scardino 1986, Stock 2000). Also, rebiopsy can help in distinguishing local from distant recurrence because serum PSA measurement does not unequivocally discriminate between these 2 events. Whole prostate glands are available for examination when salvage radical prostatectomy (or even exenteration) is performed for locally recurrent prostate cancer. This salvage procedure is uncommon, and most series in the literature are small (Miles 2000, Rogers 1995) and include patients treated with both hormonal therapy and radiotherapy.

Gross descriptions of radiation effect on prostatic tissues have not been published. Microscopically, the effects of radiation treatment in prostatic tissue can be profound **t19.5, t19.6**. For benign prostatic tissue, the classic alterations are extensive atrophy, cytologic atypia, and basal cell prominence or hyperplasia (Bostwick 1982, Cheng 1999A, Dhom 1982, Gaudin 1999, Grignon 1995, Sheaff 1997) **t19.5**. Just as

■ t19.5 Essential Histologic Changes Induced by Radiation Therapy in the Prostate

Benign prostatic epithelium
Atrophy
Nuclear atypia: Nuclear pleomorphism and nucleolar prominence
Basal cell prominence/hyperplasia

High-grade PIN
Decrease in prevalence and extent

Adenocaricnoma
Decrease in number of neoplastic glands
Poorly formed glands and single cells
Cytoplasmic vacuolization
Nuclear pyknosis

■ t19.6 Histologic Features in Benign Prostatic Tissue After Radiation Therapy[1]

Compartment	Histologic Feature	% of Cases
Epithelium		
	Atrophy	27%-99%[2]
	Cytologic atypia	77%-99%
	Basal cell hyperplasia	68%-82%
	Squamous metaplasia	0%-63%[3]
	Paneth cell-like metaplasia	31%
	Cytoplasmic vacuolization	29%
	Mucinous metaplasia	21%
	Wispy blue luminal mucin	4%-12%
	Mitotic figures	0%-rare
Stroma		
	Chronic inflammation	7%-90%
	Stromal fibrosis	90-93%
	Foreign body giant cell reaction[4]	13%-44%
	Edema, calcification	21%
	Atypical (radiation) fibroblasts	11%-25%
Vessels		
	Arterial intimal hyperplasia	11%-92%
	Arterial medial thickening/hyalinization	85%
	Arterial luminal narrowing	82%
	Atherosis	21%
	Fibrinoid necrosis and thrombosis	"occasional"

[1]Bostwick 1982, Sheaff 1997, Gaudin 1999, Cheng 1999A
[2]Three studies: 79%, 80%, 99%. One study (Bostwick 1982): 27%
[3]Two studies: 59%, 63%. Two studies: 0%, 5%
[4]To extruded corpora amylacea

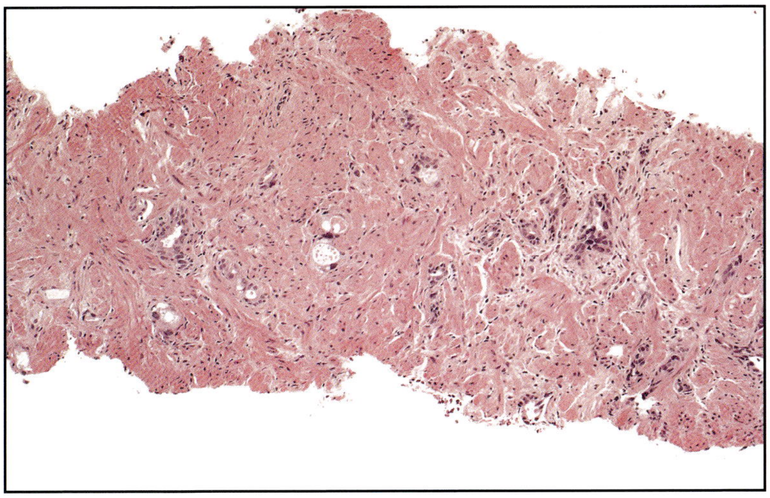

■ **i19.21** *Radiation treatment effect on benign prostatic tissue: Stromal dominance with scattered, atrophic small acini.*

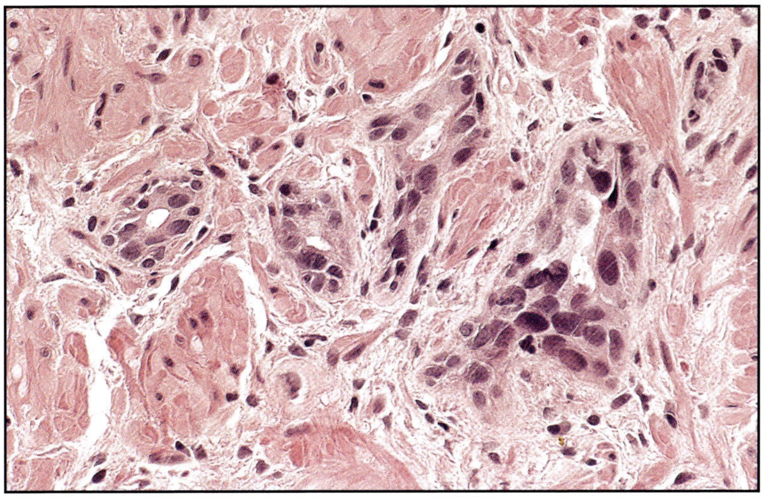

■ **i19.22** *Radiation treatment effect on benign prostatic glands: Nuclear atypia with nucleomegaly.*

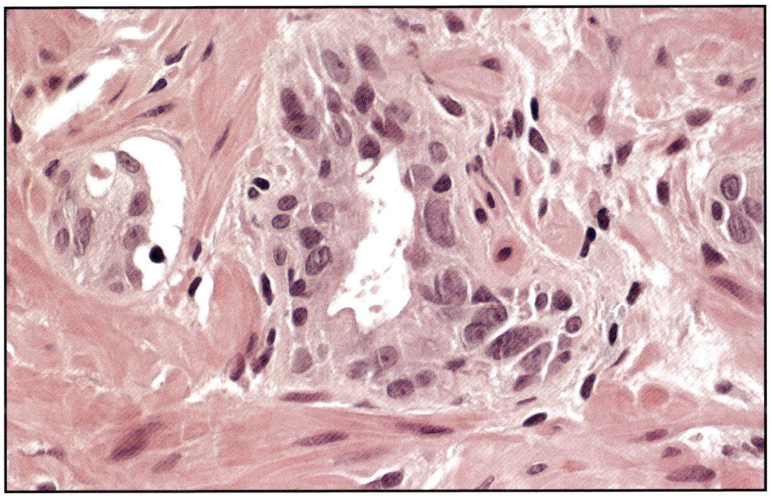

■ **i19.23** *Radiation treatment effect on benign prostatic glands: Nuclear atypia with macronucleoli.*

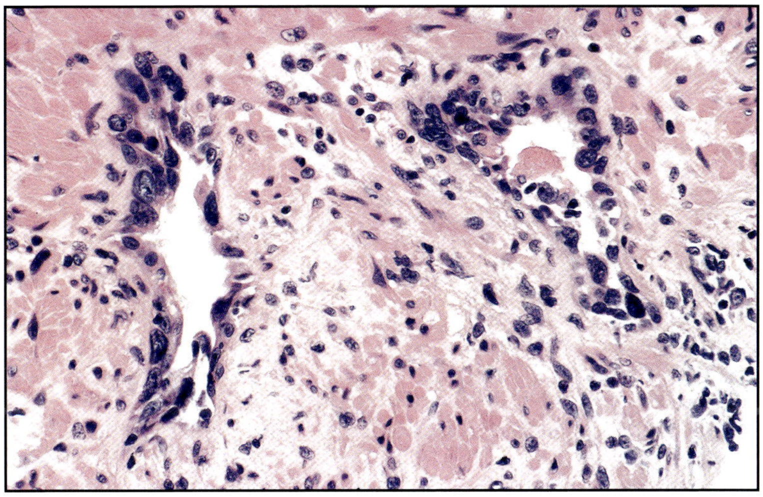

■ **i19.24** *Radiation treatment effect on benign prostatic glands: Nuclear atypia with hyperchromasia.*

for hormonal therapy, the first indication of treatment effect at low magnification is the large amount of stroma relative to a diminished number of glands, or stromal dominance **i19.21**. Both size and number of benign glands are reduced. Luminal secretory epithelial cells exhibit atrophy in the form of cytoplasm volume loss. Basal cells often are prominent or hyperplastic and often display pronounced nuclear atypia **i19.22, i19.23**. This latter feature has been called atypical basal cell hyperplasia (Cheng 1999A). The cytologic and nuclear atypia induced by radiation in benign epithelial nuclei in the prostate can mimic malignancy. Specifically, nucleomegaly and prominent nucleoli, including true macronucleoli (of several microns in diameter), can be seen in a majority of cases (Cheng 1999A). Nuclear pleomorphism is also evident, with variations in nuclear size and shape. These atypical nuclei may have a vacuolated or smudged, hyperchromatic appearance **i19.24** (Gaudin 1998). In these cases of radiation-induced nuclear atypia in benign prostatic epithelium, immunohistochemical detection of basal cells in the atypical glands can be extremely valuable in establishing a diagnosis of benign atypia **i19.25**. At the same time, shrunken and pyknotic nuclei can also present in a majority of cases (Cheng 1999A, Dhom 1982). Cytoplasmic changes include vacuolization, Paneth cell–like-metaplasia, mucinous metaplasia, and squamous metaplasia **t19.6**. The frequency of squamous metaplasia, as reported in the literature, is highly variable **t19.6**. As for hormonal therapy, this may relate to the difficulty in distinguishing immature

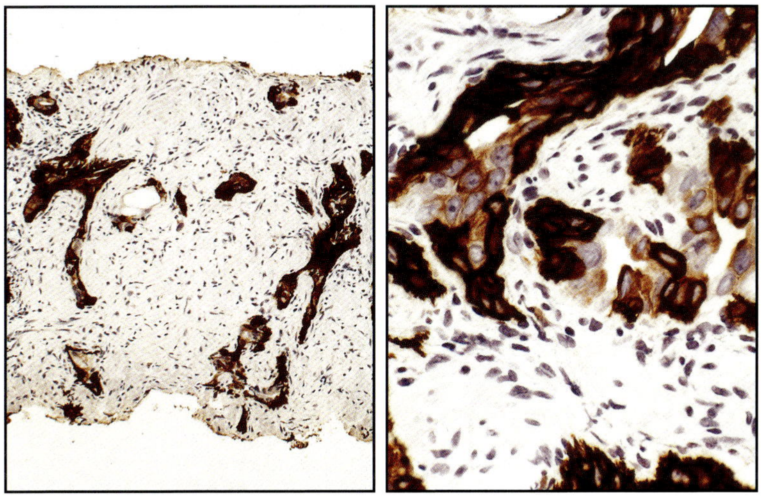

■ **i19.25** *Irradiated benign prostatic tissue: Basal cells identified in prostatic needle biopsy tissue by 34βE12 immunohistochemical stain. This immunostain is extremely valuable in difficult cases since cytological atypia are often not useful in distinguishing neoplastic nuclear atypia vs radiation-induced nuclear atypia in benign glands (low and higher magnification).*

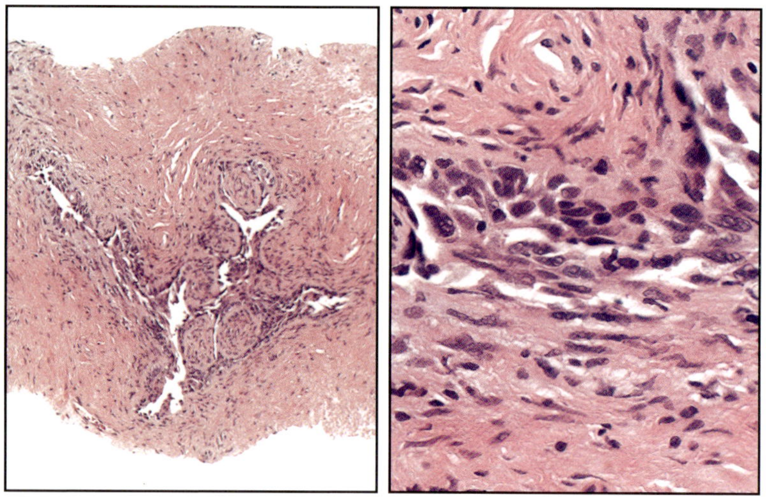

■ **i19.26** *Radiation treatment effect on benign prostatic tissue: Stromal fibrosis is present in most cases. Here the irradiated glands are distorted by the stromal fibrosis and exhibit nuclear atypia (low and higher magnification).*

squamous metaplasia from basal cell proliferation. Stromal and vascular changes are also common, with fibrosis **i19.26** and chronic inflammation evident in the stroma **t19.6**. Radiation (atypical, stellate) fibroblasts are only occasionally found. Severe vascular damage, with intimal and medial thickening, medial hyalinization, and luminal narrowing, is often noted **t19.6**.

High-grade prostatic intraepithelial neoplasia appears to be reduced in prevalence and extent after radiation therapy but can still be found in needle biopsy (Gaudin 1999) and salvage radical prostatectomy tissues (Arakawa 1995, Cheng 1999C, Wheeler 1996). The architecture of high-grade PIN (tufting, micropapillary, cribriform, and flat) does not appear to be altered by radiation therapy (Arakawa 1995, Cheng 1999C). Occasionally, basal cell prominence and cytoplasmic vacuolization may be appreciated (Cheng 1999C). The persistence of high-grade PIN after radiation therapy means that recurrent carcinoma could originate from this source, although it seems more likely that recurrent tumors derive from the initial incompletely eradicated tumor (Arakawa 1995).

Radiation-treated prostatic adenocarcinoma has a variable appearance, from cases showing no histologic changes to others that demonstrate marked alterations (Böcking 1987, Bostwick 1982, Cheng 1999A, Crook 1997, Dhom 1982, Gaudin 1998, 1999, Goldstein 1998, Grignon 1995, Helpap 1985). This heterogeneity of tumor cell responsiveness exists between patients and also in individual patients. It is more apparent in larger tissue samples and is most readily seen in radical prostatectomy specimens, where in almost all cases areas of cancer with little or no radiation effect could be identified (Cheng 1999A). The classical radiation-related histologic changes in carcinoma are a decrease in number of tumor glands, poorly formed glands and single cells, cytoplasmic vacuolization, nuclear pyknosis, and stromal fibrosis **i19.27, i19.28; t19.5**. The small amount of tumor is highlighted by one needle biopsy study in which about one third of cases had focal tumor involving <10% of needle core tissue (Cheng 1999A). The pattern of arrangement of the neoplastic glands is critical in recognition of malignancy because they are infiltrative or haphazardly disposed **i19.27, i19.28**. The individual glands of carcinoma often are distorted and poorly formed **i19.27**. Single neoplastic cells may be noticed **i19.28**. Cytologically, cytoplasmic vacuolization and nuclear pyknosis usually are present, but it is diagnostically reassuring that nuclear enlargement and prominent nucleoli are seen in most cases (Cheng 1999A). Perineural invasion by carcinoma should be specifically

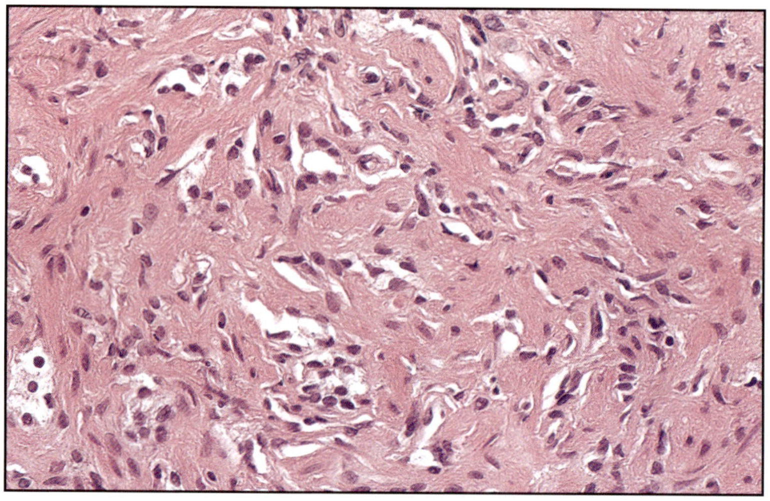

■ **i19.27** *Radiation therapy effect on prostatic adenocarcinoma: Small, irregular, atrophic malignant glands.*

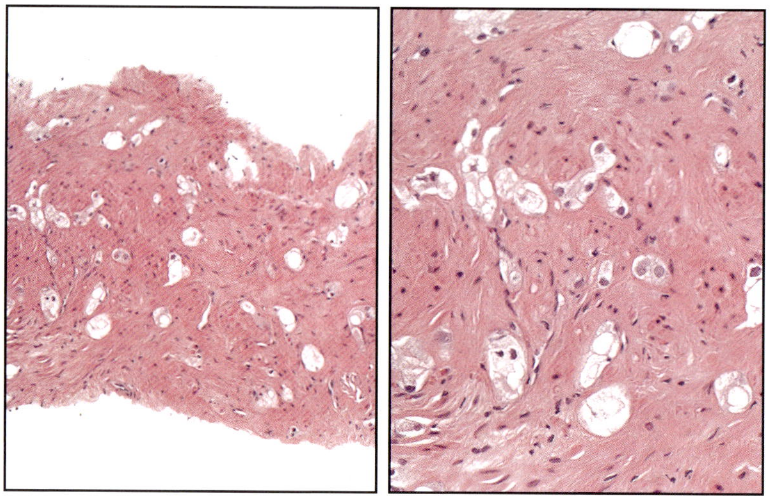

■ **i19.28** *Radiation treatment effect on prostatic adenocarcinoma: Small nests and single cells with vacuolated cytoplasm. Some of the spaces do not contain nuclei (low and higher magnification).*

sought because it can be detected up to 31% of cases in needle biopsy (Cheng 1999A).

In contrast, radiorecurrent or radioresistant prostatic adenocarcinoma in whole prostate glands resected in a salvage radical prostatectomy procedure typically is of large size (Cheng 1998, Link 1991), with extraprostatic extension. Most tumors are >3cm^3 (Cheng 1998, Link 1991, Rogers 1995), with a mean tumor volume of 11.1cm^3 (range 1.1cm^3 to 27.2cm^3) in one series (Link 1991). They are also locally extensive and usually invade outside the prostate. In the largest series of patients treated only with radiation therapy and radical prostatectomy, without hormonal therapy, 80% of cases had extraprostatic disease and fully 49% had seminal vesicle invasion (Rogers 1995).

The effect of radiation therapy on carcinoma histologic grade is variable (Grignon 1995). In cases without radiation effect, the Gleason grade remains unchanged (Crook 1997, Gaudin 1999), but in cases with radiation treatment effect, upgrading may occur. In several reports, the histologic grade (Gleason and MD Anderson Hospital grades) after radiation therapy was significantly higher than in the pretreatment carcinoma (Siders 1992, Wheeler 1993). This shift was ascribed to "dedifferentiation" of prostate cancer (Wheeler 1993) and outgrowth of a more aggressive clone. However, it probably reflects treatment effect simulating higher-grade carcinoma (Gaudin 1998, Grignon 1995).

Gleason grading should be attempted on radiation-treated carcinomas where there is no obvious treatment effect. Whether Gleason grading should be done in the face of significant radiation treatment effect is controversial (Bostwick 1999, Cheng 1999A, Gaudin 1999). In one study, the postradiation radical prostatectomy Gleason grade was an independent prognostic factor for the subset of patients in whom radiation therapy failed and who underwent radical prostatectomy (Cheng 1998). However, the current majority view, one shared by this author, is that Gleason grading should be applied, as it was in Gleason's original series, only to untreated carcinomas or, in the case of radiation therapy, to areas without radiation effect **t19.7**.

Immunohistochemical staining for basal cell high-molecular-weight cytokeratin (using, for example, antibody 34βE12) can be an extremely helpful diagnostic maneuver in evaluating atypical small glands in needle biopsy after radiation therapy **i19.25** (Brawer 1989, Cheng 1999A, Crook 1997, Gaudin 1999, Goldstein 1998, Grignon 1995). Demonstration of this cytokeratin staining in glands with atypical cells rules out recurrent or persistent adenocarcinoma. A negative result is supportive, in the correct histologic context and with appropriate controls, of a diagnosis of adenocarcinoma. Here, the best positive control is internal positive control staining of benign glands in the same needle core. No other special studies, such as determination of proliferation index or DNA ploidy status, are of diagnostic utility.

The differential diagnosis of radiation treatment effect focuses on irradiated, atypical benign glands and adenocarcinoma. Benign glands after irradiation can appear infiltrative, especially when they are atrophic and distorted by stromal sclerosis. The nuclear atypia in benign glands can be significant; indeed, in one morphometric study, the nuclear alterations (eg, increased nuclear size) in benign glands were actually greater in irradiated benign nuclei than irradiated carcinoma (Unger 1995). It has been emphasized that this nuclear atypia often assumes the form of atypical basal cell hyperplasia (Cheng 1999A). This change, which can persist for years, was recognized as the irradiation-induced alteration in benign glands that most often mimicked irradiated carcinoma (Cheng 1999A). In difficult cases such as this, staining for high-molecular-weight cytokeratin is essential. One should have a low threshold for ordering this immunostain in postirradiation needle biopsy cases. That said, this immunostain is not needed in every postirradiation needle biopsy case because some prostatic carcinomas show little or no radiation treatment effect and are not focal. Here, the diagnosis of recurrent or persistent adenocarcinoma is straightforward. A PSA immunostain has also been used to distinguish benign irradiated glands from adenocarcinoma (Crook 2000, Gaudin 1998). Irradiated benign glands often show weak or negative PSA immunoreactivity (Gaudin 1999) because they are atrophic and typically consist of atypical basal cells, whereas irradiated prostatic carcinoma maintains the same immunophenotype as nonirradiated carcinoma, with continued PSA and PSAP expression in most cases (Crook 1997, Grob 1994, Helpap 1991, Ljung 1997, Mahan 1980). However, a PSA immunostain is less informative than a high molecular weight cytokeratin immunostain.

Irradiated prostatic carcinoma, with pronounced treatment effect, can be difficult to detect, especially if it is focal. The finding of haphazardly distributed, small, distorted acini with nuclear atypia, cytoplasmic vacuolization, and absence of basal cells favors adenocarcinoma. In a small percentage of cases, a descriptive diagnosis of focal glandular atypia or "indeterminate" (Crook 2000) may be unavoidable. The definition of "indeterminate" has been either marked radiotherapy effect (Crook 2000) or glands with features of residual carcinoma with radiation effect (Prestidge 1997). This latter definition is confusing. A more logical approach would be to reserve this diagnosis for difficult cases in which, because of the presence of only a few atypical glands or marked radiation effect, a definitive diagnosis of benign or malignant cannot be made. In 2 large series, this diagnostic category constituted 7% to 33% of postirradiation biopsies (Crook 2000, Prestidge 1997). In one series, the incidence of an indeterminate diagnosis decreased over time from 33% at 1 year to 7% by nearly 4 years after radiation (Crook 2000).

Pretreatment factors that predict a clinical response to radiation therapy include clinical stage, pretreatment total serum PSA level, and pretreatment histologic grade in needle biopsy or TURP chip tissue **t19.8** (Barzell 1977, Grann 1998, Kattan 2000, 2001, Scalzo 1998, Siders 1992, Valicenti 2000). There is a suggestion in some studies that perineural invasion, amount of tumor in needle biopsy, DNA ploidy, bcl-2, p53, and proliferation index (Ki-67 labeling index or presence of any mitotic figures) might add predictive information on responsiveness (Algan 1999, Anderson 1998, Bonin 1997, Cheng 1998, Crook 2000, Gauwitz 1994, Goldstein 2002, Grann 1998, Grignon 1997, Huang 1998, Incognito 2000, Jimenez 2000, 2001, Khoo 1999, Lattanzi 1997, Mackey 1998, Scherr 1999, Song 1992, Stattin 1996). Most models incorporate at least pretreatment serum PSA level, clinical T stage, and Gleason histologic grade (Pisansky 1997, Vollmer 1999). A recently developed pretreatment nomogram uses these 3 parameters, radiation dosage, and presence or absence of hormonal therapy to predict 5-year freedom from cancer recurrence after 3-dimensional conformal radiotherapy (Kattan 2000). A similar model has been developed to predict response to brachytherapy (Kattan 2001). Many of these models harbor a degree of uncertainty in outcome prediction

■ t19.7 Handling and Reporting on Prostatic Tissues after Radiotherapy

Confirm clinical history of radiotherapy (if not provided)[1]
Histologic grading recommended only for tumor areas not showing treatment effect
Grading of degree of treatment effect not required, but WHO recommends a comment on severity and extent of treatment changes[2]
Routine high molecular weight cytokeratin immunostaining (eg, with 34βE12) not required but can be extremely useful in selected cases

[1]Radiotherapy effect can usually be suspected in histologic sections
[2]No agreement exists on method (Bostwick 1999)

■ t19.8 Factors Predictive of Clinical Response to Radiation Therapy of Prostatic Carcinoma

Pre-treatment
Serum PSA level
Clinical Stage
Histologic grade
Radiation dose
Experimental: perineural invasion, amount of tumor in needle biopsy, DNA ploidy, proliferation index, bcl-2, and p53

Post-irradiation
Presence of carcinoma in biopsy
Pathologic stage in salvage radical prostatectomy specimens
Experimental: Grade of treatment response, amount of residual tumor in needle biopsy, DNA ploidy, and proliferation index

(Vollmer 1999), suggesting that additional clinical, histologic, or molecular markers may aid in model refinement.

The frequency and clinical significance of a prostate biopsy positive for carcinoma after radiation therapy have been long debated (Grignon 1995). The frequency of a biopsy positive for carcinoma has varied from series to series (Crook 1997, 2000, Kabalin 1989, Kiesling 1980, Ljung 1996, Miller 1993, Mollenkamp 1975, Prestidge 1997, Scardino 1986, Stock 2000), with a range of 11% (Stock 2000) to 93% (Kabalin 1989). The positivity frequency depends on the characteristics of the patient population (stage, grade, serum PSA level), timing and extent of needle biopsy sampling, and dosage of radiation therapy. In the past, the significance of finding carcinoma in prostate needle biopsy after radiation was questioned because there was uncertainty about whether the treated carcinoma cells were biologically active.

It is now clear that biopsy detection of carcinoma 6 to 36 months after completion of therapy is related to clinical failure, as judged by PSA levels, distant metastases, and death from prostate cancer (Crook 2000, Freiha 1984, Goldstein 1998, Grignon 1995, Kiesling 1980, Miller 1993, Scardino 1986, Stock 2000). The clinical significance and biopsy positivity rate may relate to the timing of the biopsy after completion of radiotherapy. For patients with biopsies done at 12 to 18 months after therapy, about 30% of men have subsequent negative biopsies (Crook 2000). This has been interpreted as tumor clearance but could easily represent sampling error in which residual tumor was not sampled. Nevertheless, most authors support performance of prostate needle biopsy no earlier than 18 to 24 months after radiotherapy (Crook 2000, Gaudin 1998, Miller 1993, Scardino 1986).

Although a positive needle biopsy is one of the strongest indicators of clinical failure (along with the PSA nadir after therapy [Crook 2000]), a positive biopsy does not always herald clinical failure, and conversely, a negative biopsy does not always signal that the patient is cured. The meaning of an "indeterminate" diagnosis (Crook 2000) or a descriptive diagnosis of atypia in prostate needle biopsy after radiotherapy is just now being addressed. Follow-up biopsies after an indeterminate diagnosis have yielded variable results, with 30% to 82% being negative, 9% to 34% being indeterminate again, and 6% to 20% showing carcinoma (Crook 2000, Prestidge 1997). Prospective study of larger numbers of patients with uniform and long follow-up will be needed to substantiate these data and narrow the ranges.

Tissue-based factors after radiation treatment that predict a clinical response to radiotherapy include the presence of carcinoma in needle biopsy and, for patients who underwent radiotherapy followed by salvage radical prostatectomy, pathologic stage in the radical prostatectomy specimen (Rogers 1995) **t19.8**. Surgical margin status may also be important in this cohort of patients (Lerner 1995). For patients who undergo radical prostatectomy followed by salvage radiation therapy, conflicting data exist on whether pathologic features in the radical prostatectomy specimen predict response to subsequent radiotherapy (reviewed in Leventis 2001). Potential indicators of response to radiotherapy in treated tissues include grade of treatment response (Bôcking 1987, Crook 1997, 2000, Dhom 1982, Goldstein 1998, Helpap 1985, Soman 2001), amount of tumor in needle biopsy (Soman 2001), Gleason grade (Cheng 1998), DNA ploidy (Cheng 1998, Lerner 1995), and proliferation index (Crook 2000).

Several different methods of histologic grading of treatment effect (regressive grading or RT effect grade) have been devised (Bôcking 1987, Dhom 1982, Helpap 1985). The grading is based on the amount of residual tumor and cytologic characteristics of the treated carcinoma cells (Dhom 1982). Prediction of response to therapy using RT effect grade has been noted (Crook 1997, Goldstein 1998, Soman 2001), but in a recent large, prospective study RT effect grade did not affect clinical failure (Crook 2000). Also in the experimental category because of limited data are amount of tumor after radiation (Soman 2001) and Gleason grade after radiation (Cheng 1998). Gleason grading of carcinoma with histologic treatment effect after radiation therapy is not recommended. Potential biomarkers in radiation-treated tissue that warrant further study include DNA ploidy (Cheng 1998, Lerner 1995), proliferation index (using proliferating cell nuclear antigen or MIB-1 immunohistochemical stains), and p53. Locally recurrent tumors after irradiation can exhibit increased proliferation index and p53 protein accumulation (Grossfeld 1998), but these 2 indicators so far do not appear to be independently associated with patient outcome (Cheng 1999B, Rakozy 1999). New biomarker discovery via gene expression profiling of treated prostatic carcinoma is an important research avenue for the future.

In extremely rare cases, radiation therapy for prostatic carcinoma has been associated, with the emergence of unusual histologic variants, including sarcomatoid carcinoma and squamous cell carcinoma (see Chapter 17). A few cases of postirradiation prostatic sarcoma after external beam radiation therapy for localized prostatic adenocarcinoma have also been reported (Chapter 18). Overall, however, the risk of developing a postirradiation prostatic sarcoma is extremely low and is probably similar to, if not lower than, the cited risk of 0.03% to 0.8% for all patients treated with radiation therapy (Weiss 2001).

[19.4] Chemotherapy

Chemotherapy may be considered for patients with metastatic, hormone-refractory (androgen-independent) prostate cancer (Eisenberger 2002, Logothetis 2000, Oh 1998, Scher 2001). Although no effect on survival has been demonstrated in a prospective, randomized, controlled trial, chemotherapeutic agents may be used for palliation and to delay progression (Scher 2001). These agents include mitoxantrone, etoposide, cisplatin, estramustine, vinblastine, taxanes (paclitaxel or docetaxel), doxorubicin, mitoguazone, trimetrexate, fluorouracil, and cyclophosphamide (Logothetis 2000, Oh 1998, Scher 2001, Walther 2000). Little is known about the histomorphologic effects of these drugs on prostate cancer (Clark 2001, Matsuda 1995, Pettaway 2000) because metastatic deposits in these patients are rarely biopsied. Recently, several small trials (33 and 18 patients) of chemotherapy use have been conducted in the neoadjuvant setting before radical prostatectomy for clinical stage T1 to 3 (Pettaway 2000) and T2b/c-T3 (Clark 2001) disease. In the study on combined neoadjuvant chemotherapy and hormonal therapy, pT0 status was not achieved in any case (Pettaway 2000). That is, all radical prostatectomy specimens had residual carcinoma. In the study in which estramustine (estradiol attached to nitrogen mustard) and etoposide (a topoisomerase II inhibitor) were administered before radical prostatectomy, there was little histologic evidence in radical prostatectomy tissues of antitumor effect beyond that associated with androgen deprivation (induced by estramustine) (Clark 2001). Tumoral necrosis was not seen, and residual cancer was present in every case (no pT0 cases).

[19.5] Miscellaneous Therapies

The tissue effects of a variety of miscellaneous therapies for BPH or prostate cancer **t19.9** have been described.

t19.9 Miscellaneous Therapies for BPH and/or Prostate Cancer with Prostatic Tissue Effects

Medical therapy for BPH
Alpha-blockade (α-1 adrenoreceptor antagonists)
Phytotherapy (herbal therapy)
Minimally invasive therapy for BPH
High-intensity focused ultrasound (HIFU)*
Laser therapy*
Transurethral balloon dilation of the prostate
Hyperthermia and thermotherapy*
Transurethral electrovaporization
Intraurethral stents
Transurethral needle ablation (TUNA)
Experimental prostate cancer therapy
Cryotherapy
Gene therapy

*Also used on experimental basis to treat prostate cancer

[19.6] Medical Therapy for BPH

Alpha-blockade by use of α-adrenoreceptor antagonists is a common BPH treatment that works by relaxing prostate and bladder neck smooth muscle (Lowe 2001). Little is known of the histomorphologic effects of these antagonists, such as doxazosin, terazosin, and tamsulosin, although there is a suggestion that the former 2 drugs can induce apoptosis in prostatic epithelial and smooth muscle cells and loss of smooth muscle cells without an effect on cell proliferation (Chon 1999, Kyprianou 1998). A similar induction of apoptosis by these same 2 agents was recently observed in vitro in 2 human prostatic carcinoma cell lines (Kyprianou 2000), but it is not known whether this can occur in vivo in patients. The amount of smooth muscle in prostatic pretreatment biopsy correlates with response to terazosin (Shapiro 1992), but this is currently an experimental tool only.

Phytotherapy, or herbal therapy, is the use of plant extracts for treat disease. A variety of such extracts have been used to treat BPH, especially in Europe, including *Urtica dioica* (stinging nettle), *Secale cereale* (rye pollen), the root of *Hypoxis rooperi* (South African star grass), the fruit of *Sabal serrulata* (or *Serenoa repens,* the dwarf palm), the bark of *Pygeum africanam* (African plum), pollen extract, the seeds of *Cucurbita pepo* (pumpkin seeds), the leaves of the *Populus tremula* (aspen), and the roots of *Echinacea purpurea* (purple cone flower) (Helpap 1995, Lepor 2002, Lowe 2001, 1998, Marks 2000, Wilt 1998). Little is known of the effect of these extracts on the histologic appearance of benign and hyperplastic prostatic tissue. In one study on extracts of *Sabal serrulata* (saw palmetto), there was a reported "significant reduction in periglandular stromal edema, mucoid degeneration, intraglandular congestion and congestive prostatitis" (Helpap 1995). There was no effect on prostatic epithelium. These alterations were forwarded as an explanation for the reported clinical benefit of saw palmetto in treating BPH. A second recent investigation (Marks 2000) on the use of pills containing saw palmetto extract to treat BPH demonstrated no change in inflammation but rather a prostatic "epithelial contraction," with a decrease in the amount of epithelium and an increase in atrophy. Resolution of these reported differences in histologic alterations induced by saw palmetto and characterization of the tissue effects of all phytotherapeutic agents should be addressed as correlative science components of larger, long-term, multicenter, randomized, double-blind, placebo-controlled studies performed to ascertain the true clinical efficacy of these agents in treating BPH (Lepor 2001, Lowe 1998).

[19.7] Minimally Invasive Therapy for BPH

A number of minimally invasive therapies for BPH treatment **t19.9** have been devised as alternatives to medical therapy and TURP (although TURP remains the gold standard for clinical improvement after treatment for BPH) (Fitzpatrick 2002). Several of these therapies, namely high-intensity focused ultrasound (HIFU), laser therapy, and heat therapy, have also been used experimentally to treat prostate cancer. In many of the procedures, in contrast with TURP, tissue is not submitted for histologic examination. Nevertheless, one should be acquainted with the tissue effects of these therapies in the event that a biopsy or tissue sample is obtained after therapy.

HIFU achieves thermal tissue ablation by heating tissue with a rectal probe (McCullough 1998). HIFU induces large areas (up to 22mm in diameter) of coagulative necrosis in benign prostatic tissues (Madersbacher 1997, Susani 1993), with hemorrhagic necrosis grossly and microscopically evident at 5 to 7 days and formation of granulation tissue in 10 weeks (Susani 1993). HIFU has also been used experimentally to treat prostate cancer (Beerlage 1999A, 1999B, Chaussy 2000, Gelet 1996, 1999, Kiel 2000, Madersbacher 1995, Van Leeders 2000). As in benign prostatic tissue, coagulative necrosis of carcinomatous tissue can be achieved. However, not all tumor was ablated, and viable carcinoma remained in 30% to 70% of patients after HIFU treatment (Beerlage 1999B, Kiel 2000, Madersbacher 1995), as assessed by post-HIFU needle biopsy (Kiel 2000) or radical prostatectomy (Beerlage 1999B, Madersbacher 1995). Viable-appearing carcinoma could even be seen in HIFU-induced necrotic zones (Van Leeders 2000).

Laser therapy has also been used to treat both BPH and prostate cancer (Boni 1997, Costello 1994, Cowan 1995, Fournier 1995, McCullough 1998, Milam 1995, Pow-Sang 1995, Sulser 1997). Lasers introduced into the prostate urethra can induce prostate ablation via coagulative necrosis, incision, or contact vaporization of tissue (Fournier 1995). The morphologic effects are variable and dependent on amount of energy delivered, tissue contact (Fournier 1995), and time after treatment (Costello 1994, Cowan 1995, Pow-Sang 1995). Acutely and immediately after treatment, a brown or black eschar can be seen grossly (Cowan 1995). Periurethral coagulative necrosis and vaporization occur at low and high dosages, respectively (Cowan 1995). At 24 hours, acute inflammation and edema are noted (Costello 1994). By 1 week, there are wide zones of coagulative necrosis with a rim of inflammation and hemorrhage; dilated vessels, vascular thrombosis, and squamous metaplasia are seen adjacent to the necrotic tissue (Boni 1997, Costello 1994, Cowan 1995). Sloughing of much of the coagulated tissue is noticed at 7 weeks (Cowan 1995, Pow-Sang 1995). Granulation tissue formation, lymphocytes, macrophages, and squamous metaplasia are detected at the base of the defect (Cowan 1995). At 10 to 12 weeks, a periurethral cavity can be found (Cowan 1995,

Pow-Sang 1995), with a reepithelialized surface and a rim of inflammation and squamous metaplasia (Cowan 1995, Pow-Sang 1995). At nearly 1 year after laser therapy, ischemic change and squamous metaplasia are persistent (Costello 1994). These data are based on only a few patients, but they give one a sense of what to expect if confronted with a tissue sample from a patient treated with laser therapy.

Hyperthermia and thermotherapy use high temperatures to treat BPH or prostate cancer (Arai 1996, De La Rosette 1997, Devonec 1991, Khair 1999, Larson 1996, Mauroy 1997, McCullough 1998, Yerushalmi 1982). Heat usually is delivered to the prostate via transurethral devices that emit microwaves or radiofrequency waves (De La Rosette 1997, McCullough 1998). The tissue defect depends on the temperature achieved in the prostate and probably on tissue composition and vascularization (Arai 1996, De La Rosette 1997, Devonec 1991, Khair 1999, Larson 1996, Mauroy 1997, McCullough 1998). Heat-induced prostatic cell death can be achieved by heating BPH tissue to 45° for 30 minutes (Devonec 1991). However, much higher temperatures (up to 75°C) are necessary to create a periurethral cavity, as in laser therapy and TURP (McCullough 1998). Immediately after heat treatment, histologic evidence of coagulation necrosis and periurethral vascular thrombosis can be seen (Mauroy 1997). Small vessel thrombosis is also seen after 1 week (Devonec 1991). At an average of slightly more than 1 month after heat application, light microscopy reveals sharply circumscribed and uniform, broad areas of hemorrhagic necrosis without significant inflammation (Larson 1996). Two months after microwave heat treatment, the necrotic area exhibits signs of organization, especially at the periphery, where fibroblasts and histiocytes are seen (Larson 1996). By 1 year, there is periurethral fibrosis, scant necrosis, nonspecific chronic inflammation, and squamous metaplasia of the urethra. There is no apparent difference in the capacity of transurethral microwave thermotherapy to induce cell death in benign prostatic tissue, hyperplastic tissue, or prostatic carcinoma (Narayan 1996). Substantial but rarely complete tumoral necrosis was identified in a series of 9 patients who underwent transurethral microwave thermotherapy followed by radical prostatectomy (Khair 1999). In this small but informative series, the amount of cancer ablated by this treatment depended on prostate size, cancer volume, and amount of cancer in the transition zone (Khair 1999).

Transurethral electrovaporization of the prostate can be accomplished using heat from electrical energy delivered by a rounded rollerball or grooved electrode (McCullough 1998). Vaporization of prostatic tissue occurs when the electrode contacts and heats the tissue to >100°C. Coagulative necrosis and intravascular thrombosis are found in the bed of the tissue defect (Narayan 1996). The amount of vaporized and coagulated prostatic tissue depends, in part, on wattage, drag sped of the electrode, and type of electrode (Narayan 1996).

Transurethral needle ablation of the prostate is performed by delivery of interstitial radiofrequency waves via needles placed into the prostate through the urethra (Hourriez 1994, McCullough 1998, Zlotta 1998). This causes coagulation necrosis around the needle tips, with a lesional diameter of up to 4.5cm (Hourriez 1994, Zlotta 1998).

[19.8] Experimental Prostate Cancer Therapy

Several experimental therapies for prostate cancer, such as cryotherapy and gene therapy, have been reported to cause tissue alterations. Little is known of the prostate tissue effects of gene therapy because only a few patients have been treated (Ayala 2000). In the few patients treated with herpes simplex virus thymidine kinase gene followed by ganciclovir, tumor necrosis with loss of nuclear detail was seen (Ayala 2000). An inflammatory cell infiltrate made up of lymphocytes and macrophages was found in benign and malignant prostate tissue (Ayala 2000). Almost nothing is known of the effects on prostate cancer tissue of another experimental therapy, phytotherapy (or herbal therapy), such as saw palmetto, which is being used by patients with prostate cancer (Nam 1999).

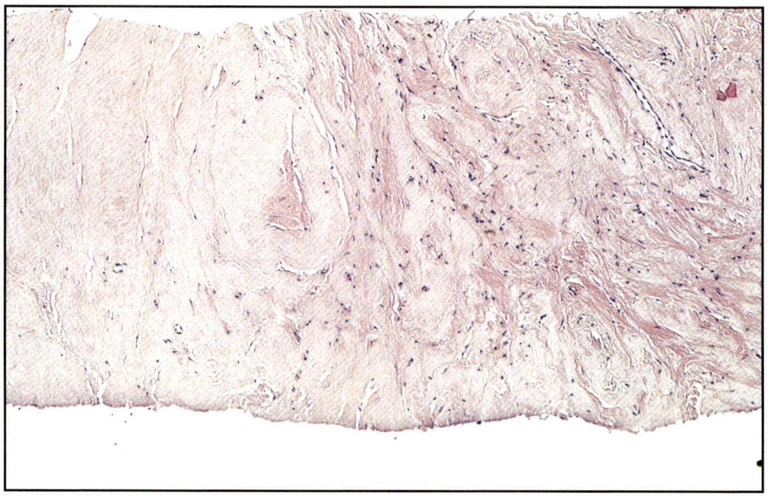

■ **i19.29** *Post cryotherapy prostate needle biopsy: Hyalinization and fibrosis, with absence of glandular elements.*

Cryotherapy of the prostate involves freezing the gland, creating an intraprostatic "ice ball" by use of transrectal ultrasound–guided placement of cryoprobes (Borkowski 1996, Colbach 1997, Donnelly 2001, Falconieri 1996, Gonder 1965, Grampsas 1995, Hansen 1973, Morgenstern 1997, Petersen 1978, Pisters 1999, Shabaik 1995, Shinohara 1997, 2002, Shuman 1997). Ultrasound can be used to monitor the size of the ice ball. Histologic changes depend on time of tissue sampling after cryotherapy. Edema and hemorrhage are seen immediately after freezing and in the first posttreatment week (Petersen 1978). Necrosis is found 10 days to 30 weeks after freezing (Petersen 1978, Shabaik 1995). Reparative alterations with stromal fibrosis, hyalinization, and inflammation predominate after 10 weeks (Petersen 1978). The most common microscopic findings in prostate needle biopsy at 5 to 48 weeks after cryotherapy include stromal fibrosis and hyalinization **i19.29**, basal cell hyperplasia, coagulative necrosis, and inflammation **t19.10**. Cryotherapy does not completely eradicate prostatic carcinoma. Residual carcinoma has been detected in 8% to 25% of

■ **t19.10 Histologic Findings in Prostate Needle Biopsy Tissue After Cryotherapy**

Histologic Feature	% of Cases[1]
Stromal fibrosis/hyalinization	53%-85%
Basal cell hyperplasia	73%
Coagulative necrosis	28%-100%
Inflammation[2]	49%
Hemorrhage/hemosiderin	24%-35%
Squamous metaplasia	21%-34%
Dystrophic calcification	13%-47%
Transitional cell metaplasia	12%
Edema	12%

[1]Data from Shabaik 1995, Borkowski 1996
[2]Usually lymphocytes and plasma cells

postcryotherapy prostate needle biopsies (Borkowski 1996, Morgenstern 1997, Shabaik 1995, Shinohara 1997, Shuman 1997). Carcinoma without treatment effect can be seen in many cases (Falconieri 1996, Shabaik 1995), and "incipient tumor regression," characterized by tumor cell–marked cytoplasmic swelling and chromatin smudging was noticed in some cases (Falconieri 1996). In cases in which the differential diagnosis is carcinoma with treatment effect versus inflamed, hyperplastic, or metaplastic benign epithelium, 34βE12 immunohistochemical detection of basal cells in benign conditions can be a useful diagnostic maneuver (Colbach 1997). Gleason grading seems feasible after prostatic cryotherapy because Gleason scores before and after cryotherapy are almost identical (Borkowski 1996, Shabaik 1995). A few radical prostatectomies have been done after cryosurgery (Donnelly 2001, Grampsas 1995, Pisters 1999), with variable results. In 10 of 15 cases, residual carcinoma was present in the whole prostate gland. In only 1 case was complete ablation of benign and malignant tissue in the entire prostate gland reported (Donnelly 2001). Cryotherapy followed by radical prostatectomy was associated with a substantial increase in morbidity, with the main problem being urinary incontinence (Pisters 1999).

References

Ahlgren G, Pedersen K, Lundberg S, et al. Tumor cell proliferation in prostate cancer after 3 months of neoadjuvant LHRH analogue treatment is a prognostic marker of recurrence after radical prostatectomy. *Urology* 54:329-324, 1999.

Algan O, Pinover WH, Hanlon AL, et al. Is there a subset of patients with PSA > or = 20 ng/ml who do well after conformal beam radiotherapy? *Radiat Oncol Investig* 7:106-110, 1999.

Anderson PR, Hanlon AL, Patchefsky A, et al. Perineural invasion and Gleason 7-10 tumors predict increased failure in prostate cancer patients with pretreatment PSA <10 ng/ml treated with conformal external beam radiation therapy. *Int J Radiat Oncol Biol Phys* 41:1087-1092, 1998.

Andriole GL, Hasan MU, Humphrey P. Finasteride induced changes in prostate histomorphology [abstract]. *J Urol* 151:507A, 1994.

Apakama I, Robinson MC, Walter NM, et al. bcl-2 overexpression combined with p53 protein accumulation correlates with hormone-refractory prostate cancer. *Br J Cancer* 74:1258-1262, 1996.

Arai Y, Fukuzawa S, Terai A, et al. Transurethral microwave thermotherapy for benign prostatic hyperplasia: relation between clinical response and prostate histology. *Prostate* 28:84-88, 1996.

Arakawa A, Song S, Scardino PT, et al. High-grade prostatic intraepithelial neoplasia in prostates removed following irradiation failure in the treatment of prostatic adenocarcinoma. *Pathol Res Pract* 191:868-872, 1995.

Armas OA, Aprikian AG, Melamed J, et al. Clinical and pathological effects of neoadjuvant total androgen ablation therapy on clinically localized prostatic adenocarcinoma. *Am J Surg Pathol* 18:979-991, 1994.

ASTROCP (American Society of Therapeutic Radiology and Oncology Consensus Panel). Consensus statements on radiation therapy of prostate cancer: guidelines for prostate re-biopsy after radiation and for radiation therapy with rising prostate-specific antigen levels after radical prostatectomy. *J Clin Oncol* 17:1155-1163, 1999.

Aus G, Brändstedt S, Häggman M, et al. Effects of 3 months' neoadjuvant hormonal treatment with a GnRH analogue (Triptorelin) prior to radical retropubic prostatectomy on prostate-specific antigen and tumor volume in prostate cancer. *Eur Urol* 26:22-28, 1994.

Aus G, Abrahamsson PA, Ahlgren G, et al. Hormonal treatment before radical prostatectomy: a 3-year follow-up. *J Urol* 159:2013-2017, 1998.

Ayala G, Wheeler TM, Shalev M, et al. Cytopathic effect of in situ gene therapy in prostate cancer. *Hum Pathol* 31:866-870, 2000.

Bainborough AR. Squamous metaplasia of prostate following estrogen therapy. *J Urol* 68:329-336, 1952.

Barzell W, Bean MA, Hilaris BS, et al. Prostatic adenocarcinoma: relationship of grade and local extent to the pattern of metastases. *J Urol* 118:278-282, 1977.

Bazinet M, Hamdy SM, Bégin LR, et al. Prognostic significance of antigenic heterogeneity, Gleason grade, and ploidy of lymph node metastases in patients with prostate cancer. *Prostate* 20:311-326, 1992.

Bazinet M, Zheng W, Begin LR, et al. Morphologic changes induced by neoadjuvant androgen ablation may result in undetection of positive surgical margins and capsular involvement by prostatic adenocarcinoma. *Urology* 49:721-725, 1997.

Beerlage HP, van Leenders GJLK, Oosterhof GON, et al. High-intensity focus ultrasound (HIFU) followed after one to two weeks by radical retropubic prostatectomy: results of a prospective study. *Prostate* 39:41-46, 1999A.

Beerlage HP, Thuroff S, Debruyne EM, et al. Transrectal high-intensity focused ultrasound using the Ablatherm device in the treatment of localized prostate carcinoma. *Urology* 54:273-277, 1999B.

Beisland HO, Sander S. Localized prostate carcinoma treated with TUR and neodymium-YAG laser irradiation. *Scand J Urol Nephrol* 138(suppl):117-119, 1991.

Bentley G, Dey J, Sakr WA, et al. Significance of the Gleason scoring system after neoadjuvant hormonal therapy. *Mol Urol* 4:125-130, 2000.

Blasko JC, Mate TP. Brachytherapy. In: Vogelzang NJ, Scardino PT, Shipley WU, et al, eds. *Genitourinary Oncology,* 2nd ed. Philadelphia: Lippincott Williams & Wilkins; 754-761, 2000.

Bôcking A, Auffermann W. Cytological grading of therapy-induced tumor regression in prostatic carcinoma: proposal of a new system. *Diagn Cytopathol* 3:108-111, 1987.

Boni RAH, Sulser T, Jochum W, et al. Laser ablation-induced changes in the prostate: findings at endorectal MR imaging with histologic correlation. *Radiology* 202:232-236, 1997.

Bonin SR, Hanlon AL, Lee WR, et al. Evidence of increased failure in the treatment of prostate carcinoma patients who have perineural invasion treated with three-dimensional conformal radiation therapy. *Cancer* 79:75-80, 1997.

Bonney WW, Schned AR, Timberlake DS. Neoadjuvant androgen ablation for localized prostatic cancer: pathology methods, surgical endpoints and meta-analysis of randomized trials. *J Urol* 160:1754-1760, 1998.

Bono AV, Pagano F, Montironi R, et al. on behalf of the Italian PROSIT Study Group. Effect of complete androgen blockade on pathologic stage and margin status of prostate cancer: progress pathology report of the Italian PROSIT study. *Urology* 57:117-121, 2001.

Borkowski P, Robinson MJ, Poppiti RJ Jr, et al. Histologic findings in postcryosurgical prostatic biopsies. *Mod Pathol* 9:807-811, 1996.

Bostwick DG, Egbert BM, Fajardo LF. Radiation injury of the normal and neoplastic prostate. *Am J Surg Pathol* 6:541-551, 1982.

Bostwick DG, Aguilina JW. Finasteride shows modest changes in prostate cancer. *J Urol Pathol* 6:83-94, 1997.

Bostwick DG, Foster CS. Predictive factors in prostate cancer: current concepts form the 1999 College of American Pathologists Conference on Solid Tumor Prognostic Factors and the 1999 World Health Organization Second International Consultation on Prostate Cancer. *Semin Urol Oncol* 17:222-272, 1999.

Bostwick DG. Immunohistochemical changes in prostate cancer after androgen deprivation therapy. *Mol Urol* 4:101-106, 2000.

Bratt O, Borg A, Kristoffersson U, et al. CAG repeat length in the androgen receptor gene is related to age at diagnosis of prostate cancer and response to endocrine therapy, but not to prostate cancer risk. *Br J Cancer* 81:672-676, 1999.

Brawer MK, Nagle RB, Pitts W, et al. Keratin immunoreactivity as an aid to the diagnosis of persistent adenocarcinoma in irradiated human prostates. *Cancer* 63:454-460, 1989.

Bullock MJ, Srigley JR, Klotz LH, et al. Pathologic effects of neoadjuvant cyproterone acetate on nonneoplastic prostate, prostatic intraepithelial neoplasia, and adenocarcinoma. A detailed analysis of radical prostatectomy specimens from a randomized trial. *Am J Surg Pathol* 26:1400-1413, 2002.

Colecchia M, Frigo B, Del Boca C, et al. Detection of apoptosis by the TUNEL technique in clinically localized prostatic cancer before and after combined endocrine therapy. *J Clin Pathol* 50:384-388, 1997.

Chaussy C, Thüroff S. High-intensity focused ultrasound in prostate cancer: results after 3 years. *Mol Urol* 4:179-182, 2000.

Cheng L, Sebo TJ, Slezak J, et al. Predictors of survival in prostate cancer patients treated with salvage radical prostatectomy after radiation therapy. *Cancer* 83:2164-2171, 1998.

Cheng L, Cheville JC, Bostwick DG. Diagnosis of prostate cancer in needle biopsies after radiation therapy. *Am J Surg Pathol* 23:1173-1183, 1999A.

Cheng L, Sebo TJ, Cheville JC, et al. p53 protein overexpression is associated with increased cell proliferation in patients with locally recurrent prostate carcinoma after radiation therapy. *Cancer* 85:1293-1299, 1999B.

Cheng L, Cheville JC, Pisansky TM, et al. Prevalence and distribution of prostatic intraepithelial neoplasia in salvage radical prostatectomy specimens after radiation therapy. *Am J Surg Pathol* 23:803-808, 1999C.

Chon JK, Borkowski A, Partin AW, et al. Alpha 1-adrenoreceptor antagonists terazosin and doxazosin induce prostate apoptosis without affecting cell proliferation in patients with benign prostatic hyperplasia. *J Urol* 161:2002-2008, 1999.

Civantos F, Marcial MA, Banks ER, et al. Pathology of androgen deprivation therapy in prostate carcinoma. *Cancer* 75:1634-1641, 1995.

Civantos F, Soloway MS, Pinto JE. Histopathological effects of androgen deprivation in prostatic cancer. *Semin Urol Oncol* 14:22-31, 1996.

Civantos F, Watson RB, Pinto JE, et al. Finasteride effect on prostatic hyperplasia and prostate cancer: a comparative clinicopathologic study of radical prostatectomies. *J Urol Pathol* 6:1-14, 1997.

Clark PE, Peereboom DM, Dreicer D, et al. Phase II trial of neoadjuvant estramustine and etoposide plus radical prostatectomy for locally advanced prostate cancer. *Urology* 57:281-285, 2001.

Colbach C, Long J, Ucci AA, et al. Immunohistochemical (IHC) properties of cryoablated prostate [abstract]. *Mod Pathol* 10:72A, 1997.

Cosar EF, Manecke R, Kwon E, et al. Histologic changes in prostate tissue following total androgen blockade (TAB) in the first twenty eight days of therapy [abstract]. *Mod Pathol* 14:105A, 2001.

Costello AJ, Bolton DM, Ellis D, et al. Histopathological changes in human prostatic adenoma following neodymium: YAG laser ablation therapy. *J Urol* 152:1526-1529, 1994.

Cote RJ, Skinner EC, Salem CE, et al. The effect of finasteride on the prostate gland in men with elevated serum prostate-specific antigen levels. *Br J Cancer* 78:413-418, 1998.

Cowan DF, Orihuela E, Motamedi M, et al. Histopathologic effects of laser radiation on the human prostate. *Mod Pathol* 8:716-721, 1995.

Crook JM, Bahadur YA, Robertson SJ, et al. Evaluation of radiation effect, tumor differentiation, and prostate specific antigen staining in sequential prostate biopsies after external beam radiotherapy for patients with prostate carcinoma. *Cancer* 79:81-89, 1997.

Crook J, Malone S, Perry G, et al. Postradiotherapy prostate biopsies: what do they really mean? Results for 498 patients. *Int J Radiat Oncol Biol Phys* 48:355-367, 2000.

Dalkin BL, Ahmann FR, Nagle R, et al. Randomized study of neoadjuvant testicular androgen ablation therapy before radical prostatectomy in men with clinically localized prostate cancer. *J Urol* 155:1357-1360, 1996.

D'Amico AV, Moul JD, Kattan MW. Emerging prognostic factors for outcome prediction in clinically localized prostate cancer: prostate-specific antigen level, race, molecular markers, and neural networks. In: Vogelzang NJ, Scardino PT, Shipley WU, et al, eds. *Comprehensive Textbook of Genitourinary Oncology.* 2nd ed. Philadelphia: Lippincott Williams & Wilkins; 680-700, 2000.

D'Amico AV, Crook J, Beard CJ, et al. Radiation therapy for prostate cancer. In: Walsh PC, Retik AB, Vaughn ED Jr, et al eds. *Campbell's Urology*, 8th ed. Philadelphia: Saunders; 3147-3170, 2002.

De La Rosette JJMCH, D'Ancona FCH, Debruyne FMJ. Current status of thermotherapy of the prostate. *J Urol* 157:430-438, 1997.

De Voot HJ, Rao BR, Geldof AA, et al. Androgen action blockade does not result in reduction in size but changes histology of the normal human prostate. *Prostate* 11:305-311, 1987.

Devonec M, Berger N, Perrin P. Transurethral microwave heating of the prostate, or from hyperthermia to thermotherapy. *J Endourol* 5:129-135, 1991.

Dhom G, Degro S. Therapy of prostatic cancer and histopathologic follow-up. *Prostate* 3:531-542, 1982.

Donnelly BJ, Saliken JC, Ali-Ridha N, et al. Histologic findings in the prostate two years following cryosurgical ablation. *Can J Urol* 8:1237-1239, 2001.

Drew PA, Murphy WM, Kubilis PS, et al. Can androgen deprivation with leuprolide be predicted from histology alone? If not, why not? *J Urol* 157:2201-2205, 1997.

Eisenberger MA, Carducci MA. Chemotherapy for hormone resistant prostate cancer. In: Walsh PC, Retik AB, Vaughn ED Jr, et al, eds. *Campbell's Urology*, 8th ed. Philadelphia: Saunders; 3209-3226, 2002.

Epstein JI, Partin AW, Shue M, et al. Histological changes in benign prostate biopsies following long-term finasteride therapy for prostatic hyperplasia. *J Urol Pathol* 10:87-95, 1999.

Eri LM, Svindland A, Tveter KJ. The effect of bicalutamide on prostate histology. *Prostate* 46:275-282, 2001.

Falconieri G, Lugnani F, Zanconati F, et al. Histopathology of the frozen prostate. The microscopic bases of prostatic carcinoma cryoablation. *Pathol Res Pract* 192:579-587, 1996.

Ferguson J, Zincke H, Ellllison E, et al. Decrease in prostatic intraepithelial neoplasia following total androgen blockade therapy. *Urology* 44:91-95, 1994.

Fergusson JD, Franks LM. The response of prostatic carcinoma to oestrogen treatment. *Br J Surg* 40:422-428, 1953.

Fitzpatrick JM, Mebust WK. Minimally invasive and endoscopic management of benign prostatic hyperplasia. In: Walsh PC, Retik AB, Vaughn ED Jr, et al, eds. *Campbell's Urology.* 8th ed. Philadelphia: Saunders; 1379-1422, 2002.

Forman JD, Oppenheim T, Liu H, et al. Frequency of residual neoplasm in the prostate following three-dimensional conformal radiotherapy. *Prostate* 23:235-243, 1993.

Fournier GR Jr, Narayan P. Laser effects on prostatic tissue: review of experimental data. *J Endourol* 9:89-92, 1995.

Franks LM. Estrogen-treated prostatic cancer. The variation in responsiveness of tumor cells. *Cancer* 13:490-501, 1960.

Freiha FS, Bagshaw MA. Carcinoma of the prostate: results of post-irradiation biopsy. *Prostate* 5:19-24, 1984.

Furr BJA, Kaisary AV. Antiandrogens. In: Kaisary AV, Murphy GP, Denis L, et al, eds. *Textbook of Prostate Cancer: Pathology, Diagnosis and Treatment.* London: Martin-Dunitz; 227-290, 1999.

Gaudin PB. Histopathologic effects of radiation and hormonal therapies on benign and malignant prostate tissues. *J Urol Pathol* 8:55-67, 1998.

Gaudin PB, Zelefsky MJ, Leibel SA, et al. Histopathologic effects of three-dimensional conformal external beam radiation therapy on benign and malignant prostate tissues. *Am J Surg Pathol* 23:1021-1031, 1999.

Gauwitz MD, Pollack A, El-Naggar AK, et al. The prognostic significance of DNA ploidy in clinically localized prostate cancer treated with radiation therapy. *Int J Radiat Oncol Biol Phys* 28:821-828, 1994.

Gelet A, Chapelon JY, Bouvier J, et al. Treatment of prostate cancer with transrectal focused ultrasound: early clinical experience. *Eur Urol* 29:174-183, 1996.

Gelet A, Chapelon JY, Bouvier R, et al. Local control of prostate cancer by transrectal high intensity focused ultrasound therapy: preliminary results. *J Urol* 161:152-162, 1999.

Gleave ME, Goldenberg SL, Jones EC, et al. Biochemical and pathological effects of 8 months of neoadjuvant androgen withdrawal before radical prostatectomy in patients with clinically confined prostate cancer. *J Urol* 155:213-219, 1996.

Gleave ME, La Bianca SE, Goldenberg SL, et al. Long-term neoadjuvant therapy prior to radical prostatectomy: evaluation of risk for biochemical recurrence at 5-year follow-up. *Urology* 56:289-294, 2000.

Goldstein NS, Martinez A, Vicini F, et al. The histology of radiation therapy effect on prostate adenocarcinoma as assessed by needle biopsy after brachytherapy boost. Correlation with biochemical failure. *Am J Clin Pathol* 110:765-775, 1998.

Goldstein NS, Kestin LL, Vicini FA, et al. The influence of percentage of preradiation needle biopsies with adenocarcinoma and total radiation dose on the pathologic response of unfavorable prostate adenocarcinoma. *J Clin Pathol* 117:927-934, 2002.

Gonder MJ, Soanes WA, Smith V. Chemical and morphologic changes in the prostate following extreme cooling. *Ann NY Acad Sci* 125:716-729, 1965.

Gormley GJ, Stoner E, Bruskewitz RC, et al. The effect of finasteride in men with benign prostatic hyperplasia. The Finasteride Study Group. *N Engl J Med* 327:1185-1191, 1992.

Grampsas SA, Miller GJ, Crawford ED. Salvage radical prostatectomy after failed transperineal cryotherapy: histologic findings from prostate whole-mount specimens correlated with intraoperative transrectal ultrasound findings. *Urology* 45:936-941, 1995.

Grann A, Gaudin PB, Raben A, et al. Pathologic features from prostate needle biopsy and prognosis after I-125 brachytherapy. *Radiat Oncol Invest* 6:170-174, 1998.

Grignon D, Troster M. Changes in immunohistochemical staining in prostatic adenocarcinoma following diethylstilbestrol therapy. *Prostate* 7:195-202, 1985.

Grignon DJ, Sakr WA. Histologic effects of radiation therapy and total androgen blockade on prostate cancer. *Cancer* 75:1837-1841, 1995.

Grignon DJ, Caplan R, Sarkar FH, et al. p53 status and prognosis of locally advanced prostatic adenocarcinoma: a study based on RTOG 8610. *J Natl Cancer Inst* 89:158-165, 1997.

Grignon DJ, Bostwick DG, Civantos F, et al. Pathologic handling and reporting of prostate tissue specimens in patients receiving neoadjuvant hormonal therapy: report of the pathology committee. *Mol Urol* 3:193-197, 1999.

Grob BM, Schellhammer PF, Brassil DN, et al. Changes in immunohistochemical staining of PSA, PAP, and TURP-27 following irradiation therapy for clinically localized prostate cancer. *Urology* 44:525-529, 1994.

Grossfeld GD, Olumi AF, Connolly JA, et al. Locally recurrent prostate tumors following either radiation therapy or radical prostatectomy have changes in K-67 labeling index, p53 and bcl-2 immunoreactivity. *J Urol* 159:1437-1443, 1998.

Hansen RI, Wanstrup J. Cryoprostatectomy. Histologic changes elucidated by serial biopsies. *Scand J Urol Nephrol* 7:100-104, 1973.

Heckel NJ, Kretschmer HL. Carcinoma of the prostate treated with diethylstilbestrol. *JAMA* 119:1087, 1942.

Hellström M, Häggman M, Brändstedt S, et al. Histopathological changes in androgen-deprived localized prostatic cancer. A study in total prostatectomy specimens. *Eur Urol* 24:461-465, 1993.

Helpap B. Treated prostatic carcinoma. Histological, immunohistochemical and cell kinetic studies. *Appl Pathol* 3:230-241, 1985.

Helpap B, Koch V. Histological and immunohistochemical findings of prostatic carcinoma after external or interstitial radiotherapy. *J Cancer Res Clin Oncol* 117:608-614, 1991.

Helpap B, Oehler U, Weisser H, et al. Morphology of benign prostatic hyperplasia after treatment with Sabal Extract IDS 89 or placebo. *J Urol Pathol* 3:175-182, 1995.

Horwitz EM, Hanks GE. Hormonal therapy combined with radiation or surgery in treatment of locally advanced non-metastatic prostate cancer. In: Vogelzang NJ, Scardino PT, Shipley WU, et al, eds. *Genitourinary Oncology.* 2nd ed. Philadelphia: Lippincott Williams & Wilkins; 783-789, 2000.

Hourriez LA, Zlotta AR, Schulman CC. Transurethral needle ablation (TUNA): histopathological, radiological and clinical studies of a new office procedure for treatment of benign prostatic hyperplasia. *Acta Urol Belg* 62:33-38, 1994.

Huang A, Gandour-Edwards R, Rosenthal SA, et al. p53 and bcl-2 immunohistochemical alterations in prostate cancer treated with radiation therapy. *Urology* 51:346-351, 1998.

Huggins C, Hodges CV. Studies on prostatic cancer: (I) The effect of estrogen and of androgen injection on serum phosphates in metastatic carcinoma of the prostate. *Cancer Res* 1:293-297, 1941A.

Huggins C, Stevens RE, Hodges CV. Studies on prostatic cancer: (II) The effects of castration on advanced carcinoma of the prostate gland. *Arch Surg* 43:209, 1941B.

Hugosson J, Abrahamsson PA, Ahlgren G, et al. The risk of malignancy in the surgical margin at radical prostatectomy reduced almost three-fold in patients given neo-adjuvant hormone treatment. *Eur Urol* 29:413-419, 1996.

Incognito LS, Cazares LH, Schellhammer PF, et al. Overexpression of p53 in prostate carcinoma is associated with improved overall survival but not predictive of response to radiotherapy. *Int J Oncol* 17:761-769, 2000.

Jimenez RE, Lu JD, Mesic J, et al. Perineural invasion as a prognostic marker in patients treated by radiation therapy (RT): a radiation therapy oncology group (RTOG) study [abstract]. *Mod Pathol* 13:103A, 2000.

Jimenez RE, Lu JD, Mesic J, et al. Mitotic figures as a prognostic marker in prostate cancer (PCa) patients treated with radiation therapy: a Radiation Therapy Oncology Group (RTOG) Study [abstract]. *Mod Pathol* 14:112A, 2001.

Jonler M, Bruskewitz RC. Prostatic histology in secondary transurethral resection of the prostate. *J Urol* 154:119-122, 1995.

Kabalin JN, Hodge KK, McNeal JE, et al. Identification of residual cancer in the prostate following radiation therapy: role of transrectal ultrasound guided biopsy and prostate specific antigen. *J Urol* 142:326-331, 1989.

Kattan MW, Zelefsky MJ, Kupelian PA, et al. Pretreatment nomogram for predicting the outcome of three-dimensional conformal radiotherapy in prostate cancer. *J Clin Oncol* 18:3352-3359, 2000.

Kattan MW, Potters L, Blasko JC, et al. Pretreatment nomogram for predicting freedom from recurrence after permanent prostate brachytherapy in prostate cancer. *Urology* 58:393-399, 2001.

Khair AA, Pacelli A, Iczkowski KA, et al. Does transurethral microwave thermotherapy have a different effect on prostate cancer than on benign or hyperplastic tissue? *Urology* 54:67-72, 1999.

Khoo VS, Pollack A, Cowen D, et al. Relationship of Ki-67 labeling index to DNA ploidy, S-phase fraction, and outcome in prostate cancer treated with radiotherapy. *Prostate* 41:166-172, 1999.

Khoury S. Testicular androgen ablation. In: Kaisary AV, Murphy GP, Denis L, et al, eds. *Textbook of Prostate Cancer. Pathology, Diagnosis and Treatment.* London: Martin Dunitz; 291-302, 1999.

Kiel HJ, Wieland WF, Rossler W. Local control of prostate cancer by transrectal HIFU-therapy. *Arch Ital Urol Androl* 72:313-319, 2000.

Kiesling VJ, McAninch JW, Goebel JL, et al. External beam radiotherapy for adenocarcinoma of the prostate: a clinical follow-up. *J Urol* 124:851-854, 1980.

Klotz LH, Goldenberg SL, Jewett M, et al. CUOG randomized trial of neoadjuvant androgen ablation before radical prostatectomy: 36-month post-treatment PSA results. *Urology* 53:757-763, 1999.

Kollerman J, Feek U, Muller H, et al. Nondetected tumor (pT0) after prolonged, neoadjuvant treatment of localized prostatic carcinoma. *Eur Urol* 38:714-720, 2000.

Kyprianou N, Litvak JP, Borkowski A, et al. Induction of prostate apoptosis by doxazosin in benign prostatic hyperplasia. *J Urol* 159:1810-1815, 1998.

Kyprianou N, Benning CM. Suppression of human prostate cancer cell growth by a1-adrenoceptor antagonists doxazosin and terazosin via induction by apoptosis. *Cancer Res* 60:4550-4555, 2000.

Labrie F, Dupont A, Cusan L, et al. Downstaging of localized prostate cancer by neoadjuvant therapy with flutamide and Lupron: the first controlled and randomized trial. *Clin Invest Med* 16:499-509, 1995.

Larson TR, Bostwick DG, Corica A. Temperature-correlated histopathologic changes following microwave thermoablation of obstructive tissue in patients with benign prostatic hyperplasia. *Urology* 47:463-469, 1996.

Lattanzi JP, Hanlon AL, Hanks GE. Early stage prostate cancer treated with radiation therapy: stratifying an intermediate risk group. *Int J Radiat Oncol Biol Phys* 38:569-573, 1997.

Lepor H, Lowe FC. Evaluation and nonsurgical management of benign prostatic hyperplasia. In: Walsh PC, Retik AB, Vaughan ED Jr, et al, eds. *Campbell's Urology.* 8th ed. Philadelphia: Saunders; 1337-1378, 2002.

Lerner SE, Blute ML, Zincke H. Critical evaluation of salvage surgery for radio-recurrent/resistant prostate cancer. *J Urol* 154:1103-1109, 1995.

Leventis AK, Shariat SF, Kattan MW, et al. Prediction of response to salvage radiation therapy in patients with prostate cancer recurrence after radical prostatectomy. *J Clin Oncol* 19:1030-1039, 2001.

Link P, Freiha FS. Radical prostatectomy after definitive radiation therapy for prostate cancer. *Urology* 37:189-192, 1991.

Ljung G, Egevad L, Norberg M, et al. Assessment of proliferation indicators in residual prostatic adenocarcinoma cells after radical external beam radiotherapy. *Prostate* 29:303-310, 1996.

Ljung G, Norberg M, Holmberg L, et al. Characterization of residual tumor cells following radiation therapy for prostatic adenocarcinoma, immunohistochemical expression of prostate-specific antigen, prostatic acid phosphatase, and cytokeratin 8. *Prostate* 31:91-97, 1997.

Logothetis CJ, Vogelzang NJ. Current treatment and investigative approaches to the management of hormone-refractory prostate cancer. In: Vogelzang NJ, Scardino PT, Shipley WU, et al, eds. *Comprehensive Textbook of Genitourinary Oncology.* 2nd ed. Philadelphia: Lippincott Williams & Wilkins; 862-869, 2000.

Lowe FC, Fagelman E. Phytotherapy in the management of benign prostatic hyperplasia: a critical review. *Urology* 58(6 Suppl 1):71-77, 2001.

Lowe FC, Dreikorn K, Borkowski A, et al. Review of recent placebo-controlled trials utilizing phytotherapeutic agents for treatment of BPH. *Prostate* 37:187-193, 1998.

Lytton B, Collins JT ,Weiss RM, et al. Results of biopsy after early stage prostate cancer treatment by implantation of ^{125}I seeds. *J Urol* 121:306-309, 1979.

Lytton B. Prostate cancer: a brief history and the discovery of hormonal ablation treatment. *J Urol* 165:1859-1862, 2001.

Mackey TJ, Borkowski A, Amin P, et al. bcl-2/bax ratio as a predictive marker for therapeutic response to radiotherapy in patients with prostate cancer. *Urology* 52:1085-1090, 1998.

Madersbacher S, Pedevilla M, Vingers L, et al. Effect of high-intensity focused ultrasound on human prostate cancer in vivo. *Cancer Res* 55:3346-3351, 1995.

Madersbacher S, Kratzik C, Marberger M. Prostatic tissue ablation by transrectal high intensity focused ultrasound: histological impact and clinical application. *Ultrason Sonochem* 4:175-179, 1997.

Mahan DE, Bruce AW, Manley PN, et al. Immunohistochemical evaluation of prostatic carcinoma before and after radiotherapy. *J Urol* 124:488-491, 1980.

Marks LS, Partin AW, Gormley GJ, et al. Prostate tissue composition and response to finasteride in men with symptomatic benign prostatic hyperplasia. *J Urol* 157:2171-2178, 1997.

Marks LS, Partin AW, Dorey FJ, et al. Long-term effects of finasteride on prostate tissue composition. *Urology* 53:574-580, 1999.

Marks LS, Partin AW, Epstein JI, et al. Effects of saw palmetto herbal blend in men with symptomatic benign prostatic hyperplasia. *J Urol* 163:1451-1456, 2000.

Matsuda H, Nonomura K, Nagamori S, et al. Clinicopathological evaluation of etoposide or estramustine phosphate in castrated patients with advanced prostatic cancer [in Japanese]. *Jpn J Urol* 86:1530-1537, 1995.

Mauroy B, Chive M, Stefaniak X, et al. Study of the effects of thermotherapy in benign prostatic hypertrophy. *Eur Urol* 32:198-208, 1997.

McConnell JD, Bruskewitz R, Walsh P, et al. The effect of finasteride on the risk on acute urinary retention and the need for surgical treatment among men with benign prostatic hyperplasia: Finasteride Long-Term Efficacy and Safety Study Group. *N Engl J Med* 338:557-563, 1998.

McCullough DL. Minimally invasive treatment of benign prostatic hyperplasia. In: Walsh PC, Retik AB, Vaughan ED Jr, et al, eds. *Campbell's Urology.* 7th ed. Philadelphia: WB Saunders; 1479-1506, 1998.

McLeod DG, Vogelzang NJ. Androgen blockade: monotherapy and quality-of-life issues. In: Vogelzang NJ, Shipley WU, Scardino PT, et al, eds. *Comprehensive Textbook of Genitourinary Oncology.* 2nd ed. Philadelphia: Lippincott Williams & Wilkins; 824-841, 2000.

Milam DF, Smith JA Jr. Laser prostatectomy devices and their tissue effects. *J Endourol* 9:85-88, 1995.

Miles BJ, Herman JR, Reiter RE, et al. Salvage radical prostatectomy for local recurrence of prostate cancer after radiation therapy. In Vogelzang NJ, Scardino PT, Shipley WU, et al, eds. *Genitourinary Urology.* 2nd ed. Philadelphia: Lippincott Williams & Wilkins; 813-822, 2000.

Miller EB, Ladaga LE, El-Mahdi AM, et al. Reevaluation of prostate biopsy after definitive radiation therapy. *Urology* 41:311-316, 1993.

Mollenkamp JS, Cooper JF, Kagan AR. Clinical experience with supervoltage radiotherapy in carcinoma of the prostate: a preliminary report. *J Urol* 113:374-377, 1975.

Montironi R, Muzzonigro G, Galluzzi CM, et al. Effect of LHRH agonist and flutamide (combination endocrine therapy) on the frequency and location of proliferating cell nuclear antigen and apoptotic bodies in prostatic hyperplasia. *J Urol Pathol* 2:161-171, 1994A.

Montironi R, Magi-Galluzzi C, Muzzonigro G, et al. Effects of combination endocrine treatment on normal prostate, prostatic intraepithelial neoplasia, and prostatic adenocarcinoma. *J Clin Pathol* 47:906-913, 1994B.

Montironi R, Diamanti L. Morphologic changes in benign prostatic hyperplasia following chronic treatment with the 5-α-reductase inhibitor finasteride. Comparison with the effect of combination endocrine therapy. *J Urol Pathol* 4:123-136, 1996A.

Montironi M, Valli M, Fabris G. Treatment of benign prostatic hyperplasia with 5-a-reductase inhibitor: morphological changes in patients who fail to respond. *J Clin Pathol* 49:324-328, 1996B.

Montironi R, Diamanti L, Santinelli A, et al, Italian PROSIT Study Group. Effect on total androgen ablation on pathologic stage and resection limit status of prostatic cancer. *Pathol Res Pract* 195:201-208, 1999.

Montironi R, Schulman CC. Pathological changes in prostate lesions after androgen manipulation. *J Clin Pathol* 51:5-12, 1998.

Moore RA, McLellan AM. A histological study of the effect of the sex hormones in the human prostate. *J Urol* 40:641-657, 1938.

Morgenstern N, Ro JY, Batts P, et al. Prostate cryotherapy: chronological post-therapy histologic changes with clinical correlation [abstract]. *Mod Pathol* 10:83A, 1997.

Murphy WM, Soloway MS, Barrows GH. Pathologic changes associated with androgen deprivation therapy for prostate cancer. *Cancer* 68:821-828, 1991.

Nam RK, Fleshner N, Rakovitch E, et al. Prevalence and patterns of use of complementary therapies among prostate cancer patients: an epidemiological analysis. *J Urol* 161:1521-1524, 1999.

Narayan P, Tewari A, Crocker B, et al. Factors affecting size and configuration of electrovaporization lesions in the prostate. *Urology* 47:679-688, 1996.

Noordzij MA, Bogdanowicz JF, van Krimpen C, et al. The prognostic value of pretreatment expression of androgen receptor and bcl-2 in hormonally treated prostate cancer patients. *J Urol* 158:1880-1884, 1997.

Oh WK, Kantoff PW. Management of hormone-refractory prostate cancer: current standards and future prospects. *J Urol* 160:1220-1229, 1998.

Palmberg C, Koivisto P, Kakkola L, et al. Androgen receptor gene amplification at primary progression predicts response to combined androgen blockade as second line therapy for advanced prostate cancer. *J Urol* 164:1992-1995, 2000.

Paterson RF, Gleave ME, Jones EC, et al. Immunohistochemical analysis of radical prostatectomy specimens after 8 months of neoadjuvant hormonal therapy. *Mol Urol* 3:297-286, 1999.

Pertschuk LP, Macchia RJ, Feldman JG, et al. Immunocytochemical assay for androgen receptors in prostate cancer: a prospective study of 63 cases with long-term follow-up. *Am Surg Oncol* 1:495-503, 1994.

Pertschuk LP, Schaeffer H, Feldman JG, et al. Immunostaining for prostate cancer androgen receptor in paraffin identifies a subset of men with a poor prognosis. *Lab Invest* 73:302-305, 1995.

Petersen DS, Milleman LA, Rose EF, et al. Biopsy and clinical course after cryosurgery for prostatic cancer. *J Urol* 120:308-311, 1978.

Pettaway CA, Pisters LL, Troncoso P, et al. Neoadjuvant chemotherapy and hormonal therapy followed by radical prostatectomy: feasibility and preliminary results. *J Clin Oncol* 18:1050-1057, 2000.

Pisansky TM, Kahn MJ, Rasp GM, et al. A multiple prognostic index predictive of disease outcome after irradiation for clinically localized prostate carcinoma. *Cancer* 79:337-344, 1997.

Pisters LL, Dinney CPN, Pettaway CA, et al. A feasibility study of cryotherapy followed by radical prostatectomy for locally advanced prostate cancer. *J Urol* 161:509-514, 1999.

Polito M, Muzzonigro G, Minardi D, et al. Effects of neoadjuvant androgen deprivation therapy on prostatic cancer. *Eur Urol* 30(suppl):26-31, 1996.

Pollack A, Troncoso P, Zagars GK, et al. The significance of DNA-ploidy and S-phase fraction in node-positive (stage D1) prostate cancer treated with androgen ablation. *Prostate* 31:21-28, 1997.

Porter AT, Hart KB. Radiation therapy in the treatment of localized/organ-confined prostate cancer. In: Kaisary AV, Murphy GP, Denis L, et al, eds. *Textbook of Prostate Cancer. Pathology, Diagnosis, and Treatment.* London: Martin Dunitz; 231-247, 1999.

Pow-Sang M, Cowan DF, Orihuela E, et al. Thermocoagulation effect of diode laser radiation in the human prostate: acute and chronic study. *Urology* 45:790-794, 1995.

Prestidge BR, Hoak DC, Grimm PD, et al. Posttreatment biopsy results following interstitial brachytherapy in early-stage prostate cancer. *Int J Radiat Oncol Biol Phys* 37:31-39, 1997.

Prins GS, Sklarew RJ, Pertschuk LP. Image analysis of androgen receptor immunostaining in prostate cancer accurately predicts response to hormonal therapy. *J Urol* 159:641-649, 1998.

Rakozy C, Grignon DJ, Li YW, et al. p53 gene alterations in prostate cancer after radiation failure and their association with clinical outcome: a molecular and immunohistochemical analysis. *Pathol Res Pract* 195:129-135, 1999.

Reuter VE. Pathological changes in benign and malignant tissue following androgen deprivation therapy. *Urology* 49(suppl 3A):16-22, 1997.

Rezek PR, Coplan MN, Woods FM, et al. Histological studies of carcinoma of the prostate treated by estrogen. *J Urol* 66:379-389, 1951.

Rittmaster RS, Norman RW, Thomas LN, et al. Evidence for atrophy and apoptosis in the prostates of men given finasteride. *J Clin Endocrinol Metab* 81:814-818, 1996.

Rogers E, Ohori M, Kassabian VS, et al. Salvage radical prostatectomy: outcome measured by serum prostate specific antigen levels. *J Urol* 153:104-110, 1995.

Ruizeveld de Winter JA, Janssen PJA, Sleddens HM, et al. Androgen receptor status in localized and locally progressive hormone refractory human prostate cancer. *Am J Pathol* 144:735-746, 1994.

Sadi MV, Walsh PC, Barrack ER. Immunohistochemical study of androgen receptors in metastatic prostate cancer. Comparison of receptor content and response to therapy. *Cancer* 67:3057-3064, 1991.

Scalzo DA, Kallakury BVS, Gaddipati RV, et al. Cell proliferation rate by MIB-1 immunohistochemistry predicts postradiation recurrence in prostatic adenocarcinomas. *Am J Clin Pathol* 109:163-168, 1998.

Scardino PT, Frankel JM, Wheeler TM, et al. The prognostic significance of post-irradiation biopsy results in patients with prostatic cancer. *J Urol* 135:510-516, 1986.

Schellhammer PF, Ladaga LE, El-Mahdi AM. Histological characteristics of prostatic biopsies after 125 iodine implantation. *J Urol* 123:700-705, 1980.

Schenken JR, Burns EL, Kahle PJ. The effect of diethylstilbestrol and diethylstilbestrol dipropionate on carcinoma of the prostate gland. II. Cytologic changes following treatment. *J Urol* 48:99-112, 1942.

Scher HI. Hyperplastic and malignant diseases of the prostate. In: Braunwald E, Hauser SL, Fauci AS, et al, eds. *Harrison's Principles of Internal Medicine.* 15th ed. New York: McGraw-Hill; 608-616, 2001.

Scherr DS, Vaughan ED Jr, Wei J, et al. Bcl-2 and p53 expression in clinically localized prostate cancer predicts response to external beam radiotherapy. *J Urol* 162:12-17, 1999.

Schned AR, Gormley EA. Florid xanthomatous pelvic lymph node reaction to metastatic prostatic adenocarcinoma. A sequela of preoperative androgen deprivation therapy. *Arch Pathol Lab Med* 120:96-100, 1996.

Schröeder FH. Hormonal therapy of prostate cancer. In: Walsh PC, Retik AB, Vaughan ED Jr, et al, eds. *Campbell's Urology.* 8th ed. Philadelphia: Saunders; 3182-3208, 2002.

Schulman CC. Neoadjuvant androgen blockade prior to prostatectomy: a retrospective study and critical review. *Prostate* 5(suppl):9-14, 1994.

Schulman CC, Debruyne FM, Forster G, et al. 4-year follow-up results of a European prospective randomized study on neoadjuvant hormonal therapy prior to radical prostatectomy in T2-3N0M0 prostate cancer. *Eur Urol* 38:706-713, 2000.

Shabaik A, Wilson S, Bidair M, et al. Pathologic changes in prostate biopsies following cryoablation therapy of prostate carcinoma. *J Urol Pathol* 3:183-193, 1995.

Shapiro E, Hartanto V, Lepor H. Anti-desmin vs. anti-actin for quantifying the area density of prostate smooth muscle. *Prostate* 20:259-267, 1992.

Sheaff MT, Baithun SI. Effects of radiation on the normal prostate gland. *Histopathology* 30:341-348, 1997.

Shinohara K, Rhee B, Presti JC Jr, et al. Cryosurgical ablation of prostate cancer: patterns of cancer recurrence. *J Urol* 158:2206-2209, 1997.

Shinohara K, Carroll PR. Cryotherapy for prostate cancer. In: Walsh PC, Retik AB, Vaughn ED Jr, et al, eds. *Campbell's Urology*. 8th ed. Philadelphia: Saunders; 3171-3181, 2002.

Shuman BA, Cohen JK, Miller RJ Jr, et al. Histological presence of viable prostatic glands on routine biopsy following cryosurgical ablation of the prostate. *J Urol* 157:552-555, 1997.

Siders DB, Lee F. Histologic changes of irradiated prostatic carcinoma diagnosed by transrectal ultrasound. *Hum Pathol* 23:344-351, 1992.

Smith DS, Murphy WM. Histologic changes in prostate carcinomas treated with leuprolide (luteinizing hormone–releasing hormone effect). Distinction from poor differentiation. *Cancer* 73:1472-1477, 1994.

Soloway MS, Civantos F, Murphy WM, et al. Androgen deprivation prior to radical prostatectomy for T2b and T3 prostate cancer. *Urology* 43(suppl 2):52-56, 1994.

Soloway MS, Sharifi R, Wajsman Z, et al. Randomized prospective study comparing radical prostatectomy alone versus radical prostatectomy preceded by androgen blockade in clinical stage B2 (T2bNxM0) prostate cancer. *J Urol* 154:424-428, 1995.

Soman A, Goldstein NS, Kestin LL, et al. Prostate needle biopsies after radiation therapy: features associated with treatment failure [abstract]. *Mod Pathol* 14:123A, 2001.

Song J, Cheng WS, Cupps RE, et al. Nuclear deoxyribonucleic acid content measured by static cytometry: important prognostic association for patients with clinically localized prostate carcinoma treated by external beam radiotherapy. *J Urol* 147:794-797, 1992.

Stattin P, Damber JE, Modig H, et al. Pretreatment p53 immunoreactivity does not infer radioresistance in prostate cancer patients. *Int J Radiat Oncol Biol Phys* 35:885-889, 1996.

Stattin P, Westin P, Damber JE, et al. Short-term cellular effects induced by castration therapy in relation to clinical outcome in prostate cancer. *Br J Cancer* 77:670-675, 1998.

Stenner J, Crawford ED. Combined androgen blockade. In: Kaisary AV, Murphy GP, Denis L, et al, eds. *Textbook of Prostate Cancer. Pathology, Diagnosis and Treatment.* London: Martin Dunitz; 303-317, 1999.

Stock RG, Stone NN, Kao J, et al. The effect of disease and treatment-related factors on biopsy results after prostate brachytherapy. Implications for treatment optimization. *Cancer* 89:1829-1834, 2000.

Sulser T, Jochum W, Huch Boni RA, et al. Laser treatment of benign prostatic hypertrophy: the correlation of histologic results to nuclear magnetic resonance imaging [in French]. *Ann Urol* 31:19-26, 1997.

Susani M, Madersbacher S, Kratzik C, et al. Morphology of tissue destruction induced by focused ultrasound. *Eur Urol* 23(suppl):34-38, 1993.

Takeda H, Akakura K, Masai M, et al. Androgen receptor content of prostate carcinoma cells estimated by immunohistochemistry is related to prognosis of patients with stage D2 prostate carcinoma. *Cancer* 77:934-940, 1996.

Tetu B, Srigley JR, Boivin JC, et al. Effect of combination endocrine therapy (LHRH agonist and flutamide) on normal prostate and prostatic adenocarcinoma. A histopathologic and immunohistochemical study. *Am J Surg Pathol* 15:111-120, 1991.

Tran TA, Jennings TA, Ross JS, et al. Pseudomyxoma ovairiilike posttherapeutic alteration in prostatic adenocarcinoma. A distinctive pattern in patients receiving neoadjuvant androgen ablation therapy. *Am J Surg Pathol* 22:347-354, 1998.

Tunn UW, Acar O, Goldschmidt AJW. Effects of androgen deprivation prior to radical prostatectomy in 375 patients. *Urol Int* 56(suppl):6-12, 1996.

Unger PD, Hoon V, Stone N, et al. Computerized interactive morphometry in the differential diagnosis of irradiated prostates. *Analyt Quant Cytol Histol* 17:100-108, 1995.

Vaillancourt L, Têtu B, Fradet Y, et al. Effect of neoadjuvant endocrine therapy (combined androgen blockade) on normal prostate and prostatic carcinoma. A randomized study. *Am J Surg Pathol* 20:86-93, 1996.

Valicenti R, Lu J, Pilepich M, et al. Survival advantage from higher-dose radiation therapy for clinically localized prostate cancer treated on the radiation therapy oncology group trials. *J Clin Oncol* 18:2740-2746, 2000.

Van de Voorde WM, Elgamal AA, van Poppel HP, et al. Morphologic and immunohistochemical changes in prostate cancer after preoperative hormonal therapy. A comparative study of radical prostatectomies. *Cancer* 74:3164-3175, 1994.

Van der Kwast TH, Têtu B, Candas B, et al. Prolonged neoadjuvant combined androgen blockade leads to further reduction of prostatic tumor volume: three versus six months of endocrine therapy. *Urology* 53:523-529, 1997.

Van Leeders GJLH, Beerlage HP, Th Ruijter E, et al. Histopathological changes associated with high-intensity focused ultrasound (HIFU) treatment for localised adenocarcinoma of the prostate. *J Clin Pathol* 53:391-394, 2000.

Van Poppel H, De Ridder D, Elgamal AA, et al. Neoadjuvant hormonal therapy before radical prostatectomy decreases the number of positive margins in stage T2 prostate cancer: interim results of a prospective randomized trial. *J Urol* 154:429-434, 1995.

Voges GE, Mottrie AM, Stöckle M, et al. Hormone therapy prior to radical prostatectomy in patients with clinical stage C prostate cancer. *Prostate* 5(suppl):4-8, 1994.

Vollmer RT, Montana GS. Predicting tumor failure in prostate carcinoma after definitive radiation therapy: limitations of models based on prostate-specific antigen, clinical stage, and Gleason score. *Clin Cancer Res* 5:2476-2484, 1999.

Walther PJ. Contemporary chemotherapeutic approaches for the treatment of hormone-refractory prostate carcinoma. *World J Urol* 18:216-221, 2000.

Weiss SW, Goldblum JR. *Enzingers and Weiss's Soft Tissue Tumors.* 4th ed. St. Louis, Mo: Mosby; 3-4, 2001.

Wheeler JA, Zagars GK, Ayala AG. Dedifferentiation of locally recurrent prostate cancer after radiation therapy. Evidence for tumor progression. *Cancer* 71:3783-3787, 1993.

Wheeler TM. Influence of irradiation and androgen ablation on prostatic intraepithelial neoplasia. *Eur Urol* 30:261-264, 1996.

Wilt TJ, Ishani A, Stark G, et al. Saw palmetto extracts for treatment of benign prostatic hyperplasia: a systematic review. *JAMA* 280:1604-1609, 1998.

Xu LL, Su YP, Labiche R, et al. Quantitative expression profile of androgen-regulated genes in prostate cancer cells and identification of prostate-specific genes. *Int J Cancer* 92:322-328, 2001.

Yang XJ, Lecksell K, Short K, et al, PLESS Study Group. Does long-term finasteride therapy affect the histologic features of benign prostatic tissue and prostate cancer on needle biopsy? *Urology* 53:696-700, 1999.

Yerushalmi A, Servadio C, Leib Z, et al. Local hyperthermia for treatment of carcinoma of the prostate: a preliminary report. *Prostate* 3:623-630, 1982.

Zlotta AR, Djavan B, Matos C, et al. Percutaneous transperineal radiofrequency ablation of prostate tumour: safety, feasibility and pathological effects on human prostate cancer. *Br J Urol* 81:265-275, 1998.

Malignant Neoplasms Mistaken for Benign Conditions

CHAPTER

20

Just as benign prostatic lesions can simulate malignancy in the prostate (Chapter 10), so can malignant proliferations in the prostate mimic benign conditions. Here, presented in tabular form **t20.1-t20.3**, are various malignancies in the prostate along with the corresponding benign entity that is most often mimicked by the cancer.

■ t20.1 Prostatic Carcinoma Patterns that Mimic Benign Conditions

Prostatic Carcinoma Pattern	Benign Condition Mimicked	References[1]
Well-differentiated adenocarcinoma	Atypical adenomatous hyperplasia (adenosis)	Bostwick 1993, Gaudin 1994, 1995
Atrophic pattern adenocarcinoma	Atrophy	Cina 1997, Egan 1997, Kaleem 1998
Cribriform adenocarcinoma	Cribriform hyperplasia	Ayala 1986, McNeal 1986, Rubin 1998
Foamy gland adenocarcinoma	Xanthoma	Nelson 1996, Sebo 1994
Inflamed prostatic adenocarcinoma	Inflammatory, reactive atypia	
Hypernephromatoid carcinoma	Granulomatous prostatitis	Presti 1991
Pseudohyperplastic carcinoma	BPH	Humphrey 1998, Levi 2000
Hormonal and radiation therapy	Histiocytes, lymphocytes, atrophy	Grignon 1995, Rentee 1997

[1]Selected references. Also see index and relevant chapters for additional references

■ t20.2 Prostatic Carcinoma Variants that Mimic Benign Conditions

Prostatic Carcinoma Variant	Benign Condition Mimicked
Prostatic duct adenocarcinoma	Prostatic urethral polyps, papillary nephrogenic adenomas
Signet ring carcinoma	Artifactual signet ring cells in benign smooth muscle cells and lymphocytes
Squamous cell carcinoma	Squamous metaplasia
Basaloid/adenoid cystic "carcinomas"	Basal cell hyperplasia
Transitional cell carcinoma	Transitional cell metaplasia
Small cell carcinoma	Benign lymphocytes
Sarcomatoid carcinoma with spindle cells	Stromal hyperplasia

References: See Chapter 17

■ t20.3 Unusual Prostatic Malignancies that Mimic Benign Conditions

Unusual Prostatic Malignancy	Benign Condition Mimicked
Leiomyosarcoma	Stromal hyperplasia, leiomyoma
Prostatic stromal sarcoma	Stromal hyperplasia, leiomyoma
Leukemia/lymphoma	Inflammation

References: see Chapter 18

References

Ayala AG, Srigley JR, Ro JY, et al. Clear cell cribriform hyperplasia of the prostate. Report of 10 cases. *Am J Surg Pathol* 10:665-671, 1986.

Bostwick DG, Srigley J, Grignon D, et al. Atypical adenomatous hyperplasia of the prostate. Morphologic criteria for its distinction from well-differentiated carcinoma. *Hum Pathol* 24:819-832, 1993.

Cina SJ, Epstein JI. Adenocarcinoma of the prostate with atrophic features. *Am J Surg Pathol* 21:289-295, 1997.

Egan AJM, Lopez-Beltran A, Bostwick DG. Prostatic adenocarcinoma with atrophic features: malignancy mimicking a benign process. *Am J Surg Pathol* 21:931-935, 1997.

Gaudin PB, Epstein JI. Adenosis of the prostate. Histologic features in transurethral resection specimens. *Am J Surg Pathol* 18:863-870, 1994.

Gaudin PB, Epstein JI. Adenosis of the prostate. Histologic features in needle biopsy specimens. *Am J Surg Pathol* 19:737-747, 1995.

Grignon DJ, Sakr WA. Histologic effects of radiation therapy and total androgen blockade on prostate cancer. *Cancer* 75:1837-1847, 1995.

Humphrey PA, Kaleem Z, Swanson PE, Vollmer RT. Pseudohyperplastic prostatic adenocarcinoma. *Am J Surg Pathol* 22:1239-1246, 1998.

Kaleem Z, Swanson PE, Vollmer RT, Humphrey PA. Prostatic adenocarcinoma with atrophic features. A study of 202 consecutive, completely embedded radical prostatectomy specimens. *Am J Clin Pathol* 109:695-703, 1998.

Levi AW, Epstein JI. Pseudohyperplastic prostatic adenocarcinoma on needle biopsy and simple prostatectomy. *Am J Surg Pathol* 24:1039-1046, 2000.

McNeal JE, Reese JH, Redwine EA, et al. Cribriform adenocarcinoma of the prostate. *Cancer* 58:1714-1749, 1986.

Nelson RS, Epstein JI. Prostatic carcinoma with abundant xanthomatous cytoplasm: foamy gland carcinoma. *Am J Surg Pathol* 20:419-426, 1996.

Presti B, Weidner N. Granulomatous prostatitis and poorly differentiated adenocarcinoma. Their distinction with the use of immunohistochemical methods. *Am J Clin Pathol* 95:330-334, 1991.

Reuter VE. Pathological changes in benign and malignant tissue following androgen deprivation therapy. *Urology* 49(suppl 3A):16-22, 1997.

Rubin MA, de La Taille A, Bagiella E, et al. Cribriform carcinoma of the prostate and cribriform prostatic intraepithelial neoplasia. Incidence and clinical implications. *Am J Surg Pathol* 22:840-848, 1998.

Sebo TJ, Bostwick DG, Farrow GM, et al. Prostatic xanthoma: a mimic of prostatic adenocarcinoma. *Hum Pathol* 25:386-389, 1994.

CHAPTER 21

Molecular Biology of Human Prostatic Carcinoma: Clinical and Pathologic Implications

[21.1] DNA Content (Ploidy) **481**

[21.2] Chromosomal Alterations **482**

[21.3] Tumor Suppressor Genes **487**

[21.4] Oncogenes **489**

[21.5] Androgen Receptor **490**

[21.6] DNA Methylation **491**

[21.7] Cell Proliferation and Cell Death (Apoptosis) **491**

[21.8] Gene Expression Profiling and Proteomics **494**

T here is a large and rapidly expanding body of knowledge regarding the molecular and cellular biology of human prostatic carcinoma. Presented in this chapter is an overview of selected molecular aberrations that have been discovered in prostatic carcinoma. The emphasis here is on human prostatic tissue, rather than in vitro cell lines or animal model systems. Although it appears likely that the expression of hundreds of genes is altered in prostatic carcinoma compared with benign prostatic tissues, not a single molecular diagnostic test is currently recommended for routine use in diagnostic or prognostic determinations in prostate carcinoma **t21.1** (Bostwick 1999, Bostwick 2000). It may be anticipated in the future that a number of molecular diagnostic and molecular pathologic tests could become important in the clinical management of prostate cancer patients. For example, once the nature of the precise genetic mutations that predispose one to prostatic carcinoma is elucidated, a blood test for such predisposition could be developed. Additionally, it is possible that gene expression profiling might identify gene expression patterns that would allow for diagnosis and/or prognostic stratification for prostatic carcinoma patients. Most desirable would be therapeutic stratification based on molecular diagnostics where the likelihood of response to a specific therapy might be predicted prior to treatment. To prove the clinical utility of potentially important molecular markers, these markers will need to be incorporated and tested in prospective, randomized controlled, clinical trials.

[21.1] DNA Content (Ploidy)

DNA ploidy refers to the number of sets of homologous chromosomes in a cell or cells **t21.2**. In prostatic carcinoma, it is well-established that there is commonly a derangement in the number of chromosomes in each cell. This abnormality in genetic instability could be due in part to defects in centrosomes, organelles that organize microtubule arrays, including mitotic spindles (Pihan 2001). The altered chromosomal number in prostatic carcinoma is reflected in cellular DNA content, which can be quantitated by flow cytometry, image cytometry, and fluorescence in situ hybridization (FISH). These techniques can be applied to formalin-fixed, paraffin-embedded tissue samples obtained by prostate needle biopsy, transurethral resection of the prostate (TURP), and radical prostatectomy. Image cytometry and FISH are best suited for characterization of a smaller number of cells in limited tissue samples, such as needle biopsy (Falkmer 1991, Ross 1996). Moreover, these two methods may be more sensitive in the detection of aneuploidy (Steilen 1994, Takahashi 1994). A major confounding factor in the measurement of DNA ploidy is a sampling problem where needle biopsy carcinoma DNA ploidy is not always concordant with DNA ploidy in carcinoma whole gland (Abou-Elella 1998, Häggman 1994, Takai 1994), in part because of the heterogeneity of DNA ploidy in an individual patient's tumor (Häggman 1994, Kucuk 1993, O'Malley 1993, Warzynski 1995). A potential problem in flow cytometry is detectable aneuploidy in ejaculatory duct and seminal vesicle epithelium (Arber 1991, Wojcik 1999).

t21.1 Prognostic Factors for Prostate Cancer: College of American Pathologists (CAP) and World Health Organization (WHO) Recommendations*

Category I: Recommended for routine reporting.†
TNM stage
Histologic grade (Gleason)
Surgical margin status
Perioperative serum PSA
Category II: Factors with promise or recommended (despite incomplete data)
DNA ploidy
Histologic type
Tumor amount in needle biopsy tissue (recommended)
Tumor amount in radical prostatectomy specimens (recommended)
Category III: Not currently recommended (due to insufficient evidence)
Genetic markers
Neuroendocrine markers
Proliferation markers, apoptosis
Perineural invasion
Vascular/lymphatic invasion
Microvessel density
Nuclear morphometry
Androgen receptors

*From Bostwick 1999 and Bostwick 2000
†Factors agreed upon by both CAP and WHO. WHO also recommends reporting WHO nuclear grade, pathologic effects of treatment and location of cancer within prostate

t21.2 DNA Ploidy in Prostatic Carcinoma

Ploidy = amount of chromosomal DNA
Methods of measurement: flow cytometry, image cytometry, FISH*
Related to Gleason grade, tumor size, pathologic stage, and clinical outcome in most univariate, but only some multivariate, analyses
Confounding factor: Ploidy heterogeneity in prostatic carcinoma
Clinical setting with strongest evidence for use: clinical stage D1 disease (regional lymph node metastasis)
Currently: not recommended for routine use

*FISH = fluorescence in situ hybridization

There are conflicting data on the value of DNA ploidy as a prognostic indicator. DNA ploidy status has been correlated with a variety of pathologic and clinical variables. At the histopathologic level, DNA ploidy has been linked to Gleason histologic grade, nuclear grade, tumor size (volume), and pathologic stage (Badalament 1996, Brinker 1999, Diaz 1999, Egawa 1996, Erbesdobler 1999, Geburek 1997, Greene 1994, Häggman 1997B, Humphrey 1991, Mora 1999, Papadoupoulos 1996, Vesalainen 1994A). Aneuploid tumors tend to be high-grade (with a Gleason score of ≥7), of larger volume, and of higher stage. However, there is a degree of overlap between diploid and nondiploid tumors in these associations. For example, some very small (<0.1 cc) peripheral-zone carcinomas can be aneuploid (Greene 1994). In tissue-based studies, DNA ploidy has also been correlated with microvessel density (Hall 1994), p53 expression (Papadoupoulos 1996), and proliferation index (Cheng 1999B, Khoo 1999, Papadoupoulos 1996).

DNA ploidy status of carcinoma in a prostate needle biopsy has been used to predict pathologic stage (Ross 1994), but overall the results are mixed. In two recent studies (Brinker 1999, Sebo 2001), DNA ploidy in needle biopsy tissue did not predict tumor volume (Sebo 2001) or pathologic stage (Brinker 1999, Sebo 2001) once the preoperative serum PSA, amount of tumor in needle biopsy tissue, and accurate needle biopsy Gleason grade were known. Additionally, in a recent survey of published nomograms, not a single model incorporated DNA ploidy in preoperative prediction of margin status, tumor volume, or pathologic stage (Ross 2001). The most widely used model to predict pretreatment pathologic stage, the "Partin Tables" (Partin 1997), uses the biopsy Gleason grade, clinical stage, and serum PSA without DNA ploidy.

DNA ploidy has been related to clinical outcomes and response to therapy, where prostate cancer patients with diploid tumors usually have a better outcome than patients with nondiploid tumors (Adolfsson 1994, Bostwick 1999). This association has strong support when ploidy is assessed in isolation as a single parameter in a univariate analysis. However, in multivariate analyses, it is not clear if DNA ploidy provides additional prognostic information beyond the standard predictors of stage and grade (Adolfsson 1994). In a recent review of 22 models used to predict outcome after radical prostatectomy or radiotherapy, only one uses DNA ploidy in the set of predictive factors (Ross 2001). In contrast to localized prostate cancer, the DNA ploidy pattern in the primary tumor or lymph node metastatic deposits appears to provide significant, additional prognostic information in the clinical setting of regional lymph node metastasis (Cheng 1998A, Cher 1996A, Pollack 1997, Stephenson 1987, Winkler 1988, Zincke 1992). DNA ploidy prognostic importance in patients with distant metastases is less certain (Jorgensen 1995, Miller 1991, Yokogi 1991). Currently, DNA ploidy is not recommended for routine reporting (Bostwick 1999, Bostwick 2000) **t21.1**.

[21.2] Chromosomal Alterations

Hereditary Prostate Cancer

Genetic abnormalities in DNA that are inherited (germline) and/or acquired (somatic) are associated with the initiation and progression of prostate cancer (Abate-Shen 2000, Bratt 2002, Brothman 1999, Dong 1997, Dorkin 1997, Elo 2001, Isaacs 1998, Konishi 1997B, Lalani 1997, Latil 1998, Ozen 2000, Visakorpi 1999). It has been estimated that about 42% of the risk for prostate cancer may be explained by heritable factors (Lichtenstein 2000), whereas virtually all established prostatic carcinomas show acquired chromosomal defects.

Inherited susceptibility to prostate cancer has been recognized for over 40 years (Woolf 1960). An autosomal dominant mode of susceptibility has been proposed (Schaid 1998), but X-linked, recessive, or imprinted components could also exist (Elo 2001). High-penetrance susceptibility genes probably cause 5%-10% of all prostate cancers (Elo 2001), whereas low-penetrance polymorphisms may be more prevalent and may thereby have an overall larger contribution to the heritable nature of some prostate cancers. A fairly large number (n = ~20) of chromosomal loci may harbor high-penetrance germline prostate cancer susceptibility genes **t21.3**, but only a few genes at these loci: *ELAC2* (Tavtigian 2001), *RNASEL* (Carpten 2002, Rökman 2002), *MSR-1* (Xu 2002), and the breast cancer susceptibility gene *BRCA2* (Gayther 2000, Tonin 1995),have been identified. Prostate cancer genetic susceptibility appears to be heterogeneous, and thus far not a single major susceptibility locus that accounts for a large proportion of inherited prostate cancer has been mapped. Indeed, the heterogeneity of mutation in different predisposition genes in different populations may be the basis for the inability of many studies to reproduce the findings of the specific high-penetrance susceptibility loci listed in **t21.3**. Prostate cancer inheritance is likely to be complex, heterogeneous, and multigenic.

Low-penetrance polymorphisms that may create susceptibility to prostate cancer include polymorphisms in CAG repeats in the androgen receptor (Casella 2001, Giovannucci 1997, Ingles 1997, Stanford 1997); vitamin D receptor gene (Blazer 2000, Correa-Cerro 1999B, Habuchi 2000A, Ingles 1997, Taylor 1996); 5α-reductase (*SRD5A2*) (Kantoff 1997, Makridakis 1999, Nam 2001); and cytochrome P450 (*CYP3A4* and *CYP17*) (Habuchi 2000B, Rebbeck 1998). That alteration of the gene expression of several of these genes might increase susceptibility to prostate cancer makes biologic sense. For example, a short CAG repeat is associated with increased transcriptional activity of the androgen receptor (Chamberlain 1994) and an increased relative risk of prostate cancer (Giovannucci 1997, Ingles 1997, Stanford 1997). Also, one missense polymorphic variant in the gene-encoding

t21.3 Chromosomal Loci Implicated as Sites of Prostate Cancer Susceptibility Genes

Chromosomal Locus	Name	Comment	References
1q24-25	*HPC1*	Accounts for about 6% of inherited prostate cancers. *HPC1*-related carcinomas slightly higher grade and stage compared to sporadic carcinomas. *RNASEL* gene mutated in limited number of families showing linkage with *HPC1*	Smith 1996, Grönberg 1997A, Grönberg 1997B, Xu 2000, Dunsmuir 1998, Carpten 2002, Rökmah 2002
1q42.2-43	*PCAP*	Not confirmed in several subsequent studies	Berthon 1998, Berry 2000B, Gibbs 1999A, Whittmore 1999
1p36	*CAPB*	Rare; found in a few families with history of brain and prostate cancer	Gibbs 1999B
8p2223		Missense mutations detected in *MSR1* gene in families with hereditary prostate cancer	Xu 2002
11	Not named	Later-onset families	Gibbs 2000
13q12-13		Germ-line *BRCA2* mutations may account for 5% of prostate cancer in familial clusters	Tonin 1995, Gayther 2000
16q23	Not named	16p had stronger linkage in subsequent analysis	Suarez 2000A, Suarez 2000B
17p	*HPC2*	*HPC2/ELAC2* gene mutation may account for 4%-5% of prostate cancer cases	Tavtigian 2001
20q13;20pter-20q11	*HPC20*	Strongest linkage with pedigrees with < 5 family members, older age	Berry 2000A, Zheng 2001
Xq27-28	*HPCX*	No strong linkage in two studies, but support from a third study	Xu 1998, Singh 2000, Peters 2001, Schleutker 2000
Others: 2q,4q,5p-5q,8,10, 12p,14, 15q, 16p, 19p			Gibbs 2000, Suarez 2000A, Hsieh 2001, Goddard 2001

steroid 5α-reductase type II (*SRD5A2*), which converts testosterone to the more active dihydrotestosterone, generates increased catalytic activity of this enzyme (Makridakis 1997) and is associated with an increased risk of advanced prostate cancer (Jaffe 2000, Makridakis 1999). Overall, however, prostate cancer inheritance risk associated with these polymorphisms has been deemed weak and not always reproducible (Elo 2001).

The genetic alterations in prostatic carcinomas that arise somatically in genetically predisposed individuals are similar to those of sporadic tumors, with common losses on 6q, 7q, 8p, 10q, 13q, and 16q, and gains at 7q, 8q, and 19p-q (Rökman 2001, Verhagen 2000). These preliminary results of a limited number of cases suggest that, for the most part, these familial prostate cancers utilize the same somatic progression pathways as sporadic prostate cancers (Rökman 2001). There were a few distinctive abnormalities in several *HPC1* and *HPCX* cases, with a loss of 3p and a gain of 6q (Verhagen 2000). Of note, allelic imbalance at *HPC1*, *PCAP*, and *CAPB* loci are low in both sporadic and familial prostatic carcinomas (Ahman 2000, Bergthorsson 2000, Dunsmuir 1998, Latil 1997), suggesting that genes at these loci are not classical tumor suppressor genes. Also apparently not important in hereditary prostate cancer is defective DNA mismatch repair, since tumoral microsatellite instability is rare (Ahman 2001). Finally, prostate carcinoma p53, bcl-2, proliferation index, and microvessel density did not differ in patients with and without a family history of prostate cancer (Bauer 1998).

There is little histopathologic difference between sporadic and hereditary prostatic carcinomas (Bastacky 1995, Bova 1998, Grönberg 1998, Hanus 1999, Keetch 1996, Kupelian 1997B, Valeri 2000), except for a slightly lower Gleason grade in hereditary prostatic carcinoma (Bastacky 1995, Grönberg 1998, Keetch 1996) and more small multifocal cancers associated with prostatic intraepithelial neoplasia in the sporadic group (Bastacky 1995). Not much is known of prostatic carcinoma phenotype (histopathologic features) associated with a specific susceptibility genotype. For *HPC1* hereditary prostatic carcinomas, the tumors were of slightly higher grade and stage compared with sporadic tumors (Grönberg 1997B). Additionally, a polymorphic variant of the *SRD5A2* gene associated with prostate cancer susceptibility (A49T genotype) has been correlated with a higher pathologic stage (Jaffe 2000). Future genotypic-phenotypic relationships should be defined based on specific abnormal genes identified at the susceptibility loci listed in **t21.3**.

Clinically, men with inherited prostate cancer present at a younger age, but the clinical stage and PSA level at presentation do not differ from sporadic prostate cancers (Valeri 2000). Because of this younger age at onset, the American Cancer Society suggests that early detection efforts (with serum PSA and digital rectal examination) begin at ages 40-45 for men with first-degree relatives diagnosed with prostate cancer at a young age (Smith 2001). Family members of men with hereditary prostate cancer are at a small but statistically significant higher risk for the development of central nervous system tumors (Walsh 1997) and possibly stomach cancer (Matikaine 2001), but not breast, ovarian, or endometrial carcinoma (Walsh 1997). The response to treatment and survival of men with inherited prostate cancer is not different, in most studies, from sporadic prostate cancer (Bova 1998, Grönberg 1998, Hanus 1999, Kupelian 1997A, Kupelian 1997B, Narain 2001). In the future, clinical correlations with specific gene alterations should provide a more precise picture of the biological and clinical significance of inherited prostate cancer.

Sporadic Prostate Cancer

Sporadic prostatic carcinomas, which constitute 90% of all prostate cancers, exhibit patterns of acquired chromosomal loss and gain that are different from those germline chromosomal alterations that predispose one to inherited prostatic carcinoma **t21.4**. Chromosomal aberrations, as detected by cytogenetics and molecular methods including Southern blotting, microsatellite analysis by polymerase chain reaction, FISH, and comparative genomic hybridization, are found in all prostate cancers (Elo 2001). Numerous heterogenous patterns of both loss and gain of chromosomes or chromosomal regions (loci) have been identified **t21.5, t21.6;** **f21.1 see p 486**. Correlations of certain chromosomal aberrations with pathologic and/or clinical endpoints have been made **t21.5, t21.6**, but further investigation will be necessary to clarify the diagnostic and prognostic significance of these genetic changes. These abnormal chromosomal loci should serve as a road map that leads to the identification of specific target genes critical for prostate cancer initiation and progression. A number of candidate genes have been suggested to be altered at these loci, but currently specific target genes for most of the chromosomal alterations are still not known (Abate-Shen 2000, Elo 2001, Isaacs 1998, Latil 1998).

The initial characterization of chromosomal abnormalities in prostatic carcinoma by classical cytogenetics was difficult due to overgrowth of fibroblasts when culturing the cancer cells (Sandberg 1992). About 25% of primary prostatic carcinomas have revealed abnormal karyotypes obtained by staining metaphase chromosomes, with clonal abnormalities involving many of the chromosomes listed in **t21.5, t21.6** (Verma 1999). Subsequently, molecular techniques have also defined numerical chromosomal aberrations and further mapped minimal common regions of chromosomal loss or gain. Moreover, a distinct advantage for FISH, microsatellite analysis by PCR, and CGH is that a paraffin-embedded tumor can be utilized. This tremendously expands the number of cases that can be assessed, allows for more precise phenotypic-genotypic (histopathologic) correlations to then be established, and requires only a small amount of tumor (including that in needle biopsy tissue) for analysis.

Loss of chromosomal DNA in prostatic carcinoma has been discovered at many loci **t21.5**. A loss of genetic material tends to predominate in earlier-stage prostate cancer, whereas DNA copy number gain is more common in hormone-refractory prostate cancer (Visakorpi 1995A). For 10 loci, the reported loss is seen in 50% of more of cases **t21.5**. The highest frequency of loss is on chromosomal arms 7q, 8p, 10q, 13q, and 16q **i21.1, i21.2**. Sites of allelic loss (also termed allelic imbalance and loss of heterozygosity [LOH]) are potential locations of recessively altered tumor suppressor genes, so much effort has been directed toward the physical definition of these

■ **t21.4 Chromosomal Abnormalities in Sporadic Prostate Cancers**

All prostatic carcinomas acquire genetic alterations
Most common* chromosomal deletions: 1p, 5q, 7q, 8p, 10q, 13q, 16q, 17p, 17q, Y
Most common* chromosomal gains: 1q, 3p, 3q, 7, 8q, 11p, 12q, 16p, 17, 18, 19, 20, 22, Xq
Some alterations associated with more aggressive cancer
Specific target genes for most of the aberrations are still not known

*At least one study with at least 50% of cases with loss or gain

■ t21.5 Chromosomal DNA Loss in Prostate Cancer

Chromosome	% Cases With Loss	Comment	Reference(s)
1p	50%		Nupponen 1998
2p	7%		Kunimi 1991
2q	18%-42%		Cher 1996B, Alers 2000, Zitzelsberger 2001, El Gedaily 2001
3p	10%-20%		Carter 1990A, Kunimi 1991, Cunningham 1996, Huang 1996
4q	18%-26%		Alers 2000, Zitzelsberger 2001, El Gedaily 2001
5q	14%-50%	Associated with higher Gleason grade	Cher 1996B, Cher 1998, Fu 2000, Alers 2000, Witte 2000, Zitzelsberger 2001, El Gedaily 2001
6q	6%-48%	No correlation with grade and stage	Visakorpi 1995A, Huang 1996, Cher 1996B, Cher 1998, Srikantan 1999, Alers 2000
7p	8%		Kunimi 1991
7q	10%-75%	Associated with higher grade, stage, and progression and lower survival	Carter 1990A, Zenklusen 1994, Takahashi 1995, Kunimi 1991, Jenkins 1998B, Witte 2000
8p	22%-91%	Some evidence for association with higher grade, stage, progression, and risk of death	Bova 1993, Sakr 1994, Trapman 1994, Emmert-Buck 1995, Visakorpi 1995, Kagan 1995, Crundwell 1996, Cunningham 1996, Huang 1996, Deubler 1997, Häggman 1997A, Jenkins 1998B, Cher 1998, Prasad 1998, Washburn 2000, El Gedaily 2001
8q	11%-25%		Trapman 1994
9p	16%		Visakorpi 1995A
9q	15%		Carter 1990A
10q	18%-62%	Linked with higher stage	Carter 1990A, Gray 1995, Kunimi 1991, Ittmann 1996, Cher 1996B, Deubler 1997, Cher 1998, Nupponen 1998, Rubin 2000, Alers 2000
11p	0-9%		Carter 1990A, Hügel 1999
11q	7%		Hügel 1999
12p	0-47%		Sakr 1994, Kunimi 1991, Kibel 1998, Hügel 1999, Kibel 2000B
12q	6%-11%		Kunimi 1991, Hügel 1999
13q	9%-75%	Some evidence for correlation with increased grade, stage, and tumor volume	Carter 1990A, Visakorpi 1995A, Kunimi 1991, Cher 1996B, Li 1998, Cher 1998, Nupponen 1998, Hyytinen 1999, Afonso 1999, Hügel 1999, Dong 2000, Alers 2000, El Gedaily 2001
15q	39%		Cher 1996B
16q	14%-83%	and progression	Osman 1997, Elo 1997, Jenkins 1998B, Cher 1998, Nupponen 1998, Elo 1999, Fu 2000, Alers 2000, Paris 2000
17p	17%-50%	Related to grade and progression after radical prostatectomy	Carter 1990A, Cher 1996B, Brooks 1996
17q	6%-70%		Gao 1995A, Gao 1995B, Kunimi 1991, Cunningham 1996, Williams 1996, Deubler 1997
18q	13%-45%	Correlated with higher stage	Visakorpi 1995A, Jenkins 1998B, Hügel 1999, Fu 2000, Padalecki 2000, Alers 2000, El Gedaily 2001
19q		Associated with increased Gleason grade	Witte 2000
21q	23%		Cunningham 1996
22q	6%-16%		Kunimi 1991, Crundwell 1996, Huang 1996, Hügel 1999
Xq	25%		Zitzelsberger 2001
Y	16%-53%		Breitkreuz 1993, Konig 1994, Alers 1995, Alers 2000, Jordan 2001

regions and identification of the candidate genes that reside there. The frequency of loss is variable, as indicated by the percentage ranges in **t21.5**, and dependent on the technique used, number and location of regions assessed, and the patient population. Heterogeneity of LOH is present not only between patients, but also within an individual patient's prostate cancer. Evidence exists to suggest that each prostate cancer has its own pattern of allelic loss (Hügel 1999) and that physically separate prostatic carcinomas within the same prostate gland can exhibit different patterns of LOH (Cheng 1998B, Macintosh 1998, Ruijter 1999).

Chromosomal gain of DNA is a common genetic event, where 13 chromosomes or chromosomal arms exhibit DNA gain in at least 50% of cases **t21.6**. The highest frequency of gain is on chromosomes 7, 8q, and 19 **t21.6**. Sites of chromosomal gain are potential locations of amplified oncogenes. Short, high-level amplifications suggestive of single amplified oncogenes are rare in primary carcinomas (Bubendorf 1999, Sattler 1999), but can be seen in metastatic cancer (Alers 2000, Bubendorf 1999). Except for chromosomes 7, 8, X, and Y, chromosomal gains have not been as well-studied as

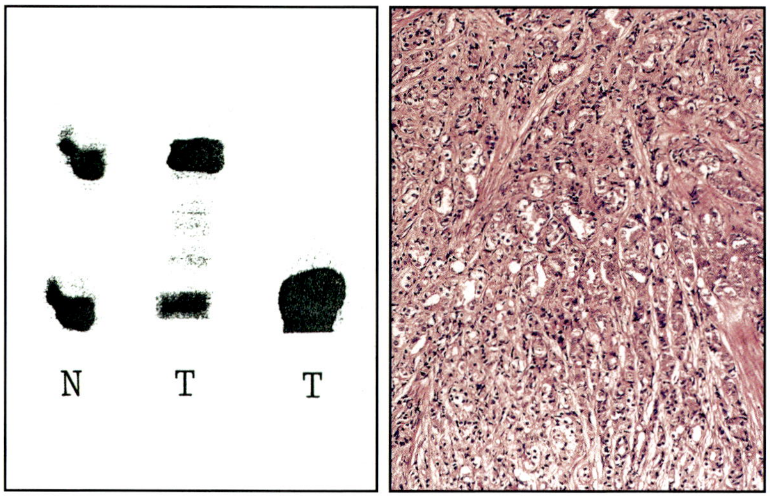

■ i21.1 *Allelic loss at chromosome 8p22 (LPL-3′ marker) in high-grade prostatic carcinoma, as determined by polymerase chain reaction amplification. There is a lost allele (band) in one tumor sample (T, far right lane), compared to normal tissue (N) and a second tumor sample (T, middle lane). DNA loss on chromosome 8p is one of the most common genetic abnormalities in prostatic carcinoma.*

■ **t21.6 Chromosomal DNA Gains in Prostate Cancer**

Chromosome	% Cases with Gain	Comment	Reference
1	36%	Associated with distant metastasis	Konig 1994, Cher 1996B
1p	38%		Zitzelsberger 2001
1q	16%-52%		Cher 1996B,Alers 2000
2p	45%		Cher 1996B
3p	56%		Sattler 1999
3q	18%-52%		Cher 1996B, Sattler 2000, Alers 2000
4	44%		Sattler 1999
5	38%		Sattler 1999
5q	38%		Cher 1998
6q	44%		Sattler 1999
7	8%-76%	Associated with increased grade, stage, and recurrence after radical prostatectomy	Bandyk 1994, Qian 1995, Takahashi 1995, Alers 1995, Gburek 1997, Alers 2000, Skacel 2001
7q	21%-40%	Correlated with increased Gleason grade and metastasis	Nupponen 1998, Jenkins 1998A, Sattler 1999, Alers 2000
8	30%-59%	Associated with increased grade and stage	Qian 1995, Takahashi 1995, Matsuura 1996, Skacel 2001
8p	9%	Amplification at 8p24	Van den Berg 1995
8q	9%-85%	Linked to grade, stage, bony metastasis and progression	Cher 1996B, Alers 1997, Nupponen 1998, Sattler 1999, Fu 2000, Alers 2000, El Gedaily 2001, Steiner 2002
9p	38%		Sattler 1999
9q	18%		Alers 2000
10	23%		Qian 1995
11p	52%		Cher 1996B
12	9%		Qian 1995
12q	25%-56%		Sattler 1999, Zitzelsberger 2001
13q	31%		Sattler 1999
15q	25%		Zitzelsberger 2001
16p	69%		Zitzelsberger 2001
17	50%		Zitzelsberger 2001
17q	23%		Alers 2000
18	63%		Konig 1994
18q	33%		Nupponen 1998
19	75%		Zitzelsberger 2001
20	50%		Zitzelsberger 2001
20q	15%		Alers 2000
22	56%		Zitzelsberger 2001
X		Associated with metastasis	Gburek 1997
Xp	16%-33%		Nupponen 1998, Alers 2000, El Gedaily 2001
Xq	21%-50%		Sattler 1999, Fu 2000, Alers 2000, El Gedaily 2001
Y	4%-28%	Associated with metastasis	Konig 1994, Qian 1995, Matsuura 1996, Gburek 1997

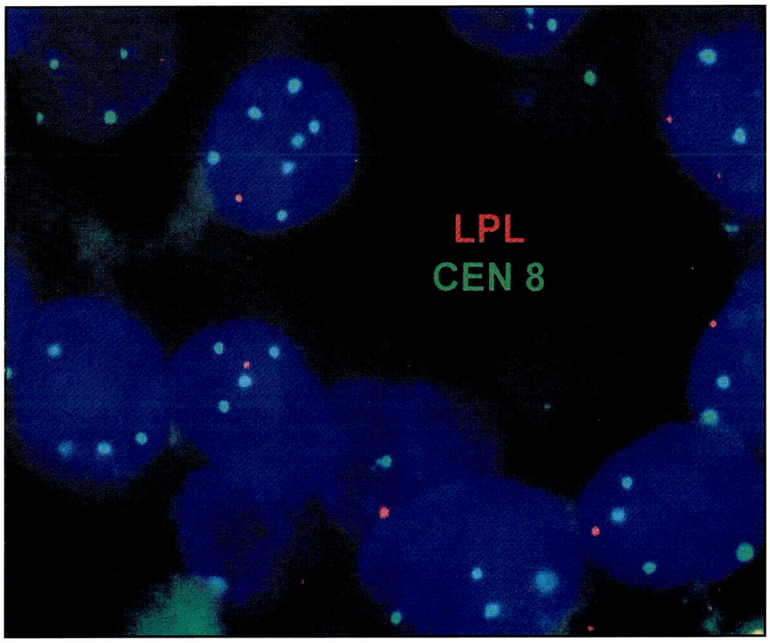

■ **i21.2** *Loss of chromosome 8p22 LPL locus in Gleason score 9 prostatic carcinoma cell nuclei demonstrated by FISH. (Courtesy of Dr Robert B Jenkins)*

losses, and therefore frequency figures are usually a single percentage number derived from a single paper **t21.6**.

Prostatic carcinoma initiation and progression are not likely to be defined by a single, linear, stereotyped pathway of carcinogenesis, but rather as the progressive accumulation of genetic damage, manifested in numerous chromosomes as loss and/or gain, that will characterize various stages of prostate cancer development. Chromosomal abnormalities can be detected at the earliest stage of prostatic neoplasia, prostatic intraepithelial neoplasia (**t11.17, p 206**). Numerical chromosomal abnormalities can be seen in up to two-thirds of high-grade PIN foci (Jenkins 1997). Small, invasive adenocarcinomas less than 0.5cc (Alers 2001) and incidentally detected transition zone carcinomas in TURP chips (Crandwell 1997) also exhibit chromosomal arm and allelic loss. With an increase in tumor volume, histologic grade, and pathologic stage, there is a progressive accumulation in the number of aberrant chromosomes per patient (Alers 2000, Alers 2001, Carter 1990A, Kunimi 1991, Saric 1999, Visakorpi 1995A). However, no single chromosomal alteration is necessary and sufficient for initiation and progression, and there is substantial heterogeneity of genetic lesions at each stage of progression and within each individual's prostate cancer. The heterogeneity can be found at the preinvasive PIN stage where different PIN foci within

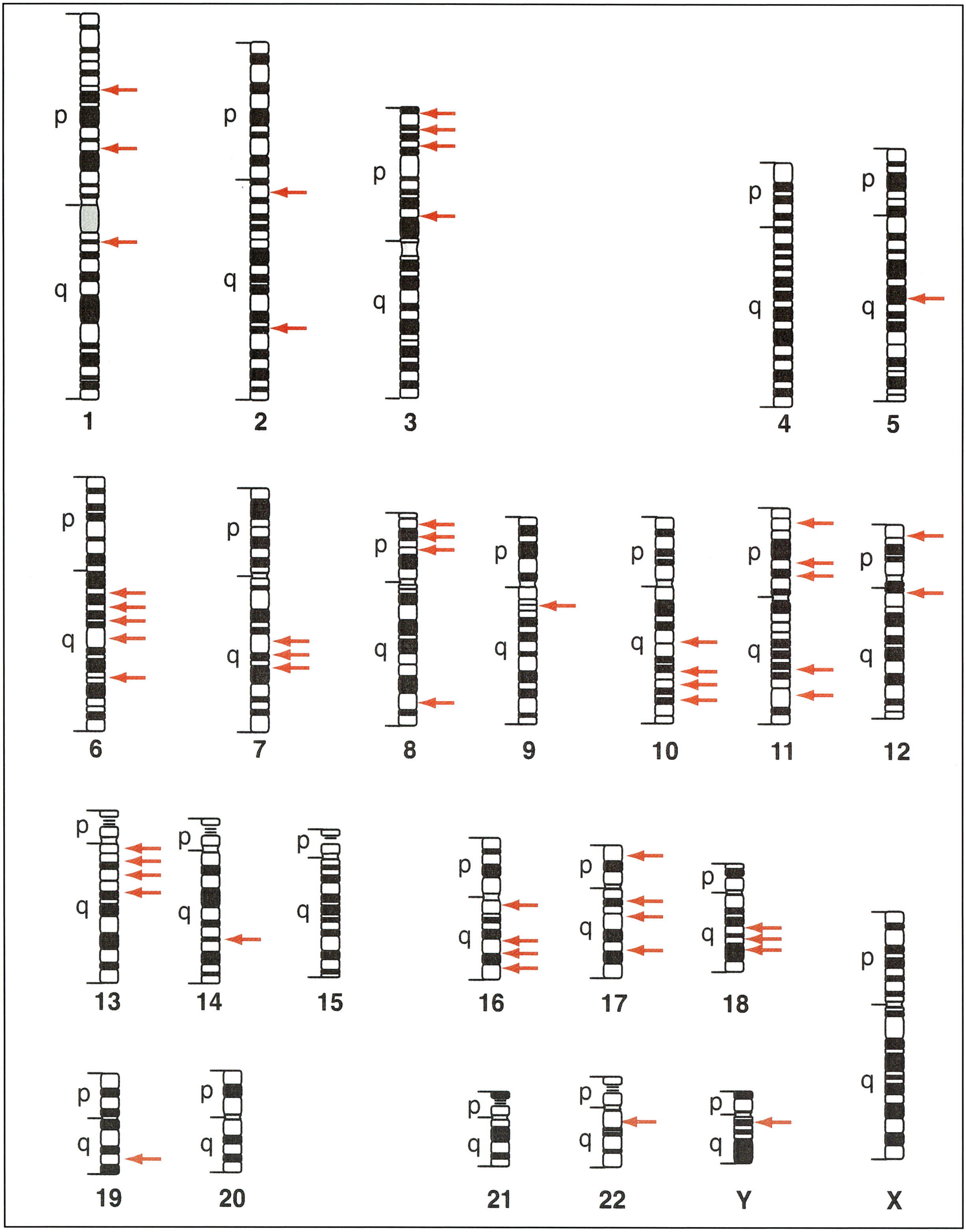

■ **f21.1** *Sites of chromosomal structural abnormalities in prostatic carcinoma. (Brothman 1999)*

the same gland were genetically diverse (Saric 1999). PIN cells share some but not all of the chromosomal aberrations of invasive carcinoma (**f11.5**, p 209). Similarly, genetic analysis of paired primary tumor and metastatic tumor deposits show similar patterns of gains and/or losses in only about one-half of cases (Cheng 1999A, Gburek 1997, Nupponen 1998). These shifting patterns of chromosomal anomalies may be related to intrinsic prostate cancer heterogeneity, overall genetic instability, and clonal divergence and evolution (Cheng 1999A). It is not clear if genomic instability in prostate cancer is related to defects in DNA mismatch repair that normally corrects replication errors: microsatellite instability (MSI), which is indicative of defects(s) in this repair mechanism, has been reported in 0%-65% of prostatic carcinomas (Crundwell 1997, 1999, Cunningham 1996, Egawa 1995, Gao 1994, Rohrbach 1999, Terrell 1995, Uchida 1995, Watanabe 1996). Associations of MSI with pathologic and clinical endpoints have also been inconsistent (Crundwell 1999, Egawa 1995, Rohrbach 1999, Uchida 1995, Watanabe 1996).

Scant data exist on the relationship of all of the chromosomal abnormalities in prostatic carcinoma and clinical outcome endpoints. Loss of genetic material on 7q, 8p, and 16q and gain on 7 and 8q have been associated with clinical progression (recurrence or patient survival) (Alers 1997, Alers 2000, Elo 1997, Elo 1999, Jenkins 1998B, Suzuki 1995, Washburn 2000), but only a few studies (Alers 2000, Jenkins 1998B, Washburn 2000) have assessed significance in multivariate analyses. In the future, specific gene alterations, rather than chromosomal loci abnormalities, should be analyzed for independent prognostic significance. Currently, genetic markers such as chromosomal abnormalities are category III prognostic factors, which at this time are not recommended for use because of insufficient evidence (Bostwick 1999, Bostwick 2000) **t21.1**.

[21.3] Tumor Suppressor Genes

Tumor suppressor genes are negative regulators or "brakes" of cell growth, where inactivation of both alleles leads to release of suppression. Those tumor suppressor genes that are commonly mutated in other cancers, such as *p53* and *Rb*, are not essential in most prostate cancers. Although a number of genes have been implicated as tumor suppressor genes in prostate cancer **t21.7**, the genes at most of the loci of chromosomal loss, where such genes may reside, have not been identified. Such loss is detectable early in PIN and is found at all stages of prostate cancer, suggesting that tumor suppressor genes may be important in the initiation and progression of prostate cancer.

■ t21.7 Tumor Suppressor Genes in Prostate Cancer

Inactivation of these genes releases the "brakes" on prostate cancer growth and spread

Only a few specific candidate tumor suppressor genes have been identified in inherited prostate carcinoma: *BRCA1, BRCA2, ELAC2*

Numerous candidate tumor suppressor genes have been identified in sporadic prostate carcinoma

Tumor suppressor genes are probably involved in initiation and progression of prostate cancer

p53

p53, a tumor suppressor gene located on chromosome 17p13.1, is the most commonly altered gene in human cancer (Humphrey 1994, Malkin 1998). The normal p53 protein appears to be a transcription factor that binds specific DNA sequences and modulates growth regulatory genes. In response to DNA damage, p53 arrests the cell cycle, allowing genomic repair or apoptosis to occur. Inactivation of p53 via missense mutations, deletions, or nonsense mutations results in cessation of arrest of the cell cycle at G1 and damaged DNA is replicated, which can result in mutation, aneuploidy, mitotic failure, and cell death (Malkin 1998). Just as in other solid tumors, most inactivating *p53* gene mutations in prostatic carcinoma are missense single-base substitutions in exons 4-11 and usually in exons 5-8 (Bookstein 1993, Chi 1994, Eastham 1995, Hall 1995, Incognito 2000, Kubota 1995B, Kunimi 1996, Massenkeil 1994, Moyret-Lalle 1995, Navone 1999, Stapleton 1997). At the protein level this point mutation can generate an amino acid substitution that results in an increased protein half-life, allowing for detection by immunohistochemical means (Humphrey 1994). In prostatic carcinoma, visualization of immunoreactive, nuclear, p53 is often, but not always, indicative of p53 gene mutation (Bookstein 1993, Heidenberg 1995, Navone 1993, Wertz 1996).

The frequency of *p53* alteration at the DNA and protein levels in prostate cancer is related to histologic grade and stage. It is uncommon that the *p53* gene is mutated and/or that the p53 protein exhibits abnormal nuclear accumulation in localized prostatic carcinoma. In one literature survey of over 1000 cases reported in 20 studies, abnormal p53 protein accumulation was detected by immunohistochemical analysis, on average, in about 16% of clinically localized prostatic carcinomas (Humphrey 1995B) **i21.3**. In metastatic deposits, particularly androgen-insensitive, bony metastasis, *p53* gene mutations and immunoreactive p53 protein can be found in up to 60% of cases (Aprikian 1994, Cheng 1999C, Dinjens 1994, Malkin 1998, McDonnell 1997, Myers 1994A, Suzuki 1996, Voeller 1994). This increased frequency of p53 abnormalities in distant metastatic sites suggests possible clonal expression with tumor spread and the aggressive nature of prostatic carcinoma cells with abnormal p53. In support of this latter notion are the reported associations of p53

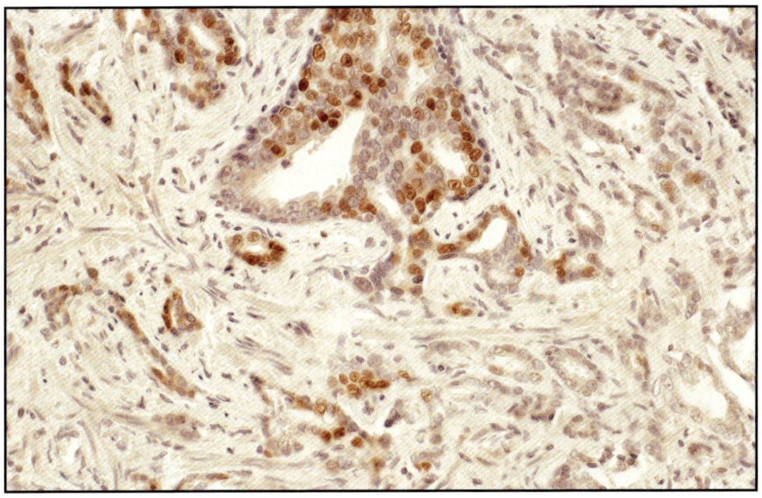

■i21.3 *p53 protein accumulation in nuclei of high-grade prostatic intraepithelial neoplasia and carcinoma, detected by immuohistochemical staining. Such increased immuoreactivity, which is often due to p53 gene mutation, is uncommon in PIN and localized prostatic carcinoma, but often found in androgen-independent, bony metastatic deposits.*

abnormalities with an increasing proliferation index (Borre 2000, Cheng 1999D); increasing histologic grade (Borre 2000, Byrne 1997, Matsushima 1997, Moul 1996B, Mydlo 1998, Ruijter 1998, Schlechte 1997, Shiraishi 1998A, Sinik 1997, Stattin 1996B); increasing stage (Aprikian 1994, Bookstein 1993, Eastham 1995, Moul 1996B, Myers 1994A, Navone 1993, Ruijter 1998, Schlechte 1997); clinical progression (Bauer 1996, Brewster 1999, Byrne 1997, Cheng 1999C, Leibovich 2000, Matsushima 1997, Moul 1996B, Osman 1999, Shurbaji 1995, Stackhouse 1999, Stricker 1996, Thomas 1993); and patient survival (Borre 2000, Grignon 1997, Kuczyk 1998, Stattin 1996B, Thomas 1993). Despite this wealth of supportive data for use of p53 as a prognostic indicator, major confounding problems include lack of a uniform definition of a positive immunohistochemical signal and heterogeneity of p53 immunoreactivity in prostatic carcinoma (Aprikian 1994, Borre 2000, Mirchandani 1995). This heterogeneity and the inherently minimal prostate gland sampling afforded by prostate needle biopsy limit practical application of p53 immunostains on carcinoma in prostate needle biopsy tissue. In one recent study that underscores this potential difficulty, immunoreactive p53 in carcinoma in needle biopsy tissue did not correlate with immunoreactive p53 in matched radical prostatectomy tissue or with recurrence after the surgery, whereas immunoreactive p53 in carcinoma in the radical prostatectomy specimens did correlate with recurrence (Stackhouse 1999). p53 is currently a category III prognostic factor. In the future, a combination of p53 abnormality with bcl-2 (Apakama 1996), Rb (Theodorescu 1997), and MDM-2 (Leite 2001) status may refine its prognostic capacity. Finally, p53 status could be important for predicting response to p53-directed therapy, such as wild-type p53 gene therapy, which is currently in clinical trials (Steiner 2000).

RB1

The retinoblastoma gene *RB1,* a prototypic tumor suppressor gene, is located at chromosome 13q14 (Newsham 1998). The encoded 110 kd protein product ($pp110^{RB}$) is a nuclear phosphoprotein involved in the negative regulation of cell proliferation (Weinberg 1995). In the prostate, the RB1 protein has been implicated as a regulator of apoptosis of prostate cells, especially in response to androgens (Abate-Shen 2000). In prostatic carcinoma, *RB1* abnormalities have been described at the gene, mRNA, and protein levels. Allelic loss on 13q, including the *RB1* region, is common in prostatic carcinoma **t21.5**, but this does not correlate with *RB1* mRNA or protein levels (Cooney 1996, Latil 1999, Li 1998), suggesting the existence of another tumor suppressor gene in this region. Gross rearrangement or mutations of the *RB1* gene are uncommon at 4% (Tricoli 1996) and 16% (Kubota 1995A), respectively. *RB* gene loss is seen more frequently after androgen deprivation therapy (Kaltz-Wittmer 2000). Loss of nuclear RB1 protein immunohistochemical reactivity has been found in about 20%-30% of cases (Cooney 1996, Theodorescu 1997, Phillips 1994B), and in one study the percentage of cells staining for RB1 protein was related to disease-specific survival after radical prostatectomy (Theodorescu 1997). In a second study, low *RB1* mRNA expression correlated with tumor grade and stage (Tricoli 1996). However, the role of *RB1* in prostate cancer is uncertain (Abate-Shen 2000, Latil 1998).

PTEN/MMAC1

PTEN (for phosphatase and tensin homolog deleted on chromosome 10), also known as *MMAC1* (for mutated in multiple advanced cancers), is a tumor suppressor gene cloned from the q23 region of chromosome 10 (Li 1997, Steck 1997). The encoded 403 amino acid protein is a tyrosine phosphatase (Myers 1997), which possibly functions in cell death and aberrant cell proliferation pathways (Abata-Shen 2000). *PTEN* inactivation is uncommon in localized, low-stage prostate cancer but is frequently inactivated in metastatic prostatic carcinomas (Cairns 1997, Dong 1998, Dong 2001, Feilotter 1998, McMenamin 1999, Myers 1997, Pesche 1998, Suzuki 1998, Teng 1997, Vlietstra 1998, Wang 1998, Whang 1998). Deletions at 10q in the region of the *PTEN* occur in 15%-55% of primary carcinomas (Cairns 1997, Dong 1998, Feilotter 1998, Pesche 1998), with gene alterations (deletions or point mutations) in 0%-24% of cases (Cairns 1997, Dong 1998, Dong 2001, Feilotter 1998, Pesche 1998, Wang 1998). *PTEN* gene mutations are much more common in metastatic sites, at an incidence of 63% (Suzuki 1998). Of interest, there was substantial *PTEN* mutational heterogeneity among different sites in the same patient, suggesting diverging genetic profiles between various clonal lineages of prostate cancer cells as they evolved during the metastatic process (Suzuki 1998). By immunohistochemical analysis, PTEN protein expression was completely absent in 20% of prostatic carcinoma cases; this loss correlated with high a Gleason grade (score of 7 or higher) and advanced pathologic stage (McMenamin 1999). It is not known if *PTEN* loss carries independent prognostic information.

Additional Putative Tumor-Suppressor Genes

Additional genes implicated as candidate tumor suppressor genes include *BRCA1*, *BRCA2*, *ELAC2*, *DCC*, *APC*, *KAI1*, *CTNNA1* (*a-catenin*), *CDH1* (*E-cadherin*), *CD44*, *WAF1/CIP1* (*p21*), *p16/CDKN2*, *HIC-1*, *KREV*, *NME1*, *NME2*, *ANX7*, *ST7*, *N33*, *NKx3.1*, *MXI1*, *CDH13*, *BBC*, *MADR2*, *DPC4*, and the Y-chromosome–specific genes *SRY* and *BY2* (Abate-Shen 2000, Latil 1998, Ozen 2000, Park 2000, Perinchery 2000, Rosen 2001, Sinclair 2000, Srivastava 2001, Vazina 2000, Visakorpi 1999, Yeh 2000, Zenklusen 2001). For many of these genes only limited data, such as location at a chromosomal region of loss and/or inactivation in prostate cancer, exist to suggest a tumor-suppressor role in prostate cancer. Functional proof of true tumor suppressor gene activity has mainly been accomplished by the transfer of chromosome segments or whole chromosomes (reviewed in Latil 1998), rather than specific genes, into prostate cancer cells. Thus most of these genes are currently only tumor suppressor gene candidates.

The few specific potential tumor suppressor genes thus far identified in hereditary prostate cancer—*BRCA1*, *BRCA2*, and *ELAC2*—appear mutated in the germline in only a small percent of inherited prostate cancer cases. The *BRCA1* breast cancer susceptibility gene on chromosome 17q21 was initially thought to confer a threefold elevated risk for inherited prostate cancer (Ford 1994), but several recent studies did not find a significant contribution of this gene to familial prostate cancer (Gayther 2000, Sinclair 2000, Vazina 2000). However, *BRCA1* could still provide tumor suppressor functions in the prostate (Rosen 2001). Of interest, *BRCA1* may modulate androgen receptor signaling (Park 2000, Yeh 2000). There is more consistent support for a role of germline mutation of the breast cancer susceptibility gene *BRCA2* on chromosome 13q12-13 as a risk factor for development of familial prostate cancer (Gayther 2000, Tonin 1995). Such mutations account for about 5% of familial prostate cancer cases (Gayther 2000). In tumor tissue, the possible functional importance of *BRCA2* is underscored by demonstration that allelic loss at *BRCA2* can be seen in about one-quarter of both familial and sporadic tumors (Edwards 1998) and in up to 71% of metastatic deposits (Hyytinen 1999). Moreover, there is the suggestion of shorter survival rates for patients with allelic loss at *BRCA2* (Edwards 1998). Finally, sequence variants in the gene *ELACA2* on chromosome 17p appear to impart for a few patients an increased risk for inherited prostate cancer (Tavtigian 2001). It is not clear how these mutations (three missense and one frameshift) might inactivate a tumor suppressor function for *ELAC2*, which is a metal-dependent hydrolase.

Interesting potential tumor suppressor genes in sporadic prostate cancer include those involved in cell cycle regulation, such as *p16*, *p21*, and *p27* (reviews in Abata-Shen 2000, Macri 1999), where inactivation of the gene or protein may lead to uncontrolled cell proliferation. Molecules that regulate these cell cycle genes, such as *KLF6*, a zinc finger transcription factor, which up-regulates p21, may also be potential tumor suppressor genes in prostate cancer (Narla 2001). Inactivation of transcription factors such as *NKx3.1*, a gene located at the frequently lost region of 8p21 in prostate cancers, and *MXI*, a Myc-binding protein, may also be important in some prostate cancers (Abate-Shen 2000). Loss of cellular adhesion by reduced expression of E-cadherin and c-CAM (Abate-Shen 2000) may lead to an enhanced capacity of prostate cancer cells to spread. A metastasis suppressor gene for prostate cancer, *KAI1*, has been identified (Dong 1995). Reduced expression of the KAI1 protein correlates with a higher Gleason grade and clinical stage (Ueda 1996). The mechanism for tumor suppression by this integral membrane protein, which is identical to CD33, has not been elucidated. CD44 is another membrane protein, encoded by a gene on chromosome 11p13, that may be involved in the suppression of prostate cancer metastasis (Gao 1997).

[21.4] Oncogenes

Oncogenes are altered forms of normal cellular genes called proto-oncogenes (Park 1998). The protein products of these proto-oncogenes are typically involved in the cell cycle, cell division, and differentiation. Activation of a proto-oncogene into an oncogene can occur by gene amplification, gene rearrangement, and point mutation (Park 1998). Of a recent list of 44 oncogenes (Park 1998), several have been implicated in human prostatic carcinoma, including *MYC, RAF, MET, RET,* and the epidermal growth factor receptor (EGFR) family-related proto-oncogenes c-*erb*B-1 (EGFR), c-*erb*B-2 (HER-2/neu; heregulin receptor), c-*erb*B-3, and c-*erb*B-4 (Abate-Shen 2000, Latil 1998, Netto 1994, Ozen 2000) **t21.8**.

■ t21.8 Oncogenes in Prostate Cancer

Oncogenes are altered normal cell genes termed proto-oncogenes
Activated oncogenes cause dysregulation of cell cycle, cell division, and differentiation
Oncogenes implicated in prostate cancer include *MYC, RAS, MET, RET,* c-*erb*B family
Oncogenes commonly mutated in other cancers, such as *MYC* and *RAS* are uncommonly altered in prostate cancer
Oncogenes probably play a more prominent role in metastatic and androgen-independent prostate cancer

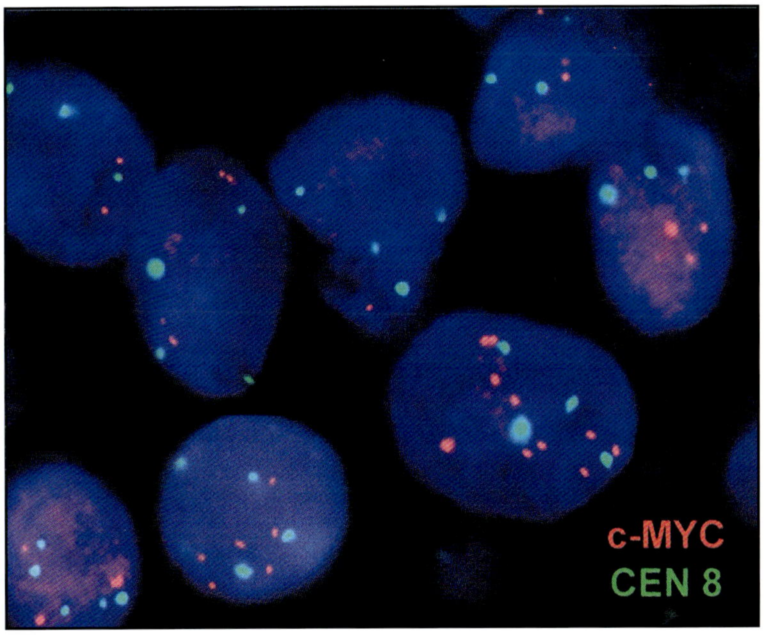

■ i21.4 *c-myc gene amplification (increased gene copy number) in prostatic carcinoma cells nuclei, as detected by FISH. (Courtesy of Dr Robert B Jenkins)*

The c-*myc* proto-oncogene, located at 8q24, encodes for a nuclear phosphoprotein that is important in the regulation of cellular proliferation and differentiation (Latil 1998, Netto 1994). High-level c-*myc* proto-oncogene amplification (that is, a substantial increase in gene copy number) has been detected in 0%-8% of primary carcinomas, with a rise to 11%-21% in metastatic deposits (Bubendorf 1999, Jenkins 1997) **i21.4**. Substantial c-*myc* amplification was associated with increasing carcinoma nuclear grade and immunohistochemical evidence of c-myc protein overexpression (Jenkins 1997). Expression of c-*myc* has been linked to higher histologic grade (Buttyan 1987), but not to cancer recurrence (Ow 1995).

The *RAS* family of proto-oncogenes (c-H-*ras*, c-k-*ras*, and N-*ras*) encode for a 21 kd membrane-associated GTPase (p21) (Bar-Sagi 1989, Bos 1989, Park 1998). RAS, as a downstream effector of growth factor receptors, is a critical regulator of cell shape, motility, and growth (Park 1998). Point mutations in *ras* proto-oncogenes result in a constitutively active *ras* oncogene. *Ras* mutations in non-Japanese prostate cancers are infrequent at an average of 5% in six studies (Carter 1990B, Gumerlock 1991, Konishi 1997A, Moul 1992, Moyret-Lalle 1995, Watanabe 1994). Higher rates of *ras* mutation are seen in Japanese prostate cancers, with 11%-24% of tumors exhibiting point mutations (Konishi 1997A, Konishi 1992, Shiraishi 1998B). It is not known to what extent population genetics versus environment account for these population differences in *ras* mutation rates (Konishi 1997A). In one investigation, the frequency of *ras* mutation appeared to increase with clinical stage (Shiraishi 1998B). High levels of p21 protein expression have been identified by immunohistochemical analysis of prostatic carcinoma (Bushman 1995, Sumiya 1990, Viola 1986), but associations with grade and stage have not been constant, and the antibody used in one study is not specific for *ras* p21 (Samowitz 1988).

Proto-oncogenes that encode certain growth factor receptors such as c-*met* (receptor for hepatocyte growth factor), *c-ret* (GDNF receptor), c-*erb*B-1 (EGFR), and c-*erb*B-2 (HER-2/neu) have been shown to be overexpressed in prostatic carcinoma, although the data for the c-*erb*B family members are conflicting. The c-MET and RET receptor proteins are overexpressed in high-grade prostatic intraepithelial neoplasia and carcinoma. In prostate cancer this overexpression is related to grade and stage (Dawson 1998, Pisters 1995, Humphrey 1995A). The mechanism of overexpression has not been established for MET and RET. The data on overexpression of the c-*erb*B-1 and c-*erb*B-2 proto-oncogenes in prostatic carcinoma are decidedly mixed. c-*erb*B-1 (EGFR) is expressed in a subset of prostatic carcinomas in some but not all studies (Cohen 1994, Harper 1995, Ibrahim 1993, Maygarden 1992, Maygarden 1994, Mellon 1992, Montone 1993, Moul 1996A, Ow 1995, Scher 1995, Turkeri 1994). There is no consistent association of EGFR expression with histologic grade (Harper 1995, Maygarden 1994, Montone 1993, Moul 1996A) or cancer recurrence (Moul 1996A, Ow 1995). Coexpression of EGFR and its ligands, including transforming growth factor-a, by prostatic carcinoma cells may represent an independent autocrine-signaling pathway (Cohen 1994, Djakiew 2000, Scher 1995), especially in metastatic, androgen-independent tumors (Scher 1995). There are also conflicting publications on the expression of c-*erb*B-2 (HER-2/neu) in prostatic carcinoma, with rates of 0%-100% reported (Ibrahim 1992, Koeppen 2001, McCann 1990, Morote 1999, Myers 1994B, Oxley 2002, Reese 2001, Ross 1993, Savinainen 2002, Signoretti 2000, Visakorpi 1992A, Ware 1991). HER-2/neu expression may increase with progression to androgen independence (Signoretti 2000), but the value of this expression measurement as a prognostic indicator is controversial. Contradictory results also exist on c-*erb*B-2 gene amplification in prostatic carcinoma, with reported incidence figures of 0%-40% (Bubendorf 1999, Kallakury 1998, Kaltz-Wittmer 2000, Mark 1999, Ross 1997, Signoretti 2000); most studies have not found amplification. These discrepancies in HER-2/neu studies in prostate cancer may derive from differences in patient populations, in tissue fixation, reagents, techniques, and definitions of positivity (Scher 2000, Sanchez 2002). Assessment of c-*erb* B-2 gene amplification and/or expression would assume greater importance if therapy directed toward the HER-2/neu protein were effective. A phase II clinical trial evaluating trastuzumab monoclonal antibody therapy directed against the HER-2/neu protein in prostate cancer has been reported (Morris 2002). The authors concluded that due to variability of HER-2 expression with clinical state, until more reliable and practical methods of sampling metastatic prostate cancer are developed to assess for HER-2/neu status, further studies to test the potential effectiveness of trastuzumab will not be feasible (Morris 2002).

[21.5] Androgen Receptor

The androgen receptor is a 910 amino acid nuclear protein that mediates androgen hormonal signals for growth, differentiation, and survival of prostatic epithelial cells (Trapman 1996). Abnormalities in the androgen receptor gene may contribute, in a subset of prostate cancer patients, to loss of androgen regulation of prostatic carcinoma cell growth and to an androgen-independent state of growth and progression **t21.9**. These abnormalities include short CAG repeats in exon 1 of the androgen receptor gene, androgen receptor gene methylation, mutations in the androgen receptor gene, and androgen receptor gene amplification.

t21.9 Androgen Receptor Gene Alterations in Prostate Cancer

Short CAG repeats in exon 1: predisposes to increased risk of prostate cancer
Methylation of 5' -regulatory region: 20%-28% of cases; could inactivate androgen receptor
Gene mutation: 15% of cases of androgen-independent, metastatic disease
Gene amplification: 13%-31% of hormone-refractory prostatic carcinomas

Shorter CAG repeat sequences in germline DNA were associated in most, but not all, studies with an increased risk of prostatic carcinoma development (Correa-Cerro 1999A, Edwards 1999, Giovannucci 1997, Hakimi 1997, Hsing 2000, Ingles 1997, Lange 2000, Nam 2000, Schoenberg 1994, Stanford 1997, Xue 2000). For men with prostatic carcinoma, short CAG repeats correlated with more aggressive disease, with linkages to higher histologic grade (Giovannucci 1997); stage (Giovannucci 1997, Hakimi 1997, Ingles 1997, Xue 2000); and fatal prostate cancer (Giovannucci 1997). Scant data exist on correlations with response to therapy; in one study, CAG repeats were not a predictor of response to radical prostatectomy, except in a subset of low-risk patients (Nam 2000). The biological basis for the increased risk of prostatic carcinoma with shorter CAG repeats is thought to be due to increased transcriptional activity of the androgen receptor when short CAG repeats are present (Beilin 2000).

DNA hypermethylation of androgen receptor promoter CpG islands is another potential transcriptional regulatory mechanism; here down-regulation of androgen receptor expression would occur (Jarrard 1998, Nakayama 2000). Aberrant methylation of the 5' regulatory region has been found in 20%-28% of prostate carcinomas, but this did not relate to clinical androgen-independence (Nakayama 2000).

Androgen receptor gene mutations causing an amino acid change or addition have been found in about 8% of patients (reviewed in Marcelli 2000). Overall, these mutations are rare in clinically localized prostatic carcinoma and can be detected in about 15% of cases of androgen-independent, metastatic disease (Taplin 2001). These mutations often seem to arise in response to selection pressure from treatment with the androgen receptor antagonists flutamide or bicalutamide (Taplin 1999, Taplin 2001). Interestingly, the function of these mutant androgen receptors appears to be altered such that they are more "promiscuous" in being activated by other ligands (Taplin 1999, Zhao 2000), including the very receptor antagonists used to initially treat the cancer (Taplin 1999).

Androgen receptor gene amplification has been identified in 13%-31% of hormone refractory prostate carcinomas (Kaltz-Wittmer 2000, Koivisto 1997, Linja 2001, Palmberg 2000, Visakorpi 1995B), whereas androgen receptor gene amplification has not been found in BPH or primary carcinomas (Linja 2001). This amplification leads to a modest twofold increase in androgen receptor RNA expression (Linja 2001). The data are mixed on the association of this gene amplification with clinical endpoints: in one study there was no correlation with clinical course (Kaltz-Wittmer 2000); in a second report, survival time was longer for patients with androgen receptor gene amplification (Koivisto 1997), whereas in a third investigation the amplification was associated with a favorable response to a second-line–combined androgen blockade, but not survival (Palmberg 2000). Amplification of the gene, with resultant increased expression, may be caused by clonal expansion, under the selection presence of hormonal therapy, where tumor cells with the amplified gene may have a growth advantage in being able to continue androgen-dependent growth in the presence of low concentrations of serum androgens (Koivisto 1997). This could be one potential mechanism of resistance to hormonal therapy. Additional possible androgen receptor–mediated hormonal-resistance mechanisms include androgen receptor mutations and activation of the androgen receptor by polypeptide growth factors (reviewed in Van der Kwast 1995).

Androgen receptor protein expression, as assessed by immunohistochemical staining, is diminished and more heterogeneous in prostatic carcinoma compared with BPH (Miyamoto 1993, Ruizeveld de Winter 1994, Sweat 1999B, Van der Kwast 1995). Eighty-five percent to 100% of prostatic carcinomas express the androgen receptor, and expression status is not related to histologic grade, stage, or whether the tumor is androgen-dependent or androgen-independent (Henshall 2001, Hobisch 1995, Magi-Galluzzi 1997, Miyamoto 1993, Prins 1998, Ruizeveld de Winter 1994, Sweat 1999A, Sweat 1999B). Heterogeneity of expression does increase with grade (Magi-Galluzzi 1997), and this finding could account, in part, for variable responses of patients with prostatic carcinoma to endocrine therapy. Conflicting results exist on whether androgen receptor expression predicts response to hormonal therapy and survival (reviewed in Sweat 1999B). Currently, androgen receptor expression analysis, including immunohistochemical staining, is not performed to predict prognosis or aid in the decision of whether to treat with hormonal therapy.

[21.6] DNA Methylation

DNA hypermethylation is capable of silencing gene expression by blocking transcription via methylation of cytosine-rich areas, termed CpG islands, in the 5' regulatory region of genes. This type of inactivation of gene expression has been found in prostatic carcinoma in the androgen receptor promoter (Jarrard 1998, Nakayama 2000), as noted above, for the glutathione S-transferase gene *GSTP1,* the E-cadherin gene, and the estrogen receptor (ER) gene (Lee 1997, Li 2000, Li 2001, Santourlidis 1999, Sasaki 2002). Glutathione S-transferase functions to detoxify carcinogens, so its inactivation could initiate and/or promote prostate carcinogenesis by increasing the vulnerability of prostatic epithelial cells to genome-damaging stresses (Nelson 2001). An alternative explanation for glutathione S-transferase protein absence in high-grade PIN and prostatic carcinoma is that it could be related more to differentiation than carcinogenesis (Cookson 1997). The degree of promoter methylation of E-cadherin, which is an epithelial cell adhesion molecule that may function as a tumor suppressor, correlated with tumor progression (Li 2001). ER gene down-regulation in prostatic carcinoma by DNA methylation also implicates a functional role for ER protein in prostatic carcinoma. Low ER expression has been correlated with a higher histologic grade and pathologic stage (Konishi 1993, Nativ 1997, Lear 2001) and a poor prognosis after hormonal therapy (Konishi 1993).

[21.7] Cell Proliferation and Cell Death (Apoptosis)

The growth of a prostate cancer is determined by the imbalance of cell proliferation and cell death. Adenocarcinoma within the prostate gland has a relatively low proliferation index, usually with a mean around 3%-7% **t21.10**. This index is significantly higher than that of benign or hyperplastic prostatic epithelium, which is typically 1% or less. There is substantial heterogeneity of proliferating cells both within individual tumors and between different cases. This is reflected in the extremely large ranges for the labeling indices given in many of the studies compiled **t21.10**. A wealth of data suggests that the proliferation index of prostatic carcinoma is highly correlated with pathologic and clinical endpoints, such as histologic grade, pathologic stage, response to therapy, and patient survival **t21.10**. However, there are confounding factors that currently limit the clinical use of cell cycle proteins as prognostic markers (Kibel 2000A). Most proliferation index studies have utilized immunohistochemical staining, especially for Ki-67 (often using monoclonal antibody MIB-1, which reacts with Ki-67 in formalin-fixed tissue sections), which detects a nuclear matrix antigen in mid-G_1 and M phases of the cell cycle (Ross 1996). Such immunostains are not quantitative and are subject to interpretation. Lack of standardization of tissue fixation and immunohistochemical technique also generates difficulty in the translation of Ki-67 immunostains into everyday practice. Heterogeneity of Ki-67 labeling and sampling problems with needle biopsy compromise the use of this marker where it is most needed—in the assessment of carcinoma in pretreatment needle core biopsy tissue. Finally, other cell cycle proteins, particularly p27 **t21.10** and p53 (Kibel 2000A), exhibit promise in the stratification of prostatic cancer patients into low- and high-risk groups. Given the molecular complexity of the cell cycle, further study of additional protein components of this machinery is clearly needed to identify potentially useful new cell cycle markers or panels of markers of clinically aggressive prostate cancer.

Apoptosis (from the Greek for falling away or off), or programmed cell death, is the active induction of cell death by a regulated pathway within the cell (Magi-Galluzzi 1998, Rudin 1998). In the prostate, there is a progressive increase in the frequency of apoptosis, as measured by apoptotic body counts or TUNEL (terminal deoxynucleotidyl transferase-mediated dUTP-biotin nick end labeling) staining, from 0.3% in benign glands to 0.7%-1.4% for high-grade PIN, to 0.4%-2.8% for primary carcinomas to 5.8% for carcinomas metastatic to regional lymph nodes (Drachenberg 1997, Kaleem 1998, Montironi 1994, Tu 1996). Limited data exist regarding correlations of the carcinoma apoptotic index with pathologic or clinical parameters. Increasing apoptotic index has been linked to a higher Gleason grade (Aihara 1994), but not pathologic stage (Brown 1996), and it has been associated with a poorer outcome for patients in two series (Aihara 1995, Stapleton 1998).

Prostate cancer cells can use multiple molecular mechanisms to evade apoptosis (Tang 1998), and those mechanisms likely contribute to the development of androgen-independent, lethal prostate cancer (Isaacs 2000). For example, prostatic carcinoma cells may overexpress apoptosis-suppressing genes, such as members of the *bcl-2* family, including *bcl-2* (Apakama 1996, Bauer 1996, Borre 1998B, Cheng 1999B, Krajewska 1996, Lipponen 1997, Matsushima 1997, McDonnell 1997, Moul 1996B, Stattin 1996A, Szostak 2001, Theodorescu 1997); *bcl-x*; and *mcl-1* (Krajewska 1996). *bcl-2* expression was increased in androgen-independent carcinoma (McDonnell 1992) and has been linked to histologic grade (Krajewska 1996, Lipponen 1997, Moul 1996B, Stattin 1996A); pathologic stage (Lipponen 1997, Matsushima 1997, Moul 1996B); and response to therapy in most, but not all, studies (Bauer 1996, Cheng 1999B, Keshgegian 1998, Lipponen 1997, Matsushima 1997, McDonnell 1997, Moul 1996B, Szostak 2001, Theodorescu 1997, Wikstrom 2000).

■ t21.10 Cell Proliferation Markers in Prostatic Carcinoma: Relationship to Pathologic and Clinical Endpoints

Study	Marker	Labeling Index in Carcinoma*	Correlations
Raymond 1988	Ki-67[†]	Benign: 4%; Carcinoma: 16%	Positive with histologic grade; trend with clinical stage
Gallee 1989	Ki-67	BPH: 0.3%; Carcinoma: 2.9% (range 0.4%-9.1%)	—
Nemoto 1990	BrdU[‡]	3.2% (range 1%-10.7%)	S-phase fraction significantly correlated with Gleason grade and pT stage
Sesterhenn 1991	AgNORs[§]	3.17/μm[†]	No relationship with grade; trend with stage
Oomens 1991	Ki-67	Benign: 1.2% (range 0%-3%) Carcinoma: 5.1% (range 1%-18%)	Decrease after androgen therapy or radiotherapy
Scrivner 1991	BrdU	1.6% (range 0.1%-29%)	Correlated with Gleason grade and DNA aneuploidy
Contractor 1991	AgNORs	4.8/nucleus	AgNOR "quotient" related to grade and survival
Sadi 1991	Ki-67	Carcinoma: 2.5% (range 1.7%-7.5%)	With > 2.5% positive nuclei, trend toward shorter time to progression after hormonal therapy
Ghazizadeh 1991	AgNORs	Carcinoma: 4.3/nucleus	Correlated with grade and stage
Kallioniemi 1991	S-phase fraction (SPF) by flow cytometry	Carcinoma: 4.2%	Linked to survival in univariate analysis
Eskelinen 1991	SPF by flow cytometry	Carcinoma: WHO grade I+II: 5% vs grade III: 12%	Positivity correlated with grade, stage, and progression, but not survival
Visakorpi 1991	SPF by flow cytometry	Carcinoma: 4.2%	Associated with grade, aneuploidy, tumor size, stage, progression, response to hormones, and survival
Masai 1992	AgNORs	Hyperplasia: 2.1/cell Carcinoma: 6.1/ cell	Correlated with T stage but not response to treatment or survival
Visakorpi 1992	S+G_2/M-phase fractions PCNA[‖], SPF	9.7% PCNA index	S+G_2/M predicted survival in multivariate analysis
Harper 1992	Ki-67	Most carcinomas ≤ 10% nuclei stained	Correlated with grade, metastasis, and survival
Thompson 1992	Ki-67	1.9% (range 0.2%-9.1%)	Associated with p53 staining, but not grade
Carroll 1993	BrdU PCNA	1.6%-3.1% 3.5%-6.0%	Poor correlation with grade, but good correlation with clinical and pathologic stage
Sakr 1993	AgNOR PCNA SPF	4.7/nucleus 8.6% (range 0%-55%) 8.5% (range 5%-13%)	AgNOR counts correlated with Gleason grade, but not SPF
McLoughlin 1993	Ki-67	Hyperplasia: 0.6% (range 0%-2.3%) Carcinoma: 4.8% (range (0%-28%)	Associated with metastatic spread, but not disease progression or hormone responsiveness
Konishi 1994	AgNOR	2.4-3.8/ nucleus	Correlated with grade, but not metastasis
Centeno 1994	SPF SPF +G_2M	5.3% (range 0.3%-23%) 11% (range 3.1%-30%)	Did not predict survival. For patients with low histologic grade and diploid tumor, both predicted local control.
Vesalainen 1994A	SPF	6.7%-7.3%	Correlated with pT stage, ploidy, Gleason score, and survival in univariate, but not multivariate, analysis
Naito 1994	PCNA	BPH: 1.3%; Carcinoma: 11.7% (range 0.3%-23%)	Positive correlation with nuclear grade, T stage, and survival in univariate, but not multivariate, analysis
Vesalainen 1994B	PCNA	19% (range 0%-99%)	PCNA index predicted T stage, Gleason score, and survival in multivariate analysis
Müller 1994	G_2M fraction by flow cytometry	6.3%	Not related to stage, but was related to nonaneuploid carcinoma recurrence
Cher 1995	BrdU Ki-67 PCNA	3.0% 3.4% 7.0%	Labeling index by all three methods correlated well with histologic grade and clinical and pathologic stage
Vesalainen 1995	Mitotic figures	Mean = 10.3 mitoses per 10 hpf (range 0-94)	Mitotic index correlated with Gleason score, progression, and survival
Brown 1996	MIB-1 (Ki-67)	7.9%-10.7%	Correlated with Gleason grade, but not pathologic stage
Tu 1996	Ki-67	"Normal": 1.1% Primary carcinoma: 4.2% Metastatic carcinoma: 22.7%	High proliferation index of metastatic prostatic carcinoma cells in lymph nodes
Bubendorf 1996	Ki-67 (MIB-1)	7.5% (range 0%-33%)	Ki-67 labeling index did not correlate with pTN stage or Gleason score, but was predictive of progression after radical prostatectomy in univariate and multivariate analyses
Moul 1996	Ki-67	38% with "staining score" of 2+ to 4+	Positive correlation with stage, grade, and recurrence after radical prostatectomy in univariate, but not multivariate, analysis
Feneley 1996	Ki-67	Median 5% (range 0%-37%)	Related to grade and stage in TURP chips
Speights 1996	MIB-1 (Ki-67)	Mean 10.9% (range 2%-33%)	Did not predict progression after radical prostatectomy
Tamboli 1996	MIB-1 (Ki-67)	Benign: 0.4 cells (range 0-2)/400× field HG-PIN: 2.5 (range 0-17)/field Carcinoma: 13.8 (range 0.3-74)/field	Significant increase from benign to PIN to carcinoma
Goel 1996	MIB-1 (Ki-67)	Benign: 0.6% (range 0-2.6) Carcinoma: 5.1% (range 1.9-20.2)	Immunopositive nuclear area by image analysis tied to Gleason grade and overall, but not cancer-free survival

■ **t21.10 Cell Proliferation Markers in Prostatic Carcinoma: Relationship to Pathologic and Clinical Endpoints (continued)**

Study	Marker	Labeling Index in Carcinoma*	Correlations
Mashal 1996	Ki-67 cyclin A cyclin B cyclin E	7.7% (range 0-97) 2.4% (range 0.2-14.3) 0.4% (range 0-29) 4.3% (range 0-98.1)	% cyclin A+B positive cells/Ki-67 was predictive of relapse after radical prostatectomy
Ahlgren 1997	SPF, G_2M by flow cytometery	6-11%	Proliferation index increased with increasing grade, and predicted survival in univariate and multivariate analyses
Coetzee 1997	Ki-67, MIB-1	Mean = 0.7%	Not significant in multivariate analysis in predicting failure after radial prostatectomy
Connolly 1997	Ki-67	1^0 mean: 3.0% Recurrent mean: 6.5%	Locally recurrent prostatic carcinoma after radial prostatectomy had higher proliferation index
Stattin 1997	Ki-67	Mean: 2.1%	Significantly related to grade, stage, and survival
Kaleem 1998	MIB-1 (Ki-67)	Mean: 5.3% (range 0%-16%)	Atrophic pattern prostate carcinomas had similar proliferation index of 4.0%
Yang 1998	p27	16% "low expressors"	Low p27, a cell cycle inhibitor, independently predicted biochemical recurrence after radical prostatectomy
Chi 1997	CDKN2	Reduced expression in 43% of primaries	CDKN2 protein = $p16^{INK4a}$ inhibits cyclins and G_1 to S-phase progression
Cote 1998	p27 (p27 Kip1)	Immunohistochemical reactivity decreased in 45% of primaries	Decreased p27 associated with grade, and probability of recurrence and survival after radical prostatectomy
Matsushima 1998	$p21^{WAF1}$	52% of carcinomas positive	p21 loss by image analysis of immunostains correlated with higher grade, and worse survival in univariate and multivariate analysis
Cheville 1998	$p27^{KIP1}$	28% "low expressors"	Low p27 expression correlated with higher Gleason score, stage, and ploidy, but not failure after surgery
Borre 1998	MIB-1	Median score 10.3% (range 0%-46%)	Correlated with grade and stage, but not survival in clinically localized cancer, by multivariate analysis
Bubendorf 1998	Ki-67	Median 7.5% in core needle biopsies	Strong relationship with Gleason grade and predicted survival in univariate and multivariate analyses
Cordon-Cardo 1998	$p27^{KIP1}$	64% primary carcinomas with low to undetectable immunoreactive p27	Predictive in multivariate analysis of relapse after radical prostatectomy
Tsihlias 1998	p27	Reduced immunostaining in most prostatic carcinomas compared to strong, uniform staining of benign epithelium	Low p27 staining predicted recurrence after radical prostatectomy
Erdamar 1999	$p27^{KIP1}$	7% labeling in metastatic carcinoma, 44% immunoreactivity in primary carcinoma, 59% in high-grade PIN, and 86% in benign epithelia	p27 labeling index not associated with grade, stage, or progression after radical prostatectomy
Aaltomaa 1999	cyclin A cyclin D	2.1% 16.3%	Cyclin A immunoreactivity related to stage, grade and cancer-related survival, but neither cyclin significant in multivariate analysis
Osman 1999	p21/WAF1	33% positive	p21-positive phenotype correlated with high Ki-67 proliferation index and decreased time to PSA relapse after radical prostatectomy
Cheng 1999	MIB-1 (Ki-67)		MIB-1 labeling index in nodal metastatic deposits correlated with Gleason score, DNA ploidy, nodal cancer volume and systemic progression-free survival
Sarkar 1999	$p21^{WAF1}$	26% positive	Immunostaining correlated with recurrence after radical prostatectomy
Nguyen 2000	p14 p15 p16	22% of cases with overexpression 17% overexpression 66% overexpression	No relationship with grade or stage
Drobnjak 2000	cyclin D1	11% positivity in primary carcinoma vs. 68% androgen	No correlation with Gleason score, neoadjuvant hormonal treatment, or relapse, but was related to high Ki-67 proliferation index
Vis 2000	MIB-1 P27Kip1	 56% low expressors	Both correlated with Gleason score and pathologic stage; low p27Kip1 independent predictor of clinical recurrence after radical prostatectomy. MIB-1 was not
Thomas 2000	p27	25% low expressors	Low p27 expression in needle biopsy tissue correlated with radical prostatectomy p27, Gleason score, pathologic stage, and higher recurrence rate after radical prostatectomy
Dunsmuir 2000	MIB-1 cyclin D1		MIB-1 and cyclin D1 correlated with grade, stage, and survival
Lacombe 2001	p21 (WAF1/CIP1)		p21 expression was associated with an increased risk of failure after radical prostatectomy
Sebo 2001	MIB-1 SPF	Mean: 3% (range 0-40%) Mean: 26% (0-74%)	In needle biopsy tissue, MIB-1 not linked to pathologic stage or tumor volume (TV); SPF related to TV
Wu 2001	p16	Not given	Loss of p16 immunoreactivity correlated with grade and distant metastasis in univariate analysis

■ **t21.10 Cell Proliferation Markers in Prostatic Carcinoma: Relationship to Pathological and Clinical End-points (continued)**

Study	Marker	Labeling Index in Carcinoma*	Correlations
Sebo 2002	MIB-1 SPF	Mean: 3% (range 0-40%) Mean: 26% (0-74%)	MIB-1 immunostain quantitation by image analysis of carcinoma needle biopsy tissue yielded proliferation index that was insignificant in univariate and multivariate analysis in predicting progression after radical prostatectomy
Cowen 2002	MIB-1	Mean: 3.2%	Mean labeling index for carcinoma in needle biopsy and TURP tissue significantly higher in stage T3/T4, Gleason score 7-10, and in patients who failed radiotherapy

*Data given as means or medians
†Ki-67: An antibody used to indirectly measure cell proliferation in immunohistochemical staining (Ross 1996)
‡BrdU: Thymidine analog 5-bromodeoxyuridine: used in an antibody assay to detect cells in S-phase (Ross 1996)
§AgNORs: Silver-stained nucleolar organized regions (Ross 1996)
||PCNA: Proliferating cell nuclear antigen, detectable by immunohistochemistry (Ross 1996)

[21.8] Gene Expression Profiling and Proteomics

DNA microarrays, made of cDNA arrays or oligonucleotide arrays (gene chips), allow for simultaneous profiling of expression patterns of thousands of genes **i21.5**. Recently, this approach has been applied to prostatic carcinoma tissues (Bull 2001, Chaib 2001, Chetcuti 2001, Dhanasekaran 2001, Ernst 2002, LaTulippe 2002, Luo 2001, Magee 2001, Rhodes 2002, Singh 2002, Stamey 2001, Varambally 2002, Welsh 2001) and has already yielded hundreds of genes that differ in expression between BPH and cancer. Both upregulated and downregulated genes have been detected. Hepsin, a transmembrane serine protease, has been consistently detected as overexpressed in these studies (Dhanasekaran 2001, Luo 2001, Magee 2001, Stamey 2001, Welsh 2001). A comparison of organ-confined and metastatic prostate carcinoma identified 55 genes that were significantly up-regulated and 480 genes that were significantly down-regulated in metastatic disease (Varambally 2002). One of the upregulated genes, E2H2, appears to be a marker of aggressive prostate cancer (Varambally 2002). Additionally, proteomic analyses to survey protein expression differences between benign and malignant prostatic cells and tissues have been launched (Meehan 2002, Praweletz 2001). Proteomic patterns can also be assessed in serum (Petricoin 2002). These global expression analyses should help in the understanding of pathways of prostate cancer initiation and progression and in identifying molecular markers for diagnostic, prognostic, and therapeutic use (Dhanasekaran 2001, Luo 2001, Magee 2001, Welsh 2001).

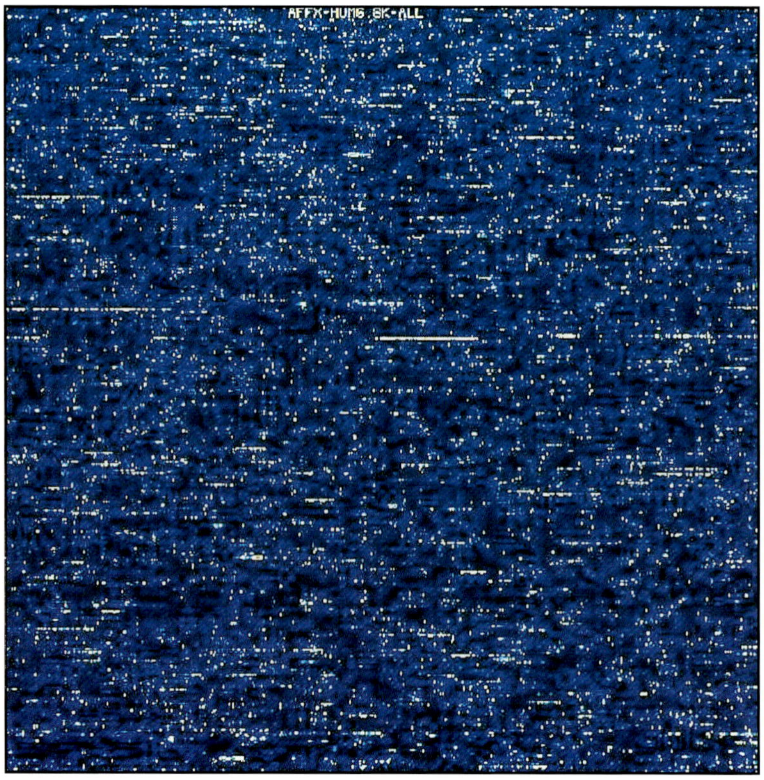

■ **i21.5** *Gene chip with hybridization intensity signals for thousands of genes. (Courtesy of Dr Mark Watson).*

References

Aaltomaa S, Eskelinen M, Lipponen P. Expression of cyclin A and D proteins in prostate cancer and their relation to clinicopathologic variables and patient survival. *Prostate* 38:175-182, 1999.

Abate-Shen C, Shen MM. Molecular genetics of prostate cancer. *Genes Dev* 14:2410-2434, 2000.

Abou-Elella AA, DeRose PB, Cohen C. Nuclear DNA ploidy of prostate carcinoma in biopsy and resection specimens. An image and flow cytometric study. *J Urol Pathol* 9:29-39, 1998.

Adolfsson J, Rönström L, Hedlund P-O, et al. The prognostic value of modal deoxyribonucleic acid in low grade, low stage untreated prostate cancer. *J Urol* 144:1404-1407, 1990.

Adolfsson J. Prognostic value of deoxyribonucleic acid content in prostate cancer: a review of current results. *Int J Cancer* 58:211-216, 1994.

Afonso A, Emmert-Buck MR, Duray PH, et al. Loss of heterozygosity on chromosome 13 is associated with advanced stage prostate cancer. *J Urol* 163:922-926, 1999.

Ahlgren G, Lindholm K, Falkmer U, et al. A DNA cytometric proliferation index improves the value of the DNA ploidy pattern as a prognosticating tool in patients with carcinoma of the prostate. *Urology* 50:379-384, 1997.

Ahlgren G, Falkmer U, Gadaleanu V, et al. Evaluation of DNA ploidy combined with a cytometric proliferation index of imprints form core needle biopsies in prostate cancer. *Eur Urol* 36:314-319, 1999.

Ahman A-K, Jonsson B-A, Damber J-E, et al. Low frequency of allelic imbalance at the prostate cancer susceptibility loci HPC1 and 1p36 in Swedish men with hereditary prostate cancer. *Genes Chromosomes Cancer* 29:292-296, 2000.

Ahman AK, Jonsson BA, Damber JE, et al. Low frequency of microsatellite instability in hereditary prostate cancer. *BJU Int* 87:334-338, 2001.

Aihara M, Truong LD, Dunn JK, et al. Frequency of apoptotic bodies positively correlates with Gleason grade in prostate cancer. *Hum Pathol* 25:797-801, 1994.

Aihara M, Scardino PT, Truong LD, et al. The frequency of apoptosis correlates with the prognosis of Gleason grade 3 adenocarcinoma of the prostate. *Cancer* 75:522-529, 1995.

Alers JA, Krijtenburg PJ, Vissers KJ, et al. Interphase cytogenetics of prostatic adenocarcinoma and precursor lesions: analysis of 25 radical prostatectomies and 17 adjuvant prostatic intraepithelial neoplasias. *Genes Chromosomes Cancer* 12:241-250, 1995.

Alers JC, Krijtenburg PJ, Rosenberg C, et al. Interphase cytogenetics of prostate tumor progression: specific chromosomal abnormalities are involved in metastasis to the bone. *Lab Invest* 77:437-448, 1997.

Alers JC, Rochat J, Krijtenburg PJ, et al. Identification of genetic markers for prostatic cancer progression. *Lab Invest* 80:931-942, 2000.

Alers JC, Krijtenburg PJ, Vis AN, et al. Molecular cytogenetic analysis of prostatic adenocarcinomas from screening studies: early cancers may contain aggressive genetic features. *Am J Pathol* 158:399-406, 2001.

Amling CL, Lerner SE, Martin SK, et al. Deoxyribonucleic acid ploidy and serum prostate specific antigen predict outcome following salvage prostatectomy for radiation refractory prostate cancer. *J Urol* 161:857-862, 1999.

Apakama I, Robinson MC, Walter NM, et al. bcl-2 overexpression combined with p53 protein accumulation correlates with hormone-refractory prostate cancer. *Br J Cancer* 74:1258-1262, 1996.

Aprikian AG, Sarkis AS, Fair WR, et al. Immunohistochemical determination of p53 protein nuclear accumulation in prostatic adenocarcinoma. *J Urol* 151:1276-1280, 1994.

Arber DA, Speights VO. Aneuploidy in benign seminal vesicle epithelium: an example of the paradox of ploidy studies. *Mod Pathol* 4:687-689, 1991.

Badalament RA, O'Toole RV, Young DC, et al. DNA ploidy and prostate-specific antigen as prognostic factors in clinically resectable prostate cancer. *Cancer* 67:3014-3023, 1991.

Badalament RA, Miller MC, Peller PA, et al. An algorithm for predicting nonorgan confined prostate cancer using the results obtained from sextant core biopsies with prostate specific antigen level. *J Urol* 156:1375-1380, 1996.

Bandyk MG, Zhao L, Troncoso P, et al. Trisomy 7: a potential cytogenetic marker of human prostate cancer progression. *Genes Chromosomes Cancer* 9:19-27, 1994.

Bar-Sagi D. *RAS* proteins: biological effects and biochemical targets (review). *Anticancer Res* 9:1427-1437, 1989.

Bastacky SI, Wojno KJ, Walsh PC, et al. Pathological features of hereditary prostate cancer. *J Urol* 153:987-992, 1995.

Bauer JJ, Sesterhenn IA, Mostofi FK, et al. Elevated levels of apoptosis regulator proteins p53 and bcl-2 are independent prognostic biomarkers in surgically treated clinically localized prostate cancer. *J Urol* 156:1511-1516, 1996.

Bauer JJ, Connelly RR, Sesterhenn IA, et al. Biostatistical modeling using traditional preoperative and pathological prognostic variables in the selection of men at high risk for disease recurrence after radical prostatectomy for prostate cancer. *J Urol* 159:929-933, 1998.

Beilin J, Ball EM, Favaloro JM, et al. Effect of androgen receptor CAG repeat polymorphism on transcriptional activity: specificity in prostate and non-prostate cell lines. *J Mol Endocrinol* 25:85-96, 2000.

Bergerheim USR, Kunimi K, Collins VP, et al. Deletion mapping of chromosomes 8, 10, and 16 in human prostatic carcinoma. *Genes Chromosome Cancer* 3:215-220, 1991.

Bergthorsson JT, Johannesdottir G, Arason A, et al. Analysis of HPC1, HPCX, and PCaP in Icelandic hereditary prostate cancer. *Hum Genet* 107:372-275, 2000.

Berner A, Waere H, Nesland JM, et al. DNA ploidy, serum prostate specific antigen, histological grade and immunohistochemistry as predictive parameters of lymph node metastases in T1-T3/M0 prostatic adenocarcinoma. *Br J Urol* 75:26-32, 1995.

Berry R, Schroeder JJ, French AJ, et al. Evidence for a prostate cancer-susceptibility locus on chromosome 20. *Am J Hum Genet* 67:82-91, 2000A.

Berry R, Shaid DJ, Smith JR, et al. Linkage analyses at the chromosome 1 loci 1q24-25 (HPC1), 1q42.2-43 (PCAP), and 1p36 (CAPB) in families with hereditary prostate cancer. *Am J Human Genet* 66:539-546, 2000B.

Berthon P, Valeri A, Cohen-Akenine A, et al. Predisposing gene for early-onset prostate cancer, localized on chromosome 1q42.4-43. *Am J Hum Genet* 62:1416-1424, 1998.

Berthorsson JT, Johannedottir G, Arason A, et al. Analysis of HPC1, HPCX, and PCaP in Icelandic hereditary prostate cancer. *Hum Genet* 107:372-375, 2000.

Blazer DG III, Umbach DM, Bostick RM, et al. Vitamin D receptor polymorphisms and prostate cancer. *Mol Carcinog* 27:18-23, 2000.

Blute ML, Nativ O, Zincke H, et al. Pattern of failure after radical retropubic prostatectomy for clinically and pathologically localized adenocarcinoma of the prostate: influence of tumor deoxyribonucleic acid ploidy. *J Urol* 142:1262-1269, 1989.

Blute ML, Bergstralh EJ, Iocca A, et al. Use of Gleason score, prostate specific antigen, seminal vesicle and margin status to predict biochemical failure after radical prostatectomy. *J Urol* 165:119-125, 2001.

Bock C, Cunningham J, McDonnell S, et al. Analysis of prostate cancer-susceptibility locus HPC20 in 172 families affected by prostate cancer. *Am J Hum Genet* 68:795-801, 2001.

Bookstein R, MacGrogan D, Hilsenbeck SG, et al. p53 is mutated in a subset of advanced-stage prostate cancers. *Cancer Res* 53:3369-3373, 1993.

Borre M, Hoyer M, Nerstrom B, et al. DNA ploidy and survival of patients with clinically localized prostate cancer treated without intent to cure. *Prostate* 36:244-249, 1998A.

Borre M, Bentzen SM, Nerstrom B, et al. Tumor cell proliferation and survival in patients with prostate cancer followed expectantly. *J Urol* 159:1609-1614, 1998B.

Borre M, Stausbol-Gron B, Overgaard J. p53 accumulation associated with bcl-2, the proliferation marker MIB-1 and survival in patients with prostate cancer subjected to watchful waiting. *J Urol* 164:716-721, 2000.

Bos JL. *RAS* oncogenes in human cancer. A review. *Cancer Res* 49:4682-4689, 1989.

Bostwick DG, Foster CS. Predictive factors in prostate cancer: Current concepts from the 1999 College of American Pathologists Conference on Solid Tumor Prognostic Factors and the 1999 World Health Organization International Consultation on Prostate Cancer. *Semin Urol Oncol* 17:222-272, 1999.

Bostwick DG, Grignon DJ, Hammond EH, et al. Prognostic factors in prostate cancer. College of American Pathologist Consensus Statement 1999. *Arch Pathol Lab Med* 124:995-1000, 2000.

Bova GS, Carter BS, Bussemakes MJG, et al. Homozygous deletion and frequent allelic loss of chromosome 8p22 loci in human prostate cancer. *Cancer Res* 53:3869-3873, 1993.

Bova GS, Partin AW, Isaacs SD, et al. Biological aggressiveness of hereditary prostate cancer: long-term evaluation following radical prostatectomy. *J Urol* 160:660-663, 1998.

Bratt O, Anderson H, Bak-Jensen E, Baldetorp B, Lundgren R. Metaphase cytogenetics and DNA flow cytometry with analysis of S-phase fraction in prostate cancer: influence on prognosis. *Urology* 47:218-224, 1996.

Bratt O. Hereditary prostate cancer. Clinical aspects. *J Urol* 168:906-913, 2002.

Breitkreuz T, Romanakis K, Lutz S, et al. Genotypic characterization of prostatic carcinoma: a combined cytogenetic, flow cytometry, and in situ DNA hybridization study. *Cancer Res* 53:4035-4040, 1993.

Brewster SF, Oxley JD, Trivella M, et al. Preoperative p53, bcl-2, CD44 and E-cadherin immunohistochemistry as predictors of biochemical relapse after radical prostatectomy. *J Urol* 161:1238-1243, 1999.

Brinker DA, Ross JS, Tran T-A, et al. Can ploidy of prostate carcinoma diagnosed on needle biopsy predict radical prostatectomy stage and grade? *J Urol* 162:2036-2040, 1999.

Brooks JD, Bova GS, Isaacs WB. Allelic loss of the retinoblastoma gene in primary human prostatic adenocarcinomas. *Prostate* 26:35-39, 1995.

Brooks JD, Bova GS, Ewing CM, et al. An uncertain role for p53 gene alterations in human prostate cancers. *Cancer Res* 56:3814-3822, 1996.

Brothman AR, Maxwell TM, Cui J, et al. Chromosomal clues to the development of prostate tumors. *Prostate* 38:303-312, 1999.

Brown C, Sauvageot J, Kahane H, et al. Cell proliferation and apoptosis in prostate cancer—correlation with pathologic stage? *Mod Pathol* 9:205-209, 1996.

Brown JA, Slezak JM, Lieber MM, et al. Fluorescence in situ hybridization aneuploidy as a predictor of clinical disease recurrence and prostate-specific antigen level 3 years after radical prostatectomy. *Mayo Clin Proceed* 74:1214-1220, 1990.

Bubendorf L, Sauter G, Moch H, et al. Ki67 labeling index: an independent predictor of progression in prostate cancer treated by radical prostatectomy. *J Pathol* 178:437-441, 1996.

Bubendorf L, Tapia C, Gasser TC, et al. Ki-67 labeling index in core needle biopsies independently predicts tumor-specific survival in prostate cancer. *Hum Pathol* 29:949-954, 1998.

Bubendorf L, Kononen J, Koivisto P, et al. Survey of gene amplifications during prostate cancer progression by high-throughput fluorescence in situ hybridization on tissue microarrays. *Cancer Res* 59:803-806, 1999.

Bull JH, Ellison G, Patel A, et al. Identification of potential diagnostic markers of prostate cancer and prostatic intraepithelial neoplasia using cDNA microarray. *Br J Cancer* 84:1512-1519, 2001.

Bushman EC, Nayak RN, Bushman W. Immunohistochemical staining of ras p21: staining in benign and malignant prostate tissue. *J Urol* 153:233-237, 1995.

Buttyan R, Sawczuk IS, Benson MC, et al. Enhanced expression of c-myc proto-oncogene in high-grade human prostate cancers. *Prostate* 11:327-337, 1987.

Byrne RL, Horne CH, Robinson MC, et al. The expression of waf-1, p53 and bcl-2 in prostatic adenocarcinoma. *Br J Urol* 79:190-195, 1997.

Cairns P, Okami K, Halachmi S, et al. Frequent inactivation of *PTEN/MMAC2* in primary prostate cancer. *Cancer Res* 57:4997-5000, 1997.

Carmichael MJ, Veltri RW, Partin AW, et al. Deoxyribonucleic acid ploidy analysis as a predictor of recurrence following radical prostatectomy for stage T2 disease. *J Urol* 153:1015-1019, 1993.

Carpten J, Nupponen N, Isaacs S, et al. Germline mutations in the ribonuclease L gene in families showing linkage with HPC1. *Nat Genet* 30:181-184, 2002.

Carroll PR, Waldman FM, Rosenau W, et al. Cell proliferation in prostatic adenocarcinoma: in vitro measurement by 5-bromodeoxyuridine incorporation and proliferating cell nuclear antigen expression. *J Urol* 149:403-407, 1993.

Carter BS, Ewing CM, Ward WS, et al. Allelic loss of chromosomes 16q and 10q in human prostate cancer. *Proc Natl Acad Sci* 87:8751-8755, 1990A.

Carter BS, Epstein JI, Isaacs WB. *ras* gene mutation in human prostate cancer. *Cancer Res* 50:6830-6832, 1990B.

Casella R, Maduro MR, Lipshultz LI, et al. Significance of the polyglutamine tract polymorphism in the androgen receptor. *Urology* 58:651-656, 2001.

Centeno BA, Zietman AL, Shipley WU, et al. Flow cytometric analysis of DNA ploidy, percent S-phase fraction, and total proliferative fraction as prognostic indicators of local control and survival following radiation therapy for prostate carcinoma. *Int J Radiat Oncol Biol Phys* 30:309-315, 1994.

Chaib H, Cockrell EK, Rubin MA, et al. Profiling and verification of gene expression patterns in normal and malignant human prostate tissues by cDNA microarray analysis. *Neoplasia* 3:43-52, 2001.

Chamberlain NL, Driver ED, Miesfeld RL. The length and location of CAG trinucleotide repeats in the androgen receptor N-terminal desmin affect transactivation function. *Nucleic Acids Res* 22:3181-3186, 1994.

Cheng L, Bergstralh EJ, Cheville JC, et al. Cancer volume of lymph node metastasis predicts progression in prostate cancer. *Am J Surg Pathol* 22:1491-1500, 1998A.

Cheng L, Song SY, Pretlow TG, et al. Evidence of independent origin of multiple tumors from patients with prostate cancer. *J Natl Cancer Inst* 90:233-237, 1998.

Cheng L, Bostwick DG, Li G, et al. Allelic imbalance in the clonal evolution of prostate carcinoma. *Cancer* 85:2017-2022, 1999A.

Cheng L, Pisansky TM, Sebo TJ, et al. Cell proliferation in prostate cancer patients with lymph node metastasis: a marker for progression. *Clin Cancer Res* 5:2820-2823, 1999B.

Cheng L, Leibovich BC, Bergstralh EJ, et al. p53 alteration in regional lymph node metastases from prostate carcinoma: a marker for progression? *Cancer* 85:2455-2459, 1999C.

Cheng L, Sebo TJ, Cheville JC, et al. p53 protein overexpression is associated with increased cell proliferation in patients with locally recurrent carcinoma after radiation therapy. *Cancer* 85:1293-1299, 1999D.

Cher ML, Chew K, Rosenau W, et al. Cellular proliferation in prostatic adenocarcinoma as assessed by bromodeoxyuridine uptake and Ki-67 and PCNA expression. *Prostate* 26:8-93, 1995.

Cher ML, Stephenson RA, James BC, et al. Cellular proliferative fraction of metastatic lymph nodes predicts survival in stage D1 (TxN+MO) prostate cancer. *J Urol* 155:1674-1677, 1996A.

Cher ML, Bova GS, Moore DH, et al. Genetic alterations in untreated metastases and androgen-independent prostate cancer detected by comparative genomic hybridization and allelotyping. *Cancer Res* 56:3091-3102, 1996B.

Cher ML, Lewis PE, Banerjee M, et al. A similar pattern of abnormal alterations in prostate cancers from African-Americans and Caucasian Americans. *Clin Cancer Res* 4:1273-1278, 1998.

Chetcuti A, Margan S, Mann S, et al. Identification of differentially expressed genes in organ-confined prostate cancer by gene expression array. *Prostate* 47:132-140, 2001.

Cheville JC, Lloyd RV, Sebo TJ, et al. Expression of $p27^{Kip1}$ in prostatic adenocarcinoma. *Mod Pathol* 11:324-328, 1998.

Chi S-G, deVere White RW, Meyers FJ, et al. p53 in prostate cancer: frequent expressed transition mutations. *J Natl Cancer Inst* 86:926-933, 1994.

Chi S-G, deVere White RW, Muenzer JT, et al. Frequent alteration of CDKN2 (*$p16^{INK4a}$/ MTS1*) expression in human primary prostate carcinomas. *Clin Cancer Res* 3:1889-1897, 1997.

Coetzee LJ, Layfield LJ, Hars V, et al. Proliferative index determination in prostatic carcinoma tissue: is there any additional prognostic value greater than that of Gleason score, ploidy and pathological stage? *J Urol* 157:214-218, 1997.

Cohen DW, Simak R, Fair WR, et al. Expression of transforming growth factor-alpha and the epidermal growth factor receptor in human prostate tissues. *J Urol* 152:2120-2124, 1994.

Connolly JA, Presti JC Jr, Cher ML, et al. Accelerated tumor proliferation rates in locally recurrent prostate cancer after radical prostatectomy. *J Urol* 158:515-518, 1997.

Contractor H, Ruschoff J, Hanisch T, et al. Silver-stained structures in prostatic carcinoma. Evaluation of diagnostic and prognostic relevance by automated image analysis. *Urol Int* 46:9-14, 1991.

Cookson MS, Reuter VE, Linkov I, et al. Glutathione S-transferase PI (GST-p) class expression by immunohistochemistry in benign and malignant prostate tissue. *J Urol* 157:673-676, 1997.

Cooney KA, Wetzel JC, Merajver SD, et al. Distinct regions of allelic regions on 13q in prostate cancer. *Cancer Res* 56:1142-1145, 1996.

Cordon-Cardo C, Koff A, Drobnjak M, et al. Distinct altered patterns of $p27^{KIP1}$ gene expression in benign prostatic hyperplasia and prostatic carcinoma. *J Natl Cancer Inst* 90:1284-1291, 1998.

Correa-Cerro L, Wohr G, Haussler J, et al. (CAG) CAA and GGN in the human androgen receptor gene are not associated with prostate cancer in a French-German population. *Eur J Hum Genet* 7:357-362, 1999A.

Correa-Cerro L, Berthon P, Haussler J, et al. Vitamin D receptor polymorphisms as markers in prostate cancer. *Hum Genet* 105:281-287, 1999B.

Cote RJ, Shi Y, Groshen S, et al. Association of p27Kip1 levels with recurrence and survival in patients with stage C prostate carcinoma. *J Natl Cancer Inst* 90:916-920, 1998.

Cowen D, Troncoso P, Khoo VS, et al. Ki-67 staining is an independent correlate of biochemical failure in prostate cancer treated with radiotherapy. *Clin Cancer Res* 8:1148-1154, 2002.

Crundwell MC, Chughtai S, Knowles M, et al. Allelic loss on chromosomes 8q, 22q, and 18q (DCC) in human prostate cancer. *Int J Cancer* 69:295-300, 1996.

Crundwell MC, Arkell DG, Gearty J, et al. Genetic alterations in incidentally diagnosed, transitional zone prostate cancer: A seven year follow-up. *J Urol* 158:1568-1575, 1997.

Crundwell MC, Morton DG, Arkell DG, et al. Genetic instability in incidentally discovered and advanced prostate cancer. *BJU Int* 84:123-127, 1999.

Cunningham JM, Shan A, Wick MJ, et al. Allelic imbalance and microsatellite instability in prostatic adenocarcinoma. *Cancer Res* 56:4475-4482, 1996.

Dahiya R, Deng G, Chen KM, et al. p53 tumour-suppressor gene mutations are mainly localized on exon 7 in human primary and metastatic prostate cancer. *Br J Cancer* 74:264-268, 1996.

Dawson DM, Lawrence EG, MacLennan GT, et al. Altered expression of RET proto-oncogene product in prostatic intraepithelial neoplasia and prostate cancer. *J Natl Cancer Inst* 90:519-523, 1998.

Deitch AD, Miller GJ, deVere White RW. Significance of abnormal diploid DNA histograms in localized prostate cancer and adjacent benign prostatic tissue. *Cancer* 72:1692-1700, 1993.

Dejter SW Jr, Moul JW, Cunningham RE, et al. Prognostic significance of DNA ploidy in carcinoma of prostate. *Urology* 33:361-366, 1998.

Deubler DA, Williams BJ, Zhu XL, et al. Allelic loss detected on chromosomes 8, 10, and 17 by fluorescence in situ hybridization using single-copy P1 probes on isolated nuclei form paraffin-embedded prostate tumors. *Am J Pathol* 150:841-850, 1997.

Dhanasekaran SM, Barrette TR, Ghosh D, et al. Delineation of prognostic biomarkers in prostate cancer. *Nature* 412:822-926, 2001.

Di Silverio F, D'Eramo G, Caponera M, et al. The prognostic value of DNA content in patients with prostatic carcinoma. *Eur Urol* 21(suppl):92-95, 1992.

Diaz JI, Mora LB, Austin P, et al. Predictability of PSA failure in prostate cancer by computerized cytometric assessment of tumoral cell proliferation. *Urology* 53:931-938, 1999.

Dinjens WN, van der Weiden MM, Schroeder FH, et al. Frequency and characterization of p53 mutations in primary and metastatic human prostate cancer. *Int J Cancer* 56:630-633, 1994.

Djakiew D. Dysregulated expression of growth factors and their receptors in the development of prostate cancer. *Prostate* 42:150-160, 2000.

Dong J-T, Lamb PW, Rinker-Schaeffer CW, et al. KAI1, a metastatic suppressor gene for prostate cancer on human chromosome 11p11.2. *Science* 268:884-886, 1995.

Dong J-T, Isaacs WB, Isaacs JT. Molecular advances in prostate cancer. *Curr Opin Oncol* 9:101-107, 1997.

Dong J-T, Sipe TW, Hyytinen ER, et al. PTEN/MMAC1 is infrequently mutated in pT2 and pT3 carcinomas of the prostate. *Oncogene* 17:1979-1982, 1998.

Dong J-T, Chen C, Stultz BG, et al. Deletion at 13q21 is associated with aggressive prostate cancers. *Cancer Res* 60:3880-3883, 2000.

Dong J-T, Li CL, Sipe TW, et al. Mutations of PTEN/MMAC1 in primary prostate cancers from Chinese patients. *Clin Cancer Res* 7:304-308, 2001.

Dorkin TJ, Robson CN, Neal DE. The molecular pathology of urological malignancies. *J Pathol* 183:380-387, 1997.

Drachenberg CB, Ioffe OB, Papadimitriou JC. Progressive increase of apoptosis in prostatic intraepithelial neoplasia and carcinoma. Comparison between in situ end-labeling of fragmented DA and detection by routine hematoxylin-eosin staining. *Arch Path Lab Med* 121:54-58, 1997.

Drobnjak M, Osman I, Scher HI, et al. Overexpression of cyclin D1 is associated with metastatic prostate cancer to bone. *Clin Cancer Res* 6:1891-1895, 2000.

Dunsmuir WD, Edwards SM, Lakhani SR, et al. Allelic imbalance in familial and sporadic prostate cancer at the putative human prostate cancer susceptibility locus, HPC1. The CRC/BPG UK Familial Prostate Cancer Study Collaborators. Cancer Research Campaign/British Prostate Group. *Br J Cancer* 78:1430-1433, 1998.

Dunsmuir WD, Gillett CE, Meyer LC, et al. Molecular markers for predicting prostate cancer stage and survival. *BJU Int* 86:869-878, 2000.

Eastham JA, Stapleton AM, Gousse AE, et al. Association of p53 mutation with metastatic prostate cancer. *Clin Cancer Res* 1:1111-1118, 1995.

Edwards SM, Dunsmuir WD, Gillett CE, et al. Immunohistochemical expression of BRCA2 protein and allelic loss at the BRCA2 locus in prostate cancer. CRC/BPG UK Familial Study Collaborators. *Int J Cancer* 78:1-9, 1998.

Edwards SM, Badzioch MD, Minter R, et al. Androgen receptor polymorphisms: association with prostate cancer risk, relapse and overall survival. *Int J Cancer* 84:458-465, 1999.

Egawa S, Uchida T, Suyama K, et al. Genomic instability of microsatellite repeats in prostate cancer: relationship to clinicopathological variables. *Cancer Res* 55:2418-2421, 1995.

Egawa S, Satoh T, Iwamura M, et al. Deoxyribonucleic acid ploidy status as no basis for pathologic stage prediction in clinically resectable prostate cancer. *Urology* 47:548-552, 1996.

El Gedaily A, Bubendorf L, Willi N, et al. Discovery of new DNA amplification loci in prostate cancer by comparative genomic hybridization. *Prostate* 46:184-190, 2001.

Elo JP, Visakorpi T. Molecular genetics of prostate cancer. *Ann Med* 33:130-141, 2001.

Elo JP, Harkönen P, Kyllönen AP, et al. Loss of heterozygosity at 16q24.1-q24.2 is significantly associated with metastatic and aggressive behavior of prostate cancer. *Cancer Res* 57:3356-3359, 1997.

Elo JP, Harkönen P, Kyllönen AP, et al. Three independently deleted regions at chromosome arm 16q in human prostate cancer: allelic loss at 16q24.1 -q24.2 is associated with aggressive behaviour of the disease, recurrent growth, poor differentiation of the tumour and poor prognosis for the patient. *Br J Cancer* 79:156-160, 1999.

Emmert-Buck MR, Vocke CD, Pozzatti RO, et al. Allelic loss on chromosome 8p12-21 in microdissected prostatic intraepithelial neoplasia. *Cancer Res* 55:2959-2962, 1995.

Erbersdobler A, Bardenhagen P, Henke RP. Numerical chromosomal anomalies in latent adenocarcinoma of the prostate. *Prostate* 38:92-99, 1999.

Erdamar S, Yang G, Harper JW, et al. Levels of expression of $p27^{KIP1}$ protein in human prostate and prostate cancer: an immunohistochemical analysis. *Mod Pathol* 12:751-755, 1999.

Ernst T, Hergenhahn M, Kenzelmann M, et al. Decrease and gain of gene expression are equally discriminatory markers for prostate carcinoma: a gene expression analysis on total and microdissected prostate tissue. *Am J Pathol* 160:2169-2180, 2002.

Eskelinen M, Lipponen P, Majapuro R, et al. DNA ploidy, S phase fraction and G_2 fraction as prognostic determinants in prostatic adenocarcinoma. *Eur Urol* 20:62-66, 1991.

Falkmer UG. Methodological aspects on flow and image cytometric nuclear DNA assessments in prostatic adenocarcinoma. *Acta Oncol* 30:201-203, 1991.

Feilotter HE, Nagai M, Boag A, et al. Analysis of PTEN and the 10q23 region in primary prostate carcinomas. *Oncogene* 16:1743-1748, 1998.

Feneley MR, Young MPA, Chinyama C, et al. Ki-67 expression in early prostate cancer and associated pathological lesions. *J Clin Pathol* 49:741-748, 1996.

Ford D, Easton DF, Bishop DT, et al. Risks of cancer in BRCA1-mutation carriers. Breast Cancer Linkage Consortium. *Lancet* 343:692-695, 1994.

Fordham MVP, Burdge AH, Matthews J, et al. Prostatic carcinoma cell DNA content measured by flow cytometry and its relation to clinical outcome. *Br J Surg* 73:400-403,1986.

Forsslund G, Esposti P-L, Nilsson B, et al. The prognostic significance of nuclear DNA content in prostatic carcinoma. *Cancer* 69:1432-1439, 1992.

Forsslund G, Nilsson B, Zetterberg A. Near tetraploid prostate carcinoma. Methodologic and prognostic aspects. *Cancer* 78:1748-1755, 1996.

Frankfurt OS, Chin JL, Englander LS, et al. Relationship between DNA ploidy, glandular differentiation, and tumor spread in human prostate cancer. *Cancer Res* 45:1418-1423, 1985.

Fu W, Bubendorf L, Willi N, et al. Genetic changes in clinically organ-confined prostate cancer by comparative genomic hybridization. *Urology* 56:880-885, 2000.

Gallee MPW, Visser-de Jong E, Ten Kate FJW, et al. Monoclonal antibody Ki-67 defined growth fraction in benign prostatic hyperplasia and prostatic cancer. *J Urol* 142:1342-1346, 1989.

Gao AC, Lou W, Dong J-T, et al. CD44 is a metastasis suppressor gene for prostatic cancer located on human chromosome 11p13. *Cancer Res* 57:846-849, 1997.

Gao X, Wu N, Grignon D, et al. High frequency of mutator phenotype in human prostatic adenocarcinoma. *Oncogene* 9:2999-3003, 1994.

Gao X, Zacharek A, Grignon DJ, et al. Localization of potential tumor suppressor loci to a <2 mb region on chromosome 17q in human prostate cancer. *Oncogene* 11:1241-1247, 1995A

Gao X, Zacharek A, Salkowski A, et al. Loss of heterozygosity of the BRCA1 and other loci on chromosome 17q in human prostate cancer. *Cancer Res* 55:1002-1005, 1995B.

Gauwitz MD, Pollack A, el-Naggar AK, et al. The prognostic significance of DNA ploidy in clinically localized prostate cancer treated with radiation therapy. *Int J Radiat Oncol Biol Phys* 28:821-828, 1994.

Gayther SA, de Foy KA, Harrington P, et al. The frequency of germ-line mutations in the breast cancer predisposition genes BRCA1 and BRCA2 in familial prostate cancer. *Cancer Res* 60:4513-4518, 2000.

Gburek BM, Kollmorgen TA, Qian J, et al. Chromosomal anomalies in stage D1 prostate adenocarcinoma primary tumors and lymph node metastases detected by fluorescence in situ hybridization. *J Urol* 157:223-227, 1997.

Gettman MT, Pacelli A, Slezak J, et al. Role of microvessel density in predicting recurrence in pathologic stage T3 prostate adenocarcinoma. *Urology* 54:479-485, 1999.

Ghazizadeh M, Sasaki Y, Oguro T, et al. Silver staining nucleolar organizer regions in prostatic lesions. *Histopathology* 19:369-372, 1991.

Gibbs M, Chakrabarti L, Stanford JL, et al. Analysis of chromosome 1q42.2-43 in 152 families with high risk of prostate cancer. *Am J Hum Genet* 64:1087-1095, 1999A.

Gibbs M, Stanford JL, McIndoe RA, et al. Evidence for a rare prostate cancer susceptibility locus at chromosome 1p36. *Am J Hum Genet* 64:776-787, 1999B.

Gibbs M, Stanford JL, Jarvik GP, et al. A genomic scan of families of prostate cancer identifies multiple regions of interest. *Am J Hum Genet* 67:100-109, 2000.

Giovannucci E, Stampfer MJ, Krithivas K, et al. The CAG repeat within the androgen receptor gene and its relationship to prostate cancer. *Proc Natl Acad Sci* 94:3320-3323, 1997.

Goddard KAB, Witte JS, Suarez BK, et al. Model-free linkage analysis with covariates confirms linkage of prostate cancer to chromosomes 1 and 4. *Am J Hum Genet* 68:1197-1206, 2001.

Goel A, Abou-Ellela A, De Rose PB, et al. The prognostic significance of proliferation in prostate cancer. Image cytometric quantitation of MIB-1. *J Urol Pathol* 4:213-225, 1996.

Gray IC, Phillips SMA, Lee SJ, et al. Loss of chromosomal region 10q23-25 in prostate cancer. *Cancer Res* 55:4800-4300, 1995.

Greene DR, Rogers E, Wessels EC, et al. Some small prostate cancers are nondiploid by nuclear image analysis: correlation of deoxyribonucleic acid ploidy status and pathological features. *J Urol* 151:1301-1307, 1994.

Grignon DJ, Caplan R, Sarkar FH, et al. p53 status and prognosis of locally advanced prostatic adenocarcinoma: a study based on RTOG 8610. *J Natl Cancer Inst* 89:158-165, 1997.

Grönberg H, Isaacs SD, Smith JR, et al. Characteristics of prostate cancer in families potentially lined to the hereditary prostate cancer 1 (HPC1) locus. *JAMA* 278:1251-1255, 1997A.

Grönberg H, Xu J, Smith JR, et al. Early age at diagnosis in families providing evidence of linkage to the hereditary prostate cancer locus (HPC1) on chromosome 1. *Cancer Res* 57:4707-4709, 1997B.

Grönberg H, Damber L, Tavelin B, et al. No difference in survival between sporadic, familial and hereditary prostate cancer. *Br J Urol* 82:564-567, 1998.

Gumerlock PH, Poonamallee UR, Meyers FJ, et al. Activated *ras* alleles in human carcinoma of the prostate are rare. *Cancer Res* 51:1632-1637, 1991.

Habuchi T, Suzuki T, Sasaki R, et al. Association of vitamin D receptor gene polymorphism with prostate cancer and benign prostatic hyperplasia in a Japanese population. *Cancer Res* 60:305-308, 2000A.

Habuchi T, Liqing Z, Suzuki T, et al. Increased risk of prostate cancer and benign prostatic hyperplasia associated with a CYP17 gene polymorphism with a gene dosage effect. *Cancer Res* 60:5710-5713, 2000B.

Häggman M, de la Torre M, Brändstedt S, et al. Pre- and postoperative DNA ploidy patterns correlated to pT-stage, histological grade and tumor volume in total prostatectomy specimens. *Scand J Urol Nephrol* 28:59-66, 1994.

Häggman MJ, Wojno KJ, Pearsall CP, et al. Allelic loss of 8p sequences in prostatic intraepithelial neoplasia and carcinoma. *Urology* 50:643-647, 1997A.

Häggman M, Nordin B, Mattson S, et al. Morphometric studies of intra-prostatic volume relationships in localized prostatic cancer. *Br J Cancer* 80:612-617, 1997B.

Hakimi JM, Schoenberg MP, Rondinelli RH, et al. Androgen receptor variants with short glutamine or glycine repeats may identify unique subpopulations of men with prostate cancer. *Clin Cancer Res* 3:1599-1608, 1997.

Hall MC, Troncoso P, Pollack A, et al. Significance of tumor angiogenesis in clinically localized prostate carcinoma treated with external beam radiotherapy. *Urology* 44:869-875, 1994.

Hall MC, Navone NM, Troncoso P, et al. Frequency and characterization of p53 mutations in clinically localized prostate cancer. *Urology* 45:470-475, 1995.

Hanus MC, Zagars GK, Pollack A. Familial prostate cancer: outcome following radiation therapy with or without adjuvant androgen ablation. *Int J Radiat Oncol Biol Phys* 43:379-383, 1999.

Harper ME, Goddard L, Wilson DW, et al. Pathological and clinical associations of Ki-67 defined growth fractions in human prostatic carcinoma. *Prostate* 21:75-84, 1992.

Harper ME, Goddard L, Glynne-Jones E, et al. Epidermal growth factor receptor expression by northern analysis and immunohistochemistry in benign and malignant prostatic tumors. *Eur J Cancer* 31:1492-1497, 1995.

Haugen OA, Mjølnerød O. DNA-ploidy as prognostic factor in prostatic carcinoma. *Int J Cancer* 45:224-228, 1990.

Hawkins CA, Bergstralh EJ, Lieber MM, et al. Influence of DNA ploidy and adjuvant treatment on progression and survival in patients with pathologic stage T3 (pT3) prostate cancer after radical retropubic prostatectomy. *Urology* 46:356-364, 1995.

Heidenberg HB, Sesterhenn IA, Gaddipati JP, et al. Alteration of the tumor suppressor gene p53 in a high fraction of hormone refractory prostate cancer. *J Urol* 154:414-421, 1995.

Henshall SM, Quinn DI, Lee CS, et al. Altered expression of androgen receptor in the malignant epithelium and adjacent stroma is associated with early relapse in prostate cancer. *Cancer Res* 61:423-427, 2001.

Hobisch A, Culig Z, Radmayr C, et al. Distant metastases from prostatic carcinoma express androgen receptor protein. *Cancer Res* 55:3068-3072, 1995.

Hsieh CL, Oakley-Girvan I, Balise RR, et al. A genome screen of families with multiple cases of prostate cancer: evidence of genetic heterogeneity. *Am J Hum Genet* 69:148-158, 2001.

Hsing AW, Gao YT, Wu G, et al. Polymorphic CAG and GGN repeat lengths in the androgen receptor gene and prostate cancer risk: a population-based care-control study in China . *Cancer Res* 60:5111-5116, 2000.

Huang S-F, Xiao S, Renshaw AA, et al. Fluorescence in situ hybridization evaluation of chromosome deletion patterns in prostate cancer. *Am J Pathol* 149:1565-1573, 1996.

Hügel A, Wernert N. Loss of heterozygosity (LOH), malignancy grade and clonality in microdissected prostate cancer. *Br J Cancer* 79:551-557, 1999.

Humphrey PA, Walther PJ, Currin SM, et al. Histologic grade, DNA ploidy, and intraglandular tumor extent as indicators of tumor progression of clinical stage B prostatic carcinoma. A direct comparison. *Am J Surg Pathol* 15:1165-1170, 1991.

Humphrey PA. p53 mutations and immunohistochemical detection, with a focus on alterations in urologic malignancies. In: Weinstein RS, Graham AR, Anderson RE, et al, eds. *Advances in Pathology and Laboratory Medicine.* Vol 7. New York: Mosby; 579-606, 1994.

Humphrey PA, Zhu X, Zarnegar R, et al. Hepatocyte growth factor and its receptor (c-MET) in prostate carcinoma. *Am J Pathol* 147:386-396, 1995A.

Humphrey PA, Swanson PE. Immunoreactive p53 protein in high-grade prostatic intraepithelial neoplasia. *Pathol Res Pract* 191:881-887, 1995B.

Hussain MH, Powell J, Zaki N, et al. Flow cytometric DNA analysis of fresh prostatic resections. Correlation with conventional prognostic parameters in patients with prostate cancer. *Cancer* 72:3012-3019, 1993.

Hyytinen E-R, Frierson HF Jr, Boyd JC, et al. Three distinct regions of allelic loss at 13q14, 13q21-22, and 13q33 in prostate cancer. *Genes Chromosomes Cancer* 25:108-114, 1999.

Ibrahim GK, MacDonald JA, Kerns BJ, et al. Differential immunoreactivity of her-2/neu oncoprotein in prostatic tissues. *Surg Oncol* 1:151-155, 1992.

Ibrahim GK, Kerns BJ, MacDonald JA, et al. Differential immunoreactivity of epidermal growth factor receptor in benign, dysplastic and malignant prostatic tissues. *J Urol* 149:170-173, 1993.

Incognito LS, Cazares LH, Schellhammer PF, et al. Overexpression of p53 in prostate carcinoma is associated with improved overall survival but not predictive of response to radiotherapy. *Int J Oncol* 17:761-769, 2000.

Ingles SA, Ross RK, Yu MC, et al. Association of prostate cancer risk with genetic polymorphisms in vitamin D receptor and androgen receptor. *J Natl Cancer Inst* 89:166-170, 1997.

Isaacs JT. Apoptosis: translating theory to therapy for prostate cancer. *J Natl Cancer Inst* 92:1367-1369, 2000.

Isaacs WB, Bova GS. Prostate cancer. In: Vogelstein B, Kinzler KW, eds. *The Genetic Basis of Human Cancer.* New York: McGraw-Hill; 653-660, 1998.

Ittmann M. Allelic loss on chromosome 10 in prostate adenocarcinoma. *Cancer Res* 56:2143-2147, 1996.

Jaffe JM, Malkowicz SB, Walker AH, et al. Association of SRD5A2 genotype and pathological characteristics of prostate tumors. *Cancer Res* 60:1626-1630, 2000.

Jarrard DF, Kinoshita H, Shi Y, et al. Methylation of the androgen receptor promoter CpG island is associated with loss of androgen receptor expression in prostate cancer cells. *Cancer Res* 58:5310-5314, 1998.

Jenkins R, Takahashi S, Delacey K, et al. Prognostic significance of allelic imbalance of chromosome arms 7q, 8p, 16q, and 18q in stage T3NOMO prostate cancer. *Genes Chromosomes Cancer* 21:131-143, 1998.

Jenkins RB, Qian J, Lieber MM, et al. Detection of c-myc oncogene amplification and chromosomal anomalies in metastatic prostatic carcinoma by fluorescence in situ hybridization. *Cancer Res* 57:524-531, 1997.

Jenkins RB, Qian J, Lee HK, et al. A molecular cytogenetic analysis of 7q31 in prostate cancer. *Cancer Res* 58:759-766, 1998.

Jones EC, McNeal J, Bruchovsky N, et al. DNA content in prostatic adenocarcinoma. A flow cytometric study of the predictive value of aneuploidy for tumor volume, percentage Gleason grade 4 and 5, and lymph node metastases. *Cancer* 66:752-757, 1990.

Jordan JJ, Hanlon AL, Al-Saleem TI, et al. Loss of the short arm of the Y chromosome in human prostate carcinoma. *Cancer Genet Cytogenet* 124:122-126, 2001.

Jorgensen T, Yogesan K, Skjorten F, et al. Histopathological grading and DNA ploidy as prognostic markers in metastatic prostatic cancer. *Br J Cancer* 71:1055-1060, 1995.

Kagan J, Stein J, Babaian RJ, et al. Homozygous deletions at 8p22 and 8p21 in prostate cancer implicate these regions as the sites for candidate tumor suppressor genes. *Oncogene* 11:2121-2126, 1995.

Kaleem Z, Swanson PE, Vollmer RT, et al. Prostatic adenocarcinoma with atrophic features. *Am J Clin Pathol* 109:695-703, 1998.

Kallakury BV, Sheehan CE, Ambros RA, et al. Correlation of p34cdc2 cyclin-dependent kinase overexpression, CD44s downregulation and HER-2/neu oncogene amplification with recurrence in prostatic adenocarcinomas. *J Clin Oncol* 16:1302-1309, 1998.

Kallioniemi O-P, Visakorpi T, Holli K, et al. Improved prognostic impact of S-phase values from paraffin-embedded breast and prostate carcinomas after correcting for nuclear slicing. *Cytometry* 12:413-421, 1991.

Kaltz-Wittmer C, Klenk U, Glaessgen A, et al. FISH analysis of gene aberrations (myc, CCND1, ERBB2, RB and AR) in advanced prostatic carcinomas before and after androgen deprivation therapy. *Lab Invest* 80:1455-1464, 2000.

Kantoff PW, Febbo PG, Giovannucci E, et al. A polymorphism of the 5 alpha-reductase gene and its association with prostate cancer: a case-control analysis. *Cancer Epidemiol Biomarkers Prev* 6:184-189, 1997.

Keetch DW, Humphrey PA, Smith D, et al. Clinical and pathological features of hereditary prostate cancer. *J Urol* 155:1841-1843, 1996.

Kelavkar UP, Cohen C, Kamitani H, et al. Concordant induction of 15-lipoxygenase-1 and mutant p53 expression in human prostate adenocarcinoma: correlation with Gleason staging. *Carcinogenesis* 21:1777-1787, 2000.

Keshgegian AA, Johnston E, Cnaan A. Bcl-2 oncoprotein positivity and high MIB-1 (Ki-67) proliferative rate are independent predictive markers for recurrence in prostate carcinoma. *Am J Clin Pathol* 110:443-449, 1998.

Khoo VS, Pollack A, Cowen D, et al. Relationship of Ki-67 labeling index to DNA-ploidy, S-phase fraction, and outcome in prostate cancer treated with radiotherapy. *Prostate* 41:166-172, 1999.

Kibel AS, Schutte M, Kern SE, et al. Identification of 12p as a region of frequent deletion in advanced prostate cancer. *Cancer Res* 58:5652-5655, 1998.

Kibel AS, Isaacs WB. G1/S cell cycle proteins as markers of aggressive prostate carcinoma. *Urology* 55:316-322, 2000A.

Kibel AS, Faith DA, Bova GS, et al. Loss of heterozygosity at 12p12-13 in primary and metastatic prostate adenocarcinoma. *J Urol* 164:192-196, 2000B.

Koeppen HKW, Wright BD, Burt AD, et al. Overexpression of HER2/neu in solid tumours: an immunohistochemical survey. *Histopathology* 38:96-104, 2001.

Koivisto P, Kononen J, Palmberg C, et al. Androgen receptor gene amplification: a possible molecular mechanisms for androgen deprivation therapy failure in prostate cancer. *Cancer Res* 57:314-319, 1997.

Konig JJ, Teubel W, van Dongen JW, et al. Loss and gain of chromosomes 1, 18, and Y in prostate cancer. *Prostate* 25:281-291, 1994.

Konishi N, Enomoto T, Buzard G, et al. K-*ras* activation and *ras* p21 expression in latent prostatic carcinomas in Japanese men. *Cancer* 69:2293-2299, 1992.

Konishi N, Nakaoka S, Hiasa Y, et al. Immunohistochemical evaluation of estrogen receptor status in benign prostatic hypertrophy and in prostate carcinoma and the relationship to efficacy at endocrine therapy. *Oncology* 50:259-263, 1993.

Konishi N, Nakaoka S, Tsuzuki T, et al. Progressive activity in latent prostate carcinoma defined by argyrophilic staining of nucleolar organizer regions (AgNOR). *Pathol Int* 44:297-302, 1994.

Konishi N, Hiasa Y, Hayashi I, et al. p53 mutations occur in clinical, but not latent, human prostate carcinoma. *Jpn J Cancer Res* 86:57-63, 1995.

Konishi N, Hiasa Y, Tsuzuki T, et al. Comparison of ras activation in prostate carcinoma in Japanese and American men. *Prostate* 30:53-57, 1997A.

Konishi N, Cho M, Yamamoto K, et al. Genetic changes in prostate cancer. *Pathol Int* 47:735-747, 1997B.

Krajewska M, Krajewski S, Epstein JI, et al. Immunohistochemical analysis of bcl-2, bax, bcl-X, and mcl-1 expression in prostate cancers. *Am J Pathol* 148:1567-1576, 1996.

Kubota Y, Fujinami K, Uemura H, et al. Retinoblastoma gene mutations in primary human prostate cancer. *Prostate* 27:314-320, 1995A.

Kubota Y, Shuin T, Uemura H, et al. Tumor suppressor gene p53 mutations in human prostate cancer. *Prostate* 27:18-24, 1995B.

Kucuk O, Demirer T, Gilman-Sachs A, et al. Intratumor heterogeneity of DNA ploidy and correlations with clinical stage and histologic grade in prostate cancer. *J Surg Oncol* 54:171-174, 1993.

Kuczyk MA, Serth J, Bokemeyer C, et al. The prognostic value of p53 for long-term and recurrence-free survival following radical prostatectomy. *Eur J Cancer* 34:679-686, 1998.

Kuhn EJ, Kurnot RA, Sesterhenn IA, et al. Expression of the *c-erb*B-2 (HER-2/neu) oncoprotein in human prostatic carcinoma. *J Urol* 150:1427-1433, 1993.

Kunimi K, Bergerheim US, Larsson IL, et al. Allelotyping of human prostatic adenocarcinoma. *Genomics* 11:530-536, 1991.

Kunimi K, Amano T, Uchibayashi T. Point mutation of the p53 gene is an infrequent event in untreated prostate cancer. *Cancer Detect Prev* 20:218-222, 1996.

Kupelian PA, Klein EA, Witte JS, et al. Familial prostate cancer: a different disease. *J Urol* 158:2197-2220, 1997A.

Kupelian PA, Kupelian VA, Witte JS, et al. Family history of prostate cancer in patients with localized prostate cancer: an independent predictor of treatment outcome. *J Clin Oncol* 15:1478-1480, 1997B.

Lacombe L, Maillette A, Meyer F, et al. Expression of p21 predicts PSA failure in locally advanced prostate cancer treated by prostatectomy. *Int J Cancer* 95:135-139, 2001.

Lalani E-N, Laniado ME, Abel PD. Molecular and cellular biology of prostate cancer. *Cancer Metastasis Rev* 16:29-66, 1997.

Lange EM, Chen H, Brierley K, et al. The polymorphic exon 1 androgen receptor CAG repeat in men with a potential inherited predisposition to prostate cancer. *Cancer Epidemiol Biomarkers Prev* 9:439-442, 2000.

Latil A, Cussenot O, Fournier G, et al. Infrequent allelic imbalance at the major susceptibility HPC1 locus in sporadic prostate tumor [letter to the editor]. *Int J Cancer* 71:1118, 1997.

Latil A, Lidereau R. Genetic aspects of prostate cancers. *Virchows Arch* 432:389-406, 1998.

Latil A, Bieche I, Pesche S, et al. Loss of heterozygosity at chromosome arm 13q and RB1 status in human prostate cancer. *Hum Pathol* 30:809-815, 1991.

LaTulippe E, Satagopan J, Smith A, et al. Comprehensive gene expression analysis of prostate cancer reveals distinct transcriptional programs associated with metastatic disease. *Cancer Res* 62:4499-4506, 2002.

Lear I, Lau K-M, Adams JY, et al. Comparative studies of the estrogen receptors β and α and the androgen receptor in normal human prostate glands, dysplasia, and in primary and metastatic carcinoma. *Am J Clin Pathol* 159:79-92, 2001.

Lee W-H, Isaacs WB, Bova GS, et al. CG island methylation changes near the *GSTP1* gene in prostatic carcinoma cells detected using the polymerase chain reaction: a new prostatic biomarker. *Cancer Epidemiol Biomark Prev* 6:443-450, 1997.

Leibovich BC, Cheng L, Weaver AL, et al. Outcome prediction with p53 immunostaining after radical prostatectomy in patients with locally advanced prostate cancer. *J Urol* 163:1756-1760, 2000.

Leite KR, Franco MF, Srougi M, et al. Abnormal expression of MDM2 in prostate carcinoma. *Mod Pathol* 14:428-436, 2001.

Leung C-S, Zbieranowski I, Demers J, et al. DNA image cytometry of prostatic carcinoma: a comparison of needle core biopsy and subsequent prostatectomy specimens. *Mod Pathol* 7:195-199, 1994.

Li C, Larsson C, Futreal A, et al. Identification of two distinct deleted regions on chromosome 13 in prostate cancer. *Oncogene* 16:481-487, 1998.

Li J, Yen C, Liaw D, et al. PTEN, a putative protein tyrosine phosphatase gene mutated in human brain, breast, and prostate cancer. *Science* 275:1943-1947, 1997.

Li L-C, Chui R, Nakajima K, Oh BR, Au HC, Dahiya R. Frequent methylation of estrogen receptor in prostate cancer: correlation with tumor progression. *Cancer Res* 60:702-706, 2000.

Li L-C, Zhao H, Nakajima K, et al. Methylation of the E-cadherin gene promoter correlates with progression of prostate cancer. *J Urol* 166:705-709, 2001.

Lichtenstein P, Holm NV, Verkasalo PK, et al. Environmental and heritable factors in the causation of cancer. Analyses of cohorts of twins from Sweden, Denmark, and Finland. *N Engl J Med* 343:78-85, 2000.

Linja MJ, Savinainen KJ, Saramaki OR, et al. Amplification and overexpression of androgen receptor gene in hormone-refractory prostate cancer. *Cancer Res* 61:3550-3555, 2001.

Lipponen P, Vesalainen S. Expression of apoptosis suppressing protein bcl-2 in prostatic adenocarcinoma is related to tumor malignancy. *Prostate* 32:9-15, 1997.

Losi L, Di Gregorio C, Brausi M, et al. Expression of p53 protein in prostate cancers of different histologic types. *Pathol Res Pract* 190:384-388, 1994.

Lundberg S, Carstensen J, Rundquist I. DNA flow cytometry and histopathological grading of paraffin-embedded prostate biopsy specimens in a survival study. *Cancer Res* 47:1973-1977, 1987.

Luo J, Duggan DJ, Chen Y, et al. Human prostate cancer and benign prostatic hyperplasia: molecular dissection by gene expression profiling. *Cancer Res* 61:4683-4688, 2001.

Macera MJ, Godec CJ, Sharma N, et al. Loss of heterozygosity of the TP53 tumor suppressor gene and detection of point mutations by the non-isotopic RNAse cleavage assay in prostate cancer. *Cancer Genet Cytogenet* 108:42-47, 1999.

Macintosh CA, Stower M, Reid N, et al. Precise microdissection of human prostate cancers reveals genotypic heterogeneity. *Cancer Res* 58:23-28, 1998.

Macri E, Loda M. Role of p27 in prostate carcinogenesis. *Cancer Metastasis Rev* 17:337-344, 1999.

Magee JA, Araki T, Patil S, et al. Expression profiling reveals hepsin overexpression in prostate cancer. *Cancer Res* 61:5692-5696, 2001.

Magi-Galluzzi C, Xu X, Hlatky L, et al. Heterogeneity of androgen receptor content in advanced prostate cancer. *Mod Pathol* 10:839-845, 1997.

Magi-Galluzzi C, Murphy M, Cangi MG, et al. Proliferation, apoptosis and cell cycle regulation in prostatic carcinogenesis. *Anal Quant Cytol Histol* 20:343-350, 1998.

Makridakis NM, Ross RK, Pike MC, et al. Association of mis-sense substitution in SRD5A2 gene with prostate cancer in African-American and Hispanic men in Los Angeles, USA. *Lancet* 354:975-978, 1999.

Makridakis N, Ross RK, Pike MC, et al. A prevalent missense substitution that modulates activity of prostatic steroid 5a-reductase. *Cancer Res* 57:1020-1022, 1997.

Malkin D. Molecular biology of p53. In: Vogelstein B, Kinzler KW, eds. *The Genetic Basis of Human Cancer.* New York: McGraw-Hill; 395-397, 1998.

Marcelli M, Ittmann M, Mariani S, et al. Androgen receptor gene mutations in prostate cancer. *Cancer Res* 60:944-949, 2000.

Mark HF, Feldman D, Das S, et al. Fluorescence in situ hybridization study of HER-2/neu oncogene amplification in prostate cancer. *Exp Mol Pathol* 66:170-178, 1999.

Masai M, Abe K, Akimoto S, et al. Argyrophilic nucleolar organizer regions in benign hyperplastic and cancerous human prostates. *Prostate* 20:1-13, 1992.

Mashal RD, Lester S, Corless C, et al. Expression of cell cycle-regulated proteins in prostate cancer. *Cancer Res* 56:4159-4163, 1996.

Massenkeil G, Oberhuber H, Hailemariam S, et al. p53 mutations and loss of heterozygosity on chromosomes 8p, 16q, 17p, and 18q are confined to advanced prostate cancer. *Anticancer Res* 14:2789-2794, 1994.

Masuda M, Takano Y, Iki M, et al. Prognostic significance of Ki-67, p53 and Bcl-2 expression in prostate cancer patients with lymph node metastases: a retrospective immunohistochemical analysis. *Pathol Int* 48:41-46, 1998.

Matikaine MP, Pukkala E, Schleutker J, et al. Relatives of prostate cancer patients have an increased risk of prostate and stomach cancers: a population-based cancer registry study in Finland. *Cancer Causes Control* 12:223-230, 2001.

Matsushima H, Kitamura T, Goto T, et al. Combined analysis with bcl-2 and p53 immunostaining predicts poorer prognosis in prostatic carcinoma. *J Urol* 158:2278-2283, 1997.

Matsushima H, Sasaki T, Goto T, et al. Immunohistochemical study of $p21^{WAF1}$ and p53 proteins in prostatic cancer and their prognostic significance. *Hum Pathol* 29:778-783, 1998.

Matsuura H, Shiraishi T, Yatani R, et al. Interphase cytogenetics of prostate cancer: fluorescence in situ hybridization (FISH) analysis of Japanese cases. *Br J Cancer* 74:1699-1704, 1996.

Maygarden SJ, Strom S, Ware JL. Localization of epidermal growth factor receptor by immunohistochemical methods in human prostatic carcinoma, prostatic intraepithelial neoplasia, and benign hyperplasia. *Arch Pathol Lab Med* 116:269-273, 1992.

Maygarden SJ, Novotny DB, Moul JW, et al. Evaluation of cathepsin D and epidermal growth factor receptor in prostate carcinoma. *Mod Pathol* 7:930-936, 1994.

McCann A, Dervan PA, Johnston PA, et al. C-erb B-2 oncoprotein expression in primary human tumors. *Cancer* 65:88-92, 1990.

McDonnell TJ, Troncoso P, Brisbay SM, et al. Expression of the proto oncogene bcl-2 in the prostate and its association with emergence of androgen-independent prostate cancer. *Cancer Res* 52:6940-6944, 1992.

McDonnell TJ, Navone NM, Troncoso P, et al. Expression of bcl-2 oncoprotein and p53 protein accumulation in bone marrow metastases of androgen independent prostate cancer. *J Urol* 157:569-574, 1997.

McIndoe RA, Stanford JL, Gibbs M, et al. Linkage analysis of 49 high-risk families does not support a common familial prostate cancer-susceptibility gene at 1q24-25. *Am J Hum Genet* 61:347-353, 1997.

McIntire TL, Murphy WM, Coon JS, et al. The prognostic value of DNA ploidy combined with histologic substaging for incidental carcinoma of the prostate gland. *Am J Clin Pathol* 89:370-373, 1988.

McLoughlin J, Foster CS, Price P, et al. Evaluation of Ki-67 monoclonal antibody as prognostic indicator for prostatic carcinoma. *Br J Urol* 72:92-97, 1993.

McMenamin ME, Soung P, Perera S, et al. Loss of PTEN expression in paraffin-embedded primary prostate cancer correlates with high Gleason score and advanced stage. *Cancer Res* 59:4291-4296, 1999.

Meehan KL, Holland JW, Dawkins HJS. Proteomic analysis of normal and malignant prostate tissue to identify novel proteins lost in cancer. *Prostate* 50:54-63, 2002.

Mellon K, Thompson S, Charlton RG, et al. p53, c-erbB-2 and the epidermal growth factor receptor in the benign and malignant prostate. *J Urol* 147:496-499, 1992.

Miller J, Horsfall DJ, Marshall VR, et al. The prognostic value of deoxyribonucleic acid flow cytometric analysis in stage D2 prostatic carcinoma. *J Urol* 145:1192-1196, 1991.

Mirchandani D, Zheng J, Miller GJ, et al. Heterogeneity in intratumor distribution of p53 mutations in human prostate cancer. *Am J Pathol* 147:92-101, 1995.

Miyamoto KK, McSherry SA, Dent GA, et al. Immunohistochemistry of the androgen receptor in human benign and malignant prostate tissue. *J Urol* 149:1015-1019, 1993.

Montgomery BT, Nativ O, Blute ML, et al. Stage B prostate adenocarcinoma. Flow cytometric DNA ploidy analysis. *Arch Surg* 125:327-331, 1990.

Montironi R, Magi-Galluzzi C, Diamanti L, et al. Proliferating cell nuclear antigen (PCNA) in prostatic invasive adenocarcinoma. Is the proliferation state in the marginal zone of the tumour higher than in the central part? *Anticancer Res* 13:129-132, 1993.

Montironi R, Magi-Galluzzi C, Muzzonigro G, et al. Effects of combination endocrine treatment on normal prostate, prostatic intraepithelial neoplasia, and prostate prostatic adenocarcinoma. *J Clin Pathol* 47:906-913, 1994.

Montone KT, Tomaszewski JE. In situ hybridization for epidermal growth factor receptor (EGFR) external domain transcripts in prostatic adenocarcinoma. *J Clin Lab Anal* 7:188-195, 1993.

Mora LB, Moscinski LC, Diaz JI, et al. Stage B prostate cancer: correlation of DNA ploidy analysis with histological and clinical parameters. *Cancer Control* 6:587-591, 1999.

Morote J, de Torres I, Caceres C, et al. Prognostic value of immunohistochemical expression of the c-erbB-2 oncoprotein in metastatic prostate cancer. *Int J Cancer* 84:421-425, 1999.

Morris MJ, Reuter VE, Kelly WK, et al. HER-2 profiling and targeting in prostate cancer. A phase II trial of trastuzumab alone and with paclitaxel. *Cancer* 94:980-986, 2002.

Moul JW, Friedrichs PA, Lance RS, et al. Infrequent *ras* oncogene mutations in human prostate cancer. *Prostate* 20:327-338, 1992.

Moul JW, Maygarden SJ, Ware JL, et al. Cathespin D and epidermal growth factor receptor immunohistochemistry does not predict recurrence of prostate cancer in patients undergoing radical prostatectomy. *J Urol* 155:982-985, 1996A.

Moul JW, Bettencourt MC, Sesterhenn IA, et al. Protein expression of p53, bcl-2, and KI-67 (MIB-1) as prognostic biomarkers in patients with surgically treated, clinically localized prostate cancer. *Surgery* 120:159-166, 1996B.

Moyret-Lalle C, Marcais C, Jacquemier J, et al. ras, p53 and HPV status in benign and malignant prostate tumors. *Int J Cancer* 64:124-129, 1995.

Müller JG, Demel S, Wirth MP, et al. DNA-ploidy, G2M-fractions and prognosis of stages B and C prostate carcinoma. *Virchows Archiv* 424:647-651, 1994.

Mydlo JH, Kral JG, Volpe M, et al. Analysis of microvessel density, androgen receptor, p53 and HER-2/neu expression and Gleason score in prostate cancer: preliminary results and therapeutic implications. *Eur Urol* 34:426-432, 1998.

Myers MP, Stolarov J, Eng C, et al. P-TEN, the tumor suppressor from chromosome 10q23 is a dual-specificity phosphatase. *Proc Natl Acad Sci* 94:9052-9057, 1997.

Myers RB, Oelschlager D, Srivastava S, et al. Accumulation of p53 protein occurs more frequently in metastatic than in localized prostatic adenocarcinoma. *Prostate* 25:243-248, 1994A.

Myers RB, Srivastava S, Oelschlager DK, et al. Expression of p160erbB-3 and p185erbB-2 in prostatic intraepithelial neoplasia and prostatic adenocarcinoma. *J Natl Cancer Inst* 96:1140-1145, 1994B.

Myers RP, Larson-Keller JJ, Bergstralh EJ, et al. Hormonal treatment at time of radical retropubic prostatectomy for stage D1 prostate cancer: results of long-term followup. *J Urol* 147:910-915, 1992.

Naito S, Sakamoto N, Kotoh S, et al. Proliferating cell nuclear antigen in needle biopsy specimens of prostatic carcinoma. *Eur Urol* 26:164-169, 1994.

Nakayama T, Watanabe M, Suzuki H, et al. Eigenetic regulation of androgen receptor gene expression in human prostate cancers. *Lab Invest* 80:1789-1976, 2000.

Nam RK, Elhaji Y, Krahn MD, et al. Significance of the CAG repeat polymorphism of the androgen receptor gene in prostate cancer progression. *J Urol* 164:567-572, 2000.

Nam RK, Toi A, Vesprini D, et al. V89L polymorphisms of type-2, 5-alpha reductase enzyme gene predicts prostate cancer presence and progression. *Urology* 57:199-204, 2001.

Narain V, Tiguert R, Banerjee M, et al. Biochemical recurrence after radical prostatectomy in Black and White American men with a positive or negative family history of prostate cancer. *J Urol* 165:474-477, 2001.

Narla G, Heath KE, Reeves HL. KLF6, a candidate tumor suppressor gene mutated in prostate cancer. *Science.* 294:2563-2566, 2001.

Nativ O, Winkler HZ, Raz Y, et al. Stage C prostatic adenocarcinoma: flow cytometric nuclear DNA ploidy analysis. *Mayo Clin Proc* 64:911-919, 1989.

Nativ O, Myers RP, Farrow GM, et al. Nuclear deoxyribonucleic acid ploidy and serum prostate specific antigen in operable prostatic adenocarcinoma. *J Urol* 144:303-306, 1990.

Nativ O, Umehara T, Colvard DS, et al. Relationship between DNA ploidy and functional estrogen receptors in operable prostate cancer. *Eur Urol* 32:96-99, 1997.

Navone NM, Troncoso P, Pisters LL, et al. p53 protein accumulation and gene mutation in the progression of human prostate carcinoma. *J Natl Cancer Inst* 85:1657-1659, 1993.

Navone NM, Labate ME, Troncoso P, et al. p53 mutations in prostate cancer bone metastases suggest that selected p53 mutants in the primary site define foci with metastatic potential. *J Urol* 161:302-308, 1999.

Nelson WG, DeMarzo AM, DeWeese TL. The molecular pathogenesis of prostate cancer. *Eur Urol* 39(suppl 4):8-11, 2001.

Nemoto R, Hattori K, Uchida K, et al. S-phase fraction of human prostate adenocarcinoma studied with in vivo bromodeoxyuridine labeling. *Cancer* 66:509-514, 1990.

Netto GJ, Humphrey PA. Molecular biologic aspects of human prostatic carcinoma. *Am J Clin Pathol* 102(suppl 1):S57-S64, 1994.

Newsham IF, Hadjistilianou T, Cavenee WK. Retinoblastoma. In: Vogelstein B, Kinzler KW, eds. *The Genetic Basis of Human Cancer.* New York: McGraw-Hill; 363-392, 1998.

Nguyen TT, Nguyen CT, Gonzales FA, et al. Analysis of cyclin-dependent kinase inhibitor expression and methylation patterns in human prostate cancers. *Prostate* 43:233-242, 2000.

Nupponen NN, Kakkola L, Koivisto P, et al. Genetic alterations in hormone-refractory recurrent prostate carcinomas. *Am J Pathol* 153:141-148, 1998.

O'Malley FP, Grignon DJ, Keeney M, et al. DNA heterogeneity in prostatic adenocarcinoma. A DNA flow cytometric mapping study with whole organ sections of prostate. *Cancer* 71:2797-2802, 1993.

Oomens EHGM, van Steenbrugge GJ, van der Kwast Th H, et al. Application of the monoclonal antibody Ki-67 on prostate biopsies to assess the proliferative cell fraction of human prostatic carcinoma. *J Urol* 145:81-85, 1991.

Osman I, Scher H, Dalbagni G, et al. Chromosome 16 in primary prostate cancer: a microsatellite analysis. *Int J Cancer* 71:580-584, 1997.

Osman I, Drobnjak M, Fazzari M, et al. Inactivation of the p53 pathway in prostate cancer: impact on tumor progression. *Clin Cancer Res* 5:2082-2088, 1999.

Ow KT, Mameghan K, Lochhead A, et al. The prognostic significance of tumor-associated markers p53, HER-2/neu, c-myc, v-k-ras, PCNA and EGFr of local and distant recurrence in localized human prostatic adenocarcinoma. *Urol Oncol* 1:144-152, 1995.

Oxley JD, Winkler MH, Gillatt DA, et al. Her-2/neu oncogene amplification in clinically localised prostate cancer. *J Clin Pathol* 55:118-120, 2002.

Ozen M, Pathak S. Genetic alterations in human prostate cancer: a review of current literature. *Anticancer Res* 20:1905-1912, 2000.

Padalecki SS, Troyer DA, Hansen MF, et al. Identification of two distinct regions of allelic imbalance on chromosome 18q in metastatic prostate cancer. *Int J Cancer* 85:654-658, 2000.

Palazzo JP, Ellison P, Petersen RO. DNA content in prostate adenocarcinoma. Correlation with Gleason score, nuclear grade and histologic subtypes. *J Urol Pathol* 1:283-292, 1993.

Palmberg C, Koivisto P, Kakkola L, et al. Androgen receptor gene amplification at primary progression predicts response to combined androgen blockade as second line therapy for advanced prostate cancer. *J Urol* 164:1992-1995, 2000.

Papadoupoulos I, Rudolph P, Wirth B, et al. p53 expression, proliferation marker Ki-S5, DNA content and serum PSA. possible biopotential markers in human prostatic cancer. *Urology* 48:261-268, 1996.

Paris PL, Witte JS, Kupelian PA, et al. Identification and fine mapping of a region showing a high frequency of allelic imbalance on chromosome 16q23.2 that corresponds to a prostate cancer susceptibility locus. *Cancer Res* 60:3645-3649, 2000.

Park JJ, Irvine RA, Buchanan G, et al. Breast cancer susceptibility gene 1 (BRCA1) is a coactivator of the androgen receptor. *Cancer Res* 60:5946-5949, 2000.

Park M. Oncogenes. In: Vogelstein B, Kinzler KW, eds. *The Genetic Basis of Human Cancer.* New York: McGraw-Hill; 205-228, 1998.

Partin AW, Kattan MW, Subong EN, et al. Combination of prostate-specific antigen, clinical stage, and Gleason score to predict pathological stage of localized prostate cancer. A multi-institutional update. *JAMA* 277:1445-1451, 1997.

Perinchery G, Sasaki M, Angan A, et al. Deletion of Y-chromosome specific genes in human prostate cancer. *J Urol* 163:1339-1342, 2000.

Pesche S, Latil A, Muzeau F, et al. *PTEN/MMAC1/TEP1* in primary prostate cancers. *Oncogene* 16:2879-2883, 1998.

Peters JM, Miles BJ, Kubus JJ, et al. Prognostic significance of the nuclear DNA content in localized prostatic adenocarcinoma. *Anal Quant Cytol Histol* 12:359-365, 1990.

Peters MAA, Jarvik GP, Janer M, et al. Genetic linkage analysis of prostate cancer families to Xq27-28. *Hum Hered* 51:107-113, 2001.

Petricoin EF, Ornstein DK, Paweletz CP, et al. Serum proteomic patterns for detection of prostate cancer. *J Natl Cancer Inst* 99:1576-1578, 2002.

Phillips SM, Morton DG, Lee SJ, et al. Loss of heterogeneity of the retinoblastoma and adenomatous polyposis susceptibility gene loci and in chromosomes 10p, 10q and 16q in human prostate cancer. *Br J Urol* 73:390-395, 1994A.

Phillips SM, Barton CM, Lee SJ, et al. Loss of retinoblastoma susceptibility gene (RBI) is a frequent and early event in prostatic tumorigenesis. *Br J Cancer* 70:1252-1257, 1994B.

Pihan GA, Purohit A, Wallace J, et al. Centrosome defects can account for cellular and genetic changes that characterize prostate cancer progression. *Cancer Res* 61:2212-2219, 2001.

Pindur A, Chakraborty S, Welch DG, et al. DNA ploidy measurements in prostate cancer: differences between image analysis and flow cytometry and clinical implications. *Prostate* 25:184-189, 1994.

Pisters LL, Troncoso P, Zhau HE, et al. c-met proto-oncogene expression in benign and malignant human prostate tissues. *J Urol* 154:293-298, 1995.

Pollack A, Zagars GK, el-Naggar AK, et al. Relationship of tumor DNA-ploidy to serum prostate-specific antigen doubling time after radiotherapy for prostate cancer. *Urology* 44:711-718, 1994.

Pollack A, Troncoso P, Zagars GK, et al. The significance of DNA-ploidy and S-phase fraction in node-positive (stage D1) prostate cancer treated with androgen ablation. *Prostate* 31:21-28, 1997.

Potter SR, Miller MC, Mangold LA, et al. Genetically engineered neural networks for predicting prostate cancer progression after radical prostatectomy. *Urology* 54:791-795, 1999.

Prasad MA, Trybus TM, Wojno KJ, et al. Homozygous and frequent deletion of proximal 8p sequences in human prostate cancers: identification of a potential tumor suppressor gene site. *Genes Chromosomes Cancer* 23:255-262, 1998.

Praweletz CP, Liotta LA, Petricoin EF III. New technologies for biomarker analysis of prostate cancer progression: laser capture microdissection and tissue proteomics. *Urology* 57(4 suppl 1):160-163, 2001.

Prins GS, Sklarew RJ, Pertschuk LP. Image analysis of androgen receptor immunostaining in prostate cancer accurately predicts response to hormonal therapy. *J Urol* 159:641-649, 1998.

Qian J, Bostwick DG, Takahashi S, et al. Chromosomal anomalies in prostatic intraepithelial neoplasia and carcinoma detected by fluorescence in situ hybridization. *Cancer Res* 55:5408-5414, 1995.

Quinn DI, Henshall SM, Head DR, et al. Prognostic significance of p53 nuclear accumulation in localized prostate cancer treated with radical prostatectomy. *Cancer Res* 60:1585-1594, 2000.

Raymond WA, Leong AS-Y, Bolt JW, et al. Growth fractions in human prostatic carcinoma determined by Ki-67 immunostaining. *J Pathol* 156:161-167, 1988.

Rebbeck TR, Jaffe JM, Walker AH, et al. Modification of clinical presentation of prostate tumors by a novel genetic variant in CYP3A4. *J Natl Cancer Inst* 90:1225-1229, 1998.

Reese DM, Small EJ, Magrane G, et al. HER2 protein expression and gene amplification in androgen-independent prostate cancer. *Am J Clin Pathol* 116:234-239, 2001.

Rhodes DR, Barrette TR, Rubin MA, et al. Meta-analysis of microarrays: interstudy validation of gene expression profiles reveals pathway dysregulation in prostate cancer. *Cancer Res* 62:4427-4433, 2002.

Ring KS, Karp FS, Olsson CA, et al. Flow cytometric analysis of localized adenocarcinoma of the prostate: the use of archival DNA analysis in conjunction with pathological grading to predict clinical outcome following radical retropubic prostatectomy. *Prostate* 17:155-164, 1990.

Ritchie AWS, Dorey F, Layfeld LJ, et al. Relationship of DNA content to conventional prognostic factors in clinically localized carcinoma of the prostate. *Br J Urol* 62:254-260, 1988.

Rohrbach H, Haas CJ, Baretton GB, et al. Microsatellite instability and loss of heterozygosity in prostatic carcinomas: comparison of primary tumors, and of corresponding recurrences after androgen-deprivation therapy and lymph-node metastases. *Prostate* 40:20-27, 1999.

Rökman A, Koivisto PA, Matikainen MP, et al. Genetic changes in familial prostate cancer by comparative genomic hybridization. *Prostate* 46:233-239, 2001.

Rökman A, Ikonen T, Seppala EN, et al. Germline alterations of the RNASEL gene, a candidate HPCI gene at 1q25, in patients and families with prostate cancer. *Am J Hum Genet* 70:1299-1304, 2002.

Rosen EM, Fan S, Goldberg ID. BRCA1 and prostate cancer. *Cancer Invest* 19:396-412, 2001.

Ross JS, Nazeer T, Church K, et al. Contribution of HER-2/neu oncogene expression to tumor grade and DNA content analysis in the prediction of prostatic carcinoma analysis. *Cancer* 72:3020-3028, 1993.

Ross JS, Figge H, Bui HK, et al. Prediction of pathologic stage and postprostatectomy disease recurrence by DNA ploidy analysis of initial needle biopsy of specimens of prostate cancer. *Cancer* 74:2811-2818, 1994.

Ross JS. *DNA Ploidy and Cell Cycle Analysis.* New York: Igaku-Shoin; 1996.

Ross JS, Sheehan C, Hayner-Buchan A, et al. Prognostic significance of HER-2/neu gene amplification status by fluorescence in situ hybridization of prostate carcinoma. *Cancer* 79:2162-2170, 1997.

Ross JS, Sheehan CE, Ambros RA, et al. Needle biopsy DNA ploidy status predicts grade shifting in prostate cancer. *Am J Surg Pathol* 23:296-301, 1999.

Ross PL, Scardino PT, Kattan MW. A catalog of prostate cancer nomograms. *J Urol* 165:1562-1568, 2001.

Rubin MA, Gerstein A, Reid K, et al. 10q23.3 loss of heterozygosity is higher in lymph node-positive (pT2-3,N+) versus lymph node negative (pT2-3,NO) prostate cancer. *Hum Pathol* 31:504-508, 2000.

Rudin CM, Thompson CG. Apoptosis and cancer. In: Vogelstein B, Kinzler KW, eds. *The Genetic Basis of Human Cancer.* New York: McGraw-Hill; 193-201, 1998.

Ruijter E, van de Kaa C, Aalders T, et al. Heterogeneous expression of E-cadherin and p53 in prostate cancer: clinical implications. *Mod Pathol* 11:276-281, 1998.

Ruijter ETG, Miller GJ, van de Kaa CA, et al. Molecular analysis of multifocal prostate cancer lesions. *J Pathol* 188:271-277, 1999.

Ruizeveld de Winter JA, Janssen PJ, Sleddens HM, et al. Androgen receptor status in localized and locally progressive hormone refractory human prostate cancer. *Am J Pathol* 144:735-746, 1994.

Sadasivan R, Morgan R, Jennings S, et al. Overexpression of Her-2/neu may be an indicator of poor prognosis in prostate cancer. *J Urol* 150:126-131, 1993.

Sadi MV, Barrack ER. Determination of growth fraction in advanced prostate cancer by Ki-67 immunostaining and its relationship to the time to tumor progression after hormonal therapy. *Cancer* 67:3065-3071, 1991.

Sakr WA, Sarkar FH, Sreepathi P, et al. Measurement of cellular proliferation in human prostate by AgNOR, PCNA, and SPF. *Prostate* 22:147-154, 1993.

Sakr WA, Macoska JA, Benson P, et al. Allelic loss in locally metastatic, multisampled prostate cancer. *Cancer Res* 54:3273-3277, 1994.

Salem CE, Tomasic NA, Elmajian DA, et al. p53 protein and gene alterations in pathological stage C prostate carcinoma. *J Urol* 158:510-514, 1997.

Samowitz WS, Paull G, Hamilton SR. Reported binding of monoclonal antibody RAP-5 formalin fixed tissue sections is not indicative of ras p21 expression. *Hum Pathol* 19:129-132, 1988.

Sanchez KM, Sweeney CJ, Mass R, et al. Evaluation of HER-2/neu expression in prostatic adenocarcinoma. A request for a standardized, organ specific methodology. *Cancer* 95:1650-1655, 2002.

Sandberg AA. Chromosomal abnormalities and related events in prostate cancer. *Hum Pathol* 23:368-380, 1992.

Santourlidis S, Florl A, Ackerman R, et al. High frequency of alterations in DNA methylation in adenocarcinoma of the prostate. *Prostate* 39:166-174, 1999.

Saric T, Brkanac Z, Troyer DA, et al. Genetic pattern of prostate cancer progression. *Int J Cancer* 81:219-224, 1999.

Sarkar FH, Li Y, Sakr WA, et al. Relationship of $p21^{WAF\ 1}$ expression with disease-free survival and biochemical recurrence in prostate adenocarcinomas (PCa). *Prostate* 40:256-260, 1999.

Sasaki M, Tanaka Y, Perinchery G, et al. Methylation and inactivation of estrogen, progesterone, and androgen receptors in prostate cancer. *J Natl Cancer Inst* 94:384-390, 2002.

Sattler H-P, Rohde V, Bonkhoff H, et al. Comparative genomic hybridization reveals DNA copy number gains to frequently occur in human prostate cancer. *Prostate* 38:79-86, 1999.

Sattler H-P, Lensch R, Rohde V, et al. Novel amplification unit at chromosome 3q25-27 in human prostate cancer. *Prostate* 45:207-215, 2000.

Savinainen KJ, Saramäki OR, Linja MJ, et al. Expression and gene copy number analysis of ERBB2 oncogene in prostate cancer. *Am J Pathol* 160:339-345, 2002.

Schaid DJ, McDonnell SK, Blute ML, et al. Evidence for autosomal dominant inheritance of prostate cancer. *Am J Hum Genet* 62:1425-1438, 1998.

Scher HI, Sarkis A, Reuter V, et al. Changing pattern of expression of the epidermal growth factor receptor and transforming growth factor alpha in the progression of prostatic neoplasms. *Clin Cancer Res* 1:545-550, 1995.

Scher HI. HER 2 in prostate cancer—a viable target or innocent bystander? *J Natl Cancer Inst* 92:1866-1888, 2000.

Schlechte HH, Schnorr D, Loning T, et al. Mutation of the tumor suppressor gene p53 in human prostate and bladder cancers—investigation by temperature gradient gel electrophoresis (TGGE). *J Urol* 157:1049-1053, 1997.

Schlechte H, Lenk SV, Loning T, et al. p53 tumour suppressor gene mutations in benign prostatic hyperplasia and prostate cancer. *Eur Urol* 34:443-440, 1998.

Schleutker J, Matikainen M, Smith J, et al. A genetic epidemiological study of hereditary prostate cancer (HPC) in Finland: frequent HPCX linkage in families with late-onset disease. *Clin Cancer Res* 6:4810-4815, 2000.

Schoenberg MP, Hakimi JM, Wang S, et al. Microsatellite mutation (CAG24→18) in the androgen receptor gene in human prostate cancer. *Biochem Biophys Res Commun* 198:74-80, 1994.

Scrivner DL, Meyer JS, Rujanavech N, et al. Cell kinetics by bromodeoxyuridine labeling and deoxyribonucleic acid ploidy in prostatic carcinoma needle biopsies. *J Urol* 146:1034-1039, 1991.

Sebo TJ, Cheville JC, Riehle DL, et al. Predicting prostate carcinoma volume and stage at radical prostatectomy by assessing needle biopsy specimens for percent surface area and cores positive for carcinoma, perineural invasion, Gleason score, DNA ploidy and proliferation, and preoperative serum prostate antigen. *Cancer* 91:2196-2204, 2001.

Sebo TJ, Cheville JC, Riehle DL, et al. Perineural invasion and MIB-1 positivity in addition to Gleason score are significant preoperative predictors of progression after radical retropubic prostatectomy for prostate cancer. *Am J Surg Pathol* 26:431-439, 2002.

Sesterhenn IA, Mostofi FK, Baker RL, et al. Image analysis of nucleoli and nucleolar organizer regions in prostatic hyperplasia, intraepithelial neoplasia, and prostatic carcinoma. *J Urogen Pathol* 1:66-74, 1991.

Shiraishi T, Watanabe M, Muneyuki T, et al. A clinicopathological study of p53, p21 (WAF/CIP1) and cyclin D1 expression in human prostate cancers. *Urol Int* 61:90-94, 1998A.

Shiraishi T, Muneyuki T, Fukutome K, et al. Mutations of ras genes are relatively frequent in Japanese prostate cancers: pointing to genetic differences between populations. *Anticancer Res* 18:2789-2792, 1998B.

Shurbaji MS, Kalbfleisch JH, Thurmond TS. Immunohistochemical detection of p53 protein as a prognostic indicator in prostate cancer. *Hum Pathol* 26:106-109, 1995.

Signoretti S, Montironi R, Manola J, et al. Her-2-neu expression and progression toward androgen independence in human prostate cancer. *J Natl Cancer Inst* 92:1918-1925, 2000.

Signoretti S, Loda M. Estrogen receptor B in prostate cancer. Brake pedal or accelerator? *Am J Pathol* 159:13-16, 2001.

Sinclair CS, Berry R, Schaid D, et al. BRCA1 and BRCA2 have a limited role in familial prostate cancer. *Cancer Res* 60:1371-1375, 2000.

Singh D, Febbo PG, Ross K, et al. Gene expression correlates of clinical prostate cancer behavior. *Cancer Cell* 1:203-209, 2002.

Singh R. No evidence of linkage to chromosome 1q42.2-43 in 131 prostate cancer families from the ACTANE consortium. Anglo, Canada, Texas, Australia, Norway, EU Biomed. *Br J Cancer* 83:1654-1658, 2000.

Sinik Z, Alkibay T, Ataoglu O, et al. Nuclear p53 overexpression in bladder, prostate, and renal carcinomas. *Int J Urol* 4:546-551, 1997.

Skacel M, Ormsby AH, et al. Aneusomy of chromosomes 7,8, and 17, and amplification of HER-2/neu and epidermal growth factor receptor in Gleason score of prostate carcinoma. A differential fluorescent in situ hybridization study of Gleason pattern 3 and 4 using tissue microarray. *Hum Pathol* 32:1392-1397, 2001.

Smith JR, Freije D, Carpten JD, et al. Maor susceptibility locus for prostate cancer on chromosome 1 suggested by a genome-wide search. *Science* 274:1371-1374, 1996.

Smith RA, von Eschenbach AC, Wender R, et al. American Cancer Society guidelines for the early detection of cancer: update for early detection guidelines of prostate, colorectal, and endometrial cancers. *CA Cancer J Clin* 51:38-75, 2001.

Speights VO Jr, Arber DA, Riggs MW, et al. Proliferative index of organ-confined prostatic adenocarcinoma determined by MIB-1. *J Urol Pathol* 4:25-30, 1996.

Srikantan V, Sesterhenn IA, Davis L, et al. Allelic loss on chromosome 6q in primary prostate cancer. *Int J Cancer* 84:331-335, 1999.

Srivastava M, Bubendorf L, Srikantan V, et al. ANX7, a candidate tumor suppressor gene for prostate cancer. *Proc Natl Acad Sci* 98:4575-4580, 2001.

Stackhouse GB, Sesterhenn IA, Bauer JJ, et al. p53 and bcl-2 immunohistochemistry in pretreatment prostate needle biopsies to predict recurrence of prostate cancer after radical prostatectomy. *J Urol* 162:2042-2045, 1999.

Stamey TA. DNA ploidy status. *Urology* 45:563-565, 1995.

Stamey TA, Warrington JA, Caldwell MC, et al. Molecular genetic profiling of Gleason grade 4/5 prostate cancers compared to benign prostatic hyperplasia. *J Urol* 166:2171-2177, 2001.

Stanford JL, Just JJ, Gibbs M, et al. Polymorphic repeats in the androgen receptor gene: molecular markers of prostate cancer risk. *Cancer Res* 57:1194-1198, 1997.

Stapleton AM, Timme TL, Gousse AE, et al. Primary human prostate cancer cells harboring p53 mutations are clonally expanded in metastases. *Clin Cancer Res* 3:1389-1397, 1997.

Stapleton AM, Zbell P, Kattan MW, et al. Assessment of the biologic markers p53, Ki-67, and apoptotic index as predictive indicators of prostate carcinoma recurrence after surgery. *Cancer* 82:168-175, 1998.

Stattin P, Damber JE, Karlberg L, et al. Bcl-2 immunoreactivity in prostate tumorigenesis in relation to prostatic intraepithelial neoplasia, grade, hormonal status, metastatic growth and survival. *Urol Res* 24:257-264, 1996A.

Stattin P, Bergh A, Karlberg L, et al. p53 immunoreactivity as prognostic marker for cancer-specific survival in prostate cancer. *Eur Urol* 30:65-72, 1996B.

Stattin P, Damber J-E, Karlberg L, et al. Cell proliferation assessed by Ki-67 immunoreactivity on formalin fixed tissues is a predictive factor for survival in prostate cancer. *J Urol* 157:219-222, 1997.

Steck PA, Pershouse MA, Jasser SA, et al. Identification of a candidate tumor suppressor gene, MMAC1, at chromosome 10q23.2 that is mutated in multiple advanced cancers. *Nat Genet* 15:356-362, 1997.

Steilen H, Ketter R, Romanakis K, et al. DNA aneuploidy in prostatic adenocarcinoma: a frequent event as shown by fluorescence in situ DNA hybridization. *Hum Pathol* 25:1306-1313, 1994.

Steiner MS, Gingrich JR. Gene therapy for prostate cancer: where are we now? *J Urol* 164:1121-1236, 2000.

Stephenson RA, James BC, Gay H, et al. Flow cytometry of prostate cancer: relationship of DNA content to survival. *Cancer Res* 47:2504-2509, 1987.

Stricker HJ, Jay JK, Linden MD, et al. Determining prognosis of clinically localized prostate cancer by immunohistochemical detection of mutant p53. *Urology* 47:366-369, 1996.

Suarez BK, Lin J, Burmester JK, et al. A genome screen of multiplex sibships with prostate cancer. *Am J Hum Genet* 66:933-944, 2000A.

Suarez BK, Lin J, Witte JS, et al. Replication linkage study for prostate cancer susceptibility genes. *Prostate* 45:106-114, 2000B.

Sumiya H, Masai M, Akimoto S, et al. Histochemical examination of expression of ras p21 protein and R1881-binding protein in human prostatic cancers. *Eur J Cancer* 26:786-789, 1990.

Suzuki H, Emi M, Komiya A, et al. Localization of a tumor suppressor gene associated with progression of a human prostate cancer within a 1.2 mb region of 8p22-p21.3. *Genes Chromosomes Cancer* 13:168-174, 1995.

Suzuki H, Komiya A, Aida S, et al. Detection of human papillomavirus DNA and p53 gene mutations in human prostate cancer. *Prostate* 28:318-324, 1996.

Suzuki H, Freije D, Nusskern DR, et al. Interfocal heterogeneity of *PTEN/MMAC1* gene alterations in multiple metastatic prostate cancer tissues. *Cancer Res* 58:204-209, 1998.

Sweat SD, Pacelli A, Bergstralh EJ, et al. Androgen receptor expression in prostate cancer lymph node metastases is predictive of outcome after surgery. *J Urol* 161:1233-1237, 1999A.

Sweat SD, Pacelli A, Bergstralh EJ, et al. Androgen receptor expression in prostatic intraepithelial neoplasia and cancer. *J Urol* 161:1229-1232, 1999B.

Szostak MJ, Kaur P, Amin P, et al. Apoptosis and bcl-2 expression in prostate cancer: significance in clinical outcome after brachytherapy. *J Urol* 165:2126-2130, 2001.

Takahashi S, Qian J, Brown JA, et al. Potential markers of prostate cancer aggressiveness detected by fluorescence in situ hybridization in needle biopsies. *Cancer Res* 54:3574-3579, 1994.

Takahashi S, Shan AL, Ritland SR, et al. Frequent loss of heterozygosity at 7q31.1 in primary prostate cancer is associated with tumor aggressiveness and progression. *Cancer Res* 55:4114-4119, 1995.

Takai K, Goellner JR, Katzmann JA, et al. Static image and flow DNA cytometry of prostatic adenocarcinoma. Studies of needle biopsy and radical prostatectomy specimens. *J Urol Pathol* 2:39-47, 1994.

Tamboli P, Amin MB, Schultz DS, et al. Comparative analysis of the nuclear proliferative index (Ki-67) in benign prostate, prostatic intraepithelial neoplasia and prostatic carcinoma. *Mod Pathol* 9:1015-1019, 1996.

Tang DG, Li L, Chopra DP, Porter AT. Extended survivability of prostate cancer cells in the absence of trophic factors: increased proliferation, evasion of apoptosis, and the role of apoptosis proteins. *Cancer Res* 58:3466-3479, 1998.

Taplin ME, Bubley GJ, Ko YJ, et al. Selection for androgen receptor gene mutations in prostate cancers treated with androgen antagonist. *Cancer Res* 59:2511-2515, 1999.

Taplin M-E, Halabi S, Rajeshkumar B, et al. Androgen receptor mutations in androgen independent prostate cancer (APICA) do not correlate with anti-androgen withdrawal response: Cancer and Leukemia Group B (CALGB) 9663 [abstract]. *Proceed Am Soc Clin Onc* 20:1738, 2001.

Tavtigian SV, Simard J, Teng DH, et al. A candidate prostate cancer susceptibility gene at chromosome 17p. *Nat Genet* 27:172-180, 2001.

Taylor JA, Hirronen A, Watson M, et al. Association of prostate cancer with vitamin D receptor gene polymorphism. *Cancer Res* 56:4108-4110, 1996.

Teng DH, Hu R Lin M, et al. *MMAC1/PTEN* mutations in primary tumor specimens and tumor cell lines. *Cancer Res* 57:5221-5225, 1997.

Terrell RB, Wille AH, Cheville JC, et al. Microsatellite instability in adenocarcinoma of the prostate. *Am J Pathol* 147:799-805, 1995.

Theodorescu D, Broder SR, Boyd JC, et al. p53, bcl-2 and retinoblastoma proteins as long-term prognostic marker in localized carcinoma of the prostate. *J Urol* 158:131-137, 1997.

Thomas DJ, Robinson M, King P, et al. p53 expression and clinical outcome in prostate cancer. *Br J Urol* 72:778-781, 1993.

Thomas GV, Shrage MI, Rosenfelt L, et al. Preoperative prostate needle biopsy p27 correlates with subsequent radical prostatectomy p27, Gleason grade and pathological stage. *J Urol* 164:1987-1991, 2000.

Thompson SJ, Mellon K, Charlton RG, et al. P53 and Ki-67 immunoreactivity in human prostate cancer and benign hyperplasia. *Br J Urol* 69:609-613, 1992.

Tinari N, Natoli C, Angelucci D, et al. DNA and S-phase fraction analysis by flow cytometry in prostate cancer. Clinicopathologic implications. *Cancer* 71:1289-1296, 1993.

Tonin P, Ghadirian P, Phelan C, et al. A large multisite cancer family is linked to BRCA2. *J Med Genet* 32:982-984, 1995.

Trapman J, Sleddens HFBM, van der Weiden MM, et al. Loss of heterozygosity of chromosome 8 microsatellite loci implicates a candidate tumor suppressor gene between the loci D8S87 and D8S33 in human prostate cancer. *Cancer Res* 54:6061-6064, 1994.

Trapman J, Brinkmann AO. The androgen receptor in prostate cancer. *Pathol Res Pract* 192:752-760, 1996.

Tricoli JV, Gumerlock PH, Yao JL, et al. Alterations of the retinoblastoma gene in human prostate adenocarcinoma. *Genes Chromosomes Cancer* 15:110-114, 1996.

Tsihlias J, Kapusta LR, DeBoer G, et al. Loss of cyclin-dependent kinase inhibitor p27 (KIP1) is a novel prognostic factor in localized human prostate adenocarcinoma. *Cancer Res* 58:542-548, 1998.

Tu H, Jacobs SC, Borkowski A, et al. Incidence of apoptosis and cell proliferation in prostate cancer: relationship with TGF-β1 and bcl-2 expression. *Int J Cancer* 69:357-363, 1996.

Turkeri LN, Sakr WA, Wykes SM, et al. Comparative analysis of epidermal growth factor receptor gene expression and protein product in benign, premalignant, and malignant prostate tissue. *Prostate* 25:199-205, 1994.

Uchida T, Wada C, Wang C, et al. Microsatellite instability in prostate cancer. *Oncogene* 10:1019-1022, 1995.

Ueda T, Ichikawa T, Tamaru J-I, et al. Expression of the KAI1 protein in benign prostatic hyperplasia and prostate cancer. *Am J Pathol* 149:1435-1440, 1996.

Uzoaru I, Rubenstein M, Mirochnik Y, et al. An evaluation of the markers p53 and Ki-67 for their predictive value in prostate cancer. *J Surg Oncol* 67:33-37, 1998.

Valeri A, Azzouzi R, Drelon E, et al. Early-onset hereditary prostate cancer is not associated with specific clinical and biological features. *Prostate* 45:66-71, 2000.

Van den Berg C, Guan X-Y, von Hoff D, et al. DNA sequence amplification in human prostate cancer identified by chromosome microdissection: potential prognostic implications. *Clin Cancer Res* 1:11-18, 1995.

van den Ouden D, Tribukait B, Blom JHM, et al. Deoxyribonucleic acid ploidy of core biopsies and metastatic lymph nodes of prostate cancer patients: impact on time to progression. *J Urol* 150:400-406, 1993.

Van der Kwast TH, Ruizeveld de Winter JA, Trapman J. Androgen receptor expression in human prostate cancer. *J Urol Pathol* 3:327-346, 1995.

Varambally S, Dhanasekaran SM, Zhou M, et al. The polycomb group protein EZH2 is involved in progression of prostate cancer. *Nature* 419:624-629, 2002.

Vazina A, Baniel J, Yaacobi Y, et al. The rate of founder Jewish mutations in BRCA1 and BRCA2 in prostate cancer patients in Israel. *Br J Cancer* 83:463-466, 2000.

Verhagen PCMS, Zhu XL, Rohr LR, et al. Microdissection, DOP-PCR, and comparative genomic hybridization of paraffin-embedded familial prostate cancers. *Cancer Genet Cytogenet* 122:43-48, 2000.

Verma RS, Manikal M, Conte RA, et al. Chromosomal basis of adenocarcinoma of the prostate. *Cancer Invest* 17:441-447, 1999.

Vesalainen S, Lipponen P, Talja M, et al. Mitotic activity and prognosis in prostatic adenocarcinoma. *Prostate* 26:80-86, 1995.

Vesalainen S, Nordling S, Lipponen P, et al. Progression and survival in prostatic adenocarcinoma: a comparison of clinical stage, Gleason grade, S-phase fraction and DNA ploidy. *Br J Cancer* 70:309-314, 1994A.

Vesalainen SLB, Lipponen PK, Talja MT, et al. Proliferating cell nuclear antigen and p53 expression as prognostic factors in T1-2MO prostatic adenocarcinoma. *Int J Cancer* 58:303-308, 1994B.

Viola MV, Fromowitz F, Oravez S, et al. Expression of ras oncogene p21 in prostate cancer. *N Engl J Med* 314:133-137, 1986.

Vis AN, Noorzij MA, Fitoz K, et al. Prognostic value of cell cycle proteins p27Kip1 and MIB-1, and the cell adhesion protein CD44s in surgically treated patients with prostate cancer. *J Urol* 164:2156-2161, 2000.

Visakorpi T, Kallioniemi O-P, Paronen IYI, et al. Flow cytometric analysis of DNA ploidy and S-phase fraction from prostatic carcinomas: implications for prognosis and response to endocrine therapy. *Br J Cancer* 64:578-582, 1991.

Visakorpi T, Kallioniemi O-P, Koivula T, et al. Expression of epidermal growth factor receptor and ERBB2 (HER-2/neu) oncoprotein in prostatic carcinomas. *Mod Pathol* 5:643-647, 1992A.

Visakorpi T. Proliferative activity determined by DNA flow cytometry and proliferating cell nuclear antigen (PCNA) immunohistochemistry as a prognostic factor in prostatic carcinoma. *J Pathol* 168:7-13, 1992B.

Visakorpi T, Kallioniemi AH, Syvänan A-C, et al. Genetic changes in primary and recurrent prostate cancer by comparative genomic hybridization. *Cancer Res* 55:342-347, 1995A.

Visakorpi T, Hyytinen E, Koivisto P, et al. In vivo amplification of the androgen receptor gene and progression of human prostate cancer. *Nat Genet* 9:401-406, 1995B.

Visakorpi T. Molecular genetics of prostate cancer. *Ann Chir Gynaecol* 88:11-66, 1999.

Vlietstra RJ, van Alewijk DC, Hermans KGL, et al. Frequent inactivation of *PTEN* in prostate cancer cell lines and xenografts. *Cancer Res* 58:2720-2723, 1998.

Voeller JH, Sugars LY, Petlow T, et al. p53 oncogene mutations in human prostate cancer specimens. *J Urol* 151:492-495, 1994.

Voges GE, Eigner EB, Ross W, et al. Pathologic parameters and flow cytometric ploidy analysis in predicting recurrence in carcinoma of the prostate. *Eur Urol* 24:132-139, 1993.

Walsh PC, Partin AW. Family history facilitates the early diagnosis of prostate carcinoma. *Cancer* 80:1871-1874, 1997.

Wang SI, Parsons R, Ittmann M. Homozygous deletion of the PTEN tumor suppressor gene in a subset of prostate adenocarcinomas. *Clin Cancer Res* 4:811-815, 1998.

Ware J, Maygarden S, Koontz W, et al. Immunohistochemical detection of c-erbB-2 protein in human benign and neoplastic prostate. *Hum Pathol* 22:254-258, 1991.

Warzynski MJ, Soechtig CE, Maatman TJ, et al. DNA heterogeneity determined by flow cytometry in prostatic adenocarcinoma—necessitating multiple site analysis. *Prostate* 27:329-335, 1995.

Washburn JG, Wojno KJ, Dey J, et al. 8pter-823 deletion is associated with racial differences in prostate cancer outcome. *Clin Cancer Res* 6:4647-4652, 2000.

Watanabe M, Shiraishi T, Yatani R, et al. International comparison on ras gene mutations in latent prostate carcinoma. *Int J Cancer* 58:174-178, 1994.

Watanabe M, Imai H, Kato H, et al. Microsatellite instability in latent prostate cancers. *Int J Cancer* 69:394-397, 1996.

Weinberg RA. The retinoblastoma protein and cell cycle control. *Cell* 81:323-330, 1995.

Welsh JB, Sapinoso LM, Su AI, et al. Analysis of gene expression identifies candidate markers and pharmacological targets in prostate cancer. *Cancer Res* 61:5974-5978, 2001.

Wertz IE, Deitch AD, Gumerlock PH, et al. Correlation of genetic and immunodetection of TP53 mutations in malignant and benign prostate tissues. *Hum Pathol* 27:573-580, 1996.

Whang YE, Wu XY, Suzuki H, et al. Inactivation of the tumor suppressor PTEN/MMAC1 in advanced human prostate cancer through loss of expression. *Proc Natl Acad Sci* 95:5246-5250, 1998.

Whittmore AS, Lin IG, Oakley-Girvan I, et al. No evidence of linkage for chromosome 1q42.2-43 in prostate cancer [letter to the editor]. *Am J Hum Genet* 65:254-256, 1999.

Wikstrom P, Wikstrom P, Lissbrant IF, et al. Evaluation of prognostic factors in prostate cancer with partial least squares analysis. *Scand J Urol Nephrol* 34:252-262, 2000.

Williams BJ, Jones E, Zhu XL, et al. Evidence for a tumor suppressor gene distal to BRCA1 in prostate cancer. *J Urol* 155:720-725, 1996.

Winkler HZ, Rainwater LM, Myers RP, et al. Stage D1 prostatic adenocarcinoma: significance of nuclear DNA ploidy patterns studied by flow cytometry. *Mayo Clin Proc* 63:103-112, 1988.

Wirth MP, Muller HA, Manseck A, et al. Value of nuclear DNA ploidy patterns in patients with prostate cancer after radical prostatectomy. *Eur Urol* 20:248-252, 1991.

Witte JS, Goddard KAB, Conti DV, et al. Genome wide scan for prostate cancer-aggressiveness loci. *Am J Hum Genet* 67:92-99, 2000.

Wojcik EM, Bassler TJ Jr, Orozco R. DNA ploidy in seminal vesicle cells. A potential diagnostic pitfall in urine cytology. *Anal Quant Cytol Histol* 21:29-34, 1999.

Woolf CM. An investigation of the familial aspects of carcinoma of the prostate. *Cancer* 13:361-364, 1960.

Wu CL, Chakravarti A, Delaney M, et al. Loss of p16 protein expression correlates with Gleason scores and distant metastasis of prostate cancer [abstract]. *Mod Pathol* 14:128A, 2001.

Xu J, Myers D, Freije D, et al. Evidence for a prostate cancer susceptibility locus on the X chromosome. *Nat Genet* 20:175-179, 1998.

Xu J, International Consortium for Prostate Cancer Genetics. Combined analysis of hereditary prostate cancer linkage to 1q24-25: results from 772 hereditary prostate cancer families from the International Consortium for Prostate Cancer Genetics. *Am J Hum Genet* 66:945-957, 2000.

Xu J, Zheng SL, Komiya A, et al. Germline mutations and sequence variants of the macrophage scavenger receptor 1 gene are associated with prostate cancer risk. *Nature Genet* 32:321-325, 2002.

Xue W, Irvine RA, Yu MC, et al. Susceptibility to prostate cancer: interaction between genotypes at the androgen receptor and prostate-specific antigen loci. *Cancer Res* 60:839-841, 2000.

Yang G, Stapleton AM, Wheeler TM, et al. Clustered p53 immunostaining: a novel pattern associated with prostate cancer progression. *Clin Cancer Res* 2:399-401, 1996.

Yang RM, Naitoh J, Murphy M, et al. Low p27 expression predicts poor disease-free survival in patients with prostate cancer. *J Urol* 159:941-945, 1998.

Yeh S, Hu YC, Rahman M, et al. Increase of androgen-induced cell death and androgen receptor transactivation by BRCA1 in prostate cancer cells. *Proc Natl Acad Sci* 97:11256-11261, 2000.

Yokogi H, Mizutani M, Ishibe T. Flow cytometric DNA analysis of stage D2 prostatic carcinoma. *Urol Int* 47:57-59, 1991.

Zenklusen JC, Thomspon JC, Troncoso P, et al. Loss of heterozygosity in human primary prostate carcinomas: a possible tumor suppressor gene at 7q31.1. *Cancer Res* 54:6370-6373, 1994.

Zenklusen JC, Conti CJ, Green ED. Mutational and functional analyses reveal ST7 is a highly conserved tumor-suppressor gene on human chromosome 7q31. *Nat Genet* 27:392-398, 2001.

Zhao XY, Malloy PJ, Krishnan AV, et al. Glucocorticoids can promote androgen-independent growth of prostate cancer cells through a mutated androgen receptor. *Nat Med* 6:703-706, 2000.

Zhau HE, Wan DS, Zhou J, et al. Expression of c-*erb*B-2 (HER-2/neu) oncoprotein in human prostate cancer tissues and cell lines. *Mol Carcinog* 5:320-327, 1992.

Zheng SL, Xu J, Isaacs SD, et al. Evidence for prostate cancer linkage to chromosome 20 in 159 hereditary prostate cancer families. *Hum Genet* 108:430-435, 2001.

Zincke H, Bergstralh EJ, Larson-Keller JJ, et al. Stage D1 prostate cancer treated by radical prostatectomy and adjuvant hormonal treatment. Evidence for favorable survival in patients with DNA diploid tumors. *Cancer* 70(suppl):311-323, 1992.

Zitzelsberger H, Engert D, Walch A, et al. Chromosomal changes during development and progression of prostate adenocarcinomas. *Br J Cancer* 84:202-208, 2001.

CHAPTER 22

Seminal Vesicles

[22.1] Embryology and Development 507
[22.2] Normal Anatomy 507
[22.3] Cysts 511
[22.4] Inflammation and Infection 512
[22.5] Calcification and Calculi 512
[22.6] Amyloid Deposits 512
[22.7] Hyperplasia 513
[22.8] Primary Benign Neoplasms 513
[22.9] Primary Neoplasms of Indeterminate (or Low) Malignant Potential 515
[22.10] Primary Malignant Neoplasms 515
[22.11] Secondary Neoplasms 516

The seminal vesicles are paired, coiled, and tubular male sex accessory glands that lie posterolateral to the base of the bladder and anterior to Denonvilliers' fascia and the rectum (Aboul-Azm 1979, Aumuller 1992, Partin 2002, Sandlow 2002, Trainer 1997, Williams 1998) **f1.1, p 4; i22.1**. The duct emanating from each seminal vesicle joins the ampulla of the vasa differentia to form the paired ejaculatory ducts, which course through the base of the prostate to the urethra **i1.1, p 4**).

The seminal vesicles were first described in 1521 by the Italian anatomist Berengario a Carpi (Aboul-Azm 1979). Initially, they were regarded as storage organs for semen. It is now known that the physiological function of the seminal vesicle is to secrete fluid that is important for sperm function (Aumuller 1992, Sandlow 2002). These secretions, which constitute the majority of the ejaculate volume, contain ions, fructose, prostaglandins, and proteins such as semenogelin, the scaffold protein for the semen coagulate and substrate for PSA. The seminal vesicle secretions seem to function specifically in nutrition and modification of sperm motility, in formation of the seminal coagulum, and possibly in immunosuppression and antibacterial actions (Aumuller 1992, Partin 2002, Sandlow 2002).

The seminal vesicles, in stark contrast to the prostate, are rarely the primary site of disease. Rather, they are most commonly involved by secondary processes, such as the spread of prostatic carcinoma into the seminal vesicles. The reason for this differential susceptibility to primary disease development is not known, but it could relate to their different embryologic origins: the seminal vesicles (and vas deferens and ejaculatory ducts) arise from the mesonephric duct (Wolffian duct), whereas the prostate is formed from the urogenital sinus.

Seminal vesicle tissue samples are usually examined as part of a radical prostatectomy specimen excised for prostate cancer. Currently, most surgeries on seminal vesicles are done as part of a radical cancer operation for pelvic neoplasms such as bladder, prostate, or urethral malignancy (Sandlow 2002). In this era, isolated seminal vesiculectomy is rarely performed. This procedure was performed in the past, mainly for tuberculosis or vesiculitis (Sandlow 2002). Directed seminal vesicle needle core biopsies have been done to attempt to stage prostatic carcinoma, but this is a low-yield procedure with a high false-negative rate (see Chapter 16). Needle core biopsy directed at a solid seminal vesicle mass is a specimen rarely received in pathology laboratories. Transurethral unroofing of seminal vesicle cysts or abscesses, and laparoscopic dissection or open dissection for chronic seminal vesiculitis or small benign tumors account for other, uncommon seminal vesicle tissue samples (Sandlow 2002). Additionally, aspirates of seminal vesicle cysts or abscesses may be encountered. Finally, inadvertently sampled seminal vesicle tissue can be seen as an incidental finding in 3% of TURP chip cases (Young 1988) and 5% of prostate needle biopsy cases (Coyne 1987, Shah 2001).

[22.1] Embryology and Development

The seminal vesicles initially appear, under androgenic stimulation, during the 12th-13th fetal week as outpouchings or bulbous swellings of the lower portion of the Wolffian ducts near the urogenital sinus (Brewster 1985, Watson 1918). Subsequently, the tubular vesicle elongates and develops numerous diverticulae, so that by birth the mucosa exhibits significant undulations. Mucosal folding and complexity increase with age, apparently until age 45 (Brewster 1985). Also at birth, secretory and basal cells can be discerned in the seminal vesicle epithelium.

[22.2] Normal Anatomy

The adult seminal vesicle measures 3.5cm-7.5cm in length and 1.2cm-2.4cm in thickness (Trainer 1997). The average weight is 7.5g (range 5.8g-8.8g) (Aumuller 1992). Basically, the seminal vesicle is an elongated, convoluted tubuloalveolar gland with branching, central ducts and a thick muscular wall **i22.2-i22.5**. The major anatomical compartments are the lumen, the mucosa, the smooth muscle wall, and surrounding soft (fibroadipose) tissue.

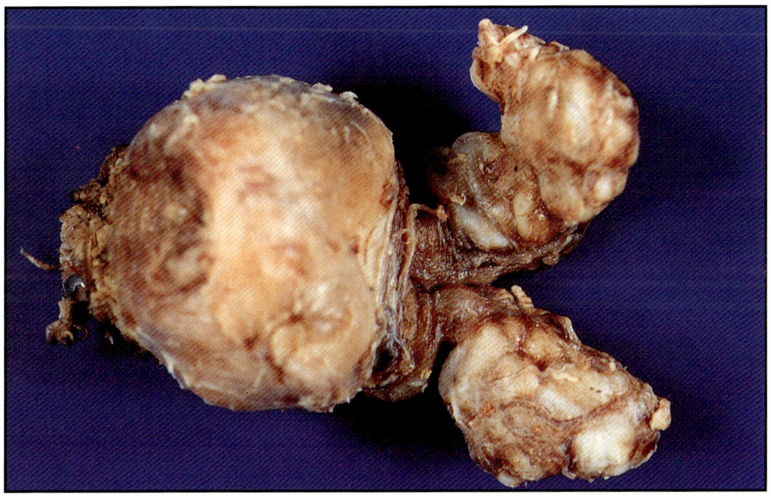

■ **i22.1** *Paired adult seminal vesicles attached to a 29g prostate in a radical prostatectomy/seminal vesiculectomy specimen. No prostatic carcinoma was detected in these grossly normal seminal vesicles.*

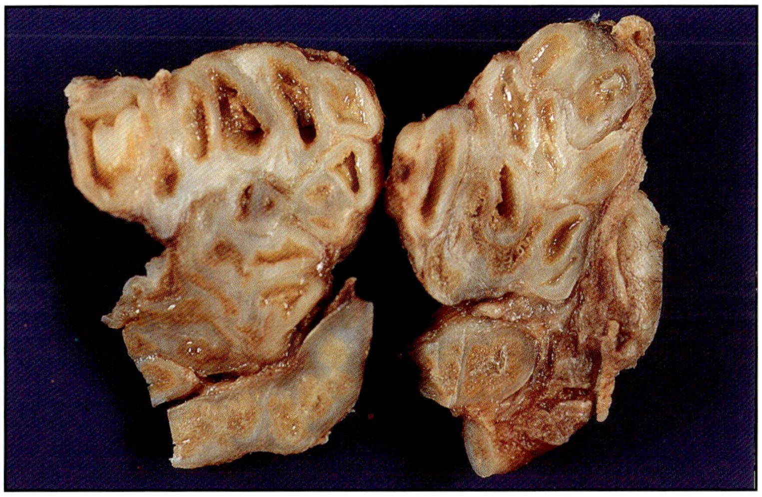

■ **i22.2** *Cut surfaces of normal adult seminal vesicles, with convolutions generating the appearance of multiple luminal spaces.*

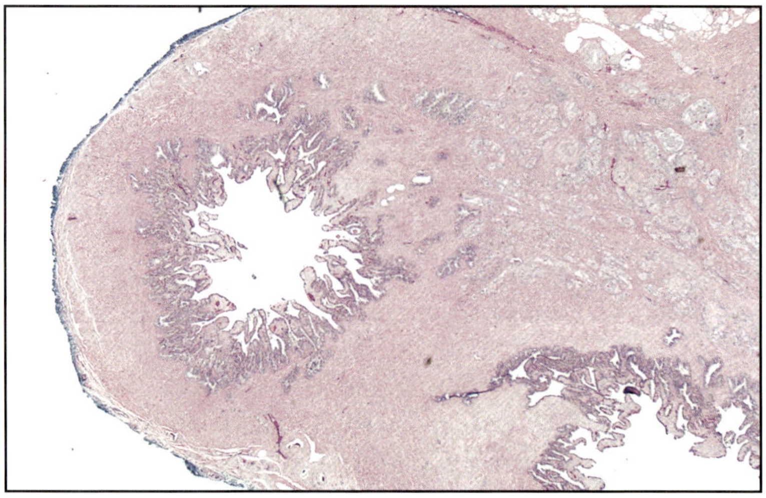

■ **i22.3** *Normal seminal vesicle: large central lumen with branching glands and muscular wall. (Mostly normal; prostatic carcinoma infiltrate can be seen on right.)*

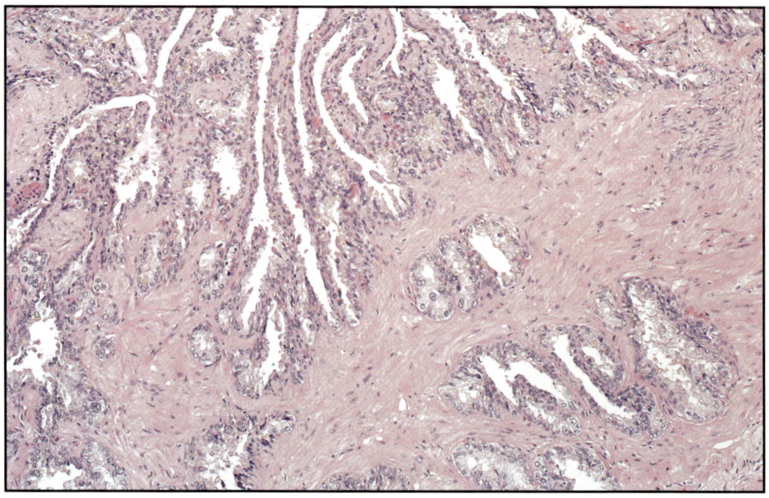

■ **i22.4** *Normal seminal vesicle: branching configuration of normal seminal vesicle glands.*

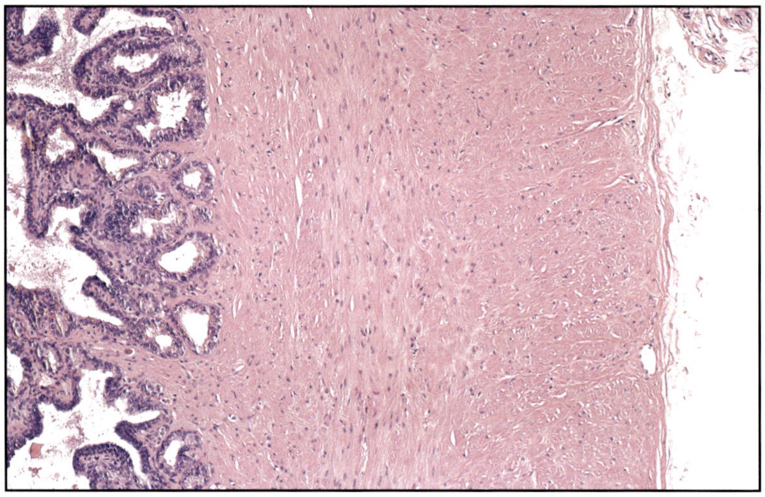

■ **i22.5** *Normal seminal vesicle glands abut a thick seminal vesicle muscular wall.*

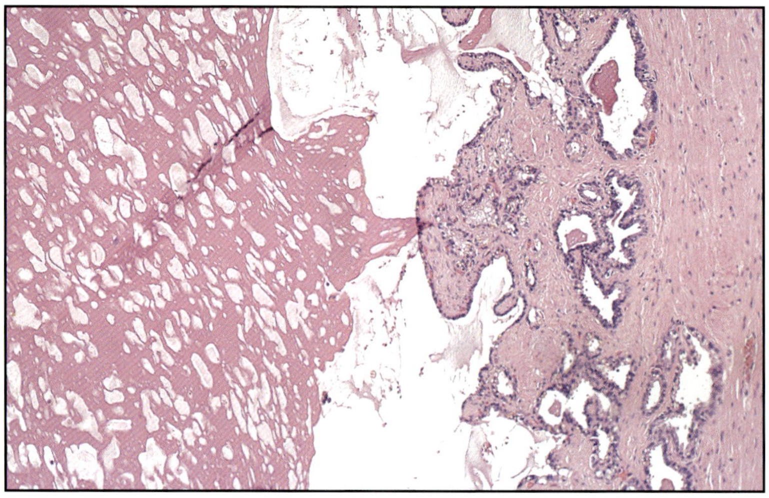

■ **i22.6** *Normal seminal vesicle: dense intraluminal secretion*

The seminal vesicle luminal capacity is about 4 cm^3 (Aumuller 1992). The lumen may contain proteinaceous fluid, sloughed epithelial cells and cellular debris, refluxed spermatozoa, and crystalloids (Amin 1996, Brewster 1985, Trainer 1997). Histologically, secretions are seen in the large majority (82%) of seminal vesicle glands (Shah 2001). The histomorphological appearance is mainly dense, eosinophilic, and platelike **i22.6**, with a minority of cases showing fluid-like eosinophilic secretions and intraluminal crystalloids (Shah 2001) **i22.7**. These crystalloids should be distinguished from prostatic crystalloids that tend to be associated with neoplastic prostatic epithelial proliferations. In contrast to prostatic crystalloids, seminal vesicle crystalloids have curved or blunt angles, associated platelike secretions, and are positive by periodic acid-Schiff histochemical staining (Shah 2001). Therefore, the presence of intraglandular crystalloids is not only not specific for prostatic carcinoma, they are not specific for prostatic glands.

The mucosa of the adult seminal vesicle displays a main, central duct with 6-8 primary branches and several secondary branches (Trainer 1997). At the periphery of the outermost extensions are small acini that may be misdiagnosed as prostatic adenocarcinoma **i22.8**. The epithelial lining of the seminal vesicle harbors columnar secretory cells and basal cells. The secretory cells characteristically contain a large amount of intracytoplasmic, golden yellow to pale brown, lipofuscin pigment, which is more abundant, coarser, larger (at 1μm-2μm), and more refractile than similar prostatic pigment (Amin 1996, Shidham 1999) **i22.9**. This pigment can be

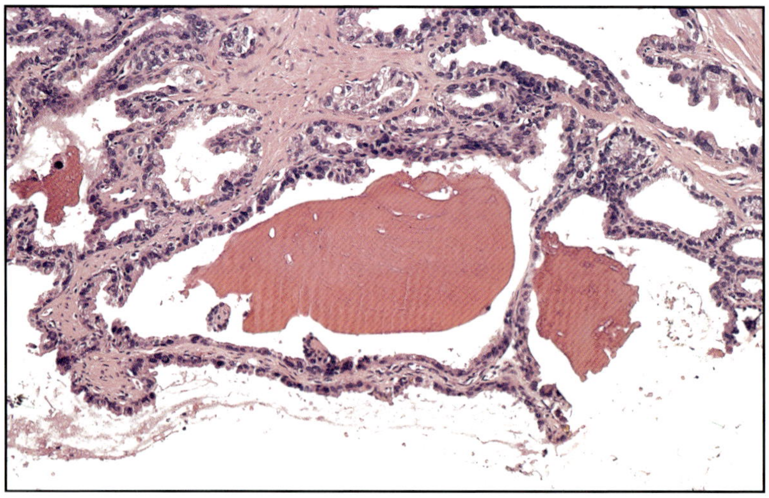

■ **i22.7** *Seminal vesicle eosinophilic luminal crystalloids.*

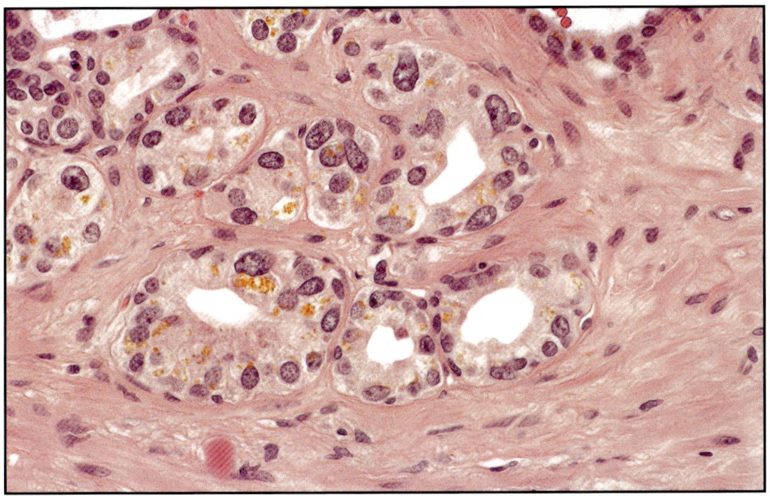

■ **i22.8** *Small normal seminal vesicle acini. Nuclear atypia may be present.*

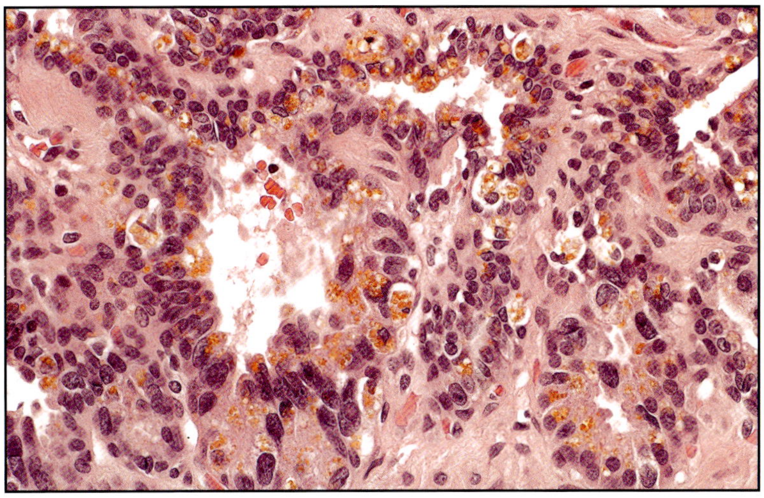

■ **i22.9** *Abundant intracytoplasmic pigment in normal seminal vesicle epithelium.*

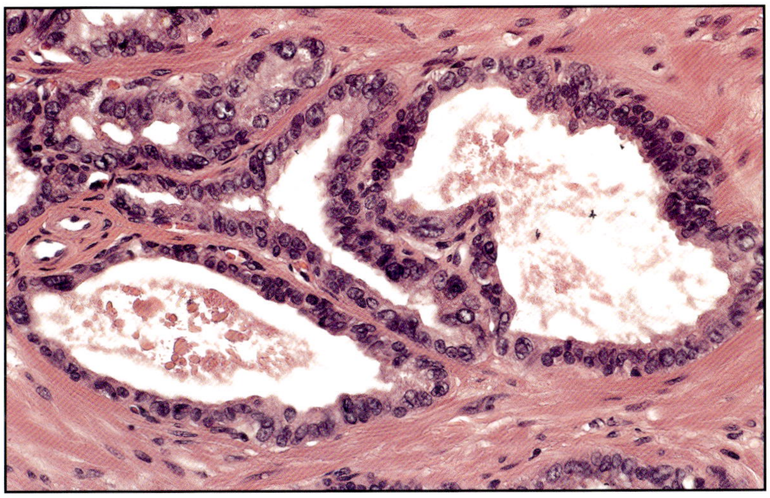

■ **i22.10** *Pigment-poor normal seminal vesicle epithelium.*

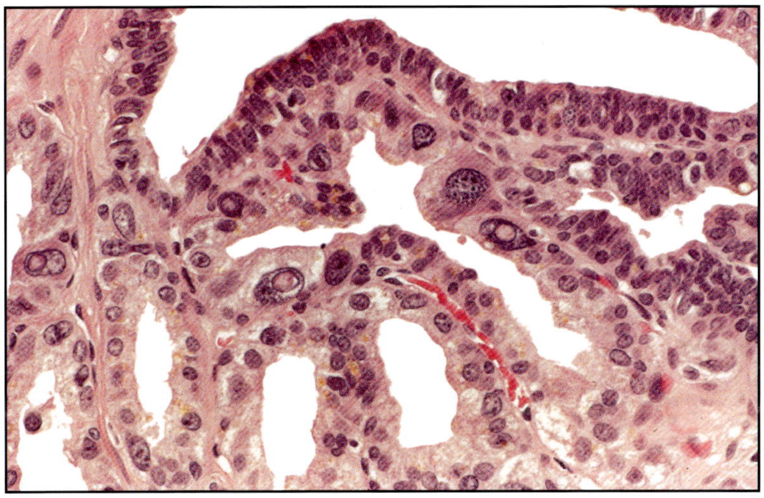

■ **i22.11** *Nuclear atypia in benign seminal vesicle epithelium. There are scattered cells with enlarged nuclei with intranuclear protrusions of cytoplasm ("inclusions").*

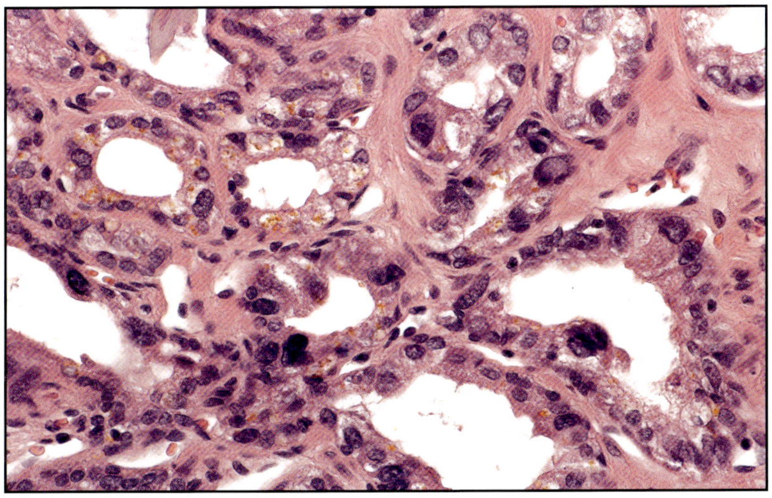

■ **i22.12** *Nuclear atypia in benign seminal vesicle epithelium: enlarged, hyperchromatic nuclei are evident.*

variable in distribution in seminal vesicle epithelium, such that it may not be present in a small sample of the epithelium **i22.10**. It is also not specific for seminal vesicle epithelium and may be seen in epithelium of the ejaculatory ducts and the ampulla of the vas deferens. Another distinctive feature of seminal vesicle secretory epithelium is the presence of scattered, peculiar, monstrous cells that exhibit nucleomegaly, nuclear hyperchromasia, and "grotesquely shaped nuclei" (Arias-Stella 1958, Kuo 1981) **i22.11, i22.12**. This pseudomalignant change is found in about 75%-100% of seminal vesicles (Kuo 1981, Shidham 1999) and appears to be age-related, being detectable in patients over 20 years of age (Arias-Stella 1958). Their mechanism of formation is not known, but the smudged chromatin suggests an age-related degenerative process; hormonal effects have also been suggested as possibly important (Arias-Stella 1958, Károlyi 1989). In addition to their alarming cytologic appearance, another potential diagnostic pitfall is that these cells are aneuploid in 7%-48% of cases (Arber 1981, Wojcik 1999). No data exist, however, to suggest that these bizarre seminal vesicle cells are dysplastic or malignant. Nuclei of the seminal vesicle epithelial cells are also characterized by intranuclear pseudoinclusions (that are actually cytoplasmic intranuclear protrusions) in 75% of cases (Shidham 1999) **i22.11**. Ultrastructurally, the columnar secretory cells have microvilli, numerous mitochondria, and a well-developed rough endoplasmic reticulum. The epithelial cells demonstrate pan-cytokeratin reactivity in the luminal cells (using antibodies AE1/AE3 and CAM 5.2), and have high molecular weight cytokeratin immunolabeling of the basal cells (De Marzo 1999).

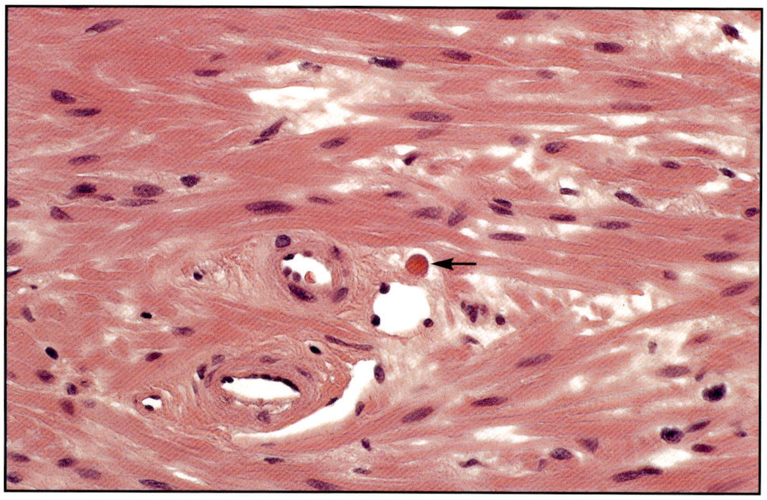

■ **i22.13** *Eosinophilic globule in seminal vesicle smooth muscle wall. This is a normal finding and is thought to represent degenerating smooth muscle cells.*

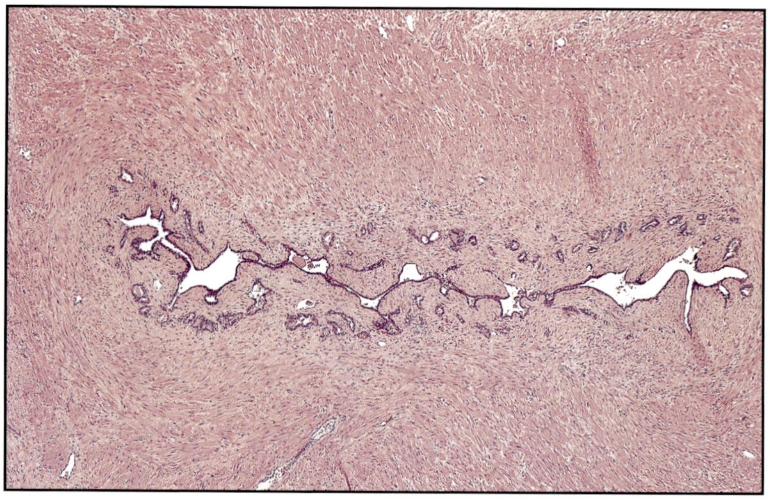

■ **i22.14** *Atrophy of seminal vesicle, with thinning of mucosa, and diminished glandular complexity.*

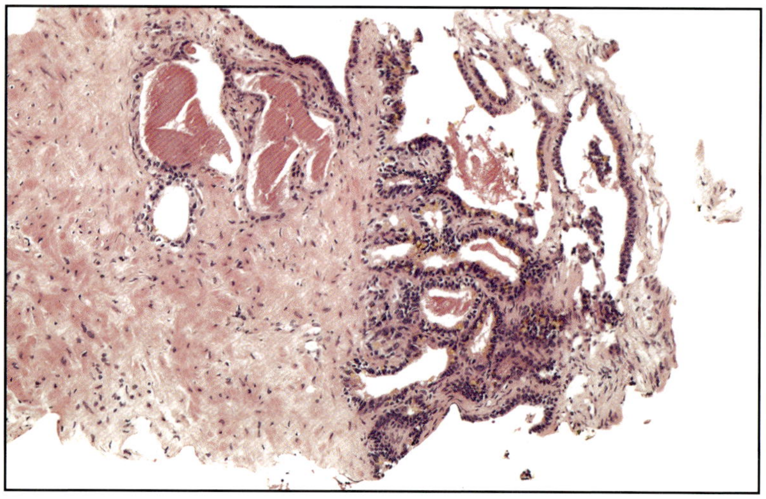

■ **i22.15** *Normal seminal vesicle or ejaculatory duct glands at tip of needle core biopsy tissue. This was inadvertent sampling: the needle biopsy was submitted as being from the prostate.*

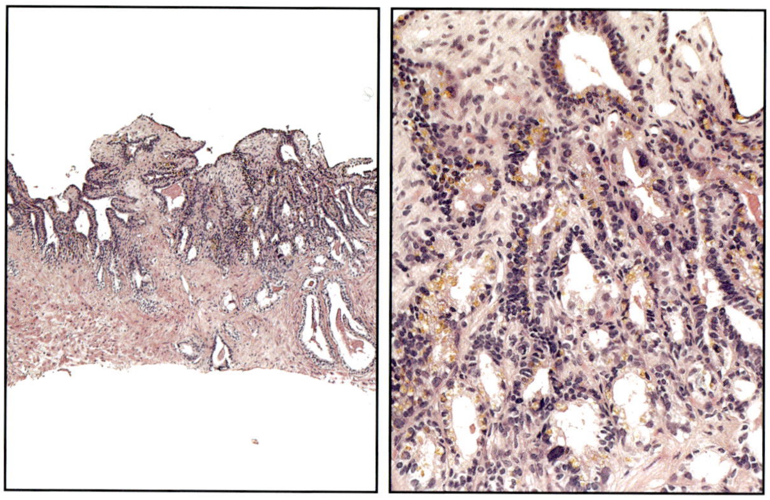

■ **i22.16** *Large amount of normal seminal vesicle in needle core biopsy tissue (low and higher magnification).*

The seminal vesicle luminal cells are negative for PSA and PSAP immunostains (De Marzo 1999, Grob 1992, Shidham 1999) as long as monoclonal antibodies are used, rather than polyclonal antibodies, which can show staining (De Marzo 1999, Varma 2002).

The smooth muscle wall of the seminal vesicle has a thin external longitudinal and thicker internal circular muscle layers (Trainer 1997) **i22.5**. Contraction of the smooth muscle fibers is mediated by adrenergic and modulatory nerve fibers (Aumuller 1992). Eosinophilic hyaline globules are often seen in the muscular wall (Kovi 1979, Kuo 1981) **i22.13** and are thought to represent degenerating smooth muscle cells (Trainer 1997). Fibroadipose tissue with nerves and blood vessels can be found at the base of the seminal vesicles. In radical prostatectomy specimens it is important to assess this soft tissue for prostatic carcinoma since extraprostatic extension at this site is a common pathway for spread into the seminal vesicles.

The blood supply to the seminal vesicle is from the vesiculodeferential artery, a branch of the umbilical artery, whereas venous drainage is via the vesiculodeferential veins and inferior vesical plexus (Sandlow 2002). The pelvic nerve and hypogastric nerve innervate the seminal vesicle, influencing secretions and muscular wall contraction (Aumuller 1992, Sandlow 2002). Lymphatic drainage is through the internal iliac lymph nodes (Sandlow 2002).

Aging of the adult seminal vesicle is associated with a decrease in seminal vesicle size (Jager 1997), atrophic flattening of the mucosa **i22.14** and individual epithelial cells, an increase in epithelial cell lipofuscin and number of monstrous nuclei, loss of muscle fibers, and hyalinization/sclerosis of the seminal vesicle wall (Aumuller 1992, Norris 1964).

Normal seminal vesicle glands may be misdiagnosed under the light microscope as prostatic intraepithelial neoplasia or prostatic adenocarcinoma. This distinction is most problematic in needle core biopsy tissue, where only a few seminal vesicle glands may be sampled **i22.15, i22.16**. Prostatic neoplastic proliferations lack the scattered monstrous cells of seminal vesicle epithelium and usually do not contain as much lipofuscin pigment. Intranuclear protrusions also favor seminal vesicle epithelium. If uncertainty still exists, negative staining for PSA and PSAP, with positive 34βE12 staining, will rule out prostatic neoplasia.

Maldevelopment

Developmental abnormalities of the seminal vesicles include agenesis, hypoplasia, fusion, duplication, ureterovesicular fistulas,

■ **t22.1 Developmental Abnormalities of Seminal Vesicles**

Agenesis
- Unilateral: Associated with ipsilateral absence of vas deferens and kidney
- Bilateral: Associated with bilateral absence of vas and cystic fibrosis

Hypoplasia
Fusion
Duplication
Ureterovesicular fistulas: Drainage of ectopic ureter into seminal vesicle
Congenital cysts: Associated with ipsilateral renal agenesis and insertion of ectopic ureters

and congenital cysts **t22.1**. Such anomalies are rare: one large series of over 10 000 postmortem examinations reported an incidence of 0.05% (cited in Meiraz 1973). For infertility patients, the incidence is higher. In two series of a combined 299 infertile patients, 6% had a seminal vesicle congenital anomaly (Dominguez 1991, Malatinsky 1987). These anomalies were mainly agenesis, or an absence of the seminal vesicles due to a failure to form. A diagnosis of agenesis can be made by radiologic means, especially ultrasound (Carter 1989, Sandlow 2002), but also by computed tomography (CT) and magnetic resonance imaging (MRI).

Agenesis of the seminal vesicles can be unilateral or bilateral. Unilateral agenesis is frequently associated with an ipsilateral absence of the vas deferens and kidney. These anomalies appear to be associated because of an embryologic insult that affects the ureteric bud and mesonephric duct prior to their separation at 7 weeks of gestation (Hall 1993). Bilateral absence of the seminal vesicles is often found in conjunction with a bilateral absence of the vas deferens in men who are carriers for the cystic fibrosis transmembrane conductance regulator (CTFR) gene mutation in cystic fibrosis (Anguiano 1994, Chillon 1995, De la Taille 1998, Holsclaw 1971, Jarvi 1998). About 60%-100% of these patients are carriers of the CTFR gene mutation (Anguiano 1994, Chillon 1995, De la Taille 1998, Jarvi 1998). A high percentage of men (80%-95%) with overt cystic fibrosis also lack bilateral vas deferens or a seminal vesicle (Holsclaw 1971). Seminal vesicle agenesis itself does not require treatment (Sandlow 2002).

Hypoplasia (Malatinsky 1987); fusion (Malatinsky 1987); duplications (Christiano 1999, Malatinsky 1987); and ureterovesicular fistulas are also rare anomalies. Only a few cases of the former three have been described. The ureteral-seminal vesicle connection is actually implantation and drainage of an ectopic ureter into the seminal vesicle (Brannan 1973, Burford 1949, Das 1980, Fuselier 1976, Goldstein 1956, Gordon 1972, Kaneti 1988, Kenney 1983, MacDonald 1986, Pasquier 1953, Riba 1946, Roehrborn 1986, Schnitzer 1965). This developmental anomaly is due to an abnormally high cranial origin of the ureteric bud on the mesonephric duct, which leads to delayed absorption and ectopic insertion of the ureter into the posterior urethra, vas deferens, seminal vesicle, or ejaculatory ducts (MacDonald 1986, Sandlow 2002). The seminal vesicle is one of the most common sites of ectopic insertion of the ureter, comprising 25%-30% of all ectopic ureteral drainage sites (Burford 1949, Goldstein 1956, Gordon 1972). The ectopic ureter often drains into a cystic seminal vesicle. Other rare forms of ectopia in seminal vesicles include vasa deferentia opening into a seminal vesicle cyst (Negi 1998) and benign prostatic tissue in a seminal vesicle wall (Salem 1996). Aberrant embryologic connections to the seminal vesicle should be distinguished from acquired fistulas involving the seminal vesicle (Carlin 1999).

[22.3] Cysts

Seminal vesicle cysts are rare **t22.2**. In one series, the clinical incidence was 0.001% (Øgreid 1979). They may be congenital or acquired because of ejaculatory duct obstruction. Congenital cysts are associated with anomalies of the ipsilateral mesonephric duct, such as ipsilateral renal agenesis (in 68% of cases (Heaney 1987)) and ureteral ectopia in the cyst (in 30% of cases (Fuselier 1976, Van den Ouden 1998)). A few examples of associated hemivertebra and single cases of associated ipsilateral testis absence and inferior vena cava duplication have also been published (Aragona 1997, Callewaert 1997, Das 1980, Sheih 1993). There are also reported linkages of seminal vesicle cysts with infertility, hematospermia, genitourinary infection, and autosomal dominant (adult) polycystic kidney disease (ADPKD) (Alpern 1991, Danaci 1998, Hendry 1998, Sandlow 2002). Up to 60% of patients with ADPKD had seminal vesicle cysts (Danaci 1998). Due to the high incidence of associated upper tract and renal abnormalities, detection of seminal vesicle cysts should prompt radiologic evaluation of the ureters and kidneys.

Most seminal vesicle cysts are small (less than 5cm), unilateral, and asymptomatic. Men with symptoms usually present in the 2nd-4th decades of life (with a range 2.5-63 years) (Phillis 1999, Van den Ouden 1998). The most frequent symptoms include dysuria, urinary frequency, perineal pain, epididymitis, postejaculatory pain, and scrotal pain (Van den Ouden 1998). A subset of patients with seminal vesicle cysts are infertile (Øgreid 1979). Most cysts are palpable by digital rectal examination (Van den Ouden 1998). A few large (10cm-11cm) cysts are palpable as suprapubic masses (Negi 1998, Phillis 1999). In the past, large cysts were termed hydrocele or hydrops of the seminal vesicle (Hart 1961). Ultrasound and MRI examinations are diagnostic (Carter 1989, Sandlow 2002). Symptomatic cysts can range from 0.5cm (Gevenois 1990) to 15cm (Heaney 1987). Treatment is usually limited to these symptomatic patients. Histopathologically, excised seminal vesicle cysts are unilocular and often show a flattened mucosa and epithelium **i22.17**, with or without ulceration (Hart 1961). Acute and chronic inflammatory cells may be present in the cyst wall, which typically is fibrotic. The cyst lumen contains red blood cells, inflammatory cells, and/or spermatozoa (Hart 1961). Only in a few cases (n = 3) has a neoplasm been discovered in a seminal vesicle cyst (Atobe 1984, Bagley 1975, Okada 1992). One 17-year-old man had a papillary adenocarcinoma that arose in a congenital seminal vesicle cyst (Okada 1992). There was no wall invasion and the patient was cancer-free 6 years after surgical excision. A second case was a 19-year-old man with a well-differentiated tubulopapillary adneocarcinoma in a seminal cyst that was apparently acquired (Atobe 1984). A third case was an apparent seminal vesicle cyst with a neoplasm of uncertain histologic type that was classified as a "mesonephroid tumor" (Bagley 1975).

■ **t22.2 Seminal Vesicle Cysts**

Rare
Congenital or acquired
Most unilateral, small, and asymptomatic in younger men
Most palpable by DRE
Ultrasound and MRI are diagnostic
Symptomatic cysts 0.5cm-15 cm in diameter
Microscopic: Unilocular, with flattened epithelium and inflamed wall

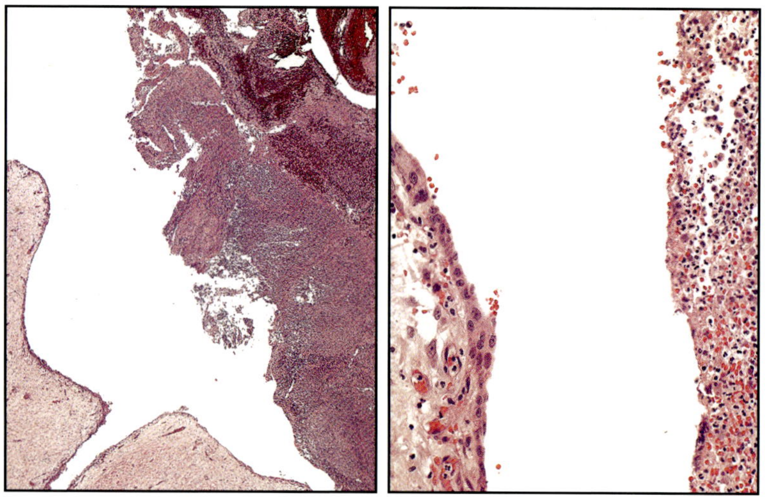

■ **i22.17** *Seminal vesicle cyst with intraluminal inflammatory exudate, hemorrhage and cellular debris (low and higher magnification).*

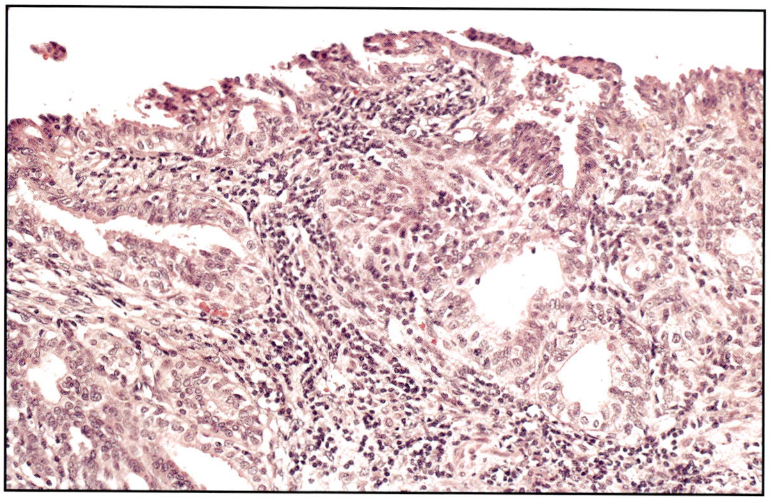

■ **i22.18** *Chronic inflammatory cell infiltrate in the seminal vesicle.*

The differential diagnosis of a seminal vesicle cyst includes congenital utricular cysts, müllerian duct cysts, ejaculatory duct cysts, vas deferens cysts, and prostatic cysts. The characteristic anatomical location and distinctive epithelial lining should together allow for the accurate identification of a seminal vesicle cyst.

[22.4] Inflammation and Infection

Inflammation of the seminal vesicles, or seminal vesiculitis, and infection of the seminal vesicles are uncommon today in the United States **t22.3**. Unlike the prostate, histologically detected inflammation in the seminal vesicle is unusual (Calams 1955) **i22.18**. Clinically, prostatitis and epididymitis predispose to seminal vesiculitis (Jensen 1988, Krishnan 1991, Williams 1998). Bacterial seminal vesiculitis associated with prostatitis is often due to bacteria from the gut (Sandlow 2002). In rare cases, abscess formation in the seminal vesicle may ensue (Eastham 1999, Jensen 1988, Kang 1989), and in one case, rupture led to acute peritonitis (Jensen 1988). Patients with diabetes mellitus, a chronic indwelling catheter, and a history of endoscopy are at higher risk for development of a seminal vesicle abscess (Williams 1998). Organisms responsible for abscesses include *Escherichia coli* (Kang 1989) and *Mycobacterium* (Eastham 1999, Kang 1989). Other specific organisms identified in a few cases as infectious agents in the seminal vesicles include cytomegalovirus (Kimura 1993), *Schistosoma* (Al Adnani 1985), and *Echinococcus* (hydatid disease) (Deklotz 1976, Pasaoglu 1997, Sagglam 1998). A case of seminal vesicle malakoplakia has also been reported (Sanchez Chapado 1995).

Inflammation of blood vessels, or vasculitis, was reported as an incidental finding in the seminal vesicle in two radical prostatectomy patients (Argani 1998). This necrotizing vasculitis was not indicative, in these two cases, of systemic vasculitis.

Acquired fistulas from the bowel or rectum/anus to the seminal vesicle can occur as a complication of inflammation from Crohn disease (Carlin 1999, Hamidinia 1984). Such fistulas have also been reported secondary to rectal carcinoma (Carlin 1999, Goldman 1989, Kollmorgen 1994) and post–open prostatectomy (Calder 2000).

■ **t22.3 Inflammation and Infection of Seminal Vesicle**

Uncommon
Predisposition: Prostatitis and epididymitis
Abscess: Associated with diabetes mellitus, indwelling catheter, and prior endoscopy
Organisms in abscess: *E Coli, Mycobacterium*
Other organisms seen: *Cytomegalovirus, Schistosoma, Echinococcus*

[22.5] Calcification and Calculi

Dystrophic calcification in the seminal vesicle is rare (George 1906, Kretschmer 1922, Marks 1942, Schned 1997, Silber 1971, Wilson 1951) and can be found in patients with diabetes and uremia. The calcification can also be a postinflammatory process (George 1906, Marks 1942) and idiopathic (Schned 1997). This calcification is often associated with calcification of the vas deferens, especially in diabetics. Histologically, the wall is most often involved, whereas calcification is rarely localized to the mucosa. Bony metaplasia has been found in a few cases (George 1906). The calcium deposition does not have known clinical significance or functional impact.

Stones are also rare in the seminal vesicle (Carachi 1997, Corriere 1997, Li 1991, Menon 1998, Sandlow 2002, White 1928, Wilkinson 1993). Stone formation here is usually secondary to obstruction and/or infection (Li 1991, Wilkinson 1993). Patients may present with perineal pain at ejaculation, hematospermia, or infertility (Corriere 1997, Sandlow 2002). The stones are smooth and hard and are composed of a nucleus of epithelial cells with a mucoid material covered with lime salts (Menon 1998). They range in size from 1mm to 3cm in greatest diameter (Corriere 1997, Menon 1998, White 1928). Treatment of symptomatic stones usually requires stone extraction via an open vesiculectomy (Sandlow 2002). Submission of seminal vesicle stone(s) for chemical analysis is not necessary.

[22.6] Amyloid Deposits

Amyloid deposits, or amyloidosis, can be detected in the seminal vesicles, most often as an incidental, localized finding in older men

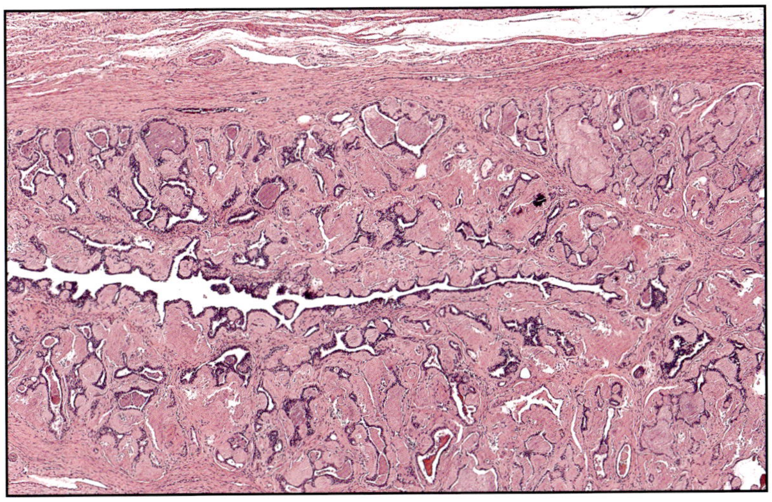

■ **i22.19** *Amyloidosis, localized, of seminal vesicle: Seminal vesicle appears atrophic at low magnification*

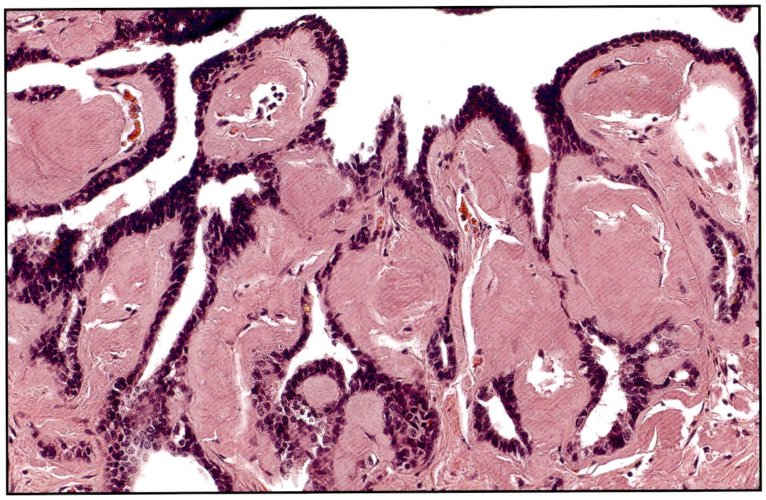

■ **i22.20** *Amyloidosis, localized, of seminal vesicle: Subepithelial nodules of amorphous amyloid.*

t22.4. The average incidence of seminal vesicle amyloidosis in seven autopsy series of 926 patients was 11% (range 1%-19%) (Bursell 1942, Coyne 1993, De Jager 1962, Goldman 1963, McDonald 1956, Pitkänen 1989, Tsutsumi 1996). The incidence is age-related, with the highest incidence of 21% in men over 75 (Pitkänen 1989). The discovery of seminal vesicle amyloidosis is usually a histologic finding without clinical manifestations (Coyne 1993, Goldman 1963), although there are rare exceptions (Carris 1976, Krane 1973). Radiologically, magnetic resonance images of seminal vesicle amyloidosis may be confused with prostatic carcinoma infiltration (Jager 1997, Ramchandani 1993). Grossly, the seminal vesicles do not typically appear abnormal, although in a few cases the seminal vesicle wall may be thickened and firm (Goldman 1963). Microscopically, the seminal vesicle involvement by amyloid is almost always bilateral, with a roughly equal amount of amyloid deposited in each seminal vesicle (Pitkänen 1989). Sections disclose a subepithelial, nodular to strandlike deposition of pink, homogenous, acellular material (Coyne 1993, Goldman 1963, Pitkänen 1989) **i22.19, i22.20**. These lumps of amyloid can cause partial or total obliteration of gland spaces (Goldman 1963). The amyloid, in the substantial majority of cases, is localized to the seminal vesicles *without* involvement of other anatomic sites or evidence of systemic amyloidosis (Coyne 1993, De Jager 1962, McDonald 1956, Pitkänen 1989). The presence of amyloid in the walls of vessels within or adjacent to the seminal vesicles suggests the existence of systemic amyloidosis (Coyne 1993, Pitkänen 1989). Histochemical staining of localized seminal vesicle amyloid reveals positivity with Congo red and crystal violet (Coyne 1993, Goldman 1963, Pitkänen 1989, Unger 1997). The Congo red staining shows a typical green birefringence and is abolished by pretreatment with potassium permanganate (Pitkänen 1989, Seidman 1989, Unger 1997). Immunohistochemical stains are positive for the P component and lactoferrin (Coyne 1993, Suess 1998, Tsutsumi 1996) and negative for AA amyloid, β-2 microglobulin, prealbumin, and kappa and lambda light chains (Coyne 1993, Unger 1997). Lactoferrin immunoreactivity could also be detected in the seminal vesicle epithelial cells, and it has been suggested that lactoferrin, derived from these cells, is a major protein constituent of localized seminal vesicle amyloidosis (Tsutsumi 1996). Another proposal is that androgen deprivation regulates amyloid protein deposition in the seminal vesicle (Unger 1997); this conjecture remains to be substantiated. In the few reported cases of systemic amyloidosis involving the seminal vesicle with or without localized amyloidosis (Coyne 1993, Pitkänen 1989, Suess 1998), immunohistochemical stains document a different type of amyloid such as a pre–albumin-transthyretin type of amyloid (Suess 1998) and AA amyloid (Coyne 1993). Thus the amyloid deposits in localized seminal vesicle amyloidosis are different morphologically (no vessel wall involvement) and biochemically from systemic types of amyloidosis. Like all forms of amyloidosis, electron microscopy of seminal vesicle amyloidosis demonstrates 7.5-10 nm rigid, linear, and nonbranching fibrils (Seidman 1989, Unger 1997).

■ **t22.4 Seminal Vesicle Amyloid**

An incidental, localized, finding in 11% of men
Increased incidence with age
Microscopic: Bilateral, subepithelial nodules or strands of amyloid
Presence of vascular wall amyloid suggests co-existing systemic amyloidosis (rare)
Typical apple-green birefrigence with Congo red stain

[22.7] Hyperplasia

Epithelial hyperplasia in the human seminal vesicle is not well-documented and no criteria exist for its diagnosis. Seminal vesicle epithelial hyperplasia has been described in int2/fibroblast growth factor-3 transgenic mice (Donjacour 1998).

A single case of fibromuscular hyperplasia of the seminal wall has been reported in a 27-year-old man who presented with perineal pain (Hatcher 1989). Adenomyomatous nodules (Young 2000) and adenomyosis (Fujisawa 1993) have also been seen in the small vesicle wall; these probably represent nodular smooth muscle hyperplasia with entrapped seminal vesicle glands.

[22.8] Primary Benign Neoplasms

Primary benign neoplasms of the seminal vesicles are quite rare, with only a few case reports published in the literature **t22.5**. Cystadenomas are the most common, with about 10 reported cases (Baschinsky 1998, Bullock 1988, Damjanov 1974, Lagalla 1993, Lundhus 1984, Mazzucchelli 1992,

■ t22.5 **Primary Seminal Vesicle Neoplasms**

Benign Neoplasms
Cystadenoma (fibroadenoma/ adenoma)
Leiomyoma
Solitary fibrous tumor
Peripheral nerve sheath tumor

Neoplasms of Indeterminate or Low Malignant Potential
Epithelial-stromal tumor (low-grade)
Adnexal tumor of probable Wolffian origin

Malignant Neoplasms
Carcinoma
- Adenocarcinoma
- Squamous cell carcinoma
- Small cell carcinoma
- Undifferentiated

Epithelial-stromal tumor (high-grade)
Sarcoma
- Fibrosarcoma
- Leiomyosarcoma
- Liposarcoma
- Angiosarcoma
- Rhabdomyosarcoma

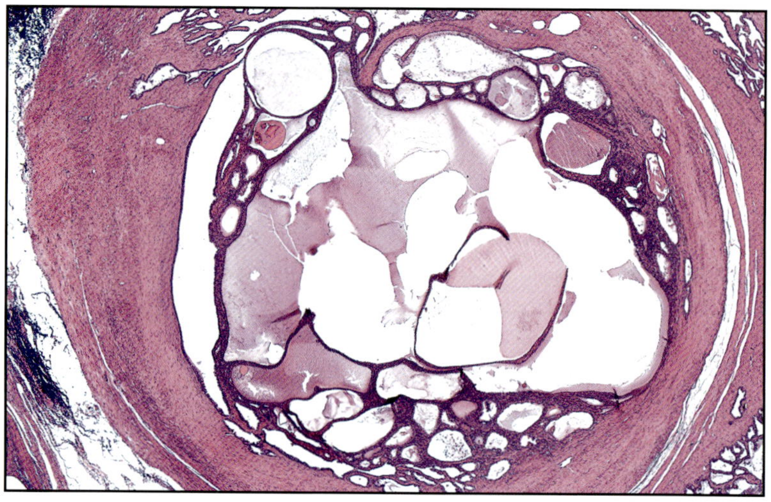

■ **i22.21** *Cystadenofibroma (cystadenomyoma) of seminal vesicle. Bilateral 1cm masses were incidental findings in a radical prostatectomy specimen. Shown here are cystically dilated benign seminal vesicle glands.*

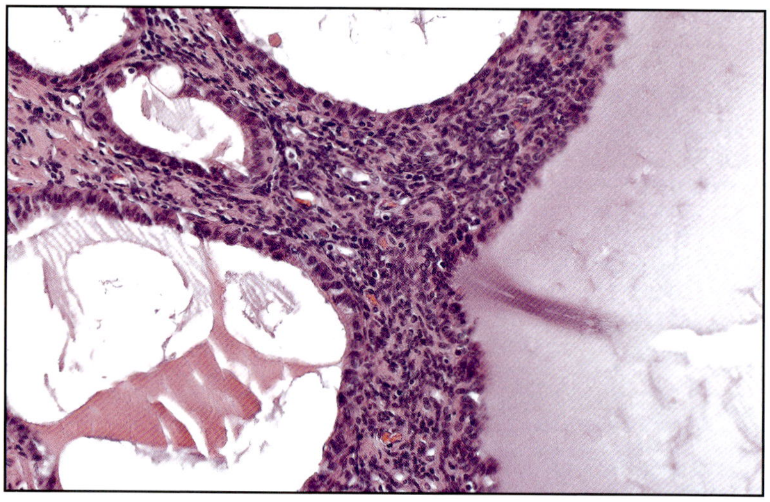

■ **i22.22** *Cystadenofibroma (cystadenomyoma) of seminal vesicle: condensed, hypercellular stroma surrounds benign seminal vesicle glands.*

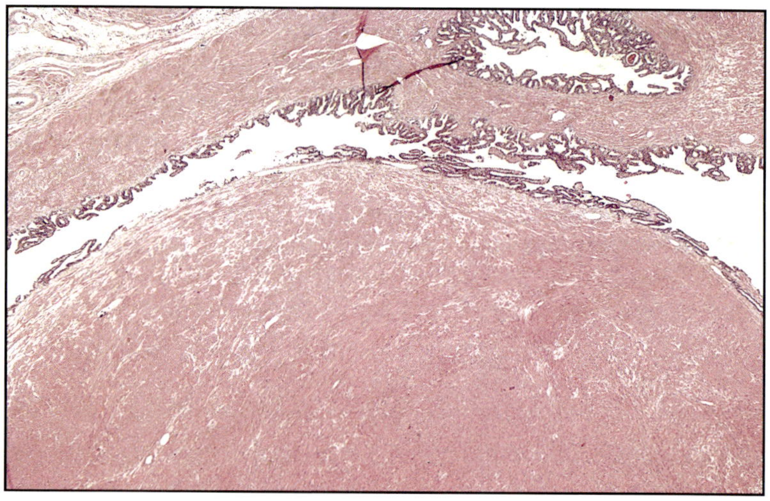

■ **i22.23** *Leiomyoma of the seminal vesicle: a smooth muscle nodule in the seminal vesicle wall.*

Peker 1997, Plaut 1944, Raghuveer 1989, Soule 1951). Many of these could be classified as benign epithelial-stromal tumors because of their biphasic nature (Young 2000). The average age at presentation is around 50 years (range 33-66). Several patients had abdominal, inguinal, or suprapubic pain; the mass can also be asymptomatic, or produce hematuria, hematospermia, fatigue, nocturia, stranguria, pollakisuria, or bladder outlet obstruction (Baschinsky 1998, Bullock 1988, Damjanov 1974, Lagalla 1993, Lundhus 1984, Mazzucchelli 1992, Peker 1997, Plaut 1944, Raghuveer 1989, Soule 1951). A supraprostatic mass was often palpable. In several cases, transrectal ultrasound, CT, and/or MRI were useful in defining the anatomic location of the mass (Baschinsky 1998, Lagalla 1993, Lundhus 1984, Peker 1997). Excision of the mass is required for definitive diagnosis. Grossly, the masses are unilateral and 3cm-15cm in greatest dimension, with smooth and lobulated outer surfaces. Cut surfaces show solid and cystic areas with smooth-walled cysts of variable size and shape, including rounded spaces and clefts. Cyst fluid is milky (Lundhus 1984) to chocolate-brown (Plaut 1944) to mucinous (Damjanov 1974, Peker 1997). Histologically, the biphasic tumor has a benign epithelial cyst surrounded by a bland fibromuscular component **i22.21, i22.22**. The simple epithelial cells lining the cysts are generally cuboidal to columnar and may be flattened in larger cysts. The cells are not stratified and do not display cytologic atypia or mitotic activity. Focal squamous epithelium has been reported in one case (Lagalla 1993) and papillary projections in another (Raghuveer 1989). The epithelial cells can contain pigment similar to that of normal seminal vesicle epithelium, but the monstrocellular atypia of that epithelium is lacking in the cyst lining (Peker 1997). The fibromuscular stroma is compromised of bland spindle cells without nuclear atypia or mitoses. Immunohistochemically, the epithelial cells are pan-cytokeratin positive (Baschinsky 1998, Peker 1997) and nonreactive for PSA and PSAP (Baschinsky 1998, Mazzucchelli 1992, Peker 1997). The stromal cells are vimentin-positive, and cytokeratin- and S-100–negative; patchy smooth muscle differentiation can be found with desmin and smooth muscle actin antibodies (Baschinsky 1998, Peker 1997). Complete surgical removal is curative.

Additional reports of benign primary neoplasm include a few cases of leiomyoma (Ahmadzadeh 1995, Bahn 1990, Gentile 1994) **i22.23** and solitary fibrous tumor (Morin 1998, Westra 2000); peripheral nerve sheath tumor (Weitzer 1998); and "benign mesenchymoma" (Islam 1979), which had benign fibromyxoid and bony elements (Islam 1979). A case reported as "mesonephric hamartoma" (Kinas 1987) may be a benign neoplasm, such as an adenomyoma, or nodular smooth muscle hyperplasia with entrapped seminal vesicle glands; the scant description generates difficulty in assessment of the nature of this mass.

[22.9] Primary Neoplasms of Indeterminate (or Low) Malignant Potential

Epithelial-stromal tumors of the seminal vesicle are rare neoplasms that span a spectrum of mixed epithelial and stromal cell proliferations that often resemble phyllodes tumors (Young 2000). At the benign end are cystadenomas, "cystomyoma" (Plaut 1944), and cystadenomas that have been termed fibroadenoma or adenomyoma (Lundhus 1984, Mazzucchelli 1992, Soule 1951, Young 2000). In an intermediate position are extraordinarily rare, low-grade epithelial-stromal tumors where cytologic atypia of the stromal component suggests low-grade malignant potential (Laurila 1992, Mazur 1987). In the clearly malignant category there is a single example published as "cystosarcoma phyllodes" (Fain 1993).

A single case of an adnexal tumor of probably Wolffian origin was reported to occur in the seminal vesicle of a 29-year-old man who suffered recurrences at 14 and 23 years after initial diagnosis (Middleton 1998). This neoplasm is viewed as being of low-grade malignant potential when it arises in the broad ligament, ovaries, and retroperitoneal of women.

[22.10] Primary Malignant Neoplasms

The most common primary malignancy in the seminal vesicles, adenocarcinoma, is exceedingly rare **t22.6**. Other reported primary malignant neoplasms include squamous cell carcinoma (Tabata 2002, Yanagisawa 2002); two high-grade epithelial-stromal tumors (Fain 1993, Laurila 1992); and a few sarcomas (Amirkhan 1994, Berger 2002, Chou 1985, Juhasz 1978, Lazarus 1946, Muentener 2000, Russo 1992, Schned 1986).

Primary carcinoma of the seminal vesicle was first described in 1925, and since that time about 50 confirmed cases have been reported (Ormsby 2000, Thiel 2002). Many cases diagnosed as primary seminal vesicle carcinoma represent a malignancy from another anatomic site. Historically, it has often been difficult to definitively establish a carcinoma as primary in the seminal vesicles, since the seminal vesicles are much more frequently involved by secondary compared with primary malignancies (Benson 1984). To qualify as a primary seminal vesicle carcinoma, specific criteria must be met (Benson 1984, Dalgaard 1956, Ormsby 1996, Young 2000) **t22.7**.

Clinically, the average mean age of men with primary seminal vesicle carcinoma is 62 (Benson 1984), with an age range of 17-90 years (Benson 1984, Okada 1992). Most patients present with urinary outlet obstructive symptomatology, including decreased stream, frequency, a sensation of incomplete bladder emptying, and dysuria (Benson 1984). A minority of men present with hematospermia. Hematuria (Benson 1984, Smith 1967) and acute urinary retention (Langham-Brown 1986) are uncommon. Almost all tumors are palpable, in a position superior to the prostate, by digital rectal examination (Benson 1984). A serum PSA level was available in only a few cases and was normal in both (Ohmori 1994, Oxley 1999). Radiologic studies, especially CT and ultrasound scans, can be useful in the assessment of the anatomic location of the mass (Kawahara 1988, Oguchi 1988, Sussman 1986). Although an IVP may reveal ureteral obstruction and an elevated bladder base in approximately 30% of patients (Benson 1984), IVP and cystoscopy may fail to reveal a mass in some cases (Ormsby 1996).

Grossly, a 2cm-13cm mass is typically centered on a single seminal vesicle (Awadalla 1968, Benson 1984, Davis 1988, Ohmori 1994, Oxley 1999, Sussman 1986). Cut surfaces are grey to grey-brown or pink (Awadalla 1968, Kindblom 1976, Tanaka 1987) and necrosis may be noted (Ormsby 1996). Bilateral involvement is evident in 9% of cases (Ormsby 1996). Rare cases are found to arise within a cyst (Atobe 1984, Okada 1992). Local infiltration into surrounding tissues, such as soft tissue, bladder, ureter, prostate, and rectum may occur (Benson 1984, Davis 1988, Oguchi 1988, Ormsby 1996). Microscopically, the carcinomas are almost all adenocarcinomas **i22.24-i22.26**. A single case of small-cell carcinoma of the seminal vesicle has been reported (Hoppin 1997). The architectural arrangements of the adenocarcinoma include papillary, solid, cribriform, and tubulopapillary **i22.24, i22.25**. Mucinous differentiation, with intracytoplasmic and/or intraluminal mucin, and clear cell features, with cleared cytoplasm and hobnail cells, may be prominent. The more solid or anaplastic areas can show a high mitotic rate (Ormsby 1996). The nuclear grade can be high, with vesicular nuclei and prominent nucleoli. The tumor cell cytoplasm lacks the lipofuscin pigment of benign epithelium. The histologic grade of these adenocarcinomas has ranged from well-differentiated (Okada 1992, Ormsby 1996) to poorly differentiated (Benson 1984, Kindblom 1976). In a few cases there was mention of an in situ neoplastic proliferation, or adenocarcinoma in situ (Davis 1988, Lathem 1975, Oxley 1999). In one case, the entire neoplasm was classified as adenocarcinoma in situ (Lathem 1975). Lymphatic channel and perineural invasion by carcinoma may be observed. Histochemical periodic acid Schiff, mucicarmine, and Alcian blue stains for mucin can be positive (Davis 1988, Oguchi 1988, Ohmori 1994, Ormsby 1996). By definition, immunohistochemical stains for PSA and PSAP are negative. In a majority of cases there is immunoreactivity for CA125 and CK7; absence of CK20 immunostaining is also characteristic (Ohmori 1994, Ormsby 2000). CEA immunopositivity may be detected (Benson 1984, Oguchi 1988, Oxley 1999). Metastatic spread occurs to regional lymph nodes, lungs, and viscera (Awadalla 1968, Ormsby 1996, Oxley 1999). Bony metastasis appears to be uncommon, and when found tends to be osteolytic (Awadalla 1968). This pattern of dissemination is different than that of prostatic carcinoma.

t22.6 Primary Adenocarcinoma of Seminal Vesicle

Rare: about 50 confirmed cases
Men (average age 62) present with bladder outlet obstruction
Palpable by DRE
Gross: 2cm-13cm mass, usually unilateral
Microscopic: Papillary, solid, cribriform, and tubulopapillary patterns
Outcome poor

t22.7 Diagnostic Criteria for Primary Seminal Vesicle Carcinoma

Microscopically-verified papillary or anaplastic carcinoma, localized mainly or exclusively to seminal vesicle
No other primary carcinoma elsewhere
Prostatic and rectal carcinomas ruled out
Negative PSA and PSAP immunostains

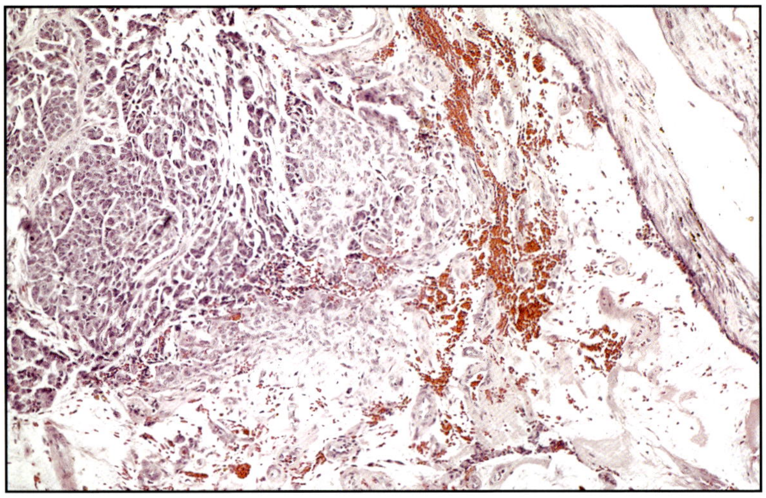

■ **i22.24** *Primary seminal vesicle: Intraluminal growth (Courtesy of Dr Tom Ulbright).*

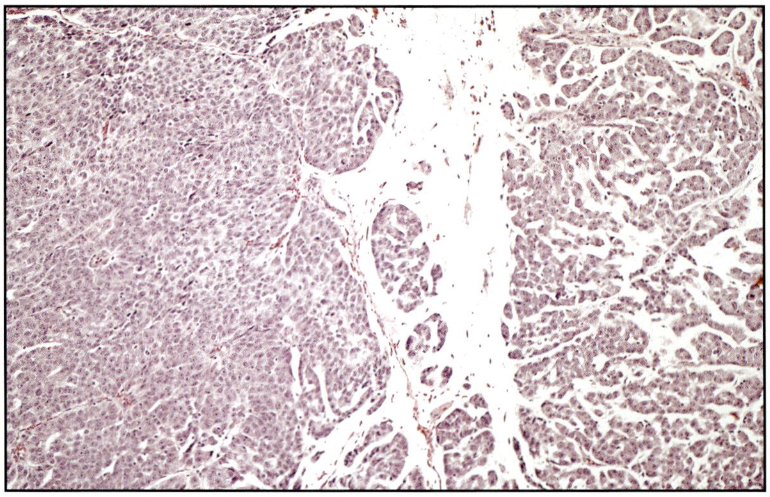

■ **i22.25** *Primary seminal vesicle adenocarcinoma: Solid growth (left) admixed with tubular and cord-like architectural configurations (right) (Courtesy of Dr Tom Ulbright).*

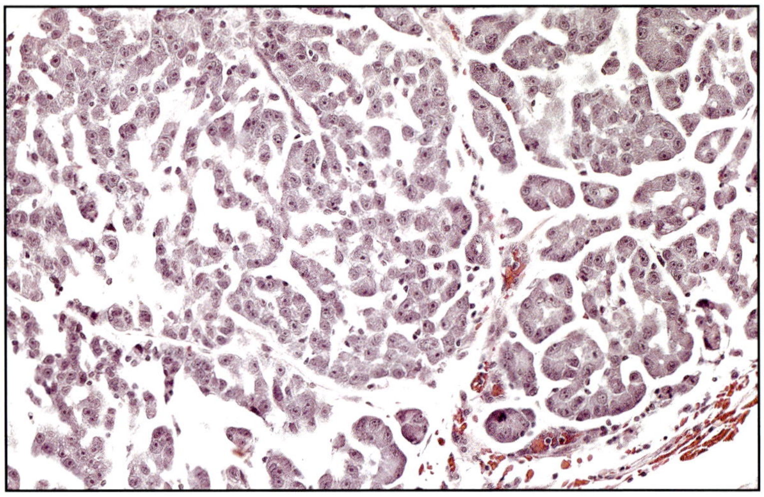

■ **i22.26** *Primary seminal vesicle adenocarcinoma: High-magnification view of tubular and cord-like arrangement of neoplastic cells (Courtesy of Dr Tom Ulbright).*

Outcome is poor, with 95% of patients dead of disease within 3 years (Ormsby 1996). There are too few cases to determine if there are any clinical or pathologic prognostic indicators. Treatment should entail surgical excision and androgen deprivation therapy (Benson 1984).

The differential diagnosis includes prostatic adenocarcinoma, transitional cell carcinoma, and colorectal adenocarcinoma. Prostatic duct adenocarcinoma with a papillary growth configuration may simulate seminal vesicle adenocarcinoma, but positive PSA and PSAP immunostains should confirm prostatic origin. Transitional cell (urothelial) carcinoma and colorectal adenocarcinoma are usually, in contrast to seminal vesicle carcinoma, CK20-positive. Anatomic location of the mass and the presence of in situ neoplasia will also aid in the determination of the site of origin.

One case of malignant epithelial-stromal tumor has been diagnosed in the seminal vesicle as cystosarcoma phyllodes (Fain 1993) or a high-grade phyllodes tumor. As in similar breast tumors, significant mitotic activity, stromal cell cytologic pleomorphism, and stromal overgrowth are histologic features that indicate malignancy. In this 61-year-old a lung metastasis was excised 4 years after the initial diagnosis.

Primary sarcomas of the seminal vesicle are even rarer than primary carcinomas of the seminal vesicles, with only a few published case reports in the literature (Amirkhan 1994, Berger 2002, Chou 1985, Juhasz 1978, Lazarus 1946, Muentener 2000, Russo 1992, Schned 1986). Primary seminal vesicle sarcomas constitute 0.1% of all adult soft tissue sarcomas (Russo 1992). Just as for many reported primary carcinomas of the seminal vesicle, rigorous documentation of seminal vesicle origin of many of the reported primary seminal vesicle sarcomas is lacking (Schned 1986). Sarcomas involving the seminal vesicle usually represent secondary spread from prostate, bladder, or retrovesical soft tissue. One should also exclude a sarcomatoid carcinoma from the prostate before diagnosing a primary sarcoma of the seminal vesicle. Leiomyosarcoma seems to be the most common type (Amirkhan 1994, Muentener 2000, Russo 1992, Sched 1986); there are isolated case reports of hemangiopericytoma (with metastasis) (Arya 2001); fibrosarcoma (Buck 1972, Williamson 1978); liposarcoma (Juhasz 1978); angiosarcoma (Chou 1985); rhabdomyosarcoma (Berger 2002); and a pleomorphic sarcoma consistent with malignant fibrous histiocytoma (Lazarus 1946).

A few "primary" germ cell tumors of the seminal vesicles have been described (Adachi 1991, Fairey 1993), but these two cases of choriocarcinoma and seminoma involvement of the seminal vesicle could represent metastasis from an undetected primary source (Young 2000), since microscopic examination of testicular tissue was not performed. Similarly, "primary" bilateral carcinoid tumors of the seminal vesicle (Soyer 1991), with extensive peritoneal metastasis, may be metastatic deposits (Young 2000).

Much remains unknown of primary seminal vesicle malignancy, mainly because of the rarity of these tumors. No predisposing factors, other than age, has been defined. In rats, seminal vesicle and prostatic adenocarcinomas can be induced with the chemical carcinogen methylnitrosourea combined with testosterone delivery (Pollard 2000). The genetic abnormalities in seminal vesicle cancers have not been characterized. Finally, possible pathways of progression have not been elucidated. That is, it is not known if hyperplasia or dysplasia (seminal vesicle intraepithelial neoplasia [SVIN]) precedes invasive primary adenocarcinoma of the seminal vesicle.

[22.11] Secondary Neoplasms

Prostatic adenocarcinoma is the neoplasm that most commonly spreads into the seminal vesicle **i21.27-i22.30; t22.8**. From 1974 to 1993, prostatic adenocarcinoma exhibited, on average, seminal vesicle

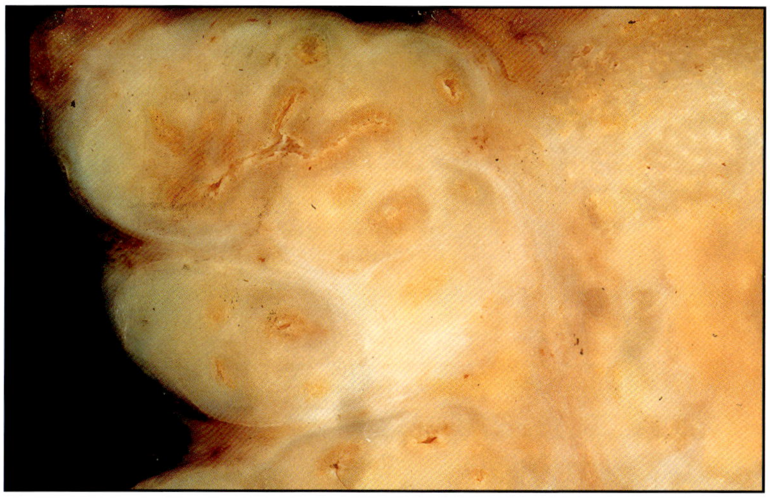

■ **i22.27** *Thickened yellow-white seminal vesicle walls with extensive adenocarcinoma of prostate.*

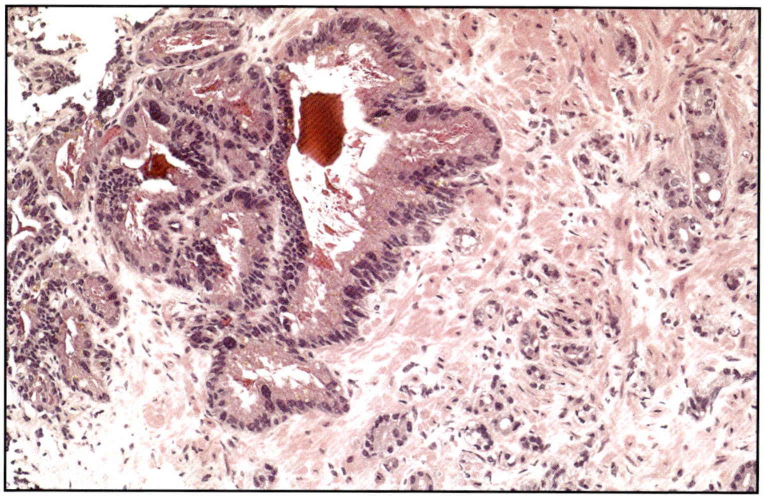

■ **i22.28** *Prostatic adenocarcinoma in wall of seminal vesicle, sampled by needle core biopsy.*

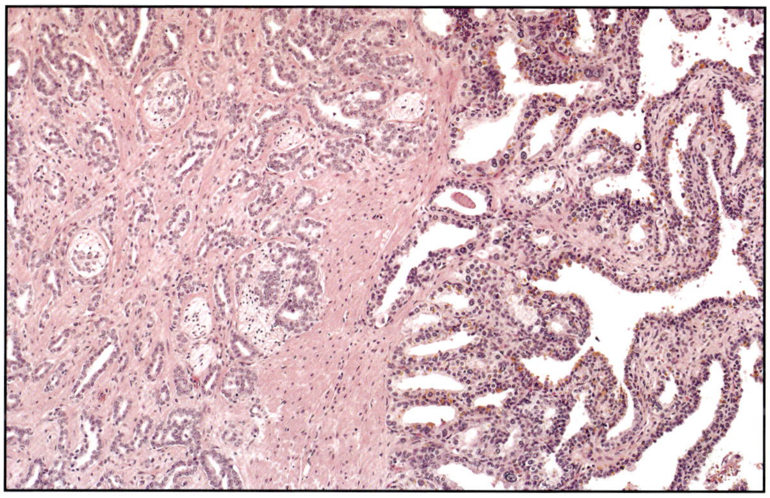

■ **i22.29** *Prostatic adenocarcinoma, usual acinar type, invading into seminal vesicle wall, in radical prostatectomy specimen.*

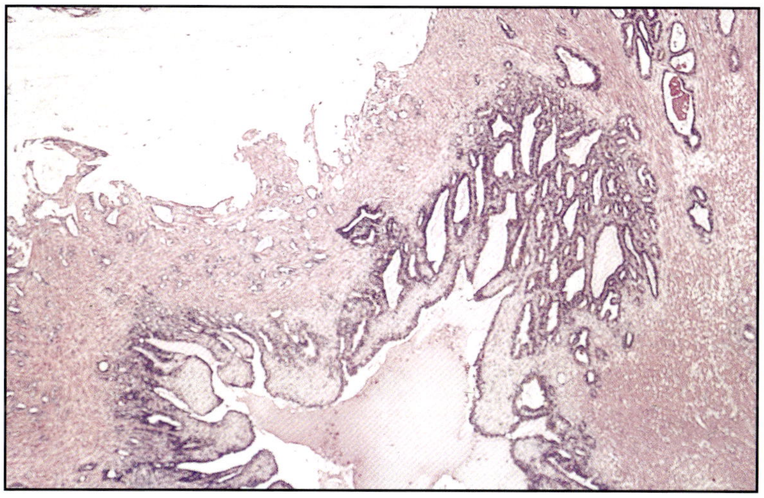

■ **i22.30** *Prostatic adenocarcinoma, mucinous type, with dissection of large pool of mucin into seminal vesicle wall.*

■ **t22.8 Secondary Neoplasms in Seminal Vesicle**

Far more common than primary tumors
Prostatic adenocarcinoma invades seminal vesicle in 12% of cases
Transitional cell carcinoma of bladder involves seminal vesicles in about 3% of cases
Other malignancies rarely involve seminal vesicle

invasion in 12% of radical prostatectomy cases, based on pooled multi-institutional data from 3485 cases (as tabulated in Jepsen 1998). The incidence is stage-dependent. For the smaller clinical stage, Tlc PSA-screen-detected prostatic carcinomas, the incidence is as low as 3% seminal vesicle involvement (Humphrey 1996). For palpable clinical stage T2 prostatic carcinoma, the incidence of seminal vesicle involvement is 14%-21% (Byar 1972, Epstein 1994, Ohori 1993), and for palpable cancer clinically outside the prostate (clinical stage T3), the incidence is 67% (Ohori 1993). [See Chapter 14 for a discussion and examples of the modes of spread **i14.134-i14.143**; **f14.4, pp 301-302**.]

Transitional carcinoma of the bladder involves the seminal vesicles much less frequently than prostate cancer, with an incidence of 3% (Ro 1987). In one-third of cases, the spread is intramucosal without stromal invasion **i22.31**, whereas in two-thirds of cases there is a direct extension from bladder wall–invasive transitional cell carcinoma (Ro 1987) **i22.32**. Colorectal carcinoma in

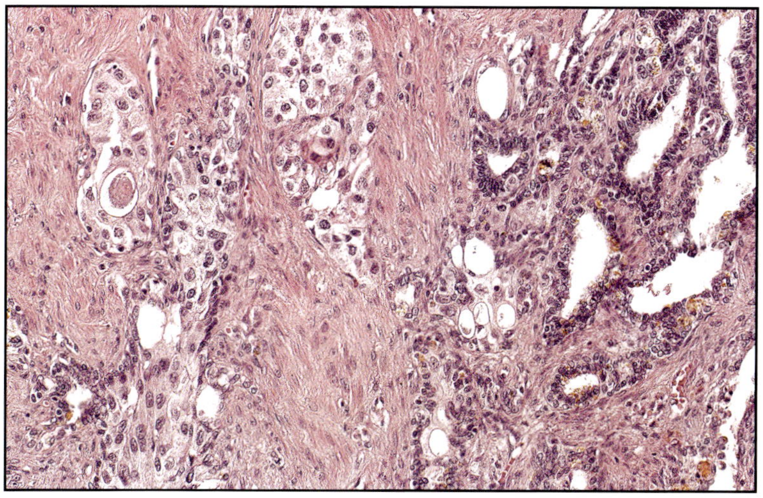

■ **i22.31** *In-situ spread of transitional cell carcinoma of bladder into seminal vesicle.*

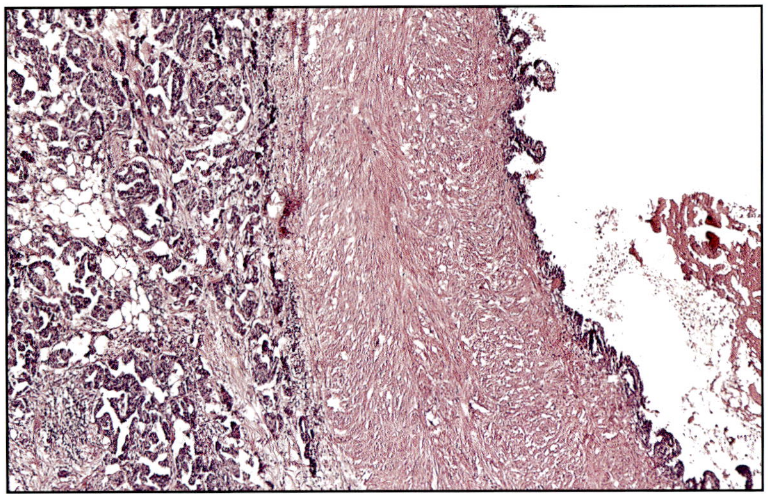

■ **i22.32** *High-grade transitional cell carcinoma of bladder extending into seminal vesicle wall by direct extension.*

advanced stages may directly extend into the seminal vesicles. There are rare reported cases of seminal vesicle metastasis of malignant melanoma (Abeshouse 1958, Berry 1953, Das Gupta 1965), renal cell carcinoma (Yamamoto 1998), and testicular mixed malignant germ cell tumors (Törnblom 1996).

References

Abeshouse BS. Primary and secondary melanoma of the genitourinary tract. *S Med J* 51:994-1006, 1958.

Aboul-Azm TE. Anatomy of the human seminal vesicles and ejaculatory ducts. *Arch Androl* 3:287-292, 1979.

Adachi Y, Rokujyo M, Kojima H, et al. Primary seminoma of the seminal vesicle: report of a case. *J Urol* 146:857-859, 1991.

Adeyoju AB, Taylor P, Payne SR. Congenital seminal vesicle cysts: an unusual but treatable cause of lower urinary tract/genital symptoms. *BJU Int* 87:901-902, 2001.

Ahmadzadeh M, Bosse A. Leiomyoma of the seminal vesicle. *Urol Int* 57:252-254, 1996.

Al Adnani MS. Schistosomiasis, metaplasia and squamous cell carcinoma of the prostate: histogenesis of the squamous cancer cells determined by localization of specific markers. *Neoplasma* 32:613-622, 1985.

Alpern MB, Dorfman RE, Gross BH, et al. Seminal vesicle cysts: association with adult polycystic kidney disease. *Radiology* 180:79-80, 1991.

Amin MB, Bostwick DG. Pigment in prostatic epithelium and adenocarcinoma: a potential source of diagnostic confusion with seminal vesicular epithelium. *Mod Pathol* 9:791-795, 1996.

Amirkhan RH, Molberg KH, Wiley EL, et al. Primary leiomyosarcoma of the seminal vesicle. *Urology* 44:132-135, 1994.

Anguiano A, Oates RD, Amos JA, et al. Congenital bilateral absence of the vas deferens: a primarily genital form of cystic fibrosis. *JAMA* 267:1794-1797, 1992.

Aragona F, D'Urso L, Valotto C, et al. Renal agenesis, ureteral ectopia into seminal vesicle, vas deferens agenesis and hemivertebra: an incomplete form of caudal regression syndrome? *Int Urol Nephrol* 29:403-410, 1997.

Arber DA, Speights VO. Aneuploidy in benign seminal vesicle epithelium: an example of the paradox of ploidy studies. *Mod Pathol* 4:687-689, 1991.

Argani P, Carter HB, Epstein JI. Isolated vasculitis of the seminal vesicle. *Urology* 52:131-133, 1998.

Arias-Stella J, Takano-Moron J. Atypical epithelial changes in seminal vesicles. *Arch Pathol* 66:761-766, 1958.

Arya M, Hayne D, Brown RSD, et al. Hemangiopericytoma of the seminal vesicle presenting with hypoglycemia. *J Urol* 166:992, 2001.

Atobe T, Naoe S, Taguchi K, et al. Primary seminal vesicle carcinoma in a 19-year-old male [in Japanese]. *Gan No Rinsho* 30:205-214, 1984.

Aumuller G, Riva A. Morphology and functions of the human seminal vesicle. *Andrologia* 24:183-196, 1992.

Awadalla O, Hunt AC, Miller A. Primary carcinoma of the seminal vesicle. *Br J Urol* 40:574-579, 1968.

Bagley DH, Javadpour N, Witebsky FG, et al. Seminal vesicle cyst containing mesonephroid tumor. *Urology* 5:147-151, 1975.

Bahn DK, Brown RK, Shei KY, et al. Sonographic findings of leiomyomas in the seminal vesicle. *J Clin Ultrasound* 18:517-519, 1990.

Baschinsky DY, Niemann TH, Maximo CB, Bahnson RR. Seminal vesicle cystadenoma: a case report and literature review. *Urology* 51:840-845, 1998.

Benson RC Jr, Clark WR, Farrow GM. Carcinoma of the seminal vesicle. *J Urol* 132:483-485, 1984.

Berger AD, Bartsch G, Horninger W. Primary rhabdomyosarcoma of the seminal vesicle. *J Urol* 168: 643, 2002.

Berry NE, Reese L. Malignant melanoma which had its first clinical manifestations in the prostate gland. *J Urol* 69:286-290, 1953.

Brannan W, Henry HH. Ureteral ectopia: report of 39 cases. *J Urol* 109:192-195, 1973.

Brewster SF. The development and differentiation of human seminal vesicles. *J Anat* 143:45-55, 1985.

Bullock KN. Cystadenoma of the seminal vesicles. *J Roy Soc Med* 81:294-295, 1988.

Buck AC, Shaw RE. Primary tumours of the retro-vesicle region with special reference to mesenchymal tumours of seminal vesicles. *Br J Urol* 44:47-50, 1972.

Burford CE, Glenn JE, Burford EH. Ureteral ectopia: a review of the literature and 2 case reports. *J Urol* 62:211-215, 1949.

Bursell S. Beitrag zur kenntis der para-amyloidase im urogenitalen system unter besonderer berücksichtigung der sog, senilen amyloidose in de sämenblaschen und ihres verhältnisses zum samenbläschenpigment. *Upsala Läkaref Forh* 47:313-331, 1942.

Byar DP, Mostofi FK. Carcinoma of the prostate: prognostic evaluation of certain pathologic features in 208 radical prostatectomies. Examined by the step-section technique. *Cancer* 30:5-13, 1972.

Calams JA. A histological search for chronic seminal vesiculitis. *J Urol* 74:638-645, 1955.

Calder JF. Seminal vesicle fistula [letter to the editor]. *Clin Radiol* 55:328, 2000.

Callewaert P, De Coster M, Vuylsteke P, et al. Anal tenesmus caused by seminal vesicle cyst. *Urology* 49:139-141, 1997.

Carachi R, Gobara D. Recurrent epididymo-orchitis in a child secondary to a stone in the seminal vesicle. *Br J Urol* 79:997, 1997.

Carlin J, Nicholson DA, Scott NA. Two cases of seminal vesicle fistula. *Clin Radiol* 54:309-311, 1999.

Carris CK, McLaughlin AP, Gittes RF. Amyloidosis of the lower genitourinary tract. *J Urol* 115:423-436, 1976.

Carter SS, Shinohara K, Lipsultz LI. Transrectal ultrasonography in disorders of the seminal vesicles and ejaculatory ducts. *Urol Clin North Am* 16:733-790, 1989.

Chillon M, Casals T, Mercier B, et al. Mutations in the cystic fibrosis gene in patients with congenital absence of the vas deferens. *N Engl J Med* 332:1475-1480, 1995.

Chou R-K, Limas C, Lange PH. Hemangiosarcoma of the seminal vesicle: case report and literature review. *J Urol* 134:371-373, 1985.

Christiano AP, Palmer JS, Chekmareva MA, et al. Duplicated seminal vesicle. *Urology* 54:162, 1999.

Cornwell GG III, Westermark GT, Pitkänen P, et al. Seminal vesicle amyloid: the first example of exocrine cell origin of an amyloid fibril precursor. *J Pathol* 167:297-303, 1992.

Corriere JN Jr. Painful ejaculation due to seminal vesicle calculi. *J Urol* 157:626, 1997.

Coyne JD, Kealy WF, Annis P. Seminal vesicle epithelium in needle biopsy specimens [letter to the editor]. *J Clin Pathol* 40:932, 1987.

Coyne JD, Kealy WF. Seminal vesicle amyloidosis: morphological, histochemical and immunohistochemical observations. *Histopathology* 22:173-176, 1993.

Dalgaard JB, Giertson JC. Primary carcinoma of the seminal vesicle: case and survey. *Acta Pathol Microbiol Scand* 39:255-267, 1956.

Damjanov I, Apic R. Cystadenoma of seminal vesicles. *J Urol* 111:808-809, 1974.

Danaci M, Akpolat T, Bastemir M, et al. The prevalence of seminal vesicle cysts in autosomal dominant polycystic kidney disease. *Nephrol Dial Transplant* 13:2825-2828, 1998.

Das Gupta T, Grabstald H. Melanoma of the genitourinary tract. *J Urol* 93:607-614, 1965.

Das S, Amar AD. Ureteral ectopia into seminal vesicle with ipsilateral renal dysgenesis and monorchia. *J Urol* 124:574-575, 1980.

Davis NS, Merguerian PA, DiMarco PL, Dvoretsky PM, Rashid H. Primary adenocarcinoma of seminal vesicle presenting as bladder tumor. *Urology* 32:466-468, 1988.

De Jager H, Stam FC. Pathology and histochemistry of amyloidosis in old age. *Gerontology* 6:19, 1962.

De la Taille A, Rigot JM, Mahe P, et al. Correlation between genito-urinary anomalies, semen analysis and *CFTR* genotype in patients with congenital bilateral absence of the vas deferens. *Br J Urol* 81:614-619, 1998.

De Marzo AM, Yang X, Nelson WG, et al. Distinguishing seminal vesicles (SV) from prostate cancer using immunohisto-chemistry (IHC) [abstract]. *Mod Pathol* 12:93A, 1999.

Deklotz RJ. Echinococcal cyst involving the prostate and seminal vesicles: a case report. *J Urol* 115:116-117, 1976.

Dominguez C, Boronat F, Cunat E, et al. Agenesis of seminal vesicles in infertile males: ultrasonic diagnosis. *Eur Urol* 20:129-132, 1991.

Donjacour AA, Thomson AA, Cunha GR. Enlargement of the ampullary gland and seminal vesicle, but not the prostate in int-2/Fgf-3 transgenic mice. *Differentiation* 62:227-237, 1998.

Donohue RE, Fauver HE. Unilateral absence of the vas deferens: a useful clinical sign. *JAMA* 261:1180-1182, 1989.

Eastham JA, Spires KS, Abreo F, et al. Seminal vesicle abscess due to tuberculosis: role of tissue culture in making the diagnosis. *South Med J* 92:328-329, 1999.

Epstein JI, Walsh PC, Carmichael M, Brendler CM. Pathologic and clinical findings to predict tumor extent of nonpalpable (stage Tlc) prostate cancer. *JAMA* 271:368-374, 1994.

Ewell GH. Seminal vesicle carcinoma. *J Urol* 88:908-912, 1963.

Fain JS, Cosnow I, King BF, et al. Cystosarcoma phyllodes of the seminal vesicle. *Cancer* 71:2055-2061, 1993.

Fairey AE, Mead GM, Murphy D, et al. Primary seminal vesicle choriocarcinoma. *Br J Urol* 71:756-757, 1993.

Fox CW Jr, Vaccaro JA, Kiesling VJ Jr, et al. Seminal vesicle abscess: the use of computerized coaxial tomography for diagnosis and therapy. *J Urol* 139:384-385, 1988.

Friedrichs R, Ebert T, Yogl TJ, et al. Use of endorectal surface coil magnetic resonance imaging for diagnosis of a multicystic seminal vesicle with ipsilateral renal agenesis. *Urol Int* 57:115-118, 1996.

Fujisawa M, Ishigami J, Kamidono S, et al. Adenomyosis of the seminal vesicle with hematospermia. *Jpn J Urol* 39:73-76, 1993.

Fuselier HA, Peters DH. Cysts of seminal vesicle with ipsilateral renal agenesis and ectopic ureters: case report. *J Urol* 116:833-835, 1976.

Gentile AT, Moseley HS, Quinn SF, Franzini D, Ditre TM. Leiomyoma of the seminal vesicle. *J Urol* 151:1027-1029, 1994.

George S. Calcification of the vas deferens and the seminal vesicles. *JAMA* 47:103-105, 1906.

Gevenois PA, Van Sinoy ML, Sintzoff SA Jr, et al. Cysts of the prostate and seminal vesicles: MR imaging findings in 11 cases. *Am J Roentgenol* 155:1021-1024, 1990.

Goldman H. Amyloidosis of seminal vesicles and vas deferens. *Arch Pathol* 75:94-110, 1963.

Goldman HS, Sapkin SL, Foote RF, Taylor JB. Seminal vesicle-rectal fistula. Report of a case. *Dis Colon Rectum* 32:67-69, 1989.

Goldstein AE, Heller E. Ectopic ureter opening into a seminal vesicle. *J Urol* 75:57-62, 1956.

Goldstein AG, Wilson ES. Carcinoma of the seminal vesicle with particular reference to the angiographic appearances. *Br J Urol* 45:211-212, 1973.

Gordon HL, Kessler R. Ectopic ureter entering the seminal vesicle associated with renal dysplasia. *J Urol* 108:389-391, 1972.

Grayhack JT. Changes with aging in human seminal vesicle fluid fructose concentration and seminal vesicle weight. *J Urol* 86:142-148, 1961.

Grob BM, Haley C, Schellhammer PF, Schlossberg SM, Wright GL Jr. The detection of prostate specific antigen, MHS-5, and other markers in invasive prostate cancer and seminal vesicle. *J Urol* 147:1435-1438, 1992.

Hall S, Oates RD. Unilateral absence of the scrotal vas deferens associated with contralateral mesonephric duct anomalies resulting in infertility: laboratory, physical and radiographic findings, and therapeutic alternatives. *J Urol* 150:1161-1164, 1993.

Hamidinia A. Recto-ejaculatory duct fistula: an usual complication of Crohn's disease. *J Urol* 131:123-124, 1984.

Hart JB. A case of cyst or hydrops of the seminal vesicle. *J Urol* 86:137-141, 1961.

Hatcher PA, Tucker JA, Carson CC. Fibromuscular hyperplasia of the seminal vesicle. *J Urol* 141:957-958, 1989.

Heaney JA, Pfister RC, Meares EM. Giant cyst of the seminal vesicle with renal agenesis. *Am J Roentgenol* 149:139-140, 1987.

Hendry WF, Rickards D, Pryor JP, et al. Seminal megavesicles with adult polycystic kidney disease. *Hum Reprod* 13:1567-1569, 1998.

Hihara T, Ohnishi H, Muraishi O, et al. MR imaging of seminal vesicle cysts associated with adult polycystic kidney disease. *Rad Med* 11:24-26, 1993.

Holsclaw DS, Perlmutter AD, Jockin H, et al. Genital abnormalities in male patients with cystic fibrosis. *J Urol* 106:568-574, 1971.

Hoppin EC, Rives RK. Small-cell carcinoma of the seminal vesicle responding to chemotherapy. *Ann Oncol* 8:503, 1997.

Humphrey PA, Keetch DW, Smith DS, et al. Prospective characterization of pathological features of prostatic carcinomas detected via serum prostate specific antigen based screening. *J Urol* 155:816-820, 1996.

Idasiak L, Kwias Z. Giant cyst of the spermatic vesicle imitating abdominal tumor. *Ginekol Pol* 63:543-545, 1992.

Indudhara R, Das K, Sharma M, et al. Seminal vesiculitis due to *Mycobacterium gastri* leading to male infertility. *Urol Int* 46:99-100, 1991.

Islam M. Benign mesenchymoma of seminal vesicles. *Urology* 13:203-205, 1979.

Jager GJ, Ruijter ET, de la Rosette JJ, et al. Amyloidosis of the seminal vesicles simulating tumor invasion of prostatic carcinoma on endorectal MR images. *Eur Radiol* 7:552-554, 1997.

Jarvi K, McCallum S, Zielenski J, et al. Heterogeneity of reproductive tract abnormalities in men with absence of the vas deferens: role of cystic fibrosis transmembrane conductance regulator gene mutations. *Fertil Steril* 70:724-728, 1998.

Jensen KH, Lundvall L. Peritonitis caused by abscess in seminal vesicle. Case report. *Acta Chir Scand* 154:245, 1988.

Jepsen JV, Bruskewitz RC. Should the seminal vesicles be resected during radical prostatectomy? *Urology* 51:12-18, 1998.

Juhasz J, Kiss P. A hitherto undescribed case of "collision tumour": liposarcoma of the seminal vesicle and prostatic carcinoma. *Int Urol Nephrol* 10:185-193, 1978.

Kaneti J, Lissmer L, Smailowitz Z, et al. Agenesis of kidney associated with malformations of the seminal vesicle. Various clinical presentations. *Int Urol Nephrol* 20:29-33, 1988.

Kang YS, Fishman EK, Kuhlman JE, et al. Seminal vesicle abscesses: spectrum of computed tomographic findings. *Urol Radiol* 11:182-185, 1989.

Károlyi P, Szentirmay Z, Krasznai G. Cytophotometric investigations on atypical epithelial cells of the human seminal vesicle. *Int Urol Nephrol* 21:399-402, 1989.

Kawahara M, Matsushima M, Matsuhashi M, et al. Primary carcinoma of the seminal vesicle. Diagnosis assisted by sonography. *Urology* 32:269-272, 1988.

Kenney PJ, Leeson MD. Congenital anomalies of the seminal vesicles: spectrum of computed tomographic findings. *Radiology* 149:247-251, 1983.

Kimura M, Maekura S, Satou T, et al. Cytomegaloviral inclusions detected in the seminal vesicle, ductus deferens and lungs in an autopsy case of lung cancer [in Japanese]. *Jpn J Clin Pathol* 41:1059-1012, 1993.

Kinas H, Kuhn MJ. Mesonephric hamartoma of the seminal vesicle: a rare cause of a retrovesical mass. *NY State J Med* 87:48-49, 1987.

Kindblom L-G, Pettersson G. Primary carcinoma of the seminal vesicle. Case report. *Acta Pathol Microbiol Scand Sect A* 84:301-305, 1976.

King BF, Hattery RR, Lieber MM, et al. Congenital cystic disease of seminal vesicle. *Radiol* 178:207-211, 1991.

Kollmorgen TA, Kollmorgen CF, Lieber MM, et al. Seminal vesicle fistula following abdominoperineal resection for recurrent adenocarcinoma of the rectum. Report of a case. *Dis Colon Rectum* 327:1325-1327, 1994.

Kovi J, Jackson MA, Akberzie ME. Unusual smooth muscle change in the prostate. *Arch Pathol Lab Med* 103:204-205, 1979.

Krane RJ, Klugo RC, Olsson CA. Seminal vesicle amyloidosis. *Urology* 2:70-72, 1973.

Kretschmer HL. Calcification of the seminal vesicles. *J Urol* 7:67-71, 1922.

Krishnan R, Heal MR. Study of seminal vesicles in acute epididymitis. *Br J Urol* 67:632-637, 1991.

Kuo T-T, Gomez LB. Monstrous epithelial cells in human epididymis and seminal vesicles. A pseudomalignant change. *Am J Surg Pathol* 5:483-490, 1981.

Lagalla R, Zappasodi F, Lo Casto A, et al. Cystadenoma of the seminal vesicle: US and CT findings. *Abdom Imaging* 18:298-300, 1993.

Langham-Brown JJ, Abercrombie GF. Carcinoma of the seminal vesicle. *Br J Urol* 58:339-340, 1986.

Lathem JE. Carcinoma of seminal vesicle. *S Med J* 68:473-474, 1975.

Laurila P, Leivo I, Makisalo H, et al. Mullerian adenosarcoma-like tumor of the seminal vesicle. *Arch Pathol Lab Med* 116:1072-1076, 1992.

Lazarus JA. Primary malignant tumors of the retrovesical region with special reference to malignant tumors of the seminal vesicles: report of a case of retro-vesical sarcoma. *J Urol* 55:190-205, 1946.

Li YK. Diagnosis and management of large seminal vesicle stones. *Br J Urol* 68:322-323, 1991.

Lundhus E, Bundgaard N, Sorensen FB. Cystadenoma of the seminal vesicle. A case report. *Scand J Urol Nephrol* 18:341-342, 1984.

Lyons O. Primary carcinoma of the left seminal vesicle. *J Urol* 13:477-484, 1925.

MacDonald GR. The ectopic ureter in men. *J Urol* 135:1269-1271, 1986.

Maheshkumar P, Harper C, Sunderland GT, Conn IG. Cystic epithelial stromal tumour of the seminal vesicle. *BJU Int* 85:1154, 2000.

Malatinsky E, Labady F, Lepies P, Zajac R, Janear M. Congenital anomalies of the seminal ducts. *Int Urol Nephrol* 19:189-194, 1987.

Marks JH, Ham DP. Calcification of vas deferens. *Am J Roentgenol* 47:859-863, 1942.

Mazur MT, Myers JL, Maddox WA. Cystic epithelial-stromal tumor of the seminal vesicle. *Am J Surg Pathol* 11:210-217, 1987.

Mazzucchelli L, Studer UE, Zimmerman A. Cystadenoma of the seminal vesicle: case report and literature review. *J Urol* 147:1621-1624, 1992.

McDonald JH, Heckel NJ. Primary amyloidosis of the lower genitourinary tract. *J Urol* 75:122-132, 1956.

Meiraz D, Fischelovitch J, Lazebnik J. Agenesis of the kidney associated with congenital malformation of the seminal vesicle. *Br J Urol* 45:541-544, 1973.

Melo AL, Oliveira RC, Turtelli CM. Seminal vesicle cyst associated with upper urinary tract malformation. Case report. *Scand J Urol Nephrol* 28:203-205, 1994.

Menon M, Parulkar BG, Drach GW. Urinary lithiasis: etiology, diagnosis, and medical management. In: Walsh PC, Retik AB, Vaughan ED Jr, Wein AJ, eds. *Campbell's Urology.* 7th ed. Philadelphia: WB Saunders; 2716-2717, 1998.

Middleton LP, Merino MJ, Popok SM, et al. Male adnexal tumour of probable Wolffian origin occurring in a seminal vesicle. *Histopathology* 33:269-274, 1998.

Morin G, Houlgatte A, Comparo P, et al. Solitary fibrous tumor of the seminal vesicles: apropos of a case [in French]. *Prog Urol* 8:92-94, 1998.

Muentener M, Hailemariam S, Dubs M, et al. Primary leiomyosarcoma of the seminal vesicle. *J Urol* 14:2027, 2000.

Negi SC, Dhiman ML, Gupta R. Larger seminal vesicle cyst obstructing the ureter of a solitary kidney. *Br J Urol* 82:446-447, 1998.

Norris HJ, Yunis E. Age changes of seminal vesicles and deferentia in diabetes. *Arch Pathol* 77:126-131, 1964.

Øgreid P, Hatteland K. Cyst of seminal vesicle associated with ipsilateral renal agenesis. *Scand J Urol Nephrol* 13:113-116, 1979.

Oguchi K, Takeuchi T, Kuriyama M, et al. Primary carcinoma of the seminal vesicle (cross-imaging diagnosis). *Br J Urol* 62:383-384, 1988.

Ohmori T, Okada K, Tabei R, et al. CA125-producing adenocarcinoma of the seminal vesicle. *Pathol Int* 44:333-337, 1994.

Ohori M, Scardino PT, Lapin SL, et al. The mechanisms and prognostic significance of seminal vesicle involvement by prostate cancer. *Am J Surg Pathol* 17:1252-1261, 1993.

Okada Y, Tanaka H, Takeuchi H, et al. Papillary adenocarcinoma in a seminal vesicle cyst associated with ipsilateral renal agenesis: a case report. *J Urol* 148:1543-1545, 1992.

Ormsby AH, Haskell R, Ruthven SE, Mylne GE. Bilateral primary seminal vesicle carcinoma. *Pathology* 28:196-200, 1996.

Ormsby AH, Haskell R, Jones D, Goldblum JR. Primary seminal carcinoma: an immunohistochemical analysis of four cases. *Mod Pathol* 13:46-51, 2000.

Oxley JD, Brett MT, Gillatt DA, Burton P. Seminal vesicle carcinoma. *Histopathology* 34:562-563, 1999.

Partin AW, Rodriguez R. The molecular biology, endocrinology, and physiology of the prostate and seminal vesicles. In: Walsh PC, Retik AB, Vaughan ED Jr, Wein AJ, eds. *Campbell's Urology.* 8th ed. Philadelphia: Saunders; 1237-1296, 2002.

Pasaoglu E, Damgaci L, Tokoglu F, et al. Hydatid cysts of the kidney, seminal vesicle and gluteus muscle. *Australas Radiol* 41:297-299, 1997.

Pasquier CM, Womack RK. Ectopic opening of ureter into seminal vesicle. *J Urol* 70:164-167, 1953.

Peker KR, Hellman BH Jr, McCammon KA, et al. Cystadenoma of the seminal vesicle. *J Urol Pathol* 6:213-221, 1997.

Phillis TM Jr, Teague JL. Seminal vesicle cyst in a child with a contralateral upper urinary tract abnormality. *BJU Int* 83:359-360, 1999.

Pitkänen P, Westermark P, Cornwell GG III, et al. Amyloid of the seminal vesicles. A distinctive and common localized form of senile amyloidosis. *Am J Pathol* 110:64-69, 1989.

Plaut A, Standard S. Cystomyoma of seminal vesicle. *Ann Surg* 119:253-261, 1944.

Pollard M, Wolter WR, Sun L. Prostate-seminal vesicle cancers induced in Noble rats. *Prostate* 43:71-74, 2000.

Rabii R, Aboutaieb R, Joual A, et al. Seminal vesicle cyst associated with homo-lateral renal agenesis and megaureter. Apropos of a case. *Ann Urol* 31:97-100, 1997.

Raghuveer CV, Nagarajan S, Aurora AL. Papillary cystadenoma of the seminal vesicle. A case report. *Indian J Pathol Microbiol* 32:314-315, 1989.

Ramchandani P, Schnall MD, LiVolsi VA, et al. Senile amyloidosis of the seminal vesicles mimicking metastatic spread of prostatic carcinoma on MR images. *Am J Roentgenol* 161:99-100, 1993.

Reddy YN, Winter CC. Cyst of the seminal vesicle: a case report and review of the literature. *J Urol* 108:134-135, 1972.

Riba LW, Schmidlapp CJ, Bosworth NL, et al. Ectopic ureter draining into the seminal vesicle . *J Urol* 56:332-338, 1946.

Riva A. Fine structure of human seminal vesicle epithelium. *J Anat* 102:71-86, 1967.

Ro JY, Ayala AG, el-Naggar A, et al. Seminal vesicle involvement by in situ and invasive transitional cell carcinoma of the bladder. *Am J Surg Pathol* 11:951-958, 1987.

Roehrborn CG, Schneider H, Rugendorff EW, et al. Embryological and diagnostic aspects of seminal vesicle cysts associated with upper urinary tract malformation. *J Urol* 135:1029-1032, 1986.

Russo P, Brady MS, Conlon K, et al. Adult urological sarcoma. *J Urol* 147:1032-1037, 1992.

Sagglam M, Tasar M, Bulakbasi N, et al. TRUS, CT and MRI findings of hydatid disease of seminal vesicles. *Eur Radiol* 8:933-935, 1998.

Salem CE, Gibbs PM, Highshaw RA, et al. Benign ectopic prostatic tissue involving the seminal vesicle in a patient with prostate cancer: recognition and implications for staging. *Urology* 48:490-493, 1996.

Sanchez Chapado M, Angulo Cuesta J, Guil Cid M, et al. Malacoplakia of the prostate and seminal vesicle. Ultrastructural study and review of the literature [in Spanish]. *Arch Esp Urol* 48:775-778, 1995.

Sandlow JL, Williams RD. Surgery of the seminal vesicles. In: Walsh PC, Retik AB, Vaughn ED Jr, Wein AJ, eds. *Campbell's Urology*. 8th ed. Philadelphia: Saunders; 3869-3885, 2002.

Schned AR, Ledbetter JS, Selikowitz SM. Primary leiomyosarcoma of the seminal vesicle. *Cancer* 57:2202-2206, 1986.

Scheinar J, Hruska F, Dusek J. Carcinoma of the seminal vesicles [in German]. *Z Urol Nephrol* 73:415-420, 1980.

Schned AR, Cozzolino DJ. Idiopathic dense calcification of the seminal vesicles. *J Urol* 157:2263, 1997.

Schnitzer B. Ectopic opening into seminal vesicle. A report of four cases. *J Urol* 93:576-581, 1965.

Seidman JD, Shmookler BM, Connolly B, et al. Localized amyloidosis of seminal vesicles: report of three cases in surgically obtained material. *Mod Pathol* 2:671-675, 1989.

Selli C, Bartoletti R, Travaglini F, et al. Surgical treatment of bilateral large seminal vesicle cysts associated with unilateral renoureteral agenesis. *Urol Int* 58:66-68, 1997.

Shabsigh R, Lerner S, Fishman IJ, et al. The role of transrectal ultrasonography in the diagnosis and management of prostatic and seminal vesicle cysts. *J Urol* 141:1206-1209, 1989.

Shah RB, Lee MW, Giraldo AA, et al. Histologic and histochemical characterization of seminal intraluminal secretions. Particular emphasis on their crystalloid morphology. *Arch Pathol Lab Med* 125:141-145, 2001.

Sheih C-P, Liao Y-J, Lin Y-W, et al. Seminal vesicle cyst associated with ipsilateral renal malformation and hemivertebra: report of 2 cases. *J Urol* 1214-1215, 1993.

Shidham VB, Lindholm PF, Kajdacsy-Balla A, et al. Prostate-specific antigen expression and lipochrome pigment granules in the differential diagnosis of prostatic adenocarcinoma versus seminal vesicle-ejaculatory duct epithelium. *Arch Pathol Lab Med* 123:1093-1097, 1999.

Silber SJ, McDonald FD. Calcification of the seminal vesicles and vas deferens in a uremic patient. *J Urol* 105:542-544, 1971.

Smith BA Jr. Carcinoma of the seminal vesicle: report of two cases. *J Urol* 72:67-76, 1954.

Smith BA Jr, Webb EA, Price WE. Carcinoma of the seminal vesicle. *J Urol* 97:743-750, 1967.

Soule EH, Dockerty MB. Cystadenoma of the seminal vesicle, a pathologic curiosity: report of a case and review of the literature concerning benign tumors of the seminal vesicle. *Mayo Clinic Proc* 26:406-414, 1951.

Soyer P, Rougier P, Gad M, et al. Primary carcinoid tumor of the seminal vesicles: CT and MR findings. *J Belge Radiol* 74:117-119, 1991.

Stenos J, Pavlakis A, Rebelakos A. Cysts of the seminal vesicle. A case report and review of the literature. *Acta Urol Bel* 3:718-723, 1985.

Suess K, Moch H, Epper R, et al. Heterogeneity of seminal vesicle amyloid. Immunohistochemical detection of lactoferrin and amyloid of the prealbumin-transthyretin type [in German]. *Pathologe* 19:115-119, 1998.

Surya BV, Washecka R, Glasser J, et al. Cysts of the seminal vesicles: diagnosis and management. *Br J Urol* 62:491-493, 1988.

Sussman SK, Dunnick NR, Silverman PM, et al. Carcinoma of the seminal vesicle: CT appearance. *J Comput Assist Tomogr* 10:519-520, 1986.

Tabata K-I, Irie A, Ishii D, Yanagisawa N, et al. Primary squamous cell carcinoma of the seminal vesicle. *Urology* 59:445, 2002.

Tanaka T, Takeuchi T, Oguchi K, et al. Primary adenocarcinoma of the seminal vesicle. *Hum Pathol* 18:200-202, 1987.

Thiel R, Effert P. Primary adenocarcinoma of the seminal vesicles. *J Urol* 168:1891-1896, 2002.

Törnblom M, Fredriksson A, Larsson P, et al. Seminal vesicle metastasis—an overlooked occurrence of testicular tumours? *Br J Urol* 77:160-162, 1996.

Trainer TD. Testis and excretory duct system. In: Sternberg SS, ed. *Histology for Pathologists.* 2nd ed. Philadelphia: Lippincott-Raven; 1032-1033, 1997.

Tsutsumi Y, Serizawa A, Hori S. Localized amyloidosis of the seminal vesicle: identification of lactoferrin immunoreactivity in the amyloid material. *Pathol Int* 46:491-497, 1996.

Unger PD, Wang Q, Gordon RE, et al. Localized amyloidosis of the seminal vesicle. Possible association with hormonally treated prostatic adenocarcinoma. *Arch Pathol Lab Med* 121:1265-1268, 1997.

Van den Ouden D, Blom JHM, Bangma C, et al. Diagnosis and management of seminal vesicle cysts associated with ipsilateral renal agenesis: a pooled analysis of 52 cases. *Eur Urol* 33:433-440, 1998.

Watson EM. The development of the seminal vesicles in man. *Am J Anat* 24:395-441, 1918.

Weitzer M, Cohen RJ. Benign peripheral nerve sheath tumor of the seminal vesicle. *Pathology* 30:80, 1998.

Westra WH, Grenko RT, Epstein JI. Solitary fibrous tumor of the lower urogenital tract: a report of five cases involving the seminal vesicles, urinary bladder, and prostate. *Hum Pathol* 31:63-68, 2000.

White JL. Stones in prostates and seminal vesicles. *Texas State J Med* 23: 581, 1928.

Wilkinson AG. Case report: calculus in the seminal vesicle. *Pediatr Radiol* 23:327, 1993.

Williamson RC, Slade N, Feneley RC. Seminal vesicle tumours. *J Roy Soc Med* 71:286-288, 1978.

Wilson LL, Marks JH. Calcification of vas deferens: its relation to diabetes mellitus and arteriosclerosis. *N Engl J Med* 245:321-325, 1951.

Winklemann M. Über lokales Amyloid der Samenblasen. *Virchow Arch Pathol Anat* 265:524-535, 1927.

Wojcik EM, Bassler TJ Jr, Orozco R. DNA ploidy in seminal vesicle cells. A potential diagnostic pitfall in urine cytology. *Analyt Quant Cytol Histol* 21: 29-34, 1999.

Yamamoto S, Mamiya Y, Noda K, et al. A case of metastasis to the seminal vesicle of renal cell carcinoma [in Japanese]. *Jpn J Urol* 89:563-566, 1998.

Yanagisawa N, Saegusa M, Yoshida T, et al. Squamous cell carcinoma arising from a seminal vesicular cyst: possible relationship between chronic inflammation and tumor development. *Pathol Int* 52:244-253, 2002.

Young RH. Pseudoneoplastic lesions of the prostate gland. *Pathol Ann* 23:109-128, 1988.

Young RH, Srigley JR, Amin MB, et al. The seminal vesicle. In: *Tumors of the Prostate Gland, Seminal Vesicles, Male Urethra, and Penis. Atlas of Tumor Pathology.* 3rd series, fascicle 20. Washington, DC: Armed Forces Institute of Pathology; 345-366, 2000.

Zenklusen HR, Weymuth G, Rist M, et al. Carcinosarcoma of the prostate in combination with adenocarcinoma of the prostate and adenocarcinoma of the seminal vesicles. A case report with immunocytochemical analysis and review of the literature. *Cancer* 66:998-1001, 1990.

Zurkirchen MA, Sulser T, Schmucki O, et al. Seminal vesicle and ipsilateral kidney failure. Report of 2 cases and review of the literature. *Urologe A* 35: 490-494, 1996.

CHAPTER 23

Prostatic Urethra

[23.1] Congenital Anomalies **523**

[23.2] Urethritis and Infection **524**

[23.3] Infarcts and Fibrosis **525**

[23.4] Urothelial Metaplasias **526**

[23.5] Prostatic Urethral Epithelial Polyps **530**

[23.6] Urothelial Hyperplasia **531**

[23.7] Benign Neoplasms **531**

[23.8] Dysplasia **532**

[23.9] Malignant Neoplasms **533**

The 15cm-20cm male urethra is comprised of 3 segments: the prostatic urethra, the membranous urethra, and the penile urethra (Reuter 1997). Commonly, an anatomical distinction is made between the proximal (posterior) urethra and the distal (anterior) urethra. In men, the "posterior" urethra is comprised of the prostatic and membranous urethra (Amin 1997B). The distinction between anterior and posterior anatomic location is important since different neoplasms tend to involve those sites. Therefore, in general, proximal urethral tumors tend to be transitional cell (urothelial) neoplasms, whereas distal urethral tumors are often squamous carcinomas (Amin 1997B, Reuter 1997).

Anatomic relationships of the 3cm-4cm prostatic urethra with surrounding prostatic tissue are presented in Chapter 1. Microscopically, the urethral mucosa can assume a flat to undulating appearance. The surface epithelial lining of the prostatic urethra is predominantly urothelial (transitional cell) **i23.1**, although prostatic epithelium may also be found. Like all urothelium, the normal epithelial lining is fragile and easily denuded **i23.2** in the course of biopsy and tissue handling. Such epithelial cell loss may raise a concern for ulceration or transitional carcinoma in situ (CIS). Unlike true erosions or ulcers, however, there is no inflammatory cell response to this iatrogenic urothelial cell loss. In partial denudation it is important to scrutinize the cytologic features of the remaining cells in order to exclude urothelial CIS.

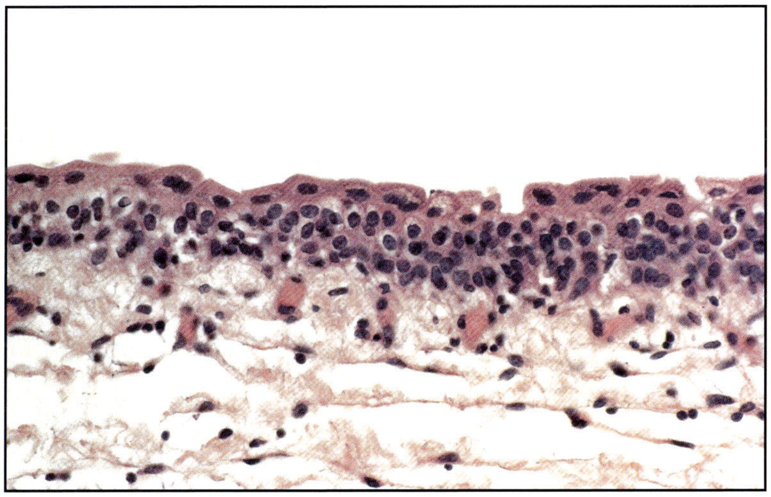

■ **i23.1** *Normal prostatic urethral urothelium with prominent cap (umbrella) cells with eosinophilic cytoplasm.*

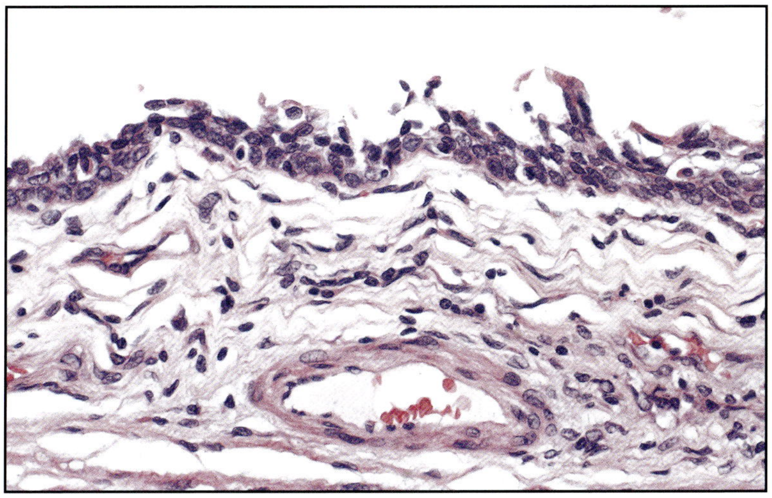

■ **i23.2** *Disrupted prostatic urethral urothelium. This artifactual change does not represent true discohesiveness as can be seen in carcinoma in situ.*

Diseases that affect the prostatic urethra, which is the conduit for urine and semen, are quite different from those that affect the substance of the prostate gland. Not surprisingly, urothelial disorders predominate in the prostatic urethra, whereas acinar disorders are by far the dominant problem in the prostatic parenchyma. Also, primary urothelial disease in the prostatic urethra is much less common than disease in the prostatic tissue itself. Yet due to the anatomic continuity of the epithelial lining of the prostatic urethra and the prostatic ducts (and ejaculatory ducts) and the merging of suburothelial connective tissue and prostate tissue, disease that affects the urethra often involves the prostate and vice versa. Another anatomical relationship that is significant in the spread of disease (particularly transitional cell carcinoma) is the direct continuity of the prostatic urothelium with the urothelium of the bladder neck.

The prostatic urethra may be directly and intentionally sampled by transurethral biopsy and resection and radical cystoprostatectomy. It may also be incidentally sampled by transrectal needle biopsy and transurethral resection or radical prostatectomy performed to treat prostatic parenchymal disease.

[23.1] Congenital Anomalies

Congenital anomalies of the prostatic urethra **t23.1** can be clinically significant but are rarely seen by surgical pathologists (Reuter 1997).

Posterior urethral valves can clinically result in renal dysfunction, hydronephrosis, vesicoureteral reflux, and vesical dysfunction (Gonzales 2002). In 1919 Young recognized three distinct types of these valves (Young 1919). Morphologically, all types are basically urothelial-lined connective tissue, tissue folds, or membranes. Management usually entails careful endoscopic destruction of the valves (Gonzales 2002), such that no tissue is submitted to the surgical pathology laboratory.

Urethral duplication usually involves the entire length of the urethra, including the prostatic urethra. It is uncommon and can present with many variations in the anatomical structure (Gonzales 2002). A portion of urethral tissue may be excised during reconstruction (Gonzales 2002).

Another rare congenital anomaly is the insertion of the ureter into the prostatic urethra (Prieto 1995).

Urethral diverticula may be congenital or acquired and are usually found in women (Jordan 2002). In men, congenital diverticula of

■ **t23.1 Congenital Anomalies of Prostatic Urethra**

Posterior urethral valves
Urethral duplication
Ectopic ureter in prostatic urethra
Diverticula
Congenital polyps
Mesonephric remnants

the prostatic urethra do occur and represent cystic change in a Müllerian duct remnant **f1.2, p 6**, in intersex disorders or an enlarged utricle associated with proximal hypospadias (Jordan 2002). If large and symptomatic, such diverticula may be surgically excised (Jordan 2002). Structures termed acquired prostatic urethral diverticula may be discovered after a prostatic abscess (Marya 1977), but since there is lack of an epithelium lining to the cavity, these are actually pseudocysts.

Congenital urethral polyps, also known as fibrous or fibroepithelial polyps, are rare, exophytic masses that protrude into the urethral lumen (Bruijnes 1985, Downs 1970, Foster 1986, Frates 1967, Hanani 1980, Kimche 1982, Madden 1986, Murphy 1982, Petersen 1992, Walker 1989, Youssif 1985). Almost all such polyps are located in the prostatic urethra. Most patients are children (with an average age of about 8 years, but the range is 1 month to 79 years) who present with obstruction, and less commonly hematuria or dysuria. The clinical diagnosis is made by the detection of a filling defect on voiding cystourethrography (Gonzales 2002). The polyp may be removed via transurethral or transvesical approaches. By urethroscopy/cystoscopy and grossly, the polyps are solitary, on a stalk, and are often a few centimeters in size (but can range up to 7cm) (Foster 1986, Walker 1989). Microscopically, the polypoid growth harbors a fibrovascular core covered by benign urothelium. Smooth muscle and nerve tissue may be found within the core. The surface lining epithelium is of normal-thickness transitional epithelium, which in a minority of cases displays squamous or intestinal (goblet cell) metaplasia (Jordan 2002). Secondary changes of inflammation and ulceration may also be observed (Reuter 1997). The microscopic differential diagnosis focuses mainly on other polypoid/papillary growths, nonneoplastic and neoplastic, of the urethra (Walker 1989) **t23.2**. A single case of recurrence has been described (Frates 1967). Some cases are morphologically indistinguishable from polypoid urethritis, and it seems likely that some fibroepithelial polyps reported in adults are actually reactive and inflammatory polyps (polypoid urethritis), rather than being of a congenital nature (Petersen 1992). Congenital fibroepithelial polyps are entirely benign, do not predispose to malignancy, and are almost always cured by simple excision.

Finally, a single case of mesonephric remnants has been reported in a urethral location (Andersen 1994). Such mesonephric remnants, with hyperplasia, have also been reported in the base of the prostate gland (Gikas 1993), periprostatic soft tissue (Gikas 1993), and bladder neck (Val-Bernal 1995). This benign small acinar proliferation could readily be misdiagnosed as adenocarcinoma and therefore qualifies as a pseudoneoplasm (see Chapter 7) (Young 1997B). Mesonephric remnants are nonreactive in PSA immunostaining (Andersen 1994), whereas lumen-forming prostatic glands, benign or malignant, with this gland-formative appearance typically would be positive.

■ **t23.2 Papillary/Polypoid Masses of the Prostatic Urethra**

Congenital urethral polyps (fibroepithelial polyps)
Papillary/polypoid urethritis
Nephrogenic "metaplasia (adenoma)"
Condyloma acuminatum
Prostatic urethral polyps
Inverted papilloma
Villous adenoma
Papillary transitional cell neoplasms
Ductal adenocarcinoma of prostate (protrudes into urethra from large prostate ducts)

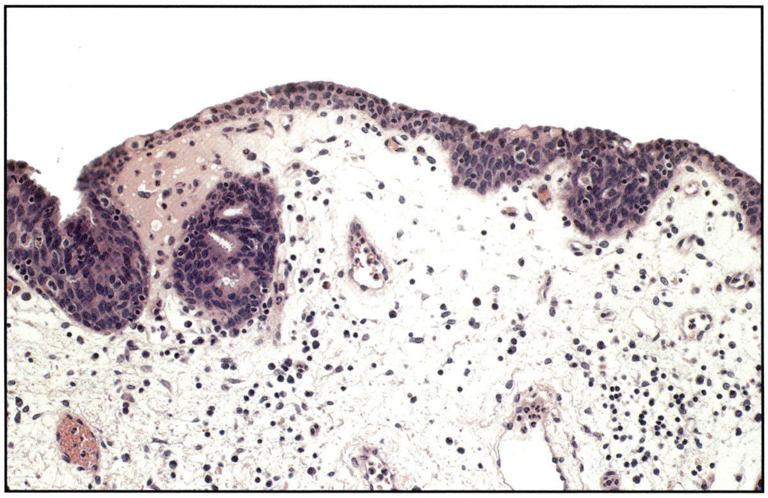

■ **i23.3** *Nonspecific chronic prostatic urethritis. Lymphocytes and plasma cells infiltrate an edematous lamina propria. Lymphocytes may be found within the urothelial lining.*

[23.2] Urethritis and Infection

A diagnosis of urethritis, including urethritis secondary to sexually transmissible microorganisms, does not typically require a biopsy. Moreover, when an inflammatory cell infiltrate is visualized in histologic sections of the urethra, the infiltrate is usually nonspecific **i23.3**, with a few important exceptions.

Human papillomavirus (HPV) infection in the male urethra usually presents as condyloma acuminata of the distal urethra or the meatus. Prostatic urethral involvement has been detected in only a few cases (Bissada 1994, DeBenedictis 1977, Libby 1985, Murphy 1983) and in these cases, such involvement was associated with extensive condylomata throughout the entire urethra. Histologically, these are most often exophytic and papillomatous growths, although a flat pattern can be seen. The condylomata are comprised of squamous epithelium with koilocytes, which may display mild to moderate koilocytic atypia (Murphy 1983). The differential diagnosis includes other papillary/polypoid growths **t23.2**, but most of these other growths lack squamous epithelium, and all others lack koilocytes. For flat condylomata, the main consideration is squamous metaplasia. For exophytic, papillomatous projections without koilocytic change, a diagnosis of squamous papilloma may be given. Although urethral condylomata often harbor HPV types 6 and 11 (Del Mistro 1987) and urethral carcinoma types 6 and 16 (Grussendorf-Conen 1987, Mevorach 1990, Weiner 1992), such genotyping is not necessary for the differential distinction between condyloma and carcinoma, as this differential is best addressed by histomorphology.

Granulomatous prostatic urethritis can be secondary to bacillus Calmette-Guérin (BCG) treatment of urothelial carcinoma. In bladder cancer patients treated with intravesical BCG, about 50% will have granulomas on posttreatment urethral biopsies (Hillyard 1988), which are used as a tool to monitor for urethral involvement by carcinoma. Histologic identification of BCG granulomatous prostatitis correlates with clinical response (Orihuela 1989). Histologically, these granulomas can be either caseating or noncaseating **i4.43-i4.47, p 90**, and are identical to granulomas seen in systemic tuberculosis, which rarely involves the prostate and urethra. The granulomas are often small, compact, and just below the urothelium, which may exhibit an associated intraepithelial lymphocytic infiltrate. In this setting of known BCG

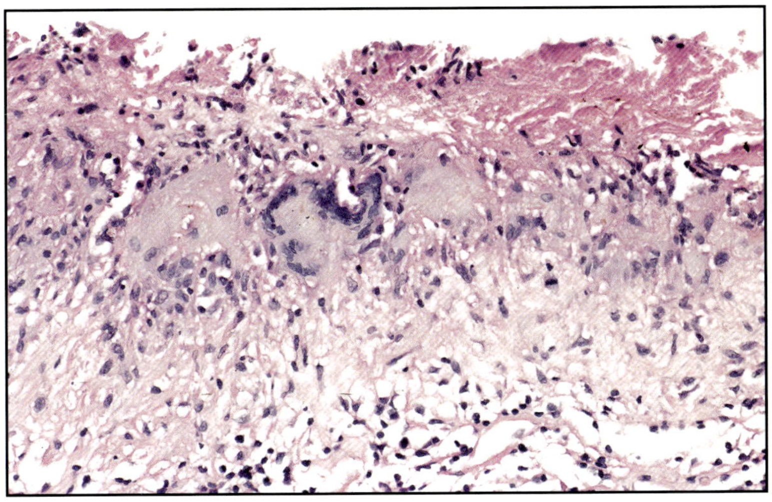

■ **i23.4** *Ulcerated prostatic urothelium, with underlying granulomatous inflammation, secondary to transurethral resection of prostate.*

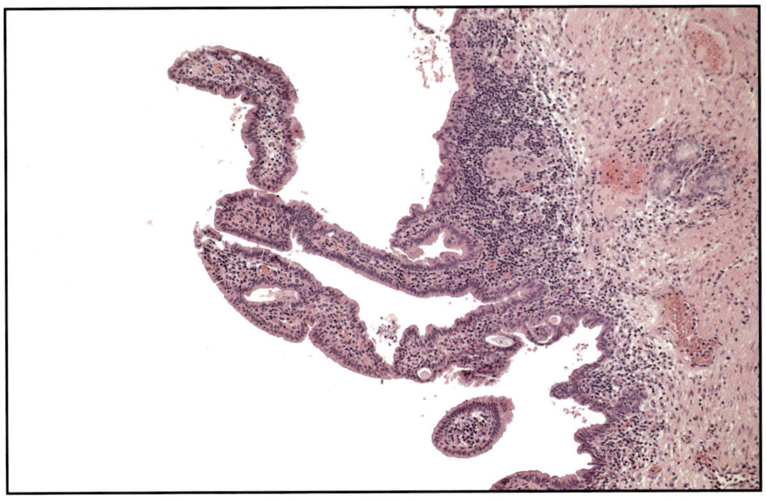

■ **i23.5** *Papillary prostatic urethritis.*

treatment, it is not necessary to stain for organisms; if staining for acid-fast bacilli is performed, these organisms will be observed in about one-half of cases. Transurethral resection of the prostate can also evoke a granulomatous response, but this mainly involves the prostatic parenchyma (see Chapter 4). Adjacent surface urothelium can become ulcerated and inflamed **i23.4**.

Malakoplakia, which is often associated with *E coli* infection, rarely involves the urethra or prostatic parenchyma, and no cases of the prostatic urethra have been reported.

Inflammation of the prostatic urethra may evoke the formation of polypoid structures, named papillary or polypoid urethritis (Schinella 1974, Walker 1989). Another label is papillary pseudotumor (proliferative papillary urethritis) (Schinella 1974). These structures are similar to the projections of papillary and polypoid cystitis in the bladder (Young 1997B). Only a few cases have been reported (Schineller 1974), and relationships with infection and benign prostatic hypertrophy have been suggested (Schineller 1974). By cystoscopy/urethroscopy a papillary lesion is seen. Histologic sections demonstrate thick, clinically inflamed edematous mucosal folds lined by normal or reactive urothelium **i23.5; t23.3**. Prostatic ducts can be found between these protrusions, but prostatic epithelium is not found within the polypoid structure itself. The main differential diagnostic concern here is with a papillary, low-grade, urothelial neoplasm and papillary ductal adenocarcinoma of the prostate. Both of these entities usually possess thin and delicate fibrovascular cores, and the ductal prostatic carcinomas will have significantly greater nuclear atypia than polypoid urethritis. Polypoid urethritis is a condition that is reversible, contingent upon removal of the inciting cause.

■ **t23.3 Papillary/Polypoid Urethritis: Microscopic Characteristics**

Thick mucosal fronds
Edematous stroma with dilated thin-walled vessels
Cuboidal to low columnar urothelial lining
Secondary ulceration, urothelial hyperplasia, squamous metaplasia possible
No prostatic epithelium in fronds
Chronic inflammatory cell infiltrate present

[23.3] Infarcts and Fibrosis

Damage to the prostatic urethra may eventuate in infarction and/or reparative fibrosis. Biopsies may be taken from fibrotic areas if a stricture or mass is formed after such damage.

Prostatic urethral infarcts are surprisingly common at autopsy, with an incidence of 12% in one series of 100 consecutive necropsies (Jones 1986). Risk factors for development of these infarcts seem to be hypotension and urethral catheterization. Histologically, edema, hemorrhage, and necrosis are noted, mainly in the anterior portion of the prostatic urethra. It is speculated that this ischemic damage could contribute to the genesis of urethral strictures (Jones 1986).

Urethral strictures most often involve the anterior urethra (meatal, penile, and bulbar urethra). Posterior (membranous and prostatic) urethral strictures, which are usually fibrotic in nature, are generally secondary to trauma (such as pelvic fracture) or treatment. Treatments that can cause prostatic urethral fibrosis and strictures include transurethral resection of the prostate, open prostatectomy, radical prostatectomy, and radiation therapy. Rarely, the posttreatment fibrosis may be complicated by a fistula. Biopsies of urethral strictures may be performed to rule out cancer as a cause for the stricture. Resection of the fibrotic tissue may be performed in some cases. Histologically, typical scar tissue and fibrosis are noted. A single case of intestinal metaplasia and dysplasia (villous adenoma) secondary to prostatic urethral stricture/inflammation has been reported (Maung 1988).

Rarely, transurethral resection of the bladder or prostate may lead to an exaggerated, reactive, spindle cell proliferation known as a postoperative spindle cell nodule (Huang 1990, Proppe 1984, Wick 1988, Young 1987). These spindle cells likely represent an exuberant fibroblastic/myofibroblastic proliferation. The original description (Proppe 1984) of eight cases of this entity included three post–transurethral resection of the prostate (TURP) cases. Although the site was designated as prostatic urethra in these cases, all three were identified in tissue from a second, repeat TURP, and no description of involvement of urothelial or suburothelial tissue was provided. These proliferative masses most likely arise from the prostatic tissue bed generated by the first TURP. Only one case is documented to involve the prostatic urethra (Huang 1990). Postoperative spindle cell nodules are benign, pseudoneoplastic spindle cell proliferations that may be mistaken for a sarcoma.

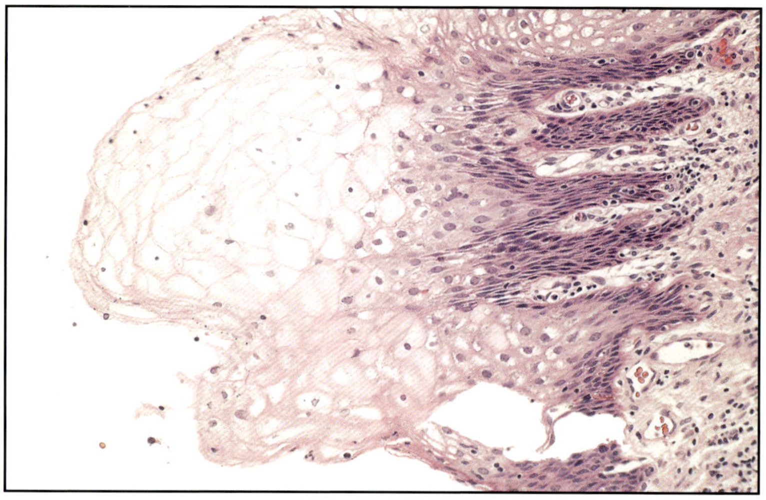

■ **i23.6** *Squamous metaplasia of prostatic urethra, with a nodular configuration. This is the glycogenated type.*

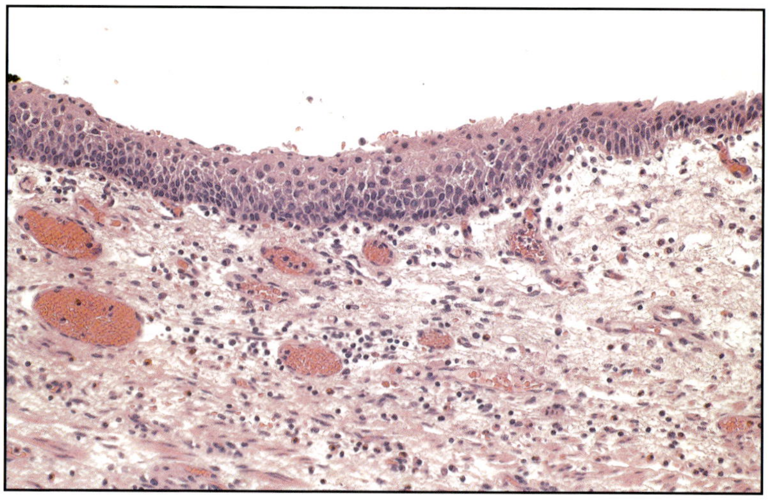

■ **i23.7** *Squamous metaplasia of prostatic urethra, associated with inflammation.*

[23.4] Urothelial Metaplasias

Like urothelium throughout the urinary tract, prostatic urethral urothelium is capable of metaplasia into squamous, columnar, and cuboidal cells (Mostofi 1954) **t23.4**.

Squamous metaplasia is a stereotyped response of the urothelium to injury: prolonged irritation, chronic inflammation, chronic infection, instrumentation, stones, radiation, and vitamin A deficiency have been linked to squamous metaplasia of the urothelium (Mostofi 1954). Squamous metaplasia of the prostatic urethra may be in direct continuity with squamous metaplasia of the bladder (Reece 1975). Squamous metaplasia and dysplasia have been viewed as precursor lesions of squamous cell carcinoma of the urethra (Amin 1997B), but the magnitude of risk of a subsequent diagnosis of squamous cell carcinoma after a diagnosis of isolated prostatic urethral squamous cell metaplasia or dysplasia has not been determined. By cystoscopy, squamous metaplasia can appear as a grayish-white plaque (leukoplakia) (Reece 1975). Histologically, the squamous metaplasia may be glycogenated **i23.6** or keratinizing and is commonly associated with an inflammatory cell infiltrate **i23.7**.

Columnar or cuboidal urothelial metaplasia may develop in von Brunn's nests, which are invaginations of urothelium into the lamina propria **i23.8**. Von Brunn's nests are commonly seen in urethral tissues and, although they are sometimes seen associated with inflammation, these nests are considered by many to be variants of normal anatomy (Kiernan 1987).

Von Brunn's nests are solid aggregates of benign urothelial cells that may be detected in a direct continuity with a surface urothelium or may be physically separate in the lamina propria **i23.8**. When numerous, the nests may be mistaken for invasive carcinoma (Young 1997B, Young 1997A). An orderly architecture, lack of stromal response, and absence of cytologic atypia (other than reactive inflammatory atypia) are useful features that point toward a diagnosis of von Brunn's nests.

Von Brunn's nests may undergo cystic change to produce urethritis cystica **i23.9** or may exhibit true glandular metaplasia or urethritis glandularis (Mostofi 1954) **i23.10, i23.11**. In urethritis cystica the cysts are lined by urothelial or cuboidal cells and contain a pink proteinaceous fluid **i23.9**. In urethritis glandularis, the columnar metaplasia is of mucous or nonmucous type (Mostofi 1954) **i23.10, i23.11**. Here, columnar cells line glandular spaces, and if mucus is absent or inconspicuous, the term typical (or nonmucous) urethritis glandularis is applied **i23.11**, whereas the presence of goblet cells and epithelium resembling colonic glands indicates urethritis glandularis of the intestinal (or mucous) type **i23.11**. Urethritis glandularis of the intestinal type is believed to be a precursor lesion in the development of adenocarcinoma (Bostwick 1984, Posso 1961, Tran 1996), although the risk imparted by the finding of pure urethritis glandularis is unknown. Nevertheless, the identification of such intestinal metaplasia should prompt a search for intestinal-type adenocarcinoma in the histologic sections.

Nephrogenic "metaplasia" is commonly designated as nephrogenic adenoma and has also been termed adenomatous metaplasia, adenomatoid metaplasia, adenomatoid tumor, and hamartoma. It has long been presumed that this is a metaplastic change in urothelium, with a resultant resemblance to renal tubules (Friedman 1950). Recently, however, the metaplastic nature of these cells has been questioned (Mazal 2002). In renal transplant patients it was shown that these nephrogenic "metaplasia" cells were actually derived from tubular cells of the kidney (Mazal 2002). It has been suggested that nephrogenic "metaplasia" or nephrogenic "adenoma" might be a kind of renal tubular satellite due to seeding, implantation, and growth of renal cells in urothelial mucosa (Mazal 2002). This type of cuboidal urothelial metaplasia is most common in the bladder (McIntire 1987, Oliva 1995, Walker 1989, Young 1997B), but cases localized to the prostatic urethra as well as cases with both bladder and urethral involvement have been reported (Berger 1981, Bhagavan 1981, Daroca 1993, Malpica 1994, Martin 1981, Walker 1983, Young 1992) **t23.5**. It has been estimated that only 4% of all cases of nephrogenic "metaplasia" occur in the prostatic urethra (McIntire 1987), and indeed only 48 cases could be extracted from the literature **t23.5**. Of these cases, three (14%) involved both the urinary bladder and prostatic urethra, and 13

■ **t23.4 Prostatic Urethral Metaplasias**

Squamous metaplasia
Urethritis cystica
Urethritis glandularis
typical type
intestinal type
Nephrogenic "metaplasia" (nephrogenic "adenoma")

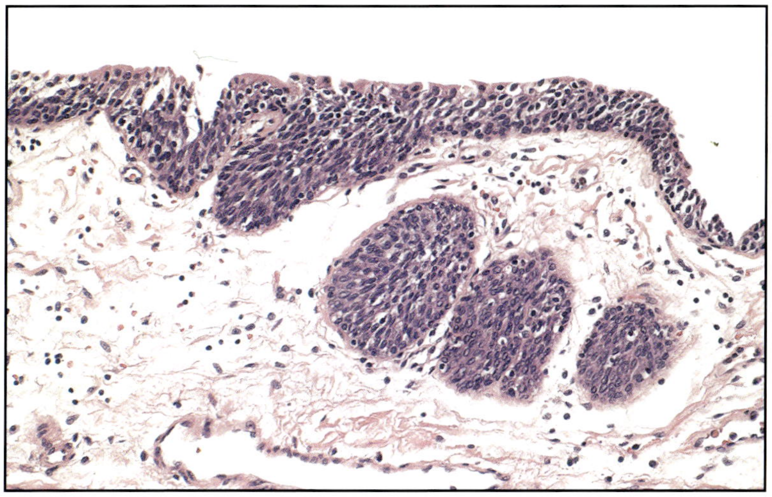

■ **i23.8** *von Brunn's nests underlying surface urothelium.*

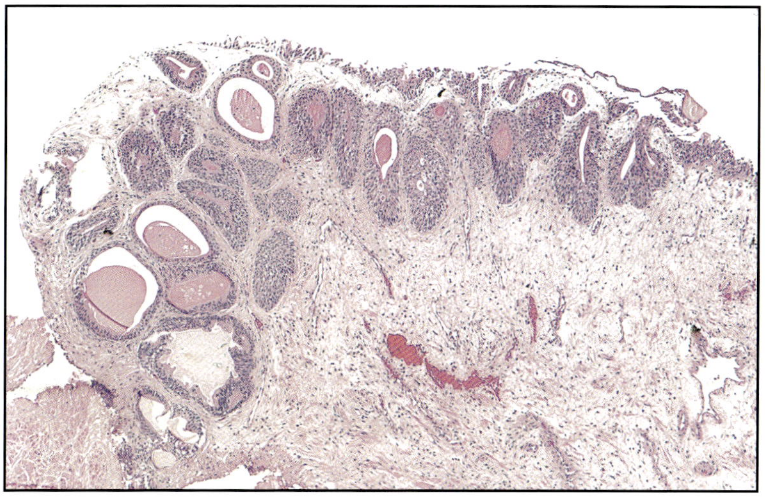

■ **i23.9** *von Brunn's nests and urethritis cystica in prostatic urethra. Note dilated gland-like structures or urethritis cystica with pink proteinaceous secretions.*

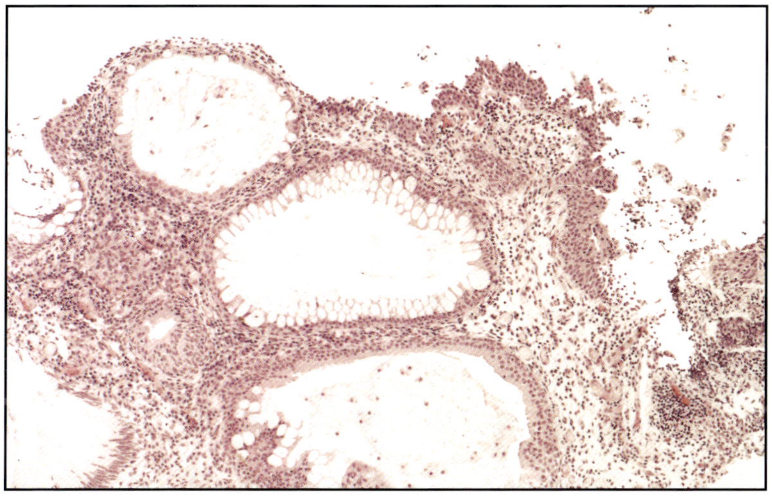

■ **i23.10** *Urethritis glandularis*

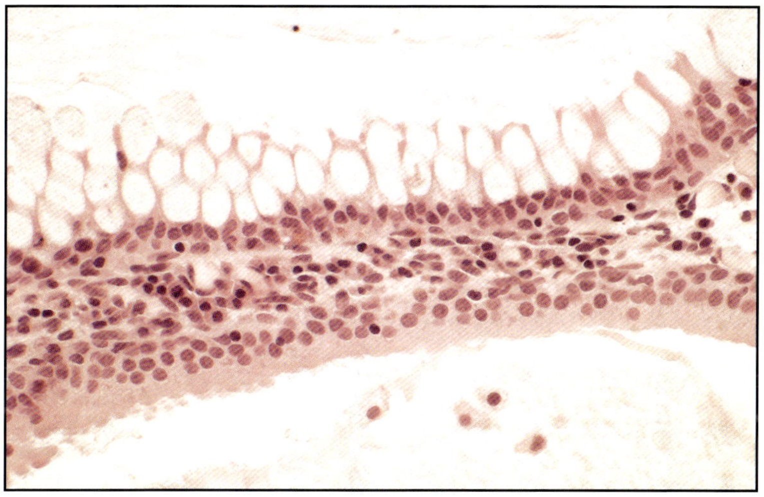

■ **i23.11** *Epithelial lining of urethritis glandularis of intestinal type (above) and usual type (below).*

■ **t23.5 Prostatic Urethral Nephrogenic "Metaplasia (Adenoma)"**

Study	No. of patients	Age	Previous history	Clinical presentation/ Cystoscopic appearance
Martin 1981	2	74	TURP	Painless hematuria/"peculiar shaggy tissue"
		64	TURP	BPH/no cystoscopic abnormality
Berger 1981	3	72[1]	Suprapubic prostatectomy	Painless gross hematuria/polyps
		76	TURP	Gross hematuria/papillary lesion
		59[1]	TURP	Dysuria, frequency, microhematuria/small papillary and cystic lesions
Bhagavan 1981	1	NA[2]	NA	NA
Walker 1983	1	70	NA	Microscopic hematuria/papillary, frond-like
Ford 1985	2	NA	TURP	NA
Young 1992	2	65[3]	TURP	Voiding difficulty/NA
		68[3]	TURP	Voiding difficulty/NA
Daroca 1993	3	66[3]	TURP	Painless gross hematuria/diffuse papillary fronds
		70[3]	—	Urinary frequency, microscopic hematuria/NA
		77[3]	TURP	Incontinence, pyuria, hematuria/0.5cm lesion
Malpica 1994	8	65[3] (Range 44-76)	4:TURP 2:TURBT[4]	7:urinary obstruction/1:urethral lesion
Allan 2001	26	66 (Range 44-76)	NA	Obstructive symptoms most common

[1]Bladder and prostatic urethra involved
[2]NA = Not available
[3]Extension into prostatic parenchyma
[4]TURBT:Transurethral resection of bladder tumor

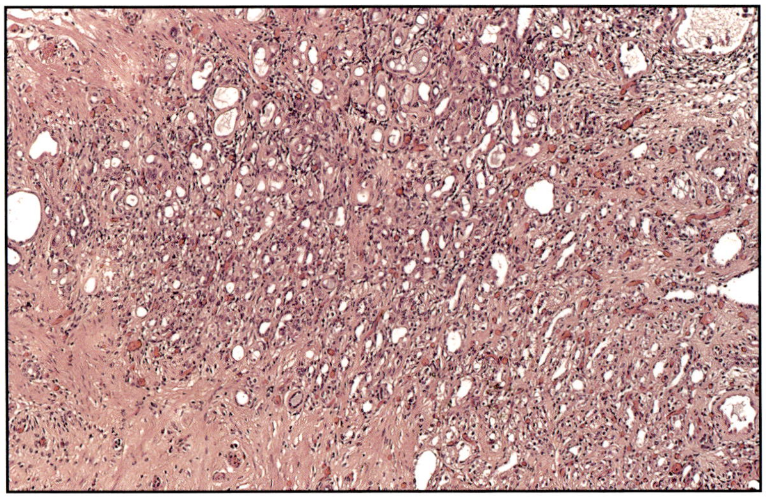

■ **i23.12** *Nephrogenic "metaplasia", tubular pattern.*

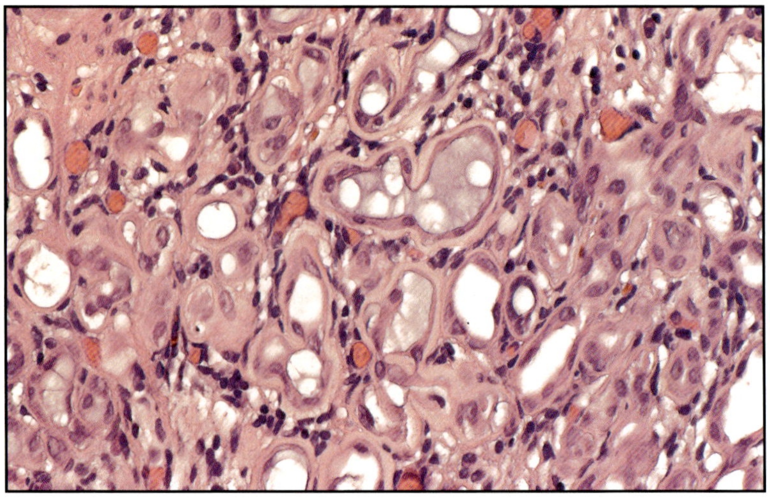

■ **i23.13** *Nephrogenic "metaplasia," tubular pattern (higher magnification of* **i23.12***).*

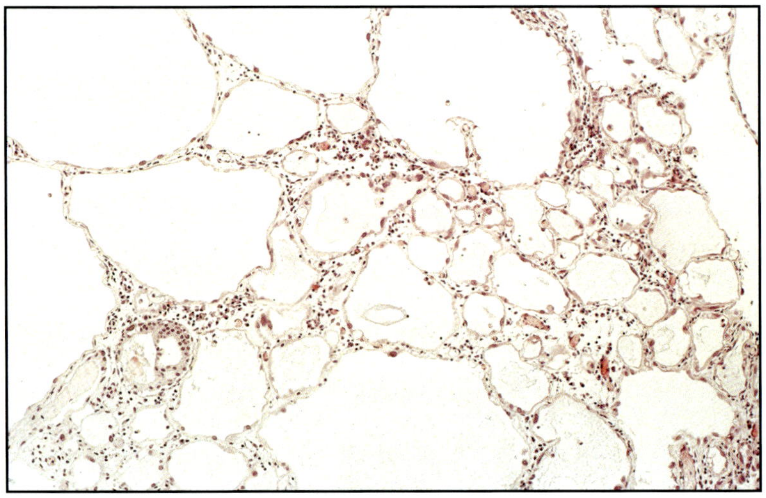

■ **i23.14** *Nephrogenic "metaplasia," cystic pattern.*

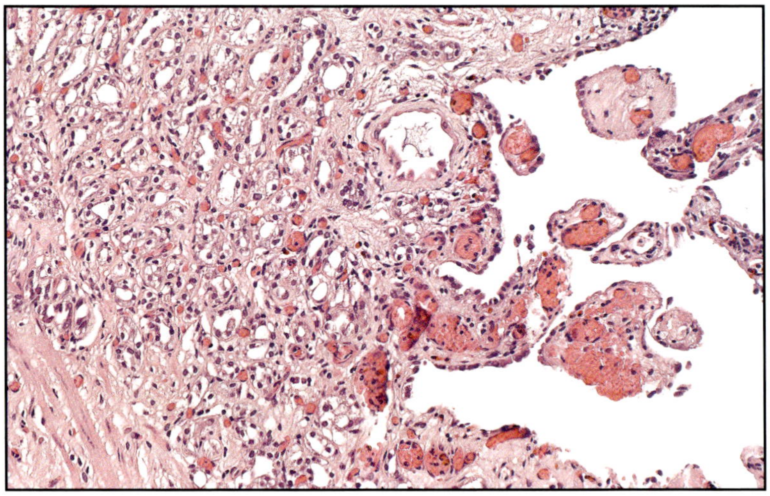

■ **i23.15** *Nephrogenic "metaplasia" with admixed surface papillary structures and underlying tubules.*

(59%) exhibited an extension into the prostatic parenchyma. Clinically, patients with prostatic urethral nephrogenic "metaplasia" are adults (with a mean age of 66) who almost always had undergone a previous surgical procedure, usually TURP. This procedure was done 1.5-10 years prior to detection of the nephrogenic "metaplasia". Hematuria and urinary obstruction are the most common clinical presentations. By cystoscopy/urethroscopy, papillary urethral lesions may often be identified and may simulate a papillary carcinoma (Young 1997B). In other cases, the nephrogenic "metaplasia" can present as an incidental, microscopic finding. Prostatic urethral lesions of nephrogenic "metaplasia" are usually quite small, with a mean size per focus of about 3mm (range 1mm-9mm) (Allan 2001). Microscopically, the classical architectural patterns are tubular **i23.12, i23.13**, cystic **i23.14**, and papillary/polypoid **i23.15; t23.6** (Allan 2001, Friedman 1950, Oliva 1995, Young 1997B). These growth configurations are often admixed **i23.15**. The tubular pattern is overall the most common one in the urinary tract and is consistently found in prostatic urethral nephrogenic "metaplasia" (Allan 2001). The tubules are usually small and round to oval **i23.13**, but cystic tubular dilatation of varying degrees may be present **i23.14**. A minority of the open tubules exhibit "thyroidization" (Allan 2001) and contain an eosinophilic, colloid-like, intraluminal material (Malpica 1994). Intraluminal wispy blue mucin can also be seen (Allan 2001). Occasionally, solid tubules or cords can be found (Allan 2001, Bhagavan 1981, Martin 1981): When sectioned obliquely, the tubules can appear elongated and can even be seen to infiltrate as single cells (Young 1992). A third kind of growth is papillary or polypoid, and surface papillary change is common (Malpica 1994). In the prostatic urethra this is an exophytic expansion, although endophytic expansion of papillary and polypoid structures into complex rarifying tubules or cysts is possible (Young 1997B). A diffuse

■ t23.6 **Nephrogenic "Metaplasia (Adenoma)": Histomorphologic Diagnosis**

Architecture:
- tubular
- cystic
- papillary/polypoid

Small round tubules to cystically dilated tubules
Surface papillary change
Architectural patterns admixed
Tubules lined by cuboidal to flattened cells with occasional "hobnail" cells
Nucleoli typically not conspicuous but may be focally prominent
Mitoses undetectable to rare

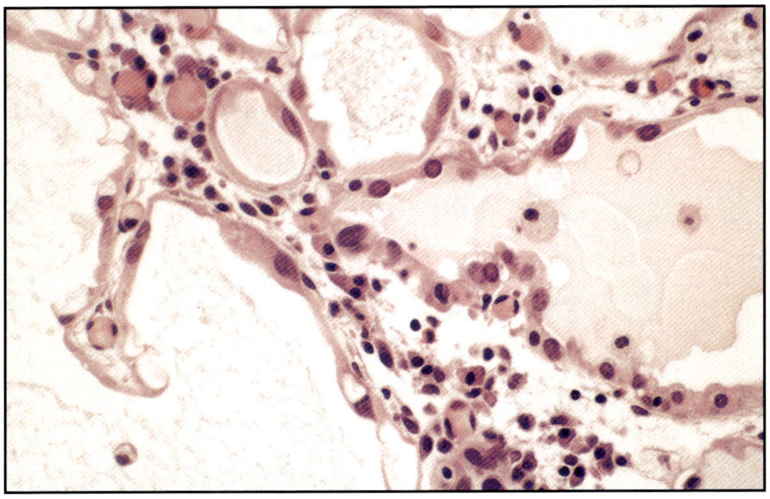

■ **i23.16** *Flattened epithelial lining cells in cystic nephrogenic "metaplasia." A slight degree of nuclear atypia (in the form of nuclear enlargement) is present, secondary to inflammation.*

pattern has been described in the urinary tract (Oliva 1995), but this pattern has not been reported in the prostatic urethra. In the tubules, the constituent metaplastic cells usually create a single-cell–lining layer and are cuboidal to flattened **i23.13, i23.16**. The flattening can generate a vascular-like appearance (Allan 2001). Distinctive "hobnail" cells can sometimes be appreciated. There is usually little nuclear atypia, although prominent nucleoli may occasionally be discerned. The cytoplasm is variable, moderate to scant, and eosinophilic or clear. Occasionally, cytoplasmic vacuolar indentation of the nucleus results in signet ring–like change (Allan 2001). Mitotic figures are absent to rare. The stromal background is not desmoplastic, but rather are often edematous; most cases display an associated acute and chronic inflammatory cell infiltrate (Allan 2001).

The most important special study is an immunohistochemistry marker panel. The most important stains are PSA, pan-cytokeratin, epithelial membrane antigen, PSAP, and carcinoembryonic antigen (CEA) **t23.7**. Focal labeling of high molecular weight cytokeratins (using antibody 34βE12) has been found (Allan 2001, Malpica 1994), along with immunopositivity for cytokeratin 7, vimentin, Leu-M1, CA-125, and CA19-9 (Allan 2001, Engelsgjerd 1999). Other special studies, including histochemical stains and electron microscopy, are not of diagnostic utility. Although basement membrane thickening has been described as a distinguishing feature of nephrogenic "metaplasia" (Epstein 1995), it is prominent in only a small minority (3%) of cases (Oliva 1995), and periodic acid Schiff (PAS) stains do not reveal basement membrane thickening in prostatic urethral nephrogenic "metaplasia" (Malpica 1994). Mucin histochemical stains (Alcian blue and PAS) exhibit focal cytoplasmic and luminal surface positivity and are also not diagnostically useful. Electron microscopy has been performed on nephrogenic "metaplasia" (Bhagavan 1981), but is not of routine diagnostic utility.

■ **t23.7 Immunophenotype of Nephrogenic "Metaplasia"**

Pan-cytokeratin +
CK7+
High molecular weight cytokeratin (detected by 34βE12) variable; negative in 44% of cases
Epithelial membrane antigen +
Carcinoembryonic antigen –
Prostate specific antigen usually negative; weak staining in up to 10% of cases
Prostate specific acid phosphatase usually negative; weak staining in up to 30% of cases

The differential diagnosis of prostatic urethral nephrogenic "metaplasia" includes both benign and malignant entities (Bhagavan 1981, Daroca 1993, Malpica 1994, Martin 1981, Young 1992). When the tubules extend into the prostate, the differential should encompass those conditions that have small tubules, such as sclerosing adenosis, atypical adenomatous hyperplasia (adenosis), atrophy, basal cell hyperplasia, and mesonephric remnant hyperplasia. Nephrogenic "metaplasia" does not possess spindled cells like the rare sclerosing adenosis of the prostate and is not a circumscribed nodule like atypical adenomatous hyperplasia. Individual tubules of nephrogenic "metaplasia" with flattened cells can easily mimic prostatic atrophy, but atrophic prostatic glands usually have a lobular arrangement, whereas nephrogenic "metaplasia" tubules appear more dispersed. Basal cell hyperplasia can present as tubules, but those are multilayered in contrast to the single-layered nephrogenic "metaplasia" tubules. Finally, the rare mesonephric remnant hyperplasia may show substantial morphologic overlap with nephrogenic "metaplasia", as both may reveal small tubules with intraluminal, eosinophilic, colloid-like material. Immunohistochemical reactions are of value in demonstrating 34βE12 positivity in all of the above-mentioned conditions, except nephrogenic "metaplasia", where the reactivity is negative or focal. Additionally, PSA and PSAP will be positive in adenosis but typically not in nephrogenic "metaplasia." Cystically dilated tubules in nephrogenic "metaplasia" may be mistaken for lymphangioma (Oliva 1995); immunopositivity of nephrogenic "metaplasia" for pan-cytokeratin, with a lack of CD31, CD34, and Factor VIII-related antigen immunoreactivity, will help establish the diagnosis of nephrogenic "metaplasia." A papillary/polypoid nephrogenic "metaplasia" could be confused with papillary polypoid urethritis, condyloma acuminatum, and prostatic urethral polyps. The finding of admixed single-cell–layered tubules will aid in the recognition of nephrogenic "metaplasia". Also, the nephrogenic metaplastic papillae are covered by a single layer of cuboidal to columnar cells compared with the multilayered epithelium of papillary/polypoid cystitis. Of interest, a case of physically combined papillary cystitis–papillary nephrogenic "metaplasia" has been reported (Oliva 1995).

Malignant proliferations that should be considered before diagnosing nephrogenic "metaplasia" include adenocarcinoma of the prostate (Daroca 1993, Malpica 1994, Young 1992) of both acinar and ductal types, papillary transitional cell carcinoma, and clear cell urethral adenocarcinoma. The presence of surface papillae, solid tubules, edematous stroma, positive 34βE12 immunoreactivity, and lack of PSA/PSAP immunostaining will all favor nephrogenic "metaplasia" over a typical small acinar adenocarcinoma of the prostate. Rarely, low-grade transitional cell carcinomas form bland-appearing nests (nested variant of transitional cell carcinoma) or tubules that may mimic nephrogenic "metaplasia" (Friedman 1950, Murphy 1992, Talbert 1989, Young 1998). Of importance, the tubules of urothelial carcinoma are multilayered with urothelial cells at the periphery. Cystic change and flattened cells (atrophic-type change) may be seen in both nephrogenic "metaplasia" and prostatic adenocarcinoma (Cina 1997, Egan 1997, Kaleem 1998). Papillary structures can be appreciated in nephrogenic "metaplasia," acinar prostatic adenocarcinoma (Humphrey 1998), ductal prostatic adenocarcinoma, and papillary transitional cell carcinoma. The papillae of nephrogenic "metaplasia" are morphologically distinguishable from these malignant proliferations, as they tend to arise from the urethral surface and possess a single-cell–lining layer of bland, cuboidal cells. The diagnostic separation of nephrogenic "metaplasia" and clear cell adenocarcinoma has historically been a challenge, particularly in small biopsies. Consideration of a combination of clinical and histologic findings are helpful in addressing this problem in the bladder (Young 1997B). Clear cell carcinoma is vanishingly rare in the prostatic urethra (Cantrell 1981, Gilcrease 1998, Oliva 1996). These patients lack a previous surgical history. Clear cell carcinomas of the urinary tract are commonly large, with a diffuse proliferation of cytologically atypical clear cells with mitotic figures readily identifiable. Cytoplasmic clearing is usually not pronounced in nephrogenic "metaplasia," and such clear cells should not form sheets or exhibit mitoses. Nephrogenic "adenomas" have a low proliferation index (mean = 2.8%, range 0%-6.5%) compared with clear cell carcinoma (mean = 23.5%, range 16.5%-25.5%), as judged by MIB-1 immunolabeling (Gilcrease 1998). This is a potentially helpful, although usually not requisite, differential diagnostic tool. A final trap is that nephrogenic "metaplasia" may contain signet ring–like cells that should not be interpreted as signet ring carcinoma (Allan 2001, Young 1997B).

Nephrogenic "metaplasia" is a benign condition without convincing evidence for premalignant status (McIntire 1987, Oliva 1995). Treatment usually entails surgical excision and fulguration. In the urinary tract in general, recurrence or persistence has been found in 37% of cases (McIntire 1987). In the largest series of prostatic urethral nephrogenic "metaplasia" with follow-up, one of eight patients experienced recurrence (Malpica 1994).

[23.5] Prostatic Urethral Epithelial Polyps

Prostatic urethral epithelial polyps are benign polypoid to papillary structures that project into the prostatic urethra **t23.8**. A variety of diagnostic labels have been affixed to this entity, including ectopic prostatic tissue, benign polyps with prostatic-type epithelium, adenomatous polyps with prostatic-type epithelium, villous polyp, papilloma, papillary adenoma, urethral adenoma, glandular polyps, and even prostatic caruncle. These polyps were initially thought to represent ectopic prostatic tissue displaced because of a developmental anomaly (Cantrell 1981), but they have also been viewed as prolapsed prostatic ducts, mucosal redundancy, metaplasia, hyperplasia, and neoplasia (Baroudy 1984, Butterick 1971, Goldstein 1981, Remick 1984, Sogbein 1989, Walker 1989, Zeid 1986). They are most likely hyperplastic, representing an exaggerated, proliferative expansion of a preexisting, normally undulating (Chan 1987) to micropapillary (Sogbein 1989) prostatic urethral mucosa.

t23.8 Prostatic Urethral Epithelial Polyps

Clinically: Younger men with hematuria
Grossly (by cystourethroscopy): Small papillary structures on verumontanum
Histologically:
- Papillae covered by benign prostatic to transitional epithelium
- Fibrovascular cores with benign prostatic acini
- Little to no inflammation

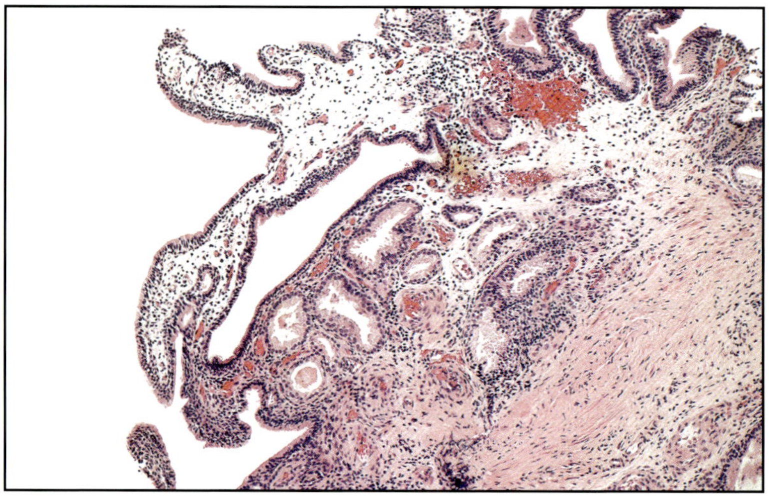

i23.17 *Prostatic urethral epithelial polyp.*

About 200 cases have been reported, and no doubt these polyps are even more common than this number might suggest. Men anywhere from 13 to 84 years of age have been diagnosed with prostatic urethral epithelial polyps. Many series, including the larger ones (Baroudy 1984, Butterick 1971, Hara 1977) have emphasized that younger adults, aged 27-41, are often affected, but it is clear that older men are affected as well. Most patients present with hematuria, but hemospermia, dysuria, and prostatism have also been chief complaints. A classical history is hematuria in a young man. By cystourethroscopy, these have been grossly characterized as small papillary or frondlike exophytic tissues or polyps that are often on the verumontanum or at its base (Butterick 1971). A few have been noted to be sessile nodules. Very few macroscopic-size measurements have been provided, but these masses usually are less than 1cm. Most appear to be single, but the polyps can be multiple and involve long segments of the urethra (Craig 1975).

Microscopically, there is papillary to polypoid growth of true fibrovascular cores lined by columnar prostatic epithelium and/or transitional epithelium **i23.17**, with embedded benign-appearing prostatic acini in the cores (Walker 1989). These acini have a typical secretory columnar cell layer with underlying basal cells. Cytologically, the secretory cells are bland without nuclear aberrations such as nucleomegaly or nucleolomegaly. No mitotic figures are evident in the epithelium. Corpora amylacea are often discovered within the prostatic glands. The fibrovascular cores usually possess little to no lymphocytic inflammation, little to no smooth muscle, and occasional ectatic vessels. Immunohistochemical evaluation has revealed strong and diffuse PSA and PSAP immunoreactivity in the surface glandular columnar cells and acini (Anjum 1997, Chan 1987, Eglen 1984, Lubin 1984, Remick 1984, Zeid 1986).

In the differential diagnosis it is important to exclude neoplastic papillary proliferations including villous adenoma, papillary transitional cell neoplasms, and ductal adenocarcinoma of the prostate (Epstein 1992). Villous adenomas of the prostatic urethra have an appearance like that of colonic villous adenomas, whereas papillary transitional cell neoplasms of the urethra would not have admixed prostatic epithelium. Prostatic ductal adenocarcinomas can also project into the prostatic urethra but have pseudostratified columnar cells with a degree of nuclear atypia ranging from mild to marked. These ductal cancers can grow within prostatic glands as in situ flat or comedo proliferations with clearly malignant lining cells or as fused papillary structures with slit-like glandular spaces. Rarely, prostatic epithelial polyps may manifest nuclear atypia in the form of stratification of elongated nuclei in cells with an increased nuclear to cytoplasmic ratio (Malpica 1994, Walker 1982, Walker 1989). The relationship of this adenomatous-like change to villous adenomas or prostatic duct adenocarcinomas is not clear, but there is a single case report of a ductal prostatic adenocarcinoma arising in a prostatic epithelial polyp that had some villous adenoma-like areas with elongated, pseudostratified nuclei (Walker 1982). Rarely, implants of papillary adenocarcinoma of the bladder may seed the prostatic urethra (Reuter 1997). Here, the clinical history and a comparison with previous biopsy slides are helpful in establishing the correct diagnosis.

Prostatic urethral epithelial polyps are benign lesions that are treated by cystoscopic excision and fulguration. Recurrences have been uncommon (n = 8) (Hara 1977, Kobayashi 1992, Mori 1995, Mostofi 1973, Zeid 1986); in the one case where the original lesion and the recurrence were compared (Mori 1995), the histologic features were the same.

[23.6] Urothelial Hyperplasia

Urothelial hyperplasia has recently been classified as flat and papillary (Epstein 1998). Flat urothelial hyperplasia was defined as "marked" thickening of the urothelium without reliance upon a specific numerical cutoff for the number of cell layers **i23.18**. No cytologic atypia should be evident in the urothelial cells (Epstein 1998). Flat urothelial hyperplasia is a nonspecific proliferation that does not possess premalignant potential (Epstein 1998). Papillary urothelial hyperplasia is more difficult to define but has been characterized as being an "undulating or papillary growth lined by urothelium of varying thickness, lacking atypia" (Epstein 1998). It lacks a well-developed fibrovascular core (Epstein 1998). Papillary urothelial hyperplasia probably in the past has been applied to some cases of papillary/polypoid urethritis. One should not confuse papillary urothelial hyperplasia with papillary urothelial neoplasia, which does have true fibrovascular cores. It is not settled whether papillary urothelial hyperplasia is a risk factor for subsequent detection of urothelial neoplasia, although data suggesting that it is a risk factor do exist (Chow 2000, Taylor 1996).

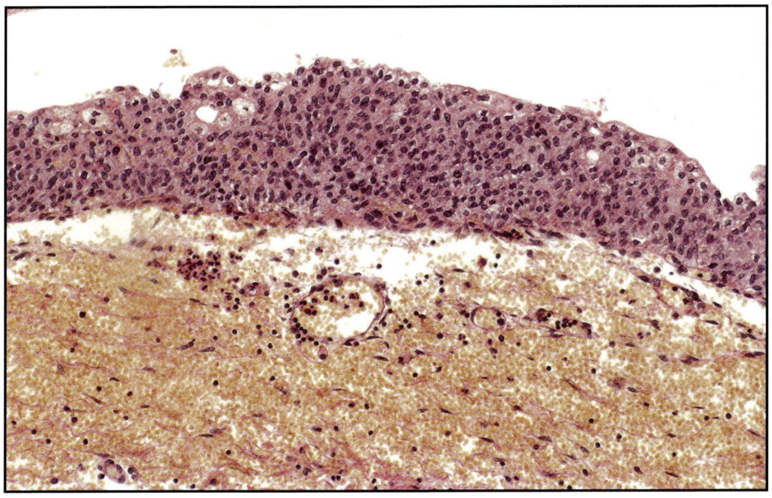

■ **i23.18** *Prostatic urethral urothelial hyperplasia, flat type.*

[23.7] Benign Neoplasms

Villous Adenoma

Villous adenomas are rare (n = 3) in the prostatic urethra (Algaba 1988, Maung 1988, Tran 1996). These adenomas have the same appearance as colonic villous adenomas, with stratification of elongated atypical nuclei, goblet cells, and mitotic figures. In one case (Tran 1996), mucinous adenocarcinoma was reported to arise from a prostatic urethral villous adenoma.

Transitional Cell (Urothelial) Papilloma

Transitional cell (urothelial) papilloma of the urothelium is in general a controversial diagnosis with some transitional cell neoplasm classification and grading systems recognizing this designation and some not (Bergkvist 1965, Epstein 1998, Murphy 1994). The incidence of transitional cell papillomas is likewise completely unsettled, with published estimates of 1%-25% of all transitional cell neoplasms (Amin 1997A, Murphy 1994). Several authorities consider transitional cell carcinoma grade 1 in the World Health Organization scheme (Reuter 1997) and other schemes (Amin 1997A) to be transitional cell papillomas. Isolated papillomas of the prostatic urethra, without urothelial tumors elsewhere in the urinary tract, are rare (Grabstald 1973). The histomorphologic features are the same as for urinary bladder transitional cell papillomas, namely the arrangement of normal-thickness urothelial cells of normal cytology on thin, single, delicate, fibrovascular stalks (Bergkvist 1965). Cytologic normality here is typified by a lack of nuclear enlargement, homogenous chromatin, no prominent nucleoli, no pleomorphism, and absent to rare mitotic figures. The differential diagnosis includes all of the diseases that produce papillary/polypoid masses in the urethra **t23.2**, with the main diagnostic problem being the distinction from papillary urethritis, papillary neoplasms of low malignant potential (Epstein 1998), and low-grade transitional cell carcinoma. Papillomas should lack the inflammation of papillary/polypoid cystitis. Various criteria have been forwarded to separate papillomas from papillary neoplasms of low malignant potential (Epstein 1998) and from low-grade transitional cell carcinoma (Bergkvist 1965, Eble 1989, Murphy 1997), but only recently has there been a convergence to a consensus on these diagnostic criteria (Epstein 1998). In this recent consensus conference, the major means of separating papilloma from papillary urothelial neoplasm of low malignant potential is that in the latter entity the urothelium is much thicker and/or nuclei are significantly enlarged (Epstein 1998). In comparison, papillary urothelial carcinoma of a low grade exhibits architectural and cytologic variation with minimal but definite nuclear pleomorphism (Epstein 1998). Transitional cell papillomas do constitute a risk factor for the development of new tumors (Murphy 1997, Reuter 1997), and therefore patients should be clinically followed in a surveillance program.

Inverted Papilloma

Inverted papillomas are also rare in the prostatic urethra (Cameron 1976, De Meester 1975, Kunze 1983, Lopez 1997, Renfer 1988, Trites 1969), and it is estimated that prostatic urethral inverted papillomas comprise only

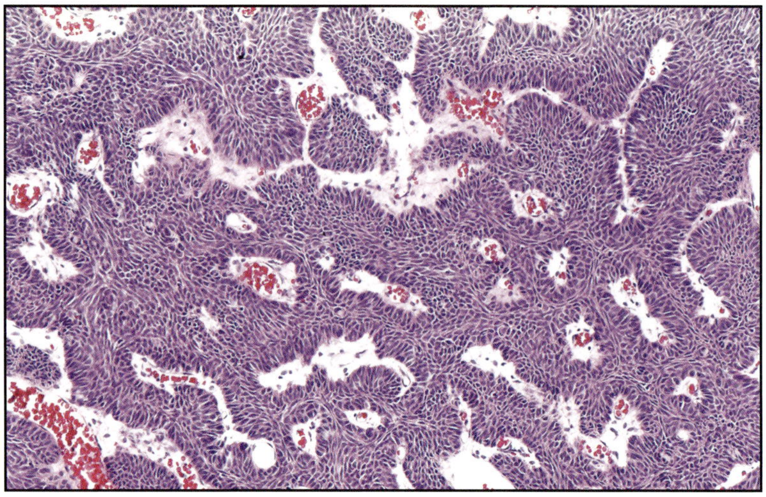

■ **i23.19** *Interdigitating columns of inverted papilloma.*

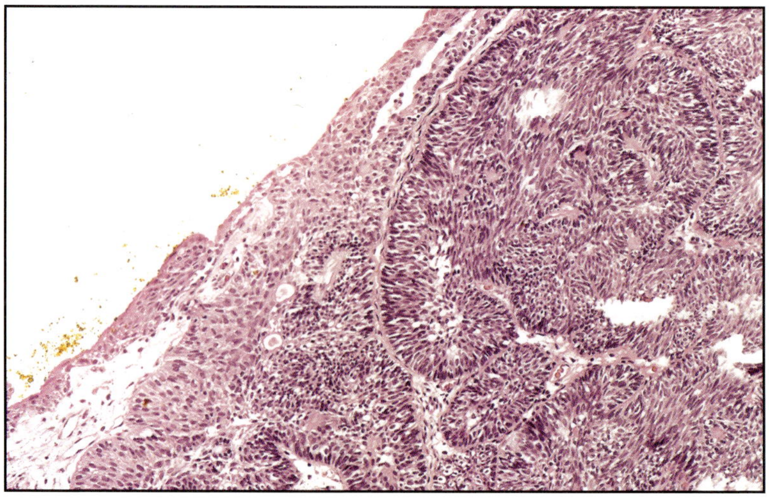

■ **i23.20** *Inverted papilloma, with suburothelial nests merging with surface urothelium.*

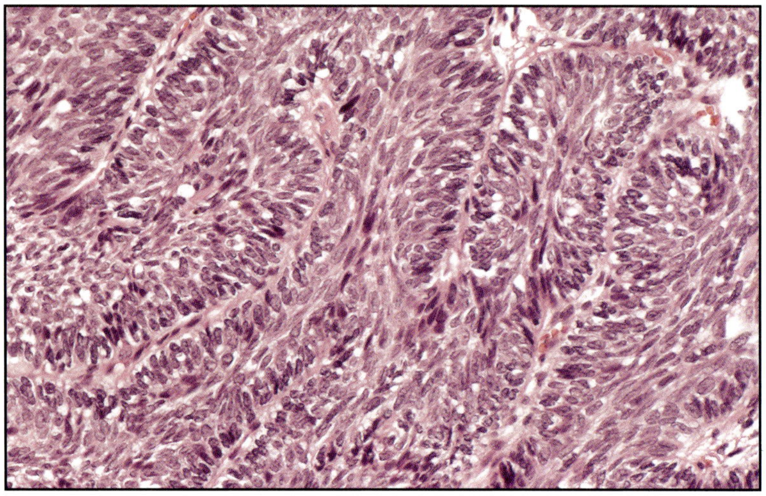

■ **i23.21** *Inverted papilloma with peripheral palisaded cells and central spindled cells.*

3.5% of all inverted papillomas of the urinary tract (Cameron 1976, Kunze 1983). Patients are usually older than 50 and present with hematuria, although a few cases have been incidental discoveries in transurethrally resected prostatic chips (Lopez 1997, Trites 1969). The endoscopic (gross) and microscopic appearances are similar to those of the more common inverted papilloma of the bladder. By urethroscopy, inverted papillomas are smooth-surfaced nodules or sessile polyps. They can range up to 2.5 cm in the urethra (Trites 1969). Histologically, the essential features are anastomosing bars and columns of urothelium **i23.19**, which are contiguous with a thinned surface epithelium **i23.20**. Nests are also seen. Trabecular and glandular subtypes, which serve diagnostic recognition purposes, have been described (Trites 1969). The moniker of inverted refers to the presence of fibrovascular tissue surrounding urothelium, rather than forming a core, as in exophytic, papillary transitional cell neoplasms. The urothelial cells are aligned perpendicular to the basement membrane at the periphery of the cellular masses, whereas cells in the center tend to spindle and stream in an orientation parallel to the basement membrane **i23.21**. Central microcyst formation, with or without glands resembling cystitis cystica and glandularis, and nonkeratizing squamous metaplasia are common. The main differential diagnostic concern is to exclude a transitional cell carcinoma with inverting or endophytic growth features. It has been emphasized that inverting carcinoma has thicker and more irregular columns of cells than inverted papilloma and that the cells do not exhibit peripheral palisading and central streaming (Eble 1997). Nuclear atypia and mitotic figures should be lacking or scarce in inverted papillomas and present in inverting carcinomas. Inverted papillomas are benign; a single recurrence in the prostatic urethra has been reported (De Meester 1975).

Hemangioma

Another benign neoplasm that has rarely been found in the prostatic urethra is the hemangioma (Furuya 1997). Leiomyomas are the most common mesenchymal neoplasm overall in the entire urethra (Reuter 1997), but have not been reported in the prostatic urethra.

[23.8] Dysplasia

The diagnostic recognition and classification of urothelial dysplasia are fraught with controversy (Amin 1997A). Very recently, urologic pathologists have formulated a new classification system called the World Health Organization/International Society of Urologic Pathologists (WHO/ISUP) Consensus Classification for urothelial atypias and proliferations (Epstein 1998) **t23.9**. Although devised for the bladder, this scheme can also be applied to all urothelium, including that of the prostatic urethra. In this scheme, intraurothelial atypias are grouped as follows:

1. Reactive atypia;
2. Dysplasia (low-grade intraurothelial neoplasia);
3. Carcinoma in situ (high-grade intraurothelial neoplasia).

It can be difficult to impossible to morphologically distinguish reactive urothelial atypia from low-grade dysplasia. Also, high-grade dysplasia morphologically merges with carcinoma in situ. Due to these difficulties, little data exist on the clinical significance of dysplasia in the prostatic urethra.

Urothelial dysplasia in the prostatic urethra is most often seen in the setting of bladder carcinoma, with an incidence of 12% in one

■ **t23.9 World Health Organization/International Society of Urologic Pathology Consensus Classification of Urothelial (Transitional Cell) Lesions of the Urinary Bladder**

I. Normal urothelium
II. Hyperplasia
  Flat
  Papillary
III. Flat lesions with atypia
  Reactive (inflammatory) atypia
  Atypia of unknown significance
  Dysplasia (low-grade intraurothelial neoplaisa)
  Carcinoma in situ (high-grade intraurothelial neoplasia)
IV. Papillary neoplasms
  Papilloma
  Inverted papilloma
  Papillary neoplasm of low malignant potential
  Papillary carcinoma, low-grade
  Papillary carcinoma, high-grade
V. Invasive neoplasms
  Lamina propria invasion
  Muscularis propria (detrusor muscle) invasion

Epstein 1998

series (Coutts 1985). Unsuspected, incidental urothelial dysplasia may be found in 1.9% (31/1615) of open or transurethral prostatectomy specimens (Bryan 1993). Of this 1.9%, seven patients (0.4%) had high-grade dysplasia, and this finding was associated with bladder carcinoma in five cases, including two patients who developed carcinoma years later. Although based on a limited number of patients, these data support the reporting high-grade prostatic urothelial dysplasia, even as an incidental finding.

[23.9] Malignant Neoplasms

Malignancy in the prostatic urethra is most often due to secondary synchronous involvement by transitional cell carcinoma of the bladder (Grabstald 1973). Primary, isolated malignancies of the prostatic urethra are rare and are typically transitional cell (urothelial) carcinomas **t23.10**, whereas more distal primary urethral carcinomas tend to be squamous cell carcinomas (Reuter 1997).

■ **t23.10 Primary Carcinoma of Prostatic Urethra**

Clinical Features
Rare
Common presentation: Hematuria, obstruction, irritative voiding

Histopathologic Features
Transitional cell carcinomas
Flat CIS, papillary, infiltrative or mixture
Low- or high-grade

Differential Diagnosis
Secondary bladder transitional cell carcinoma
Secondary prostatic ductal transitional cell carcinoma
Adenocarcinoma of prostate
Papillary/polypoid urethritis
Reactive urothelial atypia

Primary transitional cell (urothelial) carcinomas of the prostatic urethra in the absence of a bladder primary are exceedingly rare, as is highlighted by the fact that in 25 years at the M.D. Anderson Cancer Center only one patient with primary transitional cell carcinoma of the prostatic urethra was seen (Guinn 1970). Overall, only 32 cases have been reported. Twenty-seven of these cases were clinically detected (Guinn 1970, Hashimoto 1996, Kaplan 1967, Konnak 1980, Mandler 1966, Mullin 1974, Ray 1977), whereas five cases were incidentally recognized (Cohen 1996). Most patients are over 50 years of age, and many present with hematuria or obstructive urinary symptoms. Incidental primary urethral transitional cell carcinoma was found in 5/142 (3.5%) of transurethral resectates from patients with prostatic adenocarcinoma in one series compared with 0/100 patients with benign prostatic hyperplasia (Cohen 1996). A second series did not find such incidental carcinoma in 300 radical prostatectomies performed for prostatic adenocarcinoma (Reese 1992). For the five incidental carcinoma cases, the men were 66-87 years of age, three had noninvasive papillary transitional cell carcinoma (one a grade 1/3 and two grade 2/3), one patient had grade 3/3 invasive transitional cell carcinoma, and one had carcinoma in situ. The lesson from this series is that one should not ignore the prostatic urothelium when evaluating prostate tissues. Very little information is available about the histologic characteristics of clinically detected primary prostatic urethral transitional cell carcinomas, but it may be anticipated that these carcinomas would exhibit the same patterns of growth as those in the bladder (Reese 1992). Accordingly, the tumors may be papillary and noninvasive **i23.22, i23.23**, flat carcinoma in situ,

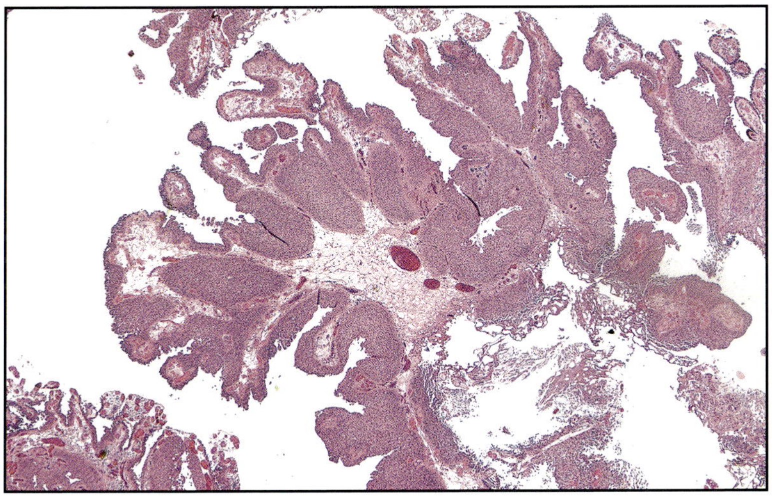

■ **i23.22** *Primary, non-invasive, papillary, prostatic urethral, transitional cell (urothelial) carcinoma, low grade.*

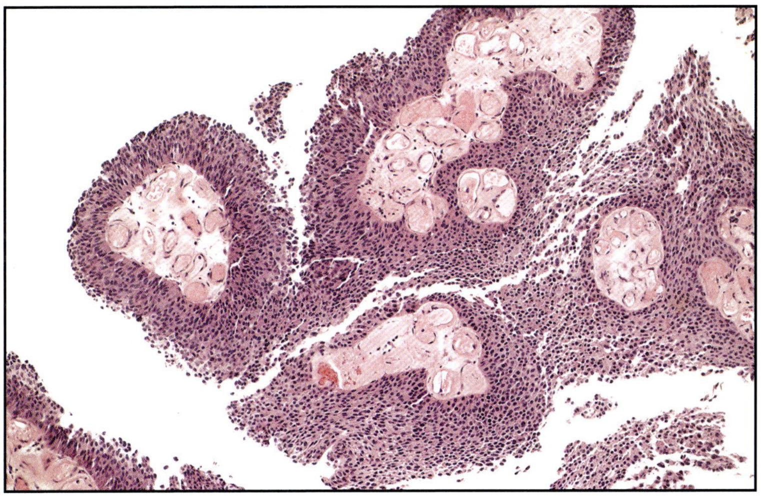

■ **i23.23** *Low-grade papillary transitional cell carcinoma (higher magnification of* **i23.22***).*

■ **t23.11 2002 TNM Staging (AJCC/UICC) of Prostatic Urethral Carcinoma**

Primary Tumor

TX	Primary tumor cannot be assessed
TO	No evidence of primary tumor
Ta	Noninvasive papillary, polypoid, or verrucous carcinoma
Tis	Carcinoma in situ
T1	Tumor invades subepithelial connective tissue
T2	Tumor invades any of the following: corpus spongiosum, prostate, periurethral muscle
T3	Tumor invades any of the following: corpus cavernosum, beyond prostatic capsule or bladder neck
T4	Tumor invades other adjacent organs

Regional Lymph Nodes (N)

NX	Regional lymph nodes cannot be assessed
NO	No regional lymph node metastasis
N1	Metastasis in a single lymph node, 2cm or less in greatest dimension
N2	Metastasis in a single node more than 2cm in greatest dimension or multiple nodes

Distant Metastasis (M)

MX	Distant metastasis cannot be assessed
MO	No distant metastasis
M1	Distant metastasis

Stage Grouping

Stage 0a	Ta	NO	MO
Stage 0is	Tis	NO	MO
Stage I	T1	NO	MO
Stage II	T2	NO	MO
Stage III	T1	N1	MO
	T2	N1	MO
	T3	NO	MO
	T3	N1	MO
StageIV	T4	NO	MO
	T4	N1	MO
	Any T	N2	MO
	Any T	Any N	M1

Greene 2002

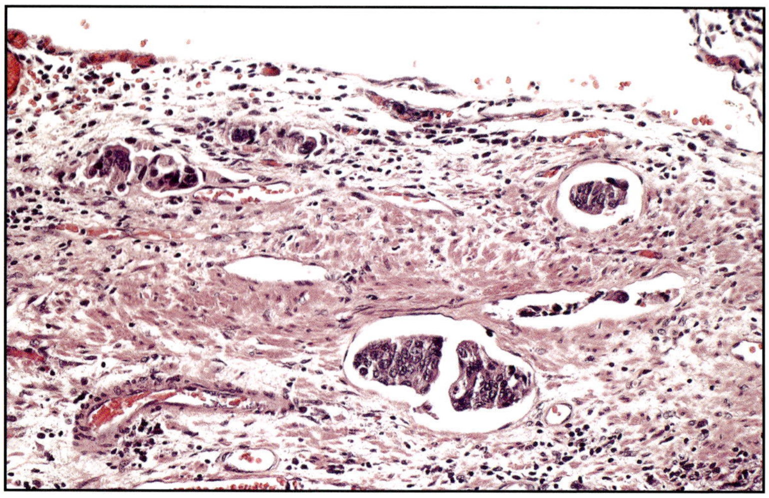

■ **i23.24** *Vascular channel invasion by prostatic urethral transitional cell carcinoma.*

infiltrating, or any combination thereof. The carcinomas may be of any grade; in one series of seven patients there were three low-grade tumors and four high-grade tumors (Mandler 1966). Staging guidelines for primary urethral carcinoma according to the American Joint Committee on Cancer (AJCC) and International Union against Cancer (UICC) recommendations are given in **t23.11** (Greene 2002).

The differential diagnosis of primary transitional cell carcinoma of the prostatic urethra includes the extension of other nonprostatic carcinomas into the prostatic urethra, involvement of the prostatic urethra by transitional cell carcinoma of the bladder, secondary transitional cell carcinoma arising in prostatic ducts, and secondary adenocarcinoma of the prostate. Benign entities that could be mistaken for papillary transitional cell carcinoma of the urethra include prostatic epithelial polyps, papillary/polypoid cystitis, and nephrogenic adenoma with papillary features._

Often it is difficult to ascertain the precise origin of a urethral carcinoma because of infiltrative growth and normal tissue destruction by the tumor (Amin 1997B, Mostofi 1992). Therefore, it may not be feasible in some cases to determine if a large, poorly differentiated transitional cell carcinoma arose from the extraprostatic urethra, large ducts of the prostate, or bladder neck. Acinar adenocarcinoma of the prostate may compress and penetrate through the prostatic urothelium, but the uniformity of the nuclei, lack of a squamoid cytoplasm, lack of urothelial dysplasia or CIS, and immunostaining for PSA and PSAP will substantiate the diagnosis of prostatic carcinoma. Papillary ductal adenocarcinoma of the prostate can grow in suburothelial ducts and erode through the urothelium or may protrude into the urethral lumen from the large prostatic ducts and can be misdiagnosed as a papillary urethral transitional carcinoma. These adenocarcinomas will also stain positively for PSA and PSAP.

Patient prognosis for primary prostatic urethral transitional cell carcinoma is linked to stage and grade of the neoplasm. The 5-year survival rate for patients with superficial disease is 87%, but it is only 37% for patients with invasive tumors (Donat 2002). For patients with noninvasive papillary urethral transitional cell carcinoma, transurethral resection and/or fulguration is sufficient treatment (Donat 2002). Biopsies of the prostate itself should be taken to evaluate for in situ and stromal spread within the substance of the prostate gland. Extensive local invasion is common and the urogenital diaphragm, rectum, prostate, and bladder may be directly invaded (Amin 1997B, Mostofi 1992). If feasible, invasive disease is treated by radical cystoprostatectomy and urethrectomy (Donat 2002). Radiation therapy and chemotherapy have also been used (Grigsby 2000, Donat 2002). Metastasis results from a propensity to invade vascular channels **i23.24**. The lymphatic drainage of the prostatic urethra is to the obturator, internal, and external iliac lymph nodes. Patients with prostatic urethral carcinoma fare worse than patients with more distal urethral carcinomas, most likely because of the advanced stage at presentation.

Histologic types of primary cancer other than transitional cell carcinoma are so rare in the prostatic urethra that their existence is mainly documented by case reports. Several cases of adenocarcinoma have been reported, including two cases of mucinous adenocarcinoma (Algaba 1988); two cases of clear cell adenocarcinoma (Konnak 1980, Oliva 1996); and single cases of papillary adenocarcinoma (Cantrell 1981) and ductal-type adenocarcinoma (Walker 1982). Squamous cell carcinoma has rarely been diagnosed as primary in the prostatic urethra (Heysek 1985). A single case of carcinosarcoma (sarcomatoid carcinoma) has been published (Oweity 2000). A few patients with primary malignant melanoma of the prostatic urethra have been seen (Weiss 1982). Last, a tumor with malignant potential, the paraganglioma, has been diagnosed in the prostatic urethra is a few patients (Badalament 1991, Boyle 1996).

t23.12 Secondary Prostatic Urethral Involvement by Transitional Cell Carcinoma of the Bladder

Reference	Type of Series	No. of Patients	No. With Involvement (%)	Type of Involvement
Farrow 1976	cystoprostatectomy	19	11 (58%)	4 CIS: urethra only; 7:urethra & prostate
Mahadevia 1986	cystoprostatectomy	20	9 (45%)	CIS (2 Pagetoid)
Bretton 1989	biopsy	264	18 (7%)	2 CIS/T1; 4 CIS/Ta; 12 CIS
Orihuela 1989	biopsy	125	15 (12%)	5 Papillary tumors; 10 CIS cases
Wood 1989	cystoprostatectomy	84	34 (40%)	Not specified
Hardeman 1990	cystoprostatectomy	86	8 (9%)	Not specified
Tobisu 1991	cystoprostatectomy	169	18 (11%)	Not specified
Sakamoto 1993	cystoprostatectomy*	134	7 (5%)	Urethral CIS only
Palou 1996	biopsy	210	18 (9%)	CIS
Esrig 1996	cystoprostatectomy	489	7 (1%)	Papillary urethral tumor only
			30 (6%)	Urethral CIS only
			37 (7%)	Only urethra
			87 (18%)	Urethra and prostate
Tobisu 1997	radical cystectomy & urethrectomy	52	23 (44%)	Not specified

*urethral CIS at 5 and/or 7 o'clock of verumontanum predicts prostatic duct and acinar involvement

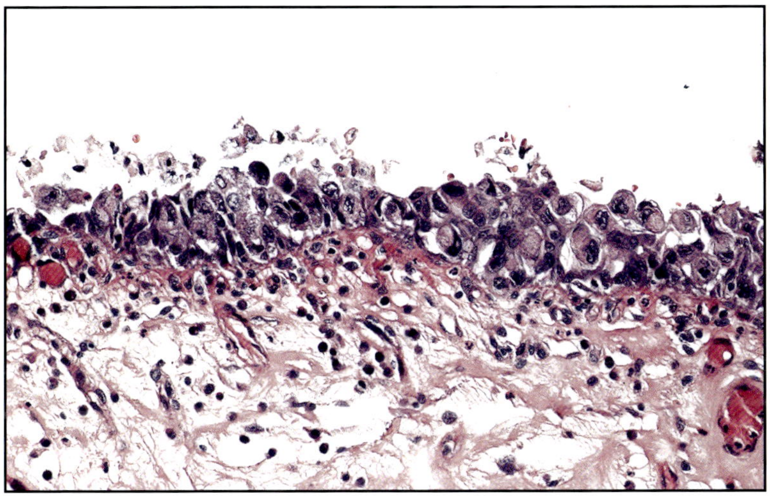

i23.25 *Carcinoma in situ of prostatic urethra: A flat, high-grade urothelial cell carcinoma.*

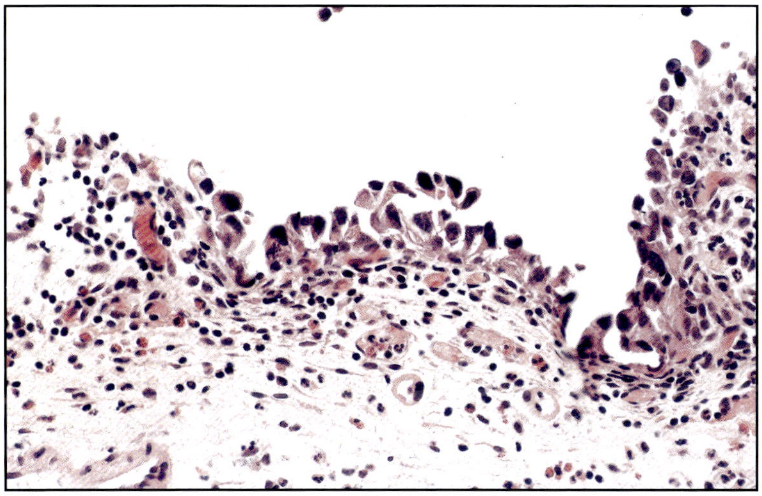

i23.26 *Carcinoma in situ of prostatic urethra with dyscohesive atypical urothelial cells, with nuclear enlargement and hyperchromasia.*

Secondary or concomitant involvement of the prostatic urethra by transitional cell carcinoma of the bladder is frequent, with up to 58% of men so affected **t23.12**. This so-called secondary involvement could represent direct extension, multifocal disease, implantation (seeding), or lymphovascular invasion. The incidence rate, which varies from 5% to 58% **t23.12**, is highly dependent on the degree of urethral sampling, with the highest rates obtained with completely embedded and mapped cystectomy/urethrectomy specimens and the lower rates with limited urethral biopsy. Grossly, secondary urethral involvement by carcinoma may not be visible; papillary tumors are more likely to be visualized than carcinoma in situ. In patients treated with BCG, inflammatory changes in the prostatic urethra secondary to BCG may be difficult to distinguish grossly from carcinoma in situ. Microscopically, direct extension of a bladder tumor into the urethra may manifest itself as pagetoid intraurothelial spread of single neoplastic cells or small clusters of neoplastic cells (Begin 1991, Ortega 1953, Tomaszewski 1985); pure carcinoma in situ **i23.25, i23.26**; noninvasive papillary tumors; or invasive carcinoma **i23.27** with or without a prostatic urethral intraurothelial component. Of these patterns of involvement, carcinoma in situ is the most common **t23.12**. In 70% of cases with prostatic urethral extension, there is also prostatic involvement (either in situ or stromal invasive disease) (Esrig 1990). Urethral carcinoma in situ at the 5 and/or 7 o'clock positions of the verumontanum seems to be highly predictive of prostatic involvement (Sakamoto 1993). Important microscopic evaluations in urethral biopsies performed in patients

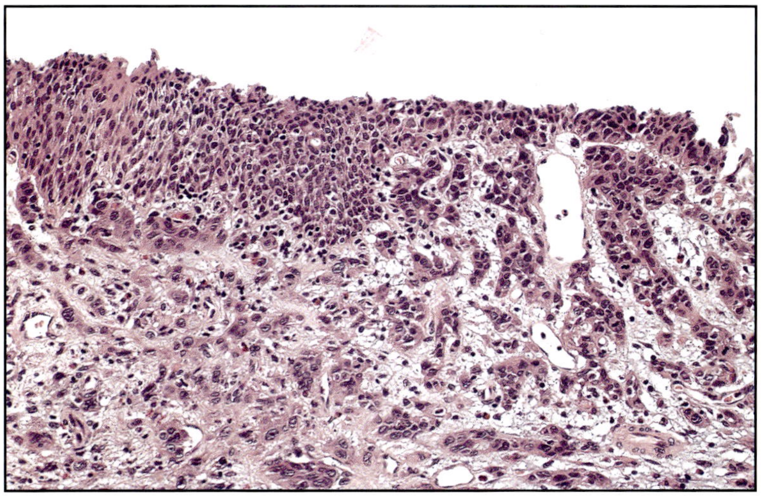

i23.27 *Invasive transitional cell carcinoma of bladder, with extension into prostatic urethra, with undermining pattern of growth. Focal carcinoma in situ is also evident.*

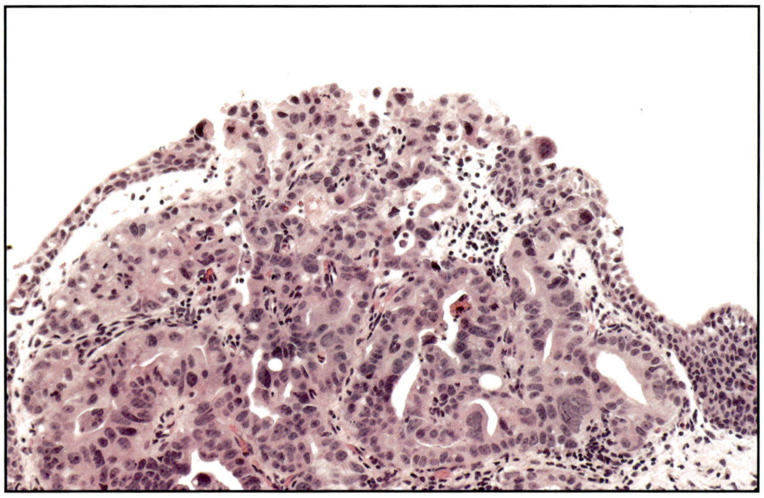

■ **i23.28** *Secondary extension of prostatic ductal adenocarcinoma into and through prostatic urethral surface urothelium.*

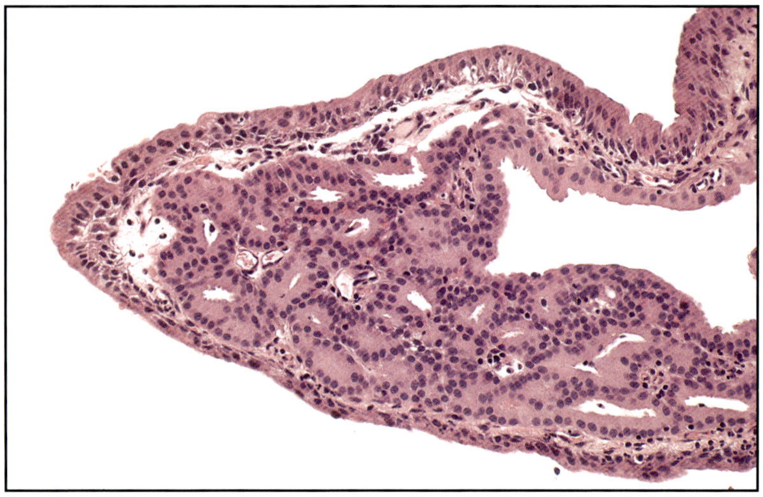

■ **i23.29** *Extension of prostatic acinar adenocarcinoma into suburothelial tissue of prostatic urethra.*

with bladder cancer include assessment for the presence of transitional cell carcinoma and extent of involvement. The anatomic structures involved (such as the urothelium, submucosa, periurethral glands, prostatic ducts and acini, prostatic stroma, and lymphovascular channels) should be specified. Patient survival is strongly linked to prostatic stromal invasion (Herr 1999). Histologic grade of the cancer should be also reported, with the WHO/ISUP scheme recommended (Epstein 1998) **t23.9**.

As previously noted, secondary involvement of the prostatic urethra can also occur in patients with primary transitional cell carcinoma of the large prostatic ducts and primary ductal adenocarcinoma of the prostate. In addition to papillary growth within the urethral lumen, intraductal and invasive growth of ductal adenocarcinomas of the prostate can be located immediately beneath the prostatic urothelium or mucosa, especially at the verumontanum (Dube 1973, Ro 1988) **i23.28**. Usual acinar adenocarcinomas of the prostate can, as previously noted, extend to prostatic urothelium **i23.29**, compress the prostatic urethra, and erode the urothelial surface, but intraurothelial involvement by prostatic adenocarcinoma cells is distinctly unusual. In the assessment of the distal "urethral margin" at the apex in radical prostatectomy specimens, a positive margin does not refer to carcinoma in the urothelium, but rather ink on the carcinoma if a "conization" of the apex is performed (Ayala 1989), or carcinoma anywhere in thin 2mm shave margins (Epstein 1993). Finally, prostatic rhabdomyosarcoma, which is mainly a childhood tumor, may involve the prostatic urethra by direct extension (Keenan 1985, Loughlin 1989). Submucosal urethral growth, which may not be visible by cystoscopy, has been reported (Loughlin 1989). As in the bladder, there may be a concentration of rhabdomyosarcoma cells immediately beneath the prostatic urothelium (Keenan 1985). This suburothelial density is known as the cambium layer. For patients with bladder/prostate rhabdomyosarcoma, careful evaluations of prostatic urethral biopsies and the urethral margin of cystectomy specimens are critical tasks (Loughlin 1989).

References

Algaba F, Matias-Guiu X, Badia F, et al. Villous adenoma of the prostatic urethra. *Eur Urol* 14:255-257, 1988.

Allan CH, Epstein JI. Nephrogenic adenoma of the prostatic urethra. A mimicker of prostate adenocarcinoma. *Am J Surg Pathol* 25:802-808, 2001.

Amin MB, Young RH. Intraepithelial lesions of the urinary bladder with a discussion of the histogenesis of urothelial neoplasia. *Semin Diagn Pathol* 14:84-97, 1997A.

Amin MB, Young RH. Primary carcinomas of the urethra. *Semin Diagn Pathol* 14:147-160, 1997B.

Andersen CB, Horn T, Rasmussen F, et al. Mesonephric remnants involving renal pelvis and prostatic urethra: a diagnostic problem towards adenocarcinoma. *Scand J Urol Nephrol* 157(suppl):119-122, 1994.

Anjum MI, Ahmed M, Shrotri W, et al. Benign polyps with prostatic-type epithelium of the urethra and urinary bladder. *Int Urol Nephrol* 29:313-317, 1997.

Ayala AG, Ro JY, Babaian R, et al. The prostatic capsule: does it exist? Its importance in staging and treatment of prostatic carcinoma. *Am J Surg Pathol* 13:21-27, 1989.

Badalament RA, Kenworthy P, Pellegrini A, et al. Paraganglioma of the urethra. *Urology* 38:76-78, 1991.

Baroudy AC, O'Connell JP. Papillary adenoma of the prostatic urethra. *J Urol* 132:120-122, 1984.

Bégin LR, Deschênes J, Mitmaker B. Pagetoid carcinomatous involvement of the penile urethra in association with high-grade transitional cell carcinoma of the urinary bladder. *Arch Pathol Lab Med*115:632-635, 1991.

Berger BW, Bhagavan SB, Reiner W, et al. Nephrogenic adenoma: clinical features and therapeutic considerations. *J Urol* 126:824-826, 1981.

Bergkvist A, Ljungqvist A, Moberger G. Classification of bladder tumors based on the cellular pattern. *Acta Chir Scand* 130:371-378, 1965.

Bhagavan BS, Tiamson EM, Wenk RE, et al. Nephrogenic adenoma of the urinary bladder and urethra. *Hum Pathol* 12:907-916, 1981.

Bissada NK, Cole AT, Fried FA. Extensive condylomata acuminata of the entire male urethra and bladder. *J Urol* 112:201-203, 1994.

Bostwick DG, Lo R, Stamey TA. Papillary adenocarcinoma of the male urethra. Case report and review of the literature. *Cancer* 54:2556-2563, 1984.

Boyle M, Gaffney EF, Thurston A. Paraganglioma of the prostatic urethra. A report of three cases and a review of the literature. *Br J Urol* 77:445-458, 1996.

Bretton PR, Herr HW, Whitmore WF Jr, et al. Intravesical bacillus Calmette-Guerin therapy for in situ transitional cell carcinoma involving the prostatic urethra. *J Urol* 141:853-856, 1989.

Bruijnes E, de Wall JG, Scholtmeijer RJ, et al. Congenital polyp of the prostatic urethra in childhood. Report of 3 cases and review of the literature. *Urol Int* 40:287-291, 1985.

Bryan RL, Newman J, Suarez V, et al. The significance of prostatic urothelial dysplasia. *Histopathology* 22:501-503, 1993.

Butterick JD, Schnitzer B, Abell MR. Ectopic prostatic tissue in urethra: a clinicopathologic entity and a significant cause of hematuria. *J Urol* 105:97-104, 1971.

Cameron KM, Lupton CH. Inverted papilloma of the lower urinary tract. *Br J Urol.* 1976;48:567-577.

Cantrell BB, Leifer G, DeKlerk DP, et al. Papillary adenocarcinoma of the prostatic urethra with clear cell appearance. *Cancer* 48:2661-2667, 1981.

Chan JKC, Chow TC, Tsui MS. Prostatic-type polyps of the lower urinary tract: three histogenetic types? *Histopathology* 11:789-801, 1987.

Chow N-H, Cairns P, Eisenberger CF, et al. Papillary urothelial hyperplasia is a clonal precursor to papillary transitional cell bladder cancer. *Int J Cancer* 89:514-518, 2000.

Cina SJ, Epstein JI. Adenocarcinoma of the prostate with atrophic features. *Am J Surg Pathol* 21:287-295, 1997.

Cohen RJ, Nixon JM, Robinson E, et al. Transitional cell carcinoma diagnosed at transurethral prostatectomy in patients with prostatic adenocarcinoma. *J Urol Pathol* 5:29-37, 1996.

Coutts AG, Grigor KM, Fowler JW. Urethral dysplasia and bladder cancer in cystectomy specimens. *Br J Urol* 57:535-541, 1985.

Craig JR, Hart WR. Benign polyps with prostatic-type epithelium of the urethra. *Am J Clin Pathol* 63:343-347, 1975.

Daroca PJ Jr, Martin AA, Reed RJ, et al. Urethral nephrogenic adenoma. A report of three cases, including a case with infiltration of the prostatic stroma. *J Urol Pathol* 1:157-172, 1993.

De Meester LJ, Farrow GM, Utz DC. Inverted papillomas of the urinary bladder. *Cancer* 36:505-513, 1975.

DeBenedictis TJ, Marmar JL, Praiss DE. Intraurethral condylomas acuminata: management and review of the literature. *J Urol* 118:767-769, 1977.

Del Mistro A, Braunstein JD, Halwer M, et al. Identification of human papillomavirus types in male urethral condylomata acuminata by in situ hybridization. *Hum Pathol* 18:936-940, 1987.

Donat SM, Cozzi PJ, Herr HW. Surgery of the penile and urethral carcinoma. In: Walsh PC, Retik AB, Vaughn ED Jr, Wein AJ, eds. *Campbell's Urology*. 8th ed. Philadelphia: Saunders; 2983-3000, 2002.

Downs RA. Congenital polyps of the prostatic urethra. A review of the literature and report of two cases. Br *J Urol* 42:76-85, 1970.

Dube VE, Farrow GM, Greene LF. Prostatic adenocarcinoma of ductal origin. *Cancer* 32:402-409, 1973.

Eble JH, Young RK. Benign and low-grade papillary lesions of the urinary bladder. *Semin Diagn Pathol* 6:351-371, 1989.

Eble JN, Young RH. Carcinoma of the urinary bladder: a review of its diverse morphology. *Semin Diagn Pathol* 14:98-108, 1997.

Egan AJM, Lopez-Beltran A, Bostwick DG. Prostatic adenocarcinoma with atrophic features: malignancy mimicking a benign process. *Am J Surg Pathol* 21:931-935, 1997.

Eglen DE, Pontius EE. Benign prostatic epithelial polyp of the urethra. *J Urol* 131:120-122, 1984.

Engelsgjerd M, Swanson PE, Wick MR, et al. Immunophenotypic profiles of nephrogenic adenocarcinoma and urethral adenocarcinoma are more similar than different [abstract]. *Mod Pathol* 12:95A, 1999.

Epstein JI. Prostatic urethral polyp vs. prostatic duct adenocarcinoma. In: *Differential Diagnosis in Pathology. Urologic Disorders.* New York: Igaku-Shoin; 134-135, 1992.

Epstein JI, Pizov G, Walsh PC. Correlation of pathologic findings with progression following radical prostatectomy. *Cancer* 71:3582-3593, 1993.

Epstein JI. Prostatic urethral lesions. In: *Prostate Biopsy Interpretation.* 2nd ed. Philadelphia: Lippincott-Raven; 261-263, 1995.

Epstein JI, Amin MB, Reuter VR, et al, the Bladder Consensus Conference Committee. The World Health Organization/International Society of Urological Pathology consensus classification of urothelial (transitional cell) lesions of the urinary bladder. *Am J Surg Pathol* 22:1435-1448, 1998.

Esrig D, Freeman JA, Elmajian DA, et al. Transitional cell carcinoma involving the prostate with a proposed staging classification for stromal invasion. *J Urol* 156:1071-1076, 1996.

Farrow GM, Utz DC, Rife CC. Morphological and clinical observations of patients with early bladder cancer treated with total cystectomy. *Cancer Res* 36:2495-2501, 1976.

Ford TF, Watson GM, Cameron KM. Adenomatous metaplasia (nephrogenic adenoma) of urothelium. An analysis of 70 cases. *Br J Urol* 57:427-433, 1985.

Foster RS, Garrett RA. Congenital posterior urethral polyps. *J Urol* 136:670-672, 1986.

Frates RE, DeLara FG. Urethral polyps in male children. *Radiology* 89:289-291, 1967.

Friedman NB, Kuhlenbeck H. Adenomatoid tumors of the bladder reproducing renal structures (nephrogenic adenomas). *J Urol* 64:657-670, 1950.

Furuya S, Ogura H, Tanaka Y, et al. Hemangioma of the prostatic urethra: hematospermia and massive postejaculatory hematuria with clot retention. *Int J Urol* 4:524-526, 1997.

Gikas PW, Del Buono EA, Epstein JI. Florid hyperplasia of mesonephric remnants involving prostate and periprostatic tissue. Possible confusion with adenocarcinoma. *Am J Surg Pathol* 17:454-460, 1993.

Gilcrease MZ, Delgado R, Vuitch F, et al. Clear cell adenocarcinoma and nephrogenic adenoma of the urethra and urinary bladder: a histopathologic and immunohistochemical comparison. *Hum Pathol* 29:1451-1456, 1998.

Glancy RJ, Gaman AJ, Rippey JJ. Polyps and papillary lesions of the prostatic urethra. *Pathology* 15:153-157, 1983.

Goldstein AMB, Bragin SD, Terry R, Yoell JH. Prostatic urethral polyps in adults: histopathologic variations and clinical manifestations. *J Urol* 126:129-131, 1981.

Gonzales ET Jr. Posterior urethral valves and other urethral anomalies. In: Walsh PC, Retik AB, Vaughan ED Jr, Wein AJ, eds. *Campbell's Urology.* 8th ed. Philadelphia: WB Saunders; 2207-2230, 2002.

Grabstald H. Tumors of the urethra in men and women. *Cancer* 32:1236-1255, 1973.

Greene FL, Page DL, Fleming ID, et al. *Urethra. AJCC Cancer Staging Manual.* 6th ed. New York: Springer Verlag; 341-343, 2002.

Grigsby PW, Herr HW. Urethral tumors. In: Vogelzang NJ, Shipley WU, Scardino PT, Coffey DS, eds. *Comprehensive Textbook of Genitourinary Oncology.* 2nd ed. Baltimore: Williams & Wilkins; 1133-1140, 2000.

Grussendorf-Conen EI, Deutz FJ, de Villiers EM. Detection of human papillomavirus-6 in primary carcinoma of the urethra in men. *Cancer* 60:1832-1835, 1987.

Guinn GA, Ayala AG. Male urethral cancer: report of 15 cases including a primary melanoma. *J Urol* 103:176-179, 1970.

Hanani Y, Hertz M, Jonas P. Congenital urethral polyp in children. *Urology* 16:162-164, 1980.

Hara S, Horie A. Prostatic caruncle: a urethral papillary tumor derived from prolapse of the prostatic duct. *J Urol* 117:303-305, 1977.

Hardeman SW, Soloway MS. Urethral recurrence following radical cystectomy. *J Urol* 144:666-669, 1990.

Hashimoto K, Ohnishi N, Katoh Y, et al. Primary transitional cell carcinoma of the prostatic urethra: a case report [in Japanese]. *Acta Urol Jpn* 42:385-387 1996.

Herr HW, Donat SM . Prostatic tumor relapse in patients with superficial bladder tumors: 15-year outcome. *J Urol* 161:1854-1857, 1999.

Heysek RV, Parsons JT, Drylie DM, et al. Carcinoma of the male urethra. *J Urol* 134:753-755, 1985.

Hillyard RW Jr, Ladaga L, Schellhammer DF. Superficial transitional cell carcinoma of the bladder associated with mucosal involvement of the prostatic urethra: results of treatment with intravesical bacillus Calmette-Guérin. *J Urol* 139:290-293, 1988.

Huang W-L, Ro JY, Grignon DJ, et al. Postoperative spindle cell nodule of the prostate and bladder. *J Urol* 143:824-826, 1990.

Humphrey PA, Kaleem Z, Swanson PE, et al. Pseudohyperplastic prostatic adenocarcinoma. *Am J Surg Pathol* 22: 1239-1246, 1998.

Jones TJ, Howie AJ. Necropsy study of infarcts of prostate and prostatic urethra. *J Clin Pathol* 39:1221-1223, 1986.

Jordan GH, Schlossberg SM, Devine CJ. Surgery of the penis and urethra. In: Walsh PC, Retik AB, Vaughan ED Jr, Wein AJ, eds. *Campbell's Urology.* 8th ed. Philadelphia: Saunders; 3886-3952, 2002.

Kaleem Z, Swanson PE, Vollmer RT, et al. Prostatic adenocarcinoma with atrophic features: a study of 202 consecutive, completely embedded radical prostatectomy specimens. *Am J Clin Pathol* 109:695-703, 1998.

Kaplan GW, Bulkley GJ, Grayhack JT. Carcinoma of the male urethra. *J Urol* 98:365-371, 1967.

Keenan DJM, Graham WH, Hayes D. Embryonal rhabdomyosarcoma of the prostatic-urethral region in an adult. *Br J Urol* 57:241, 1985.

Kiernan M, Gaffney EF. Brunn's nests and glandular metaplasia. Normal urothelial variants in the supramontanal prostatic urethra. *J Urol* 137:877-879, 1987.

Kimche D, Lask D. Congenital polyp of the prostatic urethra. *J Urol* 127:134, 1982.

Kobayashi Y, Hashimoto S, Ishikawa S, et al. Posterior urethral polyp: a recurrent case. *Acta Urol Jpn* 38:957-958, 1992.

Konnak JW. Conservative management of low grade neoplasms of the male urethra: a preliminary report. *J Urol* 123:175-177, 1980.

Kunze E, Schauer A, Schmitt M. Histology and histogenesis of two different types of inverted urothelial papillomas. *Cancer* 51:348-358, 1983.

Libby JM, Frankel JM, Scardino PT. Condyloma acuminatum of the bladder and associated urothelial malignancy. *J Urol* 134:134-136, 1985.

Lopez JI, Ereno C. Glandular-type inverted papilloma of the prostatic urethra. *Arch Anat Cytol Pathol* 45:227-229, 1997.

Loughlin KR, Retik AB, Weinstein HJ, et al. Genitourinary rhabdomyosarcoma in children. *Cancer* 63:1600-1606, 1989.

Lubin J, Mark TM, Wirtschafter AR. Papillomas of prostatic urethra with prostatic type epithelium: report of eight cases. *Mt Sinai J Med* 51:218-221, 1984.

Madden NP, Turnock RR, Rickwood AMK. Congenital polyps of the posterior urethra in neonates. *J Pediatr Surg* 21:193-194, 1986.

Mahadevia PS, Koss LG, Tar IJ. Prostatic involvement in bladder cancer. Prostate mapping in 20 cystoprostatectomy specimens. *Cancer* 58:2096-2102, 1986.

Malpica A, Ro JY, Troncoso P, et al. Nephrogenic adenoma of the prostatic urethra involving the prostate gland: a clinicopathologic and immunohistochemical study of eight cases. *Hum Pathol* 25:390-395, 1994.

Mandler JI, Pool TL. Primary carcinoma of the male urethra. *J Urol* 96:67-72, 1966.

Martin SA, Santa Cruz DJ. Adenomatoid metaplasia of prostatic urethra. *Am J Clin Pathol* 75:185-189, 1981.

Marya SKS, Kumar S, Singh S. Acquired male urethral diverticulum. *J Urol* 118:765-766, 1977.

Maung R, Kelly JK, Grace DA. Intestinal metaplasia and dysplasia of prostatic urethra secondary to stricture. *Urology* 32:361-363, 1988.

Mazal PR, Schaufler R, Altenhuber-Muller R, et al. Derivation of nephrogenic adenomas from renal tubular cells in kidney transplant recipients. *New Engl J Med* 347:653-659, 2002.

McIntire TL, Soloway MS, Murphy WM. Nephrogenic adenoma. *Urology* 29:237-241, 1987.

Mevorach RA, Cos LR, di Sant'Agnese PA, et al. Human papillomavirus type 6 in grade I transitional cell carcinoma of the urethra. *J Urol* 143:126-128, 1990.

Mori K, Spiro LH, Hecht H, et al. Recurrent intraurethral proliferation of ectopic prostatic tissue associated with hematuria. *J Urol* 114:316-318, 1995.

Mostofi FK. Potentialities of bladder epithelium. *J Urol* 71:705-714, 1954.

Mostofi FK, Price EB Jr. Tumors of the urethra. In: Firminger HI, ed. *Tumors of the Male Genital System.* Washington, DC: Armed Forces Institute of Pathology; 265-266, 1973.

Mostofi FK, Davis CJ Jr, Sesterhenn IA. Carcinoma of the male and female urethra. *Urol Clin N Am* 19:347-358, 1992.

Mullin EM, Anderson EE, Paulson DF. Carcinoma of the male urethra. *J Urol* 112:610-613, 1974.

Murphy DM, Guiney EJ. Polyp of the posterior urethra. *Eur Urol* 8:204-206, 1982.

Murphy WM, Fu YS, Lancaster WD, et al. Papillomatous structural antigens in condyloma acuminatum of the male urethra. *J Urol* 130:84-85, 1983.

Murphy WM, Deana DG. The nested variant of transitional cell carcinoma: a neoplasm resembling proliferation of Brunn's nests. *Mod Pathol* 5:240-243, 1992.

Murphy WM, Beckwith JB, Farrow GM. Tumors of the urinary bladder. In: Rosai J, Sobin LH, eds. *Tumors of the Kidney, Bladder, and Related Structures.* 3rd series, fascicle 2. Washington, DC: Armed Forces Institute of Pathology; 199, 1994.

Murphy WM. Diseases of the urinary bladder, urethra, ureters, and renal pelvises. In: Murphy WM, ed. *Urological Pathology.* 2nd ed. Philadelphia: Saunders; 75-80, 1997.

Nesbit RM. The genesis of benign polyps in the prostatic urethra. *J Urol* 87:416-418, 1962.

Oliva E, Young RH. Nephrogenic adenoma of the urinary tract: a review of the microscopic appearance of 80 cases with emphasis on unusual features. *Mod Pathol* 8:722-730, 1995.

Oliva E, Young RH. Clear cell adenocarcinoma of the urethra: a clinicopathologic analysis of 19 cases. *Mod Pathol* 9:513-520, 1996.

Orihuela E, Herr HW, Whitmore WF Jr. Conservative treatment of superficial transitional cell carcinoma of prostatic urethra with intravesical BCG. *Urology* 34:231-237, 1989.

Ortega LG, Whitemore WF Jr, Murphy AI. In situ carcinoma of the prostate with intraepithelial extension into the urethra and bladder. A Paget's disease of the urethra and bladder. *Cancer* 6:898-923, 1953.

Oweity T, Persons D, Tawfik O . Carcinosarcoma of the prostatic urethra. *J Urol Pathol* 12:199-205, 2000.

Palou J, Xavier B, Laguna P, et al. In situ transitional cell carcinoma involvement of prostatic urethra: bacillus Calmette-Guérin therapy without previous transurethral resection of the prostate. *Urology* 47:482-484,1996.

Petersen RO. Urethra. In: *Urologic Pathology.* Philadelphia: Lippincott; 395-428, 1992.

Posso MA, Berg GA, Murphy AI, et al. Mucinous adenocarcinoma of the urethra: report of a case associated with urethritis glandularis. *J Urol* 85:944-948, 1961.

Prieto Ugidos N, Marana Fernandez M, Escobal Tamayo V, et al. Ectopic ureter in prostatic urethra. Unusual discovery in an adult [in Spanish]. *Arch Esp Urol* 48:843-846, 1995.

Proppe KH, Scully RE, Rosai J. Postoperative spindle cell nodules of genitourinary tract resembling sarcomas. A report of eight cases. *Am J Surg Pathol* 8:101-108, 1984.

Ray B, Canto AR, Whitmore WF Jr. Experience with primary carcinoma of the male urethra. *J Urol* 117:591-594, 1997.

Reece RW, Koontz WN Jr. Leukoplakia of the urinary tract. A review. *J Urol* 114:165-171, 1975.

Reese JH, Freiha FS, Gelb AB, et al. Transitional cell carcinoma of the prostate in patients undergoing radical prostatectomy. *J Urol* 147:92-95, 1992.

Remick DG Jr, Kumar NB. Benign polyps with prostatic-type epithelium of the urethra and the urinary bladder. A suggestion of histogenesis based on histologic and immunohistochemical studies. *Am J Surg Pathol* 8:833-839, 1984.

Renfer LG, Kelly J, Belville WD. Inverted papilloma of the urinary tract: histogenesis, recurrence and associated malignancy. *J Urol* 140:832-834, 1988.

Reuter VE. Urethra. In: Bostwick DG, Eble JN, eds. *Urologic Surgical Pathology.* St. Louis: Mosby; 436-454, 1997.

Ro JY, Ayala AG, Wishnow KI, et al. Prostatic duct adenocarcinoma with endometrioid features: immunohistochemical and electron microscopic study. *Semin Diagn Pathol* 5:301-311, 1988.

Sakamoto N, Tsuneyoshi M, Naito S, et al. An adequate sampling of the prostate to identify prostatic involvement by urothelial carcinoma in bladder cancer patients. *J Urol.* 1993;149:318-321.

Satoh S, Ujiie T, Kubo T, et al. Prostatic epithelial polyp of the prostatic urethra. *Eur Urol* 16:92-96, 1989.

Schinella R, Thurm J, Feiner H. Papillary pseudotumor of the prostatic urethra: proliferative papillary urethritis. *J Urol* 111:38-40, 1974.

Sogbein SK, Steele AA. Papillary prostatic epithelial hyperplasia of the urethra: a cause of hematuria in young men. *J Urol* 142:1218-1220, 1989.

Stein AJ, Prioleau PG, Catalona WJ. Adenomatous polyps of the prostatic urethra: a cause of hematospermia. *J Urol* 124:298-299, 1980.

Tada K, Yamaha M, Tamura M, et al. Two cases of benign polyps of the posterior urethra (ectopic prostatic tissue). *Acta Urol Jpn* 36:717-720, 1990.

Talbert ML, Young RH. Carcinomas of the urinary bladder with deceptively benign-appearing foci: a report of three cases. *Am J Surg Pathol* 13:374-381, 1989.

Taylor DC, Bhagavan BS, Larsen MP, et al. Papillary urothelial hyperplasia. A precursor to papillary neoplasms. *Am J Surg Pathol* 20:1481-1488, 1996.

Tobisu K, Kanai Y, Sakamoto M, et al. Involvement of the anterior urethra in male patients with transitional cell carcinoma of the bladder undergoing radical cystectomy with simultaneous urethrectomy. *Jpn J Clin Oncol* 27:406-409, 1997.

Tobisu K-I, Tanaka Y, Mizutani T, et al. Transitional cell carcinoma of the urethra in men following cystectomy for bladder cancer: multivariate analysis for risk factors. *J Urol* 146:1551-1553, 1991.

Tomaszewski JE, Korat OC, LiVolsi VA, et al. Paget's disease of the urethral meatus following transitional cell carcinoma of the bladder. *J Urol* 135:368-370, 1985.

Tran KP, Epstein JI. Mucinous adenocarcinoma of urinary bladder type arising from prostatic urethra. Distinction from mucinous adenocarcinoma of the prostate. *Am J Surg Pathol* 20:1346-1350, 1996.

Trites AEW. Inverted urothelial papilloma: report of two cases. *J Urol* 101:216-219, 1969.

Val-Bernal JF, Gomez-Ortega JM. Hyperplasia of mesonephric remnants: a potential pitfall in the evaluation of prostate gland biopsy. *J Urol* 154:1138-1139, 1995.

Walker AN, Mills SE, Fechner RE, et al. Endometrial adenocarcinoma of the prostatic urethra arising in a villous polyp. A light microscopic and immunoperoxidase study. *Arch Pathol Lab Med* 106:624-627, 1982.

Walker AN, Mills SE, Fechner RE, et al. Epithelial polyps of the prostatic urethra. A light microscopic and immunohistochemical study. *Am J Surg Pathol* 7:351-356, 1983.

Walker AN, Mills SE. Papillary and polypoid tumors of the prostatic urethra. In: Damjanov I, Cohen AH, Mills SE, Young RH, eds. *Progress in Reproductive and Urinary Tract Pathology.* New York: Field and Wood Medical; 113-137, 1989.

Weiner JS, Liu ET, Walther PJ. Oncogenic human papillomavirus type 16 is associated with squamous cell cancer of the male urethra. *Cancer Res* 52:5018-5023, 1992.

Weiss J, Elder D, Hamilton R. Melanoma of the male urethra: surgical approach and pathological analysis. *J Urol* 128:382-385, 1982.

Wick MR, Brown BA, Young RH, et al. Spindle-cell proliferations of the urinary tract. An immunohistochemical study. *Am J Surg Pathol* 12:379-389, 1988.

Wood DP Jr, Montie JE, Pontes JE, et al. Transitional cell carcinoma of the prostate in cystoprostatectomy specimens removed for bladder cancer. *J Urol* 141:346-349, 1989.

Young HH, Frontz WA, Baldwin JC. Congenital obstruction of the posterior urethra. *J Urol* 3:289-365, 1918.

Young RH, Scully RE. Pseudosarcomatous lesions of the urinary bladder, prostate gland, and urethra. A report of three cases and review of the literature. *Arch Path Lab Med* 111:354-358, 1987.

Young RH. Nephrogenic adenoma of the urethra involving the prostate gland: a report of two cases of a lesion that may be confused with prostatic adenocarcinoma. *Mod Pathol* 5:617-620, 1992.

Young RH. Pseudoneoplastic lesions of the urinary bladder and urethra. A selective review with emphasis on recent information. *Semin Diagn Pathol* 14:133-146, 1997A.

Young RH. Pseudoneoplastic lesions of the urinary bladder, prostate gland, and urethra. In: Wick MR, Humphrey PA, Ritter JM, eds. *Pathology of pseudoneoplastic lesions.* Philadelphia: Lippincott-Raven; 225, 1997B.

Young RH, Oliva E. Transitional cell carcinomas of the urinary bladder that may be underdiagnosed: a report of four cases exemplifying the homology between neoplastic and non-neoplastic transitional cell lesions. *Am J Surg Pathol* 20:1448-1454, 1998.

Youssif M. Posterior urethral polyps in infants and children. *Eur Urol* 11:69-70, 1985.

Zeid M, Gaeta JF, Asirwatham JE, Suffrin G. Papillary adenoma of the prostatic urethra. *Prostate* 9:9-14, 1986.

Index

Numbers in **boldface** refer to pages on which images, figures, and tables appear.

index

A

AAH. See Atypical adenomatous hyperplasia
Abscess, prostatic, 77
Acid phosphatase. *See* Prostatic-specific acid phosphatase
Actinomycosis, 94
Acute lymphoblastic leukemia, 442, **442**
Acute myelogenous leukemia, 442, **442**
Adenocarcinoma. *See also* Prostatic carcinoma; specific types of adenocarcinoma
  adjacent to prostatic intraepithelial neoplasia, 201, **202, 259–260,** 266, 299, **299**
  admixed with inflammation, 282, **282**
  ancillary diagnostic studies in, 273–275
  around and between benign glands, **260**
  atrophic, **37,** 110–111, 282, **282, 479**
  collagenous micronodules in, 270–272, **271–272**
  cystic, 178
  diagnostic criteria for, 259–268, **259–268**
    absence of basal cells, 262–263, **263,** 273, **273,** 290, **291**
    architectural criteria, 259–262, **259–262**
    corpora amylaceum, 266, **266**
    cytoplasmic appearance, 266–267, **266–269**
    intraluminal crystalloids, 65, **65, 259,** 265–266, **265–266,** 280
    mitotic figures, **259,** 265
    nuclear atypia, 65, **65,** 263–264, **263–264,** 280, 290
    pink amorphous intraluminal secretions, **259,** 264–265, **265**
    Stout criteria, 259, **259**
    wispy blue mucin, 16, 264, **264–265,** 280
  differential diagnosis of, 123, 143, 147–148, **147,** 297
  direct extention to to seminal vesicles, 516–517, **517**
  DNA abnormalities in, 275, 287
  in edematous stroma, 260, **261**
  effect of androgen deprivation therapy on, **458**
  around ejaculatory duct, 297, **297**
  encircling blood vessels, 297, **297**
  extraprostatic extension of (capsular penetration), 278, 299–302, **299–302,** 307–308, **307**
    into periprostatic adipose tissue, 278, **279, 300**
    into prostatic urethra, **298,** 536, **536**
    into seminal vesicles, **231,** 301–303, **301–303,** 308
  fine needle aspiration biopsy in, 64–66, **64–66**
  fused microacinar, **277–278**
  glomeruloid structures in, 272–273, **272–273**
  high-grade, 262, **262–263,** 276–277, **277–278, 296**
  histopathologic features specific for carcinoma, 268–273, **268–273**
  hypernephromatoid, 266, **479**
  immunophenotyping of, **312**
  incidence at autopsy, **185**
  inflamed, **479**
  inflammatory infiltrate, 260, **261**
  intermediate-grade, 259
  invasive
    admixed with prostatic intraepithelial neoplasia, 192–193, **192–193**
    focal, **201**
    patterns of invasion, 276–279, **276–279**
    prostatic intraepithelial neoplasia with, 201, **202**
    sclerotic stromal response to, 260, **261**
  lipid accumulation of cytoplasm in, 65, **65**
  low-grade, 172
  lymphocytic infiltrate in, 282, **282**
  lymphovascular space invasion by, **261,** 270, **278,** 301–302, **302,** 309, **309**
  α-methylacyl-CoA racemase in, 274
  microacinar complexes in, 65
  microinvasive, 200–201
  minimal, **278,** 280–281, **280–281,** 283
    differential diagnosis of, 221–222, **221**
  moderately differentiated, **230,** 259, **276**
  with mucinous features, 403
  mucin-producing, **271**
  in needle core biopsy, **40,** 275–288, **275–288**
    amount of tumor in, 286–287, **287–288**
    diagnostic criteria for, 276–280, **276–279**
    differential diagnosis of, 281–285, **282–286**
    prognostic attributes, 285–288, **286**
    reporting of, 285–288, **287**
    total linear millimeters of carcinoma, 287, **287**
  nested pattern of, 297, **297**
  nodulocystic, **297**
  in open prostatectomy specimen, 289–294
    clinical, gross, and microscopic features of, 289–291, **290**
    differential diagnosis of, 292, **292**
    prognostic attributes, 292–294
    reporting of, 292–294
  patterns that mimic benign conditions, **479**
  perineural invasion by, **231, 260,** 268–270, **268–270,** 287, 301, **303,** 308–309, **308**
    circumferential extension around nerve, 268, **269,** 270
    cresentic application, 268, **269**
    intraneural invasion, 268, **269**
    knob-like configurations, 270, **270**
    peninsula pattern, 270, **270**
    perineural tracking, 268, **269, 300**
  permeation into smooth muscle, **260**
  poorly differentiated, 274
  of prostatic urethra, 534
  pseudohyperplastic, 127, 262, **262, 277,** 292, **296,** 297, **479**
    differential diagnosis of, 137–138, 160–161, **160,** 222, 290, **291**
  in radical prostatectomy specimen, 50, **51,** 294–310
    gross and microscopic features of, 294–305, **294–304**
    prognostic attributes of, 305–310, **310**
    reporting of, 305–310, **305–307**
  radiorecurrent/radioresistant, 466–467
  recurrence of, 311
  risk of recurrence of, 310
    weighted, 310
  of seminal vesicles, 515–516, **515–516**
  in skeletal muscle tissue, 279, **279,** 297, **298**
  small acinar, **14,** 147, **201, 259–261,** 276, **276–277, 279**
    autopsy-detected, 229
    differential diagnosis of, 178
  in TURP chips, 289–294, **289–291**
clinical, gross, and microscopic features of, 289–291, **290**
    differential diagnosis of, 292
    prognostic attributes, 292–294, **293**
    reporting of, 292–294, **293**
  ultrastructural characteristics of, 206, **207**
  at vesicourethral anastomotic site, 311, **313**
  well-differentiated, 259, **259,** 279–280, **279, 479**
    differential diagnosis of, 122, 137–138, 159–160, **160,** 164
Adenoid basal cell tumor, 143–145, 408
Adenoid basal proliferation of uncertain significance, 408
Adenoid cystic carcinoma. *See also* Basaloid/adenoid cystic "carcinoma"
  of Cowper's gland, 410
  of salivary glands, 408–410, **410**
Adenoid cystic-like tumor, 143, 408
Adenoid cystic tumor. *See* Adenoid basal cell tumor
Adenoid-cystic tumorlike lesion, 145
Adenoma
  of prostate, 123, 129, 143, 431–432, **431.** *See also* Nephrogenic metaplasia
  villous, of prostatic urethra, 530–531
Adenomatoid metaplasia. *See* Nephrogenic "metaplasia"
Adenomatoid prostatic tumor. *See* Sclerosing adenosis
Adenomatoid tumor. *See* Nephrogenic "metaplasia"
Adenomatous hyperplasia, 160. *See also* Atypical adenomatous hyperplasia
Adenomyoma, of seminal vesicles, 515
Adenosis. *See also* Atypical adenomatous hyperplasia
  sclerosing. *See* Sclerosing adenosis
Adenosquamous carcinoma, 406–408, **406–407**
  clinical features of, 406
  grading of, 348
  incidence of, 406
  from treated tumors, 408
Adipose tissue
  extension of adenocarcinoma into, 278, **279, 300**
  in fine needle aspirate, 62, **62**
  periprostatic, 17, **18**
    incidental sampling in needle biopsy, 35–36, **35**
  in prostatic stroma, 22, **22**
  sampled by TURP, 40

Adnexal tumor, of seminal vesicles, 515
Adrenal gland
metastasis of prostatic carcinoma to, 319
prostate specific antigen in neoplasms of, 236, **236**
African plum, 469
Age-related incidence
of atrophy, 101, **101**
of benign prostatic hyperplasia, **127**
AIDS, infectious prostatitis and, 94–95
Alkaptonuria, 169
Allelic loss, 161, **161,** 483–484, **484**
Allergic prostatitis. *See* Eosinophilic prostatitis
Alpha-blockers, 199
for benign prostatic hyperplasia, 129
effect on prostatic tissues, 469, **469**
Amebic prostatitis, 94
Aminoglutethimide, **457**
Amyloid deposits
in prostate, 169, **169**
in seminal vesicles, 512–513, **513**
Anaplastic lymphoma kinase, 434
Androgen(s)
in development of benign prostatic hyperplasia, 127–128, **127**
prostatic carcinoma and, 233
Androgen deprivation therapy
basal cell hyperplasia after, 143
cribriform hyperplasia after, 144
effect on pelvic lymph node metastases, 462, **462**
effect on prostatic carcinoma, 178, 246, 300, 305
effect on prostatic intraepithelial neoplasia, 198–199, **199**
effect on prostatic tissues, 457–463, **458–461**
grading after, 356
methods of, **457**
monitoring patient response to, 240
side effects of, 246
transitional cell metaplasia after, 119
Androgen receptor(s), 233, 464, 490–491, **490**
in benign prostatic hyperplasia, 128
Androgen receptor gene, 482, 490–491, **490**
Androgen suppression, for benign prostatic hyperplasia, 129
Angiosarcoma
of prostate, 440, **440**
of seminal vesicles, 516
Animal models
of benign prostatic hyperplasia, 128
of prostatic intraepithelial neoplasia, **206,** 209
Anterior fibromuscular stroma, 17
Antiandrogens, **457**
effects on prostatic tissues, 458, 462
Apocrine sweat gland carcinoma, prostate specific antigen in, **285**
Apoptosis
in benign prostatic hyperplasia, 128
in prostate cancer, 491, **492–494**
Aspergillus infection, 90
Atherosclerosis, of periprostatic vessels, 17, **18, 95**
Atrophy, 85, **85,** 177, **177**
biological significance of, 111
classification of, 101
cystic, 101, **193**
differential diagnosis of, 109–111, **109–111, 160,** 199, **199,** 221, **221,** 223, 282, **282,** 292, **292**
hyperplastic. *See* Postatrophic hyperplasia
incidence of, age and, 101, **101**
inflamed, 79, **79**
nuclear-cytoplasmic volume ratio in, 267–268
partial, 101, **101,** 105–106, **106–107, 111**
differential diagnosis of, 110
pathologic features of, 101–109, **101–108**
proliferation index of atrophic glands, 111
proliferative inflammatory, 101
prostatic carcinomas that mimic, **479**
sclerotic, 101, **101,** 104–105, **104, 106,** 110
simple, 101, **101–102,** 104, **104**
cystic, **101,** 104, **105–106**
noncystic, **101–102,** 102
Atypical adenomatous hyperplasia (AAH), 155–162, **156–161,** 177, **177**
allelic loss in, 161, **161**
basal cells in, 158, **158–159**
benign prostatic hyperplasia and, 156
diagnostic features of, 155, **155–156**
differential diagnosis of, 137, 147–148, **147,** 159–160, **160,** 164, **221,** 282–283, **282,** 292, **292**
extent and location of, **156**
fine needle aspiration biopsy of, 68
follow-up of, 162
histochemical analysis of, **161**
immunophenotyping of, 161, **161**
incidence of, 155, **155**
incidence of histologic features, 159, **160**
morphometric analysis of, **161**
phenotype and genotype of, **161**
prostatic carcinoma and, 161, 242
prostatic carcinomas that mimic, **479**
prostatic intraepithelial neoplasia and, 161
in TURP chips, 43
Atypical hyperplasia. *See* Atypical adenomatous hyperplasia; Focal glandular atypia; Prostatic intraepithelial neoplasia
"Atypical small acinar proliferation," 160, **160,** 224. *See also* Focal glandular atypia
Atypical stromal hyperplasia, 137
Atypical suspicious for carcinoma. *See* Focal glandular atypia
Autopsy specimen
incidence of adenocarcinoma in, **185**
prostate examination, 51, **51**
prostatic carcinoma in , 228–229, **228–229**
pathologic features of, 229–231, **230–231**

B

Bacille Calmette-Guerin (BCG) treatment
granulomatous prostatitis after, 87–89, **90,** 261
granulomatous urethritis after, 524
Bacterial prostatitis
acute, 77
chronic, 80
Basal cell(s), 8, **9–10**
absence in prostate adenocarcinoma, 262–263, **263,** 273, **273,** 290, **291**
in atypical adenomatous hyperplasia, 158, **158–159**
in fine needle aspirate, 59–60, **60**
in focal glandular atypia, 222–223
immunostaining with antibody 34βE12, 158, **158–159,** 160, **163, 195,** 222, 263, 273–274, **273–274, 465**
of prostatic epithelium
attachment to underlying basal lamina, 10–11
cell adhesion molecule in, 11
function of, 11
immunophenotyping of, 9–10, **10–11**
staining with 34βE12, 10, **11,** 85, 110, **110,** 138, **139,** 142, **142**
in prostatic intraepithelial neoplasia, 186, 194, **195,** 201, 203, 207
in sclerosing adenosis, **163**
Basal cell adenoma, 143
Basal cell carcinoma, 143, 408
Basal cell hyperplasia, 85, **85,** 135, 140–144, **140–143,** 177, **177**
after androgen deprivation, 143
atypical, 140, **140,** 142–144, 155
inflamed, 85
calcifications in, 142, **142**
cribriform, 141, **141,** 143
after cryosurgery, 143
differential diagnosis of, 109, 143, **143,** 148, 160, **160,** 199, **199,** 221, **221,** 223, 282, **282,** 292, **292**
fine needle aspiration biopsy in, 64
immunophenotyping of, 142–143
inflamed, 83–84
nodular, **140**
proliferation index for, 142
with prominent nuclei, 199, **199**
prostatic carcinomas that mimic, **479**

after radiation therapy, 143
usual, 140, **140,** 143
Basal cell prominence, 143–144
adjacent to biopsy track, 36, **37**
Basaloid/adenoid cystic "carcinoma," 143, 408–410, **408–409**
benign conditions mimicked by, **479**
clinical features of, 409
differential diagnosis of, 143, 410
grading of, 348, **348**
Basement membrane, 19
B-cell lymphoma, 444–445
BCG treatment. *See* Bacille Calmette-Guerin treatment
bcl-2 gene family, 491
Benign glandular inclusions, in pelvic lymph nodes, 177–178, **177–178,** 314
Benign prostatic hyperplasia (BPH), 5, 126–148. *See also* specific types of hyperplasia
animal models of, 128
atypical adenomatous hyperplasia and, 156
basal cell hyperplasia, 140–144, **140–143**
clinical, 127
clinical features of, 128–129, **128**
irritative symptoms, 128, **128**
obstructive symptoms, 128, **128**
cribriform hyperplasia, 144–145, **144,** 177, **177**
differential diagnosis of, 128, 160, 170–171, 290
DNA and genetic abnormalities in, 140
etiology of, 127
fibroadenomatoid nodule in, 135, **135**
fine needle aspiration biopsy in, 63–64
hereditary, 127
incidence of, 127
age-related, **127**
infarction in, 135–136
inflamed, 135, **135**
involved by high-grade carcinoma, **138**
macroscopic, 127
microscopic, 127
nodule formation, 130–131, **130–131**
pathogenesis of, 127–128
prostate specific antigen in, 128–129, 237, **237**
prostatic carcinomas that mimic, **479**
radiologic evaluation of, 129
risk factors for, **127**
squamous cell metaplasia in, 115, 125
treatment of, 129
alpha-blockers, 469, **469**
effect on prostatic tissues, 469–470, **469**
herbal therapy, 469, **469**
high-intensity focused ultrasound, 469, **469**
hyperthermia, **469,** 470
laser therapy, 469–470, **469**
minimally invasive, 469–470, **469**
open prostatectomy, 129
thermotherapy, **469,** 470
transurethral electrovaporization, **469,** 470
transurethral needle ablation, **469,** 470
transurethral resection of the prostate, 129
in TURP chips, 204
usual nodular epithelial and stromal hyperplasia, 129–140, **130–139**
vasculitis in, 94, **94–95**
Bicalutamide, **457**
Biopsy bag artifact, 39
Biopsy gun, 32, **33**
Biopty Needle and Gun, **33**
Bladder
carcinoma of
prostate involvement in, 51, 447, **447**
prostatic acid phosphatase in, **286**
prostate specific antigen in, 236, **236, 285**
treatment with BCG. *See* Bacille Calmette-Guerin treatment
clear cell adenocarcinoma of, 147
papillary adenocarcinoma of, 531
prostatic carcinoma in bladder neck, 242, **242,** 311, **311**
prostatic ectopia in, 22, **23**
sampling of bladder neck by TURP, 40
sampling of bladder neck in needle biopsy, 26, **26**
section of neck margin in radical prostatectomy specimen, 48, **48**
signet-ring carcinoma of, 405
transitional cell carcinoma of, 410, 413
involvement of prostatic urethra in, 535–536, **535**
prostate involvement in, 84, **84,** 284, **284,** 447, **447**
spread to seminal vesicles, 517, **517–518**
transitional cell lesions of, WHO classification of, 532, **533**
Blastomycosis, 90–91
Blood supply, to prostate, 19–20, **19–20**
Blue nevus, 167–169, **167–168,** 446
Bone, metastasis of prostatic carcinoma to, 234, 240–241, **241,** 244, **244,** 317–319, **317–319**
grading of metastatic deposits, 355
Bone scan
clinical staging by, 378, **378**
evaluation of metastatic carcinoma, 240–241, **241,** 317
Borderline lesions. *See* Focal glandular atypia
Bouin's solution, 37–38, **38,** 275, **275**
BPH. *See* Benign prostatic hyperplasia
Brachytherapy
effect on prostatic tissues, 464–468, **464–467**
for prostatic carcinoma, 199, 246
BRCA1 gene, 233, 488
BRCA2 gene, 233, 482, 488–489
Breast carcinoma
prostate specific antigen in, 236, **236, 285**
prostatic acid phosphatase in, **286**
prostatic carcinoma and, 233
Broders grading system, 348–349
Brucellosis, 90
Burkitt lymphoma, 445

C

CAG repeats, 482–483
Calcification
in basal cell hyperplasia, 142, **142**
of seminal vesicles, 512
Calcified corpora amylaceum, **14–15,** 16
Calculated prostate cancer volume, 384
Calculi
of prostate, 16, 80, **117**
of seminal vesicles, 512
Candida infection, 90
CAPB gene, **482,** 483
Capsule. *See* Prostatic capsule
Carcinoid tumor
of prostate, 417, **417,** 446
prostatic acid phosphatase in, **286**
of seminal vesicles, 516
Carcinoma in situ (CIS)
of prostate, 202–203
of prostatic urethra, 535, **535**
Carcinosarcoma. *See* Sarcomatoid carcinoma
Cautery artifact, in TURP chips, 43, **43, 177,** 291, **291,** 354
Cavernous nerves, 20
cDNA library, from prostatic intraepithelial neoplasia, 209
Cell adhesion molecules, in basal cells, 11
Cell cycle proteins, as prognostic indicators, 491, **492–494**
Cell proliferation
in benign prostatic hyperplasia, 128
in prostate cancer, 491, **492–494**
c-*erb*B-1 gene, 489–490
c-*erb*B-2 gene, 489–490
c-*erb*B-3 gene, 489
c-*erb*B-4 gene, 489
Chemotherapy, effect on prostatic tissues, 468
Chloroma, 442
Chondroma, 432
Chondrosarcoma, 421, 440, **440**

Choriocarcinoma, 446
Chromogranin, in neuroendocrine cells, 11
Chromosomal alterations
gain of chromosomal DNA, 484–485, **485**
in hereditary prostate cancer, 482–483
loss of chromosomal DNA, 483–484, **484–485**
as prognostic indicators, 487
in prostatic intraepithelial neoplasia, 208–209, 485–487
in sporadic prostate cancer, 483–487, **483–486**
Chromosomal number, altered, 481
Chronic lymphocytic leukemia, 441–442, **442**
Chronic myelogenous leukemia, 442, **442**
CIS. *See* Carcinoma in situ
Clear cell adenocarcinoma
of bladder, 147
of prostatic urethra, 529–530, 534
tubulocystic, 422
of urethra, 147
Clinical endpoints, relationship to histologic grade, 359–363, **359–363**
Clinical staging, 378–379, **378–379**
Cloacogenic carcinoma
differential diagnosis of, 410
prostatic acid phosphatase in, **286**
c-*met* gene, 489
c-*myc* gene, 209, **489**
Coccidioides immitis infection, 90, **91**
Collagen injections, 169
Collagenous micronodules, in adenocarcinoma, 270–272, **271–272**
Collagenous spherulosis, 169
Colloid adenocarcinoma. *See* Mucinous adenocarcinoma
Colon, incidental sampling in needle biopsy, 36, **36**
Colon/colorectal carcinoma
differential diagnosis of, 399–400, 516
extension into seminal vesicles, 517–518
involvement of prostate in, **284,** 285, 447, **447**
prostate specific antigen in, 236, **236, 285**
prostatic acid phosphatase in, **286**
Columnar metaplasia, of prostatic urethra, 526
Comedocarcinoma, 262, **262, 295, 395,** 396
Computed tomography (CT)
clinical staging by, 378, **378**
evaluation of prostatic carcinoma, 240
Condyloma acuminata, 524
Core needle biopsy. *See* Needle core biopsy
Corpora amylaceum, 13–16, **13–14**
in adenocarcinoma, 266, **266**
amyloid in, 169
in atrophic glands, 102, **103**
calcified, **14–15,** 16
in fine needle aspirate, 62, **62**
in prostatic intraepithelial neoplasia, 197, **198**
Cowper's glands, 122, **160,** 172, **172, 177**
adenoid cystic carcinoma of, 410
differential diagnosis of, 284
c-*ret* gene, 489
Cribriform adenocarcinoma, **199,** 201–202, 261–262, **261, 267,** 276, **277, 479**
differential diagnosis of, 410
Cribriform hyperplasia, 144–145, **145,** 177, **177**
after androgen deprivation therapy, 144
differential diagnosis of, 144, **144,** 284, 292, **292,** 410
prostatic carcinomas that mimic, **479**
Cryosurgery
basal cell hyperplasia after, 143
effect on prostatic tissues, 470–471, **470**
for prostatic carcinoma, 199, 247
Cryptococcus infection, 90, **91,** 95
Crystalloids
in atrophic glands, 102–103
extracellular, in adenocarcinoma, 65, **65**
intraluminal, 16
in adenocarcinoma, **259,** 265–266, **265–266,** 280
in seminal vesicles, 508, **508**
CT. *See* Computed tomography
Cuboidal metaplasia, of prostatic urethra, 526
Cushing's syndrome, with prostate cancer, 234
Cyproterone, **457**
Cyst
congenital, **5,** 6
ejaculatory duct, 5–6, **5–6**
müllerian duct, 5–6, **5–6**
retention, 6, **6,** 101
of seminal vesicle, 5–6, **5–6,** 511–512, **511–512**
utricular, 5–6, **5–6**
vas deferens, 5, **5–6**
Cystadenofibroma, of seminal vesicles, **514**
Cystadenoma, of seminal vesicles, 513–515, **514**
Cystic adenocarcinoma, 178
Cystic atrophy, 101, **193**
Cystic fibrosis, 6, 511
Cystic glandular dilatation, in benign prostatic hyperplasia, 135, **135**
Cystoprostatectomy specimen
prostatic carcinoma in, 229, **230,** 231
tissue handling and sampling, 51
Cystosarcoma phyllodes. *See also* Phyllodes tumor
of seminal vesicles, 515
Cytochrome P450, 482
Cytomegalovirus infection, 95

D

Denonvilliers' fascia, 17, **17**
Dermoid cyst, 171. *See also* Teratoma
Development
of prostate, 3–5, **4–5**
of seminal vesicles, 507
Developmental abnormalities, of prostate, 5–6, **5–6**
DHT. *See* Dihydrotestosterone
Diet, prostatic carcinoma and, 233
Digital rectal examination
clinical staging by, 378, **378**
in prostatic carcinoma, 234–235, **234–235**
Dihydrotestosterone (DHT), in benign prostatic hyperplasia, 128
Diverticula, urethral, 523–524, **523**
DNA
abnormalities
in benign prostatic hyperplasia, 140
in prostatic intraepithelial neoplasia, 208–209, **209**
methylation of, 490–491
DNA content, 80, 481–482, **481**
of adenocarcinoma, 275, 287
as prognostic indicator, 481–482
DNA microarrays, 494, **494**
DNA ploidy. *See* DNA content
Doxazosin, 469
Duct-acinar glandular system, 7–8, **8**
Ductal adenocarcinoma of prostate, **262,** 391–400, **391–398,** 530–531
benign conditions mimicked by, **479**
clinical features of, **392**
cribriform, **395, 397**
differential diagnosis of, **199,** 202, 399, 516
extension into prostatic urethra, 536, **536**
fine needle aspiration biopsy in, 68
grading of, 348, **348,** 399
incidence of, 391, **392**
metastasis of, 398, **398**
mitotic activity in, 396
mixed ductal-acinar adenocarcinoma, 393, **393**
in needle biopsy, 396, **397–398**
origin of, 400
papillary, 393, **394–395, 398**
of primary prostatic ducts, 393, **393,** 398
prognosis in, 400
prostate specific antigen in, **398–399,** 399
in radical prostatectomy specimen, 396–397, **398**

of secondary prostatic ducts, 393, **393,** 395–396, **395–396,** 398
in simple prostatectomy specimen, 396
spread of, 393, **393**
spread outside prostate gland, 398, **398**
in TURP chips, 396
Ductal-type adenocarcinoma, of prostatic urethra, 534
Dwarf palm, 469
Dysplasia, of prostatic urethra, 532–533, **533**

E

EZH2 gene, 494
Echinacea, 469
Echinococcal infection, 94
Ectomesenchymoma, 437, 440, **440**
Ectopic prostatic tissue, 22–23
in bladder, 22, **23**
in females, 22
in ovarian teratoma, 22, **22**
in prostatic urethra, 22
in retroperitoneal lipoma, 22
in testicular teratoma, 22
Ejaculatory duct, 7, 199
cells in fine needle aspirate, 61
cyst of, 5–6, **5–6**
identification of, 284
involvement by prostatic carcinoma, 243, **243**
pigment in, 13
ELAC2 gene, 482, 488
ELACA2 gene, 489
Embryology
of prostate, 3–5, **4–5**
first (bud) stage, 4, **4**
second (bud-tubule) stage, 4, **4**
third stage, 4, **4**
of seminal vesicles, 507
Embryonal hyperplasia. *See* Basal cell hyperplasia
Endodermal sinus tumor, 446
Endometrial adenocarcinoma. *See* Ductal adenocarcinoma of prostate
Endometrioid adenocarcinoma. *See* Ductal adenocarcinoma of prostate
Endometriosis
differential diagnosis of, 284
prostatic, 171, **177**
Eosinophil(s), in chronic inflammation, 83, **83**
Eosinophilic granules, in benign prostatic epithelium, 123
Eosinophilic (allergic) prostatitis, 83, 93
differential diagnosis of, 92
vasculitis in, 94, **94**
Epithelial cells
immunophenotyping of, **10**
intraluminal, 13–14, **13–14**
of prostate, release into bloodstream at needle biopsy, 36
Epithelial hyperplasia, usual, 129–140, **130–139**
differential diagnosis of, 137–138, **137,** 160, **160,** 187
immunophenotyping of, 139
Epithelial polyps, of prostatic urethra, 530–531, **530**
Epithelial-stromal tumor. *See also* Phyllodes tumor
of seminal vesicles, 515–516
Epithelium, transitional cell. *See* Transitional cell epithelium
Epithelium of prostate, 8. *See also* Basal cell(s); Luminal (secretory) cells; Neuroendocrine cells
lipofuscin in, 13
Epithelium of seminal vesicle, 13
Erythropoiesis, extramedullary, in prostate, 171, **171, 177**
Estramustine, 468
Estrogens, in benign prostatic hyperplasia, 128
Estrogen therapy
effect on prostatic tissues, 457, **457, 459,** 462
prostatic endometriosis and, 171
Etoposide, 468
Ewing's sarcoma, 417, 437, 440, **440**
Extramedullary hematopoiesis
in pelvic lymph nodes, 177, **177,** 179, 314
in prostate, 171, **171, 177**

F

Family history
of benign prostatic hyperplasia, 127, **127**
of prostatic carcinoma, 232, **232**
Fat intake, prostatic carcinoma and, 233
Female(s), prostatic ectopia in, 22
Female prostate, 3
Fetalization. *See* Basal cell hyperplasia
Fetal prostate, 4, **4**
FGA. *See* Focal glandular atypia
Fibroadenoma, of seminal vesicles, 515
Fibroepithelial nodule. *See* Sclerosing adenosis
Fibroma, 432
Fibromuscular stroma, anterior, 7, **7**
Fibromyoepithelial nodule, 135, **135**
Fibromyxoid tumor, atypical. *See* Inflammatory myofibroblastic tumor
Fibrosarcoma
of prostate, 437
of seminal vesicles, 516
Fibrosis, of prostatic urethra, 525
Fibrous histiocytoma, malignant
of prostate, 440, **440**
differential diagnosis of, 170, 437
of seminal vesicles, 516
Fibrous tumor, solitary, 432
Finasteride, **457**
for benign prostatic hyperplasia, 129
chemoprevention of prostatic carcinoma, 234, 462
effect on prostatic intraepithelial neoplasia, 199
effect on prostatic tissues, 457, 462–463
grading of prostatic carcinoma after, 356
Fine needle aspiration (FNA) biopsy, 31–32
in adenosis, 68
in basal cell hyperplasia, 64
in benign prostatic hyperplasia, 63–64
cells in
adipose cells, 62, **62**
basal cells, 59–60, **60**
bizarre benign cells, 60–61, **61**
ejaculatory duct cells, 61
neuroendocrine cells, 59
secretory epithelial cells, 59–60, **60**
seminal vesicle cells, 60–61, **61**
smooth muscle cells, 61
squamous cells, 61, **62**
transitional cells, 61
complications of, 59
corpora amylaceum in, 62, **62**
false-negative results, 59
false-positive results, 59
grading in, 349
indications for, 59
in lymphoma, 69
in malakoplakia, 63
in mesenchymal tumors, 69, **69**
in mucinous adenocarcinoma, 68
needle size for, 32
in neuroendocrine carcinoma, 69
number of specimens examined in U.S. in 2002, **31**
prophylactic antibiotics for, 59
in prostatic carcinoma, 64–66, **64–66**
grading of carcinoma, 66–67
monitoring response to therapy, 67
in prostatic duct adenocarcinoma, 68
in prostatic intraepithelial neoplasia, 67–68, **67–68**
in prostatitis, 59, 62–63, **62–63**
rectal contaminants in, 61, **61**
in sarcoma, 69, **69**

in signet-ring carcinoma, 68
in squamous cell carcinoma, 69
in transitional cell carcinoma, 68–69, **68**
Florid sinus histiocytosis, of pelvic lymph nodes, 178
Flutamide, **457**
FNA biopsy. *See* Fine needle aspiration biopsy
Foamy gland carcinoma, **267, 479**
differential diagnosis of, 178
grading of, 348, **348**
Focal glandular atypia (FGA), 218–224
basal cells in, 222–223
clinical data on patients, 219–220, **219**
diagnostic terms, 219, **219**
differential diagnosis of, 221–223, **221, 282,** 283–284
follow-up of, 223–224, **223**
histologic features of, 220–221, **220–221**
in needle biopsy, 40, 219–224, **219–224**
in open prostatectomy specimens, 224, **224**
prostate specific antigen in, **219,** 220
in TURP chips, 43, 224, **224**
Fontana-Masson stain, 167–169, **167**
Foreign body granulomatous prostatitis, **86,** 94, **94**
Foreign body histiocytosis, in pelvic lymph nodes, 177–178, **177,** 314
Formalin fixation, 37–38, 48, 275
4-glass test, 77, 80
Frozen section, of needle core biopsy, 38, **38**
Fungal infection, 90
Fused microacinar adenocarcinoma, **277–278**

G

Ganglion, prostate-associated, 20, **20–21**
Ganglioneuroma, 432
Gastric carcinoma
metastasis to prostate, 405, **447**
signet-ring, 405
Gene chips, 494, **494**
Gene expression profiles, for prostatic carcinoma, 364, 494, **494**
Gene therapy, effect on prostatic tissues, 470
Genetic abnormalities
in benign prostatic hyperplasia, 140
in prostatic carcinoma, 231
in prostatic intraepithelial neoplasia, **206,** 208–209, **209**
Germ cell tumors
differential diagnosis of, 315
metastasis to prostate, **447**
of prostate, 446
of seminal vesicles, 516
of testicles, 446
Giant cell arteritis, 94, **94**
Giant multilocular cystadenoma, 431
Glandular atypia, focal. *See* Focal glandular atypia
Gleason grading system, 286, 339–349, **339**
applied after hormonal therapy, 355–356, **355**
applied after radiation therapy, 355–356, **355**
applied to fine needle aspirates, 349
applied to metastatic deposits, 355, **355**
applied to needle core biopsy, 349–352, **349–352**
applied to open prostatectomy specimens, 292–293, **293**
applied to radical prostatectomy specimens, **351,** 354–355, **354**
applied to TURP chips, 292–293, **293,** 352–354, **353–354**
applied to whole prostate gland, 352
general approach, 340–341, **340, 342**
grade 1, 340–342, **340–342**
grade 2, 340, **340–341,** 342–343, **343–344**
grade 3, 340, **340–341,** 343–344, **343–345**
grade 4, 340, **340–341,** 344–345, **346**
grade 5, 340, **340–341,** 346–348, **347–348**
histologic variants of prostatic carcinoma, 348–349, **348**
reporting of, 364–365, **364–365**
reproducibility of, 352, **353**
staging and, 384
tutorial programs, 352
Gleason score, 286, 340–342, 349
distribution, 345, **345**
lumping of, 341, **341**
Glomeruloid structures, in adenocarcinoma, 272–273, **272–273**
Glutathione S-transferase, 491
Goserelin, **457**
Grading of prostatic carcinoma, 286
after androgen deprivation therapy, 463, **463**
Broders grading system, 348–349
ductal adenocarcinoma, 399
experimental approaches to, 363–364, **363**
by gene expression profiles, 364
Gleason system, 339–349, **339.** *See also* Gleason grading system
grade progression, 356
histologic variants, 348–349, **348**
history of, 339, **339**
after hormonal therapy, 355–356, **355,** 463
in fine needle aspiration biopsy, 66–67
metastatic deposits, 355, **355**
by nuclear abnormalities, 364
in open prostatectomy specimen, 292–293, **293**
prognosis and grade, 356–363, **356–363**
after radiation therapy, 355–356, **355,** 466–467
regressive grading, 468
relationship of histologic grade and clinical endpoints, 359–363, **359–363**
relationship of histologic grade and pathologic endpoints, 356–359, **356–358**
reporting of histologic grade, 364–365, **364–365**
signet-ring carcinoma, 404
transitional cell carcinoma, 413
in TURP chips, 292–293, **293**
WHO system, 339–340, **339–340**
Grading of prostatic intraepithelial neoplasia, 67–68, **68**
Granular cell tumor, 432
Granulocytic sarcoma, 442
Granulomatosis
lymphomatoid, 445
Wegener, 93–94, **94**
Granulomatous disease, systemic, **86,** 93–94
Granulomatous inflammation, 261
Granulomatous prostatitis
after BCG treatment, 87–89, **90,** 261
classification of, 86–87, **86**
differential diagnosis of, 274, 283
fine needle aspiration biopsy in, 63, **63**
foreign body, **86,** 94, **94**
infectious, **86,** 89–91, **90–91,** 93
Aspergillus, 90
blastomycosis, 90–91
brucellosis, 90
Candida, 90
Coccidioides immitis, 90, **91**
Cryptococcus, 90, **91,** 95
fungal, 90
herpes zoster, 91
histoplasmosis, 90
Paracoccidioides, 90
parasitic, 91
syphilis, 90
malakoplakia. *See* Malakoplakia
nonspecific, **86–89,** 87–89, 93
differential diagnosis of, 88, 92
histologic characteristics of, **87**
postbiopsy/postresection, **86,** 91–93, **91–92,** 457
prostatic carcinomas that mimic, **479**
Granulomatous urethritis, after BCG treatment, 524
Growth factors, in benign prostatic hyperplasia, 128

H

Hair, granulomatous reaction to, 94
Hamartoma. *See* Nephrogenic metaplasia
Hemangioma
of prostate, 432
of urethra, 532
Hemangiopericytoma
of prostate, **432,** 436
of seminal vesicles, 516
Hematolymphoid neoplasms, 441–446, **441–445**
differential diagnosis of, 315
incidental discovery in pelvic lymphadenectomy, 46
Hematopoiesis, extramedullary
in pelvic lymph nodes, 177, **177,** 179, 314
in prostate, 171, **171, 177**
Hemidesmosomal-associated proteins, 10–11
Hemorrhagic infarction, 136, **136–137**
Hemosiderin, 169, **169**
Hepsin, 494
HER-2/neu protein, 489–490
Herbal therapy
for benign prostatic hyperplasia, 469, **469**
effect on prostatic tissues, 469
for prostatic carcinoma, 247
Herpes zoster, prostatitis associated with, 91
HIFU. *See* High-intensity focused ultrasound
High-intensity focused ultrasound (HIFU)
for benign prostatic hyperplasia, 469, **469**
effect on prostatic tissues, 469
Hip prosthesis, 178
Histiocytosis
florid sinus, of pelvic lymph nodes, 178
foreign body, in pelvic lymph nodes, 177–178, **177,** 314
signet-ring, in pelvic lymph nodes, 177–179, **177, 179,** 314
usual, in pelvic lymph nodes, 177–178, **177,** 314
Histoplasmosis, 90
Hodgkin disease, 445–446, **447**
Hollande's solution, 37–38, 275
Hormonal therapy
effect on prostatic tissues, 403, 457–464, **457–463, 479**
grading after, 355–356, **355**
predicting response to, 464
for prostatic carcinoma, **245,** 246
monitoring response to, 67
squamous cell metaplasia after, 118, **118**
HPC1 gene, **482,** 483
HPC2 gene, **482**
HPC20 gene, **482**
HPCX gene, **482,** 483
Human papillomavirus
prostatic carcinoma and, 234
in urethra, 524
Hypernephromatoid adenocarcinoma, 20, 266, **479**
Hyperplasia
atypical. *See* Prostatic intraepithelial neoplasia
atypical adenomatous. *See* Atypical adenomatous hyperplasia
basal cell. *See* Basal cell hyperplasia
benign prostatic. *See* Benign prostatic hyperplasia
cribriform. *See* Cribriform hyperplasia
epithelial. *See* Epithelial hyperplasia
mesonephric remnant, 145–147, **145–147**
postatrophic. *See* Postatrophic hyperplasia
prostate zones affected by, **7**
of prostatic urethra, 531, **531**
of seminal vesicles, 513
stromal. *See* Stromal hyperplasia
verumontanum mucosal gland, 147–148, **148**
Hyperthermia
for benign prostatic hyperplasia, **469,** 470
effect on prostatic tissues, 470
Hypoplasia
of prostate, **5**
of seminal vesicles, 511, **511**

I

Immunohistochemical staining, 40
failure of, 223
Immunophenotyping
of adenocarcinoma, **312**
of atypical adenomatous hyperplasia, 161, **161**
of basal cell hyperplasia, 142–143
of basal cells, 9–10, **10–11**
of luminal cells, **10,** 16
of nephrogenic "metaplasia" of prostatic urethra, 529, **529**
of neuroendocrine cells, **10**
of prostatic carcinoma, **284**
of prostatic intraepithelial neoplasia, **206,** 207
of sarcomatoid carcinoma, 420, **421**
of sclerosing adenosis, 163, **164**
of small cell carcinoma, 416–417, **417**
of transitional cell carcinoma, **284,** 413
of usual epithelial hyperplasia, 139
Immunoscintigraphy, evaluation of prostatic carcinoma, 240–241
Infarction, **136–137**
in benign prostatic hyperplasia, 135–136
hemorrhagic, 136, **136–137**
prostate specific antigen in, 237, **237**
of prostatic urethra, 525
squamous cell metaplasia associated with, 116–117, **117–118, 136**
transitional cell metaplasia associated with, 119
Infection
of prostate, 76–95
of prostatic urethra, 524–525
of seminal vesicles, 512, **512**
Inflammation, 76–95. *See also* Prostatitis
admixed with adenocarcinoma, 260, **261,** 282, **282**
atrophy with, 79, **79**
in benign prostatic hyperplasia, 135, **135**
differential diagnosis of, **221, 282,** 445
histologic acute, 78–80, **78–79**
intraluminal, 78, **78–79**
neutrophilic infiltrate in, 78, **78**
histologic chronic, 80–86, **81–86**
differential diagnosis of, 84–86, **84**
dilated gland with ring of lymphocytes and plasma cells, 81, **81**
eosinophils in, 83, **83**
lymphocytes in stromal nodule, 81, **82**
lymphoplasmacytic infiltrate in stroma, 81, **81**
macrophages in, 82–83, **82**
mast cells in, 83
patterns of, **81**
perivenular lymphocytic cuffs, 81, **82**
reactive benign epithelial changes in, 83, **83**
stromal alterations in, 84
prostate specific antigen in, 237, **237**
prostate zones affected by, **7**
in prostatic carcinoma, 84, **84**
prostatic carcinomas that mimic, **479**
of seminal vesicles, 512, **512**
squamous cell metaplasia with, 79–80, **79, 83**
Inflammatory myofibroblastic tumor, 137, 170, **432,** 434
differential diagnosis of, 437, 439
Inflammatory myofibrohistiocytic proliferation. *See* Inflammatory myofibroblastic tumor
Inflammatory pseudotumor. *See* Inflammatory myofibroblastic tumor
Insulin-like growth factor 1, prostatic carcinoma and, 233
International Prostate Symptom Score (IPSS), 128
Intraductal carcinoma. *See* Carcinoma in situ
Intraductal dysplasia. *See* Prostatic intraepithelial neoplasia
Intraglandular stroma, 17
Intraluminal materials, of prostatic glands, 13–14, **13–14**
in neoplastic processes, 16
Inverted papilloma, of prostatic urethra, 531–532, **532**
IPSS. *See* International Prostate Symptom Score
Islet cell tumor, prostatic acid phosphatase in, **286**

K

KAI1 gene, 489
Kaposi's sarcoma, 170
Ketoconazole, **457**
Kidney, metastasis of prostatic carcinoma to, 319
KLF6 gene, 489

L

Laryngeal adenocarcinoma, metastasis to prostate, **447**
Laser therapy
  for benign prostatic hyperplasia, 469–470, **469**
  effect on prostatic tissues, 469–470
Leiomyoma
  of prostate, 137, 432, **432–433**
    differential diagnosis of, 432, 439
  prostatic carcinomas that mimic, **479**
  of seminal vesicles, 514, **514**
Leiomyomatous stromal nodules, 432
Leiomyosarcoma
  of prostate, 137, 421, **432,** 438–441, **438–439**
    benign conditions mimicked by, **479**
    clinical features of, 438, **438**
    differential diagnosis of, 432, 437, 439
    metastasis of, 439
  of seminal vesicles, 516
Leukemia
  acute lymphoblastic, 442, **442**
  acute myelogenous, 442, **442**
  benign conditions mimicked by, **479**
  chronic lymphocytic, 441–442, **442**
  chronic myelogenous, 442, **442**
  infiltrates in prostate, 441–442, **442**
    differential diagnosis of, 437, 442
    incidence of, 441, **441**
  metastasis to prostate, **284,** 285, 447, **447**
Leuprolide, **457**
Levator ani, **17**
Lipofuscin, 13, 167–168, 508–509
Lipoma, retroperitoneal, prostatic ectopia in, 22
Liposarcoma, of seminal vesicles, 516
Liver
  metastasis of prostatic carcinoma to, 319, **320,** 321
  prostate specific antigen in cancer of, 236, **236**
Locally advanced prostatic carcinoma, 311–313, **311–313**
Luminal (secretory) cells, of prostatic epithelium, 8, **9,** 11–12, **12**
  cleared cytoplasm of, 12, **12**
  immunophenotyping of, **10,** 16
  nuclei of, 13
  pigment in, 12–13, **13**
  prostate specific antigen in, 16, **16**
  prostatic acid phosphatase in, 16
Lung
  cancer of
    metastatic to prostate, 69, **284,** 285, **447**
    prostate specific antigen in, **285**
  metastasis of prostatic carcinoma to, 64, 319–321, **319–321**
  prostate specific antigen in tumors of, 236, **236**
Luteinizing hormone-releasing hormone analog, effect on prostatic tissues, 458, 462
Luxol fast blue stain, 168
Lycopene, prevention of prostatic carcinoma, 233
Lymphatic drainage, of prostate, 20–21, **21**
Lymph nodes
  draining prostate, 20–21, **21**
  metastasis of prostatic carcinoma to, 313–317, **313–317**
  pelvic. *See* Pelvic lymph nodes
Lymphocytes
  encirclement of nerves, 85, **85**
  signet-ring cell change in, 85, **86**
Lymphoepithelioma-like carcinoma, 422
  grading of, 348, **348**
Lymphoma. *See also* specific types
  B-cell, 444–445
  benign conditions mimicked by, **479**
  differential diagnosis of, 417, 437
  extension into prostate, 447
  fine needle aspiration biopsy in, 69
  of follicular center cell origin, 445
  prostate involvement in, 85–86, 95, **284,** 442–445, **443–445,** 447, **447**
    clinical features of, 443
    differential diagnosis of, 442, 445
    incidence of, **441**
Lymphomatoid granulomatosis, 445
Lymphovascular space, invasion by prostatic carcinoma, 243, **243, 261,** 270, **278,** 301–302, **302,** 309, **309**

M

Macrophages
  in chronic inflammation, 82–83, **82**
  in malakoplakia, 93, **93**
Magnetic resonance imaging (MRI)
  clinical staging by, 378, **378**
  evaluation of prostatic carcinoma, 240
Malakoplakia
  differential diagnosis of, 284
  of prostate, **86,** 92–93, **93, 177**
    fine needle aspiration biopsy in, 63
  of seminal vesicles, 512
  of urethra, 525
Malignant mixed mesodermal tumor. *See* Sarcomatoid carcinoma
MALToma, 444–445
Mantle cell lymphoma, 445
Mast cells, in chronic inflammation, 83
Medical castration, for prostatic carcinoma, 246
Medullary carcinoma, prostatic acid phosphatase in, **286**
Megestrol, **457**
Melanin, 13, 167, 169
Melanocytes, 169
Melanocytic neoplasms, 446
Melanoma, **167,** 168–169, 446
  differential diagnosis of, 179, 315
  metastasis to prostate, 69, **284,** 285, 446–447, **447**
  of prostatic urethra, 534
Melanosis, 167–169, **167,** 446
Melanosomes, 168
Mesenchymal tumor, fine needle aspiration biopsy in, 69, **69**
Mesenchymoma
  of prostate, 440, **440**
  of seminal vesicles, 514
Mesonephric hamartoma, of seminal vesicles, 514
Mesonephric remnant(s), **5–6,** 6
  in prosthetic urethra, **523,** 524, 529
Mesonephric remnant hyperplasia, 145–147, **145–147**
  diagnostic features of, 145, **145,** 148
  differential diagnosis of, 147, **147, 160,** 284
Mesonephroid tumor, of seminal vesicles, 511
Metal particles, foreign body histiocytosis and, 178
Metaplasia, 114–124
  mucinous. *See* Mucinous metaplasia
  nephrogenic. *See* Nephrogenic "metaplasia"
  Paneth cell-like. *See* Paneth cell-like metaplasia
  of prostatic urethra, 526–530, **526–529**
  squamous cell. *See* Squamous cell metaplasia
  stromal, 123
  transitional cell. *See* Transitional cell metaplasia
  urothelial, 115
Metaplastic carcinoma. *See* Sarcomatoid carcinoma
Metastasis, 243–245, **244**
  to prostate, 446–447, **447**
    gastric carcinoma, 405, **447**
    germ cell tumors, 446, **447**
    Hodgkin disease, **447**
    laryngeal adenocarcinoma, **447**
    leukemia/lymphoma, **284,** 285, 447, **447**

lung cancer, 69, **284,** 285, **447**
melanoma, 69, **284,** 285, 446–447, **447**
pancreatic cancer, **284,** 285, **447**
renal cell carcinoma, 447, **447**
signet-ring carcinoma, 405
squamous cell carcinoma, 408
thyroid papillary carcinoma, **447**
of prostatic carcinoma
to adrenal glands, 319
to bone, 234, 240–241, **241,** 244, **244,** 317–319, **317–319**
common sites of, **244**
distant nonbony, 319–322, **319–321**
of ductal adenocarcinoma of prostate, 398, **398**
grading of metastatic deposits, 355, **355**
to kidney, 319
of leiomyosarcoma, 439
to liver, 319, **320,** 321
to lung, 319–321, **319–321**
of mucinous adenocarcinoma, 403
osteoblastic metastasis, 64
to pelvic lymph nodes, 45–46, **45,** 234, 240–241, **241,** 244, **244,** 313–317, **313–317**
to penis, 320, **320**
to pleura, 320–321, **321**
prostatic-specific acid phosphatase in, 316
prostatic specific antigen in, 316, **316**
pulmonary metastasis, 64
to skin, 319–320, **320**
to testes, 320, **320**
of transitional cell carcinoma of prostate, 411, 413
reporting of, 322
secondary neoplasms of seminal vesicles, 516–518, **517–518**
MET gene, 489–490
Methylation, of DNA, 490–491
α-Methyl-CoA racemase, immunohistochemical reaction for, 274
Michaelis-Gutmann bodies, 93, **93**
β_2 Microglobulin, 169
Microinvasive adenocarcinoma, 200–201
Microsatellite instability, in benign prostatic hyperplasia, 140
Minimal residual cancer, 50, 298
Mitotic figures
in adenocarcinoma, **259,** 265
in ductal adenocarcinoma, 396
MMAC1 gene. See *PTEN* gene
Molecular aberrations, in prostatic carcinoma, 481–495
Monocytoid B-cell lymphoma, 445
MRI. *See* Magnetic resonance imaging
MSR-1 gene, 482
Mucin(s)
acidic, 16
neutral, 16
in prostatic intraepithelial neoplasia, 197–198, 207, **207**
wispy blue. *See* Wispy blue mucin
Mucinous adenocarcinoma, 400–403, **400–402**
clinical features of, 400, **400**
differential diagnosis of, 403
fine needle aspiration biopsy in, 68
grading of, 348, **348**
incidence of, 400
metastasis of, 403
pathologic features of, 400, **401**
prostate specific antigen in, 401, 403
prostatic-specific acid phosphatase in, 401, 403
of prostatic urethra, 534
Mucinous metaplasia, 115, 121–122, **121–122**
differential diagnosis of, 122, 172
incidence of, **121**
in postatrophic hyperplasia, 108, **108**
Mucin-producing adenocarcinoma, **271**
Mucous gland metaplasia. *See* Mucinous metaplasia
Müllerian duct cyst, 5–6, **5–6**
malignancy in, 6
Multiple myeloma, 446
MYC gene, 489
Mycobacterial prostatitis, 89–90
Myoepithelial cells, in sclerosing adenosis, 163–164, **164**
Myofibroblastic tumor, inflammatory, 170, **432,** 434
differential diagnosis of, 437, 439
Myxoid neurofibroma, 137

N

Needle core biopsy, 31–40, **32–40**
adenocarcinoma in, **40,** 275–288, **275–277**
amount of tumor in, 286–287, **287–288**
diagnostic criteria for, 276–280, **276–279**
differential diagnosis of, 281–285, **282–286**
minimal adenocarcinoma, 280–281, **280–281**
prognostic attributes, 285–288, **286**
reporting of, 285–288, **287**
total linear millimeters of carcinoma, 287, **287**
8 to 13 biopsy cores, 34
clinical goals of, **31**
ductal adenocarcinoma in, 396, **397–398**
embedding of specimen, **38,** 39
fixation of, 275, **275**
focal glandular atypia in, 40, 219–224, **219–224**
fragmentation of specimen, 38, **38**
frozen section of, 38, **38,** 275, **275**
14-gauge biopsy, 32, **33**
18-gauge biopsy, 32–40, **33–40**
complications of, 36
grading of, 349–352, **349–352**
gross examination and description of specimen, 38, **39**
handling and processing of specimen, 37–38
incidental sampling of colon or rectum, 36, **36**
incidental sampling of muscles of bladder neck, 26, **26**
incidental sampling of periprostatic adipose tissue, 35–36, **35**
needle track seeding in, 32, 36, **37**
number of specimens examined in U.S. in 2002, **31**
optimal number of cores to detect cancer, 35
paraffin block sectioning and slide preparation, 39–40, **39**
prostatic intraepithelial neoplasia in, 40, 184, **184–185,** 191, **193,** 203–204
seminal vesicle biopsy, 35, **35**
seminal vesicles in, 510, **510**
sextant biopsies, 33–34, 38
squamous cell metaplasia in, **116, 118**
ultrasound-guided transrectal, 32–40, **33–40**
Needle track seeding, in needle core biopsy, 32, 36, **37**
Nephrogenic adenoma, 399
prostatic carcinomas that mimic, **479**
Nephrogenic metaplasia, of prostate, **177,** 284. *See also* Adenoma
differential diagnosis of, 147–148, **147**
inflamed, 83
Nephrogenic "metaplasia," of prostatic urethra, 526–530, **527–529**
differential diagnosis of, 529
immunophenotyping of, 529, **529**
Nerves, adenocarcinoma around, **260**
Nerve supply, to prostate, 20, **20–21**
Neuroblastoma, 417
differential diagnosis of, 437
prostate specific antigen in, 236, **236**
Neuroendocrine carcinoma, 234, **418,** 419
differential diagnosis of, 410, 417, 442
fine needle aspiration biopsy in, 69
Neuroendocrine cells
in fine needle aspirate, 59
with large eosinophilic granules, 123
of prostatic epithelium, 11–12, **12**
immunophenotyping of, **10**
Neurofibroma, 432
myxoid, 137
Neurologic symptoms, of metastatic prostatic carcinoma, 234

Neuron-specific enolase, in neuroendocrine cells, 11
Neutrophils, acute inflammatory cell infiltrate, 78–79, **78**
Nevus, blue. *See* Blue nevus
Nevus cell aggregates, in pelvic lymph nodes, 177, **177,** 179, **179,** 314
Nilutamide, **457**
Nodular histiocytic prostatitis, 88
Nodulocystic adenocarcinoma, **297**
Nuclear atypia
  in adenocarcinoma, 263–264, **263–264,** 280, 290
  for grading of prostatic carcinoma, 364
  in prostatic intraepithelial neoplasia, 186, **186,** 188, 194–196, **196–197,** 206–207
Nucleoli
  in adenocarcinoma, 263–264, **263–264**
  prominent, in inflamed atrophy, 79
  in prostatic intraepithelial neoplasia, 188, 196

O

Ochronosis, 169
Oncocytoma, 431–432, **432**
Oncogenes, 489–490, **489**
Open (simple) prostatectomy
  retropubic, 31, 44, **44**
  suprapubic, 31, 44, **44**
Open (simple) prostatectomy specimen, 31, 44, **44**
  adenocarcinoma in, 289–294, 396
    clinical, gross, and microscopic features of, 289–291, **290**
    differential diagnosis of, 292, **292**
    frequency of incidental carcinoma detection, 289–290, **289**
    prognostic attributes, 292–294
    reporting of, 292–294
  for benign prostatic hyperplasia, 129
  focal glandular atypia in, 224, **224**
  number examined in U.S. in 2002, **31**
  prostatic intraepithelial neoplasia in, 184–185, **184,** 204
  tissue handling and sampling, 44, **44**
Orchiectomy, **457**
  grading of prostatic carcinoma after, 356
  for prostatic carcinoma, 246
Osteoblastic metastasis, of prostatic carcinoma, 64
Osteosarcoma, 420, 440
Ovarian carcinoma, prostate specific antigen in, 236, **236, 285**

P

p16 gene, 489
p21 gene, 489
p27 gene, 489
p53 gene, 487–488, **487**
p53 protein, 139–140
  in prostatic intraepithelial neoplasia, 208, **208**
  as prognostic indicator, 488
PAH. *See* Postatrophic hyperplasia
Pancreatic carcinoma
  metastasis to prostate, **284,** 285, **447**
  prostate specific antigen in, **285**
Paneth cell-like metaplasia, 115, 122–123
Paneth-like cells, of prostatic epithelium, 12
Papillary adenocarcinoma. *See also* Ductal adenocarcinoma of prostate
  of bladder, 531
  of prostatic urethra, 534
Papillary ductal adenocarcinoma. *See* Ductal adenocarcinoma of prostate
Papillary nephrogenic adenoma, prostatic carcinomas that mimic, **479**
Papillary/polyploid urethritis, 525, **525**
Papilloma, of prostatic urethra, 531–532, **532**
Paracoccidioides infection, 90
Paraganglioma
  of prostatic urethra, 534
  of prostate, 446
Paraganglion
  differential diagnosis of, 284
  prostate-associated, 20, **20–21, 177**
Paraneoplastic syndromes, in small cell carcinoma, 414
Partial atrophy, 101, **101,** 105–106, **106–107,** 110, **111**
Partin tables, 381, **382,** 482
Pathologic endpoints, relationship to histologic grade, 356–363, **356–363**
Pathologic staging, 379–381, **380**
  pretreatment models of pathologic stage, 381, **382**
PCAP gene, **482,** 483
Pelvic fascia, 17, **17**
Pelvic lymph nodes
  biopsy of, clinical staging by, 378–379, **378–379**
  ductal adenocarcinoma in, **398**
  gross description of, 46
  laparoscopic sampling of, 46
  lymphadenectomy with radical prostatectomy, 45–46, **45**
  metastasis of prostatic carcinoma to, 45–46, **45,** 234, 244, **244,** 313–317, **313–317**
    effect of androgen deprivation therapy, 462, **462**
    grading of metastatic deposits, 355
    micrometastases, 46
    reporting of, 316–317, **317**
  pseudoneoplastic lesions of, 177–179, **177–179,** 314
  sentinel node sampling, 46
Penis
  ductal adenocarcinoma metastatic to, **398**
  metastasis of prostatic carcinoma to, 320, **320**
Periglandular stomal fibroblasts, 10, **11**
Perineural invasion, by adenocarcinoma. *See* Adenocarcinoma, perineural invasion by
Peripheral nerve sheath tumor, malignant
  of prostate, 440, **440**
    differential diagnosis of, 437
  of seminal vesicles, 514
Periurethral gland carcinoma
  prostate specific antigen in, 236, **236, 285**
  prostatic acid phosphatase in, **286**
Phyllodes tumor, 137, **432,** 434–435, **434–435**
PIA. *See* Proliferative inflammatory atrophy
Pigment
  in ejaculatory duct, 13
  in epithelial cells, 12–13, **13**
  in seminal vesicles, 13
Pigmentary nevohyperplasia, prostatic. *See* Blue nevus
Pigment disorders, 167–169
Pigmented melanocytosis. *See* Blue nevus
PIN. *See* Prostatic intraepithelial neoplasia
PINATYP, 200
Pink amorphous intraluminal secretions, in adenocarcinoma, **259,** 264–265, **265**
Plasma cell granuloma. *See* Inflammatory myofibroblastic tumor
Plasma cell pseudotumor. *See* Inflammatory myofibroblastic tumor
Pleura, metastasis of prostatic carcinoma to, 320–321, **321**
PNET. *See* Primitive neuroectodermal tumor
Polyarteritis nodosa, prostatic vasculitis in, 94, **94**
Polycystic kidney disease, autosomal dominant, 511
Polyethylene, foreign body histiocytosis and, 178
Polyp, epithelial, of prostatic urethra, 530–531, **530**
Positron emission tomography, evaluation of prostatic carcinoma, 240–241
Postatrophic hyperplasia (PAH), 101, **101,** 106–109, **107–108,** 177
  clinical significance of, 111
  differential diagnosis of, 109, **160,** 282, 292, **292**
  mucinous metaplasia in, 108, **108**
  transitional cell metaplasia in, **108,** 109
Postbiopsy/postresection granulomatous prostatitis, **86, 91–92,** 92–93, 457
Postmortem examination of prostate, 51, **51.** *See also* Autopsy specimen
Postoperative spindle cell nodule, 170–171, **170, 177,** 434, 525
  differential diagnosis of, 439

Precancerous lesions. *See also* Prostatic intraepithelial neoplasia
of prostate, fine needle aspiration biopsy in, 67–68, **67–68**
Preprostatic sphincter, 7, 17
Primitive neuroectodermal tumor (PNET), 417, 437
Programmed cell death. *See* Apoptosis
Proliferation index
in atrophic glands, 111
in basal cell hyperplasia, 142
in prostatic carcinoma, 491
in prostatic epithelium, 11
in prostatic intraepithelial neoplasia, 207–208
Proliferative inflammatory atrophy (PIA), 101
Prostatectomy, 3. *See also* Cystoprostatectomy
landmarks in, 17
open. *See* Open prostatectomy
radical. *See* Radical prostatectomy
transurethral. *See* Transurethral resection of the prostate
Prostate gland
anatomy of, 3, **4**
blood supply to, 19–20, **19–20**
development of, 3–5, **4–5**
embryology of, 3–5, **4–5**
extracellular stromal matrix of, 19–20, **19–20**
functions of, 3
infantile, 5, **5**
lobes of, 3
location of, 3
lymphatic drainage of, 20–21, **21**
maldevelopment of, 5–6, **5–6**
nerve supply to, 20, **20–21**
pubertal period, 5, **5**
stroma in, 19
weight by age, **5**
zones of, 3, 7–8, **7**
central zone, 3, **4,** 7–8, **7, 9,** 13, **13**
peripheral zone, 3, **4,** 7–8, **7–9,** 13
transition zone, 3, **4,** 7–8, **7, 9,** 13
Prostate specific antigen (PSA)
in adenocarcinoma, **286**
age-specific references ranges, 129, 237–238, **237**
in benign prostatic hyperplasia, 128–129, 237, **237**
biological functions of, 236
clinical staging by, 378, **378**
complexed PSA, 237, **237**
in ductal adenocarcinoma, **398–399,** 399
in endometrium, 22
extraprostatic expression of, 236, **236**
focal glandular atypia and, **219,** 220
free PSA, 237–238, **237**
in inflammation, 237, **237**
in metastatic prostatic carcinoma, 316, **316, 319**
monitoring response to treatment, 239–240
in mucinous adenocarcinoma, 401, 403
in nonprostatic neoplasms, 285, **285**
percentage of free PSA, 129
in prostatic carcinoma, 64, 129, **234–239,** 235–240
in prostatic ectopia, 22
in prostatic infarct, 237, **237**
in prostatic intraepithelial neoplasia, 183–184, **184**
PSA density, 129, 237, **237**
PSA velocity, 129, 237, **237**
screening of, 227
in secretory cells, 16, **16**
in signet-ring carcinoma, 405–406, **405**
in small cell carcinoma, 414
structure of, 236
total serum, 238
Prostatic capsule, 17–18, **17–18**
Prostatic carcinoma, 136–137. *See also* Adenocarcinoma; Precancerous lesions; specific types of carcinoma
age-dependence of, **51,** 227, 229, 231, **231**
with androgen deprivation treatment effect, 178
atrophic, 79, **109**
atypical adenomatous hyperplasia and, 161
autopsy-detected, 228–229, **228–229**
pathologic features of, 229–231, **230–231**
breast cancer and, 233
chemoprevention of, 205, 234, 462
clinically unimportant, 238
clinical symptoms of, 234
in cystoprostatectomy specimen, 229, **230,** 231
diet and, 233
differential diagnosis of, 85, **85,** 177–179
digital rectal examination in, 234–235, **234–235**
etiology of, 231–234, **231–233**
familial, 232, 483
family history of, 232, **232**
fine needle aspiration biopsy in, 64–69, **64–69**
hereditary, 232, **232**
chromosomal alterations in, 482–483
incidence at autopsy, **51**
incidence of, 227–228, **227–228**
changes with time, 227, **227**
with inflammation, 84, **84**
"insignificant," 238
intraluminal materials in, 16
involved in benign prostatic hyperplasia, **138**
latent, 228–229, **230**
locally advanced, 311–313, **311–313**
metastatic. *See* Metastasis, of prostatic carcinoma
minimal residual cancer, 50, 298
monitoring response to therapy, fine needle aspiration biopsy, 67
mortality of, 241–245, **245**
natural history of, 241–245, **242–244**
ejaculatory duct involvement, 243, **243**
extension into bladder neck muscle, 242, **242**
extension through capsule, 242, **242,** 297, **298–299,** 299
grade progression, 356
invasion of seminal vesicles, 242, **242–243**
lymphovascular space invasion, 243, **243**
metastasis, 243–245, **244**
perineural spread, 242, **242**
patterns that mimic benign conditions, **479**
poorly differentiated, 93
potentially harmless, 239
prognostic factors for, **481**
proliferation index of, 491
prostate specific antigen in, 129, **234–239,** 235–240
prostate zones affected by, **7**
pseudohyperplastic, 127
differential diagnosis of, 160–161, 222
with pseudosarcomatous, fibrogenic stroma, 421
race and, 227–229, **228,** 233, **233**
radiologic evaluation of, 240–241, **241**
release of cells into bloodstream at needle biopsy, 36
risk factors for, 229, **229,** 231–234, **231–233**
screening for, 232, 238
stage T1c, 238, **238**
follow-up of, 239
steroid hormones and, 233
treatment of, 245–247, **245.** *See also* specific treatment modalities
brachytherapy, 199, 246
cryosurgery, 199, 247
herbal medicines, 247
hormonal therapy, **245,** 246
hormone-refractory cancer, 247
hormone therapy, 67
initial, **245**
planning of, 362
proton therapy, 246
radiation therapy, 67, 245–246, **245**
radical prostatectomy, 245–246, **245**
watchful waiting, 241, 245, **245**
Prostatic carcinoma variants, 390–422
that mimic benign conditions, **479**
Prostatic duct
adenocarcinoma of. *See* Ductal adenocarcinoma of prostate

transitional cell carcinoma of, extension into prostatic urethra, 536
Prostatic ectopia. *See* Ectopic prostatic tissue
Prostatic fascia, **17**
Prostatic fluid, composition of, 3
Prostatic intraepithelial neoplasia (PIN), 136–137, 182–210
admixed with adenocarcinoma, 192–193, **192–193,** 299, **299**
after androgen deprivation therapy, **458,** 459
atypical adenomatous hyperplasia and, 161
clinical presentation of, 183–184, **184**
diagnostic terms used for, 183, **183**
differential diagnosis of, 85, 119–120, 123, 143, **221**
fine needle aspiration biopsy in, 67–68, **67–68**
foamy gland, 189, **190**
grading of, 67–68, **68**
high-grade, 177, 183, 188–203, **188–203**
adjacent to adenocarcinoma, **259–260,** 266
animal models, **206,** 209
apocrine-like apical bleb formation in, 197, **198**
arches, 189, **191**
atrophic, 196–197, **197**
autopsy specimen, **185**
basal cells in, 194, **195,** 201, 203, 207
cDNA libraries from, 209
chromosomal abnormalities in, 208–209, 485–487
clinical management of, 203–205
corpus amylaceum in, 197, **198**
cribriform, 188, **188–189,** 196, 201–202, 209, 410
in cystic atrophy, **193**
cystification of, 194
cytoplasmic features in, 196–197, **196–197**
differential diagnosis of, 109, 199, **199, 282–283,** 283, 292, **292,** 399
distinguishing from low-grade PIN, 188, **188**
effect of androgen deprivation therapy, 198–199, **199**
effect of radiation therapy, 199, 466
flat, 188, **188–189,** 193–194, **194,** 199, 202
follow-up of, 203–205, **203**
genetic abnormalities in, **206,** 208–209, **209**
growth along fibrovascular stalks, 188, **190**
hemorrhagic and cellular debris, 202, **202**
immunophenotyping of, **206,** 207
with invasive adenocarcinoma, 201, **202**
inverted, 188, **190**
lobular, **192**
luminal contents in, 198, **198**
micropapillary, 188, **188–189,** 190, **191,** 196
mucin in, 197–198, 207, **207**
mucinous, 189, **190,** 194
natural course of, 205–206
in needle core biopsy, 40, 184, **184–185,** 191, **193,** 203–204
in open prostatectomy, 184–185, **184,** 204
with outpouching, 200, **200**
p53 protein in, 208, **208**
partial gland involvement, **191**
pigment in, 197, **198**
PINATYP, 200
proliferation indices of, 207–208
proteinaceous eosinophilic secretions in, 197
protrusion from, 222, **222**
reporting of, 205, **205**
risk factors for carcinoma, 203
Roman bridges and trabeculae, 189, **191**
signet-ring, 188, **189**
small cell neuroendocrine, **188,** 189, **190**
solid pattern, 188
tufting pattern, 188, **188–189,** 190, **191**
in TURP chips, 43, **43,** 184–185, **184,** 191, **193,** 204
ultrastructural characteristics, 206, **207**
in whole prostate glands, **184–185,** 185–186, 191–192
histologic diagnosis of, 186, **186**
low-grade, 183, 186–188, **186–187**
association with carcinoma, 187, **187**
basal cells in, 186
differential diagnosis of, 138, 187, 199, **199**
distinguishing from high-grade PIN, 188, **188**
nuclear aberrations in, 186, **186,** 188, 194–196, **196–197,** 206–207
as precursor of carcinoma, 205–209, **206–209,** 242
prostate specific antigen in, 183–184, **184**
Prostatic-specific acid phosphatase
in adenocarcinoma, 285, **286**
clinical staging by, 378, **378**
in ductal adenocarcinoma, 399
in metastatic prostatic carcinoma, 316
in mucinous adenocarcinoma, 401, 403
in nonprostatic neoplasms, 285, **286**
in prostatic carcinoma, 64, 236
in secretory cells, 16
in signet-ring carcinoma, 405–406
Prostatic stromal proliferation of uncertain malignant potential (PSPUMP), 137, 421, 432–436, **432–435**
Prostatic urethra, 7
adenocarcinoma of, **298,** 534
anatomy of, 523, **523**
benign neoplasms of, 531–532
carcinoma in situ of, 535, **535**
clear cell adenocarcinoma of, 147, 529–530
columnar/cuboidal metaplasia of, 526
congenital anomalies of, 523–524, **523–524**
diverticula of, 523–524, **523**
duplications of, 523, **523**
dysplasia of, 532–533, **533**
effect of TURP on, 525, **525**
extension of prostatic ductal adenocarcinoma into, 536, **536**
fibrosis of, 525
hemangioma of, 532
hyperplasia of, 531, **531**
infarcts of, 525
infection of, 524–525
inverted papilloma of, 531–532, **532**
involvement in prostatic adenocarcinoma, 536, **536**
involvement in transitional cell carcinoma of bladder, 535–536, **535**
involvement in transitional cell carcinoma of prostatic ducts, 536
malakoplakia of, 525
malignant neoplasms of, 533–536, **533–536**
melanoma of, 534
mesonephric remnants in, **523,** 524, 529
metaplasia of, 526–530, **526–529**
nephrogenic "metaplasia" of, 526–530, **527–529**
papillary/polypoid masses of, **524**
paraganglioma of, 534
polyps of
congenital, **523,** 524
differential diagnosis of, 399
epithelial, 530–531, **530**
prostatic carcinomas that mimic, **479**
prostatic ectopia in, 22
squamous cell carcinoma of, 533–534
squamous metaplasia of, 526, **526**
transitional cell carcinoma of, 410, 413, 530, 533–534, **533–534**
extension into prostate, 84, **84**
transitional cell papilloma of, 531
urethritis cystica of, 526, **526–527**
urethritis glandularis of, 526, **526–527**
urethritis of, 524–525, **524**
villous adenoma of, 399, 530–531
Prostatism, 128–129, **128**
Prostatitis, **177.** *See also* Inflammation
acute, fine needle aspiration biopsy in, 62, **62–63**
allergic. *See* Eosinophilic prostatitis
chronic, fine needle aspiration biopsy in, 62–63
clinical, 77
acute bacterial, 77
chronic abacterial, 80, 86
chronic bacterial, 80
classification of, 77, **77**
eosinophilic. *See* Eosinophilic prostatitis
fine needle aspiration biopsy in, 59

granulomatous, 86–94. *See also* Granulomatous prostatitis
histologic, 77
infectious
actinomycosis, 94
in AIDS, 94–95
amebic, 94
cytomegalovirus, 95
echinococcal, 94
mycobacterial, 89–90
Pseudomonas pseudomallei, 94
viral, 94
nodular histiocytic, 88
squamous cell metaplasia in, 115
xanthogranulomatous, 88, 177, **177,** 292, **292**
Prostatodynia, 77, 86
Proteinaceous eosinophilic secretions, in prostatic intraepithelial neoplasia, 197
Proteomics, 494
Proton therapy, for prostatic carcinoma, 246
Proto-oncogenes, 489
Prune belly syndrome, 5, **5**
PSA. *See* Prostate specific antigen
Pseudoadenomatoid tumor of prostate. *See* Sclerosing adenosis
Pseudoemboli, 309
Pseudohermaphroditism, male, 128
Pseudohyperplastic adenocarcinoma, 127, 262, **262, 277,** 292, **296,** 297, **479**
differential diagnosis of, 137–138, 160–161, **160,** 222, 290, **291**
Pseudolymphoma, 445
Pseudomonas pseudomallei prostatitis, 94
Pseudoneoplastic lesions
of extraprostatic tissues, 177–179, **177–179**
of prostate, 177, **177**
Pseudosarcoma. *See* Inflammatory myofibroblastic tumor
Pseudosarcomatous fibromyxoid tumor. *See* Inflammatory myofibroblastic tumor
Pseudosarcomatous lesions, 137
Pseudosarcomatous myofibroblastic proliferation. *See* Inflammatory myofibroblastic tumor
PSPUMP. *See* Prostatic stromal proliferation of uncertain malignant potential
PTEN gene, 209, 488
Puberty, 5, **5**
Pumpkin seeds, 469
Purple cone flower, 469

R

Race, prostatic carcinoma and, 227–229, **228,** 233, **233**
Racemase (α-methylacyl-CoA racemase), ~~254~~ 274
Radiation therapy
basal cell hyperplasia after, 143
clinical stage and patient outcome, 382, **382–383**
complications of, 246
damage induced in benign glands, 284
effect on prostatic intraepithelial neoplasia, 199
effect on prostatic tissues, **177, 221,** 464–468, **464–467, 479**
emergence of unusual carcinomas after, 468
grading after, 355–356, **355**
monitoring patient response to, 240
predicting response to, 467–468, **467**
for prostatic carcinoma, 245–246, **245**
monitoring response to, 67
prostatic vasculitis after, 94, **94**
squamous cell metaplasia after, 118–119
Radical prostatectomy
pelvic lymphadenectomy in, 45–46
perineal, 44–51, 246
prostate specific antigen elevation after, 240
for prostatic carcinoma, 44, 245–246, **245**
retropubic, 44–51, 246
Radical prostatectomy specimen, 31
adenocarcinoma in, 50, **51,** 294–310
gross and microscopic features of, 294–305, **294–304**
prognostic attributes, 305–310, **310**
reporting of, 305–310, **305–307**
clinical stage and patient outcome, 382–383, **382–383**
complications of, 246
cross-sections of specimen, 49–50, **50**
ductal adenocarcinoma in, 396–397, **398**
findings after diagnosis of carcinoma in TURP chips, 293, **293**
fixation of, 48
grading of carcinoma in, **351,** 354–355, **354**
gross examination and reporting, 47–48, **47**
laparoscopic, 45
number of sections to submit, 50
number of specimens examined in U.S. in 2002, **31**
sampling bladder neck margin, 48, **48**
sampling vas deferens stump margin, 49, **49**
section from distal apical (urethral) margin, 48–49, **48–49**
section of quarter of gland, **49**
slide preparation from, 49
surgical margin status of, 303–305, **303–304,** 308, **308**
tissue banking, 48
tissue handling and sampling, 44–51, **45, 47–51**
pelvic lymph nodes, 45–46, **45**
prostate gland and seminal vesicles, 46–51, **47–51**
tissues for research purposes, 48
tumor size in, 298–299, 305, **307**
whole-mount section of specimen, **49**
RAF gene, 489
ras gene, 489
RB gene, 487–488
Rectovesical fascia, 17
Rectum. *See also* Colon/colorectal carcinoma
cells in fine needle aspirate, 61, **61**
incidental sampling in needle biopsy, 36, **36**
involvement by prostatic carcinoma, 243, **243,** 311
5α-Reductase deficiency, 3, 5, **5,** 128
5α-Reductase inhibitors, effect on prostatic tissues, 457, 462–463
Regressive grading, 468
Renal cell carcinoma
metastasis to prostate, 447, **447**
prostate specific antigen in, 236, **236**
prostatic acid phosphatase in, **286**
Retention cyst, 6, **6,** 101
RET gene, 489–490
Rhabdoid tumor, malignant, 437, 440, **440**
Rhabdomyosarcoma
of prostate, 137, 417, **432,** 436–438, **436–438,** 536
alveolar, 436–437, **437**
differential diagnosis of, 437
embryonal, 436–437, **437**
incidence of, 436
staging of, 438, **438**
of seminal vesicles, 516
Rhabdosphincter. *See* Urethral sphincter, striated
RNASEL gene, 482
Rosebud, 1
Rye pollen, 469

S

Salivary gland neoplasms
adenoid cystic carcinoma, 408–410, **410**
prostate specific antigen in, 236, **236, 285,** 322
prostatic acid phosphatase in, **286**
Sarcoidosis, 93
Sarcoma, 436–442, **436, 440**
differential diagnosis of, 170, 315, 434–435
Ewing's, 417, 437, 440, **440**
Kaposi's, 170
postradiation, 441
of prostate, 137, 420–421
fine needle aspiration biopsy in, 69, **69**

of seminal vesicles, 515–516
spindle cell, 170
undifferentiated (unclassified), 440
Sarcomatoid carcinoma, 69, **69,** 137, 419–422, **419–421**
benign conditions mimicked by, **479**
clinical features of, 419, **419**
differential diagnosis of, 170, 420–421, **420–421,** 437, 439
grading of, 348, **348**
immunophenotyping of, 420, **421**
of prostatic urethra, 534
after radiation therapy, 468
after treatment of acinar adenocarcinoma, 421–422
Saw palmetto, 247, 469–470
Schistosomiasis, 91
Sclerosing adenosis, 144, 155, 162–164, **162–163,** 177, **177**
basal cells in, **163**
diagnostic attributes of, 162, **162**
differential diagnosis of, 147–148, **147, 160,** 164, 284, 292, **292**
follow-up of, 164
immunophenotyping of, 163, **164**
myoepithelial cells in, 163–164, **164**
Sclerotic atrophy, 101, **101,** 104–105, **104, 106,** 110
Screening, for prostatic carcinoma, 232, 238
Secretory epithelial cells, in fine needle aspirate, 59–60, **60**
Selenium, chemoprevention of prostatic carcinoma, 233–234
Seminal vesicles
adenocarcinoma of, 515–516, **515–516**
adnexal tumor of, 515
agenesis of, 511, **511**
amyloid deposits in, 512–513, **513**
anatomy of, 507–510, **507–510**
angiosarcoma of, 516
biopsy of, 35, **35**
clinical staging by, 378–379, **378–379**
blood supply to, 510
calcification and calculi of, 512
carcinoid of, 516
cells in fine needle aspirate, 60–61, **61**
cystadenoma of, 513–515, **514**
cystosarcoma phyllodes of, 515
cysts of, 5–6, **5–6,** 511–512, **511–512**
duplications of, 511, **511**
embryology and development of, 507
epithelial-stromal tumor of, 515–516
epithelium of, 13 ,199, 508–509, **509**
extension of colorectal carcinoma into, 517–518
fibrosarcoma of, 516
fusion of, 511, **511**
germ cell tumors of, 516
hemangiopericytoma of, 516
hyperplasia of, 513
hypoplasia of, 511, **511**
identification of, 284
infection of, 512, **512**
inflammation of, 512, **512**
intraluminal crystalloids, 508, **508**
invasion by prostatic carcinoma, 49, 242, **242–243,** 301–303, **301–303,** 308
leiomyoma of, 514, **514**
leiomyosarcoma of, 516
liposarcoma of, 516
luminal contents, 508
lymphatic drainage of, 510
malakoplakia of, 512
maldevelopment of, 510–511, **511**
malignant fibrous histiocytoma of, 516
malignant neoplasms of, **514–516,** 515–516
mesenchymoma of, 514
mesonephric hamartoma of, 514
mesonephroid tumor of, 511
mucosa of, 508
in needle core biopsy, 510, **510**
neoplasms of indeterminate or low malignant potential, **514,** 515
nerves of, 510
peripheral nerve sheath tumor of, 514
physiological functions of, 507
pigment in, 13
primary benign neoplasms of, 513–515, **514**
prostatic carcinoma metastatic to, 516–517, **517**
pseudomalignant change in, 509
in radical prostatectomy specimen, 46–51, **47–51**
rhabdomyosarcoma of, 516
sarcoma of, 515–516
secondary neoplasms of, 516–518, **517–518**
smooth muscle of, 510, **510**
spread of transitional cell carcinoma of bladder to, 517, **517–518**
squamous cell carcinoma of, 515
vasculitis of, 512
wall invasion by adenocarcinoma, **231**
Seminal vesiculectomy, 507
Seminoma, 446
Signet-ring carcinoma
of bladder, 405
of prostate, 403–406, **403–405**
benign conditions mimicked by, **479**
clinical features of, 403–404, **403**
differential diagnosis of, 85, 179, 405
fine needle aspiration biopsy in, 68
grading of, 348, **348,** 404
incidence of, 403–404
prostate specific antigen in, 405–406, **405**
prostatic-specific acid phosphatase in, 405–406
metastatic to prostate, 405
of stomach, 405
Signet-ring cell change, 405
in lymphocytes, 85, **86**
Signet-ring histiocytosis, in pelvic lymph nodes, 177–179, **177, 179,** 314
Silver-stained nucleolar organizer regions
in epithelial hyperplasia, 138
in prostatic intraepithelial neoplasia, 206–207
Simple atrophy, 101, **101–102,** 104, **104**
cystic, **101,** 104, **105–106**
noncystic, **101–102,** 102
Skeletal muscle
adenocarcinoma in, 279, **279,** 297, **298**
periprostatic, 18–19, **18–19**
sampled by TURP, 40
Skin, metastasis of prostatic carcinoma to, 319–320, **320**
Small acinar adenocarcinoma, **14,** 147, **201, 259–261,** 276, **276–277, 279**
autopsy-detected, 229
differential diagnosis of, 178
Small blue round cell tumors, 417
Small cell carcinoma, 234, 414–419, **414–418**
benign conditions mimicked by, **479**
clinical features of, 414, **415**
differential diagnosis of, 85, 417
grading of, 348, **348**
immunophenotyping of, 416–417, **417**
incidence of, 414
mixed small cell carcinoma-adenocarcinoma, 415–416, **416**
paraneoplastic syndromes in, 414
prostate specific antigen in, 414
Small lymphocytic lymphoma, 445
Small round cell tumors of childhood, 437
Smoking, prostatic cancer and, 234
Smooth muscle
cells in fine needle aspirate, 61
cells in stromal hyperplasia, **132**
periprostatic, 18–19, **18–19**
permeation by adenocarcinoma, **260**
in TURP chips, 43–44
Soft tissue tumors, 432–441, **432**
malignant, 436–441, **436**
Spherulosis, collagenous, 169
Spindle cell carcinoma. *See* Sarcomatoid carcinoma

Spindle cell nodule, postoperative, 170–171, **170, 177,** 434, 439, 525
Spindle cell sarcoma, 170
Squamous cell(s), in fine needle aspirate, 61, **62**
Squamous cell carcinoma
of prostate, 406–408, **406–407**
benign conditions mimicked by, **479**
clinical features of, 406
differential diagnosis of, 118, **118,** 408, **408**
fine needle aspiration biopsy in, 69
grading of, 348, **348**
incidence of, 406
after radiation therapy, 468
from treated tumors, 408
metastasis to prostate, 408
of prostatic urethra, 533–534
of seminal vesicles, 515
Squamous cell metaplasia, 115–119, **116–118, 177**
adjacent to biopsy track, 36, **37**
in benign prostatic hyperplasia, 115, 135
differential diagnosis of, 118, **118,** 144, 199, 408
hormonal therapy-induced, 118, **118**
immature, 115, **118**
incidence of, 115, **115**
infarct-associated, 116–117, **117–118, 136**
inflamed, 79–80, **79,** 83–84, **83**
mature, 115, **118**
in needle biopsy tract, 118, **118**
in needle core biopsy, **116**
prostatic carcinomas that mimic, **479**
of prostatic urethra, 526, **526**
in prostatitis, 115
radiation-induced, 118–119
SRD5A2 gene, 482–483
Staging of prostatic carcinoma, 235, 376–385
after androgen deprivation therapy, 463
clinical staging, 378–379, **378–379**
experimental staging procedures, 384–385, **384**
postoperative models using pathologic stage to predict response to surgery, 383, **384**
pretreatment models
of pathologic stage, 381, **382**
using clinical stage to predict response to local therapy, 383, **383**
reporting of pathologic stage, 385
stage and patient outcomes, 382–383, **382–383**
stage relationships with pathologic findings, 382, **382**
TNM system, 310, 377–381, **378, 380**
of transitional cell carcinoma, 413, **414**
using TURP chips, **42**
Whitmore-Jewett scheme, 377, **377**
Whitmore scheme, 377, **377**
Staging of prostatic urethral carcinoma, **534**
Star grass, 469
Stem cells, prostatic, 11
Stinging nettle, 469
Stones. *See* Calculi
Stout criteria, for adenocarcinoma, 259, **259**
Stricture, urethral, 525
Stromal hyperplasia
atypical, **432–433,** 433–434
differential diagnosis of, 439
leiomyomatous variant, **132**
prostatic carcinomas that mimic, **479**
usual, 129–140, **130–139**
differential diagnosis of, **137**
Stromal matrix, extracellular, of prostate, 19–20, **19–20**
Stromal metaplasia, 123
Stromal sarcoma, of prostate, **432**
benign conditions mimicked by, **479**
differential diagnosis of, 439
Surgery, effect on prostatic tissues, 457
Surgical capsule, 6
Susceptibility genes, 482, **482**
"Suspicious of malignancy," 224
Synovial sarcoma, 440, **440**
Syphilis, 90

T

Tamsulosin, 469
Teflon, granulomatous reaction to, 94, **94**
Teratoma, 171
ovarian, prostatic ectopia in, 22, **22**
testicular, prostatic ectopia in, 22
Terazosin, 469
Testes, metastasis of prostatic carcinoma to, 320, **320**
Testicular feminization, 3, 5, **5**
Testosterone, prostatic carcinoma and, 233
Thermotherapy
for benign prostatic hyperplasia, 470
effect on prostatic tissues, 470
Thyroid papillary carcinoma, metastasis to prostate, **447**
TNM staging system, 310, 377–379, **378**
pathologic staging, 379–381, **380**
of prostatic urethral carcinoma, **534**
of rhabdomyosarcoma, 438, **438**
static nature of, 384, **385**
of transitional cell carcinoma of prostate, **414**
Transcription factor Nkx3.1, 209, 489
Transitional cell carcinoma
benign conditions mimicked by, **479**
of bladder, 410, 413
involvement of prostatic urethra in, 535–536, **535**
prostate involvement in, 84, **84,** 284, **284,** 447, **447**
spread to seminal vesicles, 517, **517–518**
differential diagnosis of, 143, **199,** 202, 274, 292, **292,** 315, 399–400, 516
fine needle aspiration biopsy in, 68–69, **68**
grading of, 348, **348**
immunophenotyping of, **284,** 413
primary in prostate, 410–414, **410–413**
clinical features of, **411**
differential diagnosis of, 413, **414**
grading of, 413
metastasis of, 411, 413
staging of, 413
prostate specific antigen in, **285**
prostatic acid phosphatase in, **286**
of prostatic duct, extension into prostatic urethra, 536
of prostatic urethra, 410, 413, 530, 533–534, **533–534**
extension into prostate, 84, **84**
Transitional cell epithelium
cells in fine needle aspirate, 61
of prostate, 17, **17**
Transitional cell metaplasia, 17, 115, 119–120, **119–120, 177**
after androgen deprivation therapy, 119
differential diagnosis of, 119–120, 144, **199,** 200
incidence of, **119**
infarct-associated, 119
inflamed, 83
in postatrophic hyperplasia, **108,** 109
prostatic carcinomas that mimic, **479**
Transitional cell papilloma, of prostatic urethra, 531
Transition zone carcinoma, **193**
Transitive gland change, 200–201
Transrectal ultrasound (TRUS)
clinical staging by, 378, **378**
evaluation of prostatic carcinoma by, 240
Transurethral electrovaporization
for benign prostatic hyperplasia, **469,** 470
effect on prostatic tissues, 470
Transurethral needle ablation
for benign prostatic hyperplasia, **469,** 470
effect on prostatic tissues, 470
Transurethral resection of the prostate (TURP)
for benign prostatic hyperplasia, 129

channel, 290
clinical indications for, 40
effect on prostatic tissue, 457
effect on prostatic urethra, 525, **525**
number of specimens examined in U.S. in 2002, **31**
postbiopsy/postresection granulomatous prostatitis, 91–92, **91–92,** 457
postoperative spindle cell nodule. *See* Postoperative spindle cell nodule
post-TURP vasculitis, 94, **94**
TURP chips. *See* TURP chips
Treatment effects, 456–471. *See also* specific treatments
TRUS. *See* Transrectal ultrasound
Tumor suppressor genes, 487–489, **487**
Tumor volume-based prognostic index, 384
TURP. *See* Transurethral resection of the prostate
TURP chips, 31, 40–44, **40–43**
adenocarcinoma in, 289–294, **289–291**
clinical, gross, and microscopic features of, 289–291, **290**
differential diagnosis of, 292
frequency of incidental carcinoma detection, 289–290, **289**
prognostic attributes, 292–294, **293**
reporting of, 292–294, **293**
adenosis in, 43
adipose tissue in, 40
benign prostatic hyperplasia in, 204
bladder neck fragments in, 40
cautery artifact in, 43, **43, 177,** 291, **291,** 354
clinical staging of cancer using, **42**
diagnosis of prostate carcinoma, 42–43
ductal adenocarcinoma in, 396
fibromuscular stroma in, 40
focal glandular atypia in, 43, 224, **224**
grading of carcinoma in, 352–354, **353–354**
gross chip sampling, 43, **43**
gross examination and reporting for, 40–41, **40**
number of chips in tissue cassette, 42, **42**
numbers of chips submitted for microscopic examination, 42
prostatic intraepithelial neoplasia in, 43, **43,** 184–185, **184,** 191, **193,** 204
sectioning of paraffin blocks, 43
selection of chips for sampling, 41–42
skeletal muscle in, 40
smooth muscle in, 43–44
transition zone tissue in, 40
urethral and periurethral tissues in, 40

U

Unclassified sarcoma, 440
Undifferentiated sarcoma, 440
Ureter
ectopic, 511, **511,** 523, **523**
obstruction of, 242
Ureterovesicular fistula, 511, **511**
Urethra
membranous, 7
prostatic. *See* Prostatic urethra
tissue in TURP chips, 40
Urethral angle, 7
Urethral carcinoma, extension into prostate, 447
Urethral infection, 77
Urethral sphincter, striated, 17–18
Urethral stricture, 525
Urethral valves, posterior, 523, **523**
Urethritis, 524–525, **524**
granulomatous, 524
papillary/polyploid, 525, **525**
Urethritis cystica, 526, **526–527**
Urethritis glandularis, 526, **526–527**
Urinary bladder. *See* Bladder
Urinary incontinence, after radical prostatectomy, 246
Urinary reflux, 80
Urinary retention, 136, 237
Urinary tract infection, 77, 80
prostatic malakoplakia and, 92–93
Uroepithelium. *See* Transitional cell epithelium
Urogenital sinus, 3–4
Urography, intravenous, clinical staging by, 378, **378**
Urologic manipulations, effect on prostate specific antigen, 237
Urothelial carcinoma. *See* Transitional cell carcinoma
Urothelial dysplasia, 532–533, **533**
Usual epithelial hyperplasia. *See* Epithelial hyperplasia, usual
Usual prostatic hyperplasia, 129–140, **130–139.** *See also* Benign prostatic hyperplasia
cystic glandular dilatation in, 135, **135**
differential diagnosis of, 137, **137, 199,** 200, 292, **292,** 435
Utricular cyst, 5–6, **5–6**

V

Vanishing cancer phenomenon, 50, 298
Vasculitis
of prostate, 94, **94–95**
of seminal vesicles, 512
Vas deferens cyst, 5, **5–6**
Vas deferens stump margin, section in radical prostatectomy specimen, 49, **49**
Vasectomy, prostatic carcinoma and, 234
Verumontanum, 7, **7,** 15, **15**
Verumontanum mucosal gland hyperplasia, 147–148, **148, 177**
differential diagnosis of, 160, **160,** 284
Vesiculodeferential artery, 510
Villous adenoma, of prostatic urethra, 399, 530–531
Viral prostatitis, 94
Vitamin D, prostatic carcinoma and, 233
Vitamin D receptor gene, 482
Vitamin E, prevention of prostatic carcinoma, 233
Von Brunn's nests, 526, **527**

W

Wegener granulomatosis
prostatic granulomas in, 93–94
prostatic vasculitis in, 94, **94**
Whitmore-Jewett staging scheme, 377, **377**
Whitmore staging scheme, 377, **377**
WHO classification, of transitional cell lesions of bladder, 532, **533**
WHO grading system, 339–340, **339–340,** 349
Whole prostate gland, grading of carcinoma in, 352
Wilms' tumor, of prostate, **69,** 446
Wispy blue mucin
in adenocarcinoma, 16, 264, **264–265,** 280
in prostatic intraepithelial neoplasia, 197–198
Wolffian ducts, 5

X

Xanthogranulomatous prostatitis, 88, 177, **177**
differential diagnosis of, 292, **292**
Xanthoma
of prostate, 88
prostatic carcinomas that mimic, **479**
Xanthomatous pseudotumor. *See* Inflammatory myofibroblastic tumor

Z

Zones of the prostate gland. *See* Prostate gland.